Rapid Reference to the *Exotic Animal Formulary*, 6e

Hints for Using This Formulary, See Inside Back Cover

SIXTH EDITION

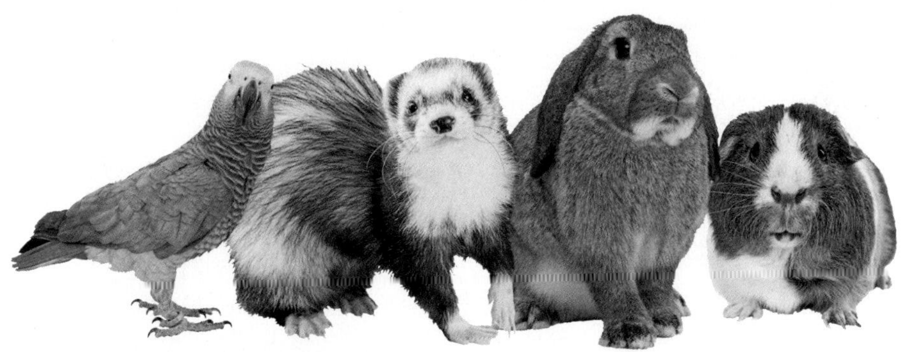

CARPENTER'S EXOTIC ANIMAL FORMULARY

Editors

JAMES W. CARPENTER, MS, DVM, DIPLOMATE ACZM

Professor
Zoological Medicine
Department of Clinical Sciences
College of Veterinary Medicine
Kansas State University
Manhattan, Kansas, USA

CRAIG A. HARMS, DVM, PHD, DIPLOMATE ACZM, DIPLOMATE ECZM (ZOO HEALTH MANAGEMENT)

Professor
Aquatic, Wildlife, and Zoo Medicine
North Carolina State University
College of Veterinary Medicine
Department of Clinical Sciences
Center for Marine Sciences and Technology
Morehead City, North Carolina, USA

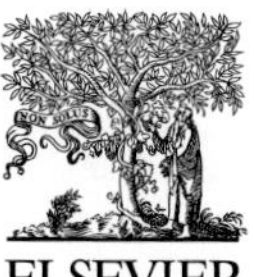

ELSEVIER

Elsevier
3251 Riverport Lane
St. Louis, Missouri 63043

CARPENTER'S EXOTIC ANIMAL FORMULARY, SIXTH EDITION

ISBN: 978-0-323-83392-9

Notice

Practitioners and researchers must always rely on their own experience and knowledge in evaluating and using any information, methods, compounds or experiments described herein. Because of rapid advances in the medical sciences, in particular, independent verification of diagnoses and drug dosages should be made. To the fullest extent of the law, no responsibility is assumed by Elsevier, authors, editors or contributors for any injury and/or damage to persons or property as a matter of products liability, negligence or otherwise, or from any use or operation of any methods, products, instructions, or ideas contained in the material herein.

Senior Content Strategist: Jennifer Catando
Senior Content Development Manager: Somodatta Roy Choudhury
Senior Content Development Specialist: Shilpa Kumar
Publishing Services Manager: Deepthi Unni
Senior Book Production Executive: Manchu Mohan
Senior Book Designer: Brian Salisbury

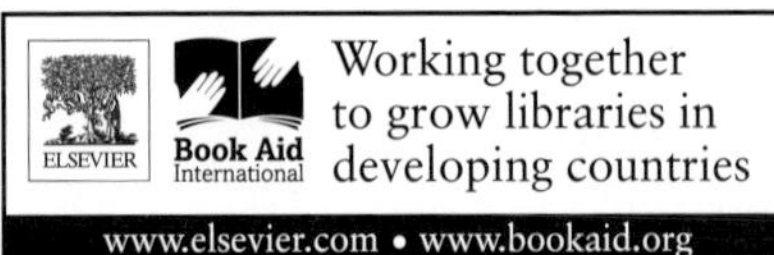

Printed in India.
Last digit is the print number: 9 8 7 6 5 4 3 2

DEDICATION

As in previous editions, this book is dedicated to the 43 interns and residents whom I've had the honor to train from 1991–2021, and who have brought great joy to my life and pride to our profession: Dr. Tess Rooney (2020–2021), Dr. Neta Ambar (2019–2020), Dr. Gail L. Huckins (2018–2019), Dr. Rob Browning (2017–2018), Dr. Louden Wright (2016–2017), Dr. Melissa R. Nau (2015–2016), Dr. Dana M. Lindemann (2014–2015), Dr. Christine Higbie (2013–2014), Dr. Katie Delk (2012–2013), Dr. Daniel V. Fredholm (2011–2012), Dr. Rodney Schnellbacher (2010–2011), Dr. Kristin Phair (2009–2010), Dr. Judilee Marrow (2008–2009), Dr. Kim Wojick (2007–2008), Dr. Julie Swenson (2006–2007), Dr. Gretchen Cole (2005–2006), Dr. Karen Wolf (2004–2005), Dr. Jessica Siegal–Willott (2003–2004), Dr. Jennifer D'Agostino (2002–2003), Dr. Adrian Mutlow (2001–2003), Dr. Nancy Boedeker (2001–2002), Dr. Robert Coke (2000–2001), Dr. Greg Fleming (1999–2000), Dr. Peter Helmer (1999–2000), Dr. Tama Cathers (1998–1999), Dr. Cornelia Ketz (1998–1999), Dr. Geoff Pye (1997–1998), Dr. Nancy Morales (1996–1998), Dr. R. Scott Larsen (1996–1997), Dr. Pilar Hayes (1995–1996), Dr. Cynthia Stadler (1995–1996), Dr. Ray Ball (1994–1996), Dr. Christine Kolmstetter (1994–1995), Dr. James K. Morrisey (1994–1995), Dr. Edward Gentz (1993–1994), Dr. Lisa Harrenstien (1993–1994), Dr. Janette Ackermann (1992–1993), Dr. Ted Y. Mashima (1992–1993), Dr. Sandra C. Wilson (1991–1992; 1992–1995), Dr. Craig A. Harms (1991–1992), Dr. Mel Shaw (1990–1992), and Dr. Mitch Finnegan (1990–1991). I am very proud of all they have accomplished and their contributions to exotic animal, wildlife, and zoo animal medicine.

I am especially grateful to Dr. Craig Harms (my 1991–1992 intern and colleague) who agreed to be co-editor of this book; this is the first time I have invited someone to serve as a collaborator on this formulary. His expertise, energy, and professionalism helped make this edition of the formulary the best yet!

This formulary is also dedicated to my family, who has patiently supported me throughout all six editions of the *Exotic Animal Formulary*.

James W. Carpenter

I am indebted to Dr. Jim Carpenter for a 1991 pre-dawn Alaska-time phone call from Kansas offering me the coveted internship in exotic, zoo, and wildlife medicine at Kansas State University, which launched me on my three decades and counting career in academic zoological medicine, putting me into a position to contribute to the present work. I am grateful to my primary mentors along the way: Dr. Carpenter (internship), Dr. Michael Stoskopf (residency), and Dr. Suzanne Kennedy-Stoskopf (PhD). My colleague and friend, Dr. Greg Lewbart, has been with me through thick and thin my entire time at North Carolina State, both in and out of work. I dedicate my efforts on this formulary to my unusually supportive family who think I work too much, but especially to my father, Ronald Harms, who passed during the final stages of this book's preparation.

Craig A. Harms

Contributors

Jeffrey R. Applegate, Jr., DVM, Diplomate ACZM
Nautilus Avian and Exotics Veterinary Specialists
Blue Jay Veterinary Consulting
Point Pleasant, New Jersey

Louisa Asseo, DVM, Diplomate ABVP
Oasis Veterinary Hospital
Martinez, California

Hugues Beaufrère, DVM, PhD, Diplomate ACZM, Diplomate ABVP (Avian), Diplomate ECZM (Avian)
Associate Professor, Zoological Companion Animal Medicine and Surgery
Department of Medicine and Epidemiology
School of Veterinary Medicine
University of California, Davis
Davis, California

James W. Carpenter, MS, DVM, Diplomate ACZM
Professor, Zoological Medicine
Department of Clinical Sciences
College of Veterinary Medicine
Kansas State University
Manhattan, Kansas

Leigh Ann Clayton, DVM, ABVP (Avian; Reptile/Amphibian), eMBA
Vice President, Animal Care
New England Aquarium
Boston, Massachusetts

Rocio Crespo, DVM, MS, DVSc, Diplomate ACPV
Professor, Poultry Health Management
Population Health and Pathobiology
College of Veterinary Medicine
North Carolina State University
Raleigh, North Carolina

Nicola Di Girolamo, DMV, MSc, PhD, Diplomate ECZM (Herpetology), Diplomate ACZM
Associate Professor, Exotic Animal Medicine
Department of Clinical Sciences
College of Veterinary Medicine
Cornell University
Ithaca, New York

Grayson A. Doss, DVM, Diplomate ACZM
Clinical Assistant Professor, Zoological Medicine
Department of Clinical Sciences
School of Veterinary Medicine
University of Wisconsin–Madison
Madison, Wisconsin

Peter Fisher, DVM, Diplomate ABVP (Exotic Companion Mammal)
Pet Care Veterinary Hospital
Virginia Beach, Virginia

Jennifer Frohlich, VMD, Diplomate ACLAM
Clinical Veterinarian
Office of Laboratory Animal Care
University of California, Berkeley
Berkeley, California

Jennifer Graham, DVM, Diplomate ABVP (Avian; Exotic Companion Mammal), Diplomate ACZM
Associate Professor, Zoological Companion Animal Medicine
Department of Clinical Sciences
Cummings School of Veterinary Medicine
Tufts University
North Grafton, Massachusetts

David Sanchez-Migallon Guzman, LV, MS, Diplomate ECZM (Avian; Small Mammal), Diplomate ACZM
Professor, Clinical Companion Zoological Medicine and Surgery
Department of Medicine and Epidemiology
School of Veterinary Medicine
University of California, Davis
Davis, California

Craig A. Harms, DVM, PhD, Diplomate ACZM, Diplomate ECZM (Zoo Health Management)
Professor, Aquatic, Wildlife, and Zoo Medicine
Center for Marine Sciences and Technology
Department of Clinical Sciences
College of Veterinary Medicine
North Carolina State University
Morehead City, North Carolina

Jill Heatley, DVM, MS, Diplomate ABVP (Avian; Reptile/Amphibian), Diplomate ACZM
Associate Professor, Zoological Medicine
Department of Small Animal Clinical Sciences
College of Veterinary Medicine and Biomedical Sciences
Texas A&M University
College Station, Texas

Cathy A. Johnson-Delaney, DVM
Medical Moderator, Exotic DVM Forum
Avian and Exotic Consulting
Edmonds, Washington

Eric Klaphake, DVM, Diplomate ACZM, Diplomate ABVP (Avian; Reptile/Amphibian)
Associate Veterinarian
Cheyenne Mountain Zoo
Colorado Springs, Colorado

Gregory A. Lewbart, MS, VMD, Diplomate ACZM, Diplomate ECZM (Zoo Health Management)
Professor, Aquatic, Wildlife, and Zoo Medicine
Department of Clinical Sciences
College of Veterinary Medicine
North Carolina State University
Raleigh, North Carolina

Jörg Mayer, Dr.Med.Vet., MSc, Diplomate ACZM, Diplomate ECZM (Small Mammal), Diplomate ABVP (Exotic Companion Mammal)
Professor, Zoological Medicine
Department of Small Animal Medicine and Surgery
College of Veterinary Medicine
University of Georgia
Athens, Georgia

Erica A. Miller, DVM
Field Operations Manager
Wildlife Futures Program
Adjunct Associate Professor
University of Pennsylvania
Kennett Square, Pennsylvania

Kristie Mozzachio, DVM, CVA, Diplomate ACVP
Mozzachio Mobile Veterinary Services
Hillsborough, North Carolina

Natalie D. Mylniczenko, MS, DVM, Diplomate ACZM
Staff Veterinarian
Disney's Animals, Science and Environment
Lake Buena Vista, Florida

Terri Parrott, DVM
President of Operations
St. Charles Veterinary Hospital
Davenport, Florida

Olivia A. Petritz, DVM, Diplomate ACZM
Assistant Professor, Exotic Animal Medicine
Department of Clinical Sciences
College of Veterinary Medicine
North Carolina State University
Raleigh, North Carolina

Nicki Rosenhagen, DVM
Wildlife Veterinarian
PAWS
Lynnwood, Washington

Kurt K. Sladky, MS, DVM, Diplomate ACZM, Diplomate ECZM (Herpetology; Zoo Health Management)
Clinical Professor, Zoological Medicine/ Special Species Health
Department of Surgical Sciences
School of Veterinary Medicine
University of Wisconsin
Madison, Wisconsin

Stephen A. Smith, MS, DVM, PhD
Professor, Aquatic, Wildlife, and Exotic Animal Medicine
Department of Biomedical Sciences & Pathobiology
Virginia-Maryland College of Veterinary Medicine
Virginia Polytechnic Institute and State University
Blacksburg, Virginia

Julie Swenson, DVM, Diplomate ACZM
Associate Veterinarian
Fossil Rim Wildlife Center
Glen Rose, Texas

Marike Visser, DVM, PhD, Diplomate ACVCP
Zoetis Inc.
Kalamazoo, Michigan

Kenneth R. Welle, DVM, Diplomate ABVP (Avian)
Clinical Assistant Professor
Department of Veterinary Clinical Medicine
University of Illinois
Urbana, Illinois

Foreword

It is my great honor and pleasure to write the foreword to the 6th edition of *Carpenter's Exotic Animal Formulary*. In this edition, Dr. James Carpenter, together with Dr. Craig Harms as co-editor, has once again produced a book of extraordinary importance to the field of exotic animal medicine. Since the first edition of the Formulary was published in 1996, it has become the indispensable source of information on pharmacologic agents used in companion exotic animal practice for veterinarians worldwide. With the publication of the 6th edition of the *Exotic Animal Formulary*, this legacy continues and is strengthened.

The first edition of the *Exotic Animal Formulary* signaled an important change in the way that veterinarians approached the use of pharmacologic agents in exotic animals. Before the Formulary, veterinarians who treated exotic pets gleaned information about drugs and dosages for use in birds, reptiles, and small mammals from a myriad of sources. Much information was anecdotal and based on personal experiences, discussions with colleagues at conferences, published case reports, or extrapolated from drugs and dosages used in dogs and cats. As companion exotic animal medicine expanded rapidly into a veterinary specialty in the early 1990s, Dr. Carpenter had the foresight to recognize that practitioners needed a centralized, collective, and evidence-based source of information about drugs used in exotic animals. With the combination of his expertise in exotic, wildlife, and zoo animal medicine, experience in pharmacokinetic studies, and attention to detail, Dr. Carpenter produced a unique and pivotal book that has become the cornerstone of an entire field. The Formulary filled the critical void of consistent, current, and comprehensive information about drugs and dosages used in exotic animal medicine, and it continues to do so with each new edition.

Since publication of the first edition, pharmacokinetic studies on a wide range of drugs used in exotic animals have been conducted and published with increasing frequency. Each subsequent edition of the Formulary has built upon the last, with updated information from the most recent pharmacokinetic studies, as well as expanded sections on biologic reference values and husbandry information. The Formulary not only compiles drugs, dosages, and biologic reference information but also provides comprehensive reference lists for the information so that readers can determine the clinical applicability on a case-by-case basis.

In this 6th edition of *Carpenter's Exotic Animal Formulary*, each chapter has been updated by top experts in species-specific fields with hundreds of new references in total. The drug tables have been completely restructured to include new doses, drug interactions, potential adverse effects, and indications and contraindications for use. Outdated drug listings and drugs that are no longer available have been removed. The index has been updated and expanded, making it easier to find drug information, and new appendices have been added. Additionally, an enhanced eBook is available on Ebooks+. Even with all of the new updates and added information, the book remains extremely well organized, compact, and user-friendly.

Referring to the Formulary for information about a drug dosage or biological data is a daily routine for any veterinarian who practices exotic animal medicine. Working in clinical practice without the Formulary at your fingertips for quick access to information is challenging for even experienced practitioners. I have owned every edition of the Formulary, and I am confident that when I look up a dosage or biologic information for a clinical case, the information is accurate, up to date, and reliable.

Carpenter's Exotic Animal Formulary **is the one book that is indispensable to companion exotic veterinary practice. For every veterinarian who strives to practice high-quality, evidence-based medicine in invertebrates, fish, amphibians, reptiles, small mammals, miniature pigs, and primates, this book is an essential, hands-on reference source that will be used daily in practice.**

Katherine Quesenberry, DVM, MPH, Diplomate ABVP (Avian Practice)
Chief Medical Officer
The Animal Medical Center
New York, New York

Preface

Welcome to the sixth edition of our formulary, currently titled *Carpenter's Exotic Animal Medicine Formulary* (compliments of Elsevier)! As many of you might recall, creating, updating, expanding, and improving the *Exotic Animal Formulary* has been one of my (JWC) life-long passions (having started it in 1991). Because medical care of exotic pets has become an integral part of most companion animal practices, *Carpenter's Exotic Animal Formulary,* 6th edition, therefore, was compiled to accommodate this rapid growth of exotic animal medicine. For this revision, 29 of the most recognized specialists in our field were invited to contribute; their role was to evaluate published drug dosages, related biologic and medical information, and references, and to select those that would be most clinically useful and relevant to the practitioner.

This edition is updated and expanded (now contains 301 tables, an increase of 46 tables from the fifth edition), and includes sections on invertebrates, fish, amphibians, reptiles, birds, backyard poultry/gamebirds/waterfowl, sugar gliders, hedgehogs, rodents, rabbits, ferrets, miniature pigs, primates, and native wildlife. The "Selected Topics for the Exotic Animal Veterinarian" has also been updated and expanded.

This book is not intended to replace existing medical resources or the use of sound medical judgment, but rather to serve as a guide in providing medical care to exotic animals. This formulary assumes that the reader has a reasonable understanding of veterinary medicine. For example, drug indications are generally listed only in unique situations. Supporting tables have been carefully selected to include those topics of major importance in clinical practice.

As in the previous five editions of this book, the selection of species, drugs, and other information used in this reference was based on an extensive review of the literature (over 3150 references are cited, an increase of 650 from the fifth edition) and our collective teaching and clinical experience. The book, therefore, is not intended to be all inclusive, but rather a handy and convenient reference for the common questions and medical situations we encounter in clinical practice.

Unfortunately, though, there are relatively few pharmacokinetic/pharmacodynamic studies on exotic companion pets for the medications we use in practice. Until more pharmacokinetic efficacy and safety studies of the drugs that we use are conducted, most dosages used in these species are based on empirical data, observations, and experience.

This book is intended to be a practical, user-friendly, quick reference for veterinary clinicians, students, and technicians working with exotic animals. We hope, therefore, that you find this formulary and accompanying tables handy to use and that it adds to the quality of the medical care you provide to your exotic animal patients. Because exotic animal practitioners face daily challenges to meet the pharmaceutical and clinical needs of their patients, our hope is that this book will be a valuable tool in helping meet these challenges.

James W. Carpenter, MS, DVM, Diplomate ACZM

Craig A. Harms, DVM, PhD, Diplomate ACZM, Diplomate ECZM (ZHM)

ACKNOWLEDGMENTS

This book would not have been possible without the invaluable assistance of many dedicated and hard-working people. Certainly, first and foremost, my appreciation goes to Dr. Craig A. Harms, who "made my day" by agreeing to serve as co-editor for this edition of the *Exotic Animal Formulary* (which has evolved into *Carpenter's Exotic Animal Formulary!*), provided editorial assistance, technical expertise, and personal encouragement. I am also greatly appreciative of the numerous contributors who unselfishly shared their expertise and gave of their time, and are largely responsible for the success of this book! I am indebted to Karissa Severud, Beth Flax, Hannah Barber, and Dr. Sarah Wilson for assistance in the preparation of this formulary; and to Dr. Brian Lubbers for reviewing and updating the antimicrobial agents (Tables 15-1 through 15-4) in Chapter 15.

I also wish to thank all those colleagues, interns and residents, and veterinary students, both national and international, who encouraged me to prepare *Carpenter's Exotic Animal Formulary*, 6th edition. This let us know that our efforts in preparing this book are appreciated by the veterinary community and provided a powerful incentive for me to continue working on this reference.

In addition, a special thanks to the strong support and encouragement from the administration and faculty at both Kansas State University and North Carolina State University while preparing this formulary.

We also thank Jennifer Catando, Shilpa Kumar, Rebecca Gruliow, Ellen M. Wurm-Cutter, Charu Bali, and Brian Salisbury, our publishing team at Elsevier, for their patience, support, and commitment to this sixth edition.

James W. Carpenter

I am particularly grateful to Dr. Jim Carpenter both for launching me on my career in zoological medicine and inviting me to take part in this sixth round of his influential, and now formally eponymous, *Carpenter's Exotic Animal Formulary* (we've been calling it the Carpenter Formulary for years). Despite his best efforts and guidance over many years, and especially the past two, I still can't match his sharp editor's eye. Special thanks to the contributors who accepted invitations, even though they knew full well that it would be more work than we let on. I thank my colleagues at the Center for Marine Sciences and Technology: Dr. Emily Christiansen, Dr. Lori Westmoreland, Dr. Maria Serrano, and Heather Broadhurst for myriad forms of support that help make it possible for me to pursue projects like this one.

Craig A. Harms

About the Editors

James W. Carpenter, MS, DVM, Diplomate ACZM, is a Professor of Zoological Medicine at the College of Veterinary Medicine, Kansas State University. He has been a clinical and research veterinarian for 48 years in the field of exotic animal, wildlife, and zoo animal medicine, and has trained 43 interns and residents. He is the author of numerous scientific papers and book chapters; is editor/co-author of the *Exotic Animal Formulary* (1996, 2001, 2005, 2013, 2018, and co-editor of the 2023 edition) and its Japanese (2002), Spanish (2006), and Portuguese (2010) translations; and was co-editor of *Ferrets, Rabbits, and Rodents: Clinical Medicine and Surgery* (2004, 2012, 2021). Dr. Carpenter is also the former Editor-in-Chief of both the *Journal of Zoo and Wildlife Medicine* (1987–1992) and the *Journal of Avian Medicine and Surgery* (1994–2020; 27 years!), served on the Wildlife Scientific Advisory Board of the Morris Animal Foundation (1998–2001; Chair, 2000–2001), the editorial board of *Seminars in Avian and Exotic Pet Medicine* (1994–2005), and the *Journal of Exotic Pet Medicine* (2006 to present), and is the Past President of the American Association of Zoo Veterinarians (1998–1999), the Association of Avian Veterinarians (2006–2007), and the American College of Zoological Medicine (2008–2009). He was awarded the Edwin J. Frick Professorship in Veterinary Medicine from the KSU College of Veterinary Medicine in 2002 and the Emil Dolensek Award by the American Association of Zoo Veterinarians in 2004. Dr. Carpenter was named the Exotic DVM of the Year for 2000 and the T.J. Lafeber Avian Practitioner of the Year for 2012. He was also named a Distinguished Alumnus of the Year by the Oklahoma State University College of Veterinary Medicine in 2009. In 2013, the Veterinary Health Center (KSU College of Veterinary Medicine) named the new veterinary facility at Manhattan's Sunset Zoo the "James W. Carpenter Clinic at Sunset Zoo." In 2016, Dr. Carpenter was awarded both the E.R. Frank Award by the KSU College of Veterinary Medicine Alumni Association for "outstanding achievements, humanitarian service, and contributions to the veterinary profession" and the KSU Distinguished Service Award for "outstanding leadership and clinical/diagnostic service to Kansas Veterinary Medical Association members." In 2019, he was the recipient of the Oxbow Quest Award for "Excellence in Small Mammal Health."

Craig A. Harms, DVM, PhD, Diplomate ACZM, Diplomate ECZM (ZHM), is a Professor of Aquatic, Wildlife and Zoo Medicine at the College of Veterinary Medicine and the Center for Marine Sciences and Technology, North Carolina State University, and Adjunct Professor in the Nicholas School of the Environment and Earth Sciences, Duke University Marine Laboratory. He is a 1989 graduate of Iowa State University College of Veterinary Medicine and worked 2 years in private practice in Eagle River and Anchorage, Alaska. He completed an internship in exotics, zoo and wildlife medicine under Dr. Carpenter at Kansas State University, a residency in zoological medicine, aquatics focus, at North Carolina State University, and a PhD in immunology, also at

North Carolina State University. Dr. Harms has been on faculty in the Department of Clinical Sciences and Center for Marine Sciences and Technology, North Carolina State University, since 1999. He has authored or co-authored over 200 scientific publications, and was co-editor of *Sea Turtle Health & Rehabilitation* (2017). He is Past President of the International Association for Aquatic Animal Medicine (2009–2010) and of the American College of Zoological Medicine (2010–2011). In 2011, he was honored with the Stange Award for Meritorious Service from the Iowa State University College of Veterinary Medicine. He moonlights as a whitewater raft guide.

Contents

Chapter 11 Ferrets

Jeffrey R. Applegate, Jr., DVM, Diplomate ACZM

Craig A. Harms, DVM, PhD, Diplomate ACZM, Diplomate ECZM (Zoo Health Management)

CHAPTER 12 Miniature Pigs

Kristie Mozzachio, DVM, CVA, Diplomate ACVP

Louisa Asseo, DVM, Diplomate ABVP

Abbreviations

• d	day
• EpiCe	epicoelomic
• h, hr	hour
• HR	heart rate
• ICe	intracoelomic
• IM	intramuscularly
• IO	intraosseous
• IP	intraperitoneally
• IPPV	intermittent positive pressure ventilation
• IV	intravenously
• IU	international units
• kg	kilogram
• L	liter
• LRS	lactated Ringer's solution
• mg	milligram
• min	minute
• mo	month
• PD	pharmacodynamic/pharmacologic data
• PK	pharmacokinetic data
• PO	orally
• prn	as needed
• q	every
• RR	respiratory rate
• SC	subcutaneously
• wk	week

DISCLAIMER

The editors and contributors attempted to verify and double-check all references, dosages, and other data contained in this book. However, despite these efforts, errors in the original sources or in the preparation of this book may have occurred. All users of this reference, therefore, should empirically evaluate all dosages to determine that they are reasonable prior to use. The publisher assumes no responsibility for and makes no warranty with respect to results obtained from the uses, procedures, or dosages listed, or for any misstatement or error, negligent or otherwise, contained in this book. In addition, the authors do not necessarily endorse specific products, procedures, or dosages reported in this book. Also, the listing of a drug or commercial product in this book does not indicate approval by the US Food and Drug Administration or the manufacturer for use in exotic animals.

Chapter 1 Invertebrates

Gregory A. Lewbart | Jeffrey R. Applegate, Jr.

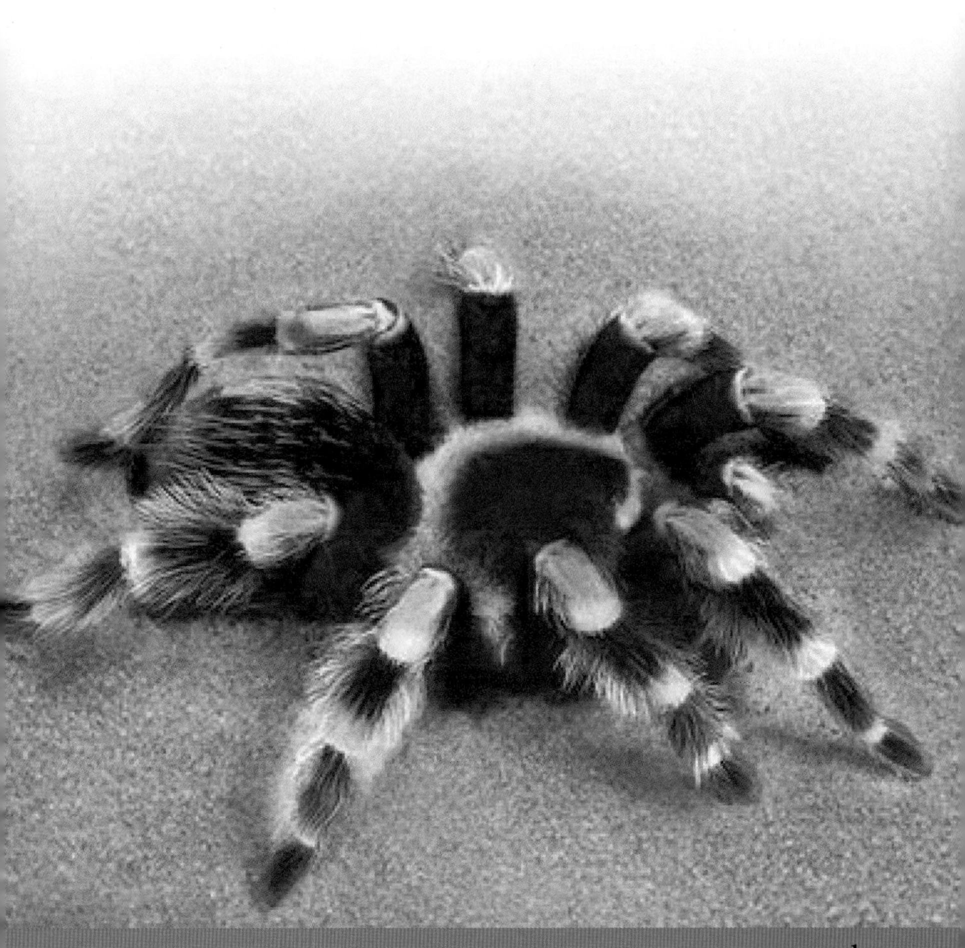

TABLE 1-1 Antimicrobial and Antifungal Agents Used in Invertebrates.[a–f]

Agent	Dosage	Comments
Amoxicillin	Topical paste applied to hard coral lesions q30d × 2 treatments[82]	Stony coral/for treating Stony Coral Tissue Loss Disease; Base 2b or proprietary "New Base" (CoreRx/Ocean Alchemists) + amoxicillin: hand mix silicone-based paste with powdered amoxicillin (Phytotechnology Laboratories; 98.1% purity) in an 8:1 (base:amoxicillin) by weight ratio; time-release products in paste regulated amoxicillin release over 3 days
Amphotericin B	1 mg/kg intrahemocoel[64]	Wax moth larvae (*Galleria mellonella*)/PK; larvae are used frequently as a model for human chemotherapeutic efficacy studies (in this case for efficacy against the fungal pathogen *Madurella mycetomatis*)
Ampicillin	100 mg/L q12h × 7 days[108]	*Acropora* sp./control of white band disease (WBD)
Benzalkonium chloride	0.5 mg/L long-term[111] 10 mg/L for 10 min[90]	Quaternary amine with broad disinfection properties, not for use on live animals
Cefovecin (Convenia, Zoetis)	8 mg/kg IV[105]	Horseshoe crab (*Limulus polyphemus*)/ single injection at the base of a lateral leg resulted in a half-life of almost 40 hr and a C_{max} of 26 µg/mL
Ceftazidime (Fortaz, Pfizer)	20 mg/kg intracardiac q72h × 3 wk[90]	Spiders/cephalosporin with good activity against gram-negative bacteria (e.g., *Pseudomonas*); appears safe, efficacy not determined
	120 mg/kg intrahemocoel[110]	Wax moth (*Galleria mellonella*) larvae/PK; given in first right proleg
Chloramphenicol	75 mg/kg PO, IM q12h × 6 days[100]	Cephalopods
	10-50 mg/L as an immersion treatment for several days[15,104,107] (prepare fresh solution with 100% water; change q24h)	Corals/reduce lighting for treated animals if possible (slows metabolic rate and may reduce stress and improve drug tolerance); rinse animals well with fresh seawater before return to primary habitat; properly treat any effluent before discharge; florfenicol may be a better alternative (risk to humans from chloramphenicol)
Ciprofloxacin	20 mg/kg intrahemocoel[110]	Wax moth (*Galleria mellonella*) larvae/PK; given in first right proleg
Doxycycline	50 mg/kg intrahemocoel[110]	Wax moth larvae/PK; given in first right proleg
Enrofloxacin	5 mg/kg IM, IV[53,100]	Cuttlefish (*Sepia officinalis*)/PK; may be applicable to other cephalopods
	10 mg/kg PO[53,100]	Cuttlefish/PK; may be applicable to other cephalopods

TABLE 1-1 Antimicrobial and Antifungal Agents Used in Invertebrates. (cont'd)

Agent	Dosage	Comments
Enrofloxacin (cont'd)	2.5 mg/L × 5 hr immersion q12-24h[53,100]	Cuttlefish/PK; may be applicable to other cephalopods
	5-6 mg/kg IV[76]	Sea hare (*Aplysia californica*)/PK; administered into the hemocoel
	5 mg/L × 24 hr immersion[21]	Manila clams (*Ruditapes philippinarum*)/ PK; decreasing temperature and/or salinity slowed elimination
	5 mg/kg IM[121]	Chinese mitten crabs (*Eriocheir sinensis*)/ PK; given between the fourth pereiopoda and parietal joint membrane
	10-20 mg/kg IM[109]	Chinese mitten crabs/PK
	10 mg/kg PO[37]	Mud crabs (*Scylla serrata*)/PK; absorption and elimination faster at higher temperatures
	10 mg/kg PO q24h × 5 days[70]	Ridgetail white prawn (*Exopalaemon carinicauda*)/PK
	10 mg/L × 24 immersion × 5 days[70]	Ridgetail white prawn/PK
	10 mg/kg IM[39]	Pacific white shrimp (*Penaeus vannamei*)/ PK
	10 mg/kg PO[91]	Giant freshwater prawn (*Macrobrachium rosenbergii*)/PK
	50 mg/kg PO × 5 days[31]	Giant freshwater prawn/PK
	5 mg/kg of feed × 5 days[91]	Giant freshwater prawn/PK
	5 mg/kg ICe[99]	Purple sea stars (*Pisaster ochraceus*)/PK
	5 mg/L immersion for 6 hr[99]	Purple sea stars/PK
	10 mg/kg ICe[89]	Green sea urchins (*Strongylocentrotus droebachiensis*)/PK
	10 mg/L immersion for 6 hr[89]	Green sea urchins/PK
	5 mg/kg IV[63]	Horseshoe crab (*Limulus polyphemus*)/PK; given in the cardiac sinus
	5 mg/kg IV[90]	Spiders
	10-20 mg/kg PO q24h[90]	Spiders
Florfenicol	10 mg/kg PO[38]	Pacific white shrimp (*Litopenaeus vannamei*)/PK; freshwater at 25°C
	100-200 mg/kg PO q12h × 6 days[97]	Pacific white shrimp/PK; both 100 and 200 mg/kg were evaluated and no deleterious effects reported
	10 mg/kg IM[42]	Ridgetail white prawn (*Exopalaemon carinicauda*)/PK; no dosing interval recommended but absorption faster and C_{max} higher than oral dose (10 mg/kg)

Continued

TABLE 1-1 Antimicrobial and Antifungal Agents Used in Invertebrates. (cont'd)

Agent	Dosage	Comments
Florfenicol (cont'd)	10 mg/kg PO q8h at 28°C and q10h at 22°C[42]	Ridgetail white prawn/PK
	10-100 mg/kg intrapericardial[12]	American lobster (*Homarus americanus*)/ safety study
Fluconazole	3 mg/kg intracardiac q4d × 6 treatments[102]	Horseshoe crabs (Limulidae)
Formalin	1-1.5 ppm immersion for 4 hr[66]	Horseshoe crabs (Limulidae)/ ectocommensals; can also be administered indefinitely (i.e., until diluted out)
Furazolidone	50 mg/L q12h for 10 min immersion[100]	Cephalopods
Imipenem	50 mg/kg intrahemocoel[110]	Wax moth (*Galleria mellonella*) larvae/PK; given in first right proleg
Iodine, Lugol's 5% solution	5-10 drops/L of seawater; use as an immersion for 10-20 min[107] Topically at full strength (5%) for 20-30 sec[107]	Corals/antiseptic; cauterize wounds; strong oxidizing agent; some corals are sensitive, including pulse corals (*Xenia* sp.), *Anthelia* spp., and star polyps (*Pachyclavularia* spp.); remove corals at first signs of stress (polyp expulsion)
Itraconazole (Sporanox, Janssen)	10 mg/kg IV q24h[3]	Horseshoe crabs (Limulidae)/PK
Lincomycin	100 mg/colony in 20 g confectioner's sugar q7d × 3 treatments[40]	Honeybees (*Apis mellifera*)/by prescription; experimental treatment of American foulbrood
	200 mg/colony in 20 g confectioner's sugar q7d × 3 treatments[40]	Honeybees/by prescription; experimental treatment of American foulbrood
	400 mg/colony in 20 g confectioner's sugar q7d × 3 treatments[40]	Honeybees/by prescription; experimental treatment of American foulbrood
Nitrofurazone	1.5 mg/L for 72 hr[106] immersion 25 mg/L q12h for 1 hr[106] immersion	Cephalopods/nitrofuran; carcinogenic; drug inactivated in bright light; water-soluble formulations preferred
Oxolinic acid	50 mg/kg PO[112]	Kuruma prawn (*Penaeus japonicus*)/PK
Oxytetracycline	91 mg/kg PO × 20 days[44]	White abalone (*Haliotis sorenseni*)/PK; effective in eliminating withering syndrome caused by a rickettsial organism
	2.6% or 4.2% in feed (dry floating and wet respectively) PO × 14 days[45]	Red abalone (*Haliotis rufescens*)/PK; effective in reducing withering syndrome mortality
	25 mg/L 30 min q48h × 3 immersion treatments[10]	Chambered nautilus (*Nautilus pompilius*)
	10 mg/kg intrasinus[113]	Tiger shrimp (*Penaeus monodon*)/PK; cooking reduced muscle levels by 30%-60% and shell levels by 20%

TABLE 1-1 Antimicrobial and Antifungal Agents Used in Invertebrates. (cont'd)

Agent	Dosage	Comments
Oxytetracycline (cont'd)	10 mg/kg intrasinus[95,22]	White shrimp (*Litopenaeus setiferus*)/PK; injection administered through the ventral arthrodial membrane between the carapace and abdomen
	100 mg/kg PO[96]	White shrimp/PK
	50 mg/kg PO[112,113]	Kuruma prawn (*Penaeus japonicus*)/PK; tiger shrimp (*Penaeus monodon*)/PK; cooking reduced muscle levels by 30%-60% and shell levels by 20%
	11 mg/kg PO, IM[93]	Giant freshwater prawn (*Macrobrachium rosenbergii*)/PK; minimum withdrawal time 8 days after cessation of treatment
	2.5-5 g/kg feed × 7 days[16]	Giant freshwater prawn/PK; minimum withdrawal time 13 days after cessation of medicated feed (21 days recommended)
	4 g/kg feed × 5 days[92]	Giant freshwater prawn/PK; minimum withdrawal time 8 days after cessation of medicated feed
	40 mg/kg IM[41]	Chinese mitten crab (*Eriocheir sinensis*)/PK
	1 g/lb of feed[85]	American lobster (*Homarus americanus*)/gaffkemia; FDA approval for food animal use
	25-50 mg/kg IV[86]	Horseshoe crabs (*Limulus polyphemus*)/PK
	10-15 mg/L q48-72h × 3-5 treatments[58]	Chocolate chip sea stars (*Poreaster nodosum*)/cutaneous ulcerations; may be applicable to other echinoderms
	200 mg/colony PO q4-5d × 3 treatments[115,116]	Honeybees (*Apis mellifera*)/for treating American and European foulbrood; withdrawal time 6 wk; should not be used on hives where honey will be consumed by humans; approved by US FDA by Veterinary Feed Directive or prescription
	700-1000 mg/colony[65]	Honeybees/for treating American and European foulbrood; withdrawal time 6 wk; should not be used on hives where honey will be consumed by humans; administered in extender sugar/vegetable shortening patties
Paromomycin	100 mg/L q12h immersion with a 25% water change × 6 days[108]	Staghorn coral (*Acropora cervicornis*)/Control of white band disease (WBD)
Silver sulfadiazine cream (Silvadene, Marion Merrill Dow)	Apply topically to lesions	Proceed with caution (biotest if possible); treatments are empirical
Sulfadimethoxine	50-100 mg/kg in feed × 14 days[85]	Penaeid shrimp (e.g., tiger shrimp, *Penaeus monodon*)

Continued

TABLE 1-1 Antimicrobial and Antifungal Agents Used in Invertebrates. (cont'd)

Agent	Dosage	Comments
Sulfadimethoxine/ ormetoprim (Romet-30, Alpharma)	42 mg/kg intrapericardial[11]	American lobster (*Homarus americanus*)/ PK; no frequency given but q3-5d may be reasonable based on half-life
Sulfamethoxazole/ trimethoprim (SMZ-TMP)	Bioencapsulated in brine shrimp PO q12h[20,69,83,84]	White shrimp (*Litopenaeus* spp.)/ PK; combine 20%-40% trimethoprim sulfamethoxazole with lipid emulsion (Selco, INVE Aquaculture) at concentration of 1:5
	100 mg/kg PO[72]	Pacific white shrimp (*Litopenaeus vannamei*)/PK; shrimp were fed 3 meals q8h with 2.0% drug/feed to reach the desired 24 hr dose
	100 mg/kg PO[46]	Swimming crab (*Portunus trituberculatus*)/ PK; 1:1 SMZ-TMP mixture more efficacious against *Vibrio* than 5:1
Terbinafine	7.14 mg/kg intrahemocoel[64]	Wax moth larvae (*Galleria mellonella*)/ PK; larvae used as model for human chemotherapeutic efficacy studies, in this case against the fungal pathogen *Madurella mycetomatis*
Tetracycline	10 mg/kg PO q24h[100]	Cephalopods
	10 mg/L bath[62,107]	Corals/efficacy questionable in saltwater; anecdotal evidence of successful treatment for bacterial infections
Thiamphenicol	10 mg/kg PO[38]	Pacific white shrimp (*Litopenaeus vannamei*)/PK; freshwater at 25°C
Trifluralin	0.01-0.1 ppm as an immersion[85]	Penaeid shrimp (e.g., tiger shrimp, *Penaeus monodon*)/larval oomycetosis
Tris EDTA and neomycin (Tricide-Neo, Molecular Therapeutics)	100 mL/L for 45 min q24h × 7 days as an immersion[58]	Cushion sea stars/cutaneous ulcers; may be applicable to other echinoderms
Tylosin (Tylan, Elanco)	200 mg/colony q7d × 3 treatments[115,116]	Honeybees (*Apis mellifera*)/ applied topically to brood chamber for control of American foulbrood (*Paenibacillus larvae*); US FDA approval by prescription; should not be used in hives where the honey will be consumed by humans
	500 mg/colony q14d × 2 treatments[98]	Honeybees/PK; sdministered in 60 g paper packs with 57 g confectioner's sugar, 3 g cherry, and the tylosin
	1.5 g/colony[2]	Honeybees/antibiotic extender patties prepared by mixing 150 g vegetable oil, 300 g of sugar and 1.5 g tylosin; for control of American foulbrood

TABLE 1-1 Antimicrobial and Antifungal Agents Used in Invertebrates. (cont'd)

Agent	Dosage	Comments
Winter savory extract (*Satureja montana*)	0.01% in microcrystalline sugar[25]	Honeybees/chalkbrood fungal disease (*Ascosphaera apis*); a number of plant aromatic oils have been tested on various diseases of honeybees[32,115,116]

[a]Not to be used with invertebrates intended for human consumption unless government approved.
[b]Preferable to treat a single animal of a species (biotest) to determine toxicity.
[c]Tank treatment: when treating the invertebrates' resident aquarium, disconnect activated carbon filtration to prevent drug removal. Many drugs adversely affect the nitrifying bacteria, so water quality should be monitored closely (especially ammonia and nitrite concentrations). Keep water well aerated when appropriate and monitor patient(s) closely. Perform water changes and reconnect filtration to remove residual drug following treatment. Discard carbon following drug removal.
[d]Bath (immersion) treatment: remove invertebrates from resident aquarium and place in container with known volume of water and concentration of therapeutic agent. Watch closely for signs of toxicity.
[e]Invertebrate species, temperature, and water quality parameters can influence the pharmacodynamics of many drugs, especially antimicrobials.
[f]Treatments are grouped by species within drug listings.

TABLE 1-2 Antiparasitic Agents Used in Invertebrates.[a-e]

Agent	Dosage	Comments
Acetic acid, glacial	3%-5% solution for 1 hr[18]	Horseshoe crabs (Limulidae)
Amitraz (Apivar, Véto-pharma)	Use as directed[75,76]	Honeybees (*Apis mellifera*)/acariasis; commercial packaging should be consulted prior to use
Diflubenzuron	0.03 mg/L for 7 days[30]	Jellyfish (*Chrysoara* spp.)/control of amphipods
Formalin	50-100 µL/L for 4 hr or 25 µL/L indefinitely[85]	Shrimp/protozoal ectoparasites; approved for use by the FDA in food animals
Formic acid	Use as directed[115,116]	Honeybees (*Apis mellifera*)/acariasis; commercial packaging should be consulted prior to use; an empty super must be used on hive during treatment
Freshwater	1-3 min dip[107]	Stony corals, some soft corals, flatworms, and other ectoparasites/ buffer to pH 8.2 and use clean, dechlorinated water; do not use on small polyp corals or xenids; biotest first, if possible, especially when attempting with a new species
Fumagillin	Use as directed[9,49,61,115,116]	Honeybees (*Apis mellifera*)/nosemosis (microsporidian parasites); commercial packaging should be consulted prior to use
Ivermectin	5 mg/kg IC[80a]	Blue crabs (*Callinectes sapidus*)/ euthanasia following eugenol anesthesia
	Stock solution of 1:1 (1% ivermectin and propylene glycol); dilute 1:50 with distilled water prior to topical use[90]	Spiders/for the treatment of individual parasitic mites; apply carefully to mites with fine paintbrush or similar implement

Continued

TABLE 1-2 Antiparasitic Agents Used in Invertebrates. (cont'd)

Agent	Dosage	Comments
Levamisole (Levasole, Schering Plough)	8 mg/L immersion for 24 hr[107]	Corals/metazoan parasites; well tolerated by *Acropora* spp., *Montipora digitata, M. capricornis, Seriatopora histrix, Stylophora pistillata*
	40 mg/L immersion for 1 hr[11a]	Corals/about 95% effective in removing *Acropora*-eating flatworms
Menthol	Use as directed[115]	Honeybees (*Apis mellifera*)/acariasis; commercial packaging should be consulted prior to use
Metronidazole	50 mg/kg intracardiac × 1 treatment[90]	Spiders/appears safe, but efficacy is unknown
	100 mg/L immersion for 16 hr[100]	Cephalopods/antiprotozoal
Milbemycin oxime (Interceptor, Novartis)	0.625 mg/L as an immersion[36,57,67]	Stony corals (*Acropora* spp.)/ "red bug" (*Tegastes acroporanus*)
	0.16 mg/L as an immersion q6-7d × 2 treatments[14]	Jellyfish (*Chrysaora* spp.)/amphipod parasites; use with caution on hydrozoans
	0.17 µg/L immersion for 6 hr q3.5d (2 × weekly) × 3 wk[23]	Stony corals (*Acropora* spp.)/copepod *Tegastes acroporanus* infestation stony corals
Oxalic acid (API-Bioxal, Véto-pharma)	Use as directed[116]	Honeybees (*Apis mellifera*)/acariasis; review commercial package instructions and regulations prior to use
Potassium permanganate	25-30 ppm for 30-60 min[85]	Penaeid shrimp (e.g., tiger shrimp, *Penaeus monodon*)/external parasiticide
Povidone iodine	0.75% solution for topical treatment[90]	Spiders/fungal infections; use water-based solution
	10% solution for topical treatment for 10 sec q24h × 30 days[10]	Chambered nautilus (*Nautilus pompilius*)/ external bacterial and nematode infection
Praziquantel	50 mg/L immersion for 1 hr[11a]	Corals/about 95% successful in removing *Acropora*-eating flatworms from coral fragments; praziquantel diluted in 100% ethanol to make a 50 g/L stock solution
Thymol	Use as directed[115,116]	Honeybees (*Apis mellifera*)/acariasis; commercial packaging should be consulted prior to use

[a]Not to be used with invertebrates intended for human consumption unless government approved.

[b]Preferable to treat a single animal of a species (biotest) to determine toxicity.

[c]Tank treatment: when treating the invertebrates' resident aquarium, disconnect activated carbon filtration to prevent drug removal. Many drugs adversely affect the nitrifying bacteria, so water quality should be monitored closely (especially ammonia and nitrite concentrations). Keep water well aerated when appropriate and monitor patient(s) closely. Perform water changes and reconnect filtration to remove residual drug following treatment. Discard carbon following drug removal.

[d]Bath (immersion) treatment: remove invertebrates from resident aquarium and place in container with known volume of water and concentration of therapeutic agent. Watch closely for signs of toxicity.

[e]Invertebrate species, temperature, and water quality parameters can influence the pharmacodynamics of many drugs.

TABLE 1-3 Chemical Restraint/Anesthetic/Analgesic Agents Used in Invertebrates.

Agent	Dosage	Comments
Alfaxalone	200 mg/kg intracardiac[51]	Tarantulas (*Grammostola rosea*)/general anesthetic
Benzocaine	100 mg/L[5,55] bath	Abalone (*Haliotis* spp.)/anesthesia; not sold as anesthetic in United States; available from chemical supply companies; do not use topical anesthetic products marketed for mammals; prepare stock solution in ethanol (benzocaine is poorly soluble in water); store in dark bottle at room temperature
	400 mg/L[29]	Leeches (*Hirudo medicinalis*)/this could be applied, with caution, to other aquatic annelids
	1 g/L[48]	Apple snails (*Pomacea paludosa*)/prepare as 1:4 w/v added to 95°C water to dissolve the benzocaine
	2.5-3 g/L[100] bath	Cephalopods/euthanasia
Butorphanol	Fish, amphibian, and reptile dosages can be employed with care	Analgesia; use with caution as dosing regimens are empirical; biotest when possible
Carbon dioxide	3%-5%[56]	Terrestrial arthropods/euthanasia; isoflurane and sevoflurane may be preferable with regard to recovery; anesthetic chamber developed/described for fruit flies (*Drosophila melanogaster*)[111]
Clove oil (eugenol)	100 mg/L (approx 0.100 mL/L)[88a]	Freshwater amphipod crustacean, *Gammarus pulex*/effective sedation but not analgesia
	0.125 mL/L (approx. 125 mg/L) immersion[47]	Crustaceans/stock solution: 100 mg/mL of eugenol by diluting 1 part clove oil with 9 parts 95% ethanol (eugenol poorly soluble in water); over-the-counter preparation (pure) available at most pharmacies contains approximately 1 g eugenol per mL clove oil
	200-400 mg/L immersion prn or intrahemocoel[121a]	Blue crabs (*C. sapidus*), red swamp crayfish (*P. clarkii*), whiteleg shrimp (*L. vannamei*)/200 and 400 mg/L doses generally comparable; minor differences among taxa; appears safe and effective in all three
	0.35 g/L immersion[48]	Apple snails (*Pomacea paludosa*)
Ethanol	5% solution[27,73]	Oligochaetes (e.g., *Lumbricus terrestris*)/ adequate anesthesia for terrestrial earthworms
	3% solution[55]	Abalone (*Haliotis* spp.)/anesthesia
	5% solution[43,56]	Aquatic gastropods/anesthesia
	1-4% solution[19]	Cuttlefish (*Sepia bandensis*), octopus (*Abdopus aculeatus, Octopus bocki*)/provided good anesthesia, usually within 5 min; dose increased by 1% increments as needed

Continued

TABLE 1-3 Chemical Restraint/Anesthetic/Analgesic Agents Used in Invertebrates. (cont'd)

Agent	Dosage	Comments
Ethanol (cont'd)	1.5%-3% solution[59]	Cuttlefish/anesthesia may not be effective for cold water cephalopods[35]
	5% solution[52]	Octopuses/general anesthesia
	10% solution[100]	Cephalopods/euthanasia
Ethanol/menthol (Listerine, McNeil-PPC)	10% in saline[120]	Aquatic gastropods/anesthesia
Isoflurane	0.5% increased to 2.0% bubbled into seawater over 40 min[119]	Common octopus (*Octopus vulgaris*)/authors[119] believe anesthetics like isoflurane are optimal drug class for cephalopod anesthesia
	2% bubbled into the water[94]	Common octopus/applied via an aquatic anesthesia delivery system
	Can be used with an anesthetic chamber	Terrestrial gastropods,[50] arachnids[27,34,74,79,90,122]/anesthesia; fast induction with possible excitatory period; anesthetic depth may not be appropriate for invasive surgery;[43] usually applied at 5% concentration for arachnids
	5% with 1 L/min oxygen[35]	Tarantulas (*Grammostola rosea*)/sedation and anesthesia (depending on the amount of time in the anesthetic chamber)
	2 mL on a cotton ball[6]	Tarantulas/place cotton ball in a 500 mL beaker with the tarantula; cotton ball should be placed/protected to avoid direct contact
Ketamine	0.025-0.1 mg/kg IV[47]	Australian giant crabs (*Pseudocarcinus gigas*)/fast induction (less than 30 sec) with an excitatory phase; dose dependent anesthetic duration of 8-40 min
	40-90 µg/g IM[17]	Crayfish (*Orconectes virilis*)/induction time less than 1 min and anesthetic duration 10 min at low dose and 2 hr at high dose
	20 mg/kg intracardiac with 200 mg/kg alfaxalone[51]	Tarantulas (*Grammostola rosea*)/results in deep plane of anesthesia
Lidocaine	0.4-1 mg/g IM[17]	Crayfish (*Orconectes virilis*)/induction time less than 2 min and anesthetic duration 5-30 min when injected into the tail
Magnesium chloride[a] ($MgCl_2 \cdot 6H_2O$)	—	6.8 or 7.5% (68 or 75 g/L, about 340 or 370 mM in deionized water) is nearly isosmotic with seawater and can be used as a stock solution
	Intracoelomic, 25-50% body weight with a 1000 mM solution[24,78]	Sea hares/short induction time (2-5 min) and good muscle relaxation
	6.8 g/L[53,55]	Cephalopods/induction time of 6-12 min in cuttlefish

TABLE 1-3 Chemical Restraint/Anesthetic/Analgesic Agents Used in Invertebrates. (cont'd)

Agent	Dosage	Comments
Magnesium chloride (cont'd)	1:3 (33%) stock solution in artificial seawater[19]	Cuttlefish (*Sepia bandensis*), octopus (*Abdopus aculeatus, Octopus bocki*)/provided good anesthesia, usually within 5 min; some required as high as a 1:1 stock solution concentration
	32.5 g/L for 20 min[52]	Octopuses
	10% solution (100 g/L) prn[100]	Cephalopods/euthanasia
	30-50 g/L[60]	Scallops (*Pecten fumatus*)/fast induction and recovery
	30 g/L for 20 min[1]	Queen conch (*Strombus gigas*)
	7.5% (75 g/L) immersion[69,81]	Polychaetes
	1:1 mixture of 7.5% (75 g/L) with seawater[58,77]	Echinoderms/concentration adjustments may be required for prolonged anesthesia
Magnesium sulfate ($MgSO_4{\cdot}7H_2O$)	4-22 g/100 mL[118]	Abalone (*Haliotis midae*)/fast induction and good recovery
Morphine	5 mg/kg intracardiac with 200 mg/kg alfaxalone[51]	Tarantulas (*Grammostola rosea*)
MS-222 (Finquel, Argent)	—	See tricaine methanesulfonate
2-phenoxyethanol	0.5-3 mL/L[118]	Abalone (*Haliotis midae*)/quick induction and short recovery
	1-2 mL/L[55]	Quick induction and short recovery
	0.15% immersion[101]	Sea cucumber (*Cucumaria miniata*)/seawater at 12°C; for relaxation prior to fixation in ethanol
	2 mL/L immersion[7]	Horseshoe crab (*Limulus polyphemus*)/most animals anesthetized within 15 min and recovered within 20 min after return to clean seawater; superior to MS-222 in same study
Potassium chloride	1 g/kg (330 mg/mL solution) IV[13]	Lobster (*Homarus americana*)/euthanasia; inject at base of second walking leg
Procaine	25 mg/kg IV[88]	Crabs/very short induction time (less than 30 sec) and prolonged anesthesia (2-3 h)
Propylene phenoxetol	1-3 mL/L of a 1% solution[55,80,87]	Oysters/anesthesia; should produce anesthesia in less than 15 min; recovery time short (under 30 min); higher doses can be used but induce deeper anesthesia; can also be used for giant clams[80]
	2 mL/L[55,114]	Echinoderms
Sevoflurane	Can be used with an anesthetic chamber at a 5% concentration[55,123]	Terrestrial arthropods/see isoflurane for details of administration; use with 1 L/min oxygen flow in tarantulas[123]

Continued

TABLE 1-3 Chemical Restraint/Anesthetic/Analgesic Agents Used in Invertebrates. (cont'd)

Agent	Dosage	Comments
Sodium bicarbonate tablets (Alka-Seltzer, Bayer)	2-4 tablets/L bath[54]	Euthanasia; generates CO_2; use when other agents unavailable; keep aquatic invertebrate in solution >10 min after respiration stops; dosage based on fish literature
Sodium pentobarbital	400 mg/L[75]	Aquatic gastropods/anesthesia; very slow onset but apparently safe; controlled drug
	1 mL/L[5]	Abalone (*Haliotis iris*)
Tricaine methanesulfonate (MS-222; Finquel, Argent)	Dosages and efficacy vary widely depending on species and application; consult taxon-specific literature[55,56]	Anesthesia; stock solution: 10 g/L, buffer acidity by adding sodium bicarbonate at 10 g/L or to saturation; store stock in dark container; shelf life of stock extended by refrigeration or freezing; discard stock that develops oily film; aerate water to prevent hypoxemia; for euthanasia keep animal in solution >20 min after respiration stops
	0.4-0.8 g/L immersion[4]	Purple sea urchin (*Arbacia punctulata*)/safe and effective
	600 mg/L[88a]	Freshwater amphipod crustacean, *Gammarus pulex*/safe analgesic and sedative effects
	1 g/L (buffered with sodium carbonate) immersion[7]	Horseshoe crab (*Limulus polyphemus*)/most animals anesthetized within 15 min and recovered within 20 min after return to clean seawater; inferior to 2-phenoxyethanol in the same study; sodium carbonate is a much stronger buffer than sodium bicarbonate (30 g MS-222 and 14 g sodium carbonate were used per 30 L seawater)
Xylazine	16-22 mg/kg IV[47]	Giant crabs (*Pseudocarcinus gigas*)/fast induction (3-5 min) and approximately 30 min anesthesia (dose dependent)
	20 mg/kg intracardiac with 200 mg/kg alfaxalone[51]	Tarantulas (*Grammostola rosea*)/results in a deep plane of anesthesia

[a]Although listed and used as an anesthetic agent, some workers do not believe it meets the criteria of a true anesthetic.[119]

TABLE 1-4 Miscellaneous Agents Used in Invertebrates.

Agent	Dosage	Comments
Barium sulfate	4 mL/15 g food[33]	Tarantulas, scorpions, millipedes, hissing cockroaches/contrast radiography; inject into a strawberry and feed to millipedes; inject into crickets and/or other prey for carnivorous invertebrates

TABLE 1-4 Miscellaneous Agents Used in Invertebrates. (cont'd)

Agent	Dosage	Comments
Benzocaine topical (Orabase, Colgate-Palmolive)	Topically[107]	Corals and potentially other aquatic invertebrates/used as a water-resistant paste; chemotherapeutics can be combined for topical therapy
Carbon, activated	75 g/40 L tank water[85]	Removal of medications and other organics from water; usually added to filter system; discard after 2 wk; 75 g ≈ 250 mL dry volume
Chlorine/chloramine neutralizer	Use as directed	See sodium thiosulfate
Diatrizoate meglumine and diatrizoate sodium (Hypaque-76, Amersham Health)	4 mL/15 g food[33]	Tarantulas, scorpions, millipedes, hissing cockroaches/contrast radiography; combine with/inject into food item and feed 1-3 hr prior to radiography
Hydrogen peroxide (3%)	0.25 mL/L water[84]	Acute environmental hypoxia; dose from fish literature
Iohexol	12 mL/kg IV[103] 15 mL PO[103]	Horseshoe crabs (*Limulus polyphemus*)/ contrast radiography
Methylmethacrylate	Apply topically as needed[28,90]	Arthropods (spiders, scorpions, insects)/ repair fractured exoskeleton; numerous references for application of surgical adhesives; consult appropriate taxon-based literature
Mineral oil	1 mL/kg PO	Insects/laxative[28]
Nitrifying bacteria	Use as directed for commercial products	Seed or improve development of biological filtration to detoxify ammonia, nitrite, and nitrate; numerous commercial preparations; do not expose products to extreme temperatures; use before expiration date
	Add material (e.g., floss, gravel) from a tank with an active biological filter and healthy animals to new tank[84]	Must evaluate risk of disease transmission with this technique
Oxygen (100%)	Fill plastic bag with O_2 containing 1/3 vol of water[54]	Acute environmental hypoxia common with transportation; close bag tightly with rubber band; keep animals in bag until normal swimming and respiratory behavior
Sodium thiosulfate	Use as directed for chlorine/ chloramine neutralizers	Active ingredient in numerous chlorine/ chloramine neutralizers; chlorine and chloramine are common additions to municipal water supplies and are toxic to many aquatic invertebrates; ammonia released by detoxification of chloramine is removed by functioning biological filter (see nitrifying bacteria) or chemical means (see zeolite)

Continued

TABLE 1-4 Miscellaneous Agents Used in Invertebrates. (cont'd)

Agent	Dosage	Comments
Sodium thiosulfate (cont'd)	10 mg/L tank water[68]	
	10 g neutralizes chlorine (up to 2 mg/L) in 1000 L water[68]	
	100 mg/L tank water[106]	Chlorine exposure
Zeolite (i.e., clinoptilite) (Ammonex, Argent)	Use as directed	Ion-exchange resin that exchanges ammonia for sodium ions; clinoptilite is an active form of zeolite; used to reduce or prevent ammonia toxicity
	20 g/L tank water[84]	

TABLE 1-5 Common Captive Invertebrate Taxa.[a]

Arthropods[b]

Chelicerates: This group includes the spiders, scorpions, and horseshoe crabs. Some common species are listed here.[90,102]
Chilean rosehair tarantula (*Grammostola rosea*).
Mexican fireleg tarantula (*Brachypelma boehmei*).
Mexican redknee tarantula (*Brachypelma smithi*).
Emperor scorpion (*Pandinus imperator*).
American horseshoe crab (*Limulus polyphemus*).
Myriapods (centipedes, millipedes):[34]
African banded millipedes (*Isulus* spp.).
Desert millipede (*Orthoporus* sp.).
Giant desert centipede (*Scolopendra heros*).
Giant train millipedes (*Spirostreptida* spp.).
Madagascar fire millipedes (*Aphistogoniulus* spp.).
Crustaceans: Decapods are a diverse group of readily recognized species including the crabs, lobsters, and shrimp. Some common examples include the banded shrimps, crayfish (numerous species), marine hermit crabs, and terrestrial hermit crabs (*Coenobita* sp.).[85]
Sea monkeys (*Artemia* sp.).[85]
Insects: Insects, sometimes referred to as the phylum Hexapoda, are an immense group of over a million described species. Some common captive insects include the beetles (Order Coleoptera), butterflies and moths (Order Lepidoptera), crickets (grey crickets [*Acheta domestica*]; black prairie crickets [*Gryllus* sp.]), honeybees (*Apis mellifera*), Madagascar hissing cockroaches (*Gromphadorhina portentosa*), and the silkworms (*Bombyx mori*).[28,34,90,115,116]

Coelenterates

Scyphozoans (jellyfishes): Although not common as pets, some individuals, and many public institutions and establishments, maintain jellyfish aquaria. Some popular species include fried egg jellies (*Phacellophora camtschatica*), moon jellies (*Aurelia aurita*), and the sea nettles (*Chrysaora* spp.).[107]
Anthozoans (anemones and corals): Numerous species of sea anemones and corals (hard and soft) are commonly maintained in reef aquaria. Frequently maintained soft coral groups include members of the families Alcyoniidae, Nephtheidae, and Xeniidae.[67] Commonly maintained scleractinian (hard coral) genera include *Acropora*, *Montipora*, and *Porites*.[67]

TABLE 1-5 Common Captive Invertebrate Taxa. (cont'd)

Echinoderms
This entirely marine phylum includes five major classes:[58] **Asteroidea:** sea stars; **Crinoidea:** feather stars, sea lilies; **Echinoidea:** sand dollars, sea biscuits, sea urchins; **Holothuroidea:** sea cucumbers; **Ophiuroidea:** basket stars, brittle stars.
Mollusks
Gastropods (nudibranchs, sea hares, slugs, and snails): This group includes a diverse array of terrestrial, freshwater, and marine species.[24,50,67] **Cephalopods** (cuttlefish, nautilus, octopuses, squid): This group includes a diverse group of marine species. Some species of octopus and the chambered nautilus (*Nautilus pompilius*) are occasionally found in home aquaria.[100] **Bivalves** (clams, mussels, oysters): This group includes a diverse group of freshwater and marine species. One of the most common reef genera is the giant clam (*Tridacna* sp.).[67,80,87]

[a]This is not a comprehensive list of taxa. The reader should be aware that taxonomy is a dynamic science and taxonomists frequently assign different taxonomic levels to the same groups depending on the anatomical, genetic, and other criteria being considered.

[b]In recent years, taxonomists have determined that crustaceans and insects are sister groups and belong to a larger common taxon, sometimes referred to as the Pancrustacea.[71]

REFERENCES

1. Acosta-Salmón H, Davis M. Inducing relaxation in the queen conch *Strombus gigas* (L.) for cultured pearl production. *Aquaculture*. 2007;262:73–77.
2. Alippi AM, Albo GN, Leniz D, et al. Comparative study of tylosin, erythromycin and oxytetracyline to control American foulbrood of honey bees. *J Apicult Res*. 1999;3-4:149–158.
3. Allender MC, Schumacher J, Milam J, et al. Pharmacokinetics of intravascular itraconazole in the American horseshoe crab (*Limulus polyphemus*). *J Vet Pharm Ther*. 2007;31:83–86.
4. Applegate JR, Dombrowski D, Christian LS, et al. Tricaine methanesulfonate (MS-222) sedation and anesthesia in the purple-spined sea urchin (*Arbacia punctulata*). *J Zoo Wildl Med*. 2016;47:1025–1033.
5. Aquilina B, Roberts R. A method for inducing muscle relaxation in the abalone, *Haliotis iris*. *Aquaculture*. 2000;190:403–408.
6. Archibald KE, Minter LJ, Lewbart GA, et al. Semen collection and characterization in the Chilean rose tarantula (*Grammostola rosea*). *Am J Vet Res*. 2014;75:929–936.
7. Archibald KE, Scott GN, Bailey KM, et al. 2-phenoxyethanol (2-PE) and tricaine methanesulfonate (MS-222) immersion anesthesia of American horseshoe crabs (*Limulus polyphemus*). *J Zoo Wild Med*. 2019;50(1):96–106.
8. Avery L, Horvitz HR. Effects of starvation and neuroactive drugs on feeding in *Caenorhabditis elegans*. *J Exp Zool*. 2000;253:263–270.
9. Bailey L. Effect of fumagillin upon *Nosema apis* (Zander). *Nature*. 1953;171:212–213.
10. Barord GJ, Ju C, Basil JA. First report of a successful treatment of a mucodegenerative disease in the chambered nautilus (*Nautilus pompilius*). *J Zoo Wild Med*. 2012;43(3):636–639.
11. Barron MG, Gedutis C, MO James. Pharmacokinetics of sulphadimethoxine in the lobster, *Homarus americanus*, following intrapericardial administration. *Xenobiotica*. 1988;18:269–276.

11a. Barton JA, Neil RC, Humphrey C, et al. Efficacy of chemical treatments for *Acropora*-eating flatworm infestations. *Aquaculture*. 2021;532:735978.
12. Basti D, Bouchard D, Lichtenwalner A. Safety of florfenicol in the adult lobster (*Homarus americanus*). *J Zoo Wild Med*. 2011;42(1):131–133.
13. Battison A, MacMillans R, MacKenzie A, et al. Use of injectable potassium chloride for euthanasia of American lobsters (*Homarus americanus*). *Comp Med*. 2000;50:545–550.
14. Boonstra JL, Koneval ME, Clark JD, et al. Milbemycin oxime (Interceptor) treatment of amphipod parasites (Hyperiidae) from several host jellyfish species. *J Zoo Wildl Med*. 2015;46:158–160.
15. Borneman EH. *Aquarium Corals: Selection, Husbandry, and Natural History*. Neptune City, NJ: T.F.H. Publications; 2001.
16. Brillantes S, Tanasomwang V, Thongrod S, et al. Oxytetracycline residues in giant freshwater prawn (*Macrobrachium rosenbergii*). *J Agri Food Chem*. 2001;49:4995–4999.
17. Brown PB, White MR, Chaille J, et al. Evaluation of three anesthetic agents for crayfish (*Orconectes virilis*). *J Shellfish Res*. 1996;15:433–435.
18. Bullis RA. Care and maintenance of horseshoe crabs for use in biomedical research. In: Stolen JS, Fletcher TC, Rowley AF, et al., eds. Fair Haven, NJ: SOS Publications; 1994. *Techniques in Fish Immunology*. 3:A9–A10.
19. Butler-Struben HM, Brophy SM, Johnson NA, et al. In vivo recording of neural and behavioral correlates of anesthesia induction, reversal, and euthanasia in cephalopod molluscs. *Front Physiol*. 2018;9:109.
20. Chair M, Nelis HJ, Leger P, et al. Accumulation of trimethoprim, sulfamethoxazole, and N-acetylsulfamethoxazole in fish and shrimp fed medicated *Artemia franciscana*. *Antimicrob Agents Chemother*. 1996;40:1649–1652.
21. Chang Z-Q, Gao A-X, Li J, et al. The effect of temperature and salinity on the elimination of enrofloxacin in the Manila clam *Ruditapes philippinarum*. *J Aquat Anim Health*. 2012;24:17–21.
22. Chiayvareesajja S, Chandumpai A, Theapparat Y, et al. The complete analysis of oxytetracycline pharmacokinetics in farmed Pacific white shrimp (*Litopenaeus vannamei*). *J Vet Pharm Ther*. 2006;29:409–414.
23. Christie BL, Raines JA. Effect of an otic milbemycin oxime formulation on *Tegastes acroporanus* infesting corals. *J Aquat Anim Health*. 2016;28:235–239.
24. Clark TR, Nossov PC, Apland JP, et al. Anesthetic agents for use in the invertebrate sea snail. *Aplysia californica. Contemp Top Lab Anim Sci*. 1996;35:75–79.
25. Colin ME, Duclos J, Larribau E, et al. Activite des huiles essentielles de Labies sur *Ascosphaera apis* et traitement d'un rucher. *Apidologie*. 1989;20:221–228.
26. Cooper EL. Transplantation immunity in annelids. *Transplantation*. 1968;6:322–337.
27. Cooper JE. Invertebrate anesthesia. *Vet Clin North Am Exot Anim Pract*. 2001;4:57–67.
28. Cooper JE, Pellett S, O'Brien M. Insects. In: Lewbart GA, ed. *Invertebrate Medicine*. 3rd ed. Oxford, UK: Wiley-Blackwell Publishing; 2022:413–437.
29. Cooper JE, Mahaffey P, Applebee K. Anaesthesia of the medicinal leech (*Hirudo medicinalis*). *Vet Rec*. 1986;118:589–590.
30. Crossley SMG, George AL, Keller CJ. A method for eradicating amphipod parasites (Hyperiidae) from host jellyfish, *Chrysaora fuscescens* (Brandt, 1835), in a closed recirculating system. *J Zoo Wild Med*. 2009;40:174–180.
31. Danyi S, Widart J, Douny C, et al. Determination and kinetics of enrofloxacin and ciprofloxacin in Tra catfish (*Pangasianodon hypophthalmus*) and giant freshwater prawn (*Macrobrachium rosenbergii*) using a liquid chromatography/mass spectrometry method. *J Vet Pharm Ther*. 2011;34:142–152.
32. Davis C, Ward W. *Control of chalkbrood disease with natural products. A report for the Rural Industries Research and Development Corporation*: RIRDC Publication; 2003:1–23 No. 03/107, RIRDC Project No. DAQ-269A.
33. Davis MR, Gamble KC, Matheson JS. Diagnostic imaging in terrestrial invertebrates: Madagascar hissing cockroach (*Gromphadorhina portentosa*), desert millipede (*Orthoporus* sp.),

emperor scorpion (*Pandinus imperator*), Chilean rosehair tarantula (*Grammostola spatulata*), Mexican fireleg tarantula (*Brachypelma boehmei*) and Mexican redknee tarantula (*Brachypelma smithi*). *Zoo Biol.* 2008;27:109–125.
34. Dombrowski D, De Voe R. Emergency care of invertebrates. *Vet Clin North Am Exot Anim Pract.* 2007;10:621–645.
35. Dombrowski D, De Voe R, Lewbart GA. Comparison of isoflurane and carbon dioxide anesthesia in rose-haired tarantulas (*Grammostola rosea*). *J Zoo Biol.* 2012;32(1):101–103.
36. Dorton D. The "cure" for red acro bugs. Formerly available at: http://www.reefs.org/forums/viewtopic.php?p=439155. Accessed Nov 14, 2016 and cited in 14, 67.
37. Fang WH, Hu LL, Yang XL, et al. Effect of temperature on pharmacokinetics of enrofloxacin in mud crab, *Scylla serrata* (Forsskal), following oral administration. *J Fish Dis.* 2008;31:171–176.
38. Fang W, Li G, Zhou S, et al. Pharmacokinetics and tissue distribution of thiamphenincol and florfenicol in Pacific white shrimp *Litopenaeus vannamei* in freshwater following oral administration. *J Aquat Anim Health.* 2013;25:83–89.
39. Fang X, Zhou J, Liu X. Pharmacokinetics and tissue distribution of enrofloxacin after single intramuscular injections in Pacific white shrimp. *J Vet Pharm Ther.* 2017;41:148–154.
40. Feldlaufera MF, Pettisa JS, Kochanskya JP, et al. Lincomycin hydrochloride for the control of American foulbrood disease of honey bees. *Apidologie.* 2001;32:547–554.
41. Feng Q, Wu GH, Liang TM, et al. Pharmacokinetics of oxytetracycline in hemolymph from the Chinese mitten crab, *Eriocheir sinensis. J Vet Pharm Ther.* 2010;34:51–77.
42. Feng Y, Zhai Q, Wang J, et al. Comparison of florfenicol pharmacokinetics in *Exopalaemon carinicauda* at different temperatures and administration routes. *J Vet Pharm Ther.* 2019;42:230–238.
43. Flores DV, Salas PJI, Vedra JPS. Electroretinography and ultrastructural study of the regenerated eye of the snail, *Cryptomphallus aspera. J Neurobiol.* 1983;14:167–176.
44. Friedman CS, Scott BB, Strenge RE, et al. Oxytetracycline as a tool to manage and prevent losses of the endangered white abalone, *Haliotis sorenseni*, caused by withering syndrome. *J Shellfish Res.* 2007;26(3):877–885.
45. Friedman CS, Trevelyan G, Robbins TT, et al. Development of an oral administration of oxytetracycline to control losses due to withering syndrome in cultured red abalone *Haliotis rufescens. Aquaculture.* 2003;224:1–23.
46. Fu G, Peng J, Wang Y, et al. Pharmacokinetics and pharmacodynamics of sulfamethoxazole and trimethoprim in swimming crabs (*Portunus trituberculatus*) and *in vitro* antibacterial activity against *Vibrio*: PK/PD of SMZ-TMP in crabs and antibacterial activity against *Vibrio. Environ Tox Pharm.* 2016;46:45–54.
47. Gardner C. Options for immobilization and killing crabs. *J Shellfish Res.* 1997;16:219–224.
48. Garr AL, Posch H, McQuillan M, et al. Development of a captive breeding program for the Florida apple snail, *Pomacea paludosa*: relaxation and sex ratio recommendations. *Aquaculture.* 2012;370-371:166–171.
49. Giacobino A, Rivero R, Molineri AI, et al. Fumagillin control of *Nosema ceranae* (Microsporidia: Nosematidae) infection in honey bee (Hymenoptera: Apidae) colonies in Argentina. *Vet Ital.* 2016;52(2):145–151.
50. Girdlestone D, Cruickshank SGH, Winlow W. The actions of three volatile anaesthetics on withdrawal responses of the pond-snail, *Lymnaea stagnalis* (L). *Comp Biochem Physiol C.* 1989;92:39–43.
51. Gjeltema J, Posner LP, Stoskopf MK. The use of injectable alphaxalone as a single agent and in combination with ketamine, xylazine, and morphine in the Chilean rose tarantula, *Grammostola rosea. J Zoo Wildl Med.* 2014;45:792–801.
52. Gleadall IG. The effects of prospective anaesthetic substances on cephalopods: summary of original data and a brief review of studies over the last two decades. *J Exp Mar Biol Ecol.* 2013;447:23–30.

53. Gore SR, Harms CA, Kukanich B, et al. Enrofloxacin pharmacokinetics in the European cuttlefish, *Sepia officinalis*, after a single i.v. injection and bath administration. *J Vet Pharm Ther.* 2005;28:433–439.
54. Gratzek JB. *Aquariology: The Science of Fish Health Management: Master Volume (Aquariology Series).* Morris Plains, NJ: Tetra Press; 1994.
55. Gunkel C, Lewbart GA. Invertebrates. In: West G, Heard D, Caulkett N, eds. *Zoo Animal and Wildlife Immobilization and Anesthesia.* Ames, IA: Blackwell; 2007:147–158.
56. Gunkel C, Lewbart GA. Anesthesia and analgesia of invertebrates. In: Fish R, Danneman P, Brown M, et al., eds. *Anesthesia and Analgesia in Laboratory Animals Animals.* St. Louis, MO: Elsevier; 2008:535–546.
57. Hadfield CA, Clayton LA, O'Neill KL. Milbemycin treatment of parasitic copepods on *Acropora* corals. *Proc 33rd East Fish Health Works.* 2008:76.
58. Harms CA. Echinoderms. In: Lewbart GA, ed. *Invertebrate Medicine.* 3rd ed. Oxford, UK: Wiley-Blackwell Publishing; 2022:579–598.
59. Harms CA, Lewbart GA, McAlarney R, et al. Surgical excision of mycotic (*Cladosporium* sp.) granulomas from the mantle of a cuttlefish (*Sepia officinalis*). *J Zoo Wildl Med.* 2006;37:524–530.
60. Heasman MP, O'Connor WA, Frazer AWJ. Induction of anaesthesia in the commercial scallop, *Pecten fumatus* Reeve. *Aquaculture.* 1995;131:231–238.
61. Higes M, Nozal MJ, Alvaro A, et al. The stability and effectiveness of fumagillin in controlling *Nosema ceranae* (Microsporidia) infection in honey bees (*Apis mellifera*) under laboratory and field conditions. *Apidologie.* 2011;42:364–377.
62. Hodgson G. Tetracycline reduces sedimentation damage to corals. *Mar Biol.* 1990;104:493–496.
63. Kirby A, Lewbart GA, Hancock-Ronemus A, et al. Pharmacokinetics of enrofloxacin and ciprofloxacin in Atlantic horseshoe crabs (*Limulus polyphemus*) after single injection. *J Vet Pharm Ther.* 2018;41:349–353.
64. Kloezen W, Parel F, Brüggemann R, et al. Amphotericin B and terbinafine but not the azoles prolong survival in *Galleria mellonella* larvae infected with *Madurella mycetomatis. Med Mycol.* 2018;56:469–478.
65. Kochansky J. Analysis of oxytetracycline in extender patties. *Apidologie.* 2000;31:517–524.
66. Landy RB, Leibovitz L. A preliminary study of the toxicity and therapeutic efficacy of formalin in the treatment of triclad turbellarid worm infestations in *Limulus polyphemus. Proc Ann Meet Soc Invert Pathol.* 1983.
67. Lehmann DW. Reef systems. In: Lewbart GA, ed. *Invertebrate Medicine.* 2nd ed. Ames, MO: Wiley-Blackwell Publishing; 2012:57–75.
68. Lewbart GA. Emergency and critical care of fish. *Vet Clin North Am Exot Anim Pract.* 1998;1:233–249.
69. Lewbart G, Riser NW. Nuchal organs of the polychaete *Parapionosyllis manca* (Syllidae). *Invert Biol.* 1996;115:286–298.
70. Liang JP, Li J, Li JT, et al. Accumulation and elimination of enrofloxacin and its metabolite ciprofloxacin in the ridgetail white prawn *Exopalaemon carinicauda* following medicated feed and bath administration. *J Vet Pharm Ther.* 2014;37:508–514.
71. Lozano-Fernandez J, Giacomelli M, Fleming JF, et al. Pancrustacean evolution illuminated by taxon-rich genomic-scale data sets with an expanded remipede sampling. *Genome Biol Evol.* 2019;11(8):2055–2070.
72. Ma R, Wang Y, Zou X, et al. Pharmacokinetics of sulfamethoxazole and trimethoprim in Pacific white shrimp, *Litopenaeus vannamei*, after oral administration of single-dose and multiple-dose. *Environ Tox Pharm.* 2017;52:90–98.
73. Marks DH, Cooper EL. *Aeromonas hydrophila* in the coelomic cavity of the earthworms *Lumbricus terrestris* and *Eisenia foetida. J Invert Pathol.* 1977;29:382–383.
74. Marnell C. Tarantula and hermit crab emergency care. *Vet Clin Exot Anim Med.* 2016;19:627–646.

75. Martins-Sousa RL, Negrao-Correa D, Bezerra FSM, et al. Anesthesia of *Biomphalaria* spp. (Mollusca, Gastropoda): sodium pentobarbital is the drug of choice. *Mem Inst Oswaldo Cruz.* 2001;96:391–392.
76. Mason SE, Papich MG, Schmale MC, et al. Enrofloxacin pharmacokinetics and sampling techniques in California sea hares (*Aplysia californica*). *J Vet Pharm Ther.* 2019;58(2):231–234.
77. McCurley RS, Kier WM. The functional morphology of starfish tube feet: the role of a crossed-fiber helical array in movement. *Biol Bull.* 1995;188:197–209.
78. McManus JM, Lu H, Chiel HJ. An in vitro preparation for eliciting and recording feeding motor programs with physiological movements in *Aplysia californica. J Vis Exp.* 2012;70:e4320.
79. Melidone R, Mayer J. How to build an invertebrate surgery chamber. *Exot DVM.* 2005;7(5):8–10.
80. Mills D, Tlili A, Norton J. Large-scale anesthesia of the silver-lip pearl oyster, *Pinctada maxima* Jameson. *J Shellfish Res.* 1997;16:573–574.
80a. Mones AB, Harms CA, Balko JA. Evaluation of intracardiac administration of potassium chloride, ivermectin, and lidocaine hydrochloride for euthanasia in anesthetized blue crabs (*Callinectes sapidus*). *Proc 53rd Int Assoc Aquat Anim Med.* 2022.
81. Müller MCM, Berenzen A, Westheide W. Regeneration experiments in *Eurythoe complanata* ("Polychaeta," Amphinomidae): reconfiguration of the nervous system and its function for regeneration. *Zoomorphology.* 2003;122:95–103.
82. Neely KL, Macaulay KA, Hower EK, et al. Effectiveness of topical antibiotics in treating corals affected by Stony Coral Tissue Loss Disease. *Peer J.* 2020;8:e9289. doi:10.7717/peerj.9289.
83. Nelis HJ, Leger F, Sorgeloos P, et al. Liquid chromatographic determination of efficacy of incorporation of trimethoprim and sulfamethoxazole in brine shrimp (*Artemia* spp.) used for prophylactic chemotherapy of fish. *Antimicrob Agents Chemother.* 1991;35:2486–2489.
84. Noga EJ. *Fish Disease: Diagnosis and Treatment.* 2nd ed. Ames, IA: Wiley-Blackwell Publishing; 2010:375–420.
85. Noga EJ, Hancock A, Bullis R. Crustaceans. In: Lewbart GA, ed. *Invertebrate Medicine.* 2nd ed. Ames, IA: Wiley-Blackwell Publishing; 2012:235–254.
86. Nolan MW, Smith SA, Jones D. Pharmacokinetics of oxytetracycline in the American horseshoe crab, *Limulus polyphemus. J Vet Pharmacol Ther.* 2007;30:451–455.
87. Norton JH, Dashorst M, Lansky TM, et al. An evaluation of some relaxants for use with pearl oysters. *Aquaculture.* 1996;144:39–52.
88. Oswald RL. Immobilization of decapod crustaceans for experimental purposes. *J Mar Biol Assoc UK.* 1977;57:715–721.
88a. Perrot-Minnot MJ, Balourdet A, Musset O. Optimization of anesthetic procedure in crustaceans: Evidence for sedative and analgesic-like effect of MS-222 using a semi-automated device for exposure to noxious stimulus. *Aquat Toxicol.* 2021;240:105981.
89. Phillips B, Harms CA, Lewbart GA, et al. Population pharmacokinetics of enrofloxacin and its metabolite ciprofloxacin in the green sea urchin (*Strongylocentrotus droebachiensis*) following intracoelomic and immersion administration. *J Zoo Wild Med.* 2016;47:175–186.
90. Pizzi R, Kennedy B. Spiders. In: Lewbart GA, ed. *Invertebrate Medicine.* 3rd ed. Oxford, UK: Wiley-Blackwell Publishing; 2022:301–347.
91. Poapolathep A, Jermnak U, Chareonsan A, et al. Dispositions and residue depletion of enrofloxacin and its metabolite ciprofloxacin in muscle tissue of giant freshwater prawns (*Macrobrachium rosenbergii*). *J Vet Pharmacol Ther.* 2009;32:229–234.
92. Poapolathep A, Poapolathep S, Imslip K, et al. Distribution and residue depletion of oxytetracycline in giant freshwater prawn (*Macrobrachium rosenbergii*). *J Food Protection.* 2008;71(4):870–873.
93. Poapolathep A, Poapolathep S, Jermnak U, et al. Muscle tissue kinetics of oxytetracyline following intramuscular and oral administration at two dosages to giant freshwater shrimp (*Macrobrachium rosenbergii*). *J Vet Pharmacol Ther.* 2008;31:517–522.

94. Polese G, Winlow W, Di Cosmo A. Dose-dependent effects of the clinical anesthetic isoflurane on *Octopus vulgaris*: a contribution to cephalopod welfare. *J Aquat Anim Health*. 2014;26(4):285–294.
95. Reed LA, Siewicki TC, Shah JC. Pharmacokinetics of oxytetracycline in the white shrimp, *Litopenaeus setiferus*. *Aquaculture*. 2004;232:11–28.
96. Reed LA, Siewicki TC, Shah C. The biopharmaceutics and oral bioavailability of two forms of oxytetracycline to the white shrimp, *Litopenaeus setiferus*. *Aquaculture*. 2006;258:42–54.
97. Ren X, Pan L, Wang L. Tissue distribution, elimination of florfenicol and its effect on metabolic enzymes and related genes expression in the white shrimp *Litopenaeus vannamei* following oral administration. *Aquaculture Res*. 2016;47:1584–1595.
98. Reynaldi F, Albo G, Avellaneda E, Rule R. Evaluation of kinetic behaviour of two preparations of tylosin administered in beehives for American foulbrood control. *Bulg J Vet Med*. 2017;20:264–270.
99. Rosenberg J, Haulena M, Phillips B, et al. Population pharmacokinetics of enrofloxacin in purple sea stars (*Pisaster ochraceus*) following an intracoelomic injection or extended immersion. *Am J Vet Res*. 2016;77:1266–1275.
100. Scimeca J, Barord G, Lewbart GA. Cephalopods. In: Lewbart GA, ed. *Invertebrate Medicine*. 3rd ed. Oxford, UK: Wiley-Blackwell Publishing; 2022:177–201.
101. Sendall K. Phenoxyethanol as a relaxant before fixation in the sea cucumber *Cucumaria miniata* (Echinodermata). *Collection Forum*. 2003;18(1-2):98–103.
102. Smith S. Horseshoe crabs. In: Lewbart GA, ed. *Invertebrate Medicine*. 3rd ed. Oxford, UK: Wiley-Blackwell Publishing; 2022:283–300.
103. Spotswood T, Smith SA. Cardiovascular and gastrointestinal radiographic contrast studies in the horseshoe crab (*Limulus polyphemus*). *Vet Radiol Ultrasound*. 2007;48:14–20.
104. Sprung J, Delbeek JC. *The Reef Aquarium: A Comprehensive Guide to the Identification and Care of Tropical Marine Invertebrates*. Vol. 2. FL: Ricordea: Coconut Grove; 1997.
105. Steeil JC, Schumacher J, George RH, et al. Pharmacokinetics of cefovecin (Convenia®) in white bamboo sharks (*Chiloscyllium plagiosum*) and Atlantic horseshoe crabs (*Limulus polyphemus*). *J Zoo Wildl Med*. 2014;45(2):389–392.
106. Stoskopf MK. Appendix V: Chemotherapeutics. In: Stoskopf MK, ed. *Fish Medicine*. Philadelphia, PA: WB Saunders; 1993:832–839.
107. Stoskopf MK, Westmoreland LS, Lewbart GA. Octocorallia, Hexacorallia, Scleractinia, and other corals. In: Lewbart GA, ed. *Invertebrate Medicine*. 3rd ed. Oxford, UK: Wiley-Blackwell Publishing; 2022:65–106.
108. Sweet MJ, Croquer A, Bythell JC. Experimental antibiotic treatment identifies potential pathogens of white band disease in the endangered Caribbean coral *Acropora cervicornis*. *Proc R Soc B*. 2014;281(1788) 2014.0094.
109. Tang J, Yang X, Zheng Z, et al. Pharmacokinetics and the active metabolite of enrofloxacin in Chinese mitten-handed crab (*Eriocheir sinensis*). *Aquaculture*. 2006;260:69–76.
110. Thomas RJ, Hamblin KA, Armstrong SJ, et al. *Galleria mellonella* as a model system to test the pharmacokinetics and efficacy of antibiotics against *Burkholderia pseudomallei*. *Int J Antimicrob Agents*. 2013:330–336.
111. Treves-Brown KM. *Applied Fish Pharmacology*. Dodrecht, Netherlands: Kluwer Academic Publishers; 2000.
112. Uno K. Pharmacokinetics of oxolinic acid and oxytetracycline in kuruma shrimp, *Penaeus japonicus*. *Aquaculture*. 2004;230:1–11.
113. Uno K, Aoki T, Kleechaya W, et al. Pharmacokinetics of oxytetracycline in black tiger shrimp, *Penaeus monodon*, and the effect of cooking on the residues. *Aquaculture*. 2006;254:24–31.
114. Van den Spiegel D, Jangoux M. Cuvierian tubules of the holothuroid *Holothuria forskali* (Echinodermata): a morphofunctional study. *Mar Biol*. 1987;96:263–275.
115. Vidal-Naquet N, Cripps C. Honey bees. In: Lewbart GA, ed. *Invertebrate Medicine*. 3rd ed. Oxford, UK: Wiley-Blackwell Publishing; 2022:439–520.

116. Vidal-Naquet N. *Honeybee Veterinary Medicine: Apis mellifera L.* Sheffield, UK: 5M Publishing; 2016:288.
117. Walcourt A, Ide D. A system for the delivery of general anesthetics and other volatile agents to the fruit fly *Drosophila melanogaster*. *J Neurosci Meth*. 1998;84:115–119.
118. White HI, Hecht T, Potgieter B. The effect of four anaesthetics on *Haliotis midae* and their suitability for application in commercial abalone culture. *Aquaculture*. 1996;140:145–151.
119. Winlow W, Polese G, Moghadam H-F, et al. Sense and insensibility—an appraisal of the effects of clinical anesthetics on gastropod and cephalopod molluscs as a step to improved welfare of cephalopods. *Front Phys*. 2018;9:1147.
120. Woodall AJ, Naruo H, Prince DJ, et al. Anesthetic treatment blocks synaptogenesis but not neuronal regeneration of cultured *Lymnaea* neurons. *J Neurophysiol*. 2003;90:2232–2239.
121. Wu G, Meng Y, Zhu X, et al. Pharmacokinetics and tissue distribution of enrofloxacin and its metabolite ciprofloxacin in the Chinese mitten-handed crab, *Eriocheir sinensis*. *Anal Biochem*. 2006;358:25–30.
121a. Wycoff S, Weineck K, Conlin S, et al. Effects of clove oil (eugenol) on proprioceptive neurons, heart rate, and behavior in model crustaceans. *Biol Faculty Publ*. 2018:145 https://uknowledge.uky.edu/biology_facpub/145?utm_source=uknowledge.uky.edu%2Fbiology_facpub%2F145&utm_medium=PDF&utm_campaign=PDFCoverPages (accessed 13 February 2022).
122. Zachariah TT, Mitchell MA, Guichard CM, et al. Isoflurane anesthesia of wild-caught goliath birdeater spiders (*Theraphosa blondi*) and Chilean rose spiders (*Grammostola rosea*). *J Zoo Wildl Med*. 2009;40:347–349.
123. Zachariah TT, Mitchell MA, Watson MK, et al. Effects of sevoflurane anesthesia on righting reflex and hemolymph gas analysis variables for Chilean rose tarantulas (*Grammostola rosea*). *Am J Vet Res*. 2014;75:521–526.

Chapter 2 Fish

Stephen A. Smith | Craig A. Harms

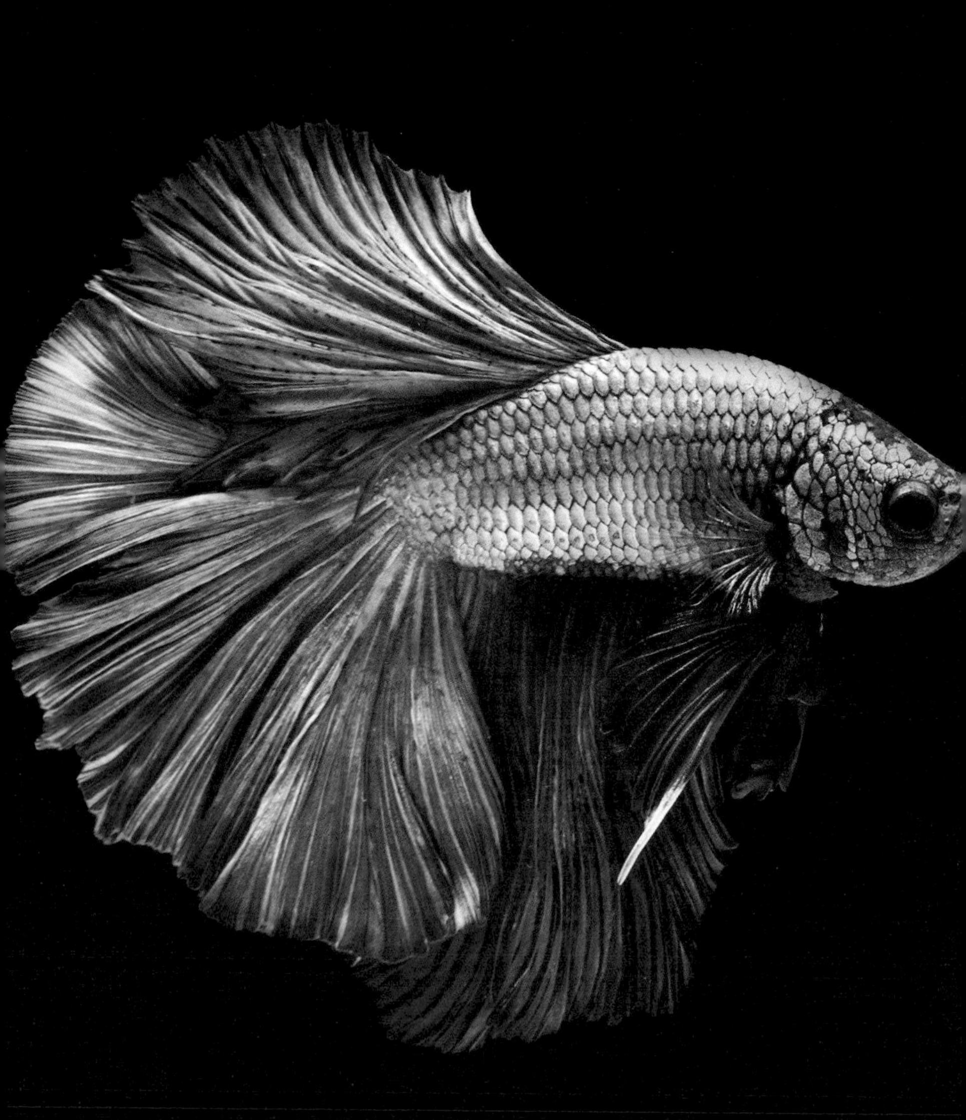

TABLE 2-1 Antimicrobial and Antifungal Agents Used in Fish.[a-h]

Agent	Dosage	Comments
Acriflavine	4 mg/L bath × 4 hr[179]	Rainbow trout/organic dye and antifungal agent
	10 mg/L bath × 4 hr[170]	Channel catfish/PK
Acyclovir	10 mg/kg ICe[25]	Koi/PD, PK; cyprinid herpesvirus 3; single dose safe, reduces cumulative mortality, but multiple doses probably required for effective treatment
Amikacin	—	Use cautiously in animals with suspected renal impairment
	5 mg/kg IM q12h[241]	
	5 mg/kg IM q72h × 3 treatments[241]	
	5 mg/kg ICe q24h × 3 days, then q48h × 2 treatments[110]	Koi
Amoxicillin	—	Infrequently indicated in ornamental fish because few pathogens are gram-positive
	12.5 mg/kg IM[21]	Atlantic salmon/PK
	25 mg/kg PO q12h[221]	
	40 mg/kg IV q24h[40]	Sea bream/PK
	80 mg/kg PO q24h × 10 days[40]	Sea bream/PK
	40-80 mg/kg q24h via feed × 10 days[150]	Sea bream/PK
	110 mg/kg/day via feed[12]	Channel catfish/PK
Ampicillin	—	Infrequently indicated in ornamental fish because few pathogens are gram-positive
	10 mg/kg q24h IM[231]	Atlantic salmon
	10 mg/kg q24h IV[169]	Striped bass
	50-80 mg/kg/day via feed × 10 days[150]	
Azithromycin (Zithromax, Zoetis)	30 mg/kg PO q24h × 14 days[50]	Chinook salmon/PK
	40 mg/kg ICe[51]	Chinook salmon/PK
Aztreonam (Azactam, Bristol-Myers Squibb)	100 mg/kg IM or ICe q48h × 7 treatments[184]	Koi/*Aeromonas salmonicida*; used by hobbyists
Benzalkonium chloride	0.5 mg/L bath long-term[231]	Quaternary amine with broad disinfection properties
	10 mg/L bath × 10 min[231]	
Bronopol (Pyceze, Novartis)	15-50 mg/L bath × 30-60 min[174,241]	Mycotic infections (eggs and fish); eggs may require the higher dose
Cefovecin (Convenia, Zoetis)	16 mg/kg SC[203]	Copper rockfish/PK; plasma levels of >1 μg/mL persisted for 7 days in adult fish

Continued

TABLE 2-1 Antimicrobial and Antifungal Agents Used in Fish. (cont'd)

Agent	Dosage	Comments
Cefovecin (Convenia, Zoetis) (cont'd)	—	Rapidly eliminated in white bamboo sharks, thus not recommended[215]
Ceftazidime (Fortaz, Zoetis)	22 mg/kg IM or ICe q72-96h × 3-5 treatments[184]	Cephalosporin with good activity against gram-negative bacteria (e.g., *Pseudomonas*)
Ceftiofur	8 mg/kg IM[44]	Species of Anabantidae, Callichthyidae, Cichlidae, and Cyprinidae
Ceftiofur crystalline free acid (CFA; Excede, Zoetis)	6.6 mg/kg IM[53]	Smooth dogfish/PK; presumed therapeutic plasma concentrations >168 hr
	20 mg/kg IM once 30 mg/kg ICe once 60 mg/kg IM once 60 mg/kg ICe once[75]	Koi/PK; concentration-time profiles unpredictable; authors do not recommend[75]
Chloramine-T	2.5-20 mg/L bath[36,231] × 60 min/day × up to 3 days[3]	Disinfectant; used to control bacterial gill disease and some ectoparasites; dosage and duration varies widely with species and water quality
	20 mg/L bath × 4 hr[142]	Rainbow trout, striped bass, yellow perch/PK
Chloramphenicol	—	Prohibited for use in food animals (risk to humans); florfenicol is an alternative
	40-182 mg/kg ICe q24h[123]	Carp/PK
	50 mg/kg PO, IM once, then 25 mg/kg q24h[221]	Rainbow trout/PK
	50 mg/kg PO q24h[34]	Rainbow trout/PK
Ciprofloxacin	15 mg/kg IM, IV[153]	Carp, African catfish, rainbow trout/PK
Danofloxacin	10 mg/kg IM once[31,138,162,236]	Amur sturgeon, koi, European sea bass, brown trout/PK
Difloxacin	10 mg/kg PO q24h[48]	Atlantic salmon/PK; plasma levels were higher in marine fish compared with freshwater fish
	10 mg/kg PO, IV once[223]	Olive flounder/PK
	20 mg/kg PO q24h × 3 days[42]	Crucian carp/PK
Diquat dibromide (Reward, Syngenta)	2-18 mg/L bath × 1-4 hr × 1-4 treatments q24-48h[1] 19-28 mg/L bath × 30-60 min × 1-3 treatments q48h[1]	Columnaris disease in freshwater fish
Doxycycline	20 mg/kg PO, IV[248]	Tilapia/PK; possible enterohepatic cycling; dosing intervals not established
Enrofloxacin (Baytril, Bayer)	—	For a review of quinolones used in fish, see Samuelsen 2006;[193] IM injections can be highly irritating to tissues[202]

TABLE 2-1 Antimicrobial and Antifungal Agents Used in Fish. (cont'd)

Agent	Dosage	Comments
Enrofloxacin (Baytril, Bayer) (cont'd)	2.5 mg/kg IV q24h[39]	Sea bream/PK; no metabolism to ciprofloxacin detected
	2.5-5 mg/L bath × 5 hr q24h × 5-7 days[134]	Red pacu/PK; change 50%-75% of water between treatments
	5 mg/kg PO, IM, ICe q24h[221]	
	5-10 mg/kg PO q24h[231]	
	5-10 mg/kg IM, ICe q48h × 7 treatments[134]	Red pacu/PK
	10 mg/kg PO q24h × 10 days[163]	Small-scaled pacu/withdrawal period (non-USA) 23 days at 27°C; ciprofloxacin detected
	10 mg/kg PO q24h[39,125,193]	Atlantic salmon, rainbow trout, sea bream/PK; no ciprofloxacin detected
	10 mg/kg PO, IV[52,118,122]	Brown trout, crucian carp, Korean catfish/PK; ciprofloxacin detected
	10 mg/kg PO via feed q24h[130,150,218]	Atlantic salmon/PK
	10 mg/kg ICe q96h × 4 treatments[132]	Koi/PK (21°C)
	20 mg/kg PO x 7 days[37]	Tra catfish
	30 mg/kg PO q24h[246]	Grass carp/prevention of resistance mutation for *Aeromonas hydrophila* strain AH10
	50 mg/kg PO q24h x 7 days[247]	Nile tilapia
	0.1% of feed × 10-14 days[130]	Oral or injectable form can be used; 0.1% feed = 1 g/kg feed; equivalent to 10 mg/kg body weight if eating 1% (10 g/kg) body weight/day
Erythromycin	—	Commonly sold as tank treatment for aquarium fish; not generally recommended because of toxicity to nitrifying bacteria[150]
	10-25 mg/kg IM, ICe[49] 10-25 mg/kg IM, ICe 1-3 × q3wk[49]	Bacterial kidney disease (salmonids); second dose for control of vertical transmission of bacterial kidney disease
	75 mg/kg PO q24h × 7 days[35]	Barramundi/*Streptococcus iniae*
	75 mg/kg PO q24h × 10 days[43]	Sea bream/PK, PD; control of *Streptococcus iniae*
	100 mg/kg q24h x 10 days[51]	Chinook salmon/PK
	100 mg/kg PO, IM q24h × 7-21 days[221,231]	
	100-200 mg/kg PO q24h × 21 days[145]	Salmonids/control of *Renibacterium salmoninarum*
	110 mg/kg PO q24h x 14 days[95]	Rainbow trout

Continued

TABLE 2-1 Antimicrobial and Antifungal Agents Used in Fish. (cont'd)

Agent	Dosage	Comments
Florfenicol (Nuflor, Merck Animal Health; Aquaflor [Veterinary Feed Directive-medicated feed], Merck Animal Health)	5-20 mg/kg PO q24h[105]	Atlantic salmon/PK
	10 mg/kg IM q24h[250]	Koi/PK; for MICs of 1-6 μg/mL)
	10 mg/kg PO q24h x 10 days[63]	Channel catfish/PK
	10-15 mg/kg PO q24h[14]	Channel catfish/PK
	10-20 mg/kg PO q24h × 10 days[194,198,199]	Cod/PK, Atlantic salmon
	10-24 mg/kg PO once[54,98]	Atlantic salmon/PK Orange-spotted grouper/PK
	10 mg/kg IV or 20 mg/kg IM once[136]	Olive flounder/PK
	10, 25, or 50 mg/kg PO q12h[251]	Gouramis/PK; for MICs of 1, 3, and 6 μg/mL, respectively
	10, 25, or 50 mg/kg PO q24h[251]	Koi/PK, for MICs of 1, 3, and 6 μg/mL, respectively
	10 or 100 mg/kg IM q12h[250]	Gouramis/PK; for MICs of 1 μg/mL or 6 μg/mL
	15 mg/kg PO via feed x 12 days[60]	Hybrid tilapia/PK
	40 mg/kg IM[255]	White-spotted bamboo sharks/PK
	40-50 mg/kg PO, IM, ICe q12-24h[133,221]	Red pacu/PK
	100 mg/kg IM q24h[199]	Atlantic salmon
Flumequine (Apoquin aqualtes, Sigma-Aldrich)	—	Gram-negative bacteria; freshwater at pH 6.8-7.2; decreased uptake in hard water; increase dose for marine fish
	22 μg/fish PO in *Artemia nauplii* q48h x 5 days, or 20 mg/L bath × 2 hr q48h × 3 treatments[230]	Sea bass larvae (40 day old)/PK
	5 mg/kg PO once[82,214]	Atlantic salmon/PK[214] Turbot, halibut, eels/PK[82]
	10 mg/kg PO q48h[81]	Cod, goldsinny wrasse/PK
	10 mg/kg PO q24h × 10 days[150]	General dose
	12-25 mg/kg PO, ICe, IV q24h[195]	Atlantic halibut/PK
	25 mg/kg PO once[237]	Atlantic cod/PK
	25 mg/kg PO once[90]	Lumpfish/PK
	25 mg/kg PO q24h x 10 days[152]	Atlantic salmon/PK
	25 mg/kg ICe q24h[197]	Corkwing wrasse/PK
	25-50 mg/kg PO q24h[186]	Atlantic salmon
	30 mg/kg IM, ICe[150]	Atlantic salmon/high antibiotic levels several days when given IM
	35 mg/kg PO via feed x 5 days[234]	Gilt-head sea bream/PK
	50-100 mg/L bath × 3-5 hr[156]	Brown trout, Atlantic salmon/PK

TABLE 2-1 Antimicrobial and Antifungal Agents Used in Fish. (cont'd)

Agent	Dosage	Comments
Formalin	—	All doses based on volumes of 100% formalin (= 37% formaldehyde solution); moderate to weak antibacterial activity;[150] caution: carcinogenic; do not use if highly toxic white precipitates of paraformaldehyde are present; some fish are very sensitive; test on small number first; monitor for respiratory distress and pale color; increased toxicity in soft, acidic water and at high temperature; treat with vigorous aeration because of oxygen depletion; toxic to plants; rapid degradation in saltwater-recirculating aquaculture systems by day 3 presumptively due to microbial digestion (biotic) or abiotic factors; testing and variable additions may be required to achieve target dose above 15 mg/L for multiple day treatments[120]
	0.23 mL/L bath × up to 60 min[150]	Eggs/mycotic (oomycete) infections; do not treat within 24 hr of hatching
	1 mL/3.8 L bath × 12-24 hr followed by 30%-70% water change, may be repeated[68]	
	1-2 mL/L bath × up to 15 min[150]	
Furazolidone	—	Nitrofuran; caution: carcinogenic; toxic to scaleless fish; absorbed from water; inactivated in bright light
	1 mg/kg PO, IV q24h[171]	Channel catfish
	25-35 mg/kg PO q24h via feed × 20 days[92]	Rainbow trout, brown trout, brook trout, cutthroat trout, not approved for fish intended for human consumption in the United States
	30 mg/kg PO[247]	Nile tilapia
	50-100 mg/kg PO q24h via feed × 10-15 days[150]	Reduced palatability at higher doses
	67.5 mg/kg PO q12h × 10 days[127]	Rainbow trout/PK; at 14°C (57°F) half-life ≈ 30 days and residue present at 40 days after 10-day treatment
	1-10 mg/L bath for ≥ 24 hr[150]	General dose
Gentamicin	1 mg/kg IM, ICe q24h[204]	Channel catfish/PK
	2 mg/kg IM, then 1 mg/kg IM at 8 and 72 hr[222]	Brown shark/PK
	2.5 mg/kg IM q72h[130]	Nephrotoxic in some species; substantial risk in species for which dosages have not been determined[178]
	3.5 mg/kg IM q24h[112]	Goldfish, toadfish/PK

Continued

TABLE 2-1 Antimicrobial and Antifungal Agents Used in Fish. (cont'd)

Agent	Dosage	Comments
Hydrogen peroxide (HP) (3%)	0.1 mL/L bath × 1 hr[189]	Swordtails/external bacteria
Hydrogen peroxide (HP) (35% PEROX-AID, Eka Chemicals)	—	One mL of 35% PEROX-AID contains 350 mg HP
	50 mg/L bath × 1 hr[167]	Channel catfish fry/columnaris disease
	50-75 mg/L bath × 1 hr[167]	Channel catfish fingerlings and adults/ columnaris disease
Iodine, potentiated (Betadine, Purdue Frederick)	Topical for wound, rinse immediately[150]	Do not use solutions combined with detergent (e.g., Betadine scrub)
	20-100 mg/L x 10 min[231]	Eggs/disinfection
Itraconazole	1-5 mg/kg PO q24h via feed × up to 7 days[221]	Systemic mycoses
Kanamycin sulfate (Kantrex, Apothecon)	20 mg/kg ICe q3d × 5 treatments[150]	Toxic to some fish
	50 mg/kg PO q24h via feed[150]	General dose
	40-640 mg/L × 2 hr bath[65]	Channel catfish
	50-100 mg/L bath q72h × 3 treatments[150]	Change 50%-75% of water between treatments; absorbed from water
Ketoconazole	2.5-10 mg/kg PO, IM, ICe × 10 days[221]	Rainbow trout/systemic mycoses
Malachite green (zinc-free)	—	Freshwater fish and eggs/mycotic and oomycete infections; caution: mutagenic, teratogenic; toxic to some fish species and to fry; increased toxicity at higher temperatures and lower pH; stains objects, especially plastic; toxic to plants; not approved for use on fish intended for human consumption
	0.1 mg/L bath q3d × 3 treatments[150]	Remove residual chemical with activated carbon after final treatment
	0.25 mg/L bath × 15 min q24h[242]	Eggs/fungal control
	0.5 mg/L bath × 1 hr[150]	Eggs of freshwater fish
	1 mg/L bath × 30-60 min[150]	Use 2 mg/L if pH is high
	1 mg/L bath × 1 hr[231]	Eggs/fungal control
	1.6 mg/L bath × 40 min q7d x 3 treatments[4]	Rainbow trout
	2 mg/L bath × 15 min q24h[231]	Eggs/fungal control
	3.2 mg/L dip q1wk × 3 treatments[4]	Rainbow trout
	10 mg/L bath × 10-30 min bath[150]	Eggs/fungal control

TABLE 2-1 Antimicrobial and Antifungal Agents Used in Fish. (cont'd)

Agent	Dosage	Comments
Malachite green (zinc-free) (cont'd)	50-60 mg/L dip × 10-30 sec[150]	General dose
	100 mg/L topical[150]	Skin lesions
Marbofloxacin	10 mg/kg PO q24 hr × 3 days at 15°C and 25°C[254]	Crucian carp/PK; half-life longer at 15°C than 25°C; increase dose in marine fish as drug binds with calcium, magnesium, and aluminum
Methylene blue	2 mg/L bath q48h × up to 3 treatments[150]	Preventing infections of freshwater eggs; toxic to nitrifying bacteria and to plants; stains plastics
Miconazole (Monistat, McNeil-PPC)	10-20 mg/kg PO, IM, ICe q24h[221]	Systemic mycoses
Nalidixic acid (NegGram, Sanofi-Aventis)	5 mg/kg PO, IM q24h[221]	Rainbow trout/PK;[109] quinolone antibiotic; gram-negative bacteria
	5 mg/kg PO, IV q24h[109]	
	20 mg/kg PO q24h[231]	General dose
	13 mg/L bath × 1-4 hr bath, repeat prn[150]	General dose
Neomycin	66 mg/L bath q3d × up to 3 treatments[150]	Commonly sold as water treatment for aquarium fish; toxic to nitrifying bacteria
Nifurpirinol	—	Nitrofuran derivative; caution: carcinogenic; toxic to scaleless fish; absorbed from water; change 50-75% of water between treatments; drug inactivated in bright light
	0.1 mg/L bath q24h × 3-5 days[150]	General dose
	0.45-0.9 mg/kg PO q24h × 5 days[150]	General dose
	4-10 mg/kg PO via feed q12h × 5 days[150]	General dose
	1-2 mg/L bath × 5 min-6 hr[150]	General dose
Nitrofurazone	—	Nitrofuran; caution: carcinogenic; toxic to scaleless fish; absorbed from water; change 50%-75% of water between treatments; drug inactivated in bright light; water-soluble formulations preferred
	2-5 mg/L bath q24h × 5-10 days[241]	General dose
	50 mg/L bath × 3 hr[30]	Gilt-head (sea) bream, Mozambique tilapia/no residues found in muscle following treatment
	100 mg/L bath × 30 min[150]	General dose
	100 mg/L bath × 6 hr[30]	Gilt-head (sea) bream, Mozambique tilapia, no residues found in muscle following treatment

Continued

TABLE 2-1 Antimicrobial and Antifungal Agents Used in Fish. (cont'd)

Agent	Dosage	Comments
Norfloxacin	10 mg/kg PO once[244]	Crucian carp, common carp/increase dose in marine fish as drug binds with calcium, magnesium, and aluminum
Oxolinic acid	—	Quinolone; active against gram-negative bacteria; increase dose in marine fish as drug binds with calcium, magnesium, and aluminum; decreased uptake in hard water
	3-10 mg/L bath × 24 hr[150]	General dose
	5-25 mg/kg PO q24h[221]	General dose
	10 mg/kg q24h PO[231]	Freshwater species/PK in many species
	10 mg/kg PO q24h via feed × 10 days[150]	General dose
	20 mg/kg PO q24h[181,182,183]	Gilt-head (sea) bream/PK; Sharpnose sea bream/PK
	25 mg/kg ICe q24h[197]	Corkwing wrasse/PK
	25 mg/kg PO q5d at 9°C[196]	Atlantic halibut/PK
	25-50 mg/kg PO q24h[231]	Marine species
	25 mg/L bath × 15 min q12h × 3 days[150]	Decreased uptake in hard water; better uptake pH <6.9
	50 mg/kg PO q24h × 5 days[32,33]	Rainbow trout/PK
Oxytetracycline	3 mg/kg IV q24h[45]	Red pacu/PK
	7 mg/kg IM q24h[45]	Red pacu/PK
	10 mg/kg IM q24h[221]	Produces high levels for several days when given IM
	20 mg/kg ICe[231]	Some salmonids
	20 mg/kg PO q8h[221]	General dose
	25-50 mg/kg IM, ICe[150]	General dose
	50 mg/kg PO once[207]	Tilapia/PK; dose acceptable for freshwater and brackish fish species but may lead to therapeutic failure in marine species[207]
	60 mg/kg IM q7d[71]	Carp/PK
	70 mg/kg PO q24h × 10-14 days[240]	General dose
	83 mg/kg PO × 10 days[26]	Walleye pike, tilapia, hybrid striped bass, summer flounder/PK
	100 mg/kg IM q24h[180]	Tench/PK
	100 mg/kg PO q24h × 5 days[251]	Yellow catfish/PK
	100 mg/kg PO q24hr × 7 days[252]	Grass carp/PK
	55-83 mg/kg PO q24h via feed × 10 days[150]	General dose

TABLE 2-1 Antimicrobial and Antifungal Agents Used in Fish. (cont'd)

Agent	Dosage	Comments
Oxytetracycline (cont'd)	75 mg/kg PO q24h via feed × 10 days[231]	General dose
	10-50 mg/L bath × 1 hr[150]	Surface bacterial infections; yellow-brown foam may develop in treatment water
	10-100 mg/L bath[150]	Use higher doses in hard water; may retreat on day 3 after 50%-75% water change; light sensitive; keep tank covered to reduce photoinactivation; decomposing drug turns dark brown-change 50% of water immediately
	400 mg/L bath x 12 hr[238]	Giant danio/PK; buffer water with sodium bicarbonate, total hardness <17.1 mg/dL
	7 mg/g of feed q24h × 10 days[240]	General dose
Potassium permanganate	2 mg/L indefinite bath[241]	Do not mix with formalin; heavily organic systems may require higher dose; test efficacy by adding the appropriate amount of $KMnO_4$ to a small amount of system water (without fish); red color should remain at least 4 hr (if not, then add $KMnO_4$ until the 4-hr test is completed); treatment durations may need to be shortened to 1-2 hr in systems with lower organic loading (e.g., moderate- to lower-intensity recirculating aquaculture systems) and for sensitive species
	5 mg/L bath × 30-60 min[150]	Freshwater fish/skin and gill bacterial infections; toxic in water with high pH; can be toxic in goldfish[219]
	1000 mg/L dip × 10-40 sec[150]	General dose
Sarafloxacin (Sarafloxacin hydrochloride, Enzo Life Sciences)	10-14 mg/kg PO q24h × 10 days[221]	Fluoroquinolone; decreased uptake in hard water; increase dose in marine fish as drug binds with calcium, magnesium, and aluminum
	10 mg/kg PO q24h[231]	Marine Atlantic salmon
	10 mg/kg PO q24h × 5-10 days[66]	Channel catfish
Silver sulfadiazine cream (Silvadene, Pfizer)	Topically q12h[130]	External bacterial (gram-positive and gram-negative) and yeast infections; keep lesion out of water 30-60 sec after application while keeping gills submerged
Sulfadimethoxine/ ormetoprim (Romet, Zoetis)	50 mg/kg PO via feed q24h × 5 days[150]	Available as a powder to add to feed and as medicated feed

Continued

TABLE 2-1 Antimicrobial and Antifungal Agents Used in Fish. (cont'd)

Agent	Dosage	Comments
Sulfadimethoxine/ ormetoprim (Romet, Zoetis) (cont'd)	3 mg/L seawater × 4 hr[150]	Medicated brine shrimp/soak brine shrimp nauplii (larvae) × 4 hr, rinse in seawater, feed immediately to fish; may also work with adult brine shrimp and other live feeds
Sulfamethoxazole (S)/ trimethoprim (T)	—	Potentiated sulfonamide; change 50-75% water between bath treatments
	20 mg/L bath × 5-12 hr q24h × 5-7 days[18]	Rainbow trout
	30 mg/kg PO q24h × 10-14 days[150]	General dose
	200 µg/mL bath × 72 hr[200]	Atlantic halibut/PK
	0.2% of feed q24h × 10-14 days[150]	General dose
	(S) 674 mg/kg + (T) 113 mg/kg of feed × 5 days[168]	Striped catfish, hybrid red tilapia/PK
Thiamphenicol	15 or 30 mg/kg PO q24h × 5 days[106]	Sea bass/PK; drug not detected in plasma or tissues at either dose on day 7; recommended withdrawal times of 5 and 6 days after last treatment, respectively
Tobramycin	2.5 mg/kg IM once, then 1 mg/kg IM q4d[222]	Brown shark/PK
Triple antibiotic ointment (polymyxin B, sulfate bacitracin, neomycin sulfate)	Topically q12h[130]	External bacterial infections; keep lesion out of water 30-60 sec following application while keeping gills submerged

[a]Not to be used in fish for human consumption.

[b]Preferable to treat a single fish of a species (biotest) to determine toxicity.

[c]Tank treatment: when treating the fishes' resident aquarium, disconnect activated carbon filtration to prevent drug removal. Many drugs adversely affect the nitrifying bacteria, so water quality should be monitored closely (especially ammonia and nitrite concentrations). Always keep water well aerated and monitor fish closely. Perform water changes and reconnect filtration to remove residual drug following treatment. Discard carbon following drug removal.[131]

[d]Bath (immersion) treatment: remove fish from resident aquarium and place in container with known volume of water and concentration of therapeutic agent. Watch closely for signs of toxicity (e.g., listing and dyspnea). Always keep water well aerated.

[e]Species of fish, temperature, and water quality parameters can influence the pharmacodynamics of many drugs, especially antimicrobials.

[f]For more information, refer to the website by Reimschuessel et al.[179] This is a comprehensive and informative resource for many drugs and other compounds used with aquatic animals.

[g]MIC = minimum inhibitory concentration.

[h]See Table 2-7 for scientific names of species listed in this table.

TABLE 2-2 Antiparasitic Agents Used in Fish.[a-e]

Agent	Dosage	Comments
Acetic acid, glacial	1-2 mL/L dip × 30-45 sec bath[150,241]	Monogeneans and crustacean ectoparasites; safe for goldfish; may be toxic to smaller tropical fish
Albendazole	5 mg/kg PO once[148]	Atlantic salmon/PK
	10 mg/kg PO once[205]	Atlantic salmon, rainbow trout, tilapia/PK
	10-50 mg/L bath × 2-6 hr[201]	Sticklebacks/treating *Glugea anomala* infection
Amprolium (A)/ salinomycin (S)	(A) 100 mg/kg/(S)70 mg/kg PO via feed[67,104]	Marine fish/*Enteromyxum leei* myxozooan infestations; reduced mortality
Chloramine-T	—	See Table 2-1 (Antimicrobial and Antifungal Agents)
Chloroquine diphosphate	10 mg/L bath, once[150] 50 mg/kg PO once[135]	Red drum/*Amyloodinium ocellatum*; monitor for 21 days, repeat prn; use activated carbon to remove drug from water
Closantel (50 mg/ mL)/mebendazole (75 mg/mL) (Supaverm, Janssen-Cilag)	1 mL/400 L bath once; may repeat in 3-7 days following a water change if necessary[241]	Koi/external monogeneans; safe and effective; reported to be highly toxic to goldfish and medaka; used in the United Kingdom for digenean trematodes of sheep
Copper sulfate	—	Marine fish/protozoan, monogenean ectoparasites; copper levels must be assessed with a commercial kit, and adjusted as needed; blue copper sulfate is copper sulfate (II) pentahydrate (= $CuSO_4 \cdot 5H_2O$); when calculating free copper 2^+ ion levels, copper sulfate pentahydrate is approximately 25% free copper; in marine systems, concentration should be increased gradually to target concentration over the course of 3-4 days; toxic to invertebrates and many plants; immunosuppressive to fish; toxic to gill tissue; may be removed by activated carbon
	Total alkalinity (TA) (mg/L)/100 = mg/L ($CuSO_4 \cdot 5H_2O$)	General dose recommendation for use in freshwater systems, for 50 < total alkalinity (TA) < 250 mg/L; not recommended for use in freshwater systems with TA <50 mg/L; chelation may be required for TA >250 mg/L[150]
	0.012 or 0.094 mg/L bath × 28 days[72]	European eels
	0.02 mg/L bath × 65 or 72 hr[73,74]	Rainbow trout
	0.1-0.2 mg/L bath[231]	Use higher dose in hard water
	Maintain free ion levels at 0.15-0.2 mg/L water until therapeutic effect[150]	
	Maintain copper levels at 0.2 mg/L water × 14-21 days[240]	Citrated copper sulfate; prepare stock solution of 1 mg/mL (3 g $CuSO_4 \cdot 5H_2O$ and 2 g citric acid monohydrate in 750 mL distilled water)

Continued

TABLE 2-2 Antiparasitic Agents Used in Fish. (cont'd)

Agent	Dosage	Comments
Copper sulfate (cont'd)	Maintain free ion levels at 0.25-1 mg/L water × 24-48 hr[84]	
	100 mg/L bath × 1-5 min[24]	Prepare stock solution of 1 mg/mL (1 g $CuSO_4 \cdot 5H_2O$ in 250 mL distilled water)
Diflubenzuron (Dimilin 25W, Chemtura)	0.01 mg/L bath × 48 hr q6d × 3 treatments[219]	Crustacean ectoparasites; inhibits chitin synthesis; drug persists in water long term; marketed for control of terrestrial insects; may need EPA restricted use pesticide license for use in the United States
Dimethyl phosphonate	—	See trichlorfon
Dimetridazole	28 mg/kg PO via feed q24h × 10 days[176]	Rainbow trout/*Ichthyophthirius multifiliis*; may be available through compounding veterinary pharmacies
	80 mg/L bath × 3 days (minimum duration)[249]	Experimental evidence suggests some control of *Cryptobia iubilans* and/or associated mortalities
Doramectin	200 µg/kg IM once[94]	Fringe-lipped peninsula carp, major South Asian carp/*Lernaea*
	200 µg/kg IM once[93]	Rohu/*Argulus*; effective but caused discoloration, lethargy, and poor appetite
	750 µg/kg PO via feed once[93]	Rohu/*Argulus*; 1000 µg/kg PO caused mortality
	1 mg/kg PO q24h × 10 days[94]	Fringe-lipped peninsula carp, major South Asian carp/*Lernaea*
Doxycycline	5 mg/kg PO × 1 then 2.5 mg/kg PO q24h × 14 days[127a]	Lumpfish/scuticociliatosis
Emamectin (SLICE, Merck Animal Health)	5 µg/kg PO q24h × 7 days[80]	Koi/*Argulus*
	50 µg/kg PO q24h × 7 days[80]	Goldfish/*Argulus*
	50 µg/kg PO q24h × 7 days[211]	Atlantic salmon/PK; sea lice (*Lepeophtheirus salmonis, Caligus elongatus, C. teres*, and *C. rogercressyi*)
	50 µg/kg PO q24h × 7 days[19,78]	Rainbow trout/*Argulus*
	50 µg/kg PO q24h × 7 days[46]	Brook trout/*Salmincola edwardsii*
Fenbendazole	1 mg/kg IV once[38]	Channel catfish/PK
	1.5 mg/L bath × 12 hr[108]	Rainbow trout
	2 mg/L bath q7d × 3 treatments[150]	Nonencysted gastrointestinal nematodes
	5 mg/kg PO × 1 dose[119]	Channel catfish/PK
	6 mg/kg PO q24h[108]	Rainbow trout
	40 mg/kg PO via feed q4d × 2 treatments[231]	Carp/*Bothriocephalus acheilognathi*
	50 mg/kg PO q24h × 2 days, repeat in 14 days[240]	

TABLE 2-2 Antiparasitic Agents Used in Fish. (cont'd)

Agent	Dosage	Comments
Fenbendazole (cont'd)	2.5 mg/g of feed × 2-3 days, repeat in 14 days[240]	
	0.2% of feed × 3 days, repeat in 14-21 days[130]	
	Bioencapsulation of brine shrimp[7]	Place 1 tablespoon of strained adult brine shrimp in 4 g fenbendazole per 500 mL volume for 30 min to achieve 15.3 µg fenbendazole per shrimp
Formalin	All doses based on volumes of 100% formalin (= 37% formaldehyde)	Protozoan, monogenean, crustacean ectoparasites. Caution: carcinogenic; do not use if highly toxic white precipitates are present; some fish are very sensitive: test on small number first, monitor for respiratory distress; increased toxicity in soft, acidic water and at high temperature; treat with aeration because of oxygen depletion; toxic to plants
	0.015-0.025 mL/L bath q48h × 3 treatments[150]	*Ichthyophthirius*; change up to 50% of water on alternate days
	0.025 ml/L (9.3 mg formaldehyde/L) bath × 144 hr[245]	Striped bass
	0.125-0.25 mL/L bath × up to 60 min, repeat q24h × 2-3 days prn[150]	When using maximum dose, treat q3d
	200 ppm bath × 1 hr[116]	Red porgy/monogeneans
	250-400 ppm bath × 1 hr followed by 5 min freshwater dip[206]	Yellow kingfish/monogeneans
	0.4 mL/L (400 ppm) bath × up to 1 hr q3d × up to 3 treatments[219]	Soft water dose
	0.5 mL/L (500 ppm) bath × up to 1 hr q3d × up to 3 treatments[219]	Hard water dose
Formalin (F)/ malachite green (M)	(F) 0.025 mL/L + (M) 0.1 mg/L bath q48h × 3 treatments[150]	Combination synergistic for *Ichthyophthirius*; change up to 50% water on alternate days; several premixed commercial products available; mutagenic and teratogenic; malachite green should never be used on fish intended for human consumption
Freshwater	3-15 min bath, repeat q7d prn[150] 4-5 min bath once[129]	Marine fish/ectoparasites; aerate well; match pH with seawater pH; monitor closely; small fish may be sensitive
Furazolidone		See Antimicrobial section

Continued

TABLE 2-2 Antiparasitic Agents Used in Fish. (cont'd)

Agent	Dosage	Comments
Hydrogen peroxide (HP) (3%; 30 mg/mL)	—	Not recommended for use in blue gourami or suckermouth catfish[189]
	5.5 mg/L (0.18 ml/L) bath × 24 hr or 7 mg/L × 1 hr[189]	Serpae tetras
	5.9 mg/L bath × 24 hr or 10 mg/L × 1 hr[189]	Tiger barbs
	6.5 mg/L bath × 1 hr[189]	Swordtails/*Ichthyobodo*
	6.5 mg/L bath × 24 hr or 20.2 mg/L × 1 hr[189]	Swordtails
	1-1.5 mL/L (30-45 mg/L) bath × 20 min[228]	Atlantic salmon/sea lice
	17.5 mL/L bath × 4-10 min once[84]	Ectoparasites; monitor closely; may be harmful to smaller fish
Hydrogen peroxide (HP) (PEROX-AID 35%, Eka Chemicals)	—	These are unlabeled experimental treatments
	75 mg/L bath × 30 min[146]	Juvenile Pacific threadfin/*Amyloodinium*
	170-560 mg/L static bath × 30 min[175]	Rainbow trout/*Ambiphrya*, *Gyrodactyus*
	300 mg/L bath × 10 min[140]	Kingfish/gill monogeneans
Ivermectin	—	Do not use; neurologic signs and death at therapeutic doses;[84,231] toxic to many species of invertebrates[231]
Levamisole	0.5 mg/kg ICe[115]	Rainbow trout/immunostimulant
	10 mg/kg IM days 1, 14, and 28[139]	Sandbar shark
	10 mg/kg PO q7d × 3 treatments[84]	Aquarium and ornamental fish/antiparasitic
	11 mg/kg IM q7d × 2 treatments[84]	Aquarium and ornamental fish/antiparasitic
	1 mg/L bath × 24 hr[224]	Eels/swimbladder nematodes
	1-2 mg/L bath × 24 hr[84]	Internal nematodes, especially larval forms
	50 mg/L bath × 2 hr[84]	Aquarium and ornamental fish/antiparasitic
	4 g/kg of feed q7d × 3 treatments[84]	External monogeneans
Lufenuron (Program, Novartis)	0.13 mg/L bath prn[184,241]	Crustacean ectoparasites
Magnesium sulfate (Epsom salt)	3% of feed x 2 days[217]	Rainbow trout/diplomonad intestinal parasite (*Spironucleus* spp.)
Malachite green	—	See Formalin for combination

TABLE 2-2 Antiparasitic Agents Used in Fish. (cont'd)

Agent	Dosage	Comments
Malachite green (cont'd)	—	Caution: mutagenic and teratogenic; toxic to some fish species (e.g., tetras) and fry; increased toxicity at higher temperatures and lower pH; toxic to plants; stains objects, especially plastic; remove residual chemical with activated carbon after last treatment; not to be used on fish intended for human consumption
	0.1 mg/L bath q3d × 3 treatments[150]	
	0.25 mg/L bath × 15 min q24h[242]	Salmonids
	1 mg/L bath × 30-60 min[150]	Use 2 mg/L if pH high
	50-60 mg/L bath × 10-30 sec[150]	
	100 mg/L topically to skin lesions[150]	Freshwater fish/protozoan ectoparasites; prepare stock solution of 3.7 mg/mL (1.4 g malachite green in 380 mL water)
Mebendazole	1 mg/L bath × 24 hr[107]	European eels/branchial monogeneans
	1 mg/L bath × 72 hr[22]	European eels/branchial monogeneans (*Pseudodactylogyrus bini* and *P. anguillae*)
	10-50 mg/L bath × 2-6 hr[201]	Sticklebacks/*Glugea anomala*
	20 mg/kg PO q7d × 3 treatments[221]	Gastrointestinal nematodes; do not administer to brood fish: embryotoxic and teratogenic
	100 mg/L bath × 10 min-2 hr[84]	Eels/monogeneans
Methylene blue	1-3 mg/L bath[150]	Freshwater fish/ectoparasites; not recommended due to poor efficacy; toxic to plants and nitrifying bacteria; stains objects
	5 mg/L bath × 24 hr[8]	Tilapia fry/trichodinids and monogeneans
Metronidazole	—	*Spironucleus* (*Hexamita*) and other internal flagellates; some external flagellates; poorly soluble in water: dissolve before adding to water or feed; change water between tank treatments
	6.6 mg/L bath q24h × 3 days[150]	
	25 mg/L bath q48h × 3 treatments[150]	
	25 mg/kg PO via feed q24h × 5-10 days[150]	Equivalent to 0.25% of feed (250 mg/100 g food) at 1% BW/day
	50 mg/kg PO via feed q24h × 5 days[239]	Freshwater angelfish/*Hexamita*, *Spironucleus*
	100 mg/kg PO via feed q24h × 3 days[150]	Equivalent to 1% of feed (1 g/100 g of food) at 1% BW/day

Continued

TABLE 2-2 Antiparasitic Agents Used in Fish. (cont'd)

Agent	Dosage	Comments
Metronidazole (cont'd)	6.25-18 mg/g of feed × 5 days[240]	
	Bioencapsulation of metronidazole in brine shrimp[6]	One Tbs of strained live adult brine shrimp is approximately 16 g wet weight (≈ 262 shrimp/g); 5 g metronidazole plus 1 Tbs brine shrimp in 500 mL saltwater for 0.25 hr will yield 9.32 µg metronidazole per shrimp (2500 µg per g of shrimp)
Niclosamide	0.055 mg/L bath × 24 hr[103]	Rainbow trout/lampricide
Piperazine	10 mg/kg PO q24h via feed × 3 days[150]	Nonencysted gastrointestinal nematodes; equivalent to 0.1% of feed at 1% BW/day
Potassium permanganate	5 mg/L bath × 30-60 min[150] 100 mg/L bath × 5-10 min[150] 1 g/L dip × 10-40 sec[150]	Freshwater fish/protozoan and crustacean ectoparasites; systems with high organic load require higher doses; toxic in water with high pH; do not mix with formalin; can be toxic in goldfish[219]; test by adding $KMnO_4$ to small sample of system water and reddish tint should remain for at least 4 hr; continue adding $KMnO_4$ until 4-hr color test reached
Praziquantel	2 mg/L bath × 2-4 hr[172]	Encysted metacercaria
	2-10 mg/L bath × up to 4 hr[240]	Monitor closely for lethargy, incoordination, loss of equilibrium
	5-10 mg/L bath × 3-6 hr, repeat in 7 days[129]	Monogenean ectoparasites, cestodes; aerate water well; some marine fish sensitive; may be toxic to *Corydoras* catfish; tank microbiome may adapt to degrade praziquantel rapidly[227]
	5 mg/kg PO q24h × 3 treatments[231]	
	5 mg/kg PO q7d via feed, × up to 3 treatments[221]	
	5 mg/kg PO, ICe, repeat in 14-21 days[129]	Cestodes, some internal digenean trematodes; can be administered via feed
	50 mg/kg PO once[150]	Adult cestodes; gavage or give 0.5% via feed at 1% BW/day
	5-12 mg/g of feed × 3 days[240]	
	Bioencapsulation of praziquantel in brine shrimp[5]	Place 1 Tbs (~15 g) of strained live adult brine shrimp and 2.5 g praziquantel per 500 mL volume for 30 min to achieve 8.6 µg praziquantel per shrimp
Pyrantel pamoate	10 mg/kg PO via feed once[221]	Gastric nematodes
Salt (as sodium chloride, seawater, or artificial sea salts)		Freshwater fish/protozoan and monogenean ectoparasites; seawater or artificial sea salts preferred; seawater is normally 30-35 g/L; use non-iodized table salts; anticaking agents in solar salts are highly toxic; species sensitivity is highly variable (some catfish species sensitive); can be toxic to plants

TABLE 2-2 Antiparasitic Agents Used in Fish. (cont'd)

Agent	Dosage	Comments
Salt (as sodium chloride, seawater, or artificial sea salts) (cont'd)	1-5 g/L indefinite bath[150]	Freshwater fish/prophylaxis or treatment of ectoparasites
	1-3 g/L bath[231]	Freshwater fish/supportive care for osmotic imbalances
	10-30 g/L bath × up to 30 min[150]	With salt-sensitive or weak fish, use lower dosage and repeat in 24 hr
	30 g/L bath × 10 min[231]	Fish >100 g only
	30-35 g/L bath × 4-5 min[129]	Safe for goldfish and koi in most cases
Thiabendazole	10-25 mg/kg PO via feed, repeat in 10 days[221]	Gastric nematodes; anorexia may be seen (more severe at higher doses), generally resolves within 2-4 days
	66 mg/kg PO once[221]	Rainbow trout
Trichlorfon (dimethyl phosphonate)	—	Caution: organophosphate, neurotoxic, avoid inhalation and skin contact; aerate water well; especially toxic to larval fish, some characins (i.e., pacu, piranha, and silver dollars); other species sensitivities; liquid form marketed for cattle is convenient to dispense
	0.25 mg/L bath × 96 hr q3d × 2 treatments	Channel catfish and other freshwater fish/ 0.5 mg/L tank water if > 27°C (80°F); treat q3d × 2 treatments for *Dactylogyrus* and other oviparous monogeneans; treat q7d × 4 treatments for anchor worms (*Lernaea*) and fish louse (*Argulus*); single treatments usually suffice for other copepods, other monogeneans, and leeches[150,179]
	0.5 mg/L bath q10d × 3 treatments[129]	Crustacean ectoparasites; change 20%-30% of water 24-48 hr following each treatment
	0.5-1 mg/L bath	Marine fish/oviparous monogeneans; treat q3d × 2 treatments; use 1 mg/L q48h × 3 treatments for turbellarians; single treatment will usually suffice for copepods (except sea lice), other monogeneans, and leeches

[a]Not to be used in fish for human consumption.

[b]Preferable to treat single fish of a species (biotest) to determine toxicity.

[c]Tank treatment: when treating the fishes' resident aquarium, disconnect activated carbon filtration to prevent drug removal; many drugs adversely affect the nitrifying bacteria, so water quality should be monitored closely (especially ammonia and nitrite concentrations); always keep water well aerated and monitor fish closely; perform water changes and reconnect filtration to remove residual drug following treatment; discard carbon following drug removal.[131]

[d]Bath (immersion) treatment: remove fish from resident aquarium and place in container with known volume of water and concentration of therapeutic agent; watch closely for signs of toxicity, e.g., listing and dyspnea; always keep water well aerated.

[e]See Table 2-7 for scientific names of species listed in this table.

TABLE 2-3 Chemical Sedation, Anesthetic, and Analgesic Agents Used in Fish.[a-e]

Agent	Dosage	Comments
Alfaxalone (Alfaxan, Jurox)	0.5 mg/L bath sedation; 5 mg/L anesthesia[17]	Goldfish/sedation and anesthesia
	5 mg/L bath induction[23]	Oscar (cichlid)/sedation and anesthesia
	10 mg/L bath induction; 1.0-2.5 mg/L maintenance[144]	Sedation and anesthesia; not recommended as an injectable agent for koi carp; may have opercular cessation at 2.5 mg/L[15]
Atipamezole (Antisedan, Zoetis)	0.2 mg/kg IM[57]	Gulf of Mexico sturgeon, black sea bass, bonnethead shark, sandbar shark/reversal agent (α_2 antagonist) for medetomidine
	IM dose dependent on previous dexmedetomidine injection (equal volume or 10x mg dose)[62]	
Benzocaine	—	Anesthetic; not sold for fish in United States; available from chemical supply companies; do not use topical anesthetic products marketed for mammals; prepare stock solution in ethanol as benzocaine is poorly soluble in water; store in dark bottle at room temperature
	15-40 mg/L bath[150]	Sedation for transport
	50-500 mg/L bath[150]	Anesthesia
	70 mg/L bath induction × 5 min, then 35 mg/L × 30 min[91]	Channel catfish/anesthesia
	100-200 mg/L bath for fish < 400 g[210]	Lumpfish/anesthesia; not suitable for fish >600 g
	1 g/L water spray[150]	Large fish/anesthesia; spray onto gills with a sprayer
Butorphanol	0.05-0.1 mg/kg IM[221]	Postoperative analgesia
	0.4 mg/kg IM once[87]	Koi/postoperative analgesia
	10 mg/kg IM once[16]	Koi/postoperative analgesia/respiratory depression at this dose; lower dosage might be warranted
Carbon dioxide	—	See Table 2-5 (Euthanasia agents)
Clove oil (also see Eugenol)	—	Clove oil consists of a mixture of eugenol, methyleugenol, isoeugenol, and other compounds; in this generic form, is not approved by the FDA for use in fish intended for human consumption
	10-15 mg/L bath[164]	Siamese fighting fish (betta)
	30 mg/L bath[124]	Pikeperch/anesthesia
	40-120 mg/L bath[129]	Stock solution: 100 mg/mL of clove oil by diluting 1 part clove oil with 9 parts 95% ethanol (eugenol is poorly soluble in water); over-the-counter preparation (pure) available at most pharmacies contains approximately 1 g eugenol per mL of clove oil; recovery may be prolonged; use lower end of this range to start; many bony fishes readily anesthetized with 25-50 mg/L

TABLE 2-3 Chemical Sedation, Anesthetic, and Analgesic Agents Used in Fish. (cont'd)

Agent	Dosage	Comments
Clove oil (also see Eugenol) (cont'd)	60 mg/L bath[165]	Walleye, northern pike, smallmouth bass, lake sturgeon/PD; anesthesia
	60 mg/L bath[59]	Cardinal tetra, freshwater angelfish/PD; anesthesia
	90 mg/L bath[59]	Banded cichlid/PD; anesthesia
	500 mg/L bath[161]	Amur catfish/PD; anesthesia; caution: this dose resulted in extremely rapid induction time of ~1 min
Dexmedetomidine	0.025-0.1 mg/kg IM once[62]	Bonnethead shark, sandbar shark/analgesia without respiratory depression
Dexmedetomidine (D)/Ketamine (K)/ Midazolam (M)	(D) 0.05-0.1 mg/kg + (K) 2-4 mg/kg + (M) 0.2 mg/kg combined IM[28]	Black sea bass/sedation; potentially fatal in red porgy
Ethanol	1%-1.5% bath[85]	Anesthetic levels difficult to control, resulting in overdose; not recommended
Etomidate	0.5-3.6 mg/L bath[173]	Golden shiners, channel catfish, striped bass/ anesthesia; lower dosage should be used with striped bass
	2-4 mg/L bath[9]	Zebrafish, black tetra, freshwater angelfish, southern platyfish/PD; anesthesia
	1-2 mL/L bath[126,187,188]	European perch, pikeperch, common carp/ anesthetic dose for commercial preparation of etomidate sold in Europe (Propiscin)
Eugenol (a purified derivative of clove oil; also see clove oil)	—	Aqui-SE contains 50% eugenol and Aqui-S20E 10% eugenol; a compound mixture of eugenol and polysorbate 80 (for solubility); lower doses (6 mg/L) will produce sedation without general anesthesia[2,231]
	10 mg/L bath[253]	Grass carp/PK, PD; sedation for transport
	10-100 mg/L bath[2]	Sedation, anesthesia
	15 or 25 mg/kg[216]	California yellowtail/anesthesia (Aqui-20E)
	17-25 mg/L bath[231]	Sedation, anesthesia
	35-55 mg/L bath[208]	Various cultured and wild marine fish species including white sea bass, California yellowtail, and California halibut/anesthesia (Aqui-20);
	50 mg/L bath[114]	Common snook/anesthesia
	60-100 mg/L bath[76]	Zebrafish/PD; anesthesia
Hydromorphone	0.2 mg/kg IM once[62]	Unicorn leatherjacket and other species/ postoperative analgesia; shorter duration of action and more potent than morphine
Isoflurane	0.5-2 mL/L bath or vaporize, then bubble in water[85]	Anesthesia; levels difficult to control resulting in overdose; also potential human exposure hazard; not recommended

Continued

TABLE 2-3 Chemical Sedation, Anesthetic, and Analgesic Agents Used in Fish. (cont'd)

Agent	Dosage	Comments
Ketamine	5-10 mg/kg IM or SC once[62]	Immobilization; generally combined with other drugs such as dexmedetomidine or midazolam
	66-88 mg/kg IM[221]	Immobilization; for short procedures; complete recovery can take >1 hr
Ketamine (K)/ medetomidine (M)[d]	(K) 1-2 mg/kg + (M) 0.05-0.1 mg/kg IM[85]	Immobilization; reverse medetomidine with atipamezole (0.2 mg/kg IM)
	(K) 6 mg/kg + (M) 0.06 mg/kg IM[57]	Gulf of Mexico sturgeon/immobilization; reversed with atipamezole (0.3 mg/kg IM)
Ketoprofen (Ketofen, Zoetis)	2 mg/kg IM once[87]	Koi/postoperative analgesia
	3 mg/kg IM, IV[69]	Rainbow trout/PK; analgesia
	8 mg/kg IM[69]	Nile tilapia/PK; analgesia
Lidocaine	<1-2 mg/kg total dose[85]	Local anesthesia; use cautiously in small fish
Medetomidine[d]	0.03-0.07 mg/kg IV[57]	See ketamine for combination; medetomidine is off market, but is available through selected compounding services
Meloxicam	1 mg/kg IM, IV once[58]	Nile tilapia/PK; rapid elimination; multiple daily treatments would be necessary
	0.5 mg/kg IM, IV q12-24h[146a]	Nursehound sharks/PK; poor oral absorption
Metomidate (Aquacalm, Syndel USA)	—	Sedation and anesthesia; gouramis may be sensitive; contraindicated in cichlids in water of pH <5
	0.06-0.2 mg/L bath[220]	Transport sedation
	0.1-1 mg/L bath[13]	
	0.5-1 mg/L bath[85]	Light sedation
	1 mg/L bath[117]	Convict cichlids/24 hr transport sedation
	1-10 mg/L bath induction; 0.1-1 mg/L maintenance[220]	Freshwater fish/anesthesia
	2.5-5 mg/L bath[85]	Heavy sedation
	2.5-5 mg/L bath induction; 0.2-0.3 mg/L maintenance[220]	Marine fish/anesthesia
	3 mg/kg IV[83]	Atlantic halibut, turbot/PK; anesthesia
	3 mg/L bath[157]	Atlantic salmon/anesthesia at 5.0-7.7°C
	5-10 mg/L bath[85]	Anesthesia; some species require 10-30 mg/L bath
	7 mg/kg PO[83]	Turbot/PK; anesthesia
	9 mg/L bath × 5 min[83]	Atlantic halibut, turbot/PK; anesthesia
Morphine	5 mg/kg IM[16]	Koi/analgesia
	6.7 mg/kg ICe[113]	Rainbow trout/PD; analgesia
	40 mg/kg IP or 17 mg/kg IV[149]	Winter flounder/analgesia; both doses caused significant bradycardia and prolonged (>48 hr) increase in cardiac output; not recommended

TABLE 2-3 Chemical Sedation, Anesthetic, and Analgesic Agents Used in Fish. (cont'd)

Agent	Dosage	Comments
MS-222 (Tricaine-S, Syndel USA)	—	See tricaine methanesulfonate
2-Phenoxyethanol	0.1-0.5 mL/L bath[231]	Carp/anesthesia
	0.15 mL/L bath[166]	Elasmobranchs (14 species)/immobilization
	0.17-0.3 mg/L bath[233]	White sea bream, sharpsnout sea bream/ anesthesia
	0.6 mL/L bath[231]	Carp/anesthesia
Propofol	2.5 mg/kg IV[143]	Spotted bamboo shark/anesthesia
	2.5 mg/L bath × up to 20 min[154]	Koi/anesthesia; immersion >20 min had prolonged recovery
	3.5-7.5 mg/kg IV[57]	Gulf of Mexico sturgeon/anesthesia
	5 mg/L bath[155]	Koi/PK; anesthesia
	7 mg/L bath[64]	Goldfish/anesthesia; induction time 7.4 min; recovery time 8.5 min
Quinaldine sulfate	—	Not sold as fish anesthetic in United States; stock solution: 10 g/L; buffer the acidity by adding sodium bicarbonate to saturation; store stock in dark container; shelf life of stock extended by refrigeration or freezing; aerate water to prevent hypoxemia; drug not metabolized and is excreted unchanged[85]
	25 mg/L bath[231]	Channel catfish, salmonids/anesthesia; do not use with largemouth bass; also not recommended for long surgical procedures
	50-100 mg/L bath induction; 15-60 mg/L maintenance[85]	Anesthesia
Robenacoxib (Onsior, Elanco)	2 mg/kg IM[177]	Rainbow trout/PK, PD; presumptive antinociceptive plasma concentration duration 3-4 days
Tricaine methanesulfonate (MS-222; Tricaine-S, Syndel USA)	—	Stock solution: 10 g/L; buffer the acidity by adding sodium bicarbonate at 10 g/L or to saturation (unbuffered solution may cause some ectoparasites to leave fish);[24] store stock in dark container; shelf life of stock extended by refrigeration or freezing; stock that develops an oily film or brown discoloration should be discarded; aerate water to prevent hypoxemia; narrower margin of safety in young fish and soft warm water
	15-50 mg/L bath[85]	Sedation, anesthesia
	25-50 ppm bath induction[62]	Mahi-mahi, bonnethead shark, other ram-ventilating fish/sedation and anesthesia
	50-100 mg/L bath induction; 50-60 mg/L maintenance[220]	Anesthesia

Continued

TABLE 2-3 Chemical Sedation, Anesthetic, and Analgesic Agents Used in Fish. (cont'd)

Agent	Dosage	Comments
Tricaine methanesulfonate (MS-222; Tricaine-S, Syndel USA) (cont'd)	100 mg/L bath[124]	Pike perch/PD; anesthesia
	100-200 mg/L bath induction; 50-100 mg/L maintenance[85]	Anesthesia
	100 mg/L and 200 mg/L bath[210]	Lumpfish/sedation and anesthesia
	1 g/L water spray[150]	Large fish/sedation and anesthesia; spray onto gills with a sprayer

[a]Not to be used in fish for human consumption.
[b]Preferable to treat single fish of a species to determine toxicity.
[c]Aerate water during anesthetic procedures; dissolved oxygen concentrations should be maintained between 6 and 10 mg/L (ppm).
[d]Medetomidine is no longer commercially available, although it can be obtained from select compounding services; a dosage is listed here as a guide for possible use with dexmedetomidine, an α_2 agonist that is the active optical enantiomer of racemic compound medetomidine; in other species, dexmedetomidine is used at 1/2 the dose of medetomidine; however, the effects of the v/v use of the two drugs may not be equivalent, so the dose of dexmedetomidine may need to be adjusted based on clinical response.
[e]See Table 2-7 for scientific names of species listed in this table.

TABLE 2-4 Miscellaneous Agents Used in Fish.[a-d]

Agent	Dosage	Comments
Ascorbic acid (vitamin C)	3-5 mg/kg IM q24h[192] 25-50 mg/kg IM, SC[62]	Dilute with appropriate fluid to decrease tissue damage due to acidity
Atropine	0.1 mg/kg IM, IV, ICe[219]	Treatment of organophosphate and chlorinated hydrocarbon toxicities
B-vitamin complex (B_1, B_2, B_6, B_{12})	10 mg/kg SC[62]	Dose is based on thiamine component
Becaplermin (Regranex, Smith & Nephew)	Topically as a thin layer × 3 min[56]	Ocean surgeonfish/light debridement of the head and lateral line erosion (HLLE) lesions recommended prior to treatment; multiple treatments not warranted; fish should be returned to habitat without predisposing factors to HLLE
Carbon, activated	75 g/40 L tank water[150]	Removal of medications and other organics from water; usually added to filter system; discard after 2 wk; 75 g ≈ 250 mL dry volume
Carp pituitary extract	0.75 mg/kg IM[231]	Female fish (<2 kg)
	1-1.5 mg/kg IM[231]	Male fish
	1.5 mg/kg IM[231]	Female fish (2-5 kg)
	2.5-3 mg/kg IM[231]	Female fish (>5 kg)

TABLE 2-4 Miscellaneous Agents Used in Fish. (cont'd)

Agent	Dosage	Comments
Carp pituitary extract (cont'd)	5 mg/kg IM, repeat in 6 hr[221]	Dose when combined with human chorionic gonadotropin (20 U/kg); hormone to stimulate release of eggs (may be given in 2 doses, 24 hr apart; the first "preparatory" dose ≤10% of the total dose); does not cause eggs to mature; do not administer unless eggs are mature
Chlorine/chloramine neutralizer	Use as directed	See also sodium thiosulfate
Dexamethasone	0.2 mg/kg IM, SC once[62]	Adjunct for shock, trauma, or chronic stress syndromes
	1-2 mg/kg IM, ICe[221]	Shock, trauma, or chronic stress
	2 mg/kg IV, ICe q12h[129]	Chlorine toxicity; may improve prognosis
Doxapram	5 mg/kg IV, ICe[219]	Respiratory stimulant
	5 mg/kg dripped over gill[62]	
Epinephrine (1:1000)	0.2-0.5 mL IM, IV, ICe, intracardiac[219]	Cardiac arrest
Furosemide	2-5 mg/kg IM, ICe q12-72h[221]	Diuretic; ascites; generalized edema; of questionable value because fish lack a loop of Henle
Glucans (MacroGard, Orffa)	—	Polysaccharides; immune stimulant
	2-10 mg/kg ICe[185,231]	Atlantic salmon
	1 g/kg of feed × 24 days fed at 3% BW[190]	Red-tailed black shark/decrease in mortalities from *Streptococcus iniae*
	2 g/kg of feed × 7 days[209]	Rainbow trout/increased nonspecific immunity
sGnRHa (salmon gonadotropin-releasing hormone analogue) + domperidone (Ovaprim, Syndel USA)	0.5 mL/kg (0.5 µL/g) IM, ICe[96,159]	Spawning aid; enhances/triggers ovulation and spermiation
Haloperidol	0.5 mg/kg IM[221]	Dopamine-blocking agent; stimulates egg release; use with luteinizing releasing hormone analog (LRH-A)
Hetastarch (hydroxyethyl starch)	0.5-1 mL/kg IV slowly[62]	Freshwater and marine fish/colloidal replacement fluid
Human chorionic gonadotropin (hCG) (Chorulon, Merck Animal Health)	—	Male and female broodfish/aid in improving spawning function; hormone to stimulate release of eggs (ovulation) and sperm (spermiation); does not cause eggs to mature: do not administer unless eggs are mature
	20 U/kg IM, repeat in 6 hr[221]	Dose when combined with carp pituitary extract (5 mg/kg)
	30 U/kg (23-232 U/kg for males; 30-828 U/kg for females) IM, repeat q6h × 1-3 treatments[27,221]	
	800-1000 U/kg IM q8h[243]	Carp

Continued

TABLE 2-4 Miscellaneous Agents Used in Fish. (cont'd)

Agent	Dosage	Comments
Hydrocortisone	1-4 mg/kg IM, ICe[221]	Adjunct for shock, trauma, or chronic stress syndromes
Hydrogen peroxide (3%)	0.25 mL/L bath[150]	Acute environmental hypoxia; see Oxygen in this section
Luteinizing releasing hormone analog (LRH-A)	2 µg/kg IM, then 8 µg/kg 6 hr later[221]	Synthetic luteinizing releasing hormone analog; stimulates egg release; does not cause eggs to mature: do not administer unless eggs are mature; administer with haloperidol or reserpine with the first injection of LRH-A in species that do not respond to LRH-A alone
Methyltestosterone	—	Masculinization of females
	30 mg/kg PO q24h × 2 or 4 days[179]	Rainbow trout/PD
	30 mg/kg PO[235]	Tilapia/PK
	40 mg/kg PO × 40 days[111]	Rainbow trout/PK
	60 mg/kg PO × 18 or 22 days[77,141]	Tilapia/PD
Nitrifying bacteria	Use as directed for commercial products	Seed or enhance development of biological filtration to detoxify ammonia and nitrite; commercial preparations; do not expose products to extreme temperatures; use before expiration date
	Add material (e.g., floss, gravel, biomedia) from system with an active biological filter and healthy fish to new or naïve system[150]	Potential risk of disease transmission with this transfer technique
Nucleotide (Aquagen, Novartis)	2 g/kg of feed at 3% BW × 24 days[190]	Red-tailed black sharks/reduced mortalities from *Streptococcus iniae*; commercial product has been discontinued
Oxygen (100%)	Fill plastic bag with O_2 containing 1/3 vol of water[129]	Acute environmental hypoxia common with transportation; close bag tightly with rubber band; keep fish in bag until normal swimming and respiratory behavior
Reserpine	50 mg/kg IM[221]	Dopamine-blocking agent; use with LRH-A to stimulate release of eggs
Salt (sodium chloride)	1-3 g/L bath[128] 3-5 g/L bath[150]	Freshwater fish/prevention of stress-induced mortality; seawater or artificial sea salts preferred; use noniodized table salts; some anticaking agents in solar salts are highly toxic; highly variable species sensitivity to salt (some catfish sensitive); toxic to some plants
	Add chloride to produce at least a 6:1 ratio (w/w) of $Cl:NO_2$ ions[150]	Treatment of nitrite toxicity; table salt = 60% Cl, artificial sea salts = 55% Cl

TABLE 2-4 Miscellaneous Agents Used in Fish. (cont'd)

Agent	Dosage	Comments
Sodium thiosulfate	Use as directed for chlorine/chloramine neutralizer products	Active ingredient in numerous chlorine/ chloramine neutralizers; chlorine and chloramine are common additions to municipal water supplies and are toxic to fish; ammonia released by detoxification of chloramine is removed by functioning biological filter (see nitrifying bacteria) or chemical means (see zeolite)
	10 mg/L water[129]	10 g neutralizes chlorine (up to 2 mg/L) from 1000 L water
	100 mg/L water[219]	Chlorine exposure
Zeolite (i.e., clinoptilolite)	Use as directed for commercial products	Ion-exchange resin that exchanges ammonia for sodium ions; clinoptilolite is an active form of zeolite; used to reduce or prevent ammonia toxicity; more effective for removal of some compounds (e.g., sulfonamides, enrofloxacin) than activated carbon[20,97,158]
	20 g/L water[150]	

[a]Not to be used in fish for human consumption.
[b]Preferable to treat single fish of a species (biotest) to determine toxicity.
[c]Bath treatment: remove fish from resident aquarium and place in container with known volume of water and concentration of therapeutic agent; watch closely for signs of toxicity, e.g., listing and dyspnea; always keep water well aerated.
[d]See Table 2-7 for scientific names of species listed in this table.

TABLE 2-5 Euthanasia Agents Used in Fish.[a,b]

A secondary method of euthanasia (physical or chemical destruction of brain function) is recommended in all instances.

Agent	Dosage	Comments
Benzocaine (benzocaine hydrochloride)	≥250 mg/L bath for at least 10 min[10]	Solution should be buffered; once the fish loses consciousness, a secondary method (double pithing, decapitation, injectable pentobarbital) should be used
Carbon dioxide	Immersion to effect[10]	Fish may become hyperactive before losing consciousness; use in a well-ventilated area; use only CO_2 from a source that allows careful regulation of concentration
Ethanol	10-30 mL 95% ethanol/L bath to effect[10]	= 1-3% ethanol; used when other agents unavailable; direct immersion in 70% or 95% ethanol not acceptable for euthanasia
Eugenol (a purified derivative of clove oil; also see clove oil)	≥17 mg/L bath to effect[10]	Concentrations up to 10 times this amount may need to be used; once the fish loses consciousness, a secondary method (double pithing, decapitation, injectable pentobarbital) should be used
Isoflurane	5-20 mL/L bath to effect[10]	Due to the volatility of this compound and risk to humans, ventilation precautions should be taken

Continued

TABLE 2-5 Euthanasia Agents Used in Fish. (cont'd)

Agent	Dosage	Comments
Ketamine	66-88 mg/kg IM[10]	Follow with a lethal pentobarbital injection
Ketamine (K)/ dexmedetomidine (D)	(K) 1-2 mg/kg + (D) 0.05-0.1 mg/kg IM[10]	Follow with a lethal pentobarbital injection
Lidocaine	400 mg/L bath to effect[29]	Adult zebrafish/solution should be buffered; response varies considerably across fish species
Pentobarbital (sodium pentobarbital)	60-100 mg/kg IV, ICe or intracardiac[10]	Often used as a secondary step for other euthanasia methods
2-phenoxyethanol	≥0.5-0.6 mL/L or 0.3-0.4 mg/L bath to effect[10]	Secondary method (double pithing, decapitation, injectable pentobarbital) should be used
Potassium chloride	10 mmol/kg (= 750 mg/kg) intracardiac[137]	Secondary method after fish is rendered insensible, not acceptable as primary method; 1-2 mmol/kg is general vertebrate dose for euthanasia[10]
Propofol	1.5-2.5 mg/kg IM[10] 5-10 mg/L bath to effect[154]	Follow with a lethal pentobarbital injection Once fish loses consciousness, a secondary method (double pithing, decapitation, injectable intracardiac pentobarbital) should be used
Quinaldine sulfate	≥100 mg/L bath to effect[10]	Solution should be buffered to prevent water from becoming acidic
Sevoflurane	5-20 mL/L bath to effect[10]	Due to the volatility of this compound and risk to humans, ventilation precautions should be taken
Sodium bicarbonate	30 g/L bath[150]	Additon to water generates CO_2; used when other agents unavailable; keep fish in solution >10 min after respiration stops then use secondary killing method; not an AVMA-approved method of euthanasia
Sodium bicarbonate tablets (Alka-Seltzer, Bayer)	2-4 tablets/L bath[68]	Additon to water generates CO_2; used when other agents unavailable; keep fish in solution >10 min after respiration stops then use secondary killing method; not an AVMA-approved method of euthanasia
Tricaine methanesulfonate (MS-222) (Tricaine-S, Syndel USA)	250-500 mg/L bath × >10 min after cessation of respiration[10] Concentrated buffered solution of MS-222 applied directly to the gills[10,86]	Buffering is required and a secondary method (double pithing, decapitation, injectable pentobarbital) should be used For use with fish that are too large for immersion; a secondary euthanasia method is required

[a]Not to be used in fish for human consumption; CO_2 euthanasia is the exception.

[b]See Table 2-7 for scientific names of species listed in this table.

TABLE 2-6 Hematologic and Serum Biochemical Values of Fish.[a,b]

Measurement	Goldfish (*Carassius auratus*)[70]	Koi (*Cyprinus carpio*)[70,160,232]
Salinity	0 ppt	0 ppt
Hematology		
PCV (%)	31 ± 7.3	35 (24-43)
RBC (10^6/μL)	1.5 ± 0.1	1.61-1.91
Hgb (g/dL)	9.1 ± 0.4	6.32-7.55
MCV (fL)	—	166-190
MCH (pg)	—	37.7-42.7
MCHC (g/dL)	—	20.4-22.9
WBC (10^3/μL)	—	19.8-28.1
Heterophils (%)	29 ± 3	8.0-13.9
Lymphocytes (%)	70 ± 5	74.5-83.7
Monocytes (%)	1 ± 0.1	2.3-3.4
Basophils (%)	—	3.5-5.6
Chemistries		
ALP (U/L)	—	12 (4-56)
ALT (U/L)	106 (97-115)	31 (9-98)
Anion gap	—	17 (14-23)
AST (U/L)	220 (111-433)	121 (40-381)
Bicarbonate (mmol/L)	—	6 (3-8)
Bile acids (μmol/L)	—	1 (0-6)
BUN (mg/dL)	28	2 (0.2-5)
Calcium (mg/dL)	9.1 (4.3-13.5)	8.7 (7.8-11.4)
Chloride (mmol/L)	—	114 (108-119)
Cholesterol (mg/dL)	—	149 (94-282)
Creatine kinase (U/L)	4515 (0-10,000)	4123 (80-9014)
Creatinine (mg/dL)	—	—
GGT (U/L)	—	1 (0-6)
Glucose (mg/dL)	35.7 (15-93)	37 (22-65)
LDH (U/L)	—	359 (41-1675)
Phosphorus (mg/dL)	8.83 (3.1-16.3)	6.1 (3.5-7.7)
Potassium (mmol/L)	2.16 (0.1-5.6)	1.4 (0-2.9)
Protein, total (g/dL)	2.03 (0.1-4.02)	3.4 (2.7-4.3)
Albumin (g/dL)	1.9 (0.3-3.2)	2 (1.4-2.7)
Globulin (g/dL)	0.69 (0.3-1.2)	0.9 (0.6-1.1)
A:G (ratio)	2.75	1.1 (0.8-1.6)
Sodium (mmol/L)	139 (126-176)	133 (110-143)
Total bilirubin (mg/dL)	—	0.5 (0.2-2)
Uric acid (mg/dL)	0.08 (0-0.2)	0.1 (0-0.5)

Continued

TABLE 2-6 Hematologic and Serum Biochemical Values of Fish. (cont'd)

Measurement	Striped bass[89,151]	Palmetto bass[101,102]
Salinity	0 ppt	0 ppt
Hematology		
PCV (%)	42 (34-48)	20-34
RBC (10^6/µL)	—	2.42-4.96
Hgb (g/dL)	—	4.2-8.4
MCV (fL)	—	65-117
MCH (pg)	—	16.2-24.8
MCHC (g/dL)	—	19-26
WBC (10^3/µL)	—	32.6-118.2
Neutrophils (10^3/µL)	—	0-6.8
Lymphocytes (small and large) (10^3/µL)	—	23.7-125.1
Monocytes (10^3/µL)	—	0-3.2
Eosinophils (%)	—	0-2.7
Chemistries		
ALP (U/L)	—	72
Anion gap	29 ± 5	24 ± 1
AST (U/L)	23 ± 6	45 ± 21
Calcium (mg/dL)	10.6 ± 0.1	11.1 ± 0.2
Chloride (mmol/L)	143 ± 2	144 ± 2
Cholesterol (mg/dL)	—	164
Creatinine (mg/dL)	0.5 ± 0	0.3 ± 0
Glucose (mg/dL)	100 ± 28	118 ± 10
LDH (U/L)	221 ± 92	164 ± 54
Osmolality (mOsm/kg)	348 ± 2	356 ± 2
Phosphorus (mg/dL)	10 ± 0.3	9.8 ± 0.2
Potassium (mmol/L)	3.9 ± 0.1	3.3 ± 0.2
Protein, total (g/dL)	3.8 ± 0.1	3.0
Albumin (g/dL)	1.1 ± 0	1.3
Globulin (g/dL)	—	1.7
A:G (ratio)	0.4 ± 0	0.76
Sodium (mmol/L)	181 ± 4	151
Total CO_2 (mmol/L)	9.5 ± 1	10.7 ± 0.9

TABLE 2-6 Hematologic and Serum Biochemical Values of Fish. (cont'd)

Measurement	[a]Red pacu[191,229]	Rainbow trout[41,100,212]
Salinity	0 ppt	0 ppt
Hematology		
PCV (%)	26 (22-32)	34.8-56.9
RBC (10^6/µL)	1.7 (1.2-2.9)	1.4-1.8
Hgb (g/dL)	—	6.4-9.5
MCV (fL)	—	192-393
MCH (pg)	—	35.3-62.4
MCHC (g/dL)	—	14.2-18.9
WBC (10^3/µL)	33.5 (13.6-52.3)	9.9 ± 1.3
Heterophils (%)	5.2 (0.3-36.7)	—
Lymphocytes (%)	84 (53-96)	—
Monocytes (%)	4.0 (0.8-11.2)	—
Eosinophils (%)	0.3 (0.3-0.7)	—
Chemistries		
Anion gap	6.9 (1.2-12.5)	—
ALP (U/L)		31
AST (U/L)	49 (0-125)	102
BUN (mg/dL)	—	—
Calcium (mg/dL)	10.8 (9.5-12.5)	2.3
Chloride (mmol/L)	139 (146-159)	137
Cholesterol (mg/dL)	—	144
Creatine kinase (U/L)	—	—
Creatinine (mg/dL)	0.3 (0.2-0.4)	0.4
Glucose (mg/dL)	—	103
Magnesium (mg/dL)		2.3
Lactate (mmol/L)	—	—
LDH (U/L)	238 (65-692)	—
Osmolality (mOsm/kg)	—	—
Phosphorus (mg/dL)	7.3 (4.1-8.9)	10.5
Potassium (mmol/L)	3.9 (2.7-5)	2.3
Protein, total (g/dL)	—	2.7
Albumin (g/dL)	0.9 (0.5-1)	1.2
Globulin (g/dL)		1.5
Sodium (mmol/L)	150 (146-159)	152
Total CO_2 (mmol/L)	7.5 (6-10)	—

Continued

TABLE 2-6 Hematologic and Serum Biochemical Values of Fish. (cont'd)

Measurement	[a]Mbuna cichlid[213]	[a]Red lionfish[11]
Salinity	0 ppt	32 ppt
Hematology		
PCV (%)	25.3 (21-29.5)	34 (27-44)
RBC ($10^6/\mu L$)	2.3 (1.7-2.7)	—
Hgb (g/L)	75 (63-91.3)	—
MCV (fL)	113.8 (95.3-132.4)	—
MCH (pg)	33.6 (26.9-40.3)	—
MCHC (g/dL)	3.0 (2.7-3.2)	—
WBC ($10^3/\mu L$)	33.2 (22.9-55.2)	—
Granulocytes ($10^3/\mu L$)	1.48 (0.3-2.4)	4.0 (2.0-8.2)
Lymphocytes ($10^3/\mu L$)	30.9 (21.2-52.4)	21.5 (7-67)
Monocytes ($10^3/\mu L$)	—	27.5 (16-51)
Eosinophils (%)	—	—
Chemistries		
ALP (U/L)	44.5 (30.1-61.9)	35 (16-66)
ALT (U/L)	59.8 (34.7-236.1)	1.0 (1.0-7.0)
Amylase (U/L)	—	1 (1-2)
AST (U/L)	12.5 (3.5-46.3)	69 (24-236)
Calcium (mg/dL)	10.4 (10.0-10.8)	10.8 (9.4-28.4)
Chloride (mmol/L)	147 (143-150)	149 (142-162)
Cholesterol (mg/dL)	410 (263-537)	159 (75-252)
Creatinine (mg/dL)	0.5 (0.3-1.1)	0.1 (0.1-0.2)
Creatine kinase (U/L)	—	860 (198-4372)
Glucose (mg/dL)	43.2 (37.9-48.6)	26.5 (10.0-49.0)
Lipase (U/L)	—	8 (2-32)
Magnesium (mg/dL)	—	3.6 (2.6-5.5)
Phosphorus (mg/dL)	4.6 (4.0-5.0)	10.7 (7.9-20.8)
Potassium (mmol/L)	3.1 (2.4-3.6)	2.9 (1.9-4.0)
Protein, total (g/dL)	3.9 (3.5-4.6)	4.0 (2.2-6.3)
Albumin (g/L)	0.9 (0.8-1.0)	1.0 (0.6-2.0)
Globulin (g/L)	2.9 (2.6-3.7)	2.9 (2.2-4.5)
A:G (ratio)	0.33	0.3 (0.2-0.5)
Sodium (mmol/L)	161 (156.3-163.4)	172 (168-177)
Triglycerides (mg/dL)	—	298 (59-661)

TABLE 2-6 Hematologic and Serum Biochemical Values of Fish. (cont'd)

Measurement	Tilapia[99,100]	[a]Channel catfish[225,226]
Salinity	0 ppt	0 ppt
Hematology		
PCV (%)	33 (27-37)	31 (27-54)
RBC (10^6/µL)	6.1 (4.8-7.8)	3 (15-41)
Hgb (g/dL)	8.2 (7.0-9.8)	7.0 (4.4-10.9)
MCV (fL)	136 (115-183)	108 (88.6-186.7)
MCH (pg)	34.9 (28.3-42.3)	—
MCHC (g/dL)	25.7 (22-29)	22 (15.7-28.7)
WBC (10^3/µL)	7.6	35.7 (8.9-124.0)
Neutrophils (10^3/µL)	1.8 (0.56-9.9)	19.0 (4.4-86.8)
Lymphocytes (total) (10^3/µL)	—	9.2 (1.4-23.6)
Lymphocytes (small) (10^3/µL)	61 (6.8-136)	—
Lymphocytes (large) (10^3/µL)	10.7 (2.9-31)	—
Monocytes (10^3/µL)	1.5 (0.4-4.3)	5.2 (0.7-14.7)
Eosinophils (10^3/µL)	0.3 (0.03-1.6)	—
Basophils (10^3/µL)	—	1.4 (0-7.1)
Thromobocytes (10^3/µL)	53 (25-85)	78 (14-147)—
Thromobocyte-like cells (10^3/µL)	1.0 (0.03-4.3)	—
Chemistries		
ALP (U/L)	26 (16-38)	—
ALT (U/L)	—	—
AST (U/L)	18 (5-124)	—
Calcium (mg/dL)	11.6 (10.4-18.9)	10.8 (9.2-13.2)
Chloride (mmol/L)	141 (136-147)	108 (80-147)
Cholesterol (mg/dL)	156 (64-299)	—
Creatinine (mg/dL)	0.2-1.1	—
Glucose (mg/dL)	52 (39-96)	35 (17-86)
Magnesium (mg/dL)	2.5 (2.3-2.8)	2.9 (2.4-4.9)
Phosphorus (mg/dL)	4.6 (3.5-7.2)	—
Potassium (mmol/L)	3.9 (3.2-4.3)	3.0 (2.1-4.8)
Protein, total (g/dL)	2.9 (2.3-3.6)	4.2 (2.6-6.6)
Albumin (g/dL)	1.2 (1.0-1.6)	—
Globulin (g/dL)	1.6 (1.3-2.1)	—
A:G (ratio)	0.75	—
Sodium (mmol/L)	150 (140-156)	141 (132-155)
Total bilirubin (mg/dL)	0 (0-0.1)	—

Continued

TABLE 2-6 Hematologic and Serum Biochemical Values of Fish. (cont'd)

Measurement	Zebrafish[147]	Iridescent shark/striped catfish[61]
Salinity	0 ppt	0 ppt
Hematology		
PCV (%)	—	30 (24-36)
RBC (10^6/µL)	3.02 (2.89-3.25)	2.27 (1.79-2.75)
Hgb (g/dL)	—	—
MCV (fL)	—	132 (106-157)
MCH (pg)	—	—
MCHC (g/dL)	—	—
WBC (10^3/µL)	—	65.3 (36.3-94.3)
Lymphocyte (% for zebrafish; 10^3/µL for iridescent shark)	83 (71-92)	39.5 (19.0-60.0)
Monocytes (% for zebrafish; 10^3/µL for iridescent shark))	9.7 (5-15)	1.6 (0-7.5)
Neutrophils (%)	7.1 (2-18)	—
Eosinophils (%)	0.15 (0-2)	—
Granulocytes (10^3/µL)	—	1.6 (4.5-18.2)
Thrombocytes (10^3/µL)	—	49.8 (26.3-73.3)
Chemistries		
ALP (U/L)	2 (0-10)	54 (33-74)
ALT (U/L)	367 (343-410)	—
AST (U/L)	—	135 20-1236)
Calcium (mg/dL)	14.7 (12.3-18.6)	12.4 (10.8-15.6)
Chloride (mmol/L)	—	124 (120-134)
Cholesterol (mg/dL)	—	145 (108-259)
Creatinine (mg/dL)	0.7 (0.5-0.9)	0.05 (0-0.09)
Glucose (mg/dL)	82 (62-91)	110 (77-155)
Magnesium (mg/dL)	—	2.7 (2.2-3.4)
Phosphorus (mg/dL)	22.3 (20.3-24.3)	6.2 (4.0-9.0)
Potassium (mmol/L)	6.8 (5.2-7.7)	4.1 (3.3-5.0)
Protein, total (g/dL)	5.2 (4.4-5.8)	36 (29-44)
Albumin (g/dL)	3.0 (2.7-3.3)	9 (7-11)
Globulin (g/dL)	—	27 (22-33)
A:G (ratio)	—	0.32 (0.27-0.39)
Sodium (mmol/L)	—	141 (135-147)

TABLE 2-6 Hematologic and Serum Biochemical Values of Fish. (cont'd)

Measurement	Shortnose sturgeon[121]	Winter flounder[47]
Salinity	0 ppt	32 ppt
Hematology		
PCV (%)	33 (26-46)	25 (19-31)
RBC (10^6/µL)	0.83 (0.65-1.09)	2.22 (1.50-3.14)
Hgb (g/dL)	7.3 (5.7-8.7)	6.0 (5.0-7.4)
MCV (fL)	400 (307-520)	116.4 (86.8-227.3)
MCH (pg)	89 (66-107.1)	27 (22-39)
MCHC (g/dL)	23 (15-30)	24.0 (10.8-28.9)
WBC (cells/µL)	60,144 (28,376-90,789)	37,500 (13,200-145,000)
Neutrophils (total)	11,153 (3,758-33,592)	3,700 (0-26,000)
Lymphocytes (small) (cells/µL)	26,243 (9,063-56,656)	31,000 (9,600-128,200)
Lymphocytes (large) (cells/µL)	5,003 (2,122-10,435)	1,800 (0-12,300)
Monocytes (cells/µL)	2,854(0-7,137)	1,000 (0-4,600)
Eosinophils (cells/µL)	536 (0-1,544)	—
Thrombocytes (cells/µL)	74,650 (32,205-122,179)	41,900 (23,000-124,800)
Thrombocyte-like cells (cells/µL)	14,504 (6,863-23,046)	—
Chemistries		
ALP (U/L)	206 (47-497)	13 (7-27)
ALT (U/L)		6 (0-40)
AST (U/L)	174 (90-311)	57 (5-318)
BUN (mg/dL)	—	7.4 (1-12)
Calcium (mg/dL)	8.3 (6.6-12.1)	12.4 (10.6-15.0)
Chloride (mmol/L)	115 (106-121)	170 (156-194)
Cholesterol (mg/dL)	83 (42-133)	(222->400)
Creatinine (mg/dL)	0.3 (0.0-1.4)	0.3 (0.1-1.0)
Glucose (mg/dL)	54 (37-74)	49 (17-224)
Magnesium (mg/dL)	2.0 (1.6-2.3)	2.3 (1.5-3.9)
Phosphorus (mg/dL)	6.5 (5.1-8.1)	9.7 (4.9-11.7)
Potassium (mmol/L)	3.3 (2.9-3.7)	0.8 (0.5-2.8)
Protein, total (g/dL)	4.0 (2.7-5.3)	3.5 (2.6-4.7)
Albumin (g/dL)	1.3 (0.8-1.7)	1.1 (0.8-1.5)
Globulin (g/dL)	2.7 (1.8-3.7)	2.4 (1.6-3.4)
Sodium (mmol/L)	135 (124-141)	184 (171-200)
Total bilirubin (mg/dL)	0.1 (0.0-0.1)	0.1 (0.1-0.3)

Continued

TABLE 2-6 Hematologic and Serum Biochemical Values of Fish. (cont'd)

Measurement	[a]Bonnethead shark[79,88]	Cownose ray[55]
Salinity	32 ppt	32 ppt
Hematology		
PCV (%)	25 (22-35)	—
RBC (10^6/µL)	—	0.51 (0.26-0.72)
WBC (10^3/µL)	51 (35-83)	0.55 (0.16-1.98)
Heterophils (10^3/µL)	10.6 (4.7-19.1)	—
Fine segmented eosinophilic granulocytes (cells/µL)	—	23 (0-72)
Fine non-segmented eosinophilic granulocytes (cells/µL)	—	12 (0-55)
Lymphocytes (cells/µL)	20.5×10^3 ($10.4\text{-}37.5 \times 10^3$)	546 (144-1881)
Monocytes (cells/µL)	1.8×10^3 ($0.47\text{-}4.6 \times 10^3$)	6 (0-26)
Eosinophils (cells/µL)	2.2×10^3 ($0.34\text{-}12.1 \times 10^3$)	—
Coarse segmented eosinophilic granulocytes (cells/µL)	—	27 (0-77)
Coarse non-segmented eosinophilic granulocytes (cells/µL)	—	22 (0-83)
Chemistries		
Anion gap	–5.8 (–15.7-+7.5)	—
ALP (U/L)		33 (22-46)
AST (U/L)	42 (15-132)	39 (15-78)
Bicarbonate (mmol/L)	3 (0-5)	—
BUN (mg/dL)	2812 (2644-2992)	1154 (1010-1270)
Calcium (mg/dL)	16.8 (15.8-18.2)	4.2 (3.75-4.85)
Chloride (mmol/L)	290 (277-304)	255 (192-290)
Cholesterol (mg/dL)	—	166 (118-321)
Creatine kinase (U/L)	82 (18-725)	—
Creatinine (µmol/L)	—	8.84
Glucose (mg/dL)	184 (155-218)	2.78 (1.94-4.0)
LDH (U/L)	<5 (<5-11)	—
Osmolality (mOsm/kg)	1094 (1056-1139)	—
Phosphorus (mg/dL)	8.8 (5.9-12.7)	5.8 (4.4-7.1)
Potassium (mmol/L)	7.3 (5.7-9.2)	1.5 (1-2.4)
Protein, total (g/dL)	2.9 (2.2-4.3)	2.9 (1.9-4.2)
Albumin (g/dL)	0.4 (0.3-0.5)	0.6 (0.5-0.8)

TABLE 2-6 Hematologic and Serum Biochemical Values of Fish. (cont'd)

Measurement	[a]Bonnethead shark[79,88]	Cownose ray[55]
Chemistries (cont'd)		
Globulin (g/dL)	2.6 (1.9-3.8)	2.2 (1.4-3.6)
A:G (ratio)	0.1 (0.1-0.2)	0.29 (0.17-0.38)
Sodium (mmol/L)	282 (273-292)	276 (208-312)
Total bilirubin (mg/dL)	—	0.2 (0.1-0.3)
Triglyceride (mmol/L)	—	9.2 (3.2-22.8)

[a]Values listed are means except where indicated with an [a], which are medians. In some cases, the data are not based on a large sample size. These values are only meant to be guidelines. Age of fish, time of year, and water temperature may all affect "normal" clinical pathological data.
[b]See Table 2-7 for scientific names of species listed in this table.

TABLE 2-7 Scientific Names of Common Names as Listed in Preceding Tables.

Common Name	Scientific Name
Angelfish, freshwater	*Pterophyllum* spp.
Barramundi	*Lates calcarifer*
Barb, tiger	*Puntigrus tetrazona*
Bass, black sea	*Centropristis striata*
Bass, European sea = sea bass	*Dicentrarchus labrax*
Bass, largemouth	*Micropterus salmoides*
Bass, palmetto	*Morone saxatilis* × *M. chrysops*
Bass, smallmouth	*Micropterus dolomieu*
Bass, striped	*Morone saxatilis*
Betta = Siamese fighting fish	*Betta splendens*
Bream, sea = gilthead sea bream	*Sparus aurata*
Bream, sharpnose sea = sharpnose sea bream = sharpsnout sea bream	*Diplodus puntazzo*
Bream, white sea	*Diplodus sargus*
Carp = common or European carp	*Cyprinus carpio*
Carp, Crucian	*Carassius carassius*
Carp, fringe-lipped peninsula	*Labeo fimbriatus*
Carp, grass	*Ctenopharyngodon idella*
Carp, major South Asian	*Catla catla*
Cichlid, banded	*Heros severus*
Cichlid, convict	*Amatitlania nigrofasciata*
Cichlid, mbuna	*Metriaclima greshakei*
Cod = Atlantic cod	*Gadus morhua*
Catfish, African	*Clarias gariepinus*
Catfish, Amur	*Silurus asotus*

Continued

TABLE 2-7 Scientific Names of Common Names as Listed in Preceding Tables. (cont'd)

Common Name	Scientific Name
Catfish, channel	*Ictalurus punctatus*
Catfish, Korean	*Silurus asotus*
Catfish, striped = iridescent shark	*Pangasianodon hypophthalmus*
Catfish, suckermouth	*Hypostomus* spp.
Catfish, tra	*Pangasianodon hypophthalmus*
Danio, giant	*Devario aequipinnatus*
Dogfish, smooth	*Mustelus canis*
Drum, red	*Sciaenops ocellatus*
Eel	*Anguilla* spp.
Eel, European	*Anguilla anguilla*
Flounder, olive	*Paralichthys olivaceus*
Flounder, winter	*Pseudopleuronectes americanus*
Koi	*Cyprinus carpio*
Goldfish	*Carassius auratus*
Gourami	*Trichogaster trichopterus*
Gourami, blue	*Trichogaster* spp.
Grouper, orange-spotted	*Epinephelus coioides*
Halibut = Atlantic halibut	*Hippoglossus hippoglossus*
Halibut, California	*Paralichthys californicus*
Kingfish, yellow = yellowtail amberjack	*Seriola lalandi*
Leatherjacket	*Aluterus monoceros*
Lionfish, red	*Pterois volitans*
Lumpfish	*Cyclopterus lumpus*
Medaka (Japanese rice fish)	*Orizias latipes*
Oscar	*Astronotus ocellatus*
Pacu, red	*Piaractus brachypomus*
Pacu, small-scaled	*Piaractus mesopotamicus*
Perch, European	*Perca fluviatilis*
Pike, northern	*Esox lucius*
Pike, walleye	*Sander vitreous*
Pike perch	*Sander lucioperca*
Piranha	e.g., *Pygocentrus nattereri*
Platyfish, southern	*Xiphophorus maculatus*
Porgy, red	*Pagrus pagrus*
Ray, cownose	*Rhinoptera bonasus*
Rockfish, copper	*Sebastes caurinus*

TABLE 2-7 Scientific Names of Common Names as Listed in Preceding Tables. (cont'd)

Common Name	Scientific Name
Rohu	*Labeo rohita*
Salmon, Atlantic	*Salmo salar*
Seabass, white	*Atractoscion nobilis*
Sea bream = gilt-head sea bream	*Sparus aurata*
Shark, bamboo	*Chiloschyllium plagiosum*
Shark, bonnethead	*Sphyrna tiburo*
Shark, iridescent = striped catfish	*Pangasianodon hypophthalmus*
Shark, nursehound	*Scyliorhinus stellaris*
Shark, red-tail black = redtail sharkminnow	*Epalzeorhynchos bicolor*
Shark, sandbar	*Carcharhinus plumbeus*
Shark, white-spotted bamboo	*Chiloschyllium plagiosum*
Shiners, golden	*Notemigonus crysoleucas*
Silver dollar	*Metynnis* spp.
Snook, common	*Centropomus undecimalis*
Stickleback	*Gasterosteus aculeatus*
Sturgeon, Amur	*Acipenser schrenckii*
Sturgeon, Gulf of Mexico	*Acipenser oxyrinchus*
Sturgeon, lake	*Acipenser fulvescens*
Sturgeon, shortnose	*Acipenser brevirostrum*
Surgeonfish, ocean	*Acanthurus bahianus*
Swordtail	*Xiphophorus* spp.
Tench	*Tinca tinca*
Tetra, cardinal	*Paracheirodon axelrodi*
Tetra, black	*Gymnocorymbus ternetzi*
Tetra, serpae	*Hyphessobrycon eques*
Threadfin, Pacific	*Polydactylus sexfilis*
Tilapia, Mozambique	*Oreochromis mossambicus*
Tilapia, Nile tilapia	*Oreochromis niloticus* and hybrids
Trout, brown	*Salmo trutta*
Trout, rainbow	*Onchorhynchus mykiss*
Turbot	*Scophthalmus maximus*
Walleye	*Sander vitreous*
Wrasse, corkwing	*Symphodus melops*
Wrasse, goldsinny	*Ctenolabrus rupestris*
Yellowtail, California	*Seriola dorsalis*
Zebrafish	*Danio rerio*

REFERENCES

1. AADAP/FDA. Web site: www.fws.gov/fisheries/aadap/inads/Diquat-INAD-10-969.html. Accessed April 28, 2021.
2. AADAP-FWS FDA INAD. Web site: www.fws.gov/fisheries/aadap/inads.html. Accessed April 28, 2021.
3. AADAP-FWS FDA INAD. Web site: www.fws.gov/fisheries/aadap/inads/Chloramine-T-INAD-9321.html. Accessed April 28, 2021.
4. Alderman DJ. Malachite green: A pharmacokinetic study in rainbow trout, *Oncorhynchus mykiss* (Walbaum). *J Fish Dis.* 1993;16:297–311.
5. Allender MC, Kastura M, George R, et al. Bioencapsulation of praziquantel in adult *Artemia*. *J Bioanal Biomed.* 2010;2:96–99.
6. Allender MC, Kastura M, George R, et al. Bioencapsulation of metronidazole in adult brine shrimp (*Artemia* sp.). *J Zoo Wildl Med.* 2011;42:241–246.
7. Allender MC, Kastura M, George R, et al. Bioencapsulation of fenbendazole in adult *Artemia*. *J Exot Pet Med.* 2012;21:207–212.
8. Aly S, Fathi M, Youssef EM, et al. Trichodinids and monogeneans infestation among Nile tilapia hatcheries in Egypt: prevalence, therapeutic and prophylactic treatments. *Aquac Int.* 2020;28:1459–1471.
9. Amend DF, Goven BA, Elliot DG. Etomidate: effective dosages for a new fish anesthetic. *Trans Am Fish Soc.* 1982;111:337–341.
10. American Veterinary Medical Association. *AVMA Guidelines for the Euthanasia of Animals: 2020 Edition*. Available at: https://www.avma.org/sites/default/files/2020-01/2020-Euthanasia-Final-1-17-20.pdf. Accessed 24 March 2021.
11. Anderson ET, Stoskopf MK, Morris JA, et al. Hematology, plasma biochemistry and tissue enzyme activities of invasive red lionfish captured off North Carolina, USA. *J Aquat Anim Health.* 2010;22:266–273.
12. Ang CY, Liu FF, Lay JO Jr, et al. Liquid chromatographic analysis of incurred amoxicillin residues in catfish muscle following oral administration of the drug. *J Agric Food Chem.* 2000;48:1673–1677.
13. Aquacalm (metomidate hydrochloride) package insert. Syndel USA, Ferndale, WA, USA.
14. Aquaflor (florfenicol) product label. Merck Animal Health, Summit, NJ, USA.
15. Bailey KM, Minter LJ, Lewbart GA, et al. Alfaxalone as an intramuscular injectable anesthetic in koi carp (*Cyprinus carpio*). *J Zoo Wildl Med.* 2014;45:852–858.
16. Baker TR, Baker BB, Johnson SM, et al. Comparative analgesic efficacy of morphine sulfate and butorphanol tartrate in koi (*Cyprinus carpio*) undergoing unilateral gonadectomy. *J Am Vet Med Assoc.* 2013;243:882–890.
17. Bauquier SH, Greenwood J, Whittem T. Evaluation of the sedative and anaesthetic effects of five different concentrations of alfaxalone in goldfish, *Carassius auratus*. *Aquaculture.* 2013;396–399:119–123.
18. Bergjso T, Bergjso HT. Absorption from water as an alternative method for the administration of sulfonamides to rainbow trout, *Salmo gairdneri*. *Acta Vet Scand.* 1978;19:102–109.
19. Bowker JD, Carty D, Bowman MP. The safety of SLICE (0.2% emamectin benzoate) administered via feed to fingerling rainbow trout. *N Am J Aquac.* 2013;75:455–462.
20. Braschi I, Blasioli S, Gigli L, et al. Removal of sulfonamide antibiotics from water: evidence of adsorption into an organophilic zeolite Y by its structural modifications. *J Hazard Mater.* 2010;178:218–225.
21. Brown AG, Grant AN. Use of amoxycillin by injection in Atlantic salmon broodstock. *Vet Rec.* 1992;131:237.
22. Buchmann K, Bjerregaard J. Mebendazole treatment of pseudodactylogyrosis in an intensive eel-culture system. *Aquaculture.* 1990;86:139–153.
23. Bugman AM, Langer PT, Hadzima E, et al. Evaluation of the anesthetic efficacy of alfaxalone in oscar fish (*Astronotus ocellatus*). *Am J Vet Res.* 2016;77:239–244.

24. Callahan HA, Noga EJ. Tricaine dramatically reduces the ability to diagnose protozoan ectoparasite (*Ichthyobodo necator*) infections. *J Fish Dis*. 2002;25:433–437.
25. Cardé EMQ, Yazdi Z, Yun S, et al. Pharmacokinetic and efficacy study of acyclovir against Cyprinid Herpesviruse 3 in *Cyprinus carpio. Front Vet Sci*. 2020;7:587952.
26. Chen CY, Getchel RG, Wooster GA, et al. Oxytetracycline residues in four species of fish after 10-day oral dosing via feed. *J Aquat Anim Health*. 2004;16:208–219.
27. Chorulon (human chorionic gonadotropin; hCG) product label. Merck Animal Health, Summit, NJ, USA.
28. Christiansen E, Mitchell JM, Harms CA, et al. Sedation of red porgy (*Pagrus pagrus*) and black sea bass (*Centropistis striata*) using ketamine, dexmedetomidine and midazolam delivered via intramuscular injection. *J Zoo Aquar Res*. 2014;2:62–68.
29. Collymore C, Banks KE, Turner PV. Lidocaine hydrochloride compared with MS222 for the euthanasia of zebrafish (*Danio rerio*). *J Am Assoc Lab Anim*. 2016;55:816–820.
30. Colorni A, Paperna I. Evaluation of nitrofurazone baths in the treatment of bacterial infections of *Sparus aurata* and *Oreochromis mossambicus. Aquaculture*. 1983;25:181–186.
31. Corum O, Corum DD, Er A, et al. Plasma and tissue disposition of danofloxacin in brown trout (*Salmo trutta fario*) after intravenous and intramuscular administrations. *Food Addit Contam Part A*. 2018;35:2340–2347.
32. Coyne R, Bergh O, Smith P, et al. A question of temperature related differences in plasma oxolinic acid concentrations achieved in rainbow trout (*Oncorhynchus mykiss*) under laboratory conditions following multiple oral dosing. *Aquaculture*. 2004;245:13–17.
33. Coyne R, Samuelsen O, Kongshaug H, et al. A comparison of oxolinic acid concentrations in farmed and laboratory held rainbow trout (*Oncorhynchus mykiss*) following oral therapy. *Aquaculture*. 2004;239:1–13.
34. Cravedi JP, Heuillet G, Peleran JC, et al. Disposition and metabolism of chloramphenicol in trout. *Xenobiotica*. 1985;15:115–121.
35. Creeper JH, Buller NB. An outbreak of *Streptococcus iniae* in barramundi (*Lates calcarifera*) in freshwater cage culture. *Aust Vet J*. 2006;84:408–411.
36. Cross DG, Hursey PA. Chloramine-T for the control of *Ichthyophthirius multifiliis* (Fouquet). *J Fish Dis*. 1973;10:789–798.
37. Danyi S, Widart J, Douny C, et al. Determination and kinetics of enrofloxacin and ciprofloxacin in tra catfish (*Pangasianodon hypophthalmus*) and giant freshwater prawn (*Macrobrachium rosenbergii*) using a liquid chromatography/mass spectrometry method. *J Vet Pharmacol Ther*. 2010;34:142–152.
38. Davis LE, Davis CA, Koritz GD, et al. Comparative studies of pharmacokinetics of fenbendazole in food-producing animals. *Vet Hum Toxicol*. 1988;30(Suppl 1):9–11.
39. della Rocca G, Di Salvo A, Malvisi J, et al. The disposition of enrofloxacin in seabream (*Sparus aurata* L.) after single intravenous injection or from medicated feed administration. *Aquaculture*. 2004;232:53–62.
40. della Rocca G, Zaghini A, Zanoni R, et al. Seabream (*Sparus aurata* L.): disposition of amoxicillin after single intravenous or oral administration and multiple dose depletion studies. *Aquaculture*. 2004;232:1–10.
41. Denton JE, Yousef MK. Seasonal changes in hematology of rainbow trout, *Salmo gairdneri*. *Comp Biochem Physiol*. 1975;51A:151–153.
42. Ding F, Cao J, Ma L, et al. Pharmacokinetics and tissue residues of difloxacin in crucian carp (*Carassius auratus*) after oral administration. *Aquaculture*. 2006;256:121–128.
43. Di Salvo A, Pellegrino RM, Cagnardi P, et al. Pharmacokinetics and residue depletion of erythromycin in gilthead seabream *Sparus aurata* L. after oral administration. *J Fish Dis*. 2014;37:797–803.
44. Dixon BA, Issvoran GS. The activity of ceftiofur sodium for *Aeromonas* spp. isolated from ornamental fish. *J Wildlife Dis*. 1992;28:453–456.

45. Doi A, Stoskopf MK, Lewbart GA. Pharmacokinetics of oxytetracycline in the red pacu (*Colossoma brachypomum*) following different routes of administration. *J Vet Pharmacol Ther.* 1998;21:364–368.
46. Duston J, Cusack RR. Emamectin benzoate: an effective in-feed treatment against the gill parasite *Salmincola edwardsii* on brook trout. *Aquaculture.* 2002;207:1–9.
47. Dye VA, Hrubec TC, Dunn JL, et al. Hematology and serum chemistry values for winter flounder (*Pleuronectes americanus*). *Int J Recirc Aquac.* 2001;2:37–50.
48. Elston RA, Drum AS, Schweitzer MG, et al. Comparative update of orally administered difloxacin in Atlantic salmon in freshwater and seawater. *J Aquat Anim Health.* 1994;6:341–348.
49. Erythromycin FWS-FDA INAD. Web site: www.fws.gov/fisheries/aadap/inads/Erythromycin-200-Injectable-INAD-12-781.html. Accessed April 28, 2021.
50. Fairgrieve WT, Masada CL, McAuley WC, et al. Accumulation and clearance of orally administered erythromycin and its derivative, azithromycin, in juvenile fall Chinook salmon *Oncorhynchus tshawytscha. Dis Aquat Org.* 2005;64:99–106.
51. Fairgrieve WT, Masada CL, Peterson ME, et al. Concentrations of erythromycin and azithromycin in mature Chinook salmon *Oncorhynchus tshawytscha* after intraperitoneal injection, and in their progeny. *Dis Aquat Org.* 2006;68:227–234.
52. Fang X, Liu X, Liu W, et al. Pharmacokinetics of enrofloxacin in allogynogenetic silver crucian carp, *Carassius auratus gibelio. J Vet Pharmacol Ther.* 2012;35:397–401.
53. Fayette MA, Rose JB, Hunter RP, et al. Naïve-pooled pharmacokinetics of ceftiofur crystalline free acid after single intramuscular administration in smooth dogfish (*Mustelus canis*). *J Zoo Wildl Med.* 2019;50:466–469.
54. Feng J-B, Huang D-R, Zhong M, et al. Pharmacokinetics of florfenicol and behaviour of its metabolite florfenicol amine in orange-spotted grouper (*Epinephelus coioides*) after oral administration. *J Fish Dis.* 2016;39:833–843.
55. Ferreira CM, Field CL, Tuttle AD. Hematological and plasma biochemical parameters of aquarium-maintained cownose rays. *J Aquat Anim Health.* 2010;22:123–128.
56. Fleming GJ, Corwin A, McCoy AJ, et al. Treatment factors influencing the use of recombinant platelet-derived growth factor (Regranex®) for head and lateral line erosion syndrome in ocean surgeonfish (*Acanthurus bahianus*). *J Zoo Wildl Med.* 2008;39:155–160.
57. Fleming GJ, Heard DJ, Francis-Floyd R, et al. Evaluation of propofol and medetomidine-ketamine for short-term immobilization of Gulf of Mexico sturgeon (*Acipenser oxyrinchus de soti*). *J Zoo Wildl Med.* 2003;34:153–158.
58. Fredholm DV, Mylniczenko ND, KuKanich B. Pharmacokinetic evaluation of meloxicam after intravenous and intramuscular administration in Nile tilapia (*Oreochromis niloticus*). *J Zoo Wildlife Med.* 2016;47:736–742.
59. Fujimoto RY, Pereira DM, Silva JCS, et al. Clove oil induces anaesthesia and blunts muscle contraction power in three Amazon fish species. *Fish Physiol Biochem.* 2018;44:245–256.
60. Gaikowski MP, Mushtaq M, Cassidy P, et al. Depletion of florfenicol amine, marker residue of florfenicol, from the edible fillet of tilapia (*Oreochromis niloticus* × *O. niloticus* and *O. niloticus* × *O. aureus*) following florfenicol administration via feed. *Aquaculture.* 2010;301:1–6.
61. Galagarza OA, Kuhn DD, Smith SA, et al. Hematologic and plasma chemistry reference intervals (RI) for cultured striped catfish (*Pangasius hypophthalmus*) in recirculating aquaculture systems. *Vet Clin Path.* 2017;46(3):457–465.
62. Gaskins J, Boylan S. Appendix C: Therapeutics for ornamental fish, tropical, bait, and other non-food fish: supportive therapy and care. In: Smith SA, ed. *Fish Diseases and Medicine.* Boca Raton, FL: CRC Press; 2019:373–377.
63. Gaunt PS. Multidose pharmacokinetics of orally administered florfenicol in the channel catfish (*Ictalurus punctatus*). *J Vet Pharmacol Therap.* 2012;36:502–506.
64. GholipourKanani H, Ahadizadeh S. Use of propofol as an anesthetic and its efficacy on some hematological values of ornamental fish *Carassius auratus. SpringerPlus.* 2013;2:76.
65. Gilmartin WG, Camp BJ, Lewis DH. Bath treatment of channel catfish with three broad-spectrum antibiotics. *J Wildl Dis.* 1976;12:555–559.

66. Gingerich WH, Meinertrz JR, Dawson VK, et al. Distribution and elimination of [14C] sarafloxacin hydrochloride from tissues of juvenile channel catfish (*Ictalurus punctatus*). *Aquaculture.* 1995;131:23–36.
67. Golomazou E, Athanassopoulou F, Karagouni E, et al. Efficacy and toxicity of orally administrated anti-coccidial drug treatment on *Enteromyxum leei* infections in sharpsnout seabream (*Diplodus puntazzo* C.). *Israeli J Aquac – Bamidgeh.* 2006;58:157–169.
68. Gratzek JB, Shotts EB, Dawe DL. Infectious diseases and parasites of freshwater ornamental fish. In: Gratzek JB, Matthews FR, eds. *Aquariology: The Science of Fish Health Management.* Morris Plains, NJ: Tetra Press; 1992:227–274.
69. Greene W, Mylniczenko ND, Storms T, et al. Pharmacokinetics of ketoprofen in Nile tilapia (*Oreochromis niloticus*) and rainbow trout (*Oncorhynchus mykiss*). *Front Vet Sci.* 2020;7:585324.
70. Groff JM, Zinkl JG. Hematology and clinical chemistry of cyprinid fish. *Vet Clin North Am Exot Anim Pract.* 1999;2:741–776.
71. Grondel JL, Nouws JFM, De Jong M, et al. Pharmacokinetics and tissue distribution of oxytetracycline in carp, *Cyprinus carpio* L., following different routes of administration. *J Fish Dis.* 1987;10:153–163.
72. Grosell MH, Hansen HJM, Rosenkilde P. Cu uptake, metabolism and elimination in fed and starved European eels (*Anguilla anguilla*) during adaptation to water-borne Cu exposure. *Comp Biochem Physiol C.* 1998;120:295–305.
73. Grosell MH, Hogstrand C, Wood CM. Cu update and turnover in both Cu- acclimated and non-acclimated rainbow trout (*Oncorhynchus mykiss*). *Aquat Toxicol.* 1997;38:257–276.
74. Grosell MH, Hogstrand C, Wood CM. Renal Cu and Na excretion and hepatic Cu metabolism in both Cu acclimated and non acclimated rainbow trout (*Oncorhynchus mykiss*). *Aquat Toxicol.* 1998;40:275–291.
75. Grosset C, Weber ES, Gehring R, et al. Evaluation of an extended-release formulation of ceftiofur crystalline-free acid in koi (*Cyprinus carpio*). *J Vet Pharmacol Ther.* 2015;38:606–615.
76. Grush J, Noakes DLG, Moccia RD. The efficacy of clove oil as an anesthetic for the zebrafish, *Danio rerio* (Hamilton). *Zebrafish.* 2004;1:46–53.
77. Guerrero RD. Use of androgens for the production of all-male *Tilapia aurea* (Steindachner). *Trans Am Fish Soc.* 1975;104:342–348.
78. Hakaalahti Y, Lankinen Y, Vaktonen T. Efficacy of emamectin benzoate in the control of *Argulus coregoni* (Crustacea: Branchiura) on rainbow trout *Oncorhynchus mykiss. Dis Aquat Org.* 2004;60(3):197–204.
79. Haman KH, Norton TM, Thomas AC, et al. Baseline health parameters and species comparisons among free-ranging Atlantic sharpnose (Rhizoprionodon terraenovae), Bonnethead (*Sphyrna tiburo*), and Spiny dogfish (*Squalus acanthias*) sharks in Georgia, Florida, and Washington, USA. *J Wildlife Dis.* 2012;48:295–306.
80. Hanson SK, Hill JE, Watson CA, et al. Evaluation of emamectin benzoate for the control of experimentally induced infestations of *Argulus* sp. in goldfish and koi carp. *J Aquat Anim Health.* 2011;23:30–34.
81. Hansen MK, Horsberg TE. Single-dose pharmacokinetics of flumequine in cod (*Gadus morhua*) and goldsinny wrasse (*Ctenolabrus rupestris*). *J Vet Pharmacol Ther.* 2000;23:163–168.
82. Hansen MK, Ingebrigtsen K, Hayton WL, et al. Disposition of 14C-flumequine in eel *Anguilla anguilla*, turbot *Scophthalmus maximus* and halibut *Hippoglossus hippoglossus* after oral and intravenous administration. *Dis Aquat Org.* 2001;47:183–191.
83. Hansen MK, Nymoen U, Horsberg TE. Pharmacokinetic and pharmacodynamic properties of metomidate in turbot (*Scophthalmus maximus*) and halibut (*Hippoglossus hippoglossus*). *J Vet Pharmacol Ther.* 2003;26:95–103.
84. Harms CA. Treatments for parasitic diseases of aquarium and ornamental fish. *Semin Avian Exot Pet Med.* 1996;5:54–63.
85. Harms CA. Anesthesia in fish. In: Fowler ME, Miller RE, eds. *Zoo and Wild Animal Medicine: Current Therapy 4.* Philadelphia, PA: Saunders; 1999:158–163.
86. Harms CA, Bakal RS. Techniques in fish anesthesia. *J Sm Exot Anim Med.* 1995;3:19–25.

87. Harms CA, Lewbart GA, Swanson CR, et al. Behavioral and clinical pathology changes in koi carp (*Cyprinus carpio*) subjected to anesthesia and surgery with and without intra-operative analgesics. *Comp Med.* 2005;55:221–226.
88. Harms CA, Ross T, Segars A. Plasma biochemistry reference values of wild bonnethead sharks, *Sphyrna tiburo*. *Vet Clin Pathol.* 2002;31:111–115.
89. Harms CA, Sullivan CV, Hodson RG, et al. Clinical pathology and histopathology characteristics of net-stressed striped bass with "red tail." *J Aquat Anim Health.* 1996;8:82–86.
90. Haughland GT, Kverme KO, Hannisdal R, et al. Pharmacokinetic data show that oxolinic acid and fluequine are absorbed and excreted rapidly from plasma and tissues of lumpfish. *Front Vet Sci.* 2019;6:394.
91. Hayton WL, Szoke A, Kemmenoe BH, et al. Disposition of benzocaine in channel catfish. *Aquat Toxicol.* 1996;36:99–113.
92. Heaton LH, Post G. Tissue residues and oral safety of furazolidone in four species of trout. *Prog Fish-Cult.* 1968;30:208–215.
93. Hemaprasanth KP, Kar B, Garnayak SK, et al. Efficacy of two avermectins, doramectin and ivermectin against *Argulus siamensis* infestation in Indian major carp, *Labeo rohita*. *Vet Parasitol.* 2012;190:297–304.
94. Hemaprasanth KP, Raghavendra A, Singh R, et al. Efficacy of doramectin against natural and experimental infections of *Lernaea cyprinacea* in carps. *Vet Parasitol.* 2008;156:261–269.
95. Hicks BD, Geraci JR. A histological assessment of damage in rainbow trout, *Salmo gairdneri* Richardson, fed rations containing erythromycin. *J Fish Dis.* 1984;7:457–465.
96. Hill JE, Kilgore KH, Pouder DB, et al. Survey of Ovaprim use as a spawning aid in ornamental fishes in the United States as administered through the University of Florida Tropical Aquaculture Laboratory. *N Am J Aquac.* 2009;71:206–209.
97. Homem V, Santos L. Degradation and removal methods of antibiotics from aqueous matrices – a review. *J Environ Manag.* 2011;92:2304–2347.
98. Horsberg TE, Hoff KA, Nordmo R. Pharmacokinetics of florfenicol and its metabolite florfenicol amine in Atlantic salmon. *J Aquat Anim Health.* 1996;8:292–301.
99. Hrubec TC, Smith SA. Differences between plasma and serum samples for the evaluation of blood chemistry values in rainbow trout, channel catfish, hybrid tilapias, and hybrid striped bass. *J Aquat Anim Health.* 1999;11:116–122.
100. Hrubec TC, Cardinale JL, Smith SA. Hematology and plasma chemistry reference intervals for cultured tilapia (*Oreochromis* hybrid). *Vet Clin Path.* 2000;29:7–12.
101. Hrubec TC, Smith SA, Robertson JL. Age-related changes in hematology and plasma chemistry values of hybrid striped bass (*Morone chrysops* × *Morone saxatilis*). *Vet Clin Path.* 2001;30:8–15.
102. Hrubec TC, Smith SA, Robertson JL, et al. Blood biochemical reference intervals for sunshine bass (*Morone chrysops* × *Morone saxatilis*) in three culture systems. *Am J Vet Res.* 1996;57:624–627.
103. Hubert TD, Bernardy JA, Vue C, et al. Residues of the lampricides 3-trifluoromethyl-4-nitrophenol and niclosamide in muscle tissue of rainbow trout. *J Agric Food Chem.* 2005;53:5342–5346.
104. Hyatt MW, Waltzek TB, Kieran EA, et al. Diagnosis and treatment of multi-species fish mortality attributed to *Enteromyxum leei* while in quarantine at a US aquarium. *Dis Aquat Org.* 2018;132:37–48.
105. Inglis V, Richards RH, Varma KJ, et al. Florfenicol in Atlantic salmon, *Salmo salar* L., parr: tolerance and assessment of efficacy against furunculosis. *J Fish Dis.* 1991;14:343–351.
106. Intorre L, Castells G, Cristofol C, et al. Residue depletion of thiamphenicol in the sea-bass. *J Vet Pharmacol Ther.* 2002;25:59–63.
107. Iosifidou EG, Haagsma N, Olling M, et al. Residue study of mebendazole and its metabolites hydroxymebendazole and amino-mebendazole in eel (*Anguilla anguilla*) after bath treatment. *Drug Metab Dispos.* 1997;25:317–320.

108. Iosifidou EG, Haagsma N, Tanck MWT, et al. Depletion study of fenbendazole in rainbow trout (*Oncorhynchus mykiss*) after oral and bath treatment. *Aquaculture*. 1997;154:191–199.
109. Jarboe H, Toth BR, Shoemaker KE, et al. Pharmacokinetics, bioavailability, plasma protein binding and disposition of nalidixic acid in rainbow trout (*Oncorhynchus mykiss*). *Xenobiotica*. 1993;23:961–972.
110. Johnson EL. *Koi Health and Disease*. Athens, GA: Reade Printers; 2006:204 pp.
111. Johnstone R, Macintosh DJ, Wright RS. Elimination of orally administered 17cr-methyltestosterone by *Oreochromis mossambicus* (tilapia) and *Salmo gairdneri* (rainbow trout) juveniles. *Aquaculture*. 1983;35:249–257.
112. Jones J, Kinnel M, Christenson R, et al. Gentamicin concentrations in toadfish and goldfish serum. *J Aquat Anim Health*. 1997;9:211–215.
113. Jones SG, Kamunde C, Lemke K, et al. The dose–response relation for the antinociceptive effect of morphine in a fish, rainbow trout. *J Vet Pharmacol Ther*. 2012;35:563–570.
114. Junior JJB, Nakagome FK, de Mello GL, et al. Eugenol as an anesthetic for juvenile common snook. *Pesq Agropec Bras Brasília*. 2013;48:1140–1144.
115. Kajita Y, Sakai M, Atsuta S, et al. The immunomodulatory effects of levamisole on rainbow trout, *Oncorhynchus mykiss*. *Fish Pathol*. 1990;25:93–98.
116. Katharios P, Papandroulakis N, Divanach P, et al. Treatment of *Microcotyle* sp. (Monogenea) on the gills of cage-cultured red porgy, *Pagrus pagrus* following baths with formalin and mebendazole. *Aquaculture*. 2006;251:167–171.
117. Kilgore KH, Hill JE, Powell JF, et al. Investigational use of metomidate hydrochloride as a shipping additive for two ornamental fishes. *J Aquat Anim Health*. 2009;21:133–139.
118. Kim MS, Lim JH, Park BK, et al. Pharmacokinetics of enrofloxacin in Korean catfish (*Silurus asotus*). *J Vet Pharmacol Ther*. 2006;29:397–402.
119. Kitzman JV, Holley JH, Huber WG, et al. Pharmacokinetics and metabolism of fenbendazole in channel catfish. *Vet Res Com*. 1990;14:217–226.
120. Knight SJ, Boles L, Stamper MA. Response of recirculating saltwater aquariums to long-term formalin treatment. *J Zoo Aquar Res*. 2016;4:77–84.
121. Knowles S, Hrubec TC, Smith SA, et al. Hematology and plasma chemistry reference intervals for cultured shortnose sturgeon (*Acipenser brevirostrum*). *Vet Clin Pathol*. 2006;35:434–440.
122. Koc F, Uney K, Atamanalp M, et al. Pharmacokinetic disposition of enrofloxacin in brown trout (*Salmo trutta fario*) after oral and intravenous administrations. *Aquaculture*. 2009;295:142–144.
123. Kozlowski F. Chloromycetin levels in the blood and some tissues of carps in the prophylactic treatment of dropsy. *Bull Vet Instit Pulway*. 1964;8:188–195.
124. Kristan J, Stara A, Polgesek M, et al. Efficacy of different anaesthetics for pikeperch (*Sander lucioperca* L.) in relation to water temperature. *Neuroendocrinol Lett*. 2014;35(Suppl. 2): 81–85.
125. Kyuchukova R, Milannova A, Pavlov A, et al. Comparison of plasma and tissue disposition of enrofloxacin in rainbow trout (*Oncorhynchus mykiss*) and common carp (*Cyprinus carpio*) after a single oral administration. *Food Addit Contam A*. 2015;32:35–39.
126. Lambooij B, Pilarczyk M, Bialowas H, et al. Anaesthetic properties of Propiscin (etomidate) and 2-phenoxyethanol in the common carp (*Cyprinus carpio* L.), neural and behavioural measures. *Aquac Res*. 2009;40:1328–1333.
127. Law FCP Total metabolic depletion and residue profile of selected drugs in trout: furazolidone. *Final FDA Report* (Contract 223-90-7016); 1994.
127a. LePage V. Personal communication. 2022.
128. Lewbart GA. Emergency pet fish medicine. In: Bonagura JD, ed. *Kirk's Current Veterinary Therapy XII: Small Animal Practice*. Philadelphia, PA: Saunders; 1995:1369–1374.
129. Lewbart GA. Emergency and critical care of fish. *Vet Clin North Am Exot Anim Pract*. 1998;1:233–249.

130. Lewbart GA. Koi medicine and management. *Suppl Comp Contin Educ Pract Vet.* 1998;20:5–12.
131. Lewbart GA. Fish supplement. In: Johnson-Delaney C, ed. *Exotic Companion Medicine Handbook.* West Palm Beach, FL: Zoological Medicine Network; 2006:1–58.
132. Lewbart GA, Butkus DA, Papich M, et al. A simple catheterization method for systemic administration of drugs to fish. *J Am Vet Med Assoc.* 2005;226:784–788.
133. Lewbart GA, Papich MG, Whitt-Smith D. Pharmacokinetics of florfenicol in the red pacu (*Piaractus brachypomus*) after single dose intramuscular administration. *J Vet Pharmacol Ther.* 2005;28:317–319.
134. Lewbart GA, Vaden S, Deen J, et al. Pharmacokinetics of enrofloxacin in the red pacu (*Colossoma brachypomum*) after intramuscular, oral and bath administration. *J Vet Pharmacol Ther.* 1997;20:124–128.
135. Lewis DH, Wenxing W, Ayers A, et al. Preliminary studies on the use of chloroquine as a systemic chemotherapeutic agent for amyloodinosis in red drum (*Sciaenops ocellatus*). *Marine Sci Suppl.* 1988;30:183–189.
136. Lim JH, Kin MS, Hwang YH, et al. Pharmacokinetics of florfenicol following intramuscular and intravenous administration in olive flounder (*Paralichthys olivaceus*). *J Vet Pharmacol Ther.* 2010;34:206–208.
137. Louis MM, Houck EL, Lewbart GA, et al. Evaluation of potassium chloride administered via three routes for euthanasia of anesthetized koi (*Cyprinus carpio*). *J Zoo Wildl Med.* 2020;51:485–489.
138. Lu TY, Yang YH, Xu LW, et al. Acute toxicity of danofloxacin in Amur sturgeon and the body residue. *J Fish Sci. China.* 2004;11:542–548.
139. MacLean RA, Fatzinger MH, Woolard KD, et al. Clearance of a dermal *Huffmanela* sp. in a sandbar shark (*Carcharhinus plumbeus*) using levamisole. *Dis Aquat Org.* 2006;73:83–88.
140. Mansell B, Powell MD, Ernst I, Nowak BF. Effects of the gill monogenean *Zeuxapta seriolae* (Meserve, 1938) and treatment with hydrogen peroxide on pathophysiology of kingfish, *Seriola lalandi* Valenciennes, 1833. *J Fish Dis.* 2005;28:253–262.
141. McGeachin RB, Robinson EH, Neil WH. Effect of feeding high levels of androgens on the sex ratio of *Oreochromis aureus*. *Aquaculture.* 1987;61:317–321.
142. Meinertz JR, Stehly GR, Greseth SL, et al. Depletion of the chloramine-T marker residue, para-toluenesulfonamide, from skin-on fillet tissue of hybrid striped bass, rainbow trout, and yellow perch. *Aquaculture.* 2004;232:1–10.
143. Miller SM, Mitchell MA, Heatley, et al. Clinical and cardiorespiratory effects of propofol in the Spotted Bamboo Shark (*Chylloscyllium plagiosum*). *J Zoo Wildlife Med.* 2005;36:673–676.
144. Minter LJ, Bailey KM, Harms CA, et al. The efficacy of alfaxalone for immersion anesthesia in koi carp (*Cyprinus carpio*). *Vet Anaesth Analg.* 2014;41:398–405.
145. Moffitt CM. Survival of juvenile Chinook salmon challenged with *Renibacterium salmoninarum* and administered oral doses of erythromycin thiocyanate for different durations. *J Aquat Anim Health.* 1992;4:119–125.
146. Montgomery-Brock D, Sato VT, Brock JA, Tamaru CS. The application of hydrogen peroxide as a treatment for the ectoparasite *Amyloodinium ocellatum* on the Pacific threadfin *Polydactylus sexfilis*. *J World Aquac Soc.* 2001;32:250–254.
146a. Morón-Elorza P, Rojo-Solis C, Álvaro-Álvarez T, et al. Pharmacokinetic studies in elasmobranchs: meloxicam administered at 0.5 mg/kg using intravenous, intramuscular, and oral routes to nursehound sharks (*Scyliorhinus stellaris*). *Front Vet Sci.* 9:845555.
147. Murtha JM, Qi M, Keller ET. Hematologic and serum biochemical values for zebrafish (*Danio rerio*). *Comp Med.* 2003;53:37–41.
148. Nafstad I, Ingebrigsten K, Langseth W, et al. Benzimidazoles for antiparasite therapy in salmon. *Acta Vet Scand Suppl.* 1991;87:302–304.
149. Newby NC, Gamperl AK, Steven D. Cardiorespiratory effects and efficacy of morphine sulfate in winter flounder (*Pseudopleuronectes americanus*). *Am J Vet Res.* 2007;68:592–597.
150. Noga EJ. *Fish Disease: Diagnosis and Treatment.* 2nd ed. Ames, IA: Wiley-Blackwell; 2010.

151. Noga EJ, Wang C, Grindem CB, et al. Comparative clinicopathological responses of striped bass and palmetto bass to acute stress. *Trans Am Fish Soc.* 1999;128:680–686.
152. Nordmo R, Riseth JMH, Varma KJ, et al. Evaluation of florfenicol in Atlantic salmon, *Salmo salar* L.: Efficacy against furunculosis due to *Aeromonas salmonicida* and cold water vibriosis due to *Vibrio salmonicida. J Fish Dis.* 1998;21:289–297.
153. Nouws JFM, Grondel JL, Schutte AR, et al. Pharmacokinetics of ciprofloxacin in carp, African catfish and rainbow trout. *Vet Quart.* 1988;10:211–216.
154. Oda A, Bailey KM, Lewbart GA, et al. Physiologic and biochemical assessments of koi carp, *Cyprinus carpio*, following immersion in propofol. *J Am Vet Med Assoc.* 2014;245:1286–1291.
155. Oda A, Messenger KM, Carajal L, et al. Pharmacokinetics and pharmacodynamic effects in koi carp (*Cyprinus carpio*) following immersion in propofol. *Vet Anaesth Analg.* 2018;45:529–538.
156. O'Grady P, Moloney M, Smith PR. Bath administration of the quinoline antibiotic flumequine to brown trout *Salmo trutta* and Atlantic salmon *S. salar. Dis Aquat Org.* 1988;4:27–33.
157. Olsen YA, Einarsdottir IE, Nilssen KJ. Metomidate anaesthesia in Atlantic salmon, *Salmo salar*, prevents plasma cortisol increase during stress. *Aquaculture.* 1995;134:155–168.
158. Otker HM, Akmehmet-Balcgoglu I. Adsorption and degradation of enrofloxacin, a veterinary antibiotic on natural zeolite. *J Hazard Mat.* 2005;122:251–258.
159. Ovaprim (salmon gonadotropin releasing hormone analog 20µg/mL plus domperidone 10 mg/mL) product label. Syndel USA, Ferndale, WA, USA.
160. Palmeiro BS, Rosenthal KL, Lewbart GA, et al. Plasma biochemical reference intervals for koi. *J Am Vet Med Assoc.* 2007;230:708–712.
161. Park I. The anesthetic effects of clove oil and MS-222 on Far Eastern catfish, *Silurus asotus. Dev Reprod.* 2019;23:183–191.
162. Parker-Graham CA, Siniard WC, Byrne BA, et al. Pharmacokinetics of danofloxacin following intramuscular administration of a single dose in koi (*Cyprinus carpio*). *Am J Vet Res.* 2020;81:708–713.
163. Paschoal JAR, Quesada SP, Goncalves LU, et al. Depletion study and estimation of the withdrawal period for enrofloxacin in pacu (*Piaractus mesopotamicus*). *J Vet Pharmacol Ther.* 2013;36:594–602.
164. Pattanasiri T, Taparhudee W, Suppakull P. Acute toxicity and anaesthetic effect of clove oil and eugenol on Siamese fighting fish, *Betta splendens. Aquacult Int.* 2017;25:163–175.
165. Peak S. Sodium bicarbonate and clove oil as potential anesthetics for nonsalmonid fishes. *N Am J Fish Manag.* 1998;18:919–924.
166. Penning MR, Vaughan DB, Fivaz K, et al. Chapter 32. Chemical immobilization of elasmobranchs at uShaka Sea World in Durban, South Africa. In: Smith M, Warmolts D, Thoney D et al., eds. *The Elasmobranch Husbandry Manual II: Recent Advances in the Care of Sharks, Rays and their Relatives.* Special Publication of the Ohio Biological Survey; 2017:504.
167. PEROX-AID (33% hydrogen peroxide) product label. Syndel USA, Ferndale, WA, USA.
168. Phu TM, Scippo M, Phuong NT, et al. Withdrawal time for sulfamethoxazole and trimethoprim following treatment of striped catfish (*Pangasianodon hypophthalmus*) and hybrid red tilapia (*Oreochromis mossambicus* × *Oreochromis niloticus*). *Aquaculture.* 2015;437:256–262.
169. Plakas SM, DePaola A, Moxey MB. *Bacillus stearothermophilis* disk assay for determining ampicillin residues in fish muscle. *J Assoc Off Anal Chem Internat.* 1991;74:910–912.
170. Plakas SM, El Said KR, Bencsath FA, et al. Pharmacokinetics, tissue distribution and metabolism of acriflavine and proflavine in the channel catfish (*Ictalurus punctatus*). *Xenobiotica.* 1998;28:605–616.
171. Plakas SM, El Said KR, Stehly GR. Furazolidone disposition after intravascular and oral dosing in the channel catfish. *Xenobiotica.* 1994;24:1095–1105.
172. Plumb JA, Rogers WA. Effect of Droncit (praziquantel) on yellow grubs *Clinostomum marginatum* and eye flukes *Diplostomum spathaceum* in channel catfish. *J Aquat Anim Health.* 1990;2:204–206.

173. Plumb JA, Schwedler TE, Limsuwan C. Experimental anesthesia of three species of freshwater fish with etomidate. *Prog Fish-Cult.* 1983;45:30–33.
174. Pottinger TG, Day JG. A *Saprolegnia parasitica* challenge system for rainbow trout: assessment of Pyceze as an anti-fungal agent for both fish and ova. *Dis Aquat Org.* 1999;36:129–141.
175. Rach JJ, Gaikowski MP, Ramsay RT. Efficacy of hydrogen peroxide to control parasitic infestations on hatchery-reared fish. *J Aquat Anim Health.* 2000;12:267–273.
176. Rapp J. Treatment of rainbow trout (*Oncorhynchus mykiss* Walb.) fry infected with *Ichthyophthirius multifiliis* by oral administration of dimetridazole. *Bull Eur Assoc Fish Pathol.* 1995;15:67–69.
177. Raulic J, Beaudry F, Beauchamp G, et al. Pharmacokinetic, pharmacodynamic and toxicology study of robenacoxib in rainbow trout (*Oncorhynchus mykiss*). *Proc Int Assoc Aquat Anim Med.* 2020.
178. Reimschuessel R, Chamie SJ, Kinnel M. Evaluation of gentamicin-induced nephrotoxicosis in toadfish. *J Am Vet Med Assoc.* 1996;209:137–139.
179. Reimschuessel R, Stewart L, Squibb E, et al. Fish Drug Analysis—Phish-Pharm: A Searchable Database of Pharmacokinetics Data in Fish. https://www.fda.gov/animal-veterinary/tools-resources/phish-pharm. Accessed April 28, 2021.
180. Reja A, Moreno L, Serrano JM, et al. Concentration-time profiles of oxytetracycline in blood, kidney and liver of tench (*Tinca tinca* L.) after intramuscular administration. *Vet Hum Toxicol.* 1996;38:344–347.
181. Rigos G, Alexis M, Typenou AE, et al. Pharmacokinetics of oxolinic acid in gilthead sea bream, *Sparus aurata* L. *J Fish Dis.* 2002;25:401–408.
182. Rigos G, Nengasa I, Alexis M, et al. Tissue distribution and residue depletion of oxolinic acid in gilthead sea bream (*Sparus aurata*) and sharpsnout sea bream (*Diplodus puntazzo*) following multiple in-feed dosing. *Aquaculture.* 2003;224:245–256.
183. Rigos G, Tyrpenou AE, Nengas I, et al. The kinetic profile of oxolinic acid in sharpsnout sea bream, *Diplodus puntazzo* (Cetti 1777). *Aquac Res.* 2004;35:1299–1304.
184. Roberts HE, Palmeiro B, Weber III ES. Bacterial and parasitic diseases of pet fish. *Vet Clin North Am Exot Anim Pract.* 2009;12:609–638.
185. Robertson B, Rorstad G, Engstad R, et al. Enhancement of non-specific disease resistance in Atlantic salmon, *Salmo salar* L., by a glucan from *Saccharomyces cerevisiae* cell walls. *J Fish Dis.* 1990;13:391–400.
186. Rogstad A, Ellingsen OF, Syvertsen C. Pharmacokinetics and bioavailability of flumequine and oxolinic acid after various routes of administration to Atlantic salmon in seawater. *Aquaculture.* 1993;110:207–220.
187. Rozynski M, Demska-Zakes K, Sikora A, et al. Impact of inducing general anesthesia with Propiscin (etomidate) on the physiology and health of European perch (*Perca fluviatilis* L.). *Fish Physiol Biochem.* 2018;44:927–937.
188. Rozynski M, Ziomek E, Demska-Zakes K, et al. Propiscin - a safe anesthetic for pikeperch (*Sander lucioperca* L). *Acta Vet Hung.* 2016;64:415–424.
189. Russo R, Curtis EW, Yanong RPE. Preliminary investigations of hydrogen peroxide treatment of selected ornamental fishes and efficacy against external bacteria and parasites in green swordtails. *J Aquat Anim Health.* 2007;19:121–127.
190. Russo R, Yanong RPE, Mitchell H. Dietary beta-glucans and nucleotides enhance resistance of redtail black shark (*Epalzeorhynchos bicolor*, fam. Cyprinidae) to *Streptococcus iniae* infection. *J World Aquac Soc.* 2006;37:298–306.
191. Sakamoto K, Lewbart GA, Smith II TM. Blood chemistry values of juvenile red pacu (*Piaractus brachypomus*). *Vet Clin Path.* 2001;30:50–52.
192. Saint-Erne N. Clinical Procedures. In: Saint-Erne N, ed. *Advanced Koi Care.* Glendale, AZ: Erned Enterprises; 2002:39–61.
193. Samuelsen OB. Pharmacokinetics of quinolones in fish: a review. *Aquaculture.* 2006; 255:55–75.

194. Samuelsen OB, Bergh O. Efficacy of orally administered florfenicol and oxolinic acid for the treatment of vibriosis in cod (*Gadus morhua*). *Aquaculture*. 2004;235:27–35.
195. Samuelsen OB, Ervik A. Single dose pharmacokinetic study of flumequine after intravenous, intraperitoneal and oral administration to Atlantic halibut (*Hippoglossus hippoglossus*) held in seawater at 9°C. *Aquaculture*. 1997;158:215–227.
196. Samuelsen OB, Ervik A. A single-dose pharmacokinetic study of oxolinic acid and vetoquinol, an oxolinic acid ester, in Atlantic halibut, *Hippoglossus hippoglossus* L., held in sea water at 9°C. *J Fish Dis*. 1999;22:13–23.
197. Samuelsen OB, Ervik A. Absorption, tissue distribution, and excretion of flumequine and oxolinic acid in corkwing wrasse (*Symphodus melops*) following a single intraperitoneal injection or bath treatment. *J Vet Pharmacol Ther*. 2001;24:111–116.
198. Samuelsen OB, Bergh O, Ervik A. Pharmacokinetics of florfenicol in cod (*Gadus morhua*) and in vitro antibacterial activity against *Vibrio anguillarum*. *Dis Aquat Org*. 2003;56:127–133.
199. Samuelsen OB, Hjeltnes B, Glette J. Efficacy of orally administered florfenicol in the treatment of furunculosis in Atlantic salmon. *J Aquat Anim Health*. 1998;10:56–61.
200. Samuelsen OB, Lunestad BT, Jelmert A. Pharmacokinetic and efficacy studies on bath - administering potentiated sulfonamides in Atlantic halibut, *Hippoglossus hippoglossus* L. *J Fish Dis*. 2003;20:287–296.
201. Schmahl G, Benini J. Treatment of fish parasites 11. Effects of different benzimadazole derivatives (albendazole, mebendazole, fenbendazole) on *Glugea anomala*, Moniez, 1887 (Microsporidia): Ultrastructural aspects and efficacy studies. *Parasitol Res*. 1998;60:41–49.
202. Scott GL, Law M, Christiansen EF, et al. Evaluation of localized inflammatory reactions secondary to intramuscular injections of enrofloxacin in striped bass (*Morone saxatilis*). *J Zoo Wildl Med*. 2020;51:46–52.
203. Seeley KE, Wolf KN, Bishop MA, et al. Pharmacokinetics of long-acting cefovecin in copper rockfish (*Sebastes caurinus*). *Am J Vet Res*. 2016;77:260–264.
204. Setser MD. Pharmacokinetics of gentamicin in channel catfish (*Ictalurus punctatus*). *Am J Vet Res*. 1985;46:2558–2561.
205. Shaikh B, Rummel N, Gieseker C, et al. Metabolism and residue depletion of albendazole in rainbow trout, tilapia, and Atlantic salmon after oral administration. *J Vet Pharmacol Ther*. 2003;26:421–428.
206. Sharp NJ, Diggles BK, Poortenaar CW, et al. Efficacy of Aqui-S, formalin and praziquantel against the monogeneans, *Benedenia seriolae* and *Zeuxapta seriolae*, infecting yellowtail kingfish *Seriola lalandi lalandi* in New Zealand. *Aquaculture*. 2004;236:67–83.
207. Sidhua PK, Smith SA, Mayer C, et al. Comparative pharmacokinetics of oxytetracycline in tilapia (*Oreochromis* spp.) maintained at three different salinities. *Aquaculture*. 2018;495:675–681.
208. Silbernagel C, Yochem P. Effectiveness of the anesthetic Aqui-S 20E in marine finfish and elasmobranchs. *J Wildl Dis*. 2016;52:S96–S103.
209. Siwicki AK, Anderson DP, Rumsey GL. Dietary intake of immunostimulants by rainbow trout affects non-specific immunity and protection against furunculosis. *Vet Immunol Immunopathol*. 1994;41:125–139.
210. Skar MW, Haugland GT, Powell MD, et al. Development of anaesthetic protocols for lumpfish (*Cyclopterus lumpus* L.): Effect of anaesthetic concentrations, sea water temperature and body weight. *PLoS ONE*. 2017;12.7:e0179344.
211. SLICE (emamectin benzoate) AADAP-FWS FDA INAD. Web site: https://www.fws.gov/Fisheries/AADAP/inads/Slice-INAD-11-370.html. Accessed April 28, 2021.
212. Smith CJ, Shaw BJ, Handy RD. Toxicity of single walled carbon nanotubes to rainbow trout (*Oncorhynchus mykiss*): respiratory toxicity, organ pathologies, and other physiological effects. *Aquat Tox*. 2007;82:94–109.
213. Snellgrove DL, Alexander LG. Haematology and plasma chemistry of the red top ice blue mbuna cichlid (*Metriaclima greshakei*). *Br J Nutr*. 2011;106:S154–S157.

214. Sohlberg S, Ingebrigtsen K, Hansen MK, et al. Flumequine in Atlantic salmon *Salmo salar*: disposition in fish held in sea water versus fresh water. *Dis Aquat Org*. 2002;49: 39–44.
215. Steeil JC, Schumacher J, George RH, et al. Pharmacokinetics of cefovecin (Convenia) in white bamboo sharks (*Chiloscyllium plagiosum*) and Atlantic horseshoe crabs (*Limulus polyphemus*). *J Zoo Wildl Med*. 2014;45:389–392.
216. Stevens BN, Gorges MA, Silbernagel C. Efficacy of two different doses of 10% eugenol in adult California yellowtail (*Seriola dorsalis*). *Aquac Res*. 2020;51:1753–1756.
217. St-Hilaire S, Price D, Taylor S, et al. Treatment of diplomonad intestinal parasites with magnesium sulphate at a commercial rainbow trout (*Oncorhynchus mykiss*) facility. *Can Vet J*. 2015;56:876–878.
218. Stoffregen DA, Chako AJ, Backman S, et al. Successful therapy of furunculosis in Atlantic salmon *Salmo salar* L. using the fluoroquinolone antimicrobial agent enrofloxacin. *J Fish Dis*. 1993;16:219–227.
219. Stoskopf MK. Appendix V: Chemotherapeutics. In: Stoskopf MK, ed. *Fish Medicine*. Philadelphia, PA: Saunders; 1993:832–839.
220. Stoskopf MK. Anesthesia of pet fishes. In: Bonagura JD, ed. *Kirk's Current Veterinary Therapy XII: Small Animal Practice*. Philadelphia, PA: Saunders; 1995:1365–1369.
221. Stoskopf MK. Fish pharmacotherapeutics. In: Fowler ME, Miller RE, eds. *Zoo and Wild Animal Medicine: Current Therapy 4*. Philadelphia, PA: Saunders; 1999:182–189.
222. Stoskopf MK, Kennedy-Stoskopf S, Arnold J, et al. Therapeutic aminoglycoside antibiotic levels in brown shark, *Carcharhinus plumbeus* (Nardo). *J Fish Dis*. 1986;9:303–311.
223. Sun M, Li J, Gai CL, et al. Pharmacokinetics of difloxacin in olive flounder *Paralichthys olivaceus* at two water temperatures. *J Vet Pharm Ther*. 2013;37:186–191.
224. Tarascheewski H, Renner C, Melhorn H. Treatment of fish parasites 3. Effects of levamisole HCl, metrifonate, fenbendazole, mebendazole, and ivermectin in *Anguillicola crassus* (nematodes) pathogenic in the air bladder of eels. *Parasitol Res*. 1988;74:281–289.
225. Tavares-Dias M, de Moraes FR. Haematological and biochemical reference intervals for farmed channel catfish. *J Fish Biol*. 2007;71:383–388.
226. Tavares-Dias M, de Moraes FR. Leukocyte and thrombocyte reference values for channel catfish (*Ictalurus punctatus* Raf), with an assessment of morphologic, cytochemical, and ultrastructural features. *Vet Clin Pathol*. 2007;36:49–54.
227. Thomas A, Dawson MR, Ellis H, et al. Praziquantel degradation in marine aquarium water. *PeerJ*. 2016;4:e1857.
228. Thomasen JM. Hydrogen peroxide as a delousing agent for Atlantic salmon. In: Boxshall GA, Defaye D, eds. *Pathogens of Wild and Farmed Fish: Sea Lice*. Chichester, England: Ellis Horwood; 1993:290–295.
229. Tocidlowski ME, Lewbart GA, Stoskopf MK. Hematologic study of red pacu (*Colossoma brachypomum*). *Vet Clin Path*. 1997;26:119–125.
230. Touraki M, Niopas I, Ladoukakis M, Karagiannis V. Efficacy of flumequine administered by bath or through medicated nauplii of *Artemia fransiscana* (L.) in the treatment of vibriosis in sea bass larvae. *Aquaculture*. 2010;306:146–152.
231. Treves-Brown KM. *Applied Fish Pharmacology (AquacultureSeries 3)*. Boston, MA: Kluwer Academic Publishers; 2000:324 pp.
232. Tripathi NK, Latimer KS, Brunley VV. Hematologic reference intervals for koi (*Cyprinus carpio*), including blood cell morphology, cytochemistry, and ultrastructure. *Vet Clin Pathol*. 2004;33:74–83.
233. Tsantilas H, Galatos AD, Athanassopoulou F, et al. Efficacy of 2-phenoxyethanol as an anaesthetic for two size classes of white sea bream, *Diplodus sargus* L., and sharp snout sea bream, *Diplodus puntazzo* C. *Aquaculture*. 2006;253:64–70.
234. Tyrpenou AE, Kotzamanis YP, Alexis NM. Flumequine depletion from muscle plus skin tissue of gilthead seabream (*Sparus aurata* L.) fed flumequine medicated feed in seawater at 18 and 24°C. *Aquaculture*. 2003;220:633–642.

235. Varadaraj K, Pandian TJ. Monosex male broods of *Oreochromis mossambicus* produced through artificial sex reversal with 17α-methyl-4 androsten-17α-ol-3-one. *Current Trends Life Sci*. 1989;15:169–173.
236. Vardali SC, Kotzamanis YP, Tyrpenou AE, et al. Danofloxacin depletion from muscle plus skin tissue of European sea bass (*Dicentrarchus labrax*) fed danofloxacin mesylate medicated feed in seawater at 16°C and 27°C. *Aquaculture*. 2017;479:534–538.
237. Vik-Mo FT, Bergh O, Samuelsen OB. Efficacy of orally administered flumequine in the treatment of vibriosis caused by *Listonella anguillarum* in Atlantic cod *Gadus morhua*. *Dis Aquat Org*. 2005;67:87–92.
238. Vorback BS, Chandasana H, Derendorf H, et al. Pharmacokinetics of oxytetracycline in the giant danio (*Devario aequipinnatus*) following bath immersion. *Aquaculture*. 2019;498:12–16.
239. Whaley J, Francis-Floyd R. A comparison of metronidazole treatments of hexamitiasis in angelfish. *Proc Int Assoc Aquat Anim Med*. 1991:110–114.
240. Whitaker BR. Preventive medicine programs for fish. In: Fowler ME, Miller RE, eds. *Zoo and Wild Animal Medicine: Current Therapy 4*. Philadelphia, PA: Saunders; 1999:163–181.
241. Wildgoose WH, Lewbart GA. Therapeutics. In: Wildgoose WH, ed. *Manual of Ornamental Fish*. 2nd ed. Gloucester, England: British Small Animal Veterinary Association; 2001:237–258.
242. Willoughby LG, Roberts RJ. Towards strategic use of fungicides against *Saprolegnia parasitica* in salmonid fish hatcheries. *J Fish Dis*. 1992;15:1–13.
243. Woynarovich E, Horvath L. *The Artificial Propagation of Warm-Water Finfishes-A Manual for Extension Fisheries*, Rome, Italy: FAO Technical Paper. 201; 1980.
244. Xu N, Ai X, Liu Y, et al. Comparative pharmacokinetics of norfloxacin nicotinate in common carp (*Cyprinus carpio*) and crucian carp (*Carassius auratus*) after oral administration. *J Vet Pharmacol Ther*. 2015;38:309–312.
245. Xu D, Rogers WA. Formaldehyde residue in striped bass muscle. *J Aquat Anim Health*. 1993;5:306–312.
246. Xu L, Wang H, Yang X, Lu L. Integrated pharmacokinetics/pharmacodynamics parameters-based dosing guidelines of enrofloxacin in grass carp *Ctenopharyngodon idella* to minimize selection of drug resistance. *BMC Vet Res*. 2013;9:126.
247. Xu W, Zhu X, Wang X, et al. Residues of enrofloxacin, furazolidone and their metabolites in Nile tilapia (*Oreochromis niloticus*). *Aquaculture*. 2006;254:1–8.
248. Yang F, Li ZL, Shan Q, Zeng ZL. Pharmacokinetics of doxycycline in tilapia (*Oreochromis aureus* × *Oreochromis niloticus*) after intravenous and oral administration. *J Vet Pharmacol Ther*. 2014;37:388–393.
249. Yanong RP, Curtis E, Russo R, et al. *Cryptobia iubilans* infection in juvenile discus. *J Am Vet Med Assoc*. 2004;224:1644–1650.
250. Yanong RPE, Curtis EW, Simmons R, et al. Pharmacokinetic studies of florfenicol in koi carp and threespot gourami *Trichogaster trichopterus* after oral and intramuscular treatment. *J Aquat Anim Health*. 2005;17:129–137.
251. Yuan J, Li RQ, Shi Y, et al. Pharmacokinetics of oxytetracycline in yellow catfish (*Pelteobagrus fulvidraco*) (Richardson, 1846) with a single and multiple-dose oral administration. *J Appl Ichthyol*. 2014;30:109–113.
252. Zhang Q, Li X. Pharmacokinetics and residue elimination of oxytetracycline in grass carp. *Ctenopharyngodon idellus*. *Aquaculture*. 2007;272:140–145.
253. Zhao D, Ke C, Liu Q, et al. Elimination kinetics of eugenol in grass carp in a simulated transportation setting. *BMC Vet Res*. 2017;13:346–351.
254. Zhu Y, Tan T, Wang C, et al. Pharmacokinetics and tissue residues of marbofloxacin in crucian carp (*Carassius auratus*) after oral administration. *Aquac Res*. 2009;40:696–709.
255. Zimmerman DM, Armstrong DL, Curro TG, et al. Pharmacokinetics of florfenicol after a single intramuscular dose in white-spotted bamboo sharks (*Chiloscyllium plagiosum*). *J Zoo Wildl Med*. 2006;37:165–173.

Chapter 3 Amphibians

Natalie D. Mylniczenko | Leigh Ann Clayton

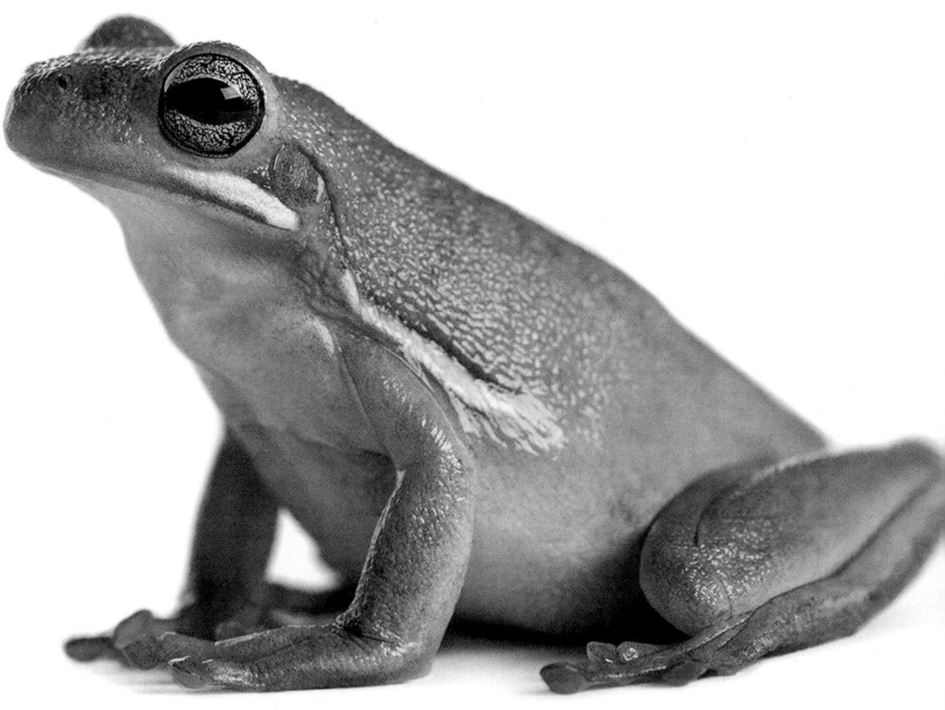

General commentary on amphibian pharmacotherapeutics:

- 1 mg/L=1 ppm=0.0001%. Where indicated, the original format is listed.
- Temperature is a critical factor in the pharmacokinetics of medications in amphibians; ensure animals are managed within the preferred active range for the species.
- Bath or immersion treatments should be in the normal water for the animal where possible, temperature managed, pH appropriate, and changed daily.
- Bath or topical drug application often has highly variable absorption.
- Subcutaneous (SC) injections in anurans are effectively lymphatic injections, the most accessible site is the dorsal lymph sac.[90]
- For all sections, the following abbreviations are used:
- Pharmacokinetic (PK) or pharmacodynamic (PD) study.
- Minimum inhibitory concentration (MIC).
- ED_{50} = dose that gives 50% analgesic effects.

TABLE 3-1 Antimicrobial Agents Used in Amphibians.

Agent	Dosage	Species/Comments
Amikacin	5 mg/kg IM q36h[90] 5-10 mg/kg SC, IM, ICe q24-48h[89]	Bullfrogs (*Lithobates catesbeianus*)/PK
Carbenicillin	100-200 mg/kg SC, IM, ICe q24h or q72h[90]	
Ceftazidime	20 mg/kg SC once[54]/PK 20 mg/kg IM q48-72h[90]	Eastern hellbenders (*Cryptobranchus alleganiensis alleganiensis*)/PK; achieved concentrations greater than MIC for 5 days[54]
Chloramphenicol	50 mg/kg SC, IM, ICe q12-24h[90] 20 mg/L bath changed daily[90]	Egyptian toads (*Sclerophrys regularis*)/PK; aplastic anemia-like findings at ~125 mg/kg PO q24h × 12 wk[28]
Ciprofloxacin	10 mg/kg PO, ICe q24h[89-91] 500-750 mg/75 L x 6-8 hr bath q24h[91]	
Doxycycline (Psittavet, Vetafarm)	5-50 mg/kg PO q24h[90] 50 mg/kg IM q7d[90]	
Enrofloxacin	5-10 mg/kg PO, SC, IM q24h[90]	Bullfrogs (*Lithobates catesbeianus*)/PK; ICe and topical routes also used but with limited data[90]
	10 mg/kg topically on thoracic dorsum[81]	Coqui frogs (*Eleutherodactylus coqui*)/PK; detectable tissue concentration for >24 hr[81]
	10 mg/kg SC, IM[29,37]	African clawed frogs (*Xenopus laevis*)/PK; no significant difference between routes;[29] suggest q24h dosing[37]
	500 mg/L × 6-8 hr bath q24h[90]	

Continued

TABLE 3-1 Antimicrobial Agents Used in Amphibians. (cont'd)

Agent	Dosage	Species/Comments
Gentamicin	2-4 mg/kg IM q72h × 4 treatments[90]	
	2.5 mg/kg IM q72h[77]	Coldwater salamander (*Necturus* sp.)/PK; supports q72h dosing at 3°C (37.4°F), more frequent dosing may be needed at higher temperature[77]
	3 mg/kg IM q24h[90]	Leopard frogs (*Lithobates pipiens*)/ PK at 22.2°C (72°F): at higher temperatures, serum concentrations will be lower[90]
	Topically to eyes[91]	Ocular infections; dilute to 2 mg/mL systemic absorption possible; monitor total mg/kg dosage to avoid toxicity[59]
Metronidazole	12-60 mg/kg topically q24h × 5-10 days[90]	
	20-50 mg/kg PO q24-48h[90]	
	50 mg/L × 24 hr bath[90]	
Ofloxacin	1 drop q2-4h × 10 days (0.3% ophthalmic solution)[89]	Keratitis; may also be applied topically to wounds
Oxytetracycline	25 mg/kg SC, IM q24h[90]	
	50 mg/kg PO q12-24h[90]	
	50-100 mg/kg IM q48h[90]	Bullfrogs (*Lithobates catesbeianus*)/ PK; especially useful in cases of chlamydiosis (use up to 30 days)[90]
	100 mg/L × 1 hr bath[91]	
	1 g/kg feed × 7 days[90]	Most useful with axolotls and *Xenopus* spp. fed in compounded pelleted diet[90]
Silver sulfadiazine	Topically q24-48h[90]	
Sulfadiazine	132 mg/kg PO q24h[90]	
Sulfamethazine	1000 mg/L bath to effect[90]	
Tetracycline	50 mg/kg PO q12h[90]	
	150 mg/kg PO q24h × 5-7 days[90]	
	167 mg/kg (5 mg/30 g) PO q12h × 7 days[90]	
Trimethoprim/ sulfadiazine	15-20 mg/kg IM q48h[90]	
Trimethoprim/ sulfamethoxazole	15 mg/kg PO q24h[91]	

TABLE 3-2 Antifungal Agents Used in Amphibians.

Agent	Dosage	Species/Comments
Amphotericin B	1 mg/kg ICe q24h[91]	Internal mycoses; acutely toxic to Majorcan midwife toads (*Alytes muletensis*) tadpoles at 8 µg/mL bath in a trial for chytridiomycosis treatment[49]
Benzalkonium chloride	0.25 mg/L × 72 hr bath[90]	*Saprolegnia* sp.
	2 mg/L × 1 hr bath q24h[91]	
Chloramphenicol	10-30 mg/L as continuous bath replaced fresh daily for up to 30 days[90]	Egyptian toad (*Sclerophrys regularis*)/PK; aplastic anemia-like findings at ~125 mg/kg PO q24h × 12 wk[28]
	20 mg/L continuous bath × 14 days[95]	Australian green frog (*Ranoidea caerulea*)/chytridiomycosis
	30 mg/L continuous bath for up to 30 days[90]	Chytridiomycosis; safe for larvae, recent metamorphs, and adults[90]
Fluconazole	60 mg/kg PO q24h[91]	
Hyperthermia, elevated enclosure temperature	30°C (86°F) × 10 days[19]	Chytridiomycosis; American bullfrog (*Lithobates catesbeianus*), northern cricket frog (*Acris crepitans*)
	37°C (98.6°F) for under 16 hr[86]	Chytridiomycosis; red-eyed tree frog (*Ranoidea chloris*)
Itraconazole	—	Chytridiomycosis;[4,18,60] some species and froglets/tadpoles are sensitive (fatalities) particularly at 0.01%; recommend testing a small number of animals in an unreported species and/or use lower doses; Sporanox Oral Solution (Janssen Pharmaceutica), for best results;[60] note: 0.0001% = 1 mg/L, 0.001% = 10 mg/L, 0.01% = 100 mg/L
	0.001% and 0.01% itraconazole bath[65]	Panamanian golden frogs (*Atelopus zeteki*)/PK; 0.001% bath exceeded MIC but was highly variable in half life[65]
	0.002% to 0.0025% (20-25 mg/L) bath x 5 min/day x 10 days[25]	Mexican axolotl (*Ambystoma mexicanum*), rough-skinned newts (*Taricha granulosa*)
	0.0025% bath x 5 min/day x 6 days[12]	Australian green tree frog (*Ranoidea caerulea*), coastal plains toad (*Incillus nebulifer*)/chytridiomycosis; authors suggest low dose reliably cures chytrid with fewer side effects than higher dose[12]
	0.005-0.01% bath x 5 min/day x 10 days[4]	Safe and effective treatment in most situations[4]
	0.01% bath x 30 min/day x 11 days[63]	Caecilians (*Geotrypetes seraphini*, *Potomotyphlus kaupii*)/chytridiomycosis
	0.01% (in buffered solution) bath × 5 min/day × 11-14 days[33]	Multiple species/chytridiomycosis; cleared chytridiomycosis by PCR 14 days post treatment; some recurrence in 6-15 mo[33]
	0.5-1.5 mg/L bath x 5 min/day × 7 days[32]	Majorcan midwife toad (*Alytes muletensis*) tadpoles/chytridiomycosis; safe; varying levels of depigmentation observed in all individuals[32]

Continued

TABLE 3-2 Antifungal Agents Used in Amphibians. (cont'd)

Agent	Dosage	Species/Comments
Itraconazole (cont'd)	50 mg/L bath x 5 min/day × 10 days (Sporanox Oral Solution, Janssen Pharmaceutica)[39]	Multiple species/chytridiomycosis; cleared chytridiomycosis in subclinical animals; confirmed with PCR[39]
Ketoconazole	Topical cream[90] 10-20 mg/kg PO q24h[90,91]	
Methylene blue	4 mg/L bath × 1 hr/day[90]	*Saprolegnia* sp.
Miconazole	Topical cream[91] 5 mg/kg ICe q24h × 14-28 days[90]	
Nystatin	Topical cream (1%)[90]	
Potassium permanganate	200 mg/L bath x 5 min/day[90]	
Terbinafine hydrochloride (Lamisil AT, Novartis)	0.005-0.01% (in distilled water) bath x 5 min/day × 5 days or 6 treatments over 10 days[10]	Various species/PK, PD; chytridiomycosis; no adverse effects noted;[10] recent studies (0.01% bath 5 min/day x 5 days) showed limited efficacy in alpine tree frogs (*Litoria verreauxii alpina*) and common eastern froglets (*Crinia signifera*)[66]
Voriconazole (VFend injectable solution, Pfizer)	1.25 µg/mL q24h topically via spray × 7 days[49]	Poison dart frogs, Iberian midwife toad (*Alytes cisternasii*)/chytridiomycosis; appeared safe in *A. cisternasii* tadpoles[49]
Voriconazole (V) + polymyxin E (P) + elevated temperature (T)	(V) 12.5 µg/mL q24h topically via spray + (P) 2000 IU/mL × 10 min bath q12h + (T) 20°C (68°F) continuous × 10 days[8]	Fire salamanders (*Salamandra salamandra*)/*Batrachochytrium salamandrivorans*; no effect of medications at 15°C (59°F)[8]

TABLE 3-3 Antiparasitic Agents Used in Amphibians.

Agent	Dosage	Species/Comments
Acriflavin	0.025% bath × 5 days[90] 500 mg/L bath for 30 min[90]	Protozoa
Benzalkonium chloride	2 mg/L bath x 1 hr/day to effect[90]	*Saprolegnia* sp.
Febantel (in combination with pyrantel pamoate and praziquantel; Drontal Plus, Bayer)	0.01 mL/1 g PO q2-3wk[60]	Create suspension from tablets for dogs at 2.25 mg/mL based on pyrantel content[60]
Fenbendazole	— 30-100 mg/kg PO[60,90,91]	Panacur 10% (100 mg/mL) (Merck) oral solution; shake well to suspend; typically needs to be diluted Variable doses and frequencies have been recommended: once to q24h × 3-5 days, repeat in 14-21 days

TABLE 3-3 Antiparasitic Agents Used in Amphibians. (cont'd)

Agent	Dosage	Species/Comments
Fenbendazole (cont'd)	Dust food items q24h x 5 days, repeat in 2-3 wk[7,60]	Houston toad (*Anaxyrus houstonensis*)/ reduced nematode egg counts; granules ground to fine dust fed q24h x 3 days for animals <20 g[7]
Formalin (10%)	—	Do not use if skin is ulcerated; may be toxic to some species[90]
	1.5 mL/L bath × 10 min/48 hr to effect[90]	Protozoans
	0.5% bath × 10 min once[90]	Monogeneans
Ivermectin	—	Caution: may cause flaccid paralysis or fatalities with overdosage;[21] caffeine or physostigmine may ameliorate effects[90]
	0.2-0.4 mg/kg IM once[90]	
	2 mg/kg topically, repeat in 2-3 wk[45]	Leopard frogs (*Lithobates pipiens*)/ nematode infections; dosage fatal if given IM[45]
	2 mg/kg topically[82]	Túngara frogs (*Engystomops pustulosus*)/ no difference compared to daily substrate changes to prevent infection by *Strongyloides*[82]
	10 mg/L × 60 min bath, repeat q14d prn[90,91]	
Levamisole	—	Caution: may cause paralysis in some species at suggested dosages;[91] caffeine or physostigmine may ameliorate effects[90]
	6.5-13.5 mg/kg topically to pelvic patch, repeat in 10 days[7]	Houston toad (*Anaxyrus houstonensis*)/ reduced nematode egg counts; diluted levamisole phosphate 136.5 mg/mL in sterile water to 13.6 mg/mL[7]
	10 mg/kg IM, ICe, topically, repeat in 2 wk[60]	Injectable formulation may be used topically[60]
	12 mg/L bath × 4 days repeated at 10-14 days[38]	African clawed frogs (*Xenopus laevis*)/ cutaneous nematodes; used ≥4.2 L of tank water/frog to deliver 50-70 mg levamisole/ frog; lower exposure not effective[38]
	100-300 mg/L × 24 hr bath, repeat in 1-2 wk[91]	
Metronidazole	10 mg/kg PO q24h × 5-10 days[91]	
	100 mg/kg PO q3d;[90] 100-150 mg/ kg PO, repeat in 2-3 wk or prn[90]	
	50 mg/L × 24 hr bath[91]	Aquatic amphibians in enclosure water
	500 mg/100 g feed × 3-4 treatments[90]	
Moxidectin (Cydectin, Wyeth-Ayerst)	200 µg/kg SC at ~ q4mo x 3 treatments[69]	Nematodes; incidentally reported in a case study[69]

Continued

TABLE 3-3 Antiparasitic Agents Used in Amphibians. (cont'd)

Agent	Dosage	Species/Comments
Moxidectin (Cydectin, Wyeth-Ayerst) (cont'd)	0.4 mg/kg divided PO and intranasal q14d x 2 treatments 0.4 mg/kg SC[68]	Archey's frog (*Leiopelma archeyi*)/PO and nasal for nasal nematode infection; SC route prophylactic use[68]
Oxfendazole	5 mg/kg PO[90]	
Oxytetracycline	25 mg/kg SC, IM q24h[90]	
	50 mg/kg PO q12h[90]	
	1 g/kg feed × 7 days[90]	
Paromomycin	50-75 mg/kg PO q24h[90]	
Piperazine	50 mg/kg PO, repeat in 2 wk[90]	
Ponazuril	30 mg/kg PO q24h × 30 days[90]	May be effective with less frequent treatments[90]
Potassium permanganate	7 mg/L × 5 min bath q24h to effect[90]	Ectoparasitic protozoa
Praziquantel	8-24 mg/kg PO, SC, ICe, topically, repeat q14d[91]	
	0.01 mL/1 g (10 mL/kg) PO q2-3wk (in combination with fenbantel and pyrantel pamoate; Drontal Plus, Bayer)[60]	Create oral suspension from tablets for dogs at 2.25 mg/mL pyrantel component[60]
	10 mg/L × 3 hr bath repeat q7-12d[91]	
Pyrantel pamoate	0.01 mL/1 g (10 mL/kg) PO q2-3wk (in combination with fenbantel and praziquantel; Drontal Plus, Bayer)[60]	Create oral suspension from tablets for dogs at 2.25 mg/mL pyrantel component[60]
Ronidazole	10 mg/kg PO q24h × 10 days[90]	Flagellated protozoa, amoebas
Salt (sodium chloride)	4-6 g/L continuous bath[90]	
	5 g/L bath up to 12 hr[48] 10 g/L bath up to 1 hr[48]	Axolotls (*Ambystoma mexicanum*)/ immediate negative clinical effects in baths >20 g/L[48]
	6 g/L × 5-10 min bath q24h × 3-5 days[90]	Ectoparasitic protozoa
	25 g/L × ≤ 10 min bath[90]	Ectoparasitic protozoa
Selamectin (Revolution, Zoetis)	6 mg/kg topically on dorsum over pelvic girdle[24]	Bullfrogs (*Lithobates catesbeianus*)/PK; keep out of water 5 min until skin dry[24]
	6 mg/kg or 60 mg/kg q7d × 3 days topically[9]	Lemur leaf frogs (*Agalynchnis lemur*)/ dissolved in isopropyl alcohol; ineffective on *Rhabdias* sp. infection even at high dose[9]
Sulfadiazine	132 mg/kg PO q24h[90]	
Sulfamethazine	1000 mg/L bath[90]	
Thiabendazole	50-100 mg/kg PO, repeat in 2 wk prn[90]	
	100 mg/L bath, repeat in 2 wk[90]	Verminous dermatitis
Trimethoprim/sulfa	3 mg/kg PO, SC, IM q24h[90,91]	Coccidiosis

TABLE 3-4 Chemical Restraint/Anesthetic/Analgesic Agents Used in Amphibians. ED_{50} = dose that gives 50% analgesic effects

Agent	Dosage	Species/Comments
Alfaxalone	5 mg/L bath for induction; 30 µL drops brachial for maintenance[51]	Mexican axolotl *(Ambystoma mexicanum)*/surgical depth; 15 min recovery, n = 1[51]
	10-17.5 mg/kg IM[62]	Bullfrogs (*Lithobates catesbeianus*)/ immobilization; not surgical depth; dose dependent time to recumbency and time to recovery; no effect by bath at 2000 mg/L for 30 min[62]
	15, 20, and 30 mg/kg IM[16]	Spanish ribbed newts (*Pleurodeles waltl*)/ sedation and muscle relaxation; higher doses resulted in decreased induction time[16]
	18 mg/kg IM, IV, ICe[36]	African clawed frogs (*Xenopus laevis*)/ deep sedation for 1-3 hr (IM, IV), 10-60 min ICe; no effect via bath at 18 mg/L[36]
	20-30 mg/kg IM[72]	Australian tree frog species/initial effect within 10 min; duration of effect 25-100 min; insufficient anesthesia as sole agent for painful procedures[72]
	200 mg/L in fresh water buffered bath[2]	Fire-bellied toads (*Bombina orientalis*)/ induction in 14 ± 4 min; variable duration of anesthesia up to 30 min; insufficient anesthesia for painful procedures[2]
Alfaxalone (A)/ midazolam (M)/ dexmedetomidine (D)	(A) 20 mg/kg + (M) 40 mg/ kg + (D) 5 mg/kg SC[93]	Blue poison dart frogs (*Dendrobates tinctorius azureus*)/gastric prolapses in several animals[93]
Alfaxalone (A)/morphine (M)	(A) 3 mg/100 mL + (M) 5 mg/100 mL bath[1]	Fire-bellied toads (*Bombina orientalis*)/ anesthetic induction and antinociception; alfaxalone at same amount with butorphanol 2.5 mg/100 mL had insufficient antinociception[1]
Atipamezole	50 mg/kg SC[93]	Blue poison dart frogs (*Dendrobates tinctorius azureus*)[93]
Benzocaine	Bath (in deionized water) to effect: 50 mg/L bath[90]	Larvae/first dissolve in ethanol or acetone[90]
	200-500 mg/L bath[90]	
	300 ppm (mg/L) bath[71]	East Asian bullfrog (*Hoplobatrachus rugulosus*)[71]
	0.1% (1 g/L, optimal), 0.5% (5 g/L), or 1% (10 g/L) bath[73]	African clawed frogs (*Xenopus laevis*)[73]
Bupivicaine	2 mg/kg topically or intra-incisional/dilute 3:1 with sodium bicarbonate solution[17]	Duration 3 hr; author recommends not exceeding 5 mg/kg total dose either topically or intraincisional[17]
Buprenorphine	38 mg/kg SC[47]	Leopard frogs (*Lithobates pipiens*)/ analgesia >4 hr; ED_{50}[47]

Continued

TABLE 3-4 Chemical Restraint/Anesthetic/Analgesic Agents Used in Amphibians. ED_{50} = dose that gives 50% analgesic effects. (cont'd)

Agent	Dosage	Species/Comments
Buprenorphine (cont'd)	50 mg/kg ICe q24h x 3 days[40]	Eastern red-spotted newts (*Notophthalmus viridescens*)/effective analgesia following limb amputation; may take >1 hr for onset[40]
	50 mg/kg ICe q24h x 2 days[46]	Axolotls (*Ambystoma mexicanum*)/no significant difference from controls during behavioral assessment at 1, 6, 12, 25, 30, and 48 hr[46]
Butorphanol	0.05, 1, or 5 mg/kg IV[78]	African clawed frogs (*Xenopus laevis*)/5 mg/kg showed some nociceptive effects[78]
	0.5 mg/L continuous bath x 3 days[40]	Eastern red-spotted newts (*Notophthalmus viridescens*)/return to normal behaviors following limb amputation; may take >1 hr for onset[40]
	0.50 or 0.75 mg/L continuous bath x 2 days, treatment refreshed at 24 hr[46]	Axolotls (*Ambystoma mexicanum*)/no significant difference from controls during behavioral assessment at 1, 6, 12, 25, 30, and 48 hr[46]
	25 mg/kg ICe[79]	Leopard frogs (*Rana pipiens*) duration 2-4 hr[79]
Clove oil (eugenol)	0.3 mL/L (≈ 310-318 mg/L)[90]	Deep anesthesia with 15 min bath; reversible gastric prolapse in 50% of leopard frogs[90]
	0.35 mL/L, used 200 mL/frog[34]	African clawed frogs (*Xenopus laevis*)/ frogs <10 g at 5 min had surgical plane of anesthesia for 15 min; frogs ~30 g at 10 min exposure to bath had surgical plane of anesthesia for 30 min[34]
	350 mg/L bath[71]	East Asian bullfrogs (*Hoplobatrachus rugulosus*)
	450 mg/L bath x 10 min exposure[53]	Tiger salamanders (*Ambystoma tigrinum*)/deep anesthesia induced in 67% (8/12); rapid induction[53]
Dexmedetomidine	40-120 mg/kg SC[47]	Leopard frogs (*Rana pipiens*)/analgesia >4 hr lower dosage and >8 hr higher dosage; ED_{50}[47]
Etomidate	15, 22.5 (optimal), or 30 mg/L bath[73]	African clawed frogs (*Xenopus laevis*)
Fentanyl	0.05, 0.25, or 0.5 mg/kg IV[78]	African clawed frogs (*Xenopus laevis*)/not analgesic[78]
	0.5 mg/kg SC[47]	Leopard frogs (*Rana pipiens*)/analgesia >4 hr; ED_{50}[47]
	0.8 µg/g SC (dorsal lymph sac)[75]	Leopard frogs (*Rana pipiens*)/analgesia; ED_{50}[75]
Flumazenil	0.05 mg/kg IM[93]	Blue poison dart frogs (*Dendrobates tinctorius azureus*)

TABLE 3-4 Chemical Restraint/Anesthetic/Analgesic Agents Used in Amphibians. ED_{50} = dose that gives 50% analgesic effects. (cont'd)

Agent	Dosage	Species/Comments
Flunixin meglumine (Banamine, Merck Animal Health)	3.3 mg/kg topically/transdermal on dorsum[67]	Marine toads (*Rhinella marina*)/PK; rapidly absorbed; plasma concentrations exceeded cattle therapeutic ranges[67]
	25 mg/kg SC[23,73]	African clawed frogs (*Xenopus laevis*)/ analgesia in an experimental setting at 24 hr; 50 mg/kg lethal in many frogs[73]
	25 mg/kg ICe[79]	Northern leopard frogs (*Lithobates pipiens*)/analgesia 2-4 hr[79]
Isoeugenol (Aqui-S; Aqui-S New Zealand) 0.54 µg/mL isoeugenol	10, 20, or 50 µL/L[74]	Brown tree frog (*Litoria ewingii*) tadpoles/ higher doses resulted in faster induction and longer recovery; 20 µL/L most suitable balance of depth and duration[74]
Isoflurane	—	For larger amphibians, inhalant anesthesia with either chamber induction or manual intubation and positive pressure ventilation can induce anesthesia; the amphibian trachea is short, use caution not to enter bronchi or perforate
	Chamber 5% induction and 2% maintenance[6]	Mountain chicken frogs (*Leptodactylus fallax*)
	0.28 mL/100 mL bath[90]	Induce in closed container
Topical mixture of isoflurane (3 mL), K-Y Jelly (3.5 mL), and water (1.5 mL)[90]	0.025 mL/g BW 0.035 mL/g BW	*Anaxyrus* spp., *Bufo* spp., African clawed frogs (*Xenopus laevis*)/induce in closed container, then remove excess[90]
Topical mixture of 1.5 parts distilled water, 3.5 parts nonspermicidal jelly, and 1.8 parts isoflurane with 2 mL spread on induction container floor[97]	Estimated dose rate of 300 µL/g[97]	American tree frogs (*Dryophytes cinereus*)/induce in closed container, then remove excess from animal; erythematous lesions and signs of systemic illness noted following application; authors do not recommend[97]
Ketamine	20-210 mg/kg IM[91]	Most species/inconsistent results
	50-150 mg/kg SC, IM[90]	Most species
	70-100 mg/kg IM[91]	Australian giant tree frogs (*Nyctimystes infrafrenatus*), Australian green tree frogs (*Ranoidea caerulea*)/15-min induction[91]
	120 mg/kg IM[88]	Two-toed amphiumas (*Amphiuma means*)/20 min induction[88]
Ketamine (K)/midazolam (M)/dexmedetomidine (D)	(K) 100 + (M) 40 + (D) 5 mg/kg[93]	Blue poison dart frogs (*Dendrobates tinctorius azureus*)/gastric prolapses in several animals[93]
Ketoprofen	1 mg/kg SC and topically[5]	Smoky jungle frogs (*Leptodactylus pentadactylus*)/PK; in plasma for 24 hr after SC or topical administration[5]

Continued

TABLE 3-4 Chemical Restraint/Anesthetic/Analgesic Agents Used in Amphibians. ED_{50} = dose that gives 50% analgesic effects. (cont'd)

Agent	Dosage	Species/Comments
Lidocaine	2 mg/kg local infiltration, dilute 3:1 with sodium bicarbonate solution, duration 30–60 min[17]	Do not exceed 5 mg/kg total dose either topically or intraincisional[17]
	5 or 50 mg/kg SC (hindleg)[83]	Bullfrogs (*Lithobates catesbeianus*)/5 mg/kg, no loss of reflex; 50 mg/kg, loss of righting reflex; resolution in 4 hr[83]
Meloxicam	0.1 mg/kg IM q24h[52]	American bullfrogs (*Lithobates catesbeianus*)/PD; decreased circulating prostaglandin E_2 (PGE2) levels measured 24 hr after muscle biopsy[52]
	0.2 mg/kg SC, topically[5]	Smoky jungle frogs (*Leptodactylus pentadactylus*)/PK; topical lacks reliable absorption; SC does not produce sustained plasma concentrations[5]
	0.4-1 mg/kg PO, SC, ICe q24h[89]	Antiinflammatory; presumptive analgesia
Meperidine	31.6 µg/g SC[75]	Northern leopard frog (*Lithobates pipiens*)/ED_{50}[75]
Metomidate hydrochloride	30 mg/L bath x 60 min[27]	Leopard frogs (*Lithobates pipiens*)/not recommended for surgical procedures[27]
Morphine	38-42 mg/kg SC[47]	Leopard frogs (*Lithobates pipiens*)/analgesia >4 hr[47]
Naltrexone	1 mg/kg SC[47]	
Propofol	10-30 mg/kg ICe[90]	Australian green tree frogs (*Ranoidea caerulea*)/use lower dosage for sedation or light anesthesia; induction within 30 min; recovery in 24 hr[90]
	35 mg/kg ICe[53,87]	Tiger salamanders (*Ambystoma tigrinum*)/surgical anesthesia in 83%; variable induction and short duration[53]
		Sonoran desert toads (*Incilius alvarius*)/sedation only; did not achieve surgical plane of anesthesia[87]
	88 mg/L bath[35]	African clawed frogs (*Xenopus laevis*)/induced for 15 min, then rinsed; death at doses over 175 mg/L[35]
	100-140 mg/kg topically[90]	Maroon-eyed tree frogs (*Agalychnis litodryas*)/for <50 g frog;[90] unpublished data; 15-20 min at 100 mg/kg dose; 10-15 min at 140 mg/kg; sedation to deep anesthesia; remove and rinse when induced
Sevoflurane (topical mixture: 1.5 parts distilled water, 3.5 parts nonspermicidal jelly, and 3 parts sevoflurane)[76,97]	37.5 µg/g of topical mixture applied to dorsum	Marine toads (*Rhinella marinus*)/loss of righting reflex within ~8 min; mean recovery time 84 +/- 47 min[76]

TABLE 3-4 Chemical Restraint/Anesthetic/Analgesic Agents Used in Amphibians. ED_{50} = dose that gives 50% analgesic effects. (cont'd)

Agent	Dosage	Species/Comments
Sevoflurane (topical mixture: 1.5 parts distilled water, 3.5 parts nonspermicidal jelly, and 3 parts sevoflurane) (cont'd)	2 mL topically[97]	American tree frogs (*Dryophytes cinereus*)/induced in closed container; recovery 44 +/− 20 min (faster than topical isoflurane jelly)[97]
Tiletamine/zolazepam (Telazol, Fort Dodge)	10-20 mg/kg IM[44,90]	Bullfrogs (*Lithobates catesbeianus*), leopard frogs (*Lithobates pipiens*)/results variable between species; rapid recovery; 50 mg/kg caused fatalities; not a good single anesthetic agent for anurans[44,90]
Tricaine meth-ane-sulfonate (MS-222) (Finquel, Argent)	—	Buffer water to a pH of 7.0-7.4; aerate; remove from the anesthetic bath after induction to prevent overdose; place terrestrial amphibians on moist materials or in shallow water for recovery (nose above the water); in some cases, anesthesia can be maintained by dripping 100-200 mg/L over the skin or by covering animal with a paper towel or gauze moistened with the anesthetic water[90]
	100-200 mg/L bath to effect[90]	Larvae/induction
	200-500 mg/L bath to effect[90]	Tadpoles, newts; induction in 15-30 min
	500 mg/L or 2000 mg/L bath[42]	Australian green tree frogs/(*Ranoidea caerulea*)/mild sedation at 500 mg/L; surgical anesthesia at 2000 mg/L
	500-2000 mg/L bath to effect[90]	Most gill-less adult species (unless very large)/induction
	1000 mg/L bath[87]	Sonoran desert toads (*Incilius alvarius*)/ keep in bath until surgical plane of anesthesia reached (13-30 min)[87]
	1000 mg/L bath[71]	East Asian bullfrogs (*Hoplobatrachus rugulosus*)[71]
	1-2 g/L bath[43]	African clawed frogs (*Xenopus laevis*)/PK, PD; 30 min (1 g/L) or 60 min (2 g/L)[43]
	0.2% (2 g/L) bath[98]	Mexican axolotl (*Ambystoma mexicanum*)/0.1% no effects at 20 min; 0.2% deeply anesthetized at 15 min for 15-20 min; at 0.4%, 90-120 min recoveries, deemed too long[98]
	2 g/L in distilled water and bicarbonate (to reach pH 6.5)[57]	Red-backed salamanders (*Plethodon cinereus*)/3-5 min induction; rapid recovery[57]
	2-3 g/L bath to effect[90,91]	Toads/15-30 min induction[90,91]
Xylazine	10 mg/kg ICe[79]	Leopard frogs (*Lithobates pipiens*)/ analgesia 12-24 hr[79]

Continued

TABLE 3-5 Euthanasia Agents Used in Amphibians.

Because of normal physiologic adaptations, unconsciousness and death should be ensured and either definitive evidence of death (e.g., absolute cessation of cardiac movement) and/or use of a secondary method (e.g., sever spinal cord, decapitation, pithing) should be considered.[3]

Agent	Dosage	Species/Comments
Benzocaine	182 mg/kg (2 cm x 1 mm of 20% gel)[80] topically	African clawed frog (*Xenopus laevis*)/loss of reflexes within 7 min, cardiac arrest of 100% within 5 hr[80]
	>250 mg/L bath[56]	
Isoflurane	Full concentration liquid on a cotton ball[55]	Keep in a sealed container
Pentobarbital sodium	60-100 mg/kg IV, ICe[3,90]	Can also be administered in lymph sacs in anurans
Pentobarbital sodium (P)/sodium phenytoin (SP)	(P) 1,100 mg/kg + (SP) 141 mg/kg ICe[80]	African clawed frogs (*Xenopus laevis*)/complete cardiac arrest within 3 hr[80]
Propofol	60-100 mg/kg ICe[90]	
Tricaine meth-ane-sulfonate (MS-222)	—	MS-222 alone is not a good euthanasia method, use secondary method; can be administered ICe or in lymph sacs in addition to bath
	5 g/L buffered solution of MS-222 × 1 hr[80]	African clawed frog (*Xenopus laevis*)
	6 g/L bath for 15 min[31]	African clawed frog (*Xenopus laevis*) larvae
	10 g/L buffered bath[90]	Most species

TABLE 3-6 Reproductive Hormones Used in Amphibians.[15,22,41]

Select Species	Protocol[a]
African clawed frog (*Xenopus laevis*)[85]	Wild type: prime with 50 U of PMSG or 50 U of hCG between 24 hr to 7 days (although priming is not essential)/induce ovulation with 2 µg/g of oLH or 500 U of hCG
	Inbred strains: 30 U of PMSG or 30 U of hCG; boost with 140 µg of oLH or 350 U of hCG
Chinese giant salamander (*Andrias davidianus*)[94]	300-1500 IU/kg hCG and 3-15 µg/kg LHRH-A2 SC; the amount of hormones can be adjusted based on the gonadal development and maturation

TABLE 3-6 Reproductive Hormones Used in Amphibians. (cont'd)

Select Species	Protocol[a]
Puerto Rican crested toad (*Peltophryne lemur*)[26]	Preinjection preparation: cooling period-slowly drop temperature to 18°C (66°F) over several days, maintain for ~3 wk; then slowly raise temperature of toads to 28°C (82°F) over 3 days; keep males and females separate under normal husbandry; soak toads in 0.01% itraconozole for 5 min daily for 5 days; "rain" can be simulated throughout the injection process and a few days prior Day 1: inject females, 5-6 hr later inject males; LHRH ethylamide 100 µg/ml in saline; females are given 0.1 µg/g SC or ICe and males are given half dose; SC or ICe Day 2: repeat if no eggs; both injections in the morning at the same time; if no eggs, repeat in the pm Day 3: morning; final attempt; do not repeat
Wyoming toad (*Bufo baxteri*)[14]	Day 1: prime with 500 IU hCG and 4 µg LHRHa SC Day 3: 100 IU hCG and 0.8 µg LHRHa SC Day 7: 500 IU hCG and 4 µg LHRHa SC Eggs produced during the fertile period (12–18 hr after hormone treatment) were fertilized in a dish with spermic urine. Males, single dose of 300 IU human chorionic gonadotrophin (hCG) SC produced spermic urine within 5-7 hr.

[a]Pregnant Mare Serum Gonadotropin (PMSG); Ovine Luteinizing Hormone (oLH); Human Chorionic Gonadotropin (hCG); Luteinizing Hormone Releasing Hormone (LHRH); Luteinizing Hormone Releasing Hormone Analogue (LHRH-A2 and LHRHa).

TABLE 3-7 Fluids and Supportive Baths Used in Amphibians.[91]

Potential fluid routes: baths, IV, IO, SC, and PO (least common).
Basic physiology: The integument actively contributes to osmoregulation, electrolytes and water are readily absorbed.[58,60,91] Ill aquatic amphibians are subject to fluid overload and electrolyte dilution. Ill terrestrial amphibians are subject to fluid loss and electrolyte increase; however, if skin disease is present, electrolytes may be low.[95]
Clinical care: Rehydration and electrolyte support via baths is appropriate; parenteral administration is needed with severe skin disease (e.g., chytridiomycosis) or in critical cases.
Fluid choice, route, and frequency: depends on natural physiology, disease condition, and clinical goal (e.g., osmolality balance or manipulation versus volume replacement). Animals may need to be weaned off fluid support. Target pH to 7.1-7.4. Formulas to create solutions from chemical salts are available, but use of common IV fluids is possible. Avoid using water without electrolytes (e.g., reverse osmosis, distilled) for baths. Dechlorinate if using tap water to make electrolyte solution for bath treatment.

Agent	Dosage	Species/Comments
General amphibian fluids: mildly hypotonic	Equal parts 5% dextrose (in water) and saline or a non-lactated electrolyte solution (e.g., Normosol-R, Hospira)[91]	Use intravenous solutions
Amphibian bath: isotonic	Normosol-R 900 ml + Dextrose 5% 100 ml[20]	Basic fluid and electrolyte bath support
Amphibian Ringer's solution (ARS): isotonic	6.6 g NaCl, 0.15 g KCl, 0.15 g $CaCl_2$, and 0.2 g $NaHCO_3$ in 1 L water[90,91]	For treating hydrocoelom and subcutaneous edema; up to 10 g/L of glucose may be added; solution must be made fresh daily[90]
Dextrose 5% solution: hypertonic	Bath[90,91]	For treating hydrocoelom and subcutaneous edema; 7.5-10% solutions may be more effective for some cases of hydrocoelom
Dextrose 50% solution	Topically to affected tissues[50]	Small amount can be applied to edematous/inflamed tissue in cases of cloacal prolapse to aid in prolapse reduction[50]
Hetastarch (6% in 0.9% saline): hypertonic	Bath not to exceed 1 hr without reassessment[90]	May help with initial treatment of hydrocoelom
Lactated Ringer's solution: slightly hypertonic (Harmann's solution, Baxter Viaflex)	50 ml/kg SC q8h x 3days, then q12h x 3 days[95]	Australian green tree frogs (*Ranoidea caerulea*)/terminal chytridiomycosis; used with chloramphenicol and hyperthermia; treatment effective[95]
0.9% NaCl: hypertonic	Bath[91]	Use intravenous solution

TABLE 3-8 Miscellaneous Agents Used in Amphibians.

Agent	Dosage	Species/Comments
Atropine	0.1 mg SC, IM as needed[90]	Organophosphate toxicosis
Budesonide	0.1 mg/kg PO q24h[20]	Repeat intestinal prolapse with inflammation; part of multimodal regime, taper over time[20]
Caffeine	Use caffeinated tea bag; steep (soak) until solution is "weak tea"; place amphibian in shallow bath, replace q6h[90]	Stimulant; may help reverse ivermectin or levamisole toxicosis, or excessively deep anesthesia
Calcium glubionate (Calcionate, 1.8 g/5 mL, Rugby Laboratories)	1 mL/kg PO q24h[90]	Nutritional secondary hyperparathyroidism
Calcium gluconate	100-200 mg/kg SC[90]	Hypocalcemic tetany
	2.3% continuous bath (with 2-3 U/mL vitamin D_3)[90]	Nutritional secondary hyperparathyroidism
Cyanoacrylate surgical adhesive (Vetbond, 3M)	Topically on wounds[91]	Produces a seal for aquatic and semiaquatic species
Dexamethasone	1.5 mg/kg SC, IM, IV[90]	Vascularizing keratitis; shock
Diphenhydramine	51 µg/g SC[75]	Northern leopard frogs (*Lithobates pipiens*)/examined for analgesic effects[75]
Haloperidol lactate	11 µg/g SC[75]	Northern leopard frogs (*Lithobates pipiens*)/examined for analgesic effects[75]
Hyperthermia, elevated temperature	Temperature increased to 28°C (82.4°F) × 14 days[95]	Australian green tree frogs (*Ranoidea caerulea*)/ chytridiomycosis; effective in conjunction with other treatments[95]
Hypertonic saline, 5% ophthalmic solution	Topically to affected tissues[50]	Cloacal prolapse; apply to edematous/inflamed tissue to aid in prolapse reduction[50]
Laxative	PO (Laxatone, Evsco)[90]	Laxative; especially for intestinal foreign bodies
Methylene blue	2 mg/mL bath to effect[91]	Nitrite and nitrate toxicoses
Nutritional supplementation[90,91] Natural diet: whole or pureed Gel diet Liquid/soft diets: Carnivore Care (Oxbow Animal Health) Emeraid Intensive Care Carnivore (Lafeber) Feline Clinical Care Liquid (Abbott) Hill's A/D (Hill's) ReptoMin slurry (Tetra) Waltham Feline Concentration (Waltham)	1%- ≥3% body weight PO q24-72h, start low and increase over time	Hand feed: as long as patient can swallow food; use headless insects or gel food; place food into the mouth Gavage feed: mix 1:1 with water if needed Puree: insect abdomens, earthworms, or pinkie mice (omit exoskeleton and skins). Supplement with vitamins and minerals: may be difficult to pass through tube; predigest with pancreatic enzymes

Continued

TABLE 3-8 Miscellaneous Agents Used in Amphibians. (cont'd)

Agent	Dosage	Species/Comments
Oxygen	100% for up to 24 hr[91]	Adjunct treatment for septicemia, toxicoses
Physostigmine (ophthalmic drops)	1 drop/50 g topically q1-2h to effect[90]	May ameliorate flaccid paralysis from ivermectin or levamisole toxicosis
Prednisolone sodium succinate	5-10 mg/kg IM, IV[91]	Shock
Sodium thiosulfate	1% solution as continuous bath to effect[91]	Halogen (e.g., chlorine) toxicoses
Vitamin A (Aquasol A Parenteral, Mayne Pharma)	Dilute 1:9 (parenteral formulation 50,000 U/mL) with sterile water; make fresh weekly; apply 1 drop from a tuberculin syringe with 27g needle to amphibians under 5 g; 1 drop from tuberculin syringe without needle is about 200 U and useful for 15-30 g BW; >30 g, 1 drop per 10 g BW; topically q24h × 14 days, then q4-7d[90]	Hypovitaminosis A (short tongue syndrome), swollen eyelids, evidence of infectious dermatitis, hydrocoelom, or simply "failing to thrive"
	Dilute 1:10 in sterile water; applied as 1 drop from 18g needle; estimated as 50 U/frog q48h or q7d[70]	Grey foam-nest tree frog (*Chiromantis xerampelina*)/weight range, 2-7 g; dosing q48h and once weekly significantly increased whole body vitamin A levels over control group and group treated with vitamin A fortified supplement dusted on crickets[70]
Vitamin A β-carotene or mixed carotenoids	PO in crickets[13]	False tomato frog (*Dyscophus guineti*)/improve skin color and increase plasma retinol concentrations[13]
Vitamin B_1	25-100 mg/kg PO, IM, ICe[90,91]	Deficiency resulting from thiaminase-containing fish
Vitamin D_3	2-3 U/mL continuous bath (with 2.3% calcium gluconate)[91]	Nutritional secondary hyperparathyroidism
	100-400 U/kg PO q24h[91]	
Vitamin E (alpha-tocopherol)	1 mg/kg PO, IM q7d[91]	
	200 U/kg feed[90]	Steatitis

TABLE 3-9 Hematologic and Serum Biochemical Values of Select Amphibians.[30]

For leukocyte totals and percentages for various species, refer to The Wildlife Leukocytes Web site at http://wildlifehematology.uga.edu/Amphibians/index.htm.

Measurement	African clawed frog (*Xenopus laevis*)[84]	American bullfrog (*Lithobates catesbeianus*)[90]	Australian green tree frog (*Ranoidea caerulea*)[96]	Japanese newt (*Cynops pyrrhogaster*)[61]	Leopard frog (*Lithobates pipiens*)[90] ♂/♀	Tiger salamander (*Ambystoma californiense*)[11]
Hematology						
PCV (%)	23-47	14-27	34-41	22-58	19-52/16-51	48
RBC (10^6/μL)	0.80-1.48	—	0.62-0.82	0.17-0.30	0.23-0.77/ 0.17-0.70	0.76
Hgb (g/dL)	6.1-15.2	4.7	8.0-10.6	—	3.8-14.6/2.7-14	11.26
MCV (fL)	31.6-62.8	—	461-602	—	722-916/730-916	3,477
MCH (pg)	6.9-22.1	—	111-148	—	182-221/182-238	872
MCHC (g/dL)	19.3-32.3	7	236-268	—	22.7-26.8/19.9-27.7	39
WBC (10^3/μL)	0.64-9.56	5.2	12.4-22.1	—	3.1-22.2/2.8-25.9	0.55
Neutrophils (%)	8 ± 1.1	22	14-27	3.1-52.9	—	25.2
Lymphocytes (%)	65.3 ± 2.7	62.9	—	0-6.8	—	48.6
Monocytes (%)	0.5	0.64	5.0-10.0	0-15.6	—	1.3
Eosinophils (%)	—	8.9	1.0-5.0	0-10.7	—	19.7
Basophils (%)	8.5 ± 1.4	2.5	0	26.3-87.7	—	4.6
Plasmacytes (%)	0.2	—	—	—	—	—
Thrombocytes (10^3/μL)	17.1	—	23.2-33.5	—	—	—

Continued

TABLE 3-9 Hematologic and Serum Biochemical Values of Select Amphibians. (cont'd)

Measurement	African clawed frog (*Xenopus laevis*)	American bullfrog (*Lithobates catesbeianus*)	Australian green tree frog (*Ranoidea caerulea*)	Japanese newt (*Cynops pyrrhogaster*)	Leopard frog (*Lithobates pipiens*) ♂/♀	Tiger salamander (*Ambystoma californiense*)
Chemistry						
ALP (U/L)	59-282	—	—	—	—	—
ALT (U/L)	10-39	—	—	—	—	—
AST (U/L)	27-1774	45	66-122		—	938
Bilirubin, total (mg/dL)	0.01-0.26	—	—	—	—	—
BUN (mg/dL)	2-10	3	—	—	—	—
Calcium (mg/dL)	5.2-12.3	8.1	10.6-13.1	—	—	9.2
Chloride (mmol/L)	73-93	77	—	—	—	—
Cholesterol (mg/dL)	56-563	—	—	—	—	—
Creatine kinase (U/L)	10-5400	—	347-705	—	—	139
Creatinine (mg/dL)	0.1-1.1	1.0	—	—	—	—
GGT (U/L)	1-19	—	—	—	—	—
Glucose (mg/dL)	18-111	—	55-78	—	—	30
LDH (U/L)	21-240	33	—	—	—	—
Phosphorus (mg/dL)	3.5-11.6	3.3	3.3-5.0	—	—	6.0
Potassium (mmol/L)	2.3-7.3	2.7	4.9-7.7		—	4.8

TABLE 3-9 Hematologic and Serum Biochemical Values of Select Amphibians. (cont'd)

Measurement	African clawed frog (*Xenopus laevis*)	American bullfrog (*Lithobates catesbeianus*)	Australian green tree frog (*Ranoidea caerulea*)	Japanese newt (*Cynops pyrrhogaster*)	Leopard frog (*Lithobates pipiens*) ♂/♀	Tiger salamander (*Ambystoma californiense*)
Protein, total (g/dL)	2.0-4.6	—	5.5-6.8	—	—	2.8
Albumin (g/dL)	0.1-2.3	1.6	—	—	—	1.2
Globulin (g/dL)	1.1-4.1	—	—	—	—	1.6
Sodium (mmol/L)	111-134	108	107-114	—	—	125
Triglyceride (mg/dL)	57-555	—	—	—	—	—
Uric acid (mg/dL)	0.1-0.4	0.1	0.2-0.7	—	—	—

TABLE 3-10 Blood Collection Sites in Amphibians.

Blood volume varies by species or genus. In general, it is safe to collect 10% of the blood volume from healthy animals (≈1% of body weight). Clinical judgment should be used in collecting blood from sick or debilitated animals.[30]

Collection Site	Species	Notes
Ventral abdominal vein	Anurans	Midline, ventral coelom, between sternum and pelvis; risk of hitting coelomic organs; visualization may be confirmed via transillumination
Lingual plexus	Anurans	Depress tongue to expose buccal surface of the oral cavity; the plexus can be visualized; sedation may be needed
Femoral vein	Anurans	Superficial vessel present along the medial aspect of the femur; runs parallel with femoral nerve; sedation may be needed
Cardiac	Multiple, including caecilians	Sedation recommended; aim needle at pectoral girdle, targeting ventricle; allow passive fill of syringe to avoid collapsing ventricle; ultrasound will help
Ventral tail vein	Urodelans	Similar to reptiles; caudal vein runs along the ventral caudal vertebrate and can be accessed via ventral or lateral approach; tail autotomy possible in some species
Facial vein/musculo-cutaneous vein	Anurans (*Ranidae*)	Collect blood just rostral or just caudal to the tympanum; insert needle in rostrocaudal direction at 30° angle to the skin; collect from hub
Lymphatic collection	Anurans	Use for bacterial culture/possible biochemical analysis; collect from dorsal or hind limb lymph sacs; easily collected if excessive lymph; hold animal with hindlimbs dependent or cerclage at pelvis if needed[64]

TABLE 3-11 General Differential Diagnoses by Predominant Signs in Pet Amphibians.[91,92]

In all cases, evaluate natural history/biology and environment/husbandry. A partial list: Housing, including substrate, enclosure furnishings/complexity for natural behavior, appropriate hiding spots, social mix (e.g., too many animals, too few, aggression), general activity around enclosure, land to water ratio, egress/ingress to water features.

Temperature and humidity throughout the enclosure.

Lighting, including photoperiod, intensity, light spectrum/type, UV exposure (e.g., present, distance to patient, quality/age of bulb).

Water quality, including source, pH, alkalinity/hardness, oxygen levels, nitrogen levels (ammonia, nitrite, and nitrates), chlorine, chloramine, salt, or nicotine in water, supersaturation.

Soil/substrate moisture (e.g., too high, too low) and pH, and how often changed.

Evaluate feeding, including food type, method of delivery, size of item, presentation, timing of feeding, supplements (type, quality, age, application); if live prey, review how it is fed and housed.

Social issues such as cage mate aggression, display of escape behaviors, breeding behavior, addition of new animals (including quarantine procedures).

Additional conditions to consider in almost all presentations include: Infectious causes include a wide range of bacteria, viruses (e.g., ranavirus), parasites (e.g., nematodes), fungal disease (e.g., chytrid).

Reproductive disease in females.

General diagnostics: Impression smears or aspirates (lesions, prolapsed tissues, masses, effusions), and cytology (direct/wet mount and stains: Diff-Quik (or similar), Gram, acid fast of lesions); cultures where indicated.

Fecal parasite exam: direct/wet mount, cytology.

Water quality, soil or substrate assessment.

Imaging: radiographs, ultrasound, and computed tomography.

Polymerase chain reaction (PCR) testing: ranavirus and chytridiomycosis.

Blood sampling and analysis; especially calcium (ionized calcium), phosphorus, cholesterol, and triglycerides; blood/lymphatic cultures.

Necropsy: consider culling if there is a group problem.

Sign	Specific Etiologic Agents to Consider
Anorexia, inappetence	Mycobacteria, chytridiomycosis, chromoblastomycosis, husbandry concerns, nutritional secondary hyperparathyroidism, hypocalcemia, ocular disease with vision impairment, geriatric/senescence, normal (i.e., estivation or hibernation cues), hypovitaminosis A (“short tongue syndrome”)
Bloat	Distinguish intestinal filling with solid material or gas versus pneumocoelom; mycobacteria, fungal infection, gastrointestinal nematodes, hypocalcemia (especially in hylid frogs), toxicosis, hypothermia, decomposition of ingesta (e.g., gastric overload, inappropriate temperatures), ruptured lung or trachea, gas supersaturation
Changes in skin color (general or focal)	*Mycobacterium* spp., chytridiomycosis, chromomycosis, *Capillaroides xenopi*; trauma, burn, or frostbite; excessive UV exposure; chemical irritation or drug reaction; dehydration or desiccation; nutritional secondary hyperparathyroidism, xanthomatosis, or hyperlipidosis
Changes in skin texture (general or focal)	As above, but also consider normal anatomy (e.g., dorsal crests in European newts, egg brood patch of Surinam toad, nuptial pads in male anurans)

Continued

Sign	Specific Etiologic Agents to Consider
Cloacal prolapse	Parasites, colitis/cloacitis, mechanical ileus, dehydration, gastric overload, intussusception, hypocalcemia, nutritional secondary hyperparathyroidism, constipation, physiologic behavior, iatrogenic (handling, sedation), straining (e.g., bladder stone, oviposition)
Excess mucus production (typically fully aquatic animals)	Protozoal overload (consider also this as a secondary to skin damage); water quality
Fluctuant mass	Abscess, helminths (e.g., immature trematodes and cestodes), subcutaneous leeches; lymphatic blockage, xanthomatosis, fluid overload, thermal injury, hypocalcemia, renal dysfunction; normal anatomy (e.g., active marsupium of *Gastrotheca* spp. females, distended lymphatic sacs of *Ceratophrys* spp.), females at certain points in the breeding cycle
Hydrocoelom or excessive fluid in lymphatic system	Mycobacteria, verminous granulomata (filarids, other helminths), hepatic failure, renal failure, hypocalcemia, toxicosis (e.g., heavy metal, poor water quality, insecticide, distilled or reverse osmosis water), xanthomatosis, neoplasia (especially ovarian, hepatic, or renal), failure to oviposit, normal (e.g., ovulation)
Lameness/mobility issues	Mycobacterial granulomas in joints, nutritional secondary hyperparathyroidism, trauma, arthritis, malnutrition (e.g., hypovitaminosis B), hypervitaminosis D, gout (rare), toxicosis (especially insecticides)
Ocular opacity	Scars, lenticular sclerosis or cataracts, corneal lipidosis/xanthomatosis, trauma, excess UV light
Sudden death (individual or groups)	Iridovirus/ranavirus, chlamydiosis, chytridiomycosis; toxicosis (water ammonia, household pesticides, chlorine, other water quality issues); electrocution, hypothermia, hyperthermia, trauma, gastric overload/impaction, stress, drowning
Weight loss	Mycobacteria, chytridiomycosis, gastrointestinal nematodes (see Table 3-13), stress/husbandry concerns, vision impairment, hypovitaminosis A ("short tongue syndrome")

TABLE 3-12 Select Disinfectants for Equipment and Cage Furniture.[60]

In order to increase the efficacy of disinfectants, rinse all organic material and debris from the surface before applying disinfectants.

Batrachochytrium dendrobatidis

- Sodium hypochlorite (household bleach) 1% for 1 min contact time
- Ethanol 70% for 1 min exposure time
- Benzalkonium chloride 1 mg/mL for 1 min contact time
- Desiccation and exposure to 50-60°C (122-140°F) heat for 30 min
- Exposure to 1:1000 quaternary ammonium compound for 30 sec

Ranavirus

- Nolvasan (chlorhexidine) 0.75% for 1 min contact time
- Sodium hypochlorite (household bleach) 3% for 1 min contact time
- Virkon S 1% for 1 min contact time
- Desiccation and exposure to 60°C (140°F) heat for 15-30 min

TABLE 3-13 Guidelines for Treatment of Pet Amphibians with Nematode Parasites.[90,91]

Overview:

Many amphibians have nematode parasites and can remain healthy with low levels of parasites; it is not always necessary or feasible to eliminate parasites from individuals or collections

Common amphibian nematodes have a direct life cycle; gastrointestinal and pulmonary nematodes are possible, both pass ova in the feces

High parasite burdens or concurrent disease can cause health concerns

Maintaining an appropriate environment, including routine cleaning and removal of feces, is an important component to preventing and treating parasite-related health issues; antiparasitics alone may not be sufficient

Stage and characterize fecal examinations to help determine if treatment is necessary:

Routine, randomly collected feces should be assessed:

Direct wet mounts and cytology

Evaluate a shift in cytology and fluctuations in nematode ova and larvae

There is often no correlation between reduction in nematode ova or larvae in feces and actual reduction in nematode numbers

Improvements in body condition score (BCS) and weight often happen when the ova or larvae counts go down and the feces has ≤5 RBC/HPF and <1 WBC/HPF

If the stool appears grossly normal:

and there are ≤5 RBC/HPF or <1 WBC/HPF, parasites may not be clinically significant

and there are >5-10 RBC/HPF or >1-5 WBC/HPF, parasites are likely clinically significant, treatment may be indicated

or there are >5 strongyle larvae/HPF on direct or float, treat

If there is diarrhea, blood, mucus, and visible nematodes present, treat

Visible nematodes alone may be environmental

Continued

TABLE 3-13 Guidelines for Treatment of Pet Amphibians with Nematode Parasites. (cont'd)

Evaluate the amphibian patient; treatment should be considered if:
Animals appear unthrifty, there are mortalities with nematodes implicated, or there are otherwise unexplained mortalities
Assess current health and BCS
if unthrifty, consider any nematode ova, larvae, or adults clinically significant; treat for nematodes appropriately in light of other clinical findings
if well fleshed, stage the fecal parasite exam; if there are low levels, treatment may not be needed
Evaluate success through return to normal weight, BCS, feces, and/or behavior and not only fecal parasite levels

REFERENCES

1. Adami C, d'Ovidio D, Casoni D. Alfaxalone-butorphanol verses alfaxalone-morphine combination for immersion anaesthesia in oriental fire-bellied toads (*Bombina orientalis*). *Lab Anim.* 2016;50:204–211.
2. Adami C, Spadavecchia C, Angeli G, et al. Alfaxalone anesthesia by immersion in oriental fire-bellied toads (*Bombina orientalis*). *Vet Anaesth Analg.* 2015;42:547–551.
3. American Veterinary Medical Association. AVMA Guidelines for the Euthanasia of Animals: 2020 Edition. Available at: https://www.avma.org/sites/default/files/2020-01/2020-Euthanasia-Final-1-17-20.pdf. Accessed November 20, 2020.
4. Baitchman EJ, Pessier AP. Pathogenesis, diagnosis, and treatment of amphibian chytridiomycosis. *Vet Clin North Am Exot Anim Pract.* 2013;16(3):669–685.
5. Balko JA, Watson MK, Papich MG, et al. Plasma concentrations of ketoprofen and meloxicam after subcutaneous and topical administration in the smoky jungle frog (*Leptodactylus pentadactylus*). *J Herpetol Med Surg.* 2018;28(3-4):89–92.
6. Barbon AR, Routh A, Lopez J. Inhalatory isoflurane anesthesia in mountain chicken frogs (*Leptodactylus fallax*). *J Zoo Wildl Med.* 2019;50(2):453–456.
7. Bianchi CM, Johnson CB, Howard LL, et al. Efficacy of fenbendazole and levamisole treatments in captive Houston toads (*Bufo [Anaxyrus] houstonensis*). *J Zoo Wildl Med.* 2014;45:564–568.
8. Blooi M, Pasmans F, Rouffaer L, et al. Successful treatment of *Batrachochytrium salamandrivorans* infections in salamanders requires synergy between voriconazole, polymyxin E and temperature. *Sci Rep.* 2015;5:11788.
9. Bodri MS. Selamectin lacks efficacy against lungworm (*Rhabdias* sp.) in the lemur leaf frog (*Hylomantis lemur*). *J Herpetol Med Surg.* 2016;26(3-4):104–107.
10. Bowerman J, Rombough C, Weinstock SR, et al. Terbinafine hydrochloride in ethanol effectively clears *Batrachochytrium dendrobatidis* in amphibians. *J Herpetol Med Surg.* 2010;20:24–28.
11. Brady S, Burgdorf-Moisuk A, Kass PH, et al. Hematology and plasma biochemistry intervals for captive-born California tiger salamanders (*Ambystoma californiense*). *J Zoo Wildl Med.* 2016;47(3):731–735.
12. Brannelly LA, Richards-Zawacki CL, Pessier AP. Clinical trials with itraconazole as a treatment for chytrid fungal infections in amphibians. *Dis Aquat Org.* 2012;101:95–104.
13. Brenes-Soto A, Dierenfeld ES. Effect of dietary carotenoids on vitamin A status and skin pigmentation in false tomato frogs (*Dyscophus guineti*). *Zoo Biol.* 2014;33:544–552.

14. Browne RK, Seratt J, Vance C, et al. Hormonal priming, induction of ovulation and in-vitro fertilization of the endangered Wyoming toad (*Bufo baxteri*). *Reprod Biol Endocrinol.* 2006;4(1):34.
15. Calatayud NE, Chai N, Gardner NR, et al. Reproductive techniques for ovarian monitoring and control in amphibians. *J Vis Exp*. 2019;May12(147). http://doi.org/10.3791/58675.
16. Cermakova E, Oliveri M, Ceplecha V, et al. Anesthesia with intramuscular administration of alfaxalone in Spanish ribbed newt (*Pleurodeles waltl*). *J Exot Pet Med.* 2020;33:23–26.
17. Chai N. Surgery in amphibians. *Vet Clin North Am Exot Anim Pract*. 2016;19(1):77–95.
18. Chai N, Whitaker BR. Amphibian chytridiomycosis. In: Divers SJ, Stahl SJ, eds. *Mader's Reptile and Amphibian Medicine and Surgery*. 3rd ed. St. Louis, MO: Elsevier; 2019:1292–1293.
19. Chatfield MWH, Richards-Zawacki CL. Elevated temperature as a treatment for *Batrachochytrium dendrobatidis* infection in captive frogs. *Dis Aquat Org*. 2011;94:235–238.
20. Clayton LA. Personal observation; 2020.
21. Clayton LA, Nelson J, Payton ME, et al. Clinical signs, management, and outcome of presumptive ivermectin overdose in a group of dendrobatid frogs. *J Herpetol Med Surg.* 2013;22(1):5–11.
22. Clulow J, Upton R, Trudeau VL, et al. Amphibian assisted reproductive technologies: moving from technology to application. In: Comizzoli P, Brown JL, Holt WV, eds. *Reproductive Sciences in Animal Conservation.* 2nd ed. Cham: Springer; 2019:413–463.
23. Coble DJ, Taylor DK, Mook DM. Analgesic effects of meloxicam, morphine sulfate, flunixin meglumine, and xylazine hydrochloride in African-clawed frogs (*Xenopus laevis*). *J Am Assoc Lab Anim Sci.* 2011;50:355–360.
24. D'Agostino JJ, West G, Boothe DM, et al. Plasma pharmacokinetics of selamectin after a single topical administration in the American bullfrog (*Rana catesbeiana*). *J Zoo Wildl Med.* 2007;38:51–54.
25. Del Valle JM, Eisthen HL. Treatment of chytridiomycosis in laboratory axolotls (*Ambystoma mexicanum*) and rough-skinned newts (*Taricha granulosa*). *Comp Med.* 2019;69(3):204–211.
26. DeVoe RS. Personal communication; 2020.
27. Doss GA, Nevarez JG, Fowlkes N, et al. Evaluation of metomidate hydrochloride as an anesthetic in leopard frogs (*Rana pipiens*). *J Zoo Wildl Med.* 2014;45:53–59.
28. El-Mofty MM, Abdelmeguid NE, Sadek IA, et al. Induction of leukaemia in chloramphenicol-treated toads. *E Mediter Health J.* 2000;6:1026–1034.
29. Felt S, Papich MG, Howard A, et al. Tissue distribution of enrofloxacin in African clawed frogs (*Xenopus laevis*) after intramuscular and subcutaneous administration. *J Am Assoc Lab Anim Sci.* 2013;52:186–188.
30. Forzán MJ, Horney BS. Amphibians. In: Heatley JJ, Russell KE, eds. *Exotic Animal Laboratory Diagnosis*. Hoboken, NJ: Wiley & Sons; 2020:347–368.
31. Galex IA, Gallant CM, D'Avignon N, et al. Evaluation of effective and practical euthanasia methods for larval African clawed frogs (*Xenopus laevis*). *J Am Assoc Lab Anim Sci.* 2020;59(3):269–274.
32. Garner TWJ, Garcia G, Carroll B, et al. Using itraconazole to clear *Batrachochytrium dendrobatidis* infection, and subsequent depigmentation of *Alytes muletensis* tadpoles. *Dis Aquat Org.* 2009;83:257–260.
33. Georoff TA, Moore RP, Rodriguez C, et al. Efficacy of treatment and long-term follow-up of *Batrachochytrium dendrobatidis* PCR-positive anurans following itraconazole bath treatment. *J Zoo Wildl Med.* 2013;44:395–403.
34. Goulet F, Hélie P, Vachon P. Eugenol anesthesia in African clawed frogs (*Xenopus laevis*) of different body weights. *J Am Assoc Lab Anim Sci.* 2010;49:460–463.
35. Guénette SA, Beaudry F, Vachon P. Anesthetic properties of propofol in African clawed frogs (*Xenopus laevis*). *J Am Assoc Lab Anim Sci.* 2008;47:35–38.
36. Hadzima E, Mitchell MA, Knotek Z, et al. Alfaxalone use in *Xenopus laevis*: comparison of IV, IM, IP, and water immersion of alfaxalone with doses of 18 mg/kg and 18 mg/L. *Proc Annu Conf Assoc Rept Amph Vet.* 2013:60–64.

37. Howard AM, Papich MG, Felt SA, et al. The pharmacokinetics of enrofloxacin in adult African clawed frogs (*Xenopus laevis*). *J Am Assoc Lab Anim Sci*. 2010;49:800–804.
38. Iglauer F, Willmann F, Hilken G, et al. Anthelmintic treatment to eradicate cutaneous capillariasis in a colony of South African clawed frogs (*Xenopus laevis*). *Lab Anim Sci*. 1997;47:477–482.
39. Jones MEB, Paddock D, Bender L, et al. Treatment of chytridiomycosis with reduced-dose itraconazole. *Dis Aquat Org*. 2012;99:243–249.
40. Koeller CA. Comparison of buprenorphine and butorphanol analgesia in the eastern red spotted newt (*Notophthalmus viridescens*). *J Am Assoc Lab Anim Sci*. 2009;48:171–175.
41. Kouba A, Vance C, Calatayud N, et al. Assisted reproductive technologies (ART) for amphibians. In: Poole VA, Grow S, eds. *Amphibian Husbandry Resource Guide*. 2nd ed. Silver Spring, MD: Association of Zoos and Aquariums; 2012:60–118.
42. Krisp AR, Hausmann JC, Sladky KK, et al. Anesthetic efficacy of MS-222 in White's tree frogs (*Litoria caerulea*). *J Herpetol Med Surg*. 2020;30(1):38–41.
43. Lalonde-Robert V, Beaudry F, Vachon P. Pharmacologic parameters of MS222 and physiologic changes in frogs (*Xenopus laevis*) after immersion at anesthetic doses. *J Am Assoc Lab Anim Sci*. 2012;51:464–468.
44. Letcher J. Evaluation of use of tiletamine/zolazepam for anesthesia of bullfrogs and leopard frogs. *J Am Vet Med Assoc*. 1995;207:80–82.
45. Letcher J, Glade M. Efficacy of ivermectin as an anthelmintic in leopard frogs. *J Am Vet Med Assoc*. 1992;200:537–538.
46. Llaniguez JT, Szczepaniak MA, Rickman BH, et al. Quantitative and qualitative behavioral measurements to assess pain in axolotls (*Ambystoma mexicanum*). *J Am Assoc Lab Anim Sci*. 2020;59(2):186–196.
47. Machin KL. Amphibian pain and analgesia. *J Zoo Wildl Med*. 1999;30:2–10.
48. Marcec R, Mitchell MA, Kirshenbaum J, et al. Clinical and physiologic effects of sodium chloride baths in axolotls, *Ambystoma mexicanum*. *Proc Annu Conf Assoc Rept Amph Vet*. 2011;1.
49. Martel A, Van Rooij P, Vercauteren G, et al. Developing a safe antifungal treatment protocol to eliminate Batrachochytrium dendrobatidis from amphibians. *Med Mycol*. 2011;49:143–149.
50. McDermott C, Hadfield K, Clayton L, et al. Cloacal prolapses in anurans: a ten-year retrospective review. *Proc Annu Conf Assoc Rept Amph Vet*. 2015:477.
51. McMillan MW, Leece EA. Immersion and branchial/transcutaneous irrigation anaesthesia with alfaxalone in a Mexican axolotl. *Vet Anaesth Analg*. 2011;38:619–623.
52. Minter LJ, Clarke EO, Gjeltema JL, et al. Effects of intramuscular meloxicam administration on prostaglandin E2 synthesis in the North American bullfrog (*Rana catesbeiana*). *J Zoo Wildl Med*. 2011;42:680–685.
53. Mitchell MA, Riggs SM, Singleton CB, et al. Evaluating the clinical and cardiopulmonary effects of clove oil and propofol in tiger salamanders (*Ambystoma tigrinum*). *J Exot Pet Med*. 2009;18:50–56.
54. Musgrave KE, Hanley CS, Papich MG. Population pharmacokinetics of ceftazidime after a single subcutaneous injection and normal oral and cloacal bacterial flora survey in eastern hellbenders (*Cryptobranchus alleganiensis alleganiensis*). *Proc Annu Conf Am Assoc Zoo Vet*. 2020;118.
55. Mylniczenko N. Personal observation; 2020.
56. Nevarez JG. Euthanasia. In: Divers SJ, Stahl SJ, eds. *Mader's Reptile and Amphibian Medicine and Surgery*. 3rd ed. St. Louis, MO: Elsevier; 2019:437–440.
57. Novarro AJ, Blackman A, Bailey SD. Tricaine methanesulfonate (MS-222) as a short-term anesthetic for the eastern red-backed salamander, *Plethodon cinereus*. *Herpetol Rev*. 2017;48(2):320–322.
58. Pessier AP. Edematous frogs, urinary tract disease, and disorders of fluid balance. *J Exot Pet Med*. 2009;18(1):4–13.
59. Pessier AP. Personal communication; 2014.
60. A Manual for Control of Infectious Diseases in Amphibian Survival Assurance Colonies and Reintroduction Programs. Version 2.0. In: Pessier AP, Mendelson JR, eds. *Apple Valley: IUCN/*

SSC Conservation Breeding Specialist Group; 2017. Available at: https://www.amphibianark.org/wp-content/uploads/2018/07/Disease-Manual-2017.pdf Accessed October 10, 2020.

61. Pfeiffer CJ, Pyle H, Asashima M. Blood cell morphology and counts in the Japanese newt (*Cynops pyrrhogaster*). *J Zoo Wildl Med.* 1990;21(1):56–64.
62. Posner LP, Bailey KM, Richardson EY, et al. Alfaxalone anesthesia in bullfrogs (*Lithobates catesbeiana*) by injection or immersion. *J Zoo Wildl Med.* 2013;44:965–971.
63. Rendle M, Tapley B, Perkins M, et al. Itraconazole treatment of *Batrachochytrium dendrobatidis* (Bd) infection in captive caecilians (*Amphibia: Gymnophiona*) and the first case of Bd in a wild neotropical caecilian. *J Zoo Aquar Res.* 2015;3(4):137–140.
64. Reynolds SJ, Christian KA, Tracy CR. Application of a method for obtaining lymph from anuran amphibians. *J Herpetol.* 2009;43(1):148–153.
65. Rifkin A, Visser M, Barrett K, et al. The pharmacokinetics of topical itraconazole in Panamanian golden frogs (*Atelopus zeteki*). *J Zoo Wildl Med.* 2017;48(2):344–351.
66. Roberts AA, Berger L, Robertson SG, et al. The efficacy and pharmacokinetics of terbinafine against the frog-killing fungus (*Batrachochytrium dendrobatidis*). *Med Mycol.* 2019;57(2):204–214.
67. Scott G, Louis MM, Balko JA, et al. Pharmacokinetics of transdermal flunixin meglumine following a single dose in marine toads (*Rhinella marina*). *Vet Med Int.* 2020;8863537.
68. Shaw S, Speare R, Lynn DH, et al. Nematode and ciliate nasal infection in captive Archey's frogs (*Leiopelma archeyi*). *J Zoo Wildl Med.* 2011;42:473–479.
69. Shilton CM, Smith DA, Crawshaw GJ, et al. Corneal lipid deposition in Cuban tree frogs (*Osteopilus septentrionalis*) and its relationship to serum lipids: an experimental study. *J Zoo Wildl Med.* 2001;32:305–319.
70. Sim RR, Sullivan KE, Valdes EV, et al. A comparison of oral and topical vitamin A supplementation in African foam-nesting frogs (*Chiromantis xerampelina*). *J Zoo Wildl Med.* 2010;41:456–460.
71. Sirimanapong W, Saetang S, Namwongprom K, et al. A comparison of 3 anesthetic agents (MS-222, benzocaine, and clove oil) in East Asian bullfrog (*Hoplobatrachus rugulosus*). *J Mahanakorn Vet Med.* 2020;15(1):43–55.
72. Sladakovic I, Johnson RS, Vogelnest L. Evaluation of intramuscular alfaxalone in three Australian frog species (*Litoria caerulea, Litoria aurea, Litorea booroolongensis*). *J Herpetol Med Surg.* 2014;24:36–42.
73. Smith BD, Vail KJ, Carroll GL, et al. Comparison of etomidate, benzocaine, and MS222 anesthesia with and without subsequent flunixin meglumine analgesia in African clawed frogs (*Xenopus laevis*). *J Am Assoc Lab An Sci.* 2018;57(2):202–209.
74. Speare R, Speare B, Muller R, et al. Anesthesia of tadpoles of the southern brown tree frog (*Litoria ewingii*) with isoeugenol (Aqui-S). *J Zoo Wildl Med.* 2014;45:492–496.
75. Stevens CW. Analgesia in amphibians: preclinical studies and clinical applications. *Vet Clin North Am Exot Anim Pract.* 2011;14(1):33–44.
76. Stone SM, Clarke-Price SC, Boesch JM, et al. Evaluation of righting reflex in cane toads (*Bufo marinus*) after topical application of sevoflurane jelly. *Am J Vet Res.* 2013;74:823–827.
77. Stoskopf MK, Arnold J, Mason M. Aminoglycoside antibiotic levels in the aquatic salamander (*Necturus necturus*). *J Zoo Anim Med.* 1987;18:81–85.
78. Strobel S, Hagedorn A, Ott S, et al. A comparison of the analgesic effects of fentanyl and butorphanol in African clawed frogs (*Xenopus laevis*) under tricaine methanesulfonate (MS222) anaesthesia. *SOJ Anesthesiol Pain Manag.* 2018;5(2):1–10.
79. Terril-Robb L, Suckow M, Grigdesby C. Evaluation of the analgesic effects of butorphanol tartrate, xylazine hydrochloride, and flunixin meglumine in leopard frogs (*Rana pipiens*). *Contemp Top Lab Anim Sci.* 1996;35:54–56.
80. Torreilles SL, McClure DE, Green SL. Evaluation and refinement of euthanasia methods for *Xenopus laevis*. *J Am Assoc Lab Anim Sci.* 2009;48:512–516.

81. Valitutto MT, Raphael BL, Calle PP, et al. Tissue concentrations of enrofloxacin and its metabolite ciprofloxacin after a single topical dose in the coqui frog (*Eleutherodactylus coqui*). *J Herpetol Med Surg.* 2013;23:69–73.
82. Wiley M, Wu J, Dawson B. A comparison of two treatments for nematode infections in the Túngara frog, *Engystomops pustulosus. J Herpetol Med Surg.* 2009;19(1):21–22.
83. Williams CJ, Alstrup AK, Bertelsen MF, et al. When local anesthesia becomes universal: pronounced systemic effects of subcutaneous lidocaine in bullfrogs (*Lithobates catesbeianus*). *Comp Biochem Physiol A: Mol Integrative Physiol.* 2017;209:41–46.
84. Wilson S, Felt S, Torreilles S, et al. Serum clinical biochemical and hematological reference ranges of laboratory-reared and wild-caught *Xenopus laevis. J Am Assoc Lab Anim Sci.* 2011;50:635–640.
85. Wlizla M, McNamara S, Horb ME. Generation and care of *Xenopus laevis* and *Xenopus tropicalis* embryos. In: Vleminckx K, ed. New York, NY: Humana Press; 2018. *Xenopus Methods and Protocols. Methods in Molecular Biology.* 1865:19–32.
86. Woodhams DC, Alford RA, Marantelli G. Emerging disease of amphibians cured by elevated body temperature. *Dis Aquat Org.* 2003;55:65–67.
87. Wojick KB, Langan JN, Mitchell MA. Evaluation of MS-222 (tricaine methanesulfonate) and propofol as anesthetic agents in Sonoran desert toads (*Bufo alvarius*). *J Herpetol Med Surg.* 2010;20:79–83.
88. Wright K. Amputation of the tail of a two-toed amphiuma, *Amphiuma means. Bull Assoc Rept Amphib Vet.* 1994;4(1):5.
89. Wright KM, Carpenter JW, DeVoe RS. Abridged formulary for amphibians. In: Mader DR, Divers SJ, eds. *Current Therapy in Reptile Medicine and Surgery.* St. Louis, MO: Elsevier; 2014:411–416.
90. Wright KM, DeVoe RS. Amphibians. In: Carpenter JW, ed. *Exotic Animal Formulary.* 4th ed. St. Louis, MO: Saunders/Elsevier; 2013:53–82.
91. Wright KM, Whitaker BR. *Amphibian Medicine and Captive Husbandry.* Malabar, FL: Krieger Publishing Co.; 2001.
92. Yaw T, Clayton L. Differential diagnoses by clinical signs-amphibians. In: Divers SJ, Stahl SJ, eds. *Mader's Reptile and Amphibian Medicine and Surgery.* 3rd ed. St. Louis, MO: Elsevier; 2019:1283–1287.
93. Yaw TJ, Mans C, Martinelli L, et al. Comparison of subcutaneous administration of alfaxalone-midazolam-dexmedetomidine with ketamine-midazolam-dexmedetomidine for chemical restraint in juvenile blue poison dart frogs (*Dendrobates tinctorius azureus*). *J Zoo Wildl Med.* 2020;50(4):868–873.
94. Yongjie W, Honglian C, Fen W. Improved method in breeding and artificial propagation for Chinese giant salamanders (*Andrias davidianus*). *J Marine Biol Aquacult.* 2017;3(2):1–5.
95. Young S, Speare R, Berger L, et al. Chloramphenicol with fluid and electrolyte therapy cures terminally ill green tree frogs (*Litoria caerulea*) with chytridiomycosis. *J Zoo Wildl Med.* 2012;43:330–337.
96. Young S, Warner J, Speare R, et al. Hematologic and plasma biochemical reference intervals for health monitoring of wild Australian tree frogs. *Vet Clin Pathol.* 2012;41:478–492.
97. Zec S, Clark-Price S, Coleman DA, et al. Loss and return of righting reflex in American green tree frogs (*Hyla cinerea*) after topical application of compounded sevoflurane or isoflurane jelly: a pilot study. *J Herpetol Med Surg.* 2014;24:72–76.
98. Zullian C, Dodelet-Devillers A, Roy S, et al. Evaluation of the anesthetic effects of MS222 in the adult Mexican axolotl (*Ambystoma mexicanum*). *Vet Med (Auckland, NZ).* 2016;7:1.

Chapter 4 Reptiles

Kurt K. Sladky | Eric Klaphake | Nicola Di Girolamo | James W. Carpenter

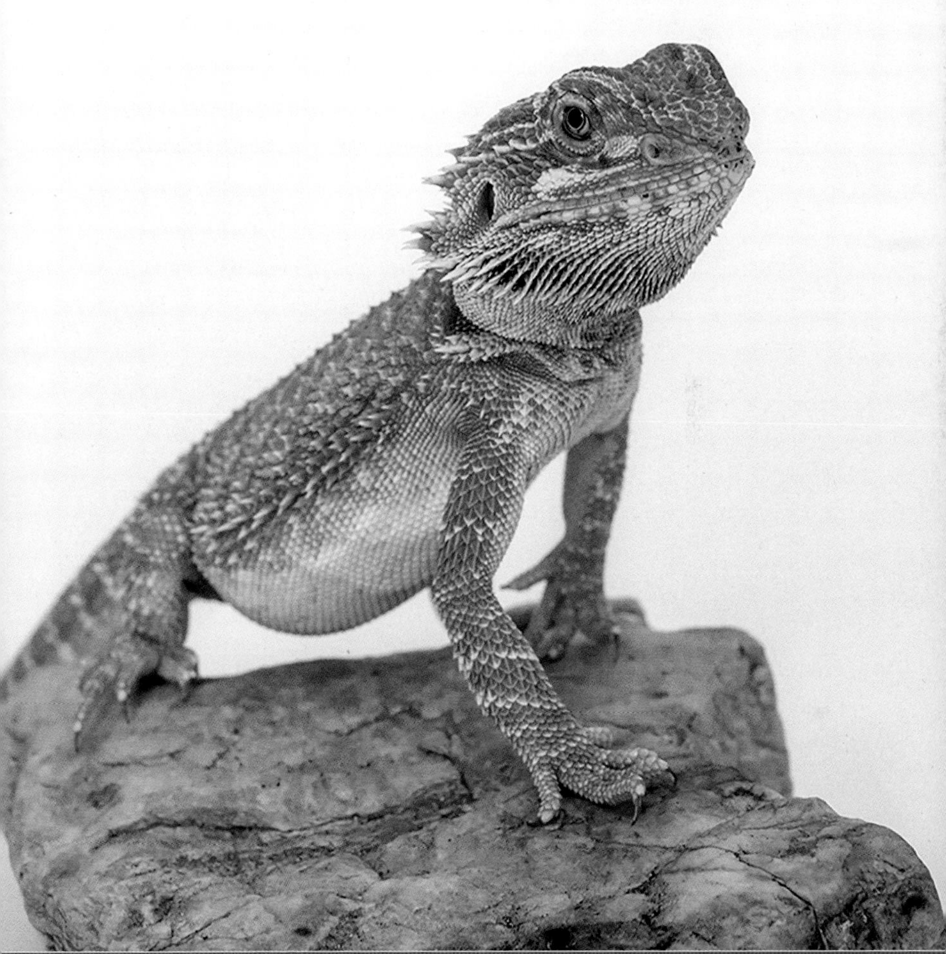

For ease of use for the Reptiles chapter, drug dosages are first listed by "most species" followed by dosages in snakes, lizards, chelonians, and crocodilians; feed and water dosages are generally listed last.

TABLE 4-1 Antimicrobial Agents Used in Reptiles.[a,b]

Agent	Dosage	Species/Comments
Amikacin	—	Potentially nephrotoxic; maintain hydration; frequently used with a penicillin or cephalosporin
	26 µg/kg/hr via osmotic infusion pump implant[77,458]	Snakes/PD; consider loading dose at time of implant
	3.48 mg/kg IM once[225]	Pythons (ball pythons)/PK
	5 mg/kg IM, then 2.5 mg/kg q72h[286]	Gopher snakes/PD; house at high end of optimum temperature range during treatment
	5 mg/kg IM then 2.5 mg/kg IM q72h[444]	Lizards
	5 mg/kg IM q48h[58]	Gopher tortoises/PK; 30°C (86°F)
	2.25 mg/kg IM q72h[218]	Alligators/PD
	50 mg/10 mL saline x 30 min nebulization q12h[243]	Most species/pneumonia; aminophylline at 25 mg/9 mL of sterile saline in nebulizer before antibiotics for bronchodilation[382]
Amoxicillin	5-10 mg/kg PO, IM q12-24h[184]	Most species/may be combined with clavulanate; may be used with an aminoglycoside (monitor hydration)
	22 mg/kg PO q12-24h[107]	Most species/use with an aminoglycoside
	5 mg/kg IM q4d[374]	Freshwater crocodiles/PK
Ampicillin	—	May use with an aminoglycoside
	10-20 mg/kg SC, IM q12h[184,243]	Most species
	50 mg/kg IM q12h[438]	Tortoise/PD
Azithromycin	10 mg/kg PO q2-7d[81,207]	Ball pythons/PK; 30°C (86°F); single-dose study; 2 wk after IV administration, one snake died from apparent nonregenerative anemia; *Mycoplasma*, *Cryptosporidium*, *Giardia*, and other susceptible organisms; location dictates dosage frequency: skin, q3d; respiratory tract, q5d; liver/kidneys, q7d; metabolites were retrieved in bile, liver, lung, kidney, and skin samples
Cefazolin	22 mg/kg IM q24h[243]	Chelonians
Cefotaxime	20-40 mg/kg IM q24h[243]	Most species/may use with an aminoglycoside
	100 mg/10 mL saline x 30 min nebulization q24h[243]	Most species/pneumonia
Cefovecin	—	Short dosing interval is likely for most reptile species[341,466]
	10 mg/kg SC q12h[466]	Green iguanas/PD; 25°C (77°F)
	8 mg/kg SC[341]	Hermann's tortoises/PK; highly variable results, $t_{1/2}$ from 12-124 hr, mean 21 hr; 22°C (72°F) + basking spot at 35°C (95°F)

TABLE 4-1 Antimicrobial Agents Used in Reptiles. (cont'd)

Agent	Dosage	Species/Comments
Cefquinome	2 mg/kg IM, IV[473]	Chelonians (red-eared sliders)/PK; half-life 27 hr (IM) and 22 hr (IV)
Ceftazidime	—	Storage: 90% strength of the ceftazidime solution is maintained for 120 hr when ceftazidime is stored in the refrigerator (4°C) and for at least 25 days when stored in the freezer (–18°C) in individual plastic tuberculin syringes of 0.2 mL;[69] in a retrospective study on susceptibility patterns of aerobic bacteria isolated from reptiles, all 11 gram-positive isolates were resistant to ceftazidime[461]
	20 mg/kg IM q48-72h[485]	Most species/retrospective study; administered to 10 lizards, 8 snakes, and 4 chelonians; unknown outcomes
	20-40 mg/kg SC, IM q48-72h[142,444,485]	Most species/chameleons use q24h
	20 mg/kg SC, IM, IV q72h[265]	Snakes/PD; 30°C (86°F); often effective against gram-negative aerobes (i.e., *Pseudomonas*)
	20 mg/kg IM, IV q60h[447]	Sea turtles/PK; 24°C (75°F); plasma concentrations were above the MIC for *Pseudomonas aeruginosa* (8 µg/mL) for at least 60 hr after IM and IV dose; 22 mg/kg may be preferred
	20 mg/kg IM q5d[69]	Turtles (box turtles, sliders, cooters)/PK; 23-24°C (73-75°F); concentrations were above 8 µg/mL for 5 days
	22 mg/kg IM q72h[211]	Sea turtles/PK; administered when turtles reached a temperature of 21-24°C (70-75°F); considering a target MIC value of 4 µg/mL, time above MIC was 100% of the dosing interval for 72 hr
Ceftiofur sodium	5 mg/kg SC, IM q24h[35]	Lizards (green iguanas)/PK; 30°C (86°F); peak plasma concentration IM significantly greater than SC; likely effective against pathogens with MIC ≤2 µg/mL
	5 mg/kg IM q24h x 18 days[188]	Lizards/treatment of *Devriesea agamarum* (causes dermatitis and septisemia);[188] in bearded dragons experimentally infected with *D. agamarum,* this dose resulted in elimination of the pathogen; in spiny-tailed lizards (*Uromastyx*) lizards with natural occurring infection, this dose resulted in clearance of the infection in 12 days
Ceftiofur crystalline-free acid (CCFA) (Excede, Pfizer)	15 mg/kg IM q24-120h[5]	Snakes (ball pythons)/PK; 26°C (79°F); dosing interval based on MIC
	5 mg/kg IM q24h[407]	Lizards (green iguanas)/PK; green iguanas; 30°C (86°F) ± 2°C; exceeded 1 µg/mL for ≈48 hr and 2 µg/mL for 24 hr
	30 mg/kg IM, SC[76]	Lizards (bearded dragons)/PK; 30°C (86°F); interval may be q10-12d
Ceftriaxone	12.5-25 mg/kg IM q48h[371]	Freshwater crocodiles/PK; AUC values increases in a dose-dependent fashion; half-life values are similar at the two dosages and around 20 hr

Continued

TABLE 4-1 Antimicrobial Agents Used in Reptiles. (cont'd)

Agent	Dosage	Species/Comments
Chloramphenicol	—	Most species/public health concern; reserve for meningitis or encephalitis caused by susceptible organisms
	40 mg/kg PO, SC, IM q24h, or 20 mg/kg PO, SC, IM q12h[142]	Most species/20 mg/kg may be given q24h in larger crocodilians
	40 mg/kg SC q24h[243]	Snakes (gopher snakes)/PD; 29°C (84°F)
	50 mg/kg SC q12-72h[78]	Snakes/PK; q12h in indigo, rat, king snakes; q24h in boids, moccasin snakes; q48h in rattlesnakes; q72h in red-bellied water snakes
Clarithromycin	—	Six months of treatment with clarithromycin resulted in complete remission of clinical signs in desert tortoises with upper respiratory tract disease (mycoplasmosis);[491] however, when clarithromycin was given orally to 10 *Mycoplasma* spp. positive tortoises without clinical signs at 20 mg/kg q48-72h for 90 days, it failed to suppress *Mycoplasma* spp. shedding in all but one of them;[391] 15 mg/kg per rectum administration did not reach 2 µg/mL[492]
	15 mg/kg PO q84h[492]	Tortoises(desert tortoises)/PD; 30-33°C (86-92°F); 2x/wk dosing maintained target levels previously recommended for the treatment of mycoplasmosis
	15 mg/kg PO q24-72h[491]	Tortoises(desert tortoises)/PK; 30-33°C (86-92°F); accumulation proven if given q24h
Chlorhexidine (Nolvasan 2%, Fort Dodge)	Topical 0.05% aqueous solution q24h[243]	All species/topical disinfection; dermatitis; infectious stomatitis; periodontal disease in lizards q24h
	Topical 0.07% (1:30 [solution:water])[243]	Most species/topical disinfection; infectious stomatitis; abscess lavage; middle ear infection flush in box turtles
Ciprofloxacin	10 mg/kg PO q48h[107]	Most species
	11 mg/kg PO q48-72h[243]	Pythons (reticulated pythons)/PD
Ciprofloxacin ophthalmic ointment or drops (Ciloxan, Alcon)	Topical[243]	All species/infectious stomatitis; gingivitis
Clarithromycin	15 mg/kg PO q84h[492]	Tortoises (desert tortoises)/PD; upper respiratory tract disease (mycoplasmosis)
Clindamycin	10 mg/kg PO, IM, IV q12h[176]	Loggerhead sea turtles/PK; 29-30°C (84-87°F); insufficient to be effective
Danofloxacin	6 mg/kg SC, IM[302]	Loggerhead sea turtles/PK; levels of danofloxacin >0.05 µg/mL were maintained for 48 hr after administration
Enrofloxacin	—	IM administration is believed to be painful and may result in tissue necrosis and sterile abscesses; in certain species may cause skin discoloration or tissue necrosis if given SC; suggest diluting with sterile NaCl before SC

TABLE 4-1 Antimicrobial Agents Used in Reptiles. (cont'd)

Agent	Dosage	Species/Comments
Enrofloxacin (cont'd)		administration; several studies show that a less frequent administration of the drug may be sufficient;[168,219,372] hyperexcitation, incoordination, diarrhea have been reported in a Galapagos tortoise[65]
	5-13 mg/kg PO, IM q24-48h[485]	Various species/retrospective study; administered to 25 lizards, 10 snakes and 2 chelonians; unknown outcomes
	10 mg/kg IM q48h[482,483,500]	Snakes (Burmese pythons, rattlesnakes, pit vipers)/PK
	10 mg/kg IM followed by 5 mg/kg IM q48h[500]	Snakes (Burmese pythons)/PK; for treatment of more enrofloxacin-sensitive gram-negative bacteria
	5 mg/kg PO, IM q24h[312]	Lizards (green iguanas)/PK; marked pharmacokinetic variability with PO administration may make parenteral administration more suitable in critically ill animals; plasma concentrations >0.2 µg/mL were obtained for variable amount of time; at the dose given, ciprofloxacin levels were below the level of quantitation of the assay
	5 mg/kg IM q24h × 27 days[188]	Bearded dragons/ineffective in treating *Devriesea agamarum* in experimentally infected animals
	10 mg/kg PO q24h × 14 days[52]	Green iguanas/effective in preventing *Salmonella* shedding in eight out of nine iguanas sensitive at 5 µg/mL
	10 mg/kg IM[409]	Lizards (bearded dragons)/PK; 24-26°C (75-79°F) and basking spot; drug diluted to 10 mg/mL and administered in the hindlimb muscle; no adverse effects noted; dose might be effective against bacteria with MIC values of 0.8–0.9 µg/mL but not sufficient for treating infections of bacteria with MIC over 0.9 µg/mL; half-life 20 hr; no effect noted on cloacal bacteria
	10 mg/kg PO[7]	Lizards (Asian house geckos)/PK; beta half-life 24 hr; result in plasma concentrations effective against susceptible bacterial species inhibited by an enrofloxacin MIC ≤0.5 µg/mL
	10 mg/kg IM q24h[206]	Monitors/PK (savannah monitor); preliminary data
	5 mg/kg IM q24-48h[376]	Chelonians (gopher tortoises)/PD
	5 mg/kg IM q12-24h[386]	Chelonians (Indian star tortoises)/PK; q12h for *Pseudomonas* and *Citrobacter*, q24h for other bacteria
	5 mg/kg IM, IV q48h[258]	Sea turtles (loggerhead sea turtles)/PK
	10 mg/kg ICe q48h[158,408]	Chelonians (Hermann's tortoises, yellow-bellied sliders)/PD; dilute with saline to 10 mg/mL
	10 mg/kg SC[168]	Chelonians (Eastern box turtles, yellow-bellied sliders, river cooters)/PK; a single SC injection resulted in plasma drug concentrations above a MIC value of 0.5 µg/mL for over 200 hr in all three species
	10-20 mg/kg PO q7d[219]	Sea turtles (loggerhead sea turtles)/PK; 25-29°C (77-84°F); tablets administered in squid; single 20 mg/kg administration calculated to be effective for bacteria with MIC =1 µg/mL for 1 wk

Continued

TABLE 4-1 Antimicrobial Agents Used in Reptiles. (cont'd)

Agent	Dosage	Species/Comments
Enrofloxacin (cont'd)	5 mg/kg IM, IV q36-72h[191,306]	Crocodilians (American alligators, estuarine crocodiles)/PK; prolonged oral absorption with effective plasma drug level only on day 3; PO pharmacokinetics not fully determined
	5 mg/kg IM, IV[372]	Crocodilians (freshwater crocodiles)/PK; single administration study; long half-life (43-44 hr) similar after IM and IV administrations
Gentamicin	—	Nephrotoxicity has been reported,[333] especially in snakes; maintain hydration; use with a penicillin or cephalosporin; injection site had no effect on pharmacokinetic parameters in red-eared sliders[204]
	2.5 mg/kg IM q72h[56]	Snakes (gopher snakes)/PD
	2.5-3 mg/kg IM, then 1.5 mg/kg q96h[200]	Snakes (blood pythons)/PK
	3 mg/kg IM q>96h[28]	Turtles (Eastern box turtles)/PK; 29°C (84°F); lower dose may be more appropriate
	6 mg/kg IM q72-96h[385]	Turtles (red-eared sliders)/PK; 24°C (75°F)
	1.75-2.25 mg/kg IM q72-96h[218]	Crocodilians (alligators)/PK; respiratory infection
Gentamicin ophthalmic ointment or drops	Topical[243]	Most species/superficial ocular infection; lesions in oral cavity
Marbofloxacin	—	In a study on yellow-bellied sliders, 2 out of 8 turtles died after one injection of marbofloxacin at 10 mg/kg ICe;[475] in Chinese soft-shelled turtles, administration of 10 mg/kg IM and PO resulted in unspecified adverse effects;[423] administration of a single dose of marbofloxacin in yellow-bellied sliders resulted in cloacal shedding of resistant *Salmonella* and *E. coli* from 48 hr from the administration, especially at lower doses (0.4 mg/kg)[475]
	10 mg/kg PO q48h[82]	Snakes (ball pythons)/PK; 30°C (86°F)
	2 mg/kg IM, IV[259]	Chelonians (red-eared sliders)/PK; room 24°C (75°F), water 28°C (82°F), basking spot 30°C (86°F); maximum plasma concentration was higher after forelimb administration; half-life after forelimb concentration was 4.6 hr
	2 mg/kg ICe[475]	Chelonians (yellow-bellied sliders)/PK; room 24°-26°C (75-79°F), water 25°C (77°F), basking spot 30°C (86°F); long half-life (25 hr)
	2 mg/kg PO[303]	Sea turtles/PK (loggerhead sea turtles); half-life 13 hr
	2 mg/kg IM, IV q24h[258]	Sea turtles (loggerhead sea turtles)/PK; water 26-28°C (79-82°F); half-life 19 hr (IM) and 15 hr (IV); IM q24h dosing likely not effective for bacteria with MIC >0.5 µg/mL
	2 mg/kg IM, IV[373]	Crocodilians (freshwater crocodiles)/PK; long half-life (2.5 days)

TABLE 4-1 Antimicrobial Agents Used in Reptiles. (cont'd)

Agent	Dosage	Species/Comments
Metronidazole	20 mg/kg PO q48h x ≥7 days[143]	Most species/anaerobes
	20 mg/kg PO q48h[254]	Yellow rat snakes/PK; 27-29°C (81-84°F); when treatment was repeated for 6 administrations, mean metronidazole plasma concentration was always higher than 4 µg/mL; should be adequate for the treatment of most anaerobic infections
	50 mg/kg PO q48h[43a]	Red rat snakes/PK; 28°C (82°F); mean metronidazole plasma concentration was higher than 6 µg/ml for 48 hr
	20 mg/kg PO q24-48h[255]	Iguanas/PK; use q24h for more resistant anaerobes
Oxytetracycline	6-10 mg/kg PO, IM, IV q24h[107,243]	Most species/may produce local inflammation at injection site
	42 mg/kg SC q6d[213]	Sea turtles (multiple species)/PK; drug was diluted prior to administration (5-20 mL/kg); plasma oxytetracycline concentrations were maintained above a MIC value of ≈4 µg/mL for ≈6 days[213]
	10 mg/kg IM, IV q5d[190]	Crocodilians (alligators)/PK; 27°C (81°F); mycoplasmosis
Piperacillin	50-100 mg/kg IM q24h[107,243]	Most species/broad-spectrum bactericidal agent; maintain hydration; may use with an aminoglycoside; is only available in combination with tazobactam
	100 mg/kg IM q48h[201]	Snakes (blood pythons)/PK
Polymyxin B sulfate, neomycin sulfate, bacitracin zinc ointment	Topical[243]	All species/rostral abrasions, dermal wounds
Povidone-iodine solution (0.05%) or ointment	Topical/lavage[63]	All species/fungal dermatitis; dermatophilosis; contaminated wound; can soak in 0.005% aqueous solution ≤1 hr q12-24h[63]
Silver sulfadiazine cream (Silvadene, Marion)	Topical q24-72h[285]	All species/broad-spectrum antibacterial for skin (i.e., wounds, burns) or oral cavity; dressing is generally not necessary
Ticarcillin (Ticar, SmithKline-Beecham)	50-100 mg/kg IM, IV q24-48h[291]	Loggerhead sea turtles/PK
Tobramycin	—	Potentially nephrotoxic; maintain hydration; potentiated by ß-lactams
Trimethoprim	—	When administered orally to red-eared sliders at 168 mg/animal, the drug was excreted unaltered within 1 hr[476]
Trimethoprim/sulfamethoxazole	30 mg/kg IM q24h[264]	Reticulated python/administered in a case of maxillary osteomyelitis together with surgical debridement; no PK studies available

Continued

TABLE 4-1 Antimicrobial Agents Used in Reptiles. (cont'd)

Agent	Dosage	Species/Comments
Trimethoprim-sulphonamide (compounded)	30 mg/kg PO q12h × 14 days[426]	Bearded dragon/administered in a case of enterococcal cholecystitis after cholecystectomy based on sensitivity testing

[a]Because reptiles are ectothermic, pharmacokinetics of drugs are influenced by ambient temperature. Antimicrobial therapy should be conducted at the upper end of the patient's preferred (selected) optimum temperature zone.
[b]See Table 15.4 for antimicrobial combination therapies, some of which are commonly used in reptiles.

TABLE 4-2 Antiviral Agents Used in Reptiles.

Agent	Dosage	Species/Comments
Acyclovir	40-80 mg/kg PO[10]	Box turtles/PK; low maximum plasma concentrations; uncertain efficacy
	80 mg/kg PO q8h or 240 mg/kg PO q24h[315]	Tortoises/herpesvirus; uncertain efficacy; unlikely to eliminate infection; combine with supportive care
	80 mg/kg PO q24h[360]	Mediterranean tortoises/decreased mortality in those infected with TeHV-3
	80 mg/kg PO q24h[86]	Australian Krefft's river turtles/herpesvirus; uncertain efficacy
	≥80 mg/kg PO q24h[144]	Marginated tortoises/PK; herpesvirus; poor oral absorption
	Topical (5% ointment) q12h[63]	All species/antiviral (i.e., herpesvirus-associated dermatitis)
Chlorhexidine solution	0.5% dilution, topical on oral lesions q24h[238]	Tortoises/herpesvirus
Famcyclovir	10-30 mg/kg PO q24h using allometric scaling[428]	Eastern box turtles/treated during outbreak of concurrent terHV-1 and ranavirus (FV-3); uncertain efficacy
Valacyclovir	40 mg/kg PO q24h[10]	Box turtles/PK; effective plasma concentrations compared to humans; uncertain efficacy or toxicity

TABLE 4-3 Antifungal Agents Used in Reptiles.

Agent	Dosage	Species/Comments
Amphotericin B	0.5 mg/kg IV q48-72h[63]	Most species/nephrotoxic; can use in combination with ketoconazole; administer slowly
	0.5-1 mg/kg IV, ICe q24-72h × 14-28 days[107]	Most species/aspergillosis
	1 mg/kg IT q24h × 14-28 days[63]	Most species/respiratory infection; dilute with water or saline
	0.1 mg/kg intrapulmonary q24h × 28 days[192]	Greek tortoises/pneumonia

TABLE 4-3 Antifungal Agents Used in Reptiles. (cont'd)

Agent	Dosage	Species/Comments
Amphotericin B (cont'd)	1 mg/kg q24h ICe × 2-4 wk[272]	Crocodilians
	5 mg/150 mL saline × 1 hr nebulization q12h × 7 days[63]	Most species/pneumonia
Chlorhexidine (Nolvasan 2%, Fort Dodge)	20 mL/g water bath[63]	Lizards/dermatophytosis
Clotrimazole (Veltrim, Haver-Lockhart; Otomax, with gentamicin and betamethasone, Schering-Plough)	Topical[402]	Most species/dermatitis; may bathe q12h with dilute organic iodine prior to use
F10 super concentrate disinfectant (Health and Hygiene, Roodeport, S Africa)	1:250 nasal flush, 0.1 mL each nare q24h[74]	Terrestrial chelonians/benzalkonium chloride/polyhexamethylene biguanide HCl
Fluconazole	5 mg/kg PO q24h[63]	Lizards/dermatophytosis
	21 mg/kg SC once, then 10 mg/kg SC 5 days later[176,177,289]	Loggerhead sea turtles/PK
Griseofulvin	15 mg/kg PO q72h[221,222,243]	Most species
	20-40 mg/kg PO q72h x 5 treatments[402]	Most species/dermatitis; limited success
Itraconazole	5 mg/kg PO q24h[305]	Most species/some hepatotoxicity noted when used for *Chrysosporium* anamorph of *Nannizziopsis vriesii*; can cause anorexia in bearded dragons without evidence of hepatotoxicity[152]
	10 mg/kg PO q24h[330]	Snakes/10 mg/kg per cloacal did not lead to therapeutic plasma or tissue concentrations in cottonmouths[271]
	5 mg/kg PO q24h[185]	Panther chameleons
	10 mg/kg PO q48h × 60 days[38]	Chameleons (Parson's)/osteomyelitis
	23.5 mg/kg PO q24h[147]	Lizards/PK (spiny lizards); following a 3-day treatment, a therapeutic plasma concentration persists for 6 days beyond peak concentration; treatment interval was not determined
	5 mg/kg PO q24h, or 15 mg/kg PO q72h[292]	Kemp's ridley sea turtles
Ketoconazole	—	May use antibiotics concomitantly to prevent bacterial overgrowth; may use concurrently with thiabendazole
	15 mg/kg q72h PO[221,222,243]	Most species
	25 mg/kg PO q24h × 21 days[217]	Snakes, turtles
	15-30 mg/kg PO q24h × 14-28 days[363]	Gopher tortoises/PK; systemic infection
	50 mg/kg PO q24h × 14-28 days[63]	Crocodilians
Malachite green	0.15 mg/L water × 1 hr bath × 14 days[107]	Dermatitis

Continued

TABLE 4-3 Antifungal Agents Used in Reptiles. (cont'd)

Agent	Dosage	Species/Comments
Miconazole (Monistat-Derm, Ortho)	Topical[402]	Most species/dermatitis; may bathe q12h with dilute organic iodine before use
Nystatin	100,000 U/kg PO q24h × 10 days[63]	Most species/enteric yeast infections; limited success
Terbinafine	Topical[233]	Use in conjunction with oral azoles for *Chrysosporium* anamorph of *Nannizziopsis vriesii;* expect long treatment calendar
	2 mg/mL solution nebulized for 30 min/day x 30 days[181]	Lake Erie watersnakes (*Nerodia* sp.)/ ophidiomycosis; terbinafine nebulization is a promosing treatment but may require multiple nebulization courses; disease may not resolve[181]
	2 mg/mL nebulization x 30 min[228]	Cottonmouths/quickly reached in vitro susceptibility concentration and maintained for at least 12 hr
	24.5 mg (75–190 mg/kg) SC implant (Melatek Implants, MELATEK L.L.C., Middleton, WI) x 7 wk[228]	Cottonmouths/quickly reached in vitro susceptibility concentration and maintained for at least 7 wk
	20 mg/kg PO[319]	Bearded dragons/PK; *Nannizziopsis quarroi* (cause cutaneous lesions, etc.); this dose would exceed the MIC concentration for *N. quarroi* for at least 24hr[319]
	3.4 mg/kg PO q24h × 15 mo[453]	Aldabra tortoises/severe phaeohyphomycosis of carapace; non-responsive to itraconazole
	15 mg/kg PO gavaged once[119]	Red-eared sliders (*Trachemys scripta*)/ PK; pilot study; q12h may be needed to meet many fungal MIC levels
Tolnaftate 1% cream (Tinactin, Schering-Plough)	Topical q12h prn[9]	Most species/dermatitis; may bathe q12h with dilute organic iodine before use
Voriconazole	—	High rate of mortality in 1-2 hr for cottonmouths at 5 mg/kg SC[271]
	10 mg/kg per cloacal 3 ×/wk × 4 wk[318]	Rattlesnakes/*Ophidiomyces ophiodiicola;* crushed in suspension (Ora-Plus, Paddock Laboratories)
	10 mg/kg PO × 47 days[427,474]	Bearded dragons for *Chrysosporium* anamorph of *Nannizziopsis vriesii*; possible hepatocellular injury
	10 mg/kg PO q24h x 10 wk[187]	Cured *Chrysosporium* anamorph of *Nannizziopsis vriesii* infection in giant girdled lizard; exceeded MIC tenfold
	10 mg/kg SC q12h x 7 days[215]	Red-eared sliders (*Trachemys scripta*)/ PK; resulted in trough concentrations considered subtherapeutic in humans but may reach MIC for some reptile fungal isolates; possible side effects seen

TABLE 4-3 Antifungal Agents Used in Reptiles. (cont'd)

Agent	Dosage	Species/Comments
Voriconazole (cont'd)	10 mg/kg PO q48h x 7 doses[498]	Western pond turtles (*Actinemys marmorata*)/PK; no adverse effects seen; observed trough plasma concentrations consistently higher than reported *Emydomyces testavorans* MIC concentrations
Voriconazole (V)/F10 super concentrate disinfectant (F10) (Health and Hygiene, Roodeport, S. Africa)	(V) 10 mg/kg PO q24h × 60 days + (F10) 1:250 dilution for 20 min bath q24h × 60 days[412]	Luthega skinks/systemic *Lecanicillium* sp. infection; nonresponsive to oral voriconazole and terbinafine ointment

TABLE 4-4 Antiparasitic Agents Used in Reptiles.

Agent	Dosage	Species/Comments
Carbaryl powder (5%)	—	If used as antiparasitical, use cautiously because it can have harmful effects, including death, on reptiles; carbaryl administered at 25 and 250 µg/g to snake-eyed lizard caused disruption in villi and prominent hemorrhage of the small intestine;[57] has been banned in some states
Chloroquine	—	Chloroquine administered at 10 mg/kg PO for 7 days was ineffective in treating blood parasites of the family Haemogregarinidae (Apicomplexa) in *Gallotia* sp. lizards[136]
Emodepside (1.98%) + praziquantel (7.94%) (Profender, Bayer)	1.12 mL/kg[323,415]	Many species/PD; nematodes; cestodes; aquatic turtles must be kept dry for 48 hr after application; appears to be safe, but needs more safety and efficacy data
	1 mL/kg once[462]	Chelonians/PD; nematodes; oxyurid eggs at day 33 after administration decreased but they were still present
Fenbendazole	—	Drug of choice for nematodes; least toxic of the benzimidazoles; may have an antiprotozoan effect; overdose may cause leukopenia; avoid in septicemic patients[345]
	25 mg/kg PO q14d[309]	Snakes (corn snakes)/hookworm; of three symptomatic snakes treated, one died, one was euthanized due to recurring prolapse, and one survived
	25-100 mg/kg PO q14d for up to 4 treatments[244]	Snakes (ball pythons)/nematodes
	40 mg/kg PO once[136]	Lizards (*Gallotia* sp.)/PD; oxyurids; no eggs were detected in nine lizards treated up to 75 days post treatment
	100 mg/kg once[151]	Tortoises/nematodes; shedding of ova continues for 30 days

Continued

TABLE 4-4 Antiparasitic Agents Used in Reptiles. (cont'd)

Agent	Dosage	Species/Comments
Fipronil (0.29%; Frontline Spray, Merial)	Apply to a cotton ball and wipe on the skin,[120] then wash off in 5 min; q7-10d prn	Most species/mites, ticks; beware of reactions to alcohol carrier; needs safety evaluation; multiple anecdotal reports of toxicity in reptiles
	4 g/animal topically[120]	Lizards (green iguana)/PD; fipronil was applied to a cotton ball and wiped on the skin, resulting in an average of 4 g fipronil/iguana; a single administration was effective in 9 out of 11 animals[120]
Halofuginone	—	Hepatotoxic and nephrotoxic effects seen in all snakes administered halofuginone in one study[165]
	110 mg/kg q7d × 5 treatments[145]	Green iguanas/PD; administered to four iguanas with cryptosporidiosis together with hyperimmune bovine colostrum and subcutaneous fluids resulted in eradication of *Cryptosporidium* after 40 days and for at least 18 months in the three iguanas that survived
Imidacloprid and moxidectin (Advantage multi/ Advocate, Bayer)	32-160 mg/kg (imidacloprid) and 8-40 mg/kg (moxidectin) topical once or q24h × 3 days[322]	Reptiles/nematodes and mites; in animals with a thick epidermis, higher dosage was needed; for nematodes, a single treatment was sufficient; for mites, treatment had to be repeated on 3 consecutive days; one Asian grass lizard out of four died after treatment; treatment should be started at low dosages to avoid side effects
	0.2 mL/kg topically q14d x 3 treatments[170]	Lizards/eliminated hookworms and pinworms; treatment did not eliminate coccidia; needs safety and pharmacokinetic evaluation
Ivermectin	—	Do not use in chelonians,[465] crocodilians, indigo snakes, or skinks;[243,246] there are multiple anecdotal and published reports of lethal ivermectin toxicity at 0.2 mg/kg SC in squamates;[46,459] ivermectin toxicity may also occur in snakes eating treated rodents;[173] ivermectin has been proven to cause flaccid paresis and death in various species of chelonians at dosages between 0.025 and 0.3 mg/kg;[465] may be safer to avoid using parenteral ivermectin in a specific species until safety study is performed
	0.2 mg/kg PO, SC, IM, repeat in 14 days[127,243]	Snakes (except indigo snakes), lizards, except skinks[243]/nematodes (including lungworms),[278] mites; can dilute with propylene glycol for oral use; colored animals may have skin discoloration at injection site; rare adverse effects reported in chameleons, possibly associated with breakdown of parasites;[25] do not use within 10 days of diazepam or tiletamine/zolazepam; rare death and occasional nervous system signs, lethargy, or inappetence have been reported;[246] used for pentastomids in one Bose's monitor lizard (repeated after 10 days)[127] and in four boa constrictors (repeated after 14 days)[278] without evidence of side effects

TABLE 4-4 Antiparasitic Agents Used in Reptiles. (cont'd)

Agent	Dosage	Species/Comments
Ivermectin (sustained release)	Topical application on areas at risk of myasis[20]	Crocodilians/myasis; a single application of a 1-10 mm layer of the product on a wound in one Nile crocodile resolved myasis
Levamisole (Levasole 13.65%, Mallinckrodt)	—	Most species/lungworms; very narrow range of safety; main advantage is that it can be administered parenterally; avoid use in debilitated animals
	10 mg/kg SC repeated in 14 days[278]	Snakes (boa constrictor)/PD; administered to four boa constrictors positive for lungworms (*Rhabdias*); only one was negative both at 28 days and 12 mo after treatment
	10 mg/kg SC, IM[63]	Chelonians (red-eared sliders)/PK; no local or systemic adverse effect was observed following administration in nine turtles; entirely absorbed following SC and IM administration; unclear effectiveness
Mebendazole	20-25 mg/kg PO, repeat in 14 days prn[243]	Most species/stronglyes, ascarids; unsure of efficacy at those dosages
	400 mg/kg PO[256]	Lizards (garden lizard *Calotes*)/PD;[256] single PO dose 100% effective against nematodes at 400 mg/kg and 1200 mg/kg; at 400 mg/kg, 84% effective against gallbladder trematodes and 58% effective against cestodes; less effective at lower dosages; unclear if safe at these doses in other species
Metronidazole	—	Protozoan (i.e., flagellates, amoebae) overgrowth; may stimulate appetite; mat cause severe neurologic signs at doses >200 mg/kg;[331] death occurred in indigo and mountain king snakes at 100 mg/kg;[243] injectable form can be administered PO; oral suspension is not available in the United States, but can be compounded; efficacy studies are lacking; dose of 100 mg/kg PO q24h for 5 days in a ball python with amebiasis was ineffective[253]
	20 mg/kg PO q48h[254]	Yellow rat snakes/PK; 27-29°C (81-84°F); when treatment was repeated for 6 administrations, mean metronidazole plasma concentration was always higher than 4 µg/mL
	50 mg/kg PO q48h[43a]	Red rat snakes/PK; 28°C (82°F); mean metronidazole plasma concentration was higher than 6 µg/mL for 48 hr
	20 mg/kg PO q24-48h[255]	Iguanas/PK; unclear effectiveness against protozoa
	40-60 mg/kg PO q7d x 2-3 doses[445]	Chameleons/flagellates; amoebae
	40-200 mg/kg PO, repeat in 14 days[326]	Geckos/ocular lesions (40 mg/kg) and subcutaneous lesions (200 mg/kg) caused by *Trichomonas*
	20 mg/kg ICe q48h[210]	Red-eared sliders/PK; ICe administration not recommended; needs further safety evaluation
	25 mg/kg PO q24h x 5 days[243]	Chelonians/amoebiasis

Continued

TABLE 4-4 Antiparasitic Agents Used in Reptiles. (cont'd)

Agent	Dosage	Species/Comments
Milbemycin	0.25-0.5 mg/kg SC prn[43]	Chelonians (red-eared sliders)/safety study; five red-eared sliders were injected and did not show adverse effects; unclear efficacy; parenteral form is not commercially available in United States; fenbendazole perferred
Oxfendazole (Benzelmin, Fort Dodge)	25 mg/kg PO once[232]	Lizards (green iguanas)/oxyurids; effective in a non-controlled study
	66 mg/kg PO once[151]	Chelonians (Hermann's tortoise)/oxyurids; may be repeated after 28 days prn
Paromomycin (Humatin, Parke Davis)	—	To date, there has not been any treatments shown to be completely effective in treating cryptosporidiosis; paromomycin, an aminoglycoside, has the most promise;[44] in reptiles with cryptosporidiosis, doses approximately 100 mg/kg q24h are likely to control clinical signs and shedding but not eradicate the organisms;[169] higher doses likely needed for eradication; limited data available on safety
	100 mg/kg PO q24h x 7 days, then 2x/wk x 3 mo[88]	Snakes/cryptosporidiosis; reduced clinical signs and oocyte shedding; does not eliminate the organism
	360 mg/kg PO 2x/wk × 6 wk[392]	Snakes/cryptosporidiosis; snake (king cobra) was subclinical at time of treatment; shedding of *Cryptosporidium* was eliminated
	360 mg/kg 2x/wk x 6 wk in food[44a]	Eastern indigo snakes/dosage was ineffective in eliminating cryptosporidiosis in naturally infected indigo snakes
	50-800 mg/kg PO q24h[44]	Leopard geckos/cryptosporidiosis; oocyst shedding subsided but resumed post treatment
	100 mg/kg PO q24h x 7 days, then q84h x 72 days[44]	Leopard geckos/cryptosporidiosis; improved condition of some animals
	300-360 mg/kg PO q48h x 14 days[364]	Lizards (gila monsters)/ cryptosporidiosis
	360 mg/kg PO q48h × 10 days[169]	Bearded dragons/intestinal cryptosporidiosis; initial treatment at 100 mg/kg q24h stopped shedding of cryptosporidia in five bearded dragons, but shedding then resumed in 3/5 bearded dragons after the daily treatment was reduced to a 2x/wk frequency; detectable excretion stopped in all individuals treated with paromomycin at 360 mg/kg q48h for 10 days; histopathology failed to reveal cryptosporidium in these lizards
	100 mg/kg PO q24h x 7 days, then q84h for 90 days[44]	Hermann's tortoises/cryptosporidiosis; controlled clinical signs and shedding
Permethrin (Provent-a-Mite, Pro Products)	Environmental treatment, 1 sec of spray/ft^2; wait until dry before returning animal to enclosure[55]	Lizards, snakes/mites; ticks; FDA approved; death reported in snakes that had permethrin applied directly on the body;[486] wash immediately if accidentally applied to skin
	Topical[54]	Tortoises/ticks

TABLE 4-4 Antiparasitic Agents Used in Reptiles. (cont'd)

Agent	Dosage	Species/Comments
Piperazine	—	Lizards (garden lizard *Calotes*)/PD;[253] single PO dose 100% effective against nematodes at 400 mg/kg and 1200 mg/kg; at 400 mg/kg, 67% effective against gallbladder trematodes and 77% effective against cestodes; less effective at lower dosages; unclear if safe at these doses in other species
	100-200 mg/kg PO[195]	Crocodilians
Ponazuril	—	Ponazuril administered at 20 mg/kg PO in red-footed tortoises did not achieve concentrations known to be effective for anticoccidial treatment in mammals;[29] tortoises showed prolonged oral absorption and a terminal elimination rate constant and half-life were not able to be determined in a study lasting 7 days[29]
	15-40 mg/kg PO q24h × 21 days[477,478]	Bearded dragons/coccidiosis
	30 mg/kg PO q48h × 2 treatments[45]	Bearded dragons/coccidiosis
	20 mg/kg PO q48h × 56 days[449]	Red-footed tortoises/intranuclear coccidiosis; two tortoises treated at these dosage became asymptomatic but did not clear the infection[449]
Praziquantel	—	See also emodepside; cestodes, trematodes
	8-10 mg/kg PO, SC, IM, repeat in 14 days[243,396]	Most species/cestodes, trematodes; higher dosages have been administered
	25 mg/kg PO q3h × 3 treatments[219a]	Loggerhead sea turtles/PK; mean plasma concentration was 90 ng/mL 48 hr after the first of 3 doses
	50 mg/kg PO × 3 times in one day[6]	Green sea turtles/PD; a 1-day course of treatment at 50 mg/kg body weight at 0, 7, and 9 hr was effective for spirorchidiasis (cardiovascular flukes); in another case, a loggerhead sea turtle that received 50 mg/kg of praziquantel developed skin lesions within 48 hr of administration[219a]
Pyrantel pamoate	5 mg/kg PO, repeat in 14 days[246]	Most species/nematodes
	25 mg/kg PO q24h x 3 days, repeat in 3 wk[142]	Most species/ascarids, hookworms, pinworms
	5 mg/kg PO, repeat in 14 days[424]	Indian star tortoises/PD; administered to 15 tortoises with oxyurids and ascarids; complete clearance of the parasites was seen on day 14 after the first treatment with no reported recurrence

Continued

TABLE 4-4 Antiparasitic Agents Used in Reptiles. (cont'd)

Agent	Dosage	Species/Comments
Pyrethrin spray (0.09%)	—	Limited published information on safety and efficacy; mortality in anole lizards reported when exposed to a solution that contained 300 mg/L of pyrethrins;[460] in one study, pyrethrins were not 100% effective in killing African tortoise ticks[54]
	Topical q7d x 2-3 treatments[123]	Most species/use water-based sprays labeled for kittens and puppies; apply with cloth; can also spray cage, wash out after 30 min; use sparingly and with caution; pyrethroids are safer (see permethrin)
Quinine sulfate	75 mg/kg SC q48h × 12 treatments[468]	Fence lizards, anole lizards/PD;[468] effective against some *Plasmodium* spp.; toxic at >100 mg/kg q24h; ineffective against exoerythrocytic forms
Spiramycin	—	Drug investigated for the treatment of cryptosporidiosis in snakes
	80 mg/kg PO q24h × 3 treatments[165]	Snakes (*Panterophis* sp.)/cryptosporidiosis resulted in negative fecal examination in two snakes, decreased oocyst shedding in two snakes, and no changes in terms of oocyst shedding in the remaining two snakes; *Cryptosporidium* was present histologically in all animals; although higher dosages have been suggested, there is limited supporting evidence for effectiveness or safety of those dosages
Spiramycin + metronidazole (Stomorgyl, Merial)	200 mg/kg PO q5d × 5 wk (given in combination with trimethoprim/ sulfadiazine)[145]	Lizards (green iguanas)/cryptosporidiosis; administered together with trimethoprim/ sulfadiazine (75 mg/kg q5d × 5 wk) to four iguanas with cryptosporidiosis; one animal died and three cleared the infection
Sulfadiazine, sulfamerazine	—	Most species/coccidia; avoid sulfa drugs in cases of dehydration, urinary calculi, or renal dysfunction[331]
	75 mg/kg PO, then 45 mg/kg q24h x 5 days[243]	Most species/coccidia
	25 mg/kg PO q24h x 21 days[243]	Snakes, lizards/coccidia
Sulfadimethoxine	50 mg/kg PO q24h x 3-5 days, then q48h prn[246]	Most species/coccidia; ensure adequate hydration and renal function
	90 mg/kg PO, IM, IV, then 45 mg/kg q24h x 5-7 days[396]	Most species/coccidia
	50 mg/kg PO q24h x 21 days[477,478]	Bearded dragons/coccidia
Sulfamethazine	25 mg/kg PO, IM, q24h x 21 days[396]	Most species/coccidia
	50 mg/kg PO q24h x 3 days, off 3 days, on 3 days[243]	Most species/coccidia

TABLE 4-4 Antiparasitic Agents Used in Reptiles. (cont'd)

Agent	Dosage	Species/Comments
Toltrazuril 5% (Baycox, Bayer)	5-15 mg/kg PO q24-48h x 3-30 days[243]	These dosages have been anecdotally suggested in other formularies, although there is limited information on safety and efficacy in any reptile species
Toltrazuril (T) + clindamycin (C)	(T) 10 mg/kg PO q24h × 3 days repeated in 7 days + (C) 5 mg/kg PO q24h × 7 days[451]	Lizards (Lawson's dragons)/ coccidiosis from *Choleoeimeria* spp.; elimination of oocysts was not impacted in a Lawson's dragon by toltrazuril in varying intervals or trimethoprim and sulfonamide; this treatment protocol, however, resulted in negative oocyst shedding
Trimethoprim-sulfonamides	—	Most species/coccidia; avoid potentiated sulfa drugs in cases of dehydration or renal dysfunction[331]
	30 mg/kg PO q24 × 2-14 days[87,243]	Most species/coccidia; although this dosage has also been suggested in other formularies, there is limited information on safety and efficacy in any reptile species
	75 mg/kg PO q5d × 5 wk (given in combination with spiramycin/ metronidazole)[145]	Lizards (green iguanas)/cryptosporidiosis; administered together with spiramycin/ metronidazole (200 mg/kg q5d × 5 wk) to four iguanas with cryptosporidiosis: one animal died and three cleared the infection

TABLE 4-5 Chemical Restraint/Anesthetic Agents Used in Reptiles.[a]

Agent	Dosage	Species/Comments
Acepromazine	0.05-0.25 mg/kg IM[243]	Most species/can be used as a preanesthetic with ketamine
	0.1-0.5 mg/kg IM[328,362]	Most species/preanesthetic; reduce by 50% if used with barbiturates
Acepromazine (A)/ propofol (P)	(A) 0.5 mg/kg IM + (P) 5 mg/kg IV; (A) 0.5 mg/kg IM + (P) 10 mg/kg IV[11]	Giant Amazon river turtles/sedation with both protocols, longer duration with higher propofol dosage
Alfaxalone (Alfaxan, Jurox)	6-9 mg/kg IV, or 9-15 mg/ kg IM[268]	Most species/good muscle relaxation; variable results; drug requires more evaluation; may have violent recovery;[30] don't use within 10 days of DMSO treatment
	6-15 mg/kg IM, IV[420]	Most species
	9 mg/kg IV[413]	Snakes, lizards/induction; not effective for blotched blue-tongued skinks
	15 mg/kg IM[328]	Lizards, chelonians/induction, 35-40 min; duration, 15-35 min; good muscle relaxation; variable results
	5 mg/kg SC[499]	Ball pythons/deeper and longer sedation when admininstered in the cranial half versus caudal half of the body

Continued

TABLE 4-5 Chemical Restraint/Anesthetic Agents Used in Reptiles. (cont'd)

Agent	Dosage	Species/Comments
Alfaxalone (Alfaxan, Jurox) (cont'd)	10-30 mg/kg IM[220]	Ball pythons/increased sedation with cranial administration and increasing dose
	15 mg/kg SC[397]	Corn snakes/moderate sedation regardless of whether administered cranial or caudal half of snake
	30 mg/kg ICe[452]	Garter snakes/sedation
	5 mg/kg IV (jugular vein)[336]	Leopard geckos/sedation for tracheal intubation; caused decreased heart rate and respiratory rate
	12 mg/kg IV[366]	Bearded dragons/rapid induction for intubation; decreased respiratory rate
	3-10 mg/kg IV[369]	Loggerhead sea turtle yearlings/rapid sedation; hypoxemia at higher doses and animals required assisted ventilation at 10 mg/kg
	5 mg/kg IV[248]	Turtles, tortoises/induction
	5 mg/kg IV[338]	Yellow-bellied sliders/increased sedation, decreased heart and respiratory rates when admininstered in the dorsal cervical sinus compared to coccydial vein
	5 mg/kg IN[66]	Red-eared sliders turtles/minimal sedation
	10-20 mg/kg IM[174,240,425]	Horsfield's tortoises (males only)/ light-to-moderate sedation with no-to-minimal analgesia; red-eared slider turtles/light sedation of short duration; PD-turtles administered 10 mg/kg at low temperature more relaxed than when warm and turtles administered 20 mg/kg at warm temperature were most relaxed
	20 mg/kg IM[212]	Red-eared sliders, Eastern painted turtles, yellow-spotted Amazon river turtles, other undocumented turtle species/anesthetic induction
	24 mg/kg ICe[171]	Red-eared sliders/surgical anesthesia with good relaxation
	3 mg/kg IV[357]	Crocodilians/induction; unpredictable results
Alfaxalone (Al)/ dexmedetomidine (De)	(Al) 30 mg/kg + (De) 0.1 mg/kg SC[388]	Brown anole lizards/surgical plane of anesthesia for approximately 30 min
Alfaxalone (Al)/ lidocaine (L)	(Al) 15 mg/kg SC + (L) 4 mg/kg IM[125]	Bearded dragons/lidocaine did not potentiate alfaxalone sedation, but did transiently increase heart rate
Alfaxalone (Al)/ medetomidine (Me)	(Al) 10 mg/kg + (Me) 0.10 mg/kg IM; (Al) 20 mg/kg + (Me) 0.05 mg/kg IM[174]	Horsfield's tortoises (males only)/ deeper sedation than alfaxalone alone with analgesia
Atipamezole (Antisedan, Zoetis)	Give same volume SC, IV, IP as medetomidine or dexmedetomidine (5x medetomidine or 10x dexmedetomidine dose in mg)[a,129,436]	Most species/medetomidine and dexmedetomidine reversal; causes severe hypotension in gopher tortoises when given IV[94]

TABLE 4-5 Chemical Restraint/Anesthetic Agents Used in Reptiles. (cont'd)

Agent	Dosage	Species/Comments
Atipamezole (Antisedan, Zoetis) (cont'd)	0.2-0.5 mg/kg IM[128]	Chelonians/shell repair 5-10 min before finished
	0.5-0.75 mg/kg IM,[386] 0.75 mg/kg SC[298]	Chelonians
	1-3 mg/kg IM[334]	Nile crocodiles
Atropine	0.01-0.04 mg/kg SC, IM, IV, ICe[63]	Most species/preanesthetic; bradycardia; rarely indicated; generally use only in profound or prolonged bradycardia; may help prevent intracardiac shunting; ineffective at this dose in green iguanas
	0.5 mg/kg IM, IV, IT, IO[331]	Most species/bradycardia, decrease secretions, CPR
	1 mg/kg IV[167]	Red-footed tortoises (females)/ decreased MAC of isoflurane by eliminating R-L shunting of blood and facilitating isoflurane distribution
Bupivicaine (0.5%)	1 mg/kg intrathecal[294]	Turtles, tortoises/spinal anesthesia
	1 mg/kg neuraxial (intrathecal)[124]	Bearded dragons/motor and sensory block in caudal part of body
	0.1 mL/10 cm carapace[27]	Green sea turtles/spinal anesthesia
Butorphanol	—	Butorphanol combinations follow; see ketamine for combinations; inadequate for analgesia
	0.4-1 mg/kg SC, IM[63]	Most species/sedation; preanesthetic
	0.5-2 mg/kg IM or 0.2-0.5 mg/kg IV, IO[33]	Most species/preanesthetic
	1-1.5 mg/kg SC, IM[63]	Lizards/administer 30 min prior to isoflurane for smooth, shorter induction
	0.2 mg/kg IM[182,386]	Chelonians/minimal sedation
Butorphanol (B)/ medetomidine (Me)[b]	(B) 0.4 mg/kg + (Me) 0.08 mg/kg IM[150]	Green tree monitors/sedation
Butorphanol (B)/ midazolam (Mi)	(B) 0.4 mg/kg + (Mi) 2 mg/kg IM[63]	Most species/preanesthetic; administer 20 min before induction
Dexmedetomidine[b] (Dexdomitor; Zoetis)	—	Dexmedetomidine combinations follow; α_2 agonist that has replaced medetomidine;[b] reverse with atipamezole
	0.2 mg/kg IM[41]	Black and white tegus/no sedation
	0.05-0.15 mg/kg IN[114]	Indian star tortoises, red-footed tortoises/no significant sedation
Dexmedetomidine (De)/ketamine (K)/ hydromorphone (H)	(De) 0.075-0.2 mg/kg + (K) 5.0-7.5 mg/kg + (H) 0.5 mg/kg IM[139]	Bearded dragons/surgical anesthesia for celioscopy; some bearded dragons required supplemental isoflurane
Dexmedetomidine (De)/ketamine (K)/ morphine (Mo)	(De) 0.075 mg/kg + (K) 8 mg/kg + (Mo) 1 mg/kg IM[321]	Gopher tortoises/anesthesia; reversed with atipamezole
Dexmedetomidine (De)/midazolam (Mi)	(De) 0.2 mg/kg + (Mi) 1 mg/kg IM[41]	Black and white tegus/moderate sedation with antinociception to a thermal noxious stimulus

Continued

TABLE 4-5 Chemical Restraint/Anesthetic Agents Used in Reptiles. (cont'd)

Agent	Dosage	Species/Comments
Dexmedetomidine (De)/midazolam (Mi)/ alfaxalone (Al)	(De) 0.05 mg/kg + (Mi) 1 mg/kg + (A) 5 mg/kg IV[21]	American alligators/significant sedation; compared sedation to (De) + (Mi) + (K); increased sedation compared to (De) + (Mi) + (K) with more apnea
Dexmedetomidine (De)/midazolam (Mi)/ ketamine (K)	(De) 0.05 mg/kg + (Mi) 0.5 mg/kg + (K) 5 mg/kg IM[406]	Bullsnakes/satisfactory sedation for minor surgical procedures
	(De) 0.1 mg/kg + (Mi) 1 mg/ kg + (K) 2-4 mg/kg SC[115,299]	Red-eared sliders, black and white tegus/deep sedation
	(De) 0.1 mg/kg + (Mi) 1 mg/kg + (K) 10 mg/kg[400]	Ornate box turtles/light anesthesia lasting ~40 min; rapid onset; smooth recovery; no adverse effects noted
	(De) 0.05 mg/kg + (Mi) 1 mg/kg + (K) 5 mg/kg IV[21]	American alligators/administered drugs in the lateral occipital venous sinus; adequate for orotracheal intubation; 5/6 (83%) alligators maintained spontaneous ventilation; slightly less sedation and less apnea compared to (De) + (Mi) + alfaxalone
Dexmedetomidine (De)/midazolam (Mi)/ketamine (K)/ alfaxalone (Al)	(De) 0.1 mg/kg + (Mi) 0.5 mg/kg + (K) 3 mg/ kg + (Al) 8.5 mg/kg IM[25]	Slider turtles/induction prior to undergoing endoscopic ovariectomy
Dexmedetomidine (De)/ tribromoethanol (Tr)	(De) 0.1 mg/kg + (Tr) 400 mg/kg SC[388]	Brown anole lizards/surgical plane of anesthesia for approximately 80 min
Dextroketamine (DK)	10 mg/kg IV, ICe[202]	Spectacled caiman/PK; mild sedation ICe
Dextroketamine (DK)/ midazolam (Mi)	(Mi) 0.5 mg/kg + (DK) 10 mg/kg IV, ICe[202]	Spectacled caiman/PK; deep sedation IV; no analgesia
Diazepam[c]	—	Diazepam has been replaced by the use of midazolam in many cases;[c] see ketamine for combinations; muscle relaxation; give 20 min prior to anesthesia; potentially reversible with flumazenil; drug interaction with ivermectin
	0.5 mg/kg IM, IV[331]	All species/seizures
	2.5 mg/kg IM, IV[403]	Most species/seizures
	0.2-0.8 mg/kg IM[63]	Snakes/use in conjunction with ketamine for anesthesia with muscle relaxation
	0.2-2 mg/kg IM, IV[420]	Snakes, lizards
	2.5 mg/kg PO[63]	Iguanas/reduce anxiety which often leads to aggression
	0.2-1 mg/kg IM [63,420]	Chelonians/use in conjunction with ketamine for anesthesia with muscle relaxation
Disoprofol	5-15 mg/kg IV to effect[63]	All species/anesthesia; similar characteristics to propofol; not available in United States
Doxapram	4-12 mg/kg IM, IV[63]	Most species/respiratory stimulant
	5 mg/kg IM, IV q10min prn[63]	Most species/respiratory stimulant; reduces recovery time; reported to partially "reverse" effects of dissociatives[269]
	20 mg/kg IM, IV, IO[331]	Most species/respiratory stimulant
	10 mg/kg[230]	Ball pythons/prevents dexmedetomidine-induced reduction of breathing frequency

TABLE 4-5 Chemical Restraint/Anesthetic Agents Used in Reptiles. (cont'd)

Agent	Dosage	Species/Comments
Doxapram (cont'd)	5-10 mg/kg IV[429]	American alligators/immediate dose-dependent increase in breathing frequency
Epinephrine (1:1000)	0.5-1 mg/kg IV, IO, IT[331]	Most species/CPR, cardiac arrest
	0.1 mg/kg IM[162]	Snapping turtles/reduction in time to spontaneous respiration after isoflurane anesthesia
	0.1 mg/kg IM[23]	Loggerhead sea turtles/more rapid recovery from isoflurane anesthesia compared to saline
	0.1 mg/kg IM[148]	American alligators/more rapid recovery from isoflurane anesthesia compared to saline
Etorphine (M-99, Wildlife Pharmaceuticals)	0.3-0.5 mg/kg IM[328] 0.3-2.75 mg/kg IM[268]	Crocodilians, chelonians/very potent narcotic; crocodilians: induction, 5-30 min; duration, 30-180 min; chelonians: induction, 10-20 min; duration, 40-120 min; not very effective in reptiles other than alligators; poor relaxation; adequate for immobilization and minor procedures; requires an antagonist; limited use because of expense and legal restrictions
Flumazenil (Romazicon, Hoffman-LaRoche)	—	All species/reversal of benzodiazepines, including diazepam and midazolam
	0.05 mg/kg SC, IM, IV[295]	All species/reversal of midazolam; extrapolated from mammals and birds
	1 mg/20 mg of zolazepam[274] IM, IV[386]	Chelonians, crocodilians/reversal of zolazepam
Fospropofol	25-50 mg/kg ICe[418]	Red-eared sliders/muscle relaxation and immobility especially at higher dosage, but prolonged recovery, and profound respiratory depression with resuscitation in 2/8 subjects; use with caution
Gallamine (Flaxedil, American Cyanamid)	0.4-1.25 mg/kg IM[63] 0.6-4 mg/kg IM[275] 0.7 mg/kg IM[335] 1.2-2 mg/kg IM[129]	Crocodiles/results in flaccid paralysis, but no analgesia; larger animals require lower dosage; reverse with neostigmine;[275] use in alligators questionable; unsafe in alligators at ≥1 mg/kg;[362] deaths reported in American alligators and false gharials[272]
	0.5-2 mg/kg IM[260]	Crocodilians
Glycopyrrolate	0.01 mg/kg SC, IM, IV[63]	Most species/preanesthetic; for excess oral or respiratory mucus; rarely indicated; generally use only in profound or prolonged bradycardia; may be preferable to atropine;[243] does not work at this dose in green iguanas[243]
Haloperidol	0.5-10 mg/kg IM q7-14d[448]	Boids/aggression management
Hyaluronidase (Wydase, Wyeth)	25 U/dose SC[273]	Crocodilians/combine with premedication, anesthetic, or reversal drugs to accelerate SC absorption

Continued

TABLE 4-5 Chemical Restraint/Anesthetic Agents Used in Reptiles. (cont'd)

Agent	Dosage	Species/Comments
Isoflurane	3-5% induction, 1-3% maintenance[63]	Most species/inhalation anesthetic of choice in reptiles; induction, 6-20 min; recovery, 30-60 min; not as smooth in reptiles compared to other animals; intubation and intermittent positive pressure ventilation advisable; may preanesthetize with low dose propofol, ketamine, etc.
	3% in 100% O_2 and 21% O_2[351]	Bearded dragons/trend toward shorter induction and recovery with 21% O_2 group compared to use of 100% O_2
	5% via chamber in 5 L O_2/min[199]	Green iguanas/15-35 min loss of righting reflex; mean MAC, 1.62%; pH 7.49
Ketamine	—	Ketamine combinations follow; muscle relaxation and analgesia may be marginal; prolonged recovery with higher doses; larger reptiles require lower dose; painful at injection site; safety is questionable in debilitated patients; avoid use in cases with renal dysfunction; snakes may be permanently aggressive after ketamine anesthesia; generally recommend use only as a preanesthetic prior to isoflurane for surgical anesthesia
	10 mg/kg SC, IM q30min[63]	Most species/maintenance of anesthesia; recovery, 3-4 hr
	20-60 mg/kg IM, or 5-15 mg/kg IV[63]	Most species/muscle relaxation improved with midazolam or diazepam[c]
	22-44 mg/kg SC, IM[63]	Most species/sedation
	55-88 mg/kg SC, IM[63]	Most species/surgical anesthesia; induction, 10-30 min; recovery, 24-96 hr
	5-10 mg/kg IM[63]	Snakes/decreases the incidence of breath-holding during chamber induction
	10-20 mg/kg IM[330,331]	Snakes/sedation
	20-60 mg/kg SC, IM[63]	Snakes/sedation; induction, 30 min; recovery, 2-48 hr
	40 mg/kg IV[1]	Hissing sand snakes/surgical plane of anesthesia for 24 min; higher doses may be fatal
	50 mg/kg IM[383]	King cobra/surgical plane of anesthesia; single case report
	60-80 mg/kg IM[63]	Snakes/light anesthesia; intermittent positive pressure ventilation may be needed at higher doses
	5-10 mg/kg IM[63]	Lizards/decreases the incidence of breath-holding during chamber induction
	20-30 mg/kg IM[63]	Iguanas/sedation (i.e., facilitates endotracheal intubation); preanesthetic; requires lower dose than other reptiles

TABLE 4-5 Chemical Restraint/Anesthetic Agents Used in Reptiles. (cont'd)

Agent	Dosage	Species/Comments
Ketamine (cont'd)	30-50 mg/kg SC, IM[63]	Lizards/sedation; variable results
	40 mg/kg IV[1]	Iguanas/sedation (i.e., facilitates endotracheal intubation); preanesthetic; requires lower dose than other reptiles
	10-20 mg/kg IM[330,331]	Chelonians/sedation
	20-60 mg/kg IM[63,203]	Chelonians/sedation; induction, 30 min; recovery, ≥24 hr; potentially dangerous in dehydrated and debilitated tortoises
	25 mg/kg IM, IV[63]	Sea turtles/sedation; used at higher doses (50-70 mg/kg); recovery times may be excessively long and unpredictable; combination of ketamine and acepromazine gives a more rapid induction and recovery
	38-71 mg/kg ICe[494]	Green sea turtles/anesthesia; induction, 2-10 min; duration, 2-10 min; recovery, <30 min
	60-90 mg/kg IM[63,328]	Chelonians/light anesthesia; induction, <30 min; recovery, hours to days; requires higher doses than most other reptiles
	20-40 mg/kg SC, IM, ICe (sedation), to 40-80 mg/kg (anesthesia)[273]	Crocodilians/induction, <30-60 min; recovery, hours to days; in larger animals, 12-15 mg/kg may permit tracheal intubation; not recommended alone in Nile crocodiles[260]
	20-100 mg/kg IM[272]	Crocodilians/lower dose for sedation, higher for anesthesia (requires intermittent positive pressure ventilation for hours)
Ketamine (K)/ acepromazine (A)	(K) 120 mg/kg + (A) 1 mg/kg IM[3]	Caspian pond turtles/stage III anesthesia; prolonged recovery
Ketamine (K)/ butorphanol (B)	See (K) dosages + (B) ≤1.5 mg/kg IM[63]	Snakes/anesthesia with improved muscle relaxation
	(K) 10-30 mg/kg + (B) 0.5-1.5 mg/kg IM[63]	Chelonians/minor surgical procedures (i.e., shell repair)
Ketamine (K)/ dexmedetomidine (De)	(K) 5-7 mg/kg + (De) 0.025-0.07 mg/kg IV[212]	Red-eared sliders, Eastern painted turtles, yellow-spotted Amazon river turtles, other undocumented turtle species/anesthetic induction
	(K) 6 mg/kg + (De) 0.03 mg/kg IV[178]	Hatchling leatherback sea turtles/ anesthesia; reversal with atipamezole (0.3 mg/kg IM, IV)
	(K) 10 mg/kg + (De) 0.05 mg/kg IM, IV[377,378]	Desert tortoises/premedication
	(K) 10 mg/kg + (De) 0.2 mg/kg IN[66]	Red-eared sliders/moderate sedation; allowed intubation; heart rate decreased
	(K) 10 mg/kg + (De) 0.2 mg/kg intracloacal[337]	Yellow-bellied sliders/minimal sedation

Continued

TABLE 4-5 Chemical Restraint/Anesthetic Agents Used in Reptiles. (cont'd)

Agent	Dosage	Species/Comments
Ketamine (K)/ diazepam (D)[c]	See (K) dosages + (D) 0.2-0.8 mg/kg IM[63]	Snakes/anesthesia with improved muscle relaxation
	(K) 44 mg/kg + (D) 0.25 mg/kg IM; (K) 44 mg/kg + (D) 0.5 mg/kg IM; (K) 22 mg/kg + (D) 0.25 mg/kg IM; (K) 22 mg/kg + (D) 0.5 mg/kg IM[4]	Greek tortoises/significant sedation with high doses of (K) + either (D) dose and low dose of (K) with high dose of (D); moderate sedation with lower doses of (K) and (D)
	(K) 60-80 mg/kg + (D) 0.2-1 mg/kg IM[63]	Chelonians/anesthesia; muscle relaxation
	(K) 120 mg/kg + (D) 2 mg/kg IM[3]	Caspian pond turtles; stage III anesthesia
Ketamine (K)/ medetomidine (Me)[b]	—	Medetomidine is no longer commercially available in the U.S., but can be compounded;[b] reverse medetomidine with atipamezole
	(K) 10 mg/kg + (Me) 0.1-0.3 mg/kg IM[108]	Most species
	(K) 5-10 mg/kg + (Me) 0.1-0.15 mg/kg IM, IV[63]	Lizards (iguanas)
	(K) 100 mg/kg + (Me) 0.2 mg/kg IM[26]	Black and white tegus/surgical anesthesia with redosing of 50% original dose every 4 hr for up to 16 hr
	(K) 3-8 mg/kg + (Me) 0.025-0.08 mg/kg IV[276]	Giant tortoises (Aldabra)
	(K) 4 mg/kg + (Me) 0.04 mg/kg IM[189]	Green sea turtles
	(K) 4-10 mg/kg + (Me) 0.04-0.14 mg/kg IM[128]	Chelonians/sedation and muscle relaxation for shell repair
	(K) 5 mg/kg + (Me) 0.05 mg/kg IV[73]	Loggerhead sea turtles/induction of anesthesia for intubation
	(K) 5 mg/kg + (Me) 0.05 mg/kg IM[352]	Tortoises (gopher)/light anesthesia; tracheal intubation; inconsistent results
	(K) 5-10 mg/kg IM + (Me) 0.1-0.15 mg/kg IM, IV[63]	Tortoises (small-medium)
	(K) 7.5 mg/kg + (Me) 0.075 mg/kg IM[352]	Tortoises (gopher)/anesthesia; tracheal intubation
	(K) 10 mg/kg + (Me) 0.1 mg/kg IM[247]	Hybrid Galapagos tortoises/sedation
	(K) 10-20 mg/kg IM + (Me) 0.15-0.3 mg/kg IM, IV[63]	Turtles (fresh water)
	(K) 15 mg/kg (also S-ketamine) + (Me) 0.1 mg/kg IM[42]	Hermann's and spur-thighed tortoises/sedation with initial bradycardia and no apparent analgesia
	(K) 5-10 mg/kg + (Me) 0.1-0.15 mg/kg IM[186]	American alligators/adults

TABLE 4-5 Chemical Restraint/Anesthetic Agents Used in Reptiles. (cont'd)

Agent	Dosage	Species/Comments
Ketamine (K)/ medetomidine (Me) (cont'd)	(K) 10-15 mg/kg + (Me) 0.15-0.25 mg/kg IM[186]	American alligators/juveniles
	(K) 15 mg/kg + (Me) 0.3 mg/kg IM[334]	Nile crocodiles/anesthetic induction; decreased heart rate and respiratory rate
Ketamine (K)/ medetomidine (Me)/ midazolam (Mi)	(K) 5 mg/kg + (Me) 0.15 mg/kg + (Mi) 1 mg/kg SC[297]	Leopard tortoises/deep sedation
Ketamine (K)/ medetomidine (Me)/ morphine (Mo)	(K) 2.5 mg/kg + (Me) 0.15 mg/kg + (Mo) 1 mg/kg SC[298]	African spurred tortoises/deep sedation and analgesia
Ketamine (K)/ medetomidine (Me)/ tramadol (T)	(K) 5 mg/kg + (Me) 0.05 mg/kg + (T) 5 mg/kg IM[410]	Green sea turtles (hatchlings)/short-term anesthesia; reversed with atipamezole; apnea with normal blood gases
Ketamine (K)/ midazolam (Mi)	(K) 20 mg/kg + (Mi) 2 mg/kg IM[12] (K) 60 mg/kg + (Mi) 2 mg/kg IM[12]	Giant Amazon river turtles/sedation with both combinations; more rapid and prolonged sedation with higher K dosage
	(K) 20-40 mg/kg + (Mi) ≤2 mg/kg IM[40]	Snapping turtles/sedation; muscle relaxation
	(K) 60-80 mg/kg + (Mi) ≤2 mg/kg IM[63]	Chelonians/anesthesia; muscle relaxation
Ketamine (K)/propofol (P)	(K) 25-30 mg/kg IM + (P) 7 mg/kg IV[63,379]	Chelonians/administer propofol ≈70-80 min post-ketamine; see propofol
Ketamine (K)/xylazine (X)	(K) 10 mg/kg + (X) 1 mg/kg IM[422]	Snake species/induction for isoflurane anesthesia; drugs administered in front half of body
	(K) 120 mg/kg + (X) 1 mg/kg IM[3]	Caspian pond turtles/stage III anesthesia but prolonged recovery
	(K) 30 mg/kg + (X) 1 mg/kg IM[61]	Broad-snouted caiman juveniles/ provided mild sedation after either forelimb or hindlimb administration
Lidocaine (0.5-2%)	Local or topical[63]	Most species/local analgesia; infiltrate to effect (e.g., 0.01 mL 2% lidocaine used for local block for IO catheter placement in iguanas);[31] often used in conjunction with chemical immobilization
	4 mg/kg IM[124]	Bearded dragons; did not potentiate alfaxalone sedation but caused transient increased heart rate
	0.158 mg/cm intrathecal (combined with epinephrine hemitartrate)[410]	Green iguana/spinal anesthesia
	2 mg/kg intrathecal (IT)[123,294]	Turtles and tortoises/surgical analgesia/ anesthesia of caudal body; bearded dragons 50-75% success rate
	0.038 mL/kg (1 mL/ 20-25 kg)[394]	Hybrid Galapagos tortoises/surgical analgesia/ anesthesia for phallectomy

Continued

TABLE 4-5 Chemical Restraint/Anesthetic Agents Used in Reptiles. (cont'd)

Agent	Dosage	Species/Comments
Medetomidine[b]	—	Medetomidine is no longer commercially available, but can be compounded;[b] reverse with atipamezole; produces poor immobilization alone; see ketamine and butorphanol for combinations
	0.1-0.15 mg/kg IM[63]	Most species
	0.06-0.15 mg/kg[419]	Lizards
	0.15 mg/kg IM[435,436]	Desert tortoises, crocodilians/sedation; incomplete immobilization; generally produces bradycardia and bradypnea
	0.04-0.15 mg/kg IM[273]	Crocodilians/need to reverse
	0.13-0.17 mg/kg IM[355,356]	Crocodilians/moderate sedation; atipamezole (0.1 mg/kg IM) for reversal
	0.5-0.75 mg/kg IM[355,356]	Crocodilians/sedation only when administered in thoracic limb (versus pelvic limb and tail); atipamezole (2.5 mg/kg) reversal
Meperidine (Mp)/ midazolam (Mi)	(Mp) 1 mg/kg + (Mi) 1 mg/ kg IM[27]	Green sea turtles/premedication
Methohexital (Brevital, Lilly)	—	Recovery time of red-sided garter snakes at 21°C (70°F), 125 min; 26°C (79°F), 86 min; 31°C (88°F), 64 min; thinner snakes had longer recovery times; if within 5 wk of parturition, mean recovery time 2x as long as nongravid; time post-feeding had no effect at 1, 3, 10 days[375]
	5-20 mg/kg SC, IV[63]	Most species/induction, 5-30 min; recovery, 1-5 hr; use at 0.125-0.5% concentration; much species variability; decrease dose 20-30% for young animals; avoid use in debilitated animals
	9-10 mg/kg SC, ICe[347]	Colubrids/induction, ≥22 min; recovery, 2-5 hr; does not produce soft tissue irritation seen with other barbiturates; may need to adjust dosage in obese snakes
Metomidate	10 mg/kg IM[108]	Snakes/profound sedation; not available in the United States
Midazolam	—	See butorphanol, ketamine for combinations; can be reversed by flumazenil
	0.1-1 mg/kg[18]	Multiple species/mild to moderate sedation
	2 mg/kg IM[63,327]	Most species/preanesthetic; increases the efficacy of ketamine; effective in snapping turtles, not in painted turtles; ball pythons moderate, short-term sedation
	1 mg/kg IM[262]	Ball pythons/reduced MAC of isoflurane
	0.5-2 mg/kg IM[63]	Lizards
	1 mg/kg IM[41]	Black and white tegus/mild sedation without antinociception to a noxious thermal stimulus
	2 mg/kg IM[48]	Green iguanas/sedation

TABLE 4-5 Chemical Restraint/Anesthetic Agents Used in Reptiles. (cont'd)

Agent	Dosage	Species/Comments
Midazolam (cont'd)	0.5-1.5 mg/kg IN[114]	Indian star tortoises, red-footed tortoises/no significant sedation
	1.5 mg/kg IM[359]	Red-eared sliders/sedation; onset, 5.5 min; duration, 82 min; recovery, 40 min; much individual variability
	2-3 mg/kg IV[178]	Hatchling leatherback sea turtles/ sedation
Naloxone	0.04-2 mg/kg SC[432,434]	Corn snakes, bearded dragons, red-eared sliders/μ-opioid agonist reversal
	4 mg/kg IM[150]	Green tree monitors/reversal of butorphanol
Neostigmine	0.03-0.25 mg/kg IM[275] 0.063 mg/kg IV[275] 0.07-0.14 mg/kg IM[335]	Crocodiles/gallamine reversal; may cause emesis and lacrimation; fast 24-48 hr before use; effects enhanced if combined with 75 mg hyaluronidase per dose when administered SC, IM[275]
Nitrous oxide	50% admixed with isoflurane[262]	Ball pythons/minimal reduction in MAC of isoflurane
Pentobarbital	—	Rarely used as an anesthetic agent in reptiles
	15-30 mg/kg ICe[328]	Snakes/induction, 30-60 min; duration, ≥2 hr; prolonged recovery (risk of occasional fatalities); venomous snakes require twice as much as nonvenomous snakes; avoid use in lizards
	10-18 mg/kg ICe[328]	Chelonians
	7.5-15 mg/kg ICe, or 8 mg/kg IM[63,238]	Crocodilians
Propofol	—	If administered in supravertebral sinus, be aware for potential submeningeal delivery;[380] see ketamine for combination; anesthesia; rapid, smooth induction; may give 15-25 min anesthesia and restraint in most species; rapid, excitement-free recovery; must be administered IV (slowly) (no inflammation if goes perivascularly); may be administered IO; dosages may be reduced by as much as 50% in premedicated (e.g., ketamine) animals; may cause apnea and bradycardia; intubation and assisted ventilation generally required; considered by many to be parenteral agent of choice for inducing anesthesia
	0.3-0.5 mg/kg/min IV, IO constant rate infusion, or 0.5-1 mg/kg IV, IO periodic bolus[420]	Most species/maintenance anesthesia; must provide respiratory and thermal support
	5-10 mg/kg IV, intra-cardiac[15,63]	Snakes
	10 mg/kg intracardiac[320]	Ball pythons/anesthetic induction for isoflurane maintenance, but prolonged recovery; mild, resolving cardiac lesions

Continued

TABLE 4-5 Chemical Restraint/Anesthetic Agents Used in Reptiles. (cont'd)

Agent	Dosage	Species/Comments
Propofol (cont'd)	15 mg/kg IV[37]	South American rattlesnakes/ anesthetic induction
	3-5 mg/kg IV, IO[183]	Lizards (iguanas)/intubation and minor diagnostic procedures; may need to give an additional dose in 3-5 min; less cardiopulmonary depression than with higher doses
	5-10 mg/kg IV, IO[34]	Iguanas/higher dose is recommended for induction for short duration procedures or intubation
	10 mg/kg IV, IO[34,108,342]	Lizards, snakes/0.25 mg/kg/min may be given for maintenance;[243] green iguanas/anesthetic induction[342]
	2 mg/kg IV[63]	Giant tortoises
	3-5 mg/kg IV supravertebral sinus[128]	Chelonians/sedation (i.e., shell repair)
	5 mg/kg IV[162]	Snapping turtles/anesthetic induction
	10 mg/kg IV (supravertebral sinus)[502]	Red-eared sliders/40-85 min anesthesia
	12-15 mg/kg IV[105,446]	Chelonians/lower dosages (5-10 mg/kg IV) may be used; 1 mg/kg/min may be given for maintenance[63]
	20 mg/kg IV (supravertebral sinus)[502]	Red-eared sliders/60-120 min anesthesia
	10-15 mg/kg IV[273]	Crocodilians/duration, 0.5-1.5 hr; maintain on gas anesthetics; experimental IM with hyaluronidase
Rocuronium (Zemuron, Organon)	0.25-0.5 mg/kg IM[231]	Box turtles/neuromuscular blocking agent; no analgesia; for intubation only and small, non-painful procedures
Sevoflurane	To effect[63,399]	Most species/anesthesia; rapid induction and recovery when intubated
Succinylcholine	—	No analgesia; narrow margin of safety; generally not recommended, but included for completeness; intermittent positive pressure ventilation generally required; paralysis occurs in 5-30 min; avoid if exposed to organophosphate parasiticides within last 30 days; administer minimal amount required to perform procedure
	0.25-1 mg/kg IM[63]	Most species
	0.75-1 mg/kg IM[63]	Large lizards
	0.25-1.5 mg/kg IM[362]	Chelonians/induction, 15-30 min; recovery, 45-90 min; facilitates intubation
	0.5-1 mg/kg IM[63]	Box turtles/induction, 20-30 min
	0.25 mg/kg IM[260]	Crocodilians
	0.4-1 mg/kg IM[362]	Alligators/rapid onset; 3-5 mg/kg in smaller animals have been used

TABLE 4-5 Chemical Restraint/Anesthetic Agents Used in Reptiles. (cont'd)

Agent	Dosage	Species/Comments
Succinylcholine (cont'd)	0.5-5 mg/kg IM[63,272]	Crocodilians/variable induction and recovery periods
Thiopental	19-31 mg/kg IV[494]	Green sea turtles/anesthesia; induction, 5-10 min; recovery, <6 hr; erratic anesthesia
Tiletamine/zolazepam (Telazol, Fort Dodge)	—	Sedation, anesthesia; severe respiratory depression possible (may need to ventilate);[243] variable results; may have prolonged recovery; use lower end of dose range in heavier species; good for muscle relaxation prior to intubation;[130,386] other anesthetic agents may be preferable
	4-5 mg/kg SC, IM[63]	Most species/sedation; induction, 9-15 min; recovery, 1-12 hr; adequate for most non-invasive procedures
	5-10 mg/kg IM[63]	Most species
	3 mg/kg IM[243,388]	Snakes/facilitates handling and intubation of large snakes; induction, 30-45 min; prolonged recovery; ball pythons short-term anesthesia with prolonged recovery
	3-5 mg/kg IM[63]	Snakes, lizards/sedation
	10-30 mg/kg IM,[328] to 20-40 mg/kg IM[63,450]	Snakes, lizards/induction, 8-20 min; recovery, 2-10 hr; variable results; longer sedation and recovery times at 22°C (72°F) than at 30°C (86°F); good sedation in boa constrictors at 25 mg/kg IM; generally need to supplement with inhalation agents for surgical anesthesia; some snakes died at 55 mg/kg
	20 mg/kg SC, IM[365]	Bearded dragons/deeper sedation if administered IM compared to SC for minor procedures
	3.5-14 mg/kg IM[328] (generally 4-8 mg/kg)	Chelonians/sedation; induction, 8-20 min; does not produce satisfactory anesthesia even at 88 mg/kg[63]
	5-10 mg/kg IM, IV[63]	Large tortoises/facilitates intubation; if light, mask with isoflurane rather than redosing
	1-2 mg/kg IM[272]	Crocodilians/recovery takes several hours
	2-10 mg/kg IM[63]	Large crocodilians/may permit intubation
	5-10 mg/kg SC, IM, ICe (sedation), 10-40 mg/kg (anesthesia)[273]	Crocodilians
	15 mg/kg IM[79]	Alligators/induction, >20 min; adequate for minor procedures
Xylazine	—	Infrequently used; variable effects; potentially reversible with yohimbine; preanesthetic for ketamine; see ketamine for combination
	0.1-1.25 mg/kg IM, IV[63]	Most species

Continued

TABLE 4-5 Chemical Restraint/Anesthetic Agents Used in Reptiles. (cont'd)

Agent	Dosage	Species/Comments
Xylazine (cont'd)	0.1-1 mg/kg IM[272]	Crocodilians/atipamezole better reversal than yohimbine
	1-2 mg/kg IM[273]	Nile crocodiles
Yohimbine (Yobine, Lloyd)	—	Xylazine reversal; rarely indicated; atipameazole commonly used to reverse all α_2 agonists

[a]Refer to Table 4.7 for other preferred injectable sedation protocols used in reptiles.

[b]Medetomidine is no longer commercially available although it can be obtained from select compounding services; dosages are listed here as a guide for possible alternative use of dexmedetomidine, an α_2 agonist that is the active optical enantiomer of racemic compound medetomidine; dexmedetomidine is generally used at ½ the dose of medetomidine but the same volume due to equivalent concentrations of the active enantiomer; both compounds tend to have similar effects.

[c]Diazepam is not soluble in aquesous solution; admixing with aquesous solutions or fluids can result in precipitation; administering SC or IM can be painful and irritating; for SC or IM administration, midazolam may be preferred.

TABLE 4-6 Analgesic (Including Antiinflammatory) Agents Used in Reptiles.

Agent	Dosage	Species/Comments
Amitriptyline hydrochloride	3 mg/kg ICe[288]	Dampened the nociceptive response to SC formalin and capsaicin injections, but not a thermal noxious stimulus
Bupivacaine	1-2 mg/kg local q4-12h prn[63]	Most species/local anesthesia; 4 mg/kg maximum dose
	1 mg/kg intrathecal[294]	Turtles, tortoises/regional analgesia/anesthesia
Buprenorphine	0.2 mg/kg SC[300]	No evidence of analgesic efficacy in red-eared sliders or other reptile species
Butorphanol	—	Recent studies call into question use of particular doses or of this drug in general in providing analgesia in reptiles, including red-eared sliders, ball pythons, corn snakes, bearded dragons, green iguanas, and black and white tegus; respiratory depression is a common side effect [237,416,432-434]
	0.4-1 mg/kg SC, IM[63]	Most species/sedation; preanesthetic; 0.2 mg/kg IM used experimentally in tortoises[63]
	1 mg/kg IM[131]	Green iguanas/ineffective for analgesia; presence of observer may affect iguana response
	20 mg/kg SC[237]	Red-eared sliders/ineffective for surgical analgesia
Carprofen	1-4 mg/kg PO, SC, IM, IV q24h, follow with half the dose q24-72h[269,316]	Most species/nonsteroidal antiinflammatory; no efficacy data in any reptile species
Dexmedetomidine	0.1-0.2 mg/kg SC[51]	Ball pythons/hermal antinociception with minimal sedation
	0.2 mg/kg IM[41]	Black and white tegus/antinociception to thermal noxious stimulus

TABLE 4-6 Analgesic (Including Antiinflammatory) Agents Used in Reptiles. (cont'd)

Agent	Dosage	Species/Comments
Etodolac	5 mg/kg PO q72h x 30 days[361]	Komodo dragons
Fentanyl	Transdermal 12 µg/h[91]	Ball pythons/PK; transdermal analgesia; using a transdermal therapeutic system; therapeutic concentrations, as defined in mammals (1 ng/mL), were reached in 4 hr and sustained throughout the study; plasma levels were higher than in mammals suggesting the potential to use smaller dosages; no adverse effects noted
	12 µg/h transdermal patch to cranial epaxial muscles[235]	Ball pythons/high plasma concentrations (above analgesic threshold in mammals); analgesic efficacy not proven in any snake species, but anecdotal evidence from certain snake clinical cases demonstrated improved condition after application of patch
	10 µg/kg/h IO constant rate infusion[426]	Bearded dragon/administered during surgical procedure
	12 µg/h transdermal patch to caudodorsal lumbar region[146]	Prehensile-tailed skinks/no side-effects reported after 24 hr when skink blood levels reached human therapeutic levels; environmental temperature can significantly affect absorption
	0.05 mg/kg SC[227]	Slider turtle species (*Trachemys dorbigni*, *Trachemys scripta elegans*); antinociceptive to interdigital forceps pinch
Flunixin meglumine	0.1-0.5 mg/kg IM q12-24h[269]	Most species/nonsteroidal antiinflammatory; use for maximum of 3 days; no evidence of efficacy
	0.5-2 mg/kg IM q12-24h[63]	Most species/nonsteroidal antiinflammatory; no evidence of efficacy
	1-2 mg/kg IM q24h x 2 treatments[441]	Lizards/post-surgical nonsteroidal antiinflammatory; no evidence of efficacy
Flurbiprofen sodium	Ophthalmic solution (0.03%); 1 drop topically in affected eye q6-12h[243]	Empirical use as a nonsteroidal antiinflammatory; some recommend q12-24h
Hydromorphone	0.5-1 mg/kg SC q24h[300]	Red-eared sliders/analgesia
	0.5 mg/kg SC[180a]	Bearded dragons, red-eared sliders/PK; determined administration frequency of q24h (bearded dragons) and q12-24h (red-eared sliders)
Ketoprofen	—	Nonsteroidal antiinflammatory
	2 mg/kg PO, SC, IM q24-48h[280,471]	Most species, green iguanas/[PK], loggerhead sea turtles/frequently used due to historical evidence of safety; no efficacy data
	2 or 20 mg/kg IM q24h × 14 days[475a]	Bearded dragons/safety; 2 mg/kg IM q24h x 14 days caused no changes in plasma biochemical or histologic parameters of renal, gastrointestinal, hepatic, or muscular systems; 20 mg/kg IM q24h x 14 days caused severe muscle necrosis of triceps but no other biologic changes; fecal occult blood was negative and clotting times were unaffected at either dosage

Continued

TABLE 4-6 Analgesic (Including Antiinflammatory) Agents Used in Reptiles. (cont'd)

Agent	Dosage	Species/Comments
Ketoprofen (cont'd)	2 mg/kg IM, IV[467]	Loggerhead sea turtles/PK; study demonstrated a single IM or IV dose had a 24 hr duration
	2 mg/kg IM q24h × up to 5 days[179]	Loggerhead sea turtles/analgesia; dosage appears safe with respect to blood clotting and blood data
Ketorolac	0.25 mg/kg IM[70]	Eastern box turtles/PK; study demonstrated a single dose had a 24 hr duration
Lidocaine (0.5-2%)	2-5 mg/kg local[63]	Most species/10 mg/kg maximum dosage
	Local or topical[63]	Most species/local analgesia; infiltrate to effect (e.g., 0.01 mL 2% lidocaine used for local block for IO catheter placement in iguanas); often used in conjunction with chemical immobilization
	0.2 mL/10 cm carapace length intrathecal[141]	Green sea turtles/cutaneous fibropapilloma excision; effective clinical analgesia
	4 mg/kg intrathecal[294]	Turtles, tortoises/regional analgesia
Lidocaine (L)/ morphine (Mo)	(L) 2 mg/kg + (Mo) 0.1 mg/kg intrathecal[378]	Desert tortoises/orchiectomy analgesia
Meloxicam	0.1-0.5 mg/kg PO, SC q24-48h[63]	Most species
	0.3 mg/kg IM q24h[354]	Ball pythons/physiologic changes not consistent with analgesia
	0.2 mg/kg PO, IV q24h[110]	Green iguanas/PK; no evidence of efficacy
	0.1 mg/kg IM, IV q24h[257]	Loggerhead sea turtles/PK; plasma concentrations not consistent with analgesia
	0.1-0.2 mg/kg PO, IM q24h x 4-10 days[128]	Chelonians/no evidence of efficacy
	0.2 mg/kg IM, IV;[472] SC q24h[377,378]	Red-eared sliders/PK; plasma concentrations consistent with therapeutic efficacy for 48 hr by IM and IV administration routes;[472] Mojave desert tortoises, post surgical nonsteroidal antiinflammatory
	0.2-0.4 mg/kg IM q24h[212]	Red-eared slider turtles, Eastern painted turtles, yellow-spotted Amazon river turtles, other undocumented turtle species/nonsteroidal anti-inflammatory; no evidence of efficacy
	0.5 mg/kg PO, IM q24h or 0.22 mg/kg IV q24h[398]	Red-eared sliders/PK; found better absorption IM vs PO;[398] after IV administration, plasma levels decreased rapidly and the elimination half-life was 7.57 hr
	1 mg/kg SC[349]	Kemp's ridleys, green sea turtles/PK; resulted in plasma concentrations >0.5 µg/mL for 12 hr for Kemp's ridleys and 120 hr for greens; administration of 2 mg/kg SC to loggerhead sea turtles resulted in adequate plasma concentrations for only 4 hr
Meperidine	5-10 mg/kg IM q12-24h[63]	Most species/analgesia; no noticeable effect in snakes even at 200 mg/kg
	20 mg/kg IM q12-24h[269]	Most species/analgesia
	2-4 mg/kg ICe q6-8h[63]	Lizards

TABLE 4-6 Analgesic (Including Antiinflammatory) Agents Used in Reptiles. (cont'd)

Agent	Dosage	Species/Comments
Meperidine (cont'd)	1-5 mg/kg IM q6-12h[229,431,480]	Turtles, crocodiles/analgesic efficacy of short duration
	2-4 mg/kg q6-12h ICe[63]	Nile crocodiles/analgesia
Methadone	3-5 mg/kg SC, IM q24h[86,431]	Aquatic turtles/analgesia
Morphine	—	No effective dose for analgesia documented in corn snakes[434]
	0.1-0.2 mg/kg intrathecal[115]	Black and white tegus
	5-10 mg/kg SC[270]	Black and white tegus/antinociceptive using a thermal noxious stimulus
	10 mg/kg IM q24h[434,488]	Bearded dragons/analgesia; ball pythons/no analgesia
	0.1-0.2 mg/kg intrathecal[294]	Turtles, tortoises/thermal analgesia for 48 hr; regional analgesia caudal body
	1 mg/kg IM q24h[212]	Red-eared sliders, Eastern painted turtle, yellow-spotted Amazon river turtle, other undocumented turtle species/analgesia
	1.5-6.5 mg/kg SC, IM q24h[431,432,434]	Red-eared sliders (long lasting respiratory depression), freshwater crocodiles, *Anolis* lizards/ may be effective thermal analgesia
	2 mg/kg SC q24h[237]	Red-eared sliders/surgical analgesia
	10 mg/kg IM[85]	Bearded dragons/antinociceptive using a thermal noxious stimulus
	0.5-4 mg/kg ICe q24h[436]	Crocodilians/analgesia
Naloxone	0.04-2 mg/kg SC[431,432,434]	Red-eared sliders, bearded dragons, corn snakes/μ-opioid agonist reversal
Oxymorphone	0.025-0.1 mg/kg IV[63] 0.05-0.2 mg/kg SC, IM q12-48h[63] 0.5-1.5 mg/kg IM[63]	Some species/analgesia; no efficacy studies; avoid in cases with hepatic or renal dysfunction; no noticeable effect in snakes, even at 1.5 mg/kg[63] See above
Pethidine	—	See meperidine
Prednisolone	2-5 mg/kg PO, IM q24-48h[269]	Most species/antiinflammatory
Proparacaine (0.5%)	Topical to eye[163,283,405,421]	Iguanas/desensitizes surface of eye; ineffective in animals with spectacles; bearded dragons/IOP by rebound tonometry;[421] Kemp's ridley sea turtles/ one drop provided 45 min duration of action;[163] do not exceed toxic dose 2 mg/kg;[63] Yacare caiman/ IOP by applanation tonometry[405]
Tapentadol	10 mg/kg IM q48-72h[156,157]	Red-eared sliders, yellow-bellied sliders/ analgesia

Continued

TABLE 4-6 Analgesic (Including AntiInflammatory) Agents Used in Reptiles. (cont'd)

Agent	Dosage	Species/Comments
Tramadol	11 mg/kg PO[166]	Bearded dragons
	5-10 mg/kg PO, SC q48-72h[22]	Red-eared sliders, sea turtles/thermal analgesia; higher doses may affect ventilation
	5-10 mg/kg PO q72h[350]	Loggerhead sea turtles/PK; plasma concentrations consistent with efficacy for 48 hr (5 mg/kg PO) or 72 hr (10 mg/kg PO)
	10 mg/kg PO q48-72h[437]	Turtles, tortoises/analgesia
	10 mg/kg IM q48-72h[159]	Yellow-bellied sliders/PK and PD comparing forelimb and hindlimb administration; analgesia; plasma concentrations consistent with analgesia in both forelimb and hindlimb

TABLE 4-7 Preferred Injectable Sedation Protocols Used in Select Reptiles.[301,400,430]

There are many individual and species differences with respect to sedative efficacy, so these combinations can be adjusted based on personal experience with individual reptile patients.
Most combinations listed are partially or fully reversible.

Snakes

A general note about snake sedation: there is recent published and anecdotal evidence that some snake species (e.g., ball pythons [*Python regius*]),[262] administered midazolam will renarcotize after administration of flumazenil: these snakes should be monitored and, if necessary, administered an additional dose of flumazenil.

Drug Protocol	Dose & Route	Comments
Alfaxalone	10-30 mg/kg SC, IM, IV	Rapid sedation if administered IV; higher doses can contribute to a surgical plane of anesthesia; not reversible
Alfaxalone (A) + midazolam (Mi)	(A) 5 mg/kg + (Mi) 0.5 mg/kg SC, IM	Moderate sedation; antagonize midazolam
Dexmedetomidine[a] (De) + ketamine (K)	(De) 0.1 mg/kg + (K) 10 mg/kg SC, IM	Moderate-to-deep sedation; antagonize dexmedetomidine
Dexmedetomidine[a] (De) + ketamine (K) + midazolam (Mi)	(De) 0.1 mg/kg + (K) 5-10 mg/kg + (Mi) 1 mg/kg SC, IM	Deep sedation; antagonize dexmedetomidine and midazolam
Dexmedetomidine[a] (De) + ketamine (K) + fentanyl (F)	(De) 0.1 mg/kg + (K) 10 mg/kg + (F) 12 mcg/h patch (snakes less than 5 kg)	Deep sedation with potential long-term analgesia; antagonize dexmedetomidine

TABLE 4-7 Preferred Injectable Sedation Protocols Used in Select Reptiles. (cont'd)

Lizards

Drug Protocol	Dose & Route	Comments
Alfaxalone	10-30 mg/kg SC, IM, IV	Rapid sedation if administered IV; higher doses can contribute to a surgical plane of anesthesia; not reversible
Dexmedetomidine[a] (De) + ketamine (K)	(De) 0.1 mg/kg + (K) 5-10 mg/kg SC, IM	Moderate sedation, which is deeper with the higher dose of ketamine; dexmedetomidine antagonized with atipamezole
Dexmedetomidine[a] (De) + midazolam (Mi)	(De) 0.1 mg/kg + (Mi) 1 mg/kg SC, IM	Moderate sedation; antagonize with atipamezole and flumazenil
Dexmedetomidine[a] (De) + ketamine (K) + midazolam (Mi)	(De) 0.05-0.1 mg/kg + (K) 5 mg/kg + (Mi) 1 mg/kg SC, IM	Moderate-to-deep sedation; antagonize dexmedetomidine and midazolam
Dexmedetomidine[a] (De) + midazolam (Mi) + hydromorphone (H)	(De) 0.05 mg/kg + (Mi) 1 mg/kg + (H) 0.5 mg/kg SC, IM	Deep sedation with analgesia
Dexmedetomidine[a] (De) + midazolam (Mi) + morphine (Mo)	(De) 0.05 mg/kg + (Mi) 1 mg/kg + (Mo) 2 mg/kg SC, IM	Deep sedation with analgesia

Chelonians

A general note about chelonian sedation, particularly tortoise species: anecdotally, some species of tortoises (or some individuals) are quite resistant to typical sedation protocols. All combinations should be administered in front half of body for best results.

Drug Protocol	Dose & Route	Comments
Dexmedetomidine[a] (De) + ketamine (K)	(De) 0.1 mg/kg + (K) 10 mg/kg SC, IM	Moderate sedation; dexmedetomidine antagonized with atipamezole
Dexmedetomidine[a] (De) + ketamine (K) + midazolam (Mi)	(De) 0.1 mg/kg + (K) 5-10 mg/kg + (Mi) 1 mg/kg SC, IM	Deeper sedation than dexmedetomidine and ketamine alone; use atipamezole and flumazenil to antagonize dexmedetomidine and midazolam, respectively
Dexmedetomidine[a] (De) + alfaxalone (A)	(De) 0.1 mg/kg + (A) 5-10 mg/kg SC, IM	Moderate sedation; dexmedetomidine antagonized with atipamzole
Dexmedetomidine[a] (De) + ketamine (K) + hydromorphone (H)	(De) 0.1 mg/kg + (K) 5 mg/kg + (H) 0.5 mg/kg SC, IM	Moderate-to-deep sedation; good analgesia for more painful procedures
Dexmedetomidine[a] (De) + ketamine (K) + morphine (Mo)	(De) 0.1 mg/kg + (K) 5 mg/kg + (Mo) 1.5 mg/kg SC, IM	Moderate-to-deep sedation; good analgesia for more painful procedures

Continued

TABLE 4-7 Preferred Injectable Sedation Protocols Used in Select Reptiles. (cont'd)

Crocodilians		
Drug Protocol	**Dose & Route**	**Comments**
Dexmedetomidine[a] (De) + ketamine (K)	(De) 0.1 mg/kg + (K) 10 mg/kg SC, IM	Moderate sedation; rapid recovery after atipamzole reversal
Dexmedetomidine[a] (De) + ketamine (K) + midazolam (Mi)	(De) 0.1 mg/kg + (K) 5 mg/kg + (Mi) 1 mg/kg SC, IM	Moderate-to-deep sedation; antagonize dexmedetomidine and midazolam
Dexmedetomidine[a] (De) + ketamine (K) + hydromorphone (H)	(De) 0.1 mg/kg + (K) 5 mg/kg + (H) 0.5 mg/kg SC, IM	Moderate-to-deep sedation with analgesia; antagonize dexmedetomidine
Dexmedetomidine[a] (De) + ketamine (K) + morphine (Mo)	(De) 0.1 mg/kg + (K) 5 mg/kg + (Mo) 2 mg/kg SC, IM	Moderate-to-deep sedation with analgesia; antagonize dexmedetomidine
Tiletamine/zolazepam (Telazol)	5-15 mg/kg SC, IM	Moderate-to-deep sedation; prolonged recoveries

Abbreviations: IM=intramuscular; SC=subcutaneous; TC=transcutaneous.

[a]Medetomidine can be substituted for dexmedetomdine in any protocol listed, but the dose should be 1.5 to 2 times the dexmedetomidine dose. When using medetomidine, increasing ketamine dose may be helpful. Atipamzole is typically administered at the same volume or 10 times the dose of dexmedetomidine; or the same volume or 5 times the dose of medetomidine. Flumazenil antagonizes midazolam and is typically dosed at 0.05 mg/kg SC or IM. In cases in which morphine or hydromorphone needs reversing, administer naloxone (0.2 mg/kg) SC or IM.

TABLE 4-8 Hormones and Steroids Used in Reptiles.

Agent	Dosage	Species/Comments
Arginine vasotocin (AVT) (Sigma Chemical)	0.01-1 µg/kg IV (preferred), ICe[274] q12-24h × several treatments	Most species/dystocias; administer 30-60 min after Ca lactate/Ca glycerophosphate; more effective in reptiles than oxytocin but not commercially available for use in animals; higher doses have been reported; 0.5 µg/kg commonly recommended

TABLE 4-8 Hormones and Steroids Used in Reptiles. (cont'd)

Agent	Dosage	Species/Comments
Calcitonin	1.5 U/kg SC q8h × 14-21 days prn[63]	Most species (e.g., iguanas)/ severe nutritional secondary hyperparathyroidism; administer after Ca supplementation; do not give if hypocalcemic
	50 U/kg IM, repeat in 14 days[63]	
	50 U/kg q7d × 2-3 doses[281]	Green iguanas/salmon calcitonin; do not give if hypocalcemic
Deslorelin acetate	—	No success with use in female reptile reproductive disease or cessation of normal egg production[67]
	4.75 mg implant SC[404]	Bearded dragons/abnormal aggression in juveniles; decreased serum testosterone; behavior ceased
Dexamethasone	0.2 mg/kg IM, IV q24h x 3 days[243]	Most species/laryngeal or pharyngeal edema and inflammation
	0.6-1.25 mg/kg IM, IV[63]	Most species/shock (septic/traumatic)
	2-4 mg/kg IM, IV, IO q24h x 3 days[395]	Most species
	0.3-1.5 mg/kg IM, IV, IO[222]	Chelonians/hyperthermia
Dexamethasone sodium phosphate	0.1-0.25 mg/kg SC, IM, IV[63]	Most species/shock (septic/traumatic)
Insulin	1-5 U/kg IM, ICe q24-72h[443]	Snakes, chelonians/doses are empirical and must be adjusted based on response to therapy and serial blood glucose; doses administered ICe may take 24-48 hr before a response is noted
	5-10 U/kg IM, ICe q24-72h[443]	Lizards, crocodilians/see above
Leuprolide acetate (Lupron Depot 1.875 mg/mL, Abbott)	0.4 mg/kg IM[239]	Iguanas/did not suppress testosterone levels in males
Levothyroxine	0.02 mg/kg PO q48h[172]	Geckos/post thyroidectomy; lifetime management
	0.02 mg/kg PO q48h[351]	Tortoises/hypothyroidism; stimulates feeding in debilitated tortoises
	0.025 mg/kg q24h in AM[137]	Tortoises/monitor T_4 levels
Methylprednisolone	1 mg/kg IV q24h[222]	Chelonians/ivermectin toxicity
Nandrolone (Deca-Durabolin, Organon)	0.5-5 mg/kg IM q7-28d[63]	Most species/hepatic lipidosis
	1 mg/kg IM q7-28d[63]	Lizards/anabolic steroid; reduces protein catabolism; may stimulate erythropoiesis

Continued

TABLE 4-8 Hormones and Steroids Used in Reptiles. (cont'd)

Agent	Dosage	Species/Comments
Oxytocin	—	Dystocias; results are variable; works well in chelonians, less so in snakes and lizards; generally administer 1 hr after Ca administration; use multiple doses with caution
	1-10 U/kg IM[63,243]	Most species/higher end of the range is commonly used; may be repeated up to 3 treatments at 90 min intervals with increasing dosage[209]
	2 U/kg IM q4-6h × 1-3 treatments[17]	Most species
	1-5 U/kg IM, repeat in 1 hr[104]	Lizards/alternatively, 5 U/kg by slow IV or IO over 4-8 hr
	1-2,[47] 2-20,[311] or 10-20[63] U/kg IM	Chelonians
	1-20 U/kg IM q90min × 3 treatments at increased doses, or 50%-100% first dose 1-12 hr later, or IO drip[456]	Chelonians
	2 U/kg IV q2h[102]	Red-eared sliders/faster onset vs IM; fewer animals required 2nd or 3rd doses vs IM route
Prednisolone	2-5 mg/kg PO, IM q12-24h[63]	Most species/analgesia (chronic pain)
	0.5 mg/kg q24h PO, SC, IM × 14 days, then q48h until PCV stable[243]	Lizards/autoimmune hemolytic anemia
	4 mg/kg q12h[161]	Parson's chameleon/autoimmune hemolytic anemia; blood transfusion from sibling; iatrogenic osteomyelitis
Prednisolone Na succinate (Solu-Delta Cortef, Pharmacia & Upjohn)	5-10 mg/kg IM, IV, IO[106]	Most species/shock; brain swelling from hyperthermia; may help reduce nephrocalcinosis
Prednisone	0.5-1 mg/kg PO, SC, IM, IV[63]	Most species/lymphoma, leukemia, myeloproliferative disease
	0.8 mg/kg q48h[150]	Most species/chronic T-lymphocytic leukemia; may combine with chlorambucil, but need to monitor uric acid levels
Stanozolol (Winstrol-V, Winthrop)	5 mg/kg IM q7d prn[63]	Most species/anabolic steroid; management of catabolic disease states

TABLE 4-9 Nutritional/Mineral/Fluid Support Used in Reptiles.[a]

Agent	Dosage	Species/Comments
Calcium	PO prn[111]	Most species/dietary sources include crushed cuttlebone, oyster shell, egg shell, tablets of Ca salts, or other commercially available products
Calcium carbonate (Rep-Cal, Rep-Cal Labs; Repti Calcium, Zoo Med; Fluker's powdered or liquid forms of calcium)	PO prn[111]	Omnivores, herbivores, insectivores/dietary Ca supplement
Calcium glubionate (Neo-Calglucon, Sandoz; Calciquid, Breckenridge Pharmaceuticals; Calcionate, Rugby)	10 mg/kg PO q12-24h prn[63]	All species/nutritional secondary hyperparathyroidism
	25-50 mg/kg PO q24h prn[296]	All species/nutritional secondary hyperparathyroidism
	360 mg/kg (1 mL/kg) PO q12-24h prn[32]	Most species/nutritional secondary hyperparathyroidism; hypocalcemia; dystocia; ensure adequate UVB exposure and proper nutrition
Calcium gluconate	50-100 mg/kg SC, IM, IV[296]	Most species/hypocalcemia (low ionized Ca); hypocalcemic muscle tremors, seizures, dystocia, or flaccid paresis in lizards; when patient is stable, switch to oral Ca; should be diluted in fluids
	100 mg/kg SC, IM, ICe q6-24h[32,316]	Most species/hypocalcemia (low ionized Ca); hypocalcemic muscle tremors, seizures, dystocia, or flaccid paresis in lizards; when patient is stable, switch to oral Ca
Calcium gluconate/ borogluconate	10-50 mg/kg SC, IM[63]	Most species/hypocalcemia; hypocalcemic dystocia
Calcium glycerophosphate/ calcium lactate (Calphosan, Glenwood)	1-5 mg/kg SC, IM[63]	Most species/hypocalcemia; hypocalcemic dystocia
	10 mg/kg SC, IM, ICe q24h x 1-7 days[63]	Lizards (iguanas)/hypocalcemia
Carnivore Care (Oxbow Animal Health)	10-20 mL/kg PO or via gavage/ esophagostomy q24-48h[63]	Carnivores/short-term nutritional support; anorexia; prepare according to directions; begin after rehydration and stable condition; more dilute in first feeding after anorexia, gradually increase concentration over 3-5 days
	30 mL/kg (3% of body weight) PO or via gavage/ esophagostomy q24h;[96] range of 2%-10% body weight PO or via gavage/esophagostomy q24h[296]	Carnivores

Continued

TABLE 4-9 Nutritional/Mineral/Fluid Support Used in Reptiles. (cont'd)

Agent	Dosage	Species/Comments
Clinicare Canine-Feline Liquid Diet (Zoetis)	Gavage prn[495]	Not a primary choice for feeding debilitated reptiles; most species/post omphalectomy; use Canine Formula for herbivores and omnivores, and Feline Formula for carnivores; initially dilute 1:1 with water and gradually increase to full strength over 48 hr; generally precede nutritional supplementation with 48-96 hr of water or electrolyte solution PO
Critical Care for Herbivores (Oxbow Animal Health)	10-20 mL/kg PO or via gavage/ esophagostomy q24-48h[63]	Herbivores/long-term nutritional support; prepare according to directions; begin after rehydration and stable condition
	30 mL/kg (3% of body weight) PO or via gavage/ esophagostomy q24h;[96] range of 2-10% body weight PO or via gavage/esophagostomy q24h[296]	Herbivores
Dextrose in water (2.5%, 5%)	PO, SC, IV, IO, ICe, EpiCe, prn[238]	All species/hyperkalemia; can mix with electrolye solutions
	Calculated water deficit IV, IO[63]	Most species/for intracellular rehydration when mentation is altered and plasma Na >160 mEq/L; for acute Na toxicosis, replace deficit in 12-24 hr; for chronic dehydration, slowly replace deficit over 48-72 hr
EmerAid Intensive Care Carnivore (Lafeber)	1st feed = 0.5% BW; 2nd feed = 1% BW; 3rd feed = 2% BW	Carnivores/nutritional support, severely debilitated, cachectic patients; prepare according to directions; use when hydrated and stable condition; greater dilution in first few feedings
	5-30 mL/kg gavage or esophagostomy tube q24-72h[63]	Carnivores
	3% BW PO or via gavage/ esophagostomy q24h;[96] range of 2-10% BW PO or via gavage/ esophagostomy q24h[296]	Carnivores
EmerAid Intensive Care Herbivore (Lafeber)	1st feed = 0.5% BW; 2nd feed = 1% BW; 3rd feed = 2% BW	Herbivores/nutritional support, severely debilitated, cachectic patients; prepare according to directions; use when hydrated and stable condition; greater dilution in first few feedings
	5-20 mL/kg gavage or esophagostomy tube q12-48h[63]	Herbivores
	3% BW PO or via gavage/ esophagostomy q24h;[96] range of 2-10% BW PO or via gavage/ esophagostomy q24h[296]	Herbivores

TABLE 4-9 Nutritional/Mineral/Fluid Support Used in Reptiles. (cont'd)

Agent	Dosage	Species/Comments
EmerAid Sustain Herbivore (Lafeber)	30 mL/kg BW daily	Herbivores/nutritional support for less debilitated patients; prepare according to directions; use when hydrated and stable condition; greater dilution in first few feedings
Emeraid Intensive Care Omnivore (Lafeber)	1st feed = 0.5% BW; 2nd feed = 1% BW; 3rd feed = 2% BW	Most species/nutritional support, severely debilitated, cachectic patients; prepare according to directions; use when hydrated and stable condition; greater dilution in first few feedings
	5-20 mL/kg gavage or esophagostomy tube q12-48h[63]	Omnivores
	3% BW PO or via gavage/ esophagostomy q24h;[96] range of 2-10% BW PO or via gavage/ esophagostomy q24h[296]	Omnivores
Hydroxyethyl starch (Hetastarch, HES)	3-5 mL/kg slow IV or IO bolus prn[63]	All species/hypoalbuminemia; hypovolemic perfusion deficits; increased capillary permeability; use with crystalloids; reduce crystalloid volume 40%-60%; max volume 20 mL/kg
Iodine	2-4 mg/kg PO q24h × 14-21 days, then q7d[63]	Herbivores/iodine deficiency (i.e., goiter); use in species fed a goitrogenic diet; can use a multivitamin-mineral mixture or iodized salt; suggested daily dietary iodine 0.03 mg/kg BW[111]
Iron dextran	12 mg/kg IM 1-2 ×/wk x 45 days[455]	Crocodilians/iron deficiency; in other species for anemia[63]
Lactated Ringer's solution (LRS)	15-40 mL/kg SC, IV, IO prn[63]	Land turtles/fluid replacement; use extracoelomically after warming the patient; avoid lactate if hepatic insufficiency
LRS + 0.9% saline (1:1 solution)	20 mL/kg/day ICe[60]	Loggerhead sea turtles/highest percentage of acid-base recovery and electrolyte balance compared to LRS, saline, or 5% dextrose in saline (1:1)
Maintenance crystalloid solution: ½-strength LRS and 2.5% dextrose	SC, IV, IO, ICe, EpiCe prn[63]	All species/maintenance fluid therapy after losses have been replaced
Multivitamin Products (ReptiVite, Zoo Med; Herptivite, RepCal; Repta-Vitamin, Fluker's; Exo-Terra; Nekton)	Dust on vegetables, fruits, or insects q84-168h[439]	Herbivores, omnivores, insectivores/pre-formed vitamin A; minerals; multivitamin
Replacement crystalloid solutions (Normosol-R, Ceva; Plasma-Lyte, Baxter)	15-25 mL/kg/d PO, SC, IV, IO, ICe, EpiCe prn[63]	All species/replacement fluid therapy; warm to 29°C (84°F)[243]
	10-30 mL/kg q24h or divided into 2-3 boluses several hr apart[238]	All species/ongoing regurgitation or severe diarrhea

Continued

TABLE 4-9 Nutritional/Mineral/Fluid Support Used in Reptiles. (cont'd)

Agent	Dosage	Species/Comments
Ringer's solution for reptiles: 1 part Normosol-R + 2 parts 2.5% dextrose in 0.45% saline or, 1 part Normosol-R + 1 part 5% dextrose + 1 part 0.9% saline	10-20 mL/kg q24h[63]	All species/hypertonic dehydration or to prevent nephrotoxicity due to aminoglycosides
	15 (large reptiles) to 25 (small reptiles) mL/kg q24h or divided into 2 doses per day[63]	All species/hypertonic dehydration; warm fluids to 28°C (82°F)
	20 mL/kg q12h[63]	Chelonians/severe dehydration
Selenium	0.028 mg/kg IM[63]	Lizards/deficiency; myopathy
Sodium chloride (0.45%)	PO, SC, IV, IO, ICe, EpiCe, prn[238]	All species/hypertonic dehydration; correct deficits over 3 days
Sodium chloride (0.9%)	SC, IV, IO, ICe, EpiCe, prn[63,238]	All species/hyperkalemia, hypercalcemia, hypochloremic metabolic alkalosis; can mix with other crystalloid solutions, particularly 5% dextrose; use SC, ICe, EpiCe routes after patient is warm
Vitamin A	—	Overdose causes epidermal sloughing; greater risk with aqueous parenteral formulation; for less severe cases, commercial formulated diets or reptile multivitamin supplements may suffice;[63,111,329] may help infectious stomatitis
	2000 U/kg PO, SC, IM q7-14d x 2-4 treatments[63]	Most species/hypovitaminosis A
	2000 U/30 g BW PO once, repeat in 7 days[175,439]	Chameleons/eye swelling, respiratory disease, hemipenile plugs, dysecdysis
	200-300 U/kg SC, IM[111]	Turtles/hypovitaminosis A; give in conjunction with PO vitamin A (2-8 U/g feed DM)
Vitamins A, D_3, E (Vital E+A+D, Stuart Products)	0.15 mL/kg IM, repeat in 21 days[63]	Most species/hypovitaminosis A, D_3, or E; product contains alcohol and may sting when administered; a product without alcohol can be compounded commercially
	0.3 mL/kg PO, then 0.06 mL/kg q7d x 3-4 treatments[63]	Box turtles/hypovitaminosis A; parenteral use may result in hypervitaminosis A and D; given PO may enhance Ca uptake
Vitamin B complex	0.3 mL/kg SC, IM q24h[63]	Most species/anorexia; hypovitaminosis B; use with caution as B_6 toxicity may occur
	25 mg thiamine/kg PO q24h x 3-7 days[63]	Most species/appetite stimulant; hypovitaminosis B
Vitamin B_1 (thiamine)	50-100 mg/kg PO, SC, IM q24h[59]	Piscivores/thiamine deficiency from thawed fish
	30 g/kg feed fish PO[63]	Crocodilians/treat or prevent deficiency
Vitamin B_{12} (cyanocobalamin)	0.05 mg/kg SC, IM[63]	Snakes, lizards/appetite stimulant

TABLE 4-9 Nutritional/Mineral/Fluid Support Used in Reptiles. (cont'd)

Agent	Dosage	Species/Comments
Vitamin C	10-20 mg/kg SC, IM q24h[138,322]	All species/empirical for hypovitaminosis C; stomatitis; skin slough in snakes; supportive therapy for bacterial infections
Vitamin D_3	—	Nutritional secondary hyperparathyroidism; hypocalcemia; deficiency and excess may result in soft tissue calcification
	1000 U/kg IM, repeat in 1 wk[63]	Most species/deficiency; use with oral calcium glubionate and carbonate, general dietary management, and UVB irradiation
	200 U/kg PO, IM q7d[32]	Lizards/PO may be safer than IM, but absorption is poor in some species[36,358]
	400 U/kg IM q7d x 3 treatments[284]	Green iguanas/nutritional secondary hyperparathyroidism; may use with calcitonin after normocalcemic; also supplement oral calcium
Vitamin E/selenium (L-Se, Schering)	1 U vitamin E/kg IM[111]	Piscivores/hypovitaminosis E; myopathy, anorexia, swollen subcutaneous nodules
	50 U vitamin E/kg + 0.025 mg selenium/kg IM[121]	Lizards/hypovitaminosis E (vitamin E/ selenium)
Vitamin K_1	0.25-0.5 mg/kg IM[63]	Most species/hypovitaminosis K_1; coagulopathies

BW: Body weight.
[a]Also see Table 4-23.

TABLE 4-10 Euthanasia Methods Used in Reptiles.[13]

When euthanizing reptiles, it is important to confirm that the heart has fully stopped functioning after applying the euthanasia technique. This is best accomplished by placing a Doppler flow probe over the heart of the reptile or using electrocardiography.

Acceptable Methods	Agents	Comments
Injectable agents	Sodium pentobarbital (most solutions contain phenytoin sodium as well; 60-100 mg/kg [≈1 mL/5 kg] IV, IC, IO, ICe)	Sedate using tiletamine-zolazepam (20-50 mg/kg SC, IM), alfaxalone (30-50 mg/kg SC, IM) or other anesthetic/analgesic prior to administering pentobarbital solution; if administering ICe, dilute pentobarbital solution by approximately 80% due to high pH of most commercial solutions
	Potassium chloride (75-150 mg/kg IV, IC, IO)	Imperative to sedate using tiletamine-zolazepam (20-50 mg/kg IM) or other anesthetic/analgesic prior to administering; unacceptable use in conscious reptiles; useful when sodium pentobarbital is unavailable or if deceased reptile's body has potential to be consumed by wildlife after euthanasia

Continued

TABLE 4-10 Euthanasia Methods Used in Reptiles. (cont'd)

Acceptable Methods	Agents	Comments
Inhaled agents	Carbon dioxide gas	While considered acceptable, injectable methods are preferred due to prolonged exposure time and potential animal distress; personnel exposure also an issue
Physical	Captive bolt or gunshot	While these are considered acceptable methods, they are not preferred; typically only used in crocodilians or other large species; knowledge of appropriate anatomic sites is imperative
Adjunctive Methods		
Physical	2-step process: sedation/ analgesia followed by decapitation or pithing	Decapitation following heavy sedation/ analgesia is acceptable in small- to medium-sized reptiles; decapitation is unacceptable in conscious reptiles; this procedure is commonly used when the brain needs preserving for research
	2-step process: sedation/ analgesia followed by exsanguination	Exsanguination following heavy sedation/ analgesia is acceptable in small-to medium-sized reptiles; exsanguination is unacceptable in conscious reptiles
Unacceptable Methods		
Physical	Hypothermia or freezing	There is no concrete evidence that reptiles exposed to freezing temperature do not experience pain and distress

Abbreviations: IV=Intravenous; IC=intracardiac; ICe=intracoelomic; IO=intraosseous; IM=intramuscular; SC=subcutaneous.

TABLE 4-11 Miscellaneous Agents Used in Reptiles.

Agent	Dosage	Species/Comments
Acetylcysteine (200 mg/mL injectable)	0.25 mL in 5 mL sterile saline for 30 min q24h[71]	Chelonian nasal discharge; given until clinical signs resolved
Activated charcoal-kaolin suspension (ToxiBan, Vet-a-Mix)	5-10 mL/kg PO q24h × 1-3 days[290]	Sea turtles/reduce exposure to brevitoxin
Allopurinol	—	Careful when giving with urine acidifiers and uricosuric drugs (probenecid)[90]
	10-20 mg/kg PO q24h[106,311,381]	Most species/gout; decreases production of uric acid;[63] long-term therapy; tortoises may respond best
	25 mg/kg PO q24h[196]	Green iguanas
	50 mg/kg PO q24h × 30 days, then q72h[251]	Chelonians/hyperuricemia

TABLE 4-11 Miscellaneous Agents Used in Reptiles. (cont'd)

Agent	Dosage	Species/Comments
Aluminum hydroxide (Amphogel, Wyeth-Ayerst)	100 mg/kg PO q12-24h[282]	Most species/hyperphosphatemia (associated with renal disease); decreases intestinal absorption of phosphorus; use cautiously in patients with gastric outlet obstruction
Amidotrizoate (Gastrografin, Squibb)	5-7.7 mL/kg PO[293]	Gastrointestinal contrast agent; reported faster transit vs barium; no risk if regurgitation
	7.5 mL/kg PO[325]	Tortoises/gastrointestinal contrast agent; give via gavage; mean transit times: 2.6 hr at 87°F (30.6°C); 6.6 hr at 71°F (21.5°C)
Aminophylline	2-4 mg/kg IM[63]	Most species/bronchodilator
Atropine	0.01-0.04 mg/kg IM, IV q8-24h[324]	Most species/dries up excess mucous secretions with infectious stomatitis
	0.1-0.2 mg/kg IM prn[63]	Most species/organophosphate toxicity
	0.2 mg/kg SC, IM[63]	Most species/respiratory distress associated with excessive secretions
Barium sulfate	5-20 mL/kg PO[62]	Most species/gastrointestinal contrast studies
	25 mL/kg PO, 35% wt:vol concentration[24]	Ball pythons/best gastrointestinal image quality
Bleomycin with high-voltage electrical pulses	1 U/cm³ intralesional, repeat in 33 days[49]	Green sea turtles/fibropapillomas; electrochemotherapy; use concurrent local anesthesia
	3.65 mg/kg (1 mg/mL) intralesional, repeat in 2 wk[261]	Yellow-bellied slider turtles/squamous cell carcinoma; post partial surgical excision
Calcium EDTA	10-40 mg/kg IM q12h[348]	Most species/heavy metal chelation; ensure hydration
Carboplatin	2.5-5 mg/kg IV, intracardiac[310]	Most species/carcinoma, osteosarcoma, mesothelioma, carcinomatosis
Carboplatin 4.6 mg implantable bead (compounded, Wedgewood Pharmacy)	≤10 mg/kg total q3wk intralesional or surgical excision sites[223]	Chameleons/squamous cell carcinoma, carcinoma; cut bead into smaller pieces to avoid overdose
Chlorambucil (Leukeran, Glaxo SmithKline)	0.1-0.2 mg/kg PO[310]	Green iguanas/successful management of lymphoma post radiation therapy
CHOP Therapy (Modified)	See original paper for full protocol details[135]	Green iguanas/successful management of lymphoma post radiation therapy
Choukroun's Platelet Rich Fibrin	0.05% body weight whole blood[71]	Elongate tortoise/nasal wound; whole blood in nonanticoagulant tube; centrifuge 6000 rpm x 7 min; 3 layers – middle layer is PRF clot, remove with sterile syringe/swab to avoid RBC's; place clot into cleaned wound; cover with antiseptic debridement gel

Continued

TABLE 4-11 Miscellaneous Agents Used in Reptiles. (cont'd)

Agent	Dosage	Species/Comments
Cimetidine	4 mg/kg PO, IM q8-12h[63]	Most species/gastric and duodenal ulceration; esophagitis; gastroesophageal reflux; may use in renal failure to increase phosphate secretion
Cisapride (Propulsid, Janssen)	0.5-2 mg/kg PO q24h[63]	Most species/motility modifier; gastrointestinal stasis; not commercially available in the United States; may be compounded; ineffective in desert tortoises at 1 mg/kg[469]
	1-4 mg/kg PO q24h until defecates[481]	Bearded dragons/constipation
Cisplatin	0.5-1 mg/kg IV (prehydrate), intracardiac, intralesional (in oil)[63]	Most species/carcinoma, osteosarcoma, infiltrative sarcoma (intralesional), mesothelioma, carcinomatosis
Cyclophosphamide	10 mg/kg SC, IM, IV, intracardiac[63]	Most species/lymphoma, leukemia, myeloproliferative tumors
Dioctyl Na sulfosuccinate	1-5 mg/kg PO[154]	Most species/constipation; use 1:20 dilution
Diphenhydramine	2 mg/kg IM q24h[290]	Sea turtles/brevitoxicosis; rapidly reduced conjunctival edema, prevented corneal ulceration
Doxorubicin	1 mg/kg IV q7d × 2 treatments, then q14d × 2 treatments, then q21d × 2 treatments[401]	Snakes/chemotherapy for sarcoma (also lymphoma, carcinoma, etc.); treatment periods variable
Enalopril	0.5-0.7 mg/kg q24h[414]	Combined with spirolactone and furosemide to briefly manage chronic heart failure in spiny-tailed monitor
Famotidine	0.5 mg/kg SC q3d[489]	Kemp's ridley sea turtles
Furosemide	2-5 mg/kg PO, IM, IV q12-24h[221,222,243]	Most species/diuretic for edema and pulmonary congestion; while lacking loop of Henle, may effect via other mechanisms
	5 mg/kg IM q24h × 1-3 days[290]	Sea turtles/intentional dehydration with brevitoxicosis; no concurrent fluids given
Hydrochlorothiazide	1 mg/kg q24-72h[106]	Lizards/promotes diuresis; monitor hydration status
Iodine compound (Conray 280, Mallinckrodt)	500 mg/kg IV, IO[106]	Lizards/IV urography; take radiographs 0, 5, 15, 30, and 60 min post injection
Iohexol (240 mg I/mL; Omnipaque, Sanofi Winthrop)	5-20 mL/kg PO[63]	Most species/gastrointestinal contrast studies; nonionic, organic iodine solution; good alternative to barium;[48] faster transit time than barium; can be diluted 1:1 with water
	75 mg/kg IV[234]	Kemp's ridley turtles (juveniles)/glomerular filtration rate assessment

TABLE 4-11 Miscellaneous Agents Used in Reptiles. (cont'd)

Agent	Dosage	Species/Comments
K-Y Jelly (Johnson & Johnson)	1-3 mL of 50% K-Y Jelly and 50% warm water/100 g[63]	Most species/enema
Lactulose	0.5 mL/kg PO q24h[222,243,442]	Lizards, chelonians/hepatic lipidosis
L-asparaginase (Elspar, Merck)	400 U/kg SC, IM, intracardiac[63]	Most species/lymphoma, leukemia, myeloproliferative tumors
Maropitant citrate (Cerenia, Zoetis)	1 mg/kg PO, SC q24h[242]	Antiemetic; antinausea; no adverse effects seen; Substance P conserved across classes
Melphalan (Alkeran, Celegene)	0.05-0.1 mg/kg PO[63]	Most species/lymphoma, leukemia, myeloproliferative tumors
Methimazole	2 mg/kg q24h × 30 days[175]	Snakes/excessive shedding from hyperthyroidism; limited effectiveness
Methotrexate	0.25 mg/kg PO, SC, IV[63]	Most species/lymphoma, leukemia, myeloproliferative tumors
Metoclopramide	0.06 mg/kg PO q24h × 7 days[103]	Most species/stimulates gastric motility
	0.05 mg/kg PO q24h × 7 days[63]	Sea turtles/intestinal motility stimulant
	0.5 mg/kg IM q24h[116]	Sea turtles/supportive care
	1-10 mg/kg PO q24h[496]	Tortoises/stimulates gastric motility; ineffective in desert tortoises at 1 mg/kg[469]
Milk thistle (*Silybum marianum*)	4-15 mg/kg PO q8-12h[222,243]	Lizards, chelonians/hepatoprotectant
Pentobarbital	60-100 mg/kg IV, ICe[13,53]	Euthanasia
Pimobendan	0.2 mg/kg PO q24h[243]	Lizards
Potassium chloride	2 mEq/kg IV, ICe[32]	Most species/euthanasia; cessation of cardiac activity; administer following a euthanasia solution
Probenecid	250 mg/kg PO q12h[370]	Most species/gout; increases uric acid excretion; can be increased prn
S-adenosylmethionine (Denosyl, Nutramax)	30 mg/kg PO q24h[340]	Savannah monitors/liver disease
Sodium bicarbonate	0.5-1 mg/kg IV[63]	Most species/hypoxic acidosis post anesthesia
Sucralfate	500-1000 mg/kg PO q6-8h[63]	Most species/oral, esophageal, gastric, and duodenal ulcers
	200 mg/kg PO q24h[490]	Green iguanas/post duodenoileal anastomosis
Tamoxifen 60-day time release pellets (Innovative Research of America)	Pellets containing 5 mg tamoxifen implants ICe[93]	Leopard geckos/inhibition of follicular development for 60 days if implanted before vitellogenesis

Continued

TABLE 4-11 Miscellaneous Agents Used in Reptiles. (cont'd)

Agent	Dosage	Species/Comments
Terbutaline	0.01-0.02 mg/kg IM[367]	Reduce bronchospasm
	Nebulization, 15-45 min/session q4-12h × 3+ days[367]	Lower respiratory tract particle size should be ≤0.5 µm, 2-10 µm for trachea; oxygen flow rates <10 kg 1-2 L/min, 5 L/min for larger reptiles; use bubble humidifier; possible adverse cardiovascular effects
Tricaine methanesulfonate (MS-222)	250-500 mg/kg ICe 1% solution followed by 0.1-1 mL 50% solution ICe or intracardiac[19,83]	Fence lizards, desert iguanas, garter snakes, house geckos, anole species/euthanasia
Vincristine	0.025 mg/kg IV[63]	Most species/lymphoma, leukemia, myeloproliferative tumors

TABLE 4-12 Hematologic and Serum Biochemical Values of Snakes.[a]

	Colubridae		
Measurement	**Common kingsnake (*Lampropeltis getula*)[64,464]**	**Corn snake (*Elaphe guttata*)[64,464]**	**Gopher snake (*Pituophis catenifer*)[287,464]**
Hematology			
PCV (%)	31 (9-47)	30 (13-50)	35 (13-49)
RBC (10^6/µL)	0.77 (0.10-1.88)	0.88 (0.40-1.60)	0.67 (0.14-1.4)
Hgb (g/dL)	—	11.5 (9.7-13.5)	9.7 (4.3-12.3)
MCV (fL)	311 (28-618)	307 (67-546)	578 (246-1571)
MCH (pg)	—	127 (110-143)	111 (81-132)
MCHC (g/dL)	—	35 (32-40)	33 (27.5-36)
WBC (10^3/µL)	7.45 (1.55-27.7)	5.93 (1.12-16.9)	7.31 (1.66-24.0)
Heterophils (10^3/µL)	1.01 (0.16-5.50)	1.24 (0.23-5.08)	1.58 (0.33-5.99)
Lymphocytes (10^3/µL)	3.92 (0.35-20.9)	2.92 (0.29-11.8)	4.06 (0.21-13.2)
Monocytes (10^3/µL)	1.98 (0.05-5.83)	0.31 (0.03-1.78)	0.14 (0.01-0.86)
Azurophils (10^3/µL)	0.24 (0-4.77)	0.42 (0.01-3.29)	0.58 (0.01-3.23)
Eosinophils (10^3/µL)	0.08 (0.02-0.37)	0.09 (0.03-0.48)	—
Basophils (10^3/µL)	0.27 (0.04-1.08)	0.19 (0.04-1.04)	0.14 (0.01-0.44)
Chemistries			
ALP (U/L)	41 (13-102)	35 (0-85)	61 (15-128)
ALT (U/L)	11 (0-50)	19 (1-57)	15 (1-70)
Amylase (U/L)	1268 (371-2671)	540 (255-2225)	711 (107-1315)
AST (U/L)	20 (4-107)	25 (4-149)	20 (5-103)
Bilirubin, total (mg/dL)	0.4 (0.1-0.7)	0.3 (0-1.0)	0.4 (0.3-0.6)

TABLE 4-12 Hematologic and Serum Biochemical Values of Snakes. (cont'd)

Colubridae			
Measurement	**Common kingsnake (*Lampropeltis getula*)**	**Corn snake (*Elaphe guttata*)**	**Gopher snake (*Pituophis catenifer*)**
BUN (mg/dL)	2 (1-10)	3 (1-6)	2.2 (1-5)
Calcium (mg/dL)	14.9 (9.1-22.2)	15.6 (11.9-19.9)	15.5 (11.0-20.0)
Chloride (mmol/L)	119 (97-141)	122 (105-139)	120 (103-138)
Cholesterol (mg/dL)	294 (75-513)	473 (267-678)	368 (118-630)
Creatine kinase (U/L)	406 (59-1909)	270 (31-967)	330 (34-1702)
Creatinine (mg/dL)	0.6 (0-1.6)	0.6 (0.2-2)	0.3 (0.1-0.6)
GGT (U/L)	9	9 (0-25)	10 (0-34)
Glucose (mg/dL)	38 (8-92)	49 (17-92)	57 (23-99)
Iron (µg/dL)	190 (30-488)	—	—
LDH (U/L)	126 (15-417)	178 (10-585)	112 (1-405)
Phosphorus (mg/dL)	3.8 (1.7-11.3)	3.7 (1.8-8.0)	3.6 (1.7-7.9)
Potassium (mmol/L)	4.6 (2.3-9.2)	4.9 (1.8-9.1)	4.8 (2.2-7.4)
Protein, total (g/dL)	6.4 (3.8-10.3)	7.0 (3.3-10.7)	6.0 (3.7-8.8)
Albumin (g/dL)[b]	1.8 (0.8-2.9)	2.1 (1.0-3.4)	2.0 (1.1-3.0)
Globulin (g/dL)[b]	4.4 (2.1-7.2)	4.7 (2.6-7.4)	4.0 (1.7-6.3)
Sodium (mmol/L)	161 (140-180)	162 (149-181)	163 (146-180)
Triglyceride (mg/dL)	—	331 (47-1118)	27 (16-37)
Uric acid (mg/dL)	4.6 (1.4-16.0)	4.4 (1.0-13.6)	4.6 (1.9-12.6)
Measurement	**Indigo snake (*Drymarchon corais*)[64,112,464]**	**Milk snake (*Lampropeltis triangulum*)[64,464]**	**Pine snake (adults) (*Pituophis ruthveni*)[160]**
Hematology			
PCV (%)	26 (10-41)	30 (10-43)	38.5 (29-43)
RBC (10^6/µL)	0.62 (0.43-0.76)	0.88 (0.36-1.45)	—
Hgb (g/dL)	9.2 (7.3-11.1)	10.4 (6.9-11.9)	—
MCV (fL)	369 (221-558)	354 (135-615)	—
MCH (pg)	258	119 (89-164)	—
MCHC (g/dL)	40 (33-46)	34 (29-45)	—
WBC (10^3/µL)	8.4 (1.5-21.6)	7.33 (1.66-23.8)	15.7 (4.9-20.7)
Heterophils (10^3/µL)	1.64 (0.14-3.94)	1.29 (0.09-5.32)	1.82 (0.6-2.7)
Lymphocytes (10^3/µL)	3.89 (0.24-14.5)	3.55 (0.61-10.33)	12.0 (3.0-17.0)
Monocytes (10^3/µL)	0.24 (0.04-2.50)	0.12 (0.03-1.19)	0.46 (0.1-1.1)
Azurophils (10^3/µL)	0.47 (0-3.51)	0.76 (0.02-6.13)	0.37 (0-1.4)
Eosinophils (10^3/µL)	—	—	0 (0-0)
Basophils (10^3/µL)	0.35 (0.03-1.09)	0.24 (0.02-0.67)	0 (0-0.2)

Continued

TABLE 4-12 Hematologic and Serum Biochemical Values of Snakes. (cont'd)

Measurement	Indigo snake (*Drymarchon corais*)	Milk snake (*Lampropeltis triangulum*)	Pine snake (adults) (*Pituophis ruthveni*)
Chemistries			
ALP (U/L)	123 (6-547)	115 (27-338)	600 (283-1434)
ALT (U/L)	10 (3-16)	8 (3-17)	—
Amylase (U/L)	—	665	—
AST (U/L)	15 (2-61)	19 (1-74)	200 (167-350)
Bilirubin, total (mg/dL)	2.1 (0.6-3.5)	0.4 (0.1-0.9)	—
BUN (mg/dL)	7 (0-22)	2 (1-14)	—
Bile Acids (mmol/L)	—	—	10 (3-15)
Calcium (mg/dL)	39 (12-97)[c]	14.9 (11.0-18.9)	4.4 (3.9-4.7)
Chloride (mmol/L)	121 (104-138)	122 (106-137)	—
Cholesterol (mg/dL)	93 (17-272)	446 (51-631)	18.6 (14.4-23.3)
Creatine kinase (U/L)	644 (68-1923)	157 (7-566)	6801 (4701-11,919)
Creatinine (mg/dL)	0.3 (0.2-0.3)	0.5 (0.3-1.1)	—
GGT (U/L)	15	8 (3-13)	70.3 (43.2-122.5)
Glucose (mg/dL)	57 (16-103)	52 (12-128)	—
LDH (U/L)	46 (28-89)	816 (18-2807)	1300 (733-2917)
Phosphorus (mg/dL)	10.1 (0.1-39.6)[c]	3.5 (1.0-7.3)	4.0 (3.4-5.3)
Potassium (mmol/L)	4.7 (2.1-7.3)	4.6 (2.2-8.1)	—
Protein, total (g/dL)	8.1 (4.2-13.1)	6.5 (3.9-10.0)	7.0 (6.5-7.7)
Albumin (g/dL)[b]	2.4 (1.0-4.3)	2.0 (0.8-3.2)	2.0 (1.8-2.2)
Globulin (g/dL)[b]	5.1 (0.7-9.2)	4.6 (2.4-6.8)	5.0 (4.7-5.8)
Sodium (mmol/L)	162 (149-175)	164 (148-180)	—
Triglyceride (mg/dL)	92 (76-118)	428 (68-1620)	—
Uric acid (mg/dL)	3.8 (0-9.1)	4.9 (1.3-15.0)	7.8 (4.5-19.7)

Measurement	Rat snake (*Elaphe obsoleta*)[64,384,464]		
Hematology			
PCV (%)	30 (12-46)		
RBC (10^6/μL)	0.83 (0.23-1.43)		
Hgb (g/dL)	9.8 (2.8-16.2)		
MCV (fL)	354 (73-636)		
MCH (pg)	121 (90-175)		
MCHC (g/dL)	31 (18-45)		

TABLE 4-12 Hematologic and Serum Biochemical Values of Snakes. (cont'd)

Measurement	Rat snake (*Elaphe obsoleta*)		
WBC (10^3/μL)	7.83 (1.02-25.2)		
Heterophils (10^3/μL)	1.20 (0.10-3.89)		
Lymphocytes (10^3/μL)	3.89 (0.41-16.1)		
Monocytes (10^3/μL)	0.48 (0.02-2.52)		
Azurophils (10^3/μL)	0.41 (0-3.50)		
Eosinophils (10^3/μL)	0.11 (0.01-0.55)		
Basophils (10^3/μL)	0.18 (0.01-0.72)		
Chemistries			
ALP (U/L)	70 (11-212)		
ALT (U/L)	10 (0-32)		
Amylase (U/L)	1337 (630-2626)		
AST (U/L)	19 (3-75)		
Bilirubin, total (mg/dL)	0.2 (0-0.8)		
BUN (mg/dL)	2 (1-12)		
Calcium (mg/dL)	15.3 (10.6-21.0)		
Chloride (mmol/L)	121 (96-146)		
Cholesterol (mg/dL)	340 (92-588)		
Creatine kinase (U/L)	228 (41-1049)		
Creatinine (mg/dL)	0.3 (0-0.8)		
GGT (U/L)	9 (1-35)		
Glucose (mg/dL)	62 (11-121)		
Iron (μg/dL)	—		
LDH (U/L)	175 (4-452)		
Lipase (U/L)	4 (3-4)		
Magnesium (mmol/L)	1.3		
Phosphorus (mg/dL)	3.8 (1.5-9.3)		
Potassium (mmolL)	5.0 (1.2-8.7)		
Protein, total (g/dL)	6.3 (3.8-10.7)		
Albumin (g/dL)[b]	2.3 (1.4-3.6)		
Globulin (g/dL)[b]	4.0 (1.5-6.6)		
Sodium (mmol/L)	164 (148-180)		
Triglyceride (mg/dL)	195 (21-1017)		
Uric acid (mg/dL)	4.1 (0.9-14.0)		

Continued

TABLE 4-12 Hematologic and Serum Biochemical Values of Snakes. (cont'd)

	Boidae		
Measurement	Boa constrictor (*Boa constrictor*)[64,72,279,464]	Emerald tree boa (*Corallus caninus*)[64,221]	Rainbow boa (*Epicrates cenchria*)[64,464]
Hematology			
PCV (%)	29 (12-40)	26 (7-44)	29 (15-44)
RBC (10^6/μL)	0.71 (0.16-1.4)	2.16 (0.54-5.05)	0.87 (0.23-1.74)
Hgb (g/dL)	8.2 (3.1-13.2)	8.2 (6.1-11.4)	10.6 (8-13.1)
MCV (fL)	395 (122-669)	237 (37-360)	314 (45-619)
MCH (pg)	117 (51-184)	120 (113-128)	160
MCHC (g/dL)	31 (21-40)	34 (30-36)	36 (33-40)
WBC (10^3/μL)	7.37 (1.47-19.6)	4.87 (0.48-11.1)	7.64 (1-21.23)
Heterophils (10^3/μL)	1.93 (0.20-6.50)	1.25 (0.18-3.64)	1.07 (0.03-3.67)
Lymphocytes (10^3/μL)	2.89 (0.34-11.9)	1.92 (0.14-5.68)	4.71 (0.1-14.1)
Monocytes (10^3/μL)	0.27 (0.03-2.38)	0.17 (0.02-1.11)	0.9 (0.03-3.06)
Azurophils (10^3/μL)	0.84 (0-4.74)	0.23 (0-3.22)	0.60 (0-2.47)
Eosinophils (10^3/μL)	0.13 (0-0.60)	0.07 (0.06-0.08)	0.11 (0.04-0.22)
Basophils (10^3/μL)	0.21 (0.03-1.01)	0.06 (0.03-0.21)	0.1 (0.02-0.27)
Chemistries			
ALP (U/L)	189 (46-652)	87 (0-236)	27 (14-37)
ALT (U/L)	11 (0-30)	7 (0-27)	4 (1-6)
Amylase (U/L)	14 (0-76)	371 (61-847)	—
AST (U/L)	15 (2-64)	23 (2-61)	18 (3-54)
Bilirubin, total (mg/dL)	0.2 (0-0.6)	0.2 (0.2-0.3)	0.4 (0-0.8)
BUN (mg/dL)	2 (0-8)	2 (1-4)	2 (1-3)
Calcium (mg/dL)	15.3 (10-20)	12.8 (8.1-17.5)	13.8 (10.2-17.5)
Chloride (mmol/L)	125 (108-138)	131 (112-149)	129 (94-158)
Cholesterol (mg/dL)	120 (46-289)	304 (77-614)	206 (140-314)
Creatine kinase (U/L)	489 (57-2099)	454 (41-1445)	95 (0-347)
Creatinine (mg/dL)	0.2 (0-0.5)	0.6 (0.4-0.9)	0.4 (0.1-0.7)
GGT (U/L)	4 (0-23)	2 (1-2)	5
Glucose (mg/dL)	34 (7-74)	27 (5-64)	36 (2-80)
Iron (μg/dL)	113 (103-122)	—	—
LDH (U/L)	149 (0-452)	128 (14-754)	401 (141-661)
Lipase (U/L)	2730	—	—
Magnesium (mmol/L)	1.5 (1.45-1.5)	—	—
Osmolarity (mOsm/L)	306	—	—

TABLE 4-12 Hematologic and Serum Biochemical Values of Snakes. (cont'd)

	Boidae		
Measurement	Boa constrictor (*Boa constrictor*)	Emerald tree boa (*Corallus caninus*)	Rainbow boa (*Epicrates cenchria*)
Phosphorus (mg/dL)	4.3 (2.4-8.6)	4.1 (1.8-8)	4.3 (1.6-7.1)
Potassium (mmol/L)	4.7 (3.1-7.3)	5 (3-8.7)	4.8 (2.4-6.7)
Protein, total (g/dL)	7.0 (4.0-10.3)	4.5 (2.6-7.2)	6.8 (4.7-8.9)
Albumin (g/dL)[b]	2.9 (1.6-4.3)	2.6 (2-3.6)	2.4 (1.1-3.6)
Globulin (g/dL)[b]	3.9 (2.0-6.8)	2.8 (1.8-3.6)	4.2 (1.9-6.5)
Sodium (mmol/L)	159 (143-173)	157 (148-167)	162 (142-181)
Triglyceride (mg/dL)	103 (3-457)	24 (10-49)	72 (64-90)
Uric acid (mg/dL)	4.0 (0.3-15.0)	4.7 (1.4-19.2)	3.6 (1.1-9.7)

Measurement	Rosy boa (*Lichanura trivirgata*)[464]		
Hematology			
PCV (%)	37 (20-54)		
RBC (10^6/μL)	—		
Hgb (g/dL)	—		
MCV (fL)	—		
MCH (pg)	—		
MCHC (g/dL)	—		
WBC (10^3/μL)	4.65 (0.57-8.73)		
Heterophils (10^3/μL)	1.67 (0.39-4.13)		
Lymphocytes (10^3/μL)	1.74 (0.18-4.92)		
Monocytes (10^3/μL)	0.10 (0.03-0.65)		
Azurophils (10^3/μL)	0.40 (0-1.68)		
Eosinophils (10^3/μL)	—		
Basophils (10^3/μL)	—		
Chemistries			
ALP (U/L)	—		
ALT (U/L)	—		
Amylase (U/L)	—		
AST (U/L)	20 (1-107)		
Bilirubin, total (mg/dL)	—		
BUN (mg/dL)	—		
Calcium (mg/dL)	13.1 (9.4-17.4)		
Chloride (mmol/L)	—		

Continued

TABLE 4-12 Hematologic and Serum Biochemical Values of Snakes. (cont'd)

Measurement	Rosy boa (*Lichanura trivirgata*)		
Cholesterol (mg/dL)	—		
Creatine kinase (U/L)	—		
Creatinine (mg/dL)	—		
GGT (U/L)	—		
Glucose (mg/dL)	37 (3-73)		
LDH (U/L)	—		
Phosphorus (mg/dL)	2.9 (0.8-6.1)		
Potassium (mmol/L)	5.9 (3.7-10.3)		
Protein, total (g/dL)	5.8 (3.7-8.3)		
Albumin (g/dL)[b]	2.1 (1.2-2.9)		
Globulin (g/dL)[b]	3.7 (2.3-4.8)		
Sodium (mmol/L)	155 (115-174)		
Triglyceride (mg/dL)	—		
Uric acid (mg/dL)	6.4 (1.9-19.0)		
Pythonidae			
Measurement	**Ball python (*Python regius*)[224,464]**	**Blood python (*Python curtus*)[64]**	**Burmese python (*Python bivittatus*)[64,464]**
Hematology			
PCV (%)	24 (10-33)	25 (15-49)	28 (13-38)
RBC (10^6/μL)	0.74 (0.31-1.16)	0.65	0.83 (0.13-1.54)
Hgb (g/dL)	7.8 (4.5-11.1)	—	9.0 (4-11)
MCV (fL)	328 (131-524)	340	319 (84-554)
MCH (pg)	102 (28-175)	—	98 (32-143)
MCHC (g/dL)	32 (24-40)	—	32 (18-44)
WBC (10^3/μL)	7.46 (2.22-21.6)	11.7 (1.13-42.5)	7.6 (2.19-24.2)
Heterophils (10^3/μL)	1.78 (0.32-6.17)	1.82 (0.31-3.99)	2.25 (0.31-5.76)
Lymphocytes (10^3/μL)	3.21 (0.35-13.8)	6.71 (0.34-33.6)	3.73 (0.46-17.4)
Monocytes (10^3/μL)	0.73 (0.01-3.26)	0.62 (0.13-2.12)	0.17 (0.02-2.13)
Azurophils (10^3/μL)	0.65 (0.01-4.12)	2.82 (0.27-6.8)	0.27 (0.01-5.89)
Eosinophils (10^3/μL)	0.10 (0.02-0.53)	0.08	0.45 (0.10-1.4)
Basophils (10^3/μL)	0.22 (0.04-1.08)	0.93 (0.32-1.83)	0.12 (0.03-0.33)
Chemistries			
ALP (U/L)	37 (11-98)	44 (8-56)	58 (4-230)
ALT (U/L)	9 (1-25)	10 (3-17)	7 (0-26)
Amylase (U/L)	1647 (383-2911)	—	3255

TABLE 4-12 Hematologic and Serum Biochemical Values of Snakes. (cont'd)

	Pythonidae		
Measurement	Ball python (*Python regius*)	Blood python (*Python curtus*)	Burmese python (*Python bivittatus*)
AST (U/L)	25 (4-97)	56 (6-209)	14 (3-65)
Bilirubin, total (mg/dL)	0.1 (0-0.2)	0.3 (0.2-0.5)	0.6 (0-2)
BUN (mg/dL)	2 (0-7)	1 (0-2)	2 (1-5)
Calcium (mg/dL)	14.7 (10.4-19.3)	14.7 (13.5-16.2)	16.1 (7.2-25.0)
Chloride (mmol/L)	121 (107-134)	131 (123-138)	118 (104-132)
Cholesterol (mg/dL)	111 (15-232)	214 (76-445)	264 (120-479)
Creatine kinase (U/L)	526 (55-2136)	668 (327-1009)	381 (39-1577)
Creatinine (mg/dL)	0.2 (0-0.7)	0.9 (0.5-1.3)	0.3 (0-1.6)
GGT (U/L)	—	8 (0-16)	25 (4-51)
Glucose (mg/dL)	25 (8-53)	30 (13-74)	24 (1-83)
LDH (U/L)	122 (4-376)	207 (49-364)	144 (12-807)
Phosphorus (mg/dL)	3.0 (1.4-7.3)	3.7 (3.1-4.5)	4.4 (2.3-9.2)
Potassium (mmol/L)	5.5 (2.4-10.0)	6.3 (3.3-11.2)	4.8 (2.6-7.0)
Protein, total (g/dL)	6.8 (3.6-9.0)	6.2 (3.6-8.1)	7.2 (4.4-11.1)
Albumin (g/dL)[b]	2.1 (1.1-3.6)	2.3 (1.6-2.8)	2.3 (1.2-3.4)
Globulin (g/dL)[b]	4.5 (2.1-6.5)	4.1 (3.1-4.9)	4.9 (1.9-7.8)
Sodium (mmol/L)	153 (137-171)	160 (155-164)	158 (145-172)
Triglyceride (mg/dL)	—	16 (13-22)	114 (16-532)
Uric acid (mg/dL)	3.0 (0.8-8.3)	4.3 (2.1-7.1)	4.3 (0.4-10.1)

	Pythonidae		
Measurement	Carpet python (*Morelia spilota* spp)[50,64,464]	Green tree python (*Morelia viridis*)[64,464]	Reticulated python (*Python reticulatus*)[64,464]
Hematology			
PCV (%)	24 (16-32)	25.3 (13-38)	26 (13-39)
RBC (10^6/μL)	0.89 (0.32-1.45)	0.85 (0.4-1.3)	0.72 (0.41-1.25)
Hgb (g/dL)	7.9 (4.9-9.7)	5.9 (4-7)	10.7 (5.2-30)
MCV (fL)	327 (260-386)	229 (208-250)	343 (176-429)
MCH (pg)	111 (86-170)	100	138 (60-186)
MCHC (g/dL)	34 (29-39)	36 (33-40)	37 (29-45)
WBC (10^3/μL)	13.4 (2.7-24.8)	7.28 (1.2-18.7)	7.48 (1.32-15.8)
Heterophils (10^3/μL)	7.13 (1.79-16.8)	1.59 (0.24-3.49)	1.92 (0.08-4.83)
Lymphocytes (10^3/μL)	2.59 (0.60-6.91)	3.46 (0.07-11.8)	2.24 (0.12-7.47)
Monocytes (10^3/μL)	0.67 (0.03-2.67)	0.61 (0.02-2.86)	1.22 (0.02-5.50)

Continued

TABLE 4-12 Hematologic and Serum Biochemical Values of Snakes. (cont'd)

	Pythonidae		
Measurement	Carpet python (*Morelia spilota* spp)	Green tree python (*Morelia viridis*)	Reticulated python (*Python reticulatus*)
Azurophils ($10^3/\mu L$)	1.09 (0.01-5.72)	0.72 (0.00-3.17)	0.10 (0.01-4.30)
Eosinophils ($10^3/\mu L$)	—	0.16 (0.1-0.22)	0.68 (0.04-1.95)
Basophils ($10^3/\mu L$)	0.16 (0-1.01)	0.17 (0.04-0.70)	0.06 (0.06-0.7)
Chemistries			
ALP (U/L)	36 (10-81)	177 (43-425)	61 (4-211)
ALT (U/L)	17 (6-78)	18 (0-52)	16 (0-51)
Amylase (U/L)	—	902 (564-1240)	1690 (416-2963)
AST (U/L)	17 (2-45)	18 (1-63)	12 (2-34)
Bilirubin, total (mg/dL)	0.5	0.2	0.3
BUN (mg/dL)	3 (2-3)	2 (0-2)	2 (1-7)
Calcium (mg/dL)	14.3 (10.9-20.5)	13.8 (9.8-17.9)	16.3 (10.9-26.6)
Chloride (mmol/L)	118 (102-131)	124 (90-153)	118 (92-141)
Cholesterol (mg/dL)	318 (126-630)	251 (72-561)	285 (81-531)
Creatine kinase (U/L)	349 (3-1230)	606 (21-1843)	351 (24-2338)
Creatinine (mg/dL)	1.3 (0.3-3.7)	0.2 (0.2-0.5)	0.2 (0.1-0.4)
GGT (U/L)	32 (9-55)	—	22
Glucose (mg/dL)	30 (3-57)	37 (1-76)	31 (1-77)
LDH (U/L)	201 (11-728)	206	313 (43-1048)
Magnesium (mmol/L)	330 (48-547)	—	—
Phosphorus (mg/dL)	4.1 (0.8-7.9)	5.1 (2.3-10.2)	5.6 (2.4-13.0)
Potassium (mmol/L)	4.9 (3.0-7.1)	5.5 (3.6-7.9)	5.0 (3.4-8.1)
Protein, total (g/dL)	7.2 (5.4-10.3)	7.2 (3.6-10.9)	7.8 (4.8-10.7)
Albumin (g/dL)[b]	2.1 (1.6-2.9)	2.0 (0.4-3.7)	2.1 (0.8-3.9)
Globulin (g/dL)[b]	5.1 (3.7-7.6)	4.9 (3.2-8.1)	5.0 (0.8-9.0)
Sodium (mmol/L)	156 (140-172)	161 (142-179)	160 (142-178)
Triglyceride (mg/dL)	30	—	45
Uric acid (mg/dL)	4.1 (0-9.3)	3.6 (0-11.0)	7.8 (3.5-17.4)

[a]Listed values are median followed by either min-max or a confidence interval in parentheses depending upon reported methods and the authors' judgment from the available evidence, unless a single value indicating n=1 or a range that is not enclosed in parentheses indicating a reported reference interval.

[b]Albumin is measured by colorimetry (e.g., bromocresol green) and globulin value is calculated unless otherwise indicated "PEP" (protein electrophoresis).

[c]Remarkably high reference ranges for Ca (mean, 159 mg/dL; range, 30-337 mg/dL) and P (mean, 35 mg/dL; range, 8-69) have also been reported.[112]

TABLE 4-13 Hematologic and Serum Biochemical Values of Lizards.[a]

Measurement	Bearded dragon (*Pogona vitticeps*)[64,113]	Blue-tongued skink (*Tiliqua scincoides*)[64,464]	Chinese (Asian) water dragon (*Physignathus cocincinus*)[313]
Hematology			
PCV (%)	30 (17-45)	28 (16-39)	35 (32-40)
RBC (10^6/μL)	1 (0.40-1.60)	0.89 (0.30-2.00)	—
Hgb (g/dL)	9.3 (4.7-14)	10.4 (6-13)	—
MCV (fL)	292 (77-506)	297 (34-441)	—
MCH (pg)	90 (16-163)	98 (44-173)	—
MCHC (g/dL)	32 (19-46)	33 (16-57)	—
WBC (10^3/μL)	6.21 (1.45-19.0)	5.93 (2.00-17.7)	13.5 (11.7-18.2)
Heterophils (10^3/μL)	2.09 (0.24-7.77)	2.24 (0.43-6.64)	5.1 (3.9-6.9)
Lymphocytes (10^3/μL)	2.77 (0.29-11.3)	1.93 (0.31-7.31)	7.2 (5.6-9.5)
Monocytes (10^3/μL)	0.25 (0.03-1.39)	0.16 (0.03-1.03)	1.1 (0.4-1.9)
Azurophils (10^3/μL)	0.11 (0.01-1.98)	0.16 (0.01-1.93)	0 (0-0.6)
Eosinophils (10^3/μL)	0.12 (0.01-0.37)	0.37 (0.02-1.50)	0.2 (0.1-0.3)
Basophils (10^3/μL)	0.26 (0.04-1.28)	0.67 (0.03-2.27)	0.5 (0.2-0.8)
Fibrinogen (mg/dL)	180 (0-300)	—	—
Chemistries			
ALP (U/L)	133 (21-569)	80 (25-159)	—
ALT (U/L)	9 (0-33)	20 (5-34)	—
Amylase (U/L)	1670(497-3430)	—	—
AST (U/L)	20 (2-90)	20 (5-80)	16.5 (8-52)
Bilirubin, total (mg/dL)	0.4 (0-1.4)	—	—
BUN (mg/dL)	2 (1-5)	2 (1-27)	—
Calcium (mg/dL)	11.9 (8.6-18)	12.7 (10.0-15.9)	12.4 (11.6-13.3)
Chloride (mmol/L)	120 (94-149)	116 (100-132)	—
Cholesterol (mg/dL)	271 (79-606)	207 (49-601)	—
Creatine kinase (U/L)	563 (33-4042)	629 (59-5570)	1747 (19-6630)
Creatinine (mg/dL)	0.2 (0-0.7)	0.3 (0.1-0.6)	—
GGT (U/L)	1 (0-21)	8	—
Glucose (mg/dL)	202 (108-333)	127 (72-202)	157 (112-243)
LDH (U/L)	347 (25-1906)	735 (364-1106)	—
Lipase (U/L)	—	364	—
Phosphorus (mg/dL)	4.4 (2.1-10.6)	4.4 (2.3-10.8)	5.7 (3.4-8.2)
Potassium (mmol/L)	4.0 (1.5-7.1)	5.1 (3.3-7.9)	4.2 (3.8-4.5)

Continued

TABLE 4-13 Hematologic and Serum Biochemical Values of Lizards. (cont'd)

Measurement	Bearded dragon (*Pogona vitticeps*)	Blue-tongued skink (*Tiliqua scincoides*)	Chinese (Asian) water dragon (*Physignathus cocincinus*)
Protein, total (g/dL)	5.0 (3.0-8.1)	6.1 (3.7-8.5)	7 (6.6-7.5)
Albumin (g/dL)[b]	2.5 (1.2-4.0)	2.1 (1.1-3.1)	2.2 (2.1-2.3)
Globulin (g/dL)[b]	2.5 (1.1-4.5)	3.9 (2.4-5.8)	4.7 (4.5-5.3)
Sodium (mmol/L)	157 (140-179)	151 (139-175)	150 (147-153)
Triglyceride (mg/dL)	261 (93-437)	—	—
Uric acid (mg/dL)	3.1 (0.5-9.8)	2.7 (0.6-9.5)	2.3 (1.9-2.7)

Measurement	Crested gecko (*Rhacodactylus ciliatus*) male[314]	Crested gecko (*Rhacodactylus ciliatus*) female[314]	Gila monster (*Heloderma suspectum*)[64,84]
Hematology			
PCV (%)	36 (23-45)	31 (24-43)	37 (22-50)
RBC (10^6/μL)	—	—	0.50 (0.22-0.67)
Hgb (g/dL)	—	—	7.4 (6.0-9.5)
MCV (fL)	—	—	812 (415-1773)
MCHC (g/dL)	—	—	21 (14-36)
WBC (10^3/μL)	15.4 (3.5-38.9)	15.4 (3.5-38.9)	4.72 (3.30-6.40)
Heterophils (10^3/μL)	1.5 (0.6-4.2)	1.5 (0.6-4.2)	2.17 (1.35-3.31)
Lymphocytes (10^3/μL)	10.7 (2.2-24.9)	10.7 (2.2-24.9)	1.54 (0.58-3.39)
Monocytes (10^3/μL)	1.9 (0.8-5.1)	1.9 (0.8-5.1)	0.07 (0-0.19)
Azurophils (10^3/μL)	—	—	0.38 (0-1.14)
Eosinophils (10^3/μL)	0 (0-0.2)	0 (0-0.2)	—
Basophils (10^3/μL)	0.3 (0-0.8)	0.3 (0-0.8)	0.57 (0.23-1.05)
Chemistries			
AST (U/L)	30 (12-84)	30 (12-84)	42 (20-66)
Bile acids (μmol/L)	43 (<35-89)	43 (<35-89)	—
Bile acids (rest; μmol/L)	—	—	16.2 (2.6-55.1)
BUN (mg/dL)	—	—	15 (6-30)
Calcium (mg/dL)	12.5 (11.8-13.9)	>20 (15.6-20.0)	12.2 (10.2-13.4)
Ionized Ca^{++} (mmol/L)	—	—	1.26 (1.09-1.50)
Creatine kinase (U/L)	489 (89-2104)	489 (89-2104)	600 (144-1812)
Glucose (mg/dL)	107 (56-180)	107 (56-180)	48 (4-109)
Phosphorus (mg/dL)	4.0 (2.6-6.2)	9.6 (3.8-18.8)	3.4 (1.1-8.6)
Potassium (mmol/L)	2.6 (1.5-4.5)	2.6 (1.5-4.5)	3.9 (2.8-4.6)
Protein, total (g/dL)	6.0 (4.9-7.7)	6.6 (5.2-8.0)	6.3 (5.4-6.9)
Albumin (g/dL)[b]	2.7 (2.3-3.2)	2.9 (2.4-3.4)	—
Albumin (PEP; g/dL)[b]	—	—	2.61 (2.14-3.23)

TABLE 4-13 Hematologic and Serum Biochemical Values of Lizards. (cont'd)

Measurement	Crested gecko (*Rhacodactylus ciliatus*) male	Crested gecko (*Rhacodactylus ciliatus*) female	Gila monster (*Heloderma suspectum*)
Globulin (g/dL)[b]	3.5 (2.6-5.2)	3.5 (2.6-5.2)	—
α-1 (PEP; g/dL)[b]	—	—	2.09 (1.48-2.60)
α-2 (PEP; g/dL)[b]	—	—	0.59 (0.44-0.76)
β (PEP; g/dL)[b]	—	—	0.58 (0.41-0.77)
γ (PEP; g/dL)[b]	—	—	0.33 (0.18-0.68)
Sodium (mmol/L)	143 (136-148)	143 (136-148)	144 (140-151)
Uric acid (mg/dL)	2.6 (0.9-6.0)	2.6 (0.9-6.0)	16.8 (9.8-24.7)

Measurement	Green iguana (*Iguana iguana*)[95,109,195,317,346,464]	Green iguana (*Iguana iguana*) male[d,180,226]	Green iguana (*Iguana iguana*) female[d,180,226]
Hematology			
PCV (%)	25-38	34 (29-39)	38 (33-44)
RBC (10^6/μL)	1-1.9	1.3 (1-1.7)	1.4 (1.2-1.8)
Hgb (g/dL)	8-12	8.6 (6.7-10.2)	10.6 (9.1-12.2)
MCV (fL)	165-305	266 (228-303)	270 (235-331)
MCH (pg)	65-105	—	—
MCHC (g/dL)	20-38	25 (23-28)	28 (25-31)
WBC (10^3/μL)	3-10	15 (11-25)	15 (8-25)
Heterophils (10^3/μL)	0.35-5.2	3.6 (1-5.4)	3.2 (0.6-6.4)
Lymphocytes (10^3/μL)	0.5-5.5	9.7 (5-16.5)	9.9 (5.2-14.4)
Monocytes (10^3/μL)	0-0.1	1.3 (0.2-2.7)	1.2 (0.4-2.3)
Azurophils (10^3/μL)	0-1.7	—	—
Eosinophils (10^3/μL)	0-1	0.1 (0-0.3)	0.1 (0-0.2)
Basophils (10^3/μL)	0-0.5	0.4 (0.1-1)	0.5 (0.2-1.2)
Fibrinogen (mg/dL)	0-300	100 (100-200)	100 (100-300)
Chemistries			
ALP (U/L)	40 (4-170)	39 (14-65)	59 (22-90)
ALT (U/L)	21 (0-97)	32 (4-76)	45 (5-96)
Amylase (U/L)	1815 (996-2988)	—	—
Anion gap (mEq/L)	—	22 (12-30)	29 (19-41)
AST (U/L)	52 (2-100)	33 (19-65)	40 (7-102)
Bile acids (rest; μmol/L)	7.5 (2.6-30.3)	—	—
Bile acids (7.5h; μmol/L)	32.5 (15.2-44.1)	—	—
Bilirubin, total (mg/dL)	0.3 (0-4.9)	0.8 (0.1-1.4)	1.5 (0.3-3.1)

Continued

TABLE 4-13 Hematologic and Serum Biochemical Values of Lizards. (cont'd)

Measurement	Green iguana (*Iguana iguana*)	Green iguana (*Iguana iguana*) male	Green iguana (*Iguana iguana*) female
BUN (mg/dL)	2 (0-10)	—	—
Calcium (mg/dL)	12 (6-18)[c]	11.3 (8.6-14.1)	12.5 (10.8-14)
Ionized Ca^{++} (mmol/L)	1.01-1.62	—	—
Chloride (mmol/L)	117 (102-130)	119 (115-124)	121 (113-129)
Cholesterol (mg/dL)	104-333[c]	161 (82-214)	255 (204-347)
Creatine kinase (U/L)	1876 (174-8768)[c]	—	—
Creatinine (mg/dL)	0.5 (0.2-1.3)	—	—
CO_2 (mEq/L)	—	19.9 (15.2-24.7)	19 (16-23)
Estradiol (pg/mL)	—	79 (36-162)	270 (81-512)
GGT (U/L)	3 (0-10)	—	—
Glucose (mg/dL)	169-288	166 (70-244)	170 (105-258)
Iron (µg/dL)	88-133	—	—
LDH (U/L)	617 (36-7424)[c]	—	—
Lipase (U/L)	21 (17-24)	—	—
Magnesium (mmol/L)	1.2-2.0	—	—
Phosphorus (mg/dL)	5 (2.5-21)[c]	5.3 (3.2-7.6)	6.3 (2.8-9.3)
Potassium (mmol/L)	1.3-3	4 (2.8-6.1)	3.6 (2-5.8)
Protein, total (g/dL)	5.4 (4.1-7.4)[c]	5.4 (4.4-6.5)	6.1 (4.9-7.6)
Albumin (g/dL)[b]	2.1-2.8	2 (1.3-3)	2.4 (1.5-3)
Albumin (PEP; g/dL)[b]	1.8 (1.4-3.1)	—	—
Globulin (g/dL)[b]	2.5-4.3[c]	3.5 (2.5-4.4)	3.8 (2.8-5.2)
α-1 (PEP; g/dL)[b]	0.9 (0.4-1.2)	—	—
α-2 (PEP; g/dL)[b]	—	—	—
β (PEP; g/dL)[b]	2.2 (1.6-3.8)[c]	—	—
γ (PEP; g/dL)[b]	0.3 (0.1-0.4)	—	—
A:G (ratio)	0.5 (0.41-0.78)	0.6 (0.4-0.9)	0.7 (0.3-1)
Sodium (mmol/L)	158-183	157 (152-162)	163 (156-172)
Testosterone (ng/mL)	—	10.2 (2.2-15.7)	0.26 (0.07-0.35)
Triglyceride (mg/dL)	383 (7-1323)[c]	—	—
Uric acid (mg/dL)	2.6 (0-8.2)[c]	2.7 (1.5-5.8)	3.6 (0.9-6.7)
Vitamin D_3 (25-OH; nmol/L)	51-393[c]	—	—

TABLE 4-13 Hematologic and Serum Biochemical Values of Lizards. (cont'd)

Measurement	Green iguana (*Iguana iguana*) juvenile[d,180]	Leopard gecko (*Eublepharis macularius*)[80]	Panther chameleon (*Furcifur pardalis*)[64,464]
Hematology			
PCV (%)	38 (30-47)	31 (21-40)	31 (17-46)
RBC (10^6/μL)	1.4 (1.3-1.6)	—	0.83 (0.42-1.6)
Hgb (g/dL)	9.6 (9.2-10.1)	—	—
MCV (fL)	—	—	330 (200-418)
WBC (10^3/μL)	16 (8-22)	—	9.92 (0.47-25.1)
Heterophils (10^3/μL)	2.2 (1-3.8)	—	2.68 (0.09-6.64)
Lymphocytes (10^3/μL)	12.9 (6.2-17.2)	—	5.98 (0.21-16.8)
Monocytes (10^3/μL)	0.4 (0.3-0.6)	—	—
Azurophils (10^3/μL)	—	—	0.46 (0-2.29)
Eosinophils (10^3/μL)	0.3 (0-0.4)	—	—
Basophils (10^3/μL)	0.5 (0.1-0.7)	—	0.13 (0.03-0.92)
Fibrinogen (mg/dL)	100 (100-300)	—	—
Chemistries			
ALP (U/L)	—	—	32 (1-109)
AST (U/L)	41 (13-72)	29 (11-65)	23 (2-70)
Bile acids (μmol/L)	—	2.0 (0.6-37.5)	
Calcium (mg/dL)	14.3 (12.1-23.2)	25 (14->37) (♀)	10.9 (7.1-14.6)
Creatine kinase (U/L)	—	430 (0-3701)	367 (47-1474)
Glucose (mg/dL)	273 (131-335)	—	319 (174-465)
Phosphorus (mg/dL)	7.7 (4.3-9)	5.6 (1.5-16.4)	9.8 (2.1-17.5)
Potassium (mmol/L)	—	6.6 (2.4-8.0)	5.5 (1.1-10.0)
Protein, total (g/dL)	5 (4.2-6.1)	6.6 (2.4-8.0)	5.9 (3.3-8.5)
Albumin (g/dL)[b]	2.3 (2-2.8)	—	2.6 (1.2-4.1)
Globulin (g/dL)[b]	2.7 (2.2-3)	—	3.2 (2.0-4.4)
A:G (ratio)	0.8 (0.7-0.9)	—	—
Sodium (mmol/L)	—	—	143 (127-159)
Uric acid (mg/dL)	3.3 (0.7-5.7)	2.1 (0.5-6.6)	5.1 (0-12.9)

Measurement	Prehensile-tailed skink (*Corucia zebrata*)[464,497]	Savannah monitor (*Varanus exanthematicus*)[64,464]	Spiny-tailed lizard (*Uromastyx* spp)[64,339]
Hematology			
PCV (%)	32 (21-43)	34 (16-51)	29 (4.9-44.5)
RBC (10^6/μL)	1.59 (0.91-2.28)	1.23 (0.63-1.58)	0.78 (0.33-4.1)

Continued

TABLE 4-13 Hematologic and Serum Biochemical Values of Lizards. (cont'd)

Measurement	Prehensile-tailed skink (*Corucia zebrata*)	Savannah monitor (*Varanus exanthematicus*)	Spiny-tailed lizard (*Uromastyx* spp)
Hgb (g/dL)	9.3 (5.7-12.0)	10.5 (6.2-13.2)	9.9 (3.3-17.4)
MCV (fL)	213 (126-311)	284 (229-382)	415 (119-614)
MCH (pg)	61 (35-91)	94 (89-99)	133 (12-203)
MCHC (g/dL)	28 (19-35)	32 (26-38)	33 (22-41)
Thrombocytes (10^3/μL)	—	—	958 (290-2290)
WBC (10^3/μL)	11.5 (3.4-31.2)	4.67 (0.10-10.9)	3.1 (1-8.1)
Heterophils (10^3/μL)	3.66 (0.70-10.6)	1.58 (0.03-4.55)	2 (0.59-5.36)
Lymphocytes (10^3/μL)	3.87 (0.50-16.2)	1.87 (0.06-4.88)	0.99 (0.27-4.05)
Monocytes (10^3/μL)	0.68 (0.07-4.55)	0.42 (0.01-2.32)	0.04 (0-0.5)
Azurophils (10^3/μL)	0.11 (0.02-4.28)	0.02 (0-0.69)	—
Eosinophils (10^3/μL)	0.45 (0.05-1.48)	—	0.04 (0-0.2)
Basophils (10^3/μL)	1.26 (0.10-5.30)	0.15 (0.07-0.28)	0.03 (0-0.33)
Fibrinogen (mg/dL)	—	156 (100-300)	—
Chemistries			
ALP (U/L)	118 (33-344)	20 (4-101)	31 (5.9-139)
ALT (U/L)	6 (1-20)	70 (7-374)	11 (2.4-35)
Amylase (U/L)	792 (255-1971)	—	134
AST (U/L)	14 (3-54)	26 (5-80)	73 (29-172)
Bilirubin, total (mg/dL)	0.2 (0-0.5)	0.1 (0-0.3)	0.3 (0.1-0.7)
BUN (mg/dL)	1 (0-4)	1 (0-5)	0.56 (0-3)
Calcium (mg/dL)	11.8 (8.9-15.2)	13.6 (10.8-16.5)	9.9 (7.2-13.2)
Chloride (mmol/L)	124 (107-138)	115 (93-133)	126 (111-135)
Cholesterol (mg/dL)	97 (39-265)	116 (49-231)	161 (64-295)
Creatine kinase (U/L)	234 (26-1319)	1529 (7-6624)	1778 (141-10 k)
Creatinine (mg/dL)	0.3 (0-0.6)	8.7 (0-67)	0.4 (0.1-3)
GGT (U/L)	2 (0-11)	7 (1-11)	0.8 (0-5.0)
Glucose (mg/dL)	107 (35-171)	108 (54-163)	200 (68-356)
LDH (U/L)	183 (28-625)	427 (29-3699)	209 (22-899)
Lipase (U/L)	25 (8-63)	—	—
Magnesium (mmol/L)	—	1.6	1.7 (1.1-5.1)
Osmolarity (mOsm/L)	—	332 (319-345)	—
Phosphorus (mg/dL)	4.3 (2.3-9.8)	4.2 (0.8-7.7)	4.5 (1.3-10)
Potassium (mmol/L)	5.0 (2.9-8.1)	4.9 (3.0-6.9)	3.7 (3-4.6)
Protein, total (g/dL)	5.8 (4.1-8.3)	6.6 (3.4-9.8)	4 (2.6-7.4)

TABLE 4-13 Hematologic and Serum Biochemical Values of Lizards. (cont'd)

Measurement	Prehensile-tailed skink (*Corucia zebrata*)	Savannah monitor (*Varanus exanthematicus*)	Spiny-tailed lizard (*Uromastyx* spp)
Albumin (g/dL)[b]	2.3 (1.4-3.4)	2.0 (0.6-3.3)	2 (1.2-3.1)
Albumin (PEP; g/dL)[b]	—	3.2 (3.1-3.3)	—
Globulin (g/dL)[b]	3.5 (2.3-5.0)	4.6 (1.4-7.9)	2.9 (2.2-4.6)
Sodium (mmol/L)	160 (145-177)	156 (142-169)	173 ± 4
Triglyceride (mg/dL)	48 (12-309)	135 (17-476)	175 (111-238)
Uric acid (mg/dL)	1.8 (0.3-5.0)	6.5 (2.0-14.6)	2.94 (0.3-7.3)

Measurement	Tegu lizard (*Tupinambus* spp)[e,64,470]	Veiled chameleon (*Chameleo calyptratus*)[464]	Water monitor (*Varanus salvator*)[64,464]
Hematology			
PCV (%)	25 ± 2.6	24 (12-37)	34 (20-47)
RBC (10^6/μL)	0.96 ± 0.14	—	0.98 (0.42-1.42)
Hgb (g/dL)	11.4 ± 1.6	—	10.5 (9.8-11.5)
MCV (fL)	261 ± 23	—	335 (227-595)
MCH	119 ± 12.5		140 (104-177)
MCHC (g/dL)	45.6 ± 3.4	—	33 (30-40)
WBC (10^3/μL)	16.8 ± 2.5	6.30 (1.20-21.0)	9.49 (2.9-18.8)
Heterophils (10^3/μL)	2.2 ± 0.45	2.35 (0.50-8.32)	4.30 (0.16-8.44)
Lymphocytes (10^3/μL)	7.5 ± 0.58	2.18 (0.07-10.8)	2.84 (0.3-7.98)
Monocytes (10^3/μL)	1 ± 0.41	—	0.81 (0.06-3.38)
Azurophils (10^3/μL)	1.8 ± 0.56	0.50 (0-2.75)	0.75 (0.01-3.72)
Eosinophils (10^3/μL)	4.1 ± 0.11	—	—
Basophils (10^3/μL)	0.4 ± 0.01	—	0.11 (0.06-0.14)
Fibrinogen (mg/dL)	133 (0-200)	—	500 (200-700)
Chemistries			
ALP (U/L)	160 ± 85	—	176 (14-405)
ALT (U/L)	33 ± 24	—	19 (1-93)
Amylase (U/L)	—	—	1021 (265-1868)
AST (U/L)	18 ± 14	397 (93-967)	24 (2-58)
Bilirubin, total (mg/dL)	0.3 ± 0.2	—	0.1 (0-0.3)
BUN (mg/dL)	1 ± 1	—	2 (1-5)
Calcium (mg/dL)	12.2 ± 0.8	11.9 (8.7-14.5)	14.0 (9.8-18.2)
Chloride (mmol/L)	121 ± 7	—	111 (97-124)
Cholesterol (mg/dL)	206 ± 67	—	78 (22-126)

Continued

TABLE 4-13 Hematologic and Serum Biochemical Values of Lizards. (cont'd)

Measurement	Tegu lizard (*Tupinambus* spp)	Veiled chameleon (*Chameleo calyptratus*)	Water monitor (*Varanus salvator*)
Creatine kinase (U/L)	641 ± 568	1873 (5-8905)	772 (176-1818)
Creatinine (mg/dL)	0.3 ± 0.1	—	0.5 (0-1)
GGT (U/L)	7	—	24 (7-48)
Glucose (mg/dL)	128 ± 30	270 (125-444)	98 (29-170)
Iron (μg/dL)	—	—	242 (111-429)
LDH (U/L)	540 ± 537	—	157 (34-1288)
Magnesium (mmol/L)	—	—	1.3 (1.1-1.4)
Phosphorus (mg/dL)	5.6 ± 2.1	8.4 (4.4-16.1)	5.2 (2.9-8.9)
Potassium (mmol/L)	2.4 ± 1.4	6.5 (3.5-12.0)	4.6 (3.5-6.1)
Protein, total (g/dL)	6.6 ± 1.3	6.4 (4.4-10.9)	7.0 (5.1-9.8)
Albumin (g/dL)[b]	3.6 ± 0.7	3.1 (1.4-4.2)	2.4 (1.4-3.4)
Albumin (PEP; g/dL)[b]	—	—	3.1 (3-3.2)
Globulin (g/dL)[b]	2.9 ± 1.2	3.3 (2.0-5.9)	4.7 (2.0-7.3)
α-1 (PEP; g/dL)[b]	—	—	0.1
α-2 (PEP; g/dL)[b]	—	—	0.9 (0.8-1)
β (PEP; g/dL)[b]	—	—	0.9
γ (PEP; g/dL)[b]	—	—	4.7 (2.6-6.8)
Sodium (mmol/L)	159 ± 4	144 (132-169)	156 (143-170)
Triglyceride (mg/dL)	31	—	35 (6-78)
Uric acid (mg/dL)	3.2 ± 2	5.6 (0-21.9)	4.7 (1-12.2)

[a]Listed values are median followed by either min-max or a confidence interval in parentheses depending upon reported methods and the authors' judgment from the available evidence, unless a single value indicating n=1 or a range that is not enclosed in parentheses indicating a reported reference interval.
[b]Albumin is measured by colorimetry (e.g., bromocresol green) and globulin value is calculated unless otherwise indicated "PEP" (protein electrophoresis).
[c]Can be elevated in gravid females.[236,346]
[d]These data were obtained from iguanas housed outdoors with unfiltered sunlight.
[e]Adults.

TABLE 4-14 Hematologic and Serum Biochemical Values of Chelonians.[a]

Measurement	African spurred tortoise (*Centrochelys sulcata*)[64,464]	Aldabra tortoise (*Aldabrachelys gigantea*)[464]	Desert tortoise (*Gopherus agassizii*)[8,75,97,164]
Hematology			
PCV (%)	28 (9-43)	22 (11-34)	15-39
RBC (10^6/μL)	0.61 (0.08-1.15)	0.45 (0.13-0.77)	0.28-1.34
Hgb (g/dL)	7.7 (2.4-13.1)	7.1 (3.8-10.5)	3.6-10.3
MCV (fL)	418 (156-678)	469 (195-742)	197-688

TABLE 4-14 Hematologic and Serum Biochemical Values of Chelonians. (cont'd)

Measurement	African spurred tortoise (*Centrochelys sulcata*)	Aldabra tortoise (*Aldabrachelys gigantea*)	Desert tortoise (*Gopherus agassizii*)
MCH (pg)	116 (2.1-193)	154 (63-244)	39-189
MCHC (g/dL)	30 (20-40)	32 (21-42)	19-35
WBC (10^3/μL)	4.41 (0.87-13.23)	5.45 (1.54-17.5)	0.97-10.9
Heterophils (10^3/μL)	1.92 (0.23-7.43)	3.17 (0.69-8.79)	0.49-7.3
Lymphocytes (10^3/μL)	1.41 (0.17-6.06)	1.52 (0.11-5.53)	0-3.8
Monocytes (10^3/μL)	0.01 (0.01-0.37)	0.14 (0.02-0.79)	0-0.57
Azurophils (10^3/μL)	0.04 (0-0.84)	0.04 (0-0.68)	0-0.9
Eosinophils (10^3/μL)	0.10 (0.01-0.43)	0.13 (0.01-0.44)	0-0.95
Basophils (10^3/μL)	0.12 (0.01-0.36)	0.11 (0.02-0.40)	0-4.3
Fibrinogen (mg/dL)	—	100 (0-200)	—
Chemistries			
ALP (U/L)	36 (10-70)	64 (15-142)	43-176
ALT (U/L)	9 (0-33)	3 (0-22)	21 (0-66)
Amylase (U/L)	1359 (399-2240)	947 (144-3266)	—
AST (U/L)	108 (34-401)	59 (19-155)	41-106
Bile acid (μmol/L)	—	—	0-5.4
Bilirubin, total (mg/dL)	0.1 (0-0.7)	0.4 (0.1-1.2)	0-0.9
BUN (mg/dL)	3 (1-6)	18 (4-43)	0-4
Calcium (mg/dL)	11.4 (7.8-21.2)	11.7 (8.5-42.7)	9.3-14.7
Chloride (mmol/L)	109 (93-124)	93 (86-104)	94-112
Cholesterol (mg/dL)	129 (36-283)	229 (69-564)	56-233
Creatine kinase (U/L)	407 (31-2088)	59 (11-380)	2262 (944-3880)
Creatinine (mg/dL)	0.3 (0.1-0.4)	0.2 (0-0.4)	0.11-0.37
GGT (U/L)	14 (3-19)	—	—
Glucose (mg/dL)	107 (55-220)	43 (12-85)	92-165
Iron (μg/dL)	81 (80-82)	—	—
LDH (U/L)	977 (140-3264)	473 (131-1077)	25-250
Magnesium (mmol/L)	—	—	1.1 (0.9-1.2)
Phosphorus (mg/dL)	3.8 (1.5-6.5)	3.9 (1.9-13)	1-6.3
Potassium (mmol/L)	6.1 (3.3-11.9)	5.5 (3.8-8.1)	3.5-4.7
Protein, total (g/dL)	3.8 (1.2-6.3)	5.3 (2.5-7.7)	3-4.6
Albumin (g/dL)[b]	1.5 (0-2.3)	1.6 (0.7-3.0)	1.2-2.2
Globulin (g/dL)[b]	2.3 (0.4-3.8)	3.7 (1.0-5.5)	1.2-2.6
α-1 (PEP; g/dL)[b]	—	—	1

Continued

TABLE 4-14 Hematologic and Serum Biochemical Values of Chelonians. (cont'd)

Measurement	African spurred tortoise (*Centrochelys sulcata*)	Aldabra tortoise (*Aldabrachelys gigantea*)	Desert tortoise (*Gopherus agassizii*)
α-2 (PEP; g/dL)[b]	—	—	1
β (PEP; g/dL)[b]	—	—	0.6
Sodium (mmol/L)	139 (125-154)	128 (119-141)	122-139
Triglyceride (mg/dL)	163 (53-388)	425 (17-1010)	0-425
Urea (mg/dL)	—	—	—
Uric acid (mg/dL)	4.6 (0.6-10.4)	1.5 (0.2-3.4)	2.7-7.2
Vitamin A (µg/mL)	—	—	0.2-0.6
Zinc (ppm)	—	—	0.4-3.7

Measurement	Eastern box turtle (*Terrapene carolina*)[64,98,134,236,464]	Galapagos tortoise (*Chelonoidis nigra*)[464]	Gopher tortoise (*Gopherus polyphemus*)[463]
Hematology			
PCV (%)	24 (8-37)	18 (7-29)	23 (15-30)
RBC (10^6/µL)	0.56 (0.08-1.03)	0.40 (0.16-0.63)	0.54 (0.24-0.91)
Hgb (g/dL)	6.8 (2.6-11.0)	5.5 (3.3-8.9)	6.4 (4.2-8.6)
MCV (fL)	396 (117-750)	535 (266-769)	—
MCH (pg)	110 (30-207)	160 (100-239)	—
MCHC (g/dL)	29 (14-43)	31 (24-38)	—
WBC (10^3/µL)	5.48 (1.34-15.9)	4.57 (0.71-17.5)	15.7 (10-22)
Heterophils (10^3/µL)	1.61 (0.15-6.4)	1.57 (0.10-6.76)	4.7 (1-12.5)[d]
Lymphocytes (10^3/µL)	1.61 (0.15-9.82)	1.45 (0.04-6.56)	8.9 (3.2-17.4)[d]
Monocytes (10^3/µL)	0.19 (0.18-0.80)	0.08 (0.02-0.33)	1.1 (0.3-2.9)[d]
Azurophils (10^3/µL)	0.03 (0-0.80)	0.03 (0-0.52)	—
Eosinophils (10^3/µL)	0.47 (0.42-3.01)	0.09 (0.02-0.40)	—
Basophils (10^3/µL)	0.55 (0.4-2.14)	0.34 (0.03-1.38)	0.94 (0.2-2.4)[d]
Chemistries			
ALP (U/L)	77 (20-225)	77 (27-235)	39 (11-71)
ALT (U/L)	6 (0-20)	3 (0-18)	15 (2-57)
Amylase (U/L)	1033 (87-2526)	22 (3-41)	—
AST (U/L)	64 (14-191)	40 (16-122)	136 (57-392)
Bilirubin, total (mg/dL)	0.1 (0.1-0.4)	0.3 (0-0.8)	0.02 (0-0.1)
BUN (mg/dL)	52 (6-121)	12 (3-35)	30 (1-130)
Calcium (mg/dL)	10.5 (6.8-23.2)[c]	10.4 (6.6-17.8)	12 (10-14)
Chloride (mmol/L)	106 (89-121)	98 (83-112)	102 (35-128)
Cholesterol (mg/dL)	205 (42-483)	172 (42-450)	76 (19-150)

TABLE 4-14 Hematologic and Serum Biochemical Values of Chelonians. (cont'd)

Measurement	Eastern box turtle (*Terrapene carolina*)	Galapagos tortoise (*Chelonoidis nigra*)	Gopher tortoise (*Gopherus polyphemus*)
Creatine kinase (U/L)	153 (23-747)	592 (35-2378)	160 (32-628)
Creatinine (mg/dL)	0.2 (0-0.5)	0.2 (0-0.4)	0.3 (0.1-0.4)
GGT (U/L)	—	4 (0-11)	—
Glucose (mg/dL)	48 (23-114)	98 (35-312)	75 (55-128)
Iron (µg/dL)	—	73 (8-593)	—
LDH (U/L)	307 (20-1032)	469 (71-1212)	273 (18-909)
Magnesium (mmol/L)	—	—	2.1 (1.7-2.4)
Phosphorus (mg/dL)	3.5 (1.7-7.5)	3.7 (2.0-8.0)	2.1 (1-3.1)
Potassium (mmol/L)	4.7 (3.1-9.4)	4.8 (3.4-7.2)	5 (2.9-7)
Protein, total (g/dL)	3.20 (3.10-3.90)	4.7 (1.8-7.9)	3.1 (1.3-4.6)
Protein, total (male; g/dL)	3.00 (1.80-5.20)	—	—
Protein, total (female; g/dL)	4.00 (2.20-6.20)	—	—
Haptoglobin	0.25 (0.27-0.38)	—	—
Albumin (g/dL)[b]	2.2 (1.2-3.2)	1.6 (0.4-2.7)	1.5 (0.5-2.6)
Pre-alb (PEP; g/dL)[b]	0 (0-0.002)	—	—
Albumin (PEP; g/dL)[b]	0.71-0.85	—	—
Globulin (g/dL)[b]	3.4 (2.5-4.7)	3.1 (1.1-5.5)	—
α-1 (PEP; g/dL)[b]	0.25 (0.25-0.30)	—	—
α-2 (PEP; g/dL)[b]	0.80 (0.76-0.92)	—	—
β (PEP; g/dL)[b]	1.27 (1.27-1.55)	—	—
γ (PEP; g/dL)[b]	0.26 (0.27-0.32)	—	—
A:G ratio	0.27-0.31	—	—
Sodium (mmol/L)	139 (120-155)	130 (119-140)	138 (127-148)
α-tocopherol (µg/dL)	—	2 (1-2)	—
Triglyceride (mg/dL)	—	271 (29-1345)	—
Free T_3	—	29	—
Uric acid (mg/dL)	0.7 (0.1-2.9)	1.7 (0.1-4.0)	3.5 (0.9-8.5)

Measurement	Green sea turtle (*Chelonia mydas*)[132,454,464]	Hawksbill sea turtle (*Eretmochelys imbri cata*)[e,464,487]	Hermann's tortoise (*Testudo hermanni*)[16,39]
Hematology			
PCV (%)	33 (23-45)	13-41	23 (11-40)
RBC (10^6/µL)	0.52 (0.21-0.97)	—	0.8 (0.4-1.0)
Hgb (g/dL)	10.7	—	8.4 (4.1-13.5)

Continued

TABLE 4-14 Hematologic and Serum Biochemical Values of Chelonians. (cont'd)

Measurement	Green sea turtle (*Chelonia mydas*)	Hawksbill sea turtle (*Eretmochelys imbricata*)	Hermann's tortoise (*Testudo hermanni*)
MCV (fL)	717 (320-1429)	—	310 (231.6-383.7)
MCH (pg)	55	—	100 (47-144.3)
MCHC (g/dL)	36	—	32.5 (17.4-45.7)
WBC (10^3/μL)	9.98 (3.76-21.7)	—	9.4 (2.4-15.3)
Heterophils (10^3/μL)	6.69 (1.57-15.7)	—	2.3 (0-5)
Lymphocytes (10^3/μL)	2.14 (0.94-4.34)	—	4.4 (0.2-8.5)
Monocytes (10^3/μL)	0.91 (0.23-1.81)	—	0.5 (0-1.2)
Azurophils (10^3/μL)	—	—	—
Eosinophils (10^3/μL)	0.12 (0-0.48)	—	0.97 (0-2.5)
Basophils (10^3/μL)	0.13 (0-1.94)	—	0.1 (0-0.2)
Chemistries			
ALP (U/L)	6-67	7-80	392 (122-606)
ALT (U/L)	32 (3-241)	1-23	1 (1-12.5)
Amylase (U/L)	534	—	—
AST (U/L)	74-245	74-245	74 (0-359)
Bilirubin, total (mg/dL)	0.03-0.2	0-10	—
BUN (mg/dL)	64 (13.9-173)	7-34	—
Calcium (mg/dL)	8-8.8	2.6-11.6	12.9 (4.8-20.5)
Chloride (mmol/L)	101-121	106-134	101 (92-111)
Cholesterol (mg/dL)	221 (142-354)	—	—
Creatine kinase (U/L)	326-2729	14-6008	168 (0-732)
Creatinine (mg/dL)	0.25 (0.1-1.6)	—	0.16 (0.03-0.3)
GGT (U/L)	6 (0-21)	—	—
Glucose (mg/dL)	67-178	79-162	68 (15-120)
Iron (μg/dL)	362 (117-600)	6-67	—
LDH (U/L)	75-477	—	395 (0-800)
Magnesium (mmol/L)	2.4-6.1	1.7-3.6	—
Phosphorus (mg/dL)	4.9-11.1	1.9-8.7	3.1 (0.6-5.5)
Potassium (mmol/L)	3-7.1	3.0-5.3	5.6 (3.5-7.7)
Protein, total (g/dL)	2.1-6.2	1.3-5.1	4.3 (2.6-6.1)
Albumin (g/dL)[b]	0.7-1.8	0.3-1.4	1.8 (0.8-2.6)
Globulin (g/dL)[b]	1.5-4.7	0.8-4.8	—
Sodium (mmol/L)	139-158	146-159	130 (116-143)
Triglyceride (mg/dL)	492 (124-932)	—	—
Urea (mg/dL)	—	—	3.75 (0-11.1)
Uric acid (mg/dL)	1.1 (0-2.7)	0.6 (0-1.8)	2.6 (0-5.2)

TABLE 4-14 Hematologic and Serum Biochemical Values of Chelonians. (cont'd)

Measurement	Indian star tortoise (*Geochelone elegans*)[64,464]	Leopard tortoise (*Stigmochelys pardalis*)[64,464]	Loggerhead sea turtle (*Caretta caretta*)[92,464]
Hematology			
PCV (%)	23 (14-38)	23 (8-37)	32 (18-40)
RBC (10^6/μL)	0.37 (0.24-0.55)	0.52 (0.15-1.06)	0.52 (0.22-1.22)
Hgb (g/dL)	7.9 (6.9-8.5)	16.1 (8.8-28)	10.7
MCV (fL)	—	488 (179-833)	416 (82-1027)
MCH (pg)	—	83	55
MCHC (g/dL)	27 (26-28)	44 (42-46)	36
WBC (10^3/μL)	6.71 (1.35-27.9)	4.24 (0.6-10.0)	9.00 (5.00-12.50)
Heterophils (10^3/μL)	2.56 (0.24-10.9)	1.92 (0.11-4.87)	3.67 (0.35-7.16)
Lymphocytes (10^3/μL)	2.83 (0.20-15.4)	1.61 (0.05-4.74)	2.72 (0.30-4.83)
Monocytes (10^3/μL)	0.20 (0.02-0.75)	0.08 (0.02-0.62)	0.96 (0.22-1.84)
Azurophils (10^3/μL)	0.05 (0.01-0.87)	0.02 (0-0.51)	—
Eosinophils (10^3/μL)	0.26 (0.03-1.51)	0.15 (0.02-0.37)	1.15 (0.45-2.10)
Basophils (10^3/μL)	0.49 (0.09-1.79)	0.11 (0.01-0.34)	—
Chemistries			
ALP (U/L)	72 (20-164)	107 (21-278)	64 (11-254)
ALT (U/L)	4 (0-14)	8	—
Amylase (U/L)	1235	—	—
AST (U/L)	54 (14-152)	54 (5-119)	154 (10-480)
Bilirubin, total (mg/dL)	0.2 (0-0.5)	0.1	—
BUN (mg/dL)	3 (0-9)	12 (1-36)	105 (19-162)
Calcium (mg/dL)	11.7 (7.6-21.2)	11.8 (6.5-18.3)	6.9 (2.2-11.5)
Chloride (mmol/L)	100 (88-112)	104 (90-119)	118 (103-137)
Cholesterol (mg/dL)	115 (15-255)	111 (9-239)	—
Creatine kinase (U/L)	374 (22-2644)	359 (223-704)	899 (258-3586)
Creatinine (mg/dL)	0.3 (0.2-0.5)	0.6	—
GGT (U/L)	4 (0-5)	—	—
Glucose (mg/dL)	76 (37-186)	75 (10-152)	120 (66-177)
Iron (μg/dL)	—	—	—
LDH (U/L)	438 (12-863)	446 (346-546)	—
Lipase (U/L)	5	—	—
Phosphorus (mg/dL)	3.6 (1.4-9.4)	2.7 (1.1-5.2)	9.3 (3.7-14.0)
Potassium (mmol/L)	4.8 (2.0-7.7)	5.4 (2.3-8.8)	3.9 (2.7-5.1)
Protein, total (g/dL)	4.7 (2.2-7.6)	3.3 (1.9-6.2)	3.3 (1.2-6.9)
Albumin (g/dL)[b]	1.7 (0.4-3.0)	1.6 (0.3-2.9)	1.5 (0.7-2.6)
Globulin (g/dL)[b]	2.9 (1.3-4.6)	2.6 (0.6-4.6)	2.2 (0.2-4.9)

Continued

TABLE 4-14 Hematologic and Serum Biochemical Values of Chelonians. (cont'd)

Measurement	Indian star tortoise (*Geochelone elegans*)	Leopard tortoise (*Stigmochelys pardalis*)	Loggerhead sea turtle (*Caretta caretta*)
Sodium (mmol/L)	127 (117-137)	132 (115-148)	153 (142-164)
Triglyceride (mg/dL)	60 (27-110)	—	—
Uric acid (mg/dL)	3.3 (0.2-7.9)	2.5 (0.5-6.6)	0.5 (0-1.2)

Measurement	Ornate box turtle (*Terrapene ornata*)[64,464]	Pacific pond turtle (*Actinemys marmorata*)[464]	Painted turtle (*Chrysemys picta*)[149,216,464]
Hematology			
PCV (%)	23 (10-37)	24 (7-42)	25 (6-43)
RBC ($10^6/\mu L$)	0.62 (0.46-0.8)	0.69 (0.24-1.20)	0.57 (0.41-0.68)
Hgb (g/dL)	7.2 (6-9)	7.6 (3.0-12.6)	11.2 (10.7-11.7)
MCV (fL)	408 (350-463)	377 (200-634)	271 (183-365)
MCH (pg)	122 (108-136)	107 (19-186)	—
MCHC (g/dL)	33 (31-33)	27 (18-42)	—
WBC ($10^3/\mu L$)	5.76 (1.2-13.4)	5.94 (1.02-17.0)	9.49 (0.40-23.2)
Heterophils ($10^3/\mu L$)	2.01 (0.10-5.9)	1.83 (0.14-5.52)	2.30 (0.17-8.39)
Lymphocytes ($10^3/\mu L$)	2.19 (0.10-7.60)	2.46 (0.22-8.48)	2.60 (0.01-7.07)
Monocytes ($10^3/\mu L$)	0.13 (0.02-0.74)	—	—
Azurophils ($10^3/\mu L$)	0.03 (0-0.13)	0.04 (0-0.43)	0.05 (0-0.26)
Eosinophils ($10^3/\mu L$)	0.23 (0.03-1.32)	0.37 (0.02-1.81)	—
Basophils ($10^3/\mu L$)	0.25 (0.02-0.92)	0.62 (0.05-2.09)	1.95 (0.04-5.91)
Chemistries			
ALP (U/L)	61 (14-139)	—	208
ALT (U/L)	30 (25-33)	—	—
Amylase (U/L)	691 (2-1893)	—	—
AST (U/L)	61 (11-141)	105 (26-228)	132 (45-284)
Bilirubin, total (mg/dL)	0.3 (0.1-0.4)	—	0.1
BUN (mg/dL)	60 (4-154)	—	37
Calcium (mg/dL)	10.3 (6.2-17.5)	10.0 (7.0-14.5)	11.7 (5.5-19.1)
Chloride (mmol/L)	108 (93-124)	—	96 (73-109)
Cholesterol (mg/dL)	201 (20-469)	—	—
Creatine kinase (U/L)	196 (0-777)	242 (63-747)	352 (35-1608)
Creatinine (mg/dL)	1 (0.2-2.4)	—	—
Glucose (mg/dL)	67 (13-120)	53 (4-113)	63 (10-133)
LDH (U/L)	362 (300-424)	—	412

TABLE 4-14 Hematologic and Serum Biochemical Values of Chelonians. (cont'd)

Measurement	Ornate box turtle (*Terrapene ornata*)	Pacific pond turtle (*Actinemys marmorata*)	Painted turtle (*Chrysemys picta*)
Magnesium (mmol/L)	—	—	2.4
Phosphorus (mg/dL)	3.3 (1.9-5.8)	3.6 (1.9-6.6)	3.6 (1.7-7.2)
Potassium (mmol/L)	4.7 (2.4-8.2)	4.3 (2.3-7.1)	3.6 (2.2-11.6)
Protein, total (g/dL)	4.0 (1.4-6.6)	4.4 (1.8-7.0)	4.4 (1.8-7.7)
Albumin (g/dL)[b]	1.5 (0.2-2.8)	1.7 (0.7-2.7)	1.3 (0-2.7)
Globulin (g/dL)[b]	2.4 (0.6-4.3)	2.8 (1.0-4.6)	3.0 (0.1-5.9)
Sodium (mmol/L)	141 (129-154)	135 (123-147)	137 (119-146)
Uric acid (mg/dL)	0.6 (0-1.9)	0.9 (0-3.1)	0.7 (0.1-1.8)

Measurement	Ploughshare tortoise (*Astrochelys yniphora*) (juveniles)[277]	Radiated tortoise (*Astrochelys radiata*)[344,464,501]	Red-footed tortoise (*Chelonoidis carbonaria*)[64,464]
Hematology			
PCV (%)	26 (20-28)	10-51	25 (6-38)
RBC (10^6/μL)	—	0.3-1.1	0.46 (0.14-0.19)
Hgb (g/dL)	—	5.6 (4-8)	7.5 (7-7.9)
MCV (fL)	—	454 (319-571)	482 (22-940)
MCH (pg)	—	108 (82-133)	136 (123-149)
MCHC (g/dL)	—	28 (26-33)	31 (29-32)
WBC (10^3/μL)	5.9 (2.1-9.5)	2.5-14	6.51 (1.15-20.0)
Heterophils (10^3/μL)	1.7 (0-3.8)	0.7-8	1.67 (0.16-7.26)
Lymphocytes (10^3/μL)	2.1 (0.1-4.5)	0.4-5.8	1.89 (0.12-9.10)
Monocytes (10^3/μL)	0.3 (0-0.8)	0.02-0.5	0.16 (0.02-0.58)
Azurophils (10^3/μL)	—	0-0.82	0.05 (0-0.87)
Eosinophils (10^3/μL)	0.08 (0-0.4)	0.03-0.82	0.17 (0.02-0.80)
Basophils (10^3/μL)	1.1 (0.-2.8)	0.1-2.5	0.92 (0.03-3.48)
Fibrinogen (mg/dL)	—	117 (100-200)	—
Chemistries			
ALP (U/L)	—	72-392	60 (6-145)
ALT (U/L)	—	0-17	7 (0-18)
Amylase (U/L)	—	—	—
AST (U/L)	59 (19.3-100.4)	25-348	130 (20-406)
Bile acid (μmol/L)	21.1 (0.3-41.6)	0.3-31.3	—
Bilirubin, total (mg/dL)	—	0-0.5	0.5 (0.1-1.1)
BUN (mg/dL)	—	2-34	14 (1-34)

Continued

TABLE 4-14 Hematologic and Serum Biochemical Values of Chelonians. (cont'd)

Measurement	Ploughshare tortoise (*Astrochelys yniphora*) (juveniles)	Radiated tortoise (*Astrochelys radiata*)	Red-footed tortoise (*Chelonoidis carbonaria*)
Calcium (mg/dL)	12.4 (8.4-16)	8.6-18	12.2 (7.1-24.1)
Chloride (mmol/L)	—	91-112	99 (81-111)
Cholesterol (mg/dL)	—	56-154	121 (10-257)
Creatine kinase (U/L)	217 (0-695)	33-5666	695 (54-3593)
Creatinine (mg/dL)	—	0.1-0.5	0.4 (0.2-1.3)
GGT (U/L)	—	5 (0-11)	28 (7-130)
Glucose (mg/dL)	—	21-93	67 (13-154)
Iron (μg/dL)	—	60	107
LDH (U/L)	—	213-6444	638 (118-1644)
Lipase (U/L)	—	5-50	—
Phosphorus (mg/dL)	0.9 (0.2-1.6)	2.5-7	3.5 (1.0-8.3)
Potassium (mmol/L)	—	3.1-5.8	5.5 (2.8-9.4)
Protein, total (g/dL)	3.4 (2.6-4.2)	3-6.6	4.7 (1.9-7.4)
Albumin (g/dL)[b]	1.2 (0.6-1.8)	0.6-2.4	1.6 (0-3.0)
Albumin (PEP; g/dL)[b]	—	0.9-2.4	—
Globulin (g/dL)[b]	—	1.4-3.2	3.1 (0.2-4.8)
α-1 (PEP; g/dL)[b]	—	0.1-0.5	—
α-2 (PEP; g/dL)[b]	—	0.6-1.9	—
β (PEP; g/dL)[b]	—	0.6-1.5	—
γ (PEP; g/dL)[b]	—	0.4-0.9	—
Sodium (mmol/L)	—	121-146	130 (117-143)
Triglyceride (mg/dL)	—	26-303	246 (28-480)
Uric acid (mg/dL)	0.8 (0.1-1.5)	0.3 (0-0.6)	0.6 (0.1-2.1)

Measurement	Russian tortoise (*Testudo horsfieldii*)[249,308]	Sliders (*Trachemys scripta* spp.)[64,89,149,216,464]	Wood turtle (*Glyptemys insculpta*)[464]
Hematology			
PCV (%)	23 (22-34)	26 (8-44)	25 (9-41)
RBC (10^6/μL)	—	0.84 (0.33-2.21)	—
Hgb (g/dL)	—	11.1 (10-12.2)	—
MCV (fL)	—	409 (179-697)	—
MCH (pg)	—	108	—
MCHC (g/dL)	—	30	—

TABLE 4-14 Hematologic and Serum Biochemical Values of Chelonians. (cont'd)

Measurement	Russian tortoise (*Testudo horsfieldii*)	Sliders (*Trachemys scripta* spp.)	Wood turtle (*Glyptemys insculpta*)
WBC (10^3/µL)	8.5 (5-12.5)	6.73 (1.0-19.4)	5.20 (0.8-20.0)
Heterophils (10^3/µL)	3.7 (1.3-4.6)	2.33 (0.18-5.86)	—
Lymphocytes (10^3/µL)	4.7 (3.6-7.6)	2.28 (0.03-6.90)	3.15 (0.59-13.0)
Monocytes (10^3/µL)	0.01 (0-0.02)	0.18 (0.04-0.65)	—
Azurophils (10^3/µL)	0.05 (0.03-0.12)	0.05 (0-0.48)	0.08 (0-1.11)
Eosinophils (10^3/µL)	0.05 (0.02-0.06)	0.52 (0.01-3.06)	—
Basophils (10^3/µL)	0.05 (0.02-0.08)	1.07 (0.01-3.56)	—
Chemistries			
ALP (U/L)	498 (181-1188)	113 (30-372)	71 (21-268)
ALT (U/L)	1 (0-2)	14 (1-66)	—
Amylase (U/L)	—	493 (411-535)	—
AST (U/L)	20 (12-32)	141 (44-358)	79 (14-212)
Bilirubin, total (mg/dL)	0.015 (0-0.09)	0.2 (0.1-0.5)	—
BUN (mg/dL)	12 (4-17)	23 (2-64)	—
Calcium (mg/dL)	13.2 (9.9-19.5)	12.6 (6.5-22.6)	11.8 (6.3-29.4)
Ionized calcium (mmol/L)	1.28 (1-1.6)	—	—
Chloride (mmol/L)	—	98 (88-112)	—
Cholesterol (mg/dL)	109 (25-210)	162 (106-227)	—
Creatine kinase (U/L)	123 (6-344)	516 (108-2125)	—
Creatinine (mg/dL)	—	0.3 (0.2-0.5)	—
GGT (U/L)	—	7 (0-21)	—
GLDH (U/L)	1 (0.6-1.5)	—	—
Glucose (mg/dL)	59 (40-86)	54 (21-143)	53 (13-108)
Iron (µg/dL)	—	—	—
LDH (U/L)	—	1713 (371-5763)	—
Lipase (U/L)	—	6 (1-15)	—
Magnesium (mmol/L)	—	1.1	—
Phosphorus (mg/dL)	2.6 (1.3-3.9)	4.0 (1.8-8.8)	3.2 (1.6-10)
Potassium (mmol/L)	5.3 (1.9-7.2)	3.8 (2.4-7.5)	—
Protein, total (g/dL)	3 (2.5-4.6)	4.8 (1.1-8.8)	4.7 (1.5-6.5)
Albumin (g/dL)[b]	1.6 (1.2-2.3)	1.8 (0.6-3.3)	—
Globulin (g/dL)[b]	1.4 (1.3-2.3)	3.2 (1.1-5.9)	—

Continued

TABLE 4-14 Hematologic and Serum Biochemical Values of Chelonians. (cont'd)

Measurement	Russian tortoise (*Testudo horsfieldii*)	Sliders (*Trachemys scripta* spp.)	Wood turtle (*Glyptemys insculpta*)
Sodium (mmol/L)	138 (131-149)	134 (123-147)	—
Triglyceride (mg/dL)	—	304 (30-664)	—
Uric acid (mg/dL)	1.2 (0.8-3.9)	0.8 (0.1-1.9)	1.0 (0-4.1)

[a]Listed values are median followed by either min-max or a confidence interval in parentheses depending upon reported methods and the authors' judgment from the available evidence, unless a single value indicating n=1, or a range that is not enclosed in parentheses indicating a reported reference interval.
[b]Albumin is measured by colorimetry (e.g., bromocresol green) and globulin value is calculated unless otherwise indicated "PEP" (protein electrophoresis).
[c]Can be elevated in gravid females[236,346]
[d]Calculated from data.
[e]Juveniles.

TABLE 4-15 Hematologic and Serum Biochemical Values of Crocodilians.[a]

Measurement	American alligator (*Alligator mississippiensis*)[64,464]	Dwarf caiman (*Paleosuchus palpebrosus*)[64,464]
Hematology		
PCV (%)	24 (9-39)	22 (12-35)
RBC (10^6/μL)	0.57 (0.21-1.3)	0.66 (0.43-0.89)
Hgb (g/dL)	7.8 (4.0-12.2)	7.7 (6.2-8.8)
MCV (fL)	430 (122-786)	362 (180-535)
MCH (pg)	135 (37-246)	98
MCHC (g/dL)	32 (18-45)	33 (23-38)
WBC (10^3/μL)	6.39 (2.03-21.3)	6 (2.1-14.7)
Heterophils (10^3/μL)	2.51 (0.50-8.19)	2.95 (0.51-7.73)
Lymphocytes (10^3/μL)	2.21 (0.29-12.1)	2.10 (0.28-9.66)
Monocytes (10^3/μL)	0.31 (0.04-2.04)	0.10 (0.02-0.44)
Azurophils (10^3/μL)	0.05 (0.01-1.25)	0.04 (0.01-0.73)
Eosinophils (10^3/μL)	0.22 (0.03-1.02)	0.12 (0.03-0.43)
Basophils (10^3/μL)	0.71 (0.04-3.23)	0.15 (0.04-0.46)
Fibrinogen (mg/dL)	267 ± 115	100 (0-200)
Chemistries		
ALP (U/L)	34 (12-105)	13 (2-26)
ALT (U/L)	37 (8-92)	37 (5-74)
Amylase (U/L)	58 (25-1067)	47 (25-234)
AST (U/L)	246 (111-539)	88 (36-218)
Bilirubin, total (mg/dL)	0.2 (0-0.8)	0.2 (0-0.6)
BUN (mg/dL)	2 (1-18)	2 (0-4)

TABLE 4-15 Hematologic and Serum Biochemical Values of Crocodilians. (cont'd)

Measurement	American alligator (*Alligator mississippiensis*)	Dwarf caiman (*Paleosuchus palpebrosus*)
Calcium (mg/dL)	11.2 (8.1-15.1)	10.4 (8.1-13.8)
Chloride (mmol/L)	112 (94-123)	121 (99-144)
Cholesterol (mg/dL)	108 (32-291)	115 (29-241)
Creatine kinase (U/L)	911 (145-7408)	1926 (89-9228)
Creatinine (mg/dL)	0.3 (0-0.7)	0.3 (0-0.6)
Glucose (mg/dL)	88 (34-177)	64 (13-146)
LDH (U/L)	346 (13-1726)	1269 (62-4058)
Osmolarity (mOsm/L)	—	303 (301-304)
Phosphorus (mg/dL)	4.3 (1.6-9.9)	4.4 (2.0-9.7)
Potassium (mmol/L)	3.8 (2.4-5.3)	4.3 (3.0-6.3)
Protein, total (g/dL)	5.1 (2.6-7.8)	5.4 (2.6-7.8)
Albumin (g/dL)[b]	1.5 (0.4-2.6)	1.4 (0.6-2.7)
Albumin (PEP; g/dL)[b]	—	2.2 (1.8-2.5)
Globulin (g/dL)[b]	3.3 (0.7-5.5)	4.0 (1.8-6.2)
Sodium (mmol/L)	147 (134-160)	151 (134-167)
Triglyceride (mg/dL)	83 (7-505)	92 (9-174)
Uric acid (mg/dL)	1.3 (0.2-4.0)	2.1 (0.4-5.6)

[a]Listed values are median followed by either min-max or a confidence interval in parentheses depending upon reported methods and the authors' judgment from the available evidence, unless a single value indicating n=1, or a range that is not enclosed in parentheses indicating a reported reference interval.
[b]Albumin is measured by colorimetry (e.g., bromocresol green) and globulin value is calculated unless otherwise indicated "PEP" (protein electrophoresis).

TABLE 4-16 Plasma Protein Electrophoresis Values of Healthy, Captive Green Iguanas (*Iguana iguana*).[a]

Analyte	Units	Subadult Males (n=20)[a-c]	Adult Females (n=14)[c,d,155]
Total protein	g/L (g/dL)	56.0-69.5; 62.6 ± 4.9 (5.6-6.95; 6.26 ± 0.49)	40.9-74.1; 56.7 ± 12.0
Albumin	g/L (g/dL)	17.2-24.6; 20.9 ± 2.1 (1.72-2.46; 2.09 ± 0.21)	13.9-30.6; 19.3 ± 4.6
Total globulin	g/L (g/dL)	34.9-49.0; 41.7 ± 4.7 (3.49-4.90; 4.17 ± 0.47)	—
α_1-globulins	g/L (g/dL)	1.5-7.6; 2.5 ± 1.3 (0.15-0.76; 0.25 ± 0.13)	4.2-12.3; 8.8 ± 2.6
α_2-globulins	g/L (g/dL)	5.0-9.5; 6.5 ± 1.6 (0.50-0.95; 0.65 ± 0.16)	—

Continued

TABLE 4-16 Plasma Protein Electrophoresis Values of Healthy, Captive Green Iguanas (*Iguana iguana*). (cont'd)

Analyte	Units	Subadult Males (n=20)	Adult Females (n=14)
β_1-globulins	g/L (g/dL)	12.1-20.9; 15.3 ± 3.6 (1.21-2.09; 1.53 ± 0.36)	15.9-37.5; 25.3 ± 8.0
β_2-globulins	g/L (g/dL)	5.1-16.3; 8.3 ± 4.2 (0.51-1.63; 0.83 ± 0.42)	—
γ-globulins	g/L (g/dL)	2.6-13.9; 5.1 ± 3.4 (0.26-1.39; 0.51 ± 0.34)	1.2-7.4; 4.0 ± 2.9
Albumin:globulin	—	0.37-0.64; 0.51 ± 0.08	0.41-0.78; 0.57 ± 0.14

[a]Unpublished data determined in clinical pathology laboratory, University of Georgia, Athens, Georgia, USA.
[b]Analyses performed using heparinized plasma, agarose gel plates.
[c]Data presented as range followed by mean ± SD.
[d]Analyses performed using heparinized plasma and cellulose acetate plates, and quantified by densitometry.
From Divers SJ, Camus MS. Lizards. In: Heatley JJ, Russell KE, eds. *Exotic Animal Laboratory Diagnosis.* Hoboken, NJ: Wiley Blackwell; 2020:319-346.

TABLE 4-17 Arterial and Venous Blood Gas Values for 37°C in 15 Conscious Green Iguanas (*Iguana iguana*) Breathing Room Air.[197]

Analyte	Units	Arterial[a]	Venous[a]
pH	—	7.29 ± 0.11 (7.38 ± 0.12)	7.31[b] (7.36 ± 0.13)
pCO_2	mm Hg	42 ± 9 (32 ± 7)	49[b] (36 ± 7)
pO_2	mm Hg	81 ± 19 (54 ± 15) [94 ± 21 (64 ± 16)]	46 ± 23 (30 ± 15)
Lactate	mmol/L	2.7 ± 1.1	2.3[b]
Bicarbonate	mmol/L	20 ± 4	22 ± 5
Total CO_2	mmol/L	22 ± 4	24 ± 5
Base excess	mmol/L	-6.3 ± 5.5	-5 ± 6
SaO_2	%	92 ± 6 [95 ± 3]	84[c] [49[b]]
SpO_2[c]	%	86 ± 6	—
RR[d]	breaths/min	28 ± 6	27 ± 6

[a]Data presented as mean ± SD unless indicated otherwise; values in parentheses are corrected for a body temperature of 30°C; when afternoon values were significantly different, they are listed in brackets.
[b]Values are reported as medians.
[c]SpO_2 = oxygen saturation measured by pulse oximetry.
[d]RR = respiration rate.
From Divers SJ, Camus MS. Lizards. In: Heatley JJ, Russell KE, eds. *Exotic Animal Laboratory Diagnosis.* Hoboken, NJ: Wiley Blackwell; 2020:319-346.

TABLE 4-18 Results of Blood Gas Analysis Performed with the i-STAT Handheld Analyzer (Zoetis) and Different Cartridges in Select Reptiles.

Parameter	Eastern box turtles (*Terrapene carolina carolina*)[a,2]		Hermann's tortoises (*Testudo hermanni*)[b,100]	Eastern rat snakes (*Panterophis alleghaniensis*)[b,68]	Common chameleons (*Chamaeleo chamaeleon*)[c,118]
Season	Spring	Summer	Spring	Various	Summer
Temperature correction	Results corrected based on air temperature	Results corrected based on air temperature	Results not corrected for patient temperature	Results not corrected for patient temperature	Results not corrected for patient temperature
Number of animals	37-38	40-41	24	17	17
pH	7.18-7.84	7.00-7.78	7.17-7.52	6.94-7.74	7.1 (6.9-7.5)
PO_2 (mmHg)	18-87	8-97	44-133	—	98 (61-180)
PCO_2 (mmHg)	15.1-64.9	16.5-74.7	35.7-99.1	11.6-78.5	39.0 (20.5-69.6)
HCO_3(mmol/L)	22.6-41.8	20.4-40.6	—	8.6-45.3	18.1 (5.6-44.7)
TCO_2 (mmol/L)	24-43	20-43	—	8.9-47.5	16.0 (6.0-38.0)
Lactate (mmol/L)	1.23-11.78	2.45-12.16	—	2.66-20.1	—
Base excess (mmol/L)	-7-11	-13-14	—	—	16 (8-25)

[a]Reference intervals.
[b]Ranges.
[c]Median (range).

TABLE 4-19 Environmental, Dietary, and Reproductive Characteristics of Reptiles.[63,390]

Species	Environmental Preference		Diet[d]	Method of Reproduction[e]	Gestation/Incubation Period (days)[f]
	Temperature[a-c]	Relative humidity (%)			
Snakes					
Ball (royal) python (*Python regius*)	25-30°C (77-86°F)	70-80 (use humidity box)[g]	C	Ov	90
Boa constrictor (*Boa constrictor*)	28-34°C (82-93°F)	50-70 (use humidity box)[g]	C	V	120-240
Corn snake (*Pantherophis guttatus*)	21-29°C (70-85°F)	50-70 (use humidity box)[g]	C	Ov	56-70
Garter snake (*Thamnophis sirtalis*)	22-30°C (72-86°F)	60-80 (use humidity box)[g]	C	V	90-110
King snake (*Lampropeltis getulus*)	23-30°C (73-86°F)	50-70 (use humidity box)[g]	Op/c	Ov	50-60
Sand boa (*Eryx* sp.)	25-30°C (77-86°F)	20-30	C	V	120-180
Lizards					
Bearded dragon (*Pogona vitticeps*)	21-35°C (70-95°F)	— (use humidity box)[g]	I-young H–adult	Ov	65-90
Crested gecko (*Correlophus ciliatus*)	25-28°C (77-82°F)	50-70 (use humidity box)[g]	F/i	Ov	60-150
Leopard gecko(*Eublepharis macularius*)	25-30°C (77-86°F)	20-30 (use humidity box)[g]	I	Ov	55-60

TABLE 4-19 Environmental, Dietary, and Reproductive Characteristics of Reptiles. (cont'd)

	Environmental Preference				
Species	Temperature[a-c]	Relative humidity (%)	Diet[d]	Method of Reproduction[e]	Gestation/Incubation Period (days)[f]
Uromastyx/spiny-tailed lizard (*Uromastyx* sp)	26-49°C (80-120°F) Large cage for gradient	— (use humidity box)[g]	H/seeds	Ov	60-80
Veiled chameleon (*Chameleo calyptratus*)	20-30°C (75-95°F)	50-70 need good ventilation	I	Ov	200
Water dragon (*Physignathus cocincinus*)	25-34°C (77-93°F)	80-90 need water with filter[h]	I/om	Ov	90
Chelonians					
Common box turtle (*Terrapene carolina*)	24-29°C (75-84°F)	60-80 (use humidity box)[g]	C/f	Ov	50-90
Desert tortoise (*Gopherus agassizii*)	25-30°C (77-86°F)	— (use humidity box)[g]	H	Ov	84-120
Greek tortoise (*Testudo graeca*)	20-27°C (68-81°F)	30-50 (use humidity box)[g]	H/om	Ov	60
Painted turtle (*Chrysemys picta*)	23-28°C (73-82°F)	80-90 need water with filter[h]	H/I/o	Ov	47-99
Red-eared slider (*Trachemys scripta elegans*)	22-30°C (72-86°F)	80-90 need water with filter[h]	C	Ov	59-93
Russian tortoise (*Agrionemys horsfieldii*)	21-32°C (70-90°F)	— (use humidity box)[g]	H	Ov	56-84

Continued

TABLE 4-19 Environmental, Dietary, and Reproductive Characteristics of Reptiles.[63,390] (cont'd)

Species	Environmental Preference				
	Temperature[a-c]	Relative humidity (%)	Diet[d]	Method of Reproduction[e]	Gestation/Incubation Period (days)[f]
Crocodilian					
American alligator (*Alligator mississippiensis*)	30-35°C (86-95°F)	80-90 need water with filter[h]	C/p	Ov	62-65

RH, Relative humidity; *C*, carnivorous; *F*, frugivorous; *H*, herbivorous; *I*, insectivorous; *O*, molluscavorous; *Om*, omnivorous; *Op*, ophiophagus; *P*, piscivorous; *V*, viviparous; *Ov*, oviparous.

[a]Temperatures shown are ideal ambient daytime temperature gradients. These should be allowed to fall by approximately 5°C (9°F) during the night. "Hot-spot" temperatures should generally be 5°C (9°F) greater than the highest temperature shown.

[b]Preferred daytime temperature range for other commonly housed captive snakes are: rosy boa (*Lichanura trivirgata*): 27-29.5°C (81-85°F); green tree python (*Morelia viridis*): 24-28°C (75-82°F); carpet python (*Morelia spilota*): 27-29.5°C (81-85°F); corn snake (*Elaphe guttata*): 25-30°C (77-86°F); yellow rat snake (*Elaphe obsoleta*): 25-29°C (77-84°F); gopher/bullsnake (*Pituophis melanoleucus*): 25-29°C (77-84°F).

[c]Preferred daytime temperature range for other commonly housed captive lizards are: day gecko (*Pheluma* sp.): 29.5°C (85°F); chameleons (montane) (*Chamaeleo* spp.): 21-27°C (70-81°F); chameleons (lowland) (*Chamaeleo* spp.): 27-29°C (81-84°F); bearded dragon (*Pogona vitticeps*): 26.7-29.5°C (80-85°F); blue-tongued skink (*Tiliqua* sp.): 27-29.5°C (81-85°F); monitor lizards (*Varanus* spp.): 29-31°C (84-88°F); tegus (*Tupinambis* spp.): 27-30°C (81-86°F).

[d]Uppercase letters denote principal dietary requirements; lowercase denotes secondary preference.

[e]Temperature-dependent.

[f]Can have long hatch times dependent on incubation parameters.

[g]This simulates humid underground burrow. Use dark-colored plastic container with cut entrance, moistened paper towels or sphagnum moss.

[h]Need to set up water component like fish tank with proper filter (use one for koi or turtles), pump, water quality testing, dechlorinator.

TABLE 4-20 Urinalysis Values of Chelonians.[153,208,250,252]

Measurement	Normal Values	Abnormal Values
Specific gravity	1.003-1.014 (mean, 1.008)	Up to 1.034
pH	Herbivores: alkaline Omnivores: 5-8	Acidic[a]
Color	Colorless to pale yellow with white urates	Dark yellow, yellow-brown, yellow-green
Turbidity	Clear	Cloudy
Protein	Trace proteinuria	Increased proteinuria
Glucose	Glucosuria up to 30 mg/dL	Glucosuria can be higher than 50 mg/dL with anorexia
Renal casts	None	Various types present
Calcium, phosphorus, ammonia, urea, creatinine	Detectable in urine	Significantly increased in urine of *Testudo* spp. with renal disease
AST, CK, LDH	Detectable in urine	Significantly increased in urine of *Testudo* spp. with renal disease
Crystals	Amorphous urates/ ammonium biurates	Many other crystals found in renal failure; uric acid crystals in gout; bilirubin and tyrosine crystals in liver disease

[a]May be associated with hibernation, anorexia, and improper diet.

TABLE 4-21 Electrocardiogram Measurement Reference Values (range) (Lead II) in Select Reptiles.[a,b]

	Boa constrictor					
Species	Unanes-thetized	Metofane	Pento-barbital	Snakes	Lizards	American alligator
Sample size	6	6	12	101	321	10
Heart rate	11-42	11-37	5-34	22-136	45-230	—
SV-P interval	—	0.24-1.3	0.40-0.60	0.29	0.19	—
SV duration	—	0.04-0.35	0.04-0.18	—	—	—
P amplitude	—	—	—	Inconsistent	Inconsistent	Inconsistent
P duration	0.06-0.1	0.05-0.2	0.04-0.11	0.02-0.07	0.02-0.06	Inconsistent
PR interval	0.38-0.90	0.04-1.04	0.35-0.56	0.26	0.16	Inconsistent
R amplitude	—	—	—	Inconsistent	Inconsistent	0.03-0.43
QRS duration	0.1-0.24	0.1-0.2	0.11-0.16	0.02-0.12	0.02-0.14	0.064-0.148
T amplitude	—	—	—	Inconsistent	Inconsistent	0.06-0.18
QT interval	0.8-2.0	0.84-1.74	1.16-2.40	0.30-1.36	0.18-1.30	0.93-1.45
MEA	—	—	—	96	95	60-108

[a]Amplitude in mV, duration in sec, MEA (mean electrical axis) in degrees.
[b]Room temperature was 22-26°C during ECG recording.
From Beaufrère H, Schilliger L, Pariaut R. Cardiovascular system. In: Mitchell MA, Tully TN Jr, eds. *Current Therapy in Exotic Pet Pratice.* St. Louis: Elsevier; 2016:151-220, with permission from Elsevier.

TABLE 4-22 Electrocardiographic Measurements of the Bearded Dragon (*Pogona vitticeps*) Recorded at 25 mm/sec and 0.5 mV/cm.[a]

Measurement	Mean or [Median]	Range	Standard Deviation or [IQR][b]
Weight (g)	335	66-517	140
Age (month)	—	4-30	—
Snout-vent length (cm)	18.9	11.5-23.0	3.0
Cloacal temperature (°C)	32.7	27.7-37.9	2.0
Ambient temperature (°C)	—	26 & 35	—
Heart rate (beats/minute)	90	24-170	39
R-R interval (mS)	[723]	353-2520	[533-1020]
P wave duration (mS)	56	30-100	13
P wave amplitude (mV)	0.03	0.01-0.06	0.01
P-R interval (mS)	145	75-253	38
SV wave duration (mS)	[57.5]	30-125	[50-67]
SV wave amplitude (mV)	0.03	0.01-0.07	0.01
SV-R interval (mS)	243	130-440	62
QRS duration (mS)	85	60-120	15
R wave amplitude (mV)	0.23	0.08-0.57	0.11
S wave amplitude (mV)	0.04	0.01-0.13	0.02
Q-T interval (mS)	355	120-980	139
T wave amplitude (mV)	0.04	0.01-0.14	0.02
MEA[c]	—	+60-+110	—

[a]Hunt C, unpublished data.
[b]IQR, Interquartile range.
[c]MEA, Mean electrical axis.
From Schilliger L, Girling S. Cardiology. In: Divers SJ, Stahl SJ, eds. *Mader's Reptile and Amphibian Medicine and Surgery.* 3rd ed. St. Louis, MO: Elsevier; 2019:669-698, with permission from Elsevier.

TABLE 4-23 Select Products and Guidelines Used in Force-Feeding Anorectic or Debilitated Reptiles.[a,b]

Agent	Guidelines	Species/Comments
Alfalfa pellets (e.g., iguana or rabbit pellets) or powder (Alfalfa Powder, NOW Foods)	Blend (1:4) with electrolyte solution or water; 20-30 mL/kg PO q48h (lizards) to q84h (chelonians)[63]	Herbivorous reptiles/administer via gavage or esophagostomy tube; may clog feeding tube; for iguanas, may gavage equal volume of water on alternate days until patient is stable and eating; soaked pellets can also be hand-fed (especially by owner)
Baby foods	Vegetable; blend in with other food sources[63]	Herbivorous reptiles/administer via gavage; for some species, some fruit baby food can be added
	Meat (small amount); blend in with other food sources[63]	Omnivorous species/ administer by gavage

TABLE 4-23 Select Products and Guidelines Used in Force-Feeding Anorectic or Debilitated Reptiles. (cont'd)

Agent	Guidelines	Species/Comments
Commercial dry or moist diets, which are genera specific (e.g., Fluker's, Zilla, Tetra, Zoo Med, etc.)	Blend (1:4) with electrolyte solution or water; 20-30 mL/kg or 3% body weight PO q48h (lizards) to q72h (chelonians)[63]	Herbivorous, omnivorous, insectivorous reptiles/administer via gavage or esophagostomy tube; may clog feeding tube; for iguanas, may gavage equal volume of water on alternate days until patient is stable and eating; soaked pellets can also be hand-fed (especially by owner)
Dog/cat food, canned (a/d, Hill's; Maximum-Calorie, Iams; Nutritional Recovery Formula, Eukanuba)	30 mL/kg PO q7-14d[245]	Carnivorous species/administer via gavage; although low protein (8.5%), some concern over high purine and vitamin A levels (probably OK unless concurrent renal disease); in dehydrated animals, dilute 1:1 with physiological solution, pediatric oral human electrolyte solution (Pedialyte, Ross), or Gatorade (Gatorade); once stabilized, small whole animals (lubricated with egg white) can be force-fed
Electrolyte solutions (Pedialyte, Ross; Gatorade, Gatorade)	15-25 mL/kg PO q24h[63]	Anecdotal most species/no data with respect to costs/benefits
Emeraid Intensive Care Omnivore, Herbivore, Carnivore & Piscivore Formulas (Lafeber)	Mix as labeled, generally to pancake batter consistency, feed small amount to start (see bag suggestion) once daily	Herbivorous, omnivorous, insectivorous, carnivorous, piscivorous reptiles/administer via gavage or esophagostomy tube; may clog feeding tube; typically follow the general feeding sequence: first feed, 1% body weight; second feed, 2% body weight; third feed, 3% body weight
High-protein powders (Carnivore Care, Oxbow Pet Products; Emeraid Carnivore, Lafeber)	Mix as labeled, generally to pancake batter consistency, feed small amount to start (see bag suggestion) once daily	Insectivorous and carnivorous species/ once reconstituted, can be mixed 1:1 with an alfalfa or timothy product for true omnivorous reptiles; administer via gavage
Vetark Professional Oxbow Critical Care Formula (CCF) Powder	Mix as labeled	Herbivorous, omnivorous reptiles/ administer via gavage or esophagostomy tube; may clog feeding tube

[a]General guidelines for force-feeding: generally provide nutrition following rehydration of patient; needs may vary with specific disease (e.g., low protein with renal disease); force-feeding volumes are frequently started at a low/modest level and gradually brought up to the desired level (for patients with severe disease/cachexia, transition should be very gradual); concurrent to with force-feeding and hydrating a patient, highly palatable food items should be provided for voluntary food intake.

[b]Dietary fiber supplements (alfalfa pellets or powder; barley powder; purified cellulose) should be an integral part of enteral therapy for herbivorous reptiles.

TABLE 4-24 Guidelines for Tracheal/Pulmonary and Colonic Lavage in Reptiles.[30,307,337]

Snakes	
Tracheal/pulmonary lavage	Although the procedure can be performed under manual restraint, sedation or anesthesia may reduce stress; pass red rubber catheter through glottis to premeasured distance; infuse with 5-10 mL/kg of tepid (29°C, 85°F), sterile 0.9% saline; massage and rock the snake's body to loosen debris; aspirate
Colonic lavage	Pass lubricated soft red rubber catheter into cloaca; infuse with 10-20 mL/kg of tepid (29°C, 85°F), sterile saline; massage coelomic cavity and gently aspirate
Lizards	
Tracheal/pulmonary lavage	General anesthesia is typically necessary; if possible, intubate with sterile endotracheal tube; pass sterile catheter inside lumen (premeasure distance to sample site); infuse 5-10 mL/kg of tepid (29°C, 85°F), sterile 0.9% saline and aspirate several times; not all fluid will be recovered
Colonic lavage	Pass lubricated soft red rubber catheter into cloaca without excessive force; infuse 10 mL/kg of tepid (29°C, 85°F), sterile saline and gently aspirate several times
Chelonians	
Tracheal/pulmonary lavage	Sedation or anesthesia usually necessary; intubate with sterile endotracheal tube if possible; if unilateral, pass radiomarked catheter into affected lung; may be helpful to bend it in the direction of the lung prior to insertion, though location cannot be ensured without orthogonal radiographic evidence of placement; infuse with tepid (29°C, 85°F), sterile saline at 5-10 mL/kg; gently aspirate
Colonic lavage	Pass lubricated red rubber catheter into cloaca; infuse with tepid (29°C, 85°F), sterile saline at no more than 10 mL/kg; gently aspirate; repeat several times

TABLE 4-25 Preferred Injection Sites in Reptiles.[a,301]

Chelonians	
Subcutaneous	Drug administration sites include the subcutaneous tissues just under the skin between the neck and forelimbs
Intramuscular	Drug administration sites include the caudal forelimbs and lateral pectoral muscles just ventral to the forelimbs
Intravenous	Drug administration sites include the jugular, brachial, or ventral coccygeal veins
Lizards	
Subcutaneous	Drug administration sites include the subcutaneous tissues just under the skin on the dorsum overlying the epaxial muscles; administer only in the cranial half of the body
Intramuscular	Drug administration sites include the forelimbs and epaxial muscles; administer only in the cranial half of the body

TABLE 4-25 Preferred Injection Sites in Reptiles. (cont'd)

Intravenous	Drug administration sites include the ventral coccygeal and ventral abdominal veins
Intraosseous	Drug administration requires intraosseous catheterization of the distal femur or proximal tibia
Snakes	
Subcutaneous	Drug administration sites include the subcutaneous tissues just under the skin on the dorsum overlying the epaxial muscles; administer only in the cranial half of the body
Intramuscular	Drug administration sites include the epaxial muscles; administer only in the cranial half of the body
Intravenous	Drug administration sites include the ventral coccygeal vein and the palatine veins in the oral cavity of larger species
Crocodilians	
Subcutaneous	Drug administration sites include the subcutaneous tissues just under the skin on the dorsum while avoiding the osteoderms; administer only in the cranial half of the body
Intramuscular	Drug administration sites include the forelimbs and epaxial muscles while avoiding the osteoderms; administer only in the cranial half of the body
Intravenous	Drug administration sites include the ventral coccygeal and the occipital sinus
Intraosseous	Drug administration requires intraosseous catheterization of the distal femur or proximal tibia

[a]Slightly modified from original.

TABLE 4-26 Venipuncture Sites Commonly Used in Reptiles.[a,63,101,117,133,193,198,389,457,479]

Snakes	
Ventral caudal vein	Ventral aspect of tail caudal to cloaca under central scute; avoid hemipenes and anal sacs, can be difficult to collect from in boas, pythons, anacondas; in rare cases, may lead to tail necrosis/paresis
Heart	Dorsal recumbency; insertion of needle under central abdominal scale at 45° angle caudal to heart; pericardial fluid contamination can occur; this procedure is likely painful and can result in myocardial laceration and cardiovascular collapse
Palatine vein	Best on large boids; leave snake body on floor with restrainers; slightly elevated head; use spatulas to hold mouth open; bend needle; no holdoff; watch catching hand on teeth; nothing to rest hands on; cotton swab to hold off
Lizards	
Ventral caudal vein	Ventral aspect of vertebral body under center of middle scale; avoid hemipenes and anal sacs; this vein can also be approached laterally by inserting needle under lateral process of vertebral body aiming toward midline; ventral approach may, in rare cases, lead to tail necrosis/paresis
Ventral abdominal vein	Vein is located on caudal to middle midline within inner surface of abdominal wall; insert 25-g needle (bent at 45° angle) cranially, at acute angle to skin and in midline of abdomen, just caudal to umbilicus; avoid urinary bladder in species with them
Jugular vein	Veins are lateral and deep; insert needle caudal to tympanum; best tried in larger animals; transillumination in chameleons and other small lizards

Continued

TABLE 4-26 Venipuncture Sites Commonly Used in Reptiles. (cont'd)

Chelonians	
Jugular vein	Lymphatic contamination can be a concern with most locations of phlebotomy in chelonians; jugular, however, considered less likely
	Right vein often larger than left; runs level with tympanum to base of neck with head extended; may require sedation
Subcarapacial vein and plexus	The sinus accessed with patient's head either extended or retracted; depending on conformation of carapace, needle may be bent up to 60° and positioned in midline just caudal to skin insertion of dorsal aspect of neck and ventral aspect of cranial rim of carapace; needle is advanced in caudodorsal direction, with slight negative pressure; can cause significant internal hemorrhage or paresis in some cases
Dorsal caudal vein	Close to carapace, dorsal to dorsal aspect of vertebral body; lymph dilution common; can flip large chelonians on carapace to access to reduce restraint needed
Brachial vein/plexus	Near triceps tendon at lateral aspect of radiohumeral joint (elbow); foreleg grasped/extended; triceps tendon palpated near caudal aspect of elbow joint; needle inserted ventral to tendon with syringe perpendicular to forearm
Interdigital vessels of rear flippers	Adult leatherback sea turtles, about 2.5 cm deep, near phalangeal junctions, best at P1-P2; along side of phalanx, 20°-30° angle to flipper surface
Crocodilians	
Ventral caudal vein	Ventral aspect of vertebral body under center of middle scale; avoid hemipenes and anal sacs; this vein can also be approached laterally by inserting needle under lateral process of vertebral body aiming toward midline; ventral approach may in rare cases lead to tail necrosis/paresis
Supravertebral vein	Position needle in dorsal midline, just caudal to occiput and perpendicular to skin surface; slowly advance needle with slight negative pressure; excessive penetration can cause spinal trauma

[a]Generally recommended to collect only 0.7% body weight (0.7 mL total in 100 g animal) in healthy reptiles, less in debilitated animals.

TABLE 4-27 Sites Commonly Used for Intravenous Catherization in Reptiles.[99]

Snakes	
Ventral tail vein	With the animal in dorsal recumbency, an area of the tail is disinfected; depending on the size of the animal and operator preferences, different levels of the tail can be used, making sure to avoid going too cranial, close to the hemipenes in males; the skin is entered at a 15- to 30-degree angle to ensure parallelism between the catheter and the vein; a blood flush can be observed in the back of the catheter when the majority of the catheter is already inserted in the tail; if this is not the case (i.e., the blood flush is observed with most of the catheter outside of the tail), it may not be possible to slide the remaining part of the teflon cathether in the vessel; the catheter in this case is secured to the tail with tape

TABLE 4-27 Sites Commonly Used for Intravenous Catherization in Reptiles. (cont'd)

Lizards	
Ventral abdominal vein	With the animal in dorsal recumbency, the vein can be entered percutaneously on the abdominal midline cranial to the umbilical scar; the catheter is passed almost parallel to the abdomen and directed cranially; in certain instances, flattening the abdominal skin during the process helps in contacting the vein
Cephalic vein	This vessel can be used for catheterization of large lizards, such as adult iguanas; the vein typically employed for catheterization is not located on the dorsal surface of the distal foreleg as in mammals, but is on the medial surface, in between the muscles extensor carpi ulnaris and flexor digitorum longus; a skin incision is generally required for visualization of this vessel; the catheter can be secured with standard tape
Chelonians	
Jugular vein	The chelonian is placed in lateral recumbency, with the neck extended and the head slightly flexed laterally to increase exposure of side of the neck that is directed toward the operator; the jugular vein is often visible after compression is applied at the celomic inlet; if the vein is not visible, latero-lateral maneuvering of the head may aid in the visualization of the vessel; the catheter is placed in a craniocaudal direction; once the catheter is placed in site, two wings are made with tape and the catheter is secured to the skin either with sutures or glue; wraps around the neck of chelonians should be avoided since it may result in asphyxiation

TABLE 4-28 Fluid Therapy in Reptiles.[368]

Please refer to Table 4.9 for additional fluid specifics, including dosing.

Osmolarity

- Normal reptile osmolarity is similar to mammals, but there are some species that vary, particularly some crocodilians
- Generally, hypo- and hyperosmolar fluids should be avoided
- Calculated osmolarity is a poor reflection of actual or measured osmolarity in at least American alligators and bearded dragons

General Fluid Therapy

- Therapy should be goal directed
- Maintenance fluid rates range from 10-15 mL/kg/day (also correct for dehydration deficits)
- Replace at rate lost—acute vs chronic; with 72-96 hours as the fastest recommended
- Fluids can be given oral, cloacal (soak in shallow bath), ICe, SC, IV, IO; latter two preferred
- ICe has significant risks and should only be used by experienced individuals
- Environmental humidity can be important to managing hydration in reptiles
- Well-hydrated chelonians in captivity urinate q48h with volumes of 0.5-3% of body weight
- IV access in reptiles, excepting the palatine vein in large snakes, may require cutdown; options include cephalic and ventral coccygeal vein in squamates; however the latter has risk of inducing distal tail necrosis
- IO catheters in lizards can be used, including femur, tibia, and humerus
- IV cutdowns for jugular access in snakes (right > left); 4-7 scutes cranial to heartbeat, 1-2 scales laterally to ventral scute
  - IV access for chelonians is ideally the jugular vein; IO placement in the humerus, femur, and gular plastron are secondary options. Recent evidence suggests the plastrocarapatial bridge is a less than ideal option

Continued

TABLE 4-28 Fluid Therapy in Reptiles. (cont'd)

Crystalloids & Colloids

- Reptiles are reported to tolerate blood lactate levels as high as 20 mmol/L, so lactated crystalloids are not as concerning in certain scenarios as mammals
- Hypertonic crystalloids may be more useful in reptiles due to the higher intracellular content in reptiles; however, do monitor for hemolysis and phlebitis
- A 3-5 mL/kg bolus of a colloid over 30-60 minutes may be given as long as patient is closely assessed
- Hydroxylethyl starch (HES) may be used, but caution is advised as having been recently banned in Europe for coagulopathies and acute renal injury in mammals, including humans

Whole Blood

- Recommended with acute severe hemmorhage and life-threatening anemia
  - Ideally a sibling used, secondarily at least same species
  - Transfusion rates of 10-15 mL/kg over 24 hours at rate of 5-10 mL/kg/hr
  - Keep blood cool, then warm to 25-30°C within 6 hours of collection
- Aseptic technique critical
- Citrate-phosphate-dextrose adenine (CPDA) at 1:9 ratio or heparin at 5-10 units/mL of blood can be used
- Up to 10% of blood donor volume can be used
- Homologous and heterologous tranfusions have been used
- Complications have been rarely reported in reptiles
- Blood filters, as used for mammals and birds, are recommended (18-u filter)
- Standard cross-matching between donor and receipient are recommended; however, a first and single donation does not seem to induce severe reactions in reptiles

TABLE 4-29 Treatment of Dystocia in Reptiles.[a,25,48,102,122,343,457]

Etiologies

- Poor environmental conditions (improper thermal environment, lack of suitable nesting substrate, shallow nesting substrate; underground obstructions [e.g., roots or buried rocks], disturbance, lack of visual security, etc)
- Social factors (e.g., competition, fighting, recent introduction of male)
- Dietary imbalances (e.g., calcium deficiency, hypovitaminosis A), malnutrition
- Endocrine imbalances
- Nutritional secondary hyperparathyroidism
- Uterine inertia
- Dehydration
- Renal disease
- Egg yolk coelomitis
- Cystic or cloacal calculi
- Infections (e.g., uterus)
- Anatomic anomalies of the reproductive tract, eggs, pelvis, or shell of chelonians
- Other (substrate ingestion, overfeeding, other illness, inadequate exercise)

Diagnosis

- History and clinical signs (prolonged anorexia, lethargy, posterior paresis, straining/tenesmus, increased pacing/seeking, excavating nests without oviposition, straining to pass eggs, passage of a few eggs but not a full clutch, fluid discharge from cloaca)
- Knowledge of normal egg retention time or usual season for laying
- Physical examination (gentle palpation of inguinal or prefemoral fossa or caudal coelom; eggs may not be palpable)
- CBC (anemia, elevated or decreased WBCs)
- Plasma biochemical analysis (hyperproteinemia, elevated ALP activity, hypercalcemia [total calcium elevated], hypocalcemia [ionized Ca <1 mmol/L])

TABLE 4-29 Treatment of Dystocia in Reptiles. (cont'd)

- Coelomic effusion aspirate and cytology—carefully avoid aspirating from the urinary bladder, oviducts, or eggs when collecting coelomic fluid samples
- Radiography (chelonian eggs have a calcified outer shell and appear radiographically similar to avian eggs; lizards and snakes generally have soft-shelled eggs with soft tissue density on radiographs); radiography typically does not allow identification of the location of the eggs
- Computed tomography - better than radiographs because it enables one to identify the location of the eggs
- Cystoscopy (chelonians) - cystoscopy should be performed in any chelonian with presence of eggs on radiographs to ascertain whether any egg is ectopic in the urinary bladder
- Ultrasound
- Coelioscopy - particularly to confirm coelomitis, salpingitis, or oviduct rupture; determine whether early surgical management is appropriate

Treatment

- If patient is stable, provide proper environmental conditions (appropriate thermal environment, humidity, nesting site, substrate material, substrate depth, and substrate moisture; minimal stimulus; isolation)
- Handle gently and infrequently
- Tepid (~29°C; ~85°F) water soak, 30-60 min q24h
- Rehydration - fluid therapy prn; do not administer fluids intracoelomically
- Alert, strong, stable, responsive females that are eating well will often oviposit without further therapy if given sufficient time
- Dextrose (SC, IV) may be of value in some cases
- Calcium (see Table 4.9; only if hypocalcemic; low Ca^{++} not generally a problem in snakes)
  - Ca glycerophosphate/Ca lactate (Calphosan, Glenwood) (5 mg each/mL): 5 mg/kg SC, IM
  - Ca gluconate: 100-200 mg/kg SC, IM
- Oxytocin[b] (see Table 4.8)
  - Generally administer 1 hr after Ca++ injection
  - 1-10 U/kg IM, ICe in lizards and snakes (results are variable); 1-20 U/kg IM, IV, ICe for chelonians; IV administration was faster than IM administration in red eared sliders
  - Repeat dose q1h; response is more rapid after IV administration in turtles
- Arginine vasotocin[c] (Sigma Chemical) (alternative to oxytocin) (see Table 4.8)
  - 0.01-1 µg/kg IV (preferred), ICe
- Dinoprostone gel (Prepodil, Upjohn)
  - 0.9 mg/kg intracloacally followed 20 minutes later by prostaglandin $F_{2\alpha}$ (Lutalyse, Zoetis) 0.6 mg/kg IM
- Propranolol
  - 1 mg/kg followed by prostaglandin $F_{2\alpha}$ 0.025 mg/kg[d]
- Prostaglandin $F_{2\alpha}$ (Lutalyse, 5 mg/mL)
  - 1.5 mg/kg SC in turtles
  - Efficacy may improve if given 20 minutes after an alpha-2 agonist (dexmedetomidine 0.035 mg/kg or xylazine 8 mg/kg)
- Lubricate cloaca with water soluble gel
- Manual massage may be useful in some situations — avoid causing oviduct rupture or prolapse
- If eggs are not laid with medical treatment, depending on the purpose of the animal (pet rather than breeding animal), ovariosalpingectomy or salpingotomy should be advised
- Considering that dystocia is typically a recurring problem, depending on the comfort level of the veterinary team, ovariosalpingectomy should be advised in affected animals once stabilized

[a]Although most reptiles are oviparous, some, including garter snakes, water snakes, boas (not pythons), vipers, Jackson's chameleons, horned lizards, and Solomon Island prehensile-tailed skinks are viviparous.

[b]Use only if *no* evidence of obstructive dystocia or broken eggs.

[c]Appears to be more effective than oxytocin in many reptiles, but it is not commercially available for use in animals.

[d]Effective in healthy *Sceloporus* sp.; did not induce oviposition in iguanas; may be effective in chelonians.

TABLE 4-30 Treatment of Metabolic Bone Diseases in Reptiles.[241]

Etiologies

- Improper Ca:P ratio; lack of dietary Ca
- Lack of vitamin D_3
- Lack of UVA and UVB light spectrum
- Renal disease
- Other: low ambient temperature, protein deficiency, small intestinal disease, parathyroid disease, etc.

Clinical Signs

- Lethargy, reluctance to move
- Poor appetite or anorexia
- Weight loss or poor weight gain
- Softening of the mandible; shortened/rounded mandible and maxilla; symmetrical swelling of the mandible (fibrous osteodystrophy)
- Fibrous osteodystrophy of the long bones of the legs
- Difficulty in lifting body off ground when walking
- Pathologic fractures
- Ataxia, paresis, or paralysis of the rear legs due to collapsed vertebrae or vertebral luxation
- Osteoporosis
- Hypocalcemic muscle fasciculations and seizures
- Soft shell in chelonians
- Constipation
- Inability to evert/replace hemipenes

Diagnosis

- Dietary and environmental history
- Clinical signs
- Physical examination
- Radiography
- Serum Ca:P ratio; usually inverse (1:2+) with renal etiology
- Uric acid levels
- Ionized calcium levels
- Calcidiol (25-hydroxyvitamin D) levels (Michigan State University)
- UV meter readings of enclosure; sun exposure or UVB bulb
- Dual-energy x-ray absorptiometry (DEXA) scan
- Determination of glomerular filtration rate
- Renal nuclear medicine
- Renal biopsy

Treatment

- Provide species-correct environmental temperature ranges for day and night
- Correct diet as needed; usually changing to improve calcium:phosphorus ratio
- Use species-appropriate UVA/UVB lighting arrangement
- Use fluorescent or mercury vapor bulbs, or light-emitting plasma lamps; taking outside for supervised exposure to natural sunlight is encouraged, but watch for overheating or attempts to escape/jump; many wild reptiles may bask at edges of 10:00 AM – 4:00 PM time of day
- Provide areas to hide, as corneal and skin burns can occur
- In general:
    - Desert-dwelling diurnal lizards/chelonians, high UVB levels (10% or full unfiltered sun, 4 hr)
    - Diurnal arboreal lizards/semiaquatic basking chelonians, moderate levels of UVB (5%, 3 hr)
    - Diurnal terrestrial lizards/chelonians from forested environment, low levels of UVB (5%, 2 hr)
    - Nocturnal lizards, low levels of UVB (2%, 1 hr)—focus more on oral vitamin D_3
    - Snakes seem to get adequate levels of calcium/cholecalciferol from ingestion of whole vertebrate prey (or earthworms); exceptions are diamond and green tree pythons, indigo snakes, some aquatic species, rough/smooth green snakes, other arboreal, diurnal snakes

TABLE 4-30 Treatment of Metabolic Bone Diseases in Reptiles. (cont'd)

- Albino (amelanistic), hypomelanistic, snow, blizzard, pastel, tangerine, lavender, yellow, pied, anerythristic, leucistic, xanthochromistic, or any other genetic mutants with less than normal levels of melanin are more susceptible to UV light burns of the eyes and dorsal skin, so lower levels of UV supplementation (if any) should be provided, oral vitamin D_3 may need to be considered
- Force-feeding (following rehydration) (see Table 4.23)
  - Use species-appropriate diet; especially useful for immature animals as maintenance until improving and closer to adult size; esophageal feeding tube usually needed for chelonians to avoid beak fractures
- Ca supplementation options (see Table 4.9)—best to use human products
  - Calcium carbonate (400 mg calcium/g product)
  - Calcium citrate (210 mg calcium/g product)
  - Calcium phosphate
- Maintain hydration
  - Fluid therapy, as needed
  - Soak in warm water (shallow) for 10-20 min q12-24h to encourage drinking and defecation (caution: head may need to be supported; do not leave unattended)
- Vitamin D_3 (see Table 4.9)
  - Best source is UVA/UVB exposure from sun or appropriate lamp
  - Some species may benefit from judicious oral supplementation
- Gut-load invertebrates (crickets, roaches) on high calcium diet (high calcium leafy greens, Mazuri Hi-Ca Cricket Diet) for several days before feeding to insectivores
  - Nontoxic, wild-caught insects and invertebrates are often some of the best sources of high calcium and other nutrients but likely seasonal
- Feed high-calcium invertebrates such as phoenix worms, snails, and earthworms when appropriate for diet in insectivores
- Dusting invertebrates may be beneficial, but they often remove dust quickly; can make unpalatable; be careful with dusts containing vitamins; avoid those with phosphorus
- Feed only leafy greens and other high-calcium plants for herbivores, minimizing thicker vegetables and avoiding most fruits
- In mammals, condition considered painful; appropriate analgesics may be warranted
- Both short-term and long-term prognosis is often guarded at best
- Other
  - Handle gently
  - Remove climbing branches to prevent injuries

TABLE 4-31 Select Sources of Diets and Other Commercial Products for Reptiles.[a,b]

Food and Supplements		
Chewy	800-672-4399	https://www.chewy.com/b/reptile-1025
Fluker Farms	800-735-8537	www.flukerfarms.com
JurassiPet	706-343-6060/ 866-587-7389	www.jurassipet.com
Mazuri	833-462-9874	www.mazuri.com
National Geographic/ PetSmart	888-839-9638	http://natgeo.petsmart.com
Oxbow Animal Health	800-249-0366	www.oxbowanimalhealth.com
Pretty Pets	800-356-5020	www.prettybird.com

Continued

TABLE 4-31 Select Sources of Diets and Other Commercial Products for Reptiles. (cont'd)

Reliable Protein Products	480-361-3940	www.zoofood.com
Repashy Superfoods	855-737-2749	www.store.repashy.com
Rep-Cal	800-406-6446	www.repcal.com
Reptiles Lounge	321-745-7373	www.reptileslounge.com
Reptile Supply	888-833-8242	www.reptilesupply.com
San Francisco Bay Brand	510-792-7200	http://sfbb.com
Sticky Tongue Farms	Unpublished	www.stickytonguefarms.com
Tetra Fauna	800-526-0650	www.tetra-fish.com
T-Rex Products	800-991-8739	www.t-rexproducts.com
Wombaroo	(08)83911713(Aust)	www.wombaroo.com.au/reptiles
Zilla	888-255-4527	www.zilla-rules.com
Zoo Med Laboratories	888-496-6633	www.zoomed.com

Live/Frozen Foods for Carnivores

American Rodent Supply	317-527-7076	www.americanrodent.com	Frozen mice, rats, chicks
Backwater Reptiles	916-740-9758	www.Backwaterreptiles.com	Frozen mice, rats
Big Apple Herp	561-397-3977	www.bigappleherp.com	Frozen mice, rats, chicks, quail, rabbits
Big Cheese Rodents	817-926-3300	www.bigcheeserodents.com	Frozen mice, rats, chicks
Frozen Rodents	734-972-5324	www.frozenrodents.com	Frozen mice, rats, rabbits, and chicks
The Gourmet Rodent	352-472-9189	www.gourmetrodent.com	Frozen mice, rats, rabbits, and chicks
Hoosier Mouse Supply	317-831-1219	www.hoosiermousesupply.com	Live (local) and frozen mice, rats, rabbits
Layne Laboratories, Inc	Unpublished	www.laynelabs.com	Frozen mice, rats
Mack Natural Reptile Food	888-372-9570	www.macksnaturalreptilefood.com	Frozen mice, rats
Reptilinks	720-841-8762	www.reptilinks.com	Rats, mice, chicken and quail chicks

TABLE 4-31 Select Sources of Diets and Other Commercial Products for Reptiles. (cont'd)

Rodent Pro	812-867-7598	www.rodentpro.com	Frozen mice, rats, rabbits, guinea pigs, chicks, quail, hamsters, gerbils
Live Foods for Insectivores			
Arbico Organics	800-827-2847	www.arbico-organics.com	Live Tiny Wigglers, Tiny Wasp, Cocoon Capers, many other insects
Backwater Reptiles	916-740-9758	www.Backwaterreptiles.com	Crickets, roaches, hornworms, mealworms, superworms, silkworms, waxworms, nightcrawlers, blackworms, ants, fly larvae
Bassett's Cricket Ranch	800-634-2445	www.bcrcricket.com	Crickets, mealworms
Big Apple Herp	561-397-3977	www.bigappleherp.com	Butterworms, mealworms, waxworms, nightcrawlers, crickets, hornworms, superworms, isopods
Fluker Farms	800-735-8537	www.flukerfarms.com	Crickets, mealworms, superworms, cockroaches, fruit flies, soldier worms, hornworms
Ghann's Cricket Farm	800-476-2248	www.ghann.com	Crickets, soldier fly larvae, mealworms, superworms, waxworms, Phoenix worms, roaches
Grubco	800-222-3563	www.grubco.com	Crickets, superworms, mealworms, fly larvae, waxworms, Mighty Mealys, hornworms, red worms, nightcrawlers
Josh's Frogs	800-691-8178	www.joshsfrogs.com	Fruit flies, mealworms, hornworms, soldier fly larvae, roaches, rice flour beetles, millipedes, butterworms, waxworms, others
Knutson's	800-248-9318	www.knutsonlivebait.com	Night crawlers, crickets, mealworms, waxworms
Millbrook Cricket Farm	800-654-3506	www.millbrookcrickets.com	Crickets, superworms
Mulberry Farms	760-731-6088	www.mulberryfarms.com	Silkworm larvae, soldier fly larvae, mealworms, superworms, waxworms, roaches, hornworms
Premium Crickets	234-738-3663	www.premiumcrickets.com	Superworms, waxworms, crickets

Continued

TABLE 4-31 Select Sources of Diets and Other Commercial Products for Reptiles. (cont'd)

Rainbow Mealworms	800-777-9676	www.rainbowmealworms.net	Crickets, mealworms, cockroaches, hornworms, superworms, fruit flies, Phoenix worms
Reptile Food	Unpublished	www.reptilefood.com	Mealworms, giant mealworms, zophobas worms, waxworms, nightcrawlers, red worms, fruit flies, crickets
Reptile Supply	888-833-8242	www.reptilesupply.com	Crickets, dubia roaches, NutriGrubs, hornworms, superworms, mealworms, waxworms, soldierfly larvae, butterworms
Rodent Pro	812-867-7598	www.rodentpro.com	Crickets, mealworms, waxworms, superworms, nightcrawlers, calciworms, red wigglers, flies, hornworms
The Phoenix Worm Store	Unpublished	www.phoenixworm.com	Phoenix worms
Timberline Fresh	800-423-2248	http://timberlinefresh.com	Crickets, superworms, hornworms, waxworms, mealworms, hornworms, CalciWorms, fruit flies
Top Hat Cricket Farm	800-638-2555	www.tophatcrickets.com	Crickets, mealworms, superworms, hornworms, waxworms
Lights			
Arcadia	Unpublished	www.arcadiareptile.com	Ultraviolet, D3
Chewy	800-672-4399	https://www.chewy.com/b/reptile-1025	Wide variety of lighting and fixtures
Exo Terra	800-724-2436	www.exo-terra.com	Ultraviolet, visible, infrared/heat
Fluker Farms	800-735-8537	www.flukerfarms.com	Incandescent, heat
General Electric	800-435-4448	www.gelighting.com	Incandescent, heat
Josh's Frogs	800-691-8178	www.joshsfrogs.com	Ultraviolet, Mega-Ray, incandescent, solar meters
LLL Reptile	888-547-3784	http://lllreptile.com	UVB, mercury vapor
Mac Industries, Inc	252-241-4584	www.reptileuv.com	Brightrite halogen, self-ballasted lamps, heat projector lamps, reptileUV, metal halide, fluorescent
Pangea Reptile LLC	Unpublished	www.pangeareptile.com	UVB

TABLE 4-31 Select Sources of Diets and Other Commercial Products for Reptiles. (cont'd)

Philips	800-555-0050	www.lighting.philips.com	Incandescent, heat
Reptiles Lounge	321-745-7373	www.reptileslounge.com.	Wide variety of lighting and fixtures
Reptile Supply	888-833-8242	www.reptilesupply.com	UV bulbs, day bulbs, night bulbs, fixtures
Sylvania	978-777-1900	www.sylvania.com	350BL blacklights, fluorescent, incandescent, ballasts, halogen
The Bean Farm	877-708-5882	www.beanfarm.com	UVB, infrared, mercury vapor, fluorescent
T-Rex Products	800-991-8739	www.t-rexproducts.com	UVB, heat
Zilla	888-255-4527	www.zilla-rules.com	Incandescent, heat, UVB fluorescent, halogen
Zoo Med Laboratories	888-496-6633	www.zoomed.com	Incandescent, heat, mercury vapor UVB, fluorescent UVB
Heating Devices			
Arcadia	Unpublished	www.arcadiareptile.com	Ceramic heaters, halogen
Big Apple Pet Supply	800-922-7753	www.bigappleherp.com	Ceramic bulbs, heat mats, heat tape, incandescent bulbs
Chewy	800-672-4399	https://www.chewy.com/b/reptile-1025	Wide variety of heating devices
Fluker Farms	800-735-8537	www.flukerfarms.com	Under-cage heat pads
Helix Controls	760-726-4464	www.helixcontrols.com	Thermostats, heat tape, heat panels
Josh's Frogs	800-691-8178	www.joshsfrogs.com	Heat pads, water heaters, heat rocks, basking bulbs, ceramic heat emitters
LLL Reptile	888-547-3784	http://lllreptile.com	Pearlco conical ceramic heat emitters, heat bulbs, heat pads, heat rocks
Pangea Reptile LLC	Unpublished	www.pangeareptile.com	Basking lamps, infrared, halogen, Solar Glo
Reptiles Lounge	321-745-7373	www.reptileslounge.com	Wide variety of heating devices
Reptile Supply	888-833-8242	www.reptilesupply.com	Basking bulbs, heat mats, night heat, misc. heaters, fixtures
The Bean Farm	877-708-5882	www.beanfarm.com	Heat tape, heat pads, cords, ceramic heaters
Zilla	800-255-4527	www.zilla-rules.com	Conical ceramic heat emitters, thermostats, heat mats, aquatic reptile heater, digital temperature controller

Continued

TABLE 4-31 Select Sources of Diets and Other Commercial Products for Reptiles. (cont'd)

Zoo Med Laboratories	888-496-6633	www.zoomed.com	Thermostats, rheostats, heat pads, tape, cables, cermaic heat emitter, rock heater, under tank heater
Humidity Devices			
Chewy	800-672-4399	https://www.chewy.com/b/reptile-1025	Foggers, misters, humidity monitors
Exo Terra (Hagen)	800-724-2436	www.exo-terra.com	Ultrasonic fogger, Monsoon rainfall
Humidifirst	561-752-1936	www.humidifirst.com	Mist-Pac ultrasonic humidifiers
Pangea Reptile LLC	Unpublished	www.pangeareptile.com	Mistiking misting system, Monsoon systems, Repti Fogger
Reptiles Lounge	321-745-7373	www.reptileslounge.com	Misters, foggers
Reptile Supply	888-833-8242	www.reptilesupply.com	Foggers, misters
Zoo Med Laboratories	888-496-6633	www.zoomed.com	Multiport fogger, Repti Fogger, Reptirain automatic misting machine, HygroTherm humidity controller
Environmental Sensing and Monitoring Devices			
Chewy	800-672-4399	https://www.chewy.com/b/reptile-1025	Thermostats, thermometers, hygrometers, timers
Exo Terra (Hagen)	800-724-2436	www.exo-terra.com	Remote digital thermometers, hygrometers
Fluke Process Instruments	800-227-8074	www.flukeprocessinstruments.com	Digital infrared thermometer
Josh's Frogs	800-691-8178	www.joshsfrogs.com	Solar meters, thermostats, hygrometers
LLL Reptile	888-547-3784	http://lllreptile.com	thermometers, thermostats, timers
Onset Computer Corp	800-564-4377	www.onsetcomp.com	Relative humidity, temperature
Pangea Reptile LLC	Unpublished	www.pangeareptile.com	Digital thermometer, humidity monitors
Raytek	800-227-8074	www.raytek.com	Digital infrared thermometer
Reptiles Lounge	321-745-7373	www.reptileslounge.com	Thermometers, thermostats, humidity monitors
Reptile Supply	888-833-8242	www.reptilesupply.com	Thermometers, hygrometers, thermostats, timers

TABLE 4-31 Select Sources of Diets and Other Commercial Products for Reptiles. (cont'd)

Solartech	800-798-3311	www.solarmeter.com	Solarmeter 6.2 UVB meter, visible and infrared meter
The Bean Farm	877-708-5882	www.beanfarm.com	Thermostats, hygrometers
Zilla	800-255-4527	www.zilla-rules.com	Digital infrared thermometer, thermometer-hygrometer
Zoo Med Laboratories	888-496-6633	www.zoomed.com	HygroTherm humidity/heat monitor and controller, ReptiTemp rheostat, many thermometer and humidity gauges

[a]Many pet stores sell live frozen food for reptiles, and many of the products listed.
[b]Numerous sources of information were used to compile this table, particularly Internet sources.

TABLE 4-32 Known and Potential Reptile Toxins.[126]

Antiparasitic Drugs	Comments
Fenbendazole	Particular issue at high doses for any species; Fea's vipers (*Azemiops feae*), Hermann's tortoises (*Testudo hermanni*)
Ivermectin	Chelonians, ball pythons (*Python regius*), Central American skinks (genus *Mabuya*), Parson's chameleons (*Calumma parsonii*), panther chameleons (*Furcifer pardalis*), Solomon Island skinks (*Corucia zebrata*), Nile crocodiles (*Crocodylus niloticus*); use with caution in all reptiles; avoid in gravid individuals, small species, and neonates
Metronidazole	Issue with high dose or frequency; consider effect on gastrointestinal microflora in herbivorous species
Antimicrobial Drugs	
Amphotericin B	As with mammals; avoid with renal disease
Chloramphenicol	As with mammals; pancytopenia, hemorhagic, appetite suppressive
Enrofloxacin	IM/SC causes muscle/tissue necrosis because of pH 10—requires dilution of 1:1000 to neutralize
Fluconazole, itraconazole, ketoconazole	As with mammals; avoid with hepatic disease
Gentamicin/amikacin	As with mammals; renotoxic and ototoxic
Griseofulvin	As with mammals; can be teratogenic
Venomous and Poisonous Animals	
Snake venom	Seem resistant to self-envenomation and more resistant to same species envenomation, though fatalities can occur; ophiphagic species can have improved resistance but not always; most envenomations occur during feeding and courtship
Lizard venom	Usually conspecifics; no issues noted
Bufotoxins	From toad genus *Bufo*; possible as in mammals, but not reported; bufophagic species may have some resistance

Continued

TABLE 4-32 Known and Potential Reptile Toxins. (cont'd)

Antiparasitic Drugs	Comments
Fire ants (*Solenopsis richteri, S. invicta*)	Invasive species in USA; bites/stings can be issue with wild and captive outdoor housed reptiles
Fireflies (*Photinus* spp.), monarch butterflies (*Donaeus plexxipus*), queen butterflies (*Donaeus gillipus*), lygaeid bugs (*Oncopeltus fasciatus*)	Lethal in bearded dragons (*Pogona vitticeps*); other reptiles will avoid, spit out, or regurgitate these species if eaten

Plants

Contact Poison Control for plants not on list or consult more comprehensive listings; only known reptile toxicities listed here. Reptile species variability, season, locale of plant, how plant is processed, and other factors can affect toxicity significantly.

Select Plants

Azaleas (*Rhododendron penthatera* sp., *Rhododendron tusutsusi* sp.)	Green iguana (*Iguana iguana*)—one death, one recovery
Marijuana (*Cannibis sativa*)	Green iguana (*Iguana iguana*)—ingestion of processed product
Oak (*Quercus* spp.)	African spur-thighed tortoise (*Centrochelys sulcata*)—death
Red cap mushroom (*Amanita pantherina*)	Green iguana (*Iguana iguana*); box turtles may be resistant as seen eating them in wild
Tobacco (*Nicotiana* spp.)	Green iguana (*Iguana iguana*), African spur-thighed tortoise (*Centrochelys sulcata*); ingestion of processed product—death

REFERENCES

1. Abidoye EO, Effiong U, Yusuf PO, et al. Effect of ketamine hydrochloride induced anaesthesia on *Psammophis sibilans*. *Nigerian Vet J*. 2017;38:178–182.
2. Adamovicz L, Leister K, Byrd J, et al. Venous blood gas in free-living Eastern box turtles (*Terrapene carolina carolina*) and effects of physiologic, demographic and environmental factors. *Conserv Physiol*. 2018;6(1):coy041.
3. Adel M, Sadegh AB, Arizza V, et al. Anesthetic efficacy of ketamine-diazepam, ketamine-xylazine, and ketamine–acepromazine in Caspian pond turtles (*Mauremys caspica*). *Indian J Pharmacol*. 2017;49:93–97.
4. Adetunji VE, Ogunsola J, Adeyemo OK. Evaluation of diazepam-ketamine combination for immobilization of African land tortoise (*Testudo graeca*). *Sokoto J Vet Sci*. 2019;17:78–81.
5. Adkesson MJ, Fernandez-Varon E, Cox S, et al. Pharmacokinetics of a long-acting ceftiofur formulation (ceftiofur crystalline free acid) in the ball python (*Python regius*). *J Zoo Wildl Med*. 2011;42:444–450.
6. Adnyana W, Ladds PW, Blair D. Efficacy of praziquantel in the treatment of green sea turtles with spontaneous infection of cardiovascular flukes. *Aust Vet J*. 1997;75:405–407.
7. Agius JE, Kimble B, Govendir M, et al. Pharmacokinetic profile of enrofloxacin and its metabolite ciprofloxacin in Asian house geckos (*Hemidactylus frenatus*) after single-dose oral administration of enrofloxacin. *Vet Anim Sci*. 2020:100–116.
8. Alleman AR, Jacobson ER, Raskin RE. Morphologic and cytochemical characteristics of blood cells from the desert tortoise (*Gopherus agassizii*). *Proc Annu Conf Assoc Rept Amph Vet*. 1996:51–55.

9. Allen DG, Pringle JK, Smith D. *Handbook of Veterinary Drugs*. Philadelphia, PA: JB Lippincott; 1993:534–567.
10. Allender MC, Mitchell MA, Yarborough J, et al. Pharmocokinetics of a single oral dose of acyclovir and valacyclovir in North American box turtles (*Terrapene* sp.). *J Vet Pharmacol Therap*. 2012;36:205–208.
11. Alves-Junior JRF, Bosso ACS, Andrade MB, et al. Association of acepromazine with propofol in giant Amazon river turtles *Podocnemis expansa* breed in captivity. *Acta Cir Bras*. 2012;27:552–556.
12. Alves-Junior JRF, Bosso ACS, Andrade MB, et al. Association of midazolam with ketamine in giant Amazon river turtles *Podocnemis expansa* reared in captivity. *Acta Cir Bras*. 2012;27:144–147.
13. American Veterinary Medical Association. AVMA Guidelines for the Euthanasia of Animals: 2020 Edition. Available at: https://www.avma.org/sites/default/files/2020-01/2020-Euthanasia-Final-1-17-20.pdf. Accessed August 15, 2021.
14. Anderson NL, Wack RF. Basic husbandry and medicine of pet reptiles. In: Birchard SJ, Sherding RG, eds. *Saunders Manual of Small Animal Practice*. 2nd ed. Philadelphia, PA: WB Saunders; 2000:1539–1567.
15. Anderson NL, Wack RF, Calloway L. Cardiopulmonary effects and efficacy of propofol as an anesthetic agent in brown tree snakes, *Boiga irregularis*. *Bull Assoc Rept Amph Vet*. 1999;9:9–15.
16. Andreani G, Carpenè E, Cannavacciuolo A, et al. Reference values for hematology and plasma biochemistry variables, and protein electrophoresis of healthy Hermann's tortoises (*Testudo hermanni* spp.). *Vet Clin Pathol*. 2014;43(4):573–583.
17. Antinoff N, Bauck L, Boyer TH, et al. *Exotic Animal Formulary*. 2nd ed. Lakewood, CO: AAHA Press; 1999.
18. Arnett-Chinn ER, Hadfield CA, Clayton LA. Review of intramuscular midazolam for sedation in reptiles at the National Aquarium, Baltimore. *J Herp Med Surg*. 2016;26:59–63.
19. Ascher JM, Bates W, Ng J, et al. Assessment of xylazine for euthanasia of anoles (*Anolis carolinensis* and *Anolis distichus*). *J Am Assoc Lab Anim Sci*. 2012;51:83–87.
20. Avni-Magen N, Eshar D, Friedman M, et al. Retrospective evaluation of a novel sustained-release ivermectin varnish for treatment of wound myiasis in zoo-housed animals. *J Zoo Wildl Med*. 2018;49(1):201–205.
21. Aymen J, Queiroz-Williams P, Hampton CCE, et al. Comparison of ketamine-dexmedetomidine-midazolam versus alfaxalone-dexmedetomidine–midazolam administered intravenously to American alligators (*Alligator mississippiensis*). *J Herp Med Surg*. 2021;31:132–140.
22. Baker BB, Sladky KK, Johnson SM. Evaluation of the analgesic effects of oral and subcutaneous tramadol administration in red-eared slider turtles. *J Am Vet Med Assoc*. 2011;238:220–227.
23. Balko JA, Gatson BJ, Cohen EB, et al. Inhalant anesthetic recovery following intramuscular epinephrine in the loggerhead sea turtle (*Caretta caretta*). *J Zoo Wildl Med*. 2018;49:680–688.
24. Banzato T, Russo E, Finotti L, et al. Development of a technique for contrast radiographic examination of the gastrointestinal tract in ball pythons (*Python regius*). *Am J Vet Res*. 2012;73:996–1001.
25. Bardi E, Antolini G, Lubian E, et al. Comparison of lateral and dorsal recumbency during endoscope-assisted oophorectomy in mature pond sliders (*Trachemys scripta*). *Animals*. 2020;10:1451–1459.
26. Barrillot B, Roux J, Arthaud S, et al. Intramuscular administration of ketamine medetomidine assures stable anaesthesia needed for long-term surgery in the Argentine tegu *Salvator merianae*. *J Zoo Wildl Med*. 2018;49:291–296.
27. Baruffaldi LC, da Silva A, Sellera FP, et al. Spinal anesthesia in a green turtle (*Chelonia mydas*) for surgical removal of cutaneous fibropapillomatosis. *J Agri Vet Sci*. 2016;9:83–86.
28. Beck K, Loomis M, Lewbart G, et al. Preliminary comparison of plasma concentrations of gentamicin injected into the cranial and caudal limb musculature of the Eastern box turtle (*Terrapene carolina carolina*). *J Zoo Wildl Med*. 1995;26:265–268.

29. Benge SL, Heinrichs MT, Crevasse SE, et al. A preliminary analysis of prolonged absorption rate of ponazuril in red-footed tortoises, *Chelonoidis carbonaria*. *J Zoo Wildl Med*. 2018;49(3):802–805.
30. Bennett RA. A review of anesthesia and chemical restraint in reptiles. *J Zoo Wildl Med*. 1991;22:282–303.
31. Bennett RA. Clinical, diagnostic, and therapeutic techniques. *Proc Annu Conf Assoc Rept Amph Vet*. 1998:35–40.
32. Bennett RA. Management of common reptile emergencies. *Proc Annu Conf Assoc Rept Amph Vet*. 1998:67–72.
33. Bennett RA, Divers SJ, Schumacher J, et al. Roundtable: anesthesia. *Bull Assoc Rept Amph Vet*. 1999;9:20–27.
34. Bennett RA, Schumacher J, Hedjazi-Haring K, et al. Cardiopulmonary and anesthetic effects of propofol administered intraosseously to green iguanas. *J Am Vet Med Assoc*. 1998;212:93–98.
35. Benson KG, Tell LA, Young LA, et al. Pharmacokinetics of ceftiofur sodium after intramuscular or subcutaneous administration in green iguanas (*Iguana iguana*). *Am J Vet Res*. 2003;64:1278–1282.
36. Bernard JB, Oftedal OT, Citino SB, et al. The response of vitamin D-deficient green iguanas (*Iguana iguana*) to artificial ultraviolet light. *Proc Annu Conf Am Assoc Zoo Vet*. 1991:147–150.
37. Bertelsen MF, Buchanan R, Jensen HM, et al. Assessing the influence of mechanical ventilation on blood gases and blood pressure in rattlesnakes. *Vet Anaesth Analg*. 2015;42:386–393.
38. Bicknese E, Pessier A, Boedeker N. Successful treatment of fungal osteomyelitis in a Parson's chameleon (*Calumma parsonii*) using surgical and anti-fungal treatments. *Proc Annu Conf Assoc Rept Amph Vet*. 2008;86.
39. Bielli M, Nardini G, Di Girolamo N, et al. Hematological values for adult eastern Hermann's tortoise (*Testudo hermanni boettgeri*) in semi-natural conditions. *J Vet Diagn Invest*. 2015;27(1):68–73.
40. Bienzle D, Boyd CJ. Sedative effects of ketamine and midazolam in snapping turtles. *J Zoo Wildl Med*. 1992;23:201–204.
41. Bisetto SP, Melo CF, Carregaro AB. Evaluation of sedative and antinociceptive effects of dexmedetomidine, midazolam and dexmedetomidine-midazolam in tegus (*Salvator merianae*). *Vet Anaesth Analg*. 2018;45:320–328.
42. Bochmann M, Wenger S, Hatt J-M. Preliminary clinical comparison of anesthesia with ketamine/medetomidine and s-ketamine/medetomidine in *Testudo* spp. *J Herp Med Surg*. 2018;28:40–46.
43. Bodri MS, Hruba SJ. Safety of milbemycin (A3-A4 oxime) in chelonians. *J Zoo Wildl Med*. 1993:171–174.
43a. Bodri MS, Rambo TM, Wagner RA, et al. Pharmacokinetics of metronidazole administered as a single oral bolus to red rat snakes, *Elaphe guttata*. *J Herpetol Med Surg*. 2006;16:15–19.
44. Bogan JE. Gastric cryptosporidiosis in snakes: a review. *J Herp Med Surg*. 2019;29(3-4):71–86.
44a. Bogan JE, Hoffman M, Dickenson F, et al. Evaluation of paromomycin treatment for *Cryptosporidium serpentis* infection in eastern indigo snakes (*Drymanchon couperi*). *J Herp Med Surg*. 2021;31(4):307–314.
45. Bogoslavsky B. The use of ponazuril to treat coccidiosis in eight inland bearded dragons (*Pogona vitticeps*). *Proc Annu Conf Assoc Rept Amph Vet*. 2007;8-9.
46. Boyer DM. Adverse ivermectin reaction in the prehensile-tailed skink, *Corucia zebrata*. *Bull Assoc Rept Amph Vet*. 1992;2:6.
47. Boyer TH. Emergency care of reptiles. *Semin Avian Exot Pet Med*. 1994;3:210–216.
48. Bressan TF, Sobreira T, Carregaro AB. Use of rodent sedation tests to evaluate midazolam and flumazenil in green iguanas (*Iguana iguana*). *J Am Assoc Lab Anim Sci*. 2019;58:810–816.
49. Brunner CHM, Dutra G, Silva CB, et al. Electrochemotherapy for the treatment of fibropapillomas in *Chelonia mydas*. *J Zoo Wild Med*. 2014;45:213–218.
50. Bryant GL, Fleming PA, Twomey L, et al. Factors affecting hematology and plasma biochemistry in the southwest carpet python (*Morelia spilota imbricata*). *J Wildl Dis*. 2012;48:282–294.

51. Bunke L, Sladky KK, Johnson SM. Antinociceptive efficacy and respiratory effects of dexmedetomidine in ball pythons (*Python regius*). *Am J Vet Res*. 2018;79:718–726.
52. Burnham BR, Atchley DH, DeFusco RP, et al. The use of enrofloxacin to prevent shedding of *Salmonella* from green iguanas, *Iguana iguana*. *J Herp Med Surg*. 2002;12:10–13.
53. Burns RB, McMahan W. Euthanasia methods for ectothermic vertebrates. In: Bonagura JD, ed. *Kirk's Current Veterinary Therapy XII: Small Animal Practice*. Philadelphia, PA: WB Saunders; 1995:1379–1381.
54. Burridge B, Burridge MJ, Peter TF, et al. Evaluation of safety and efficacy of acaricides for control of the African tortoise tick (*Amblyomma marmoreum*) on leopard tortoises (Geochelone pardalis). *J Zoo Wildl Med*. 2002;33(1):52–57.
55. Burridge A, Burridge MJ, Simmons LA, et al. Control of an exotic tick (*Aponomma komodoense*) infestation in a Komodo dragon (*Varanus komodoensis*) exhibit at a zoo in Florida. *J Zoo Wildl Med*. 2004;35(2):248–249.
56. Bush M, Smeller JM, Charache P, et al. Biological half-life of gentamicin in gopher snakes. *Am J Vet Res*. 1978;39:171–173.
57. Cakici O, Akat E. Histopathological effects of carbaryl on digestive system of snake-eyed lizard, Ophisops elegans. *Bull Environ Contam Toxicol*. 2012;88(5):685–690.
58. Caligiuri R, Kollias GV, Jacobson E, et al. The effects of ambient temperature on amikacin pharmacokinetics in gopher tortoises. *J Vet Pharm Therapeut*. 1990;13:287–291.
59. Calvert I. Nutritional problems. In: Girling SJ, Raiti P, eds. *BSAVA Manual of Reptiles*. 2nd ed. Quedgeley, UK: British Small Animal Veterinary Association; 2004:289–308.
60. Camacho M, del Pino Quintana M, Calabuig P, et al. Acid-base and plasma biochemical changes using crystalloid fluids in stranded juvenile loggerhead sea turtles (*Caretta caretta*). *Plos One*. 2015;10:1371–1381.
61. Campagnol D, Lemos FR, Silva ELF, et al. Comparacao da contencao farmacologica com cetamina e xilazina, administradas pela via intramuscular no membro toracico ou pelvico, em jacares-do-papo-amarelo juvenis. *Pesq Vet Bras*. 2014;34:675–681.
62. Carpenter JW. Radiographic imaging of reptiles. *Proc North Am Vet Conf*. 1998:873–875.
63. Carpenter JW, Klaphake E, Gibbons PM, et al. Reptile formulary. In: Divers SJ, Stahl SJ, eds. *Mader's Reptile and Amphibian Medicine and Surgery*. 3rd ed. St. Louis, MO: Elsevier; 2019:1191–1211.
64. Carpenter JW, Whitaker BR, Gibbons PM, et al. Hematology and biochemistry tables. In: Divers SJ, Stahl SJ, eds. *Mader's Reptile and Amphibian Medicine and Surgery*. 3rd ed. St. Louis, MO: Elsevier; 2019:333–350.
65. Casares M, Enders F. Enrofloxacin side effects in a Galapagos tortoise (*Geochelone elephantopus nigra*). *Proc Annu Conf Am Assoc Zoo Vet*. 1996:446–448.
66. Cermakova E, Ceplecha V, Knotek Z. Efficacy of two methods of intranasal administration of anaesthetic drugs in red-eared terrapins (*Trachemys scripta elegans*). *Vet Med*. 2017;62:87–93.
67. Cermakova E, Oliveri M, Knotkova Z, et al. Effect of a GnRH agonist (deslorelin) on ovarian activity in leopard geckos (*Eublepharis macularius*). *Vet Med (Praha)*. 2019;64:228–230.
68. Cerreta AJ, Cannizzo SA, Smith DC, et al. Venous hematology, biochemistry, and blood gas analysis of free-ranging Eastern copperheads (*Agkistrodon contortrix*) and Eastern ratsnakes (*Pantherophis alleghaniensis*). *PLoS One*. 2020;15(2):e0229102.
69. Cerreta AJ, Lewbart GA, Dise DR, et al. Population pharmacokinetics of ceftazidime after a single intramuscular injection in wild turtles. *J Vet Pharmacol Ther*. 2018;41:495–501.
70. Cerreta AJ, Masterson CA, Lewbart GA, et al. Pharmacokinetics of ketorolac in wild Eastern box turtles (*Terrapene carolina carolina*) after single intramuscular administration. *Vet Pharm Therap*. 2019;42:154–159.
71. Chen TY, Deem S. Clinical management of an intranasal abscess in a captive elongate tortoise (*Indotestudo elongata*) by using modified Choukroun's platelet-rich fibrin. *J Herpetol Med Surg*. 2019;29:87–91.
72. Chiodini RJ, Sundberg JP. Blood chemical values of the common boa constrictor (*Constrictor constrictor*). *Am J Vet Res*. 1982;43:1701–1702.

73. Chittick EJ, Stamper MA, Beasley JF, et al. Medetomidine, ketamine, and sevoflurane for anesthesia of injured loggerhead sea turtles: 13 cases (1996-2000). *J Am Vet Med Assoc.* 2002;221:1019–1025.
74. Chitty JR. Use of a novel disinfectant agent in reptile respiratory disease. *Proc Annu Conf Assoc Rept Amph Vet.* 2003:65–67.
75. Christopher MM, Berry KH, Wallis IR, et al. Reference intervals and physiologic alterations in hematologic and biochemical values of free-ranging desert tortoises in the Mojave Desert. *J Wildl Dis.* 1999;35:212–238.
76. Churgin SM, Musgrave KE, Cox SK, et al. Pharmacokinetics of subcutaneous versus intramuscular administration of ceftiofur crystalline-free acid to bearded dragons (*Pogona vitticeps*). *Am J Vet Res.* 2014;75:453–459.
77. Clancy MM, Newton AL, Sykes JM. Management of osteomyelitis caused by *Salmonella enteritica* subsp. *houtenae* in a Taylor's cantil (*Agkistrodon bilineatus taylori*) using amikacin delivered via osmotic pump. *J Zoo Wildl Med.* 2016;47:691–694.
78. Clark CH, Rogers ED, Milton JL. Plasma concentrations of chloramphenicol in snakes. *Am J Vet Res.* 1985;46:2654–2657.
79. VL Clyde, Cardeilhac PT, Jacobson ER. Chemical restraint of American alligators (*Alligator mississippiensis*) with atracurium or tiletamine-zolazepam. *J Zoo Wildl Med.* 1994;25:525–530.
80. Cojean O, Alberton S, Froment R, et al. Determination of leopard gecko (*Eublepharis macularius*) packed cell volume and plasma biochemistry reference intervals and reference values. *J Herp Med Surg.* 2020;3:156–164.
81. Coke RL, Hunter RP, Isaza R, et al. Pharmacokinetics and tissue concentrations of azithromycin in ball pythons (*Python regius*). *Am J Vet Res.* 2003;64:225–228.
82. Coke RL, Isaza R, Koch DE, et al. Preliminary single-dose pharmacokinetics of marbofloxacin in ball pythons (*Python regius*). *J Zoo Wildl Med.* 2006;37:6–10.
83. Conroy CJ, Papenfuss T, Parker J, et al. Use of tricaine methanesulfonate (MS222) for euthanasia of reptiles. *J Am Assoc Lab Anim Sci.* 2009;48:28–32.
84. Cooper-Bailey K, Smith SA, Zimmerman K, et al. Hematology, leukocyte cytochemical analysis, plasma biochemistry, and plasma electrophoresis of wild-caught and captive bred Gila monsters (*Heloderma suspectum*). *Vet Clin Pathol.* 2011;40:316–323.
85. Couture EL, Monteirob BP, Aymen J, et al. Validation of a thermal threshold nociceptive model in bearded dragons (*Pogona vitticeps*). *Vet Anaesth Analg.* 2017;44:676–683.
86. Cowan ML, Raidal SR, Peters A. Herpesvirus in a captive Australian Krefft's river turtle (*Emydura macquarii krefftii*). *Aust Vet J.* 2015;93:46–49.
87. Cranfield MR, Graczyk TK. Experimental infection of elaphid snakes with *Cryptosporidium serpentis* (Apicomplexa: Cryptosporidiidae). *J Small Anim Pract.* 2018;59(11):704–713.
88. Cranfield MR, Graczyk TK. Cryptosoporidiosis. In: Mader DR, ed. *Reptile Medicine and Surgery.* 2nd ed. St. Louis, MO: Saunders/Elsevier; 2006:756–762.
89. Crawshaw GJ, Holz P. Comparison of plasma biochemical values in blood and blood-lymph mixtures from red-eared sliders, *Trachemys scripta elegans. Bull Assoc Rept Amph Vet.* 1996;6:7–9.
90. Dallwig R. Allopurinol. *J Exot Pet Med.* 2010;19:255–257.
91. Darrow BG, Myers GE, KuKanich B, et al. Fentanyl transdermal therapeutic system provides rapid systemic fentanyl absorption in two ball pythons (Python regius). *J Herp Med Surg.* 2016;26:94–99.
92. Deem SL, Norton TM, Mitchell M, et al. Comparison of blood values in foraging, nesting, and stranded loggerhead turtles (*Caretta caretta*) along the coast of Georgia, USA. *J Wildl Dis.* 2009;45:41–56.
93. DeNardo DF, Helminski G. Birth control in lizards? Therapeutic inhibition of reproduction. *Proc Annu Conf Assoc Rept Amph Vet.* 2000:65–66.
94. Dennis PM, Heard DJ. Cardiopulmonary effects of a medetomidine-ketamine combination administered intravenously in gopher tortoises. *J Am Vet Med Assoc.* 2002;220:1516–1519.

95. Dennis PM, Bennett RA, Harr KE, et al. Plasma concentration of ionized calcium in healthy iguanas. *J Am Vet Med Assoc*. 2001;219:326–328.
96. DeVoe R. Nutritional support of reptile patients. *Vet Clin Exot Anim*. 2014;17:249–261.
97. Dickinson VM, Jarchow JL, Trueblood MH. Hematology and plasma biochemistry reference range values for free-ranging desert tortoises in Arizona. *J Wildl Dis*. 2002;38:143–153.
98. Diethelm G, Stein G. Hematologic and blood chemistry values in reptiles. In: Mader DR, ed. *Reptile Medicine and Surgery*. 2nd ed. St. Louis, MO: Saunders/Elsevier; 2006:1103–1118.
99. Di Girolamo N. Intravenous catheter placement in reptiles. *Proc ExoticsCon*. 2021:406–410.
100. Di Girolamo N, Ferlizza E, Selleri P, et al. Evaluation of point-of-care analysers for blood gas and clinical chemistry in Hermann's tortoises (*Testudo hermanni*). *J Small Anim Pract*. 2018;59(11):704–713.
101. Di Giuseppe M, Morici M, Martinez Silvestre A, et al. Jugular vein venipuncture technique in small lizard species. *J Small Anim Pract*. 2017;58:249.
102. Di Ianni F, Parmigiani E, Pelizzone I, et al. Comparison between intramuscular and intravenous administration of oxytocin in captive-bred red-eared sliders (*Trachemys scripta elegans*) with nonobstructive egg retention. *J Exot Pet Med*. 2014;23(1):79–84.
103. Divers SJ. Constipation in snakes with particular reference to surgical correction in a Burmese python (*Python molurus bivittatus*). *Proc Annu Conf Assoc Rept Amph Vet*. 1996:67–69.
104. Divers SJ. Medical and surgical treatment of pre-ovulatory ova stasis and post-ovulatory egg stasis in oviparous lizards. *Proc Annu Conf Assoc Rept Amph Vet*. 1996:119–123.
105. Divers SJ. The use of propofol in reptile anesthesia. *Proc Annu Conf Assoc Rept Amph Vet*. 1996:57–59.
106. Divers SJ. Clinician's approach to renal disease in lizards. *Proc Annu Conf Assoc Rept Amph Vet*. 1997:5–11.
107. Divers SJ. Empirical doses of antimicrobial drugs commonly used in reptiles. *Exot DVM*. 1998;1:23.
108. Divers SJ, Stahl SJ. *Mader's Reptile and Amphibian Medicine and Surgery*. 3rd ed. St. Louis, MO: Elsevier; 2019.
109. Divers SJ, Redmayne G, Aves EK. Haematological and biochemical values of 10 green iguanas (*Iguana iguana*). *Vet Rec*. 1996;138:203–205.
110. Divers SJ, Papich MG, McBride M, et al. Pharmacokinetics of meloxicam following intravenous and oral administration in green iguanas (*Iguana iguana*). *Am J Vet Res*. 2010;71:1277–1283.
111. Donoghue S. Nutrition. In: Mader DR, ed. *Reptile Medicine and Surgery*. 2nd ed. St. Louis, MO: Saunders/Elsevier; 2006:251–298.
112. Drew ML. Hypercalcemia and hyperphosphatemia in indigo snakes (*Drymarchon corais*) and serum biochemical reference values. *J Zoo Wildl Med*. 1994;25:48–52.
113. Ellman MM. Hematology and plasma chemistry of the inland bearded dragon, *Pogona vitticeps*. *Bull Assoc Rept Amph Vet*. 1997;7:10–12.
114. Emery L, Parsons G, Gerhardt L, et al. Sedative effects of intranasal midazolam and dexmedetomidine in 2 species of tortoises (*Chelonoidis carbonaria* and *Geochelone platynota*). *J Exot Pet Med*. 2014;23:380–383.
115. Epstein J, Doss G, Yaw T, et al. Diagnosis and successful medical management of a colonic, urate enterolith in an Argentine black and white tegu (*Salvator merianae*). *J Herpetol Med Surg*. 2020;30:21–27.
116. Erlacher-Reid CD, Norton TM, Harms CA, et al. Intestinal and cloacal strictures in free-ranging and aquarium-maintained green sea turtles (*Chelonia mydas*). *J Zoo Wildl Med*. 2013;44:408–429.
117. Eshar D, Lapid R, Head V. Transilluminated jugular blood sampling in the common chameleon (*Chamaeleo chamaeleon*). *J Herpetol Med Surg*. 2018;28:19–22.
118. Eshar D, Ammersbach M, Shacham B, et al. Venous blood gases, plasma biochemistry, and hematology of wild-caught common chameleons (*Chamaeleo chamaeleon*). *Can J Vet Res*. 2018;82:106–114.

119. Eshar D, KuKanich B, Avni-Magen N, et al. Terbinafine pharmacokinetics following single dose oral administration in red-eared slider turtles (*Trachemys scripta elegans*): a pilot study. *J Zoo Wildl Med.* 2021;52:520–528.
120. Farmaki R, Simou C, Papadopoulos E, et al. Effectiveness of a single application of 0.25% fipronil solution for the treatment of hirstiellosis in captive green iguanas (*Iguana iguana*): an open label study. *Parasitol.* 2013;140:1144–1148.
121. Farnsworth RJ, Brannian RE, Fletcher KC, et al. A vitamin E-selenium responsive condition in a green iguana. *J Zoo Anim Med.* 1986;17:42–43.
122. Feldman M, Feldman E. New methods to induce egg laying in turtles. *Proc 14th Annu Symp Cons Biol Tortoises Freshwater Turtles.* 2016:26.
123. Ferreira TH, Mans C. Evaluation of neuraxial anesthesia in bearded dragons (*Pogona vitticeps*). *Vet Anaesth Analg.* 2019;46(1):126–134.
124. Ferreira TH, Fink DM, Mans C. Evaluation of neuraxial administration of bupivacaine in Q1 bearded dragons (*Pogona vitticeps*). *Vet Anaesth Analg.* 2021;48(5):798–803.
125. Ferreira TH, Mans C, Di Girolamo N. Evaluation of the sedative and physiological effects of intramuscular lidocaine in bearded dragons (*Pogona vitticeps*) sedated with alfaxalone. *Vet Anaesth Analg.* 2019;46(4):496–500.
126. Fitzgerald KT, Martinez-Silvestre A. Toxicology. In: Divers SJ, Stahl SJ, eds. *Mader's Reptile and Amphibian Medicine and Surgery.* 3rd ed. St. Louis, MO: Elsevier; 2019:977–991.
127. Flach EJ, Riley J, Mutlow AG, et al. Pentastomiasis in Bosc's monitor lizards (*Varanus exanthematicus*) caused by an undescribed Sambonia species. *J Zoo Wildl Med.* 2000;31:91–95.
128. Fleming G. Clinical technique: chelonian shell repair. *J Exot Pet Med.* 2008;17:246–258.
129. Fleming GJ. Capture and chemical immobilization of the Nile crocodile (*Crocodylus niloticus*) in South Africa. *Proc Annu Conf Assoc Rept Amph Vet.* 1996:63–66.
130. Fleming GJ. Crocodilian anesthesia. *Vet Clin North Am Exot Anim Pract.* 2001;4:119–145.
131. Fleming GJ, Robertson SA. Assessments of thermal antinociceptive effects of butorphanol and human observer effect on quantitative evaluation of analgesia in green iguanas (*Iguana iguana*). *Am J Vet Res.* 2012;73:1507–1511.
132. Flint M, Morton JM, Limpus CJ, et al. Development and application of biochemical and haematological reference intervals to identify unhealthy green sea turtles (*Chelonia mydas*). *Vet J.* 2010;185:299–304.
133. Florida Iguana and Tortoise Breeders. How to Draw Blood from a Large Tortoise. Available at: https://www.youtube.com/watch?v=pIZzsyD551Y . Accessed December 14, 2020.
134. Flower JE, Byrd J, Cray C, et al. Plasma electrophoretic profiles and hemoglobin binding protein reference intervals in the Eastern box turtle (*Terrapene carolina carolina*) and influences of age, sex, season, and location. *J Zoo Wildl Med.* 2014;45:836–842.
135. Folland DW, Johnston MS, Thamm DH, et al. Diagnosis and management of lymphoma in a green iguana (*Iguana iguana*). *J Am Vet Med Assoc.* 2011;239:985–991.
136. Foronda P, Santana-Morales MA, Orós J, et al. Clinical efficacy of antiparasite treatments against intestinal helminths and haematic protozoa in *Gallotia caesaris* (lizards). *Exp Parasitol.* 2007;116(4):361–365.
137. Franco KH, Hoover JP. Levothyroxine as a treatment for presumed hypothyroidism in an adult male African spurred tortoise (*Centrochelys* [formerly *Geochelone*] *sulcata*). *J Herpetol Med Surg.* 2009;19:42–44.
138. Fraser MA, Girling SJ. Dermatology. In: Girling SJ, Raiti P, eds. *BSAVA Manual of Reptiles.* 2nd ed. Quedgeley, UK: British Small Animal Veterinary Association; 2004:184–198.
139. Frei S, Sanchez-Migallon Guzman D, Kass PH, et al. Evaluation of a ventral and a left lateral approach to coelioscopy in bearded dragons (*Pogona vitticeps*). *Am J Vet Res.* 2020;81:267–275.
140. Fudge AM. Laboratory reference ranges for selected avian, mammalian, and reptilian species. In: Fudge AM, ed. *Laboratory Medicine: Avian and Exotic Pets.* Philadelphia, PA: WB Saunders; 2000:375–400.
141. Futema F, de Carvalho FM, Werneck MR. Spinal anesthesia in green sea turtles (*Chelonia mydas*) undergoing surgical removal of cutaneous fibropapillomas. *J Zoo Wildl Med.* 2020;51:357–362.

142. Funk RS. A formulary for lizards, snakes, and crocodilians. *Vet Clin North Am Exot Anim Pract.* 2000;3:333–358.
143. Funk RS, Diethelm G. Reptile formulary. In: Mader DR, ed. *Reptile Medicine and Surgey.* 2nd ed. St. Louis, MO: Saunders/Elsevier; 2006:1119–1139.
144. Gaio C, Rossi T, Villa R, et al. Pharmacokinetics of acyclovir after a single oral administration in marginated tortoises, *Testudo marginata. J Herpetol Med Surg.* 2007;17:8–11.
145. Gałęcki R, Sokół R. Treatment of cryptosporidiosis in captive green iguanas (*Iguana iguana*). *Vet Parasitol.* 2018;252:17–21.
146. Gamble KC. Plasma fentanyl concentrations achieved after transdermal fentanyl patch application in prehensile-tailed skinks, *Corucia zebrata. J Herpetol Med Surg.* 2008;18:81–85.
147. Gamble KC, Alvarado TP, Bennett CL. Itraconazole plasma and tissue concentrations in the spiny lizard (*Sceloporus* sp.) following once-daily dosing. *J Zoo Wildl Med.* 1997;28:89–93.
148. Gatson BJ, Goe A, Granone TD, et al. Intramuscular epinephrine results in reduced anesthetic recovery time in American alligators (*Alligator mississippiensis*) undergoing isoflurane anesthesia. *J Zoo Wildl Med.* 2017;48:55–61.
149. Gaumer A, Goodnight CJ. Some aspects of the hematology of turtles as related to their activity. *Am Midland Nat.* 1957;58:332–340.
150. Georoff TA, Stacy NI, Newton AN, et al. Diagnosis and treatment of chronic T-lymphocytic leukemia in a green tree monitor (*Varanus prasinus*). *J Herpetol Med Surg.* 2009;19:106–114.
151. Giannetto S, Brianti E, Poglayen G, et al. Efficacy of oxfendazole and fenbendazole against tortoise (*Testudo hermanni*) oxyurids. *Parasitol Res.* 2007;100:1069–1073.
152. Gibbons PM. Advances in reptile clinical therapeutics. *J Exot Pet Med.* 2014;23:21–38.
153. Gibbons PM, Horton SJ, Brandl SR. Urinalysis in box turtles, *Terrapene* spp. *Proc Annu Conf Assoc Rept Amph Vet.* 2000:161–168.
153a. Carpenter JW, Gibbons PM, Whitaker BR, et al. Hematology and biochemistry tables. In: Divers SJ, Stahl SJ, eds. *Mader's Reptile and Amphibian Medicine and Surgery.* 3rd ed. St. Louis, MO: Elsevier; 2019:333–350.
154. Gillespie D. Reptiles. In: Birchard SJ, Sherding RG, eds. *Saunders Manual of Small Animal Practice.* Philadelphia, PA: WB Saunders; 1994:1390–1411.
155. Gimenez M, Saco Y, Pato R, et al. Plasma protein electrophoresis of *Trachemys scripta* and *Iguana iguana. Vet Clin Pathol.* 2010;39:227–235.
156. Giorgi M, De Vito V, Owen H, et al. PK/PD evaluations of the novel atypical opioid tapentadol in red-eared slider turtles. *Med Weter.* 2014;70:530–535.
157. Giorgi M, Lee H-K, Rota S, et al. Pharmacokinetic and pharmacodynamics assessments of tapentadol in yellow-bellied slider turtles (*Trachemys scripta scripta*) after a single intramuscular injection. *J Exot Pet Med.* 2015;24:317–325.
158. Giorgi M, Rota S, Giorgi T, et al. Blood concentrations of enrofloxacin and the metabolite ciprofloxacin in yellow-bellied slider turtles (*Trachemys scripta scripta*) after a single intracoelomic injection of enrofloxacin. *J Exot Pet Med.* 2013;22:192–199.
159. Giorgi M, Salvadori M, De Vito V, et al. Pharmacokinetic/pharmacodynamics assessments of 10 mg/kg tramadol intramuscular injection in yellow-bellied slider turtles (*Trachemys scripta scripta*). *J Vet Pharmacol Therap.* 2015;38:488–496.
160. Giori L, Stacy NI, Ogle M, et al. Hematology, plasma biochemistry, and hormonal analysis of captive Louisiana pine snakes (*Pituophis ruthveni*): effects of intrinsic factors and analytical methodology. *Comp Clin Path.* 2020;29(1):145–154.
161. Girling SJ, Hynes B. Cardiovascular and haemopoietic systems. In: Girling SJ, Raiti P, eds. *BSAVA Manual of Reptiles.* 2nd ed. Quedgeley, UK: 2004 British Small Animal Veterinary Association; 2012:243–260.
162. Goe A, Shmalberg J, Gatson B, et al. Epinephrine or GV-26 electrical stimulation reduces inhalant anesthetic recovery time in common snapping turtles (*Chelydra serpentina*). *J Zoo Wildl Med.* 2016;47:501–507.
163. Gornik KR, Pirie CG, Marrion RM, et al. Baseline corneal sensitivity and duration of action of proparacaine in rehabilitated juvenile Kemp's ridley sea turtles (*Lepidochelys kempii*). *J Herp Med Surg.* 2015;25:116–121.

164. Gottdenker NL, Jacobson ER. Effect of venipuncture sites on hematologic and clinical biochemical values in desert tortoises (*Gopherus agassizii*). *Am J Vet Res.* 1995;56:19–21.
165. Graczyk TK, Cranfield MR, Hill SL. Therapeutic efficacy of halofuginone and spiramycin treatment against *Cryptosporidium serpentis* (Apicomplexa: Cryptosporidiidae) infections in captive snakes. *Parasitol Res.* 1996;82(2):143–148.
166. Greenacre CB, Massi K, Schumacher JP, et al. Comparative antinociception of various opioids and non-steroidal anti-inflammatory medications versus saline in the bearded dragon (*Pogona vitticeps*) using electrostimulation. *Proc Annu Conf Rept Amph Vet.* 2008;87.
167. Greunz EM, Williams C, Ringgaard S, et al. Elimination of intracardiac shunting provides stable gas anesthesia in tortoises. *Sci Rep.* 2018;8:17124. doi:10.1038/s41598-018-35588-w.
168. Griffioen JA, Lewbart GA, Papich MG. Population pharmacokinetics of enrofloxacin and its metabolite ciprofloxacin in clinically diseased or injured Eastern box turtles (*Terrapene carolina carolina*), yellow-bellied sliders (*Trachemys scripta scripta*), and river cooters (*Pseudemys concinna*). *J Vet Pharmacol Ther.* 2020;43:222–230.
169. Grosset C, Villeneuve A, Brieger A, et al. Cryptosporidiosis in juvenile bearded dragons (*Pogona vitticeps*): effects of treatment with paromomycin. *J Herpetol Med Surg.* 2011;21:10–15.
170. Groza A, Mederle N, Darabus G. Advocate-therapeutical solution in parasitical infestation in frillneck lizard (*Chlamydosaurus kingii*) and bearded dragon (*Pogona vitticeps*). *Lucrari Stiintifice - Universitatea Stiinte Agricole Banatului Timisoara Med Vet.* 2009;42:105–108.
171. Hackenbroich C, Failing K, Axt-Findt U, et al. Alphaxalone-alphadolone anesthesia in *Trachemys scripta elegans* and its influence on respiration, circulation and metabolism. *Proc 2nd Conf Euro Assoc Zoo Wildl Vet.* 1998:431–436.
172. Hadfield CA, Clayton LA, Clancy MM. Proliferative thyroid lesions in three diplodactylid geckos: *Nephrurus amyae*, *Nephrurus levis*, and *Oedura marmorata*. *J Zoo Wildl Med.* 2012;43:131–140.
173. Hahn A, D'Agostino J, Cole GA. Secondary ivermectin poisoning in South American green snakes (*Philodryas baroni*). *Vet Rec.* 2014;2:e000053.
174. Hansen LL, Bertelsen MF. Assessment of the effects of intramuscular administration of alfaxalone with and without medetomidine in Horsfield's tortoises (*Agrionemys horsfieldii*). *Vet Anaesth Analg.* 2013;40:68–75.
175. Harkewicz KA. Dermatologic problems of reptiles. *Semin Avian Exot Pet Med.* 2002;11:151–161.
176. Harms CA, Lewbart GA, Beasley J. Medical management of mixed nocardial and unidentified fungal osteomyelitis in a Kemp's ridley sea turtle, *Lepidochelys kempii*. *J Herpetol Med Surg.* 2002;12:21–26.
177. Harms CA, Cranston EA, Papich MG, et al. Pharmacokinetics of clindamycin in loggerhead sea turtles (*Caretta caretta*) after a single intravenous, intramuscular, or oral dose. *J Herpetol Med Surg.* 2011;21:113–119.
178. Harms CA, Piniak WED, Eckert SA, et al. Sedation and anesthesia of hatchling leatherback sea turtles (*Dermochelys coriacea*) for auditory evoked potential measurement in air and in water. *J Zoo Wildl Med.* 2014;45:86–92.
179. Harms CA, Ruterbories LK, Stacy NI, et al. Safety of multiple-dose intramuscular ketoprofen treatment in loggerhead turtles (*Caretta caretta*). *J Zoo Wildl Med.* 2021;52(1):126–132.
180. Harr KE, Alleman AR, Dennis PM, et al. Morphologic and cytochemical characteristics of blood cells and hematologic and plasma biochemical reference ranges in green iguanas. *J Am Vet Med Assoc.* 2001;218:915–921.
180a. Hawkins SJ, Cox S, Yaw TJ, et al. Pharmacokinetics of subcutaneous administered hydromorphone in bearded dragons (*Pogona vitticeps*) and red-eared slider turtles (*Trachemys scripta elegans*. *Vet Anaesth Analg.* 2019;46(3):352–359.
181. Haynes E, Allender MC, Stanford K, et al. Controlled clinical trial using terbinafine nebulization to treat wild Lake Erie watersnakes (*Nerodia sipedon insularum*) with natural ophidiomycosis. *Proc Annu Conf Am Assoc Zoo Vet.* 2019:65.

182. Heard DJ. Principles and techniques of anesthesia and analgesia for exotic practice. *Vet Clin North Am Small Anim Pract.* 1993;23:1301–1327.
183. Heard DJ. Advances in reptile anesthesia and medicine. *Proc Annu Conf Assoc Avian Vet/Avian Speciality Advanced Prog/Small Mam Rept Prog.* 1998:113–119.
184. Hedley J. *BSAVA Small Animal Formulary: Exotic Pets.* Quedgeley, UK: British Small Animal Veterinary Association; 2020.
185. Heatley J, Mitchell M, Williams J, et al. Fungal periodontal osteomyelitis in a chameleon, *Furcifer pardalis. J Herpetol Med Surg.* 2001;11:7–12.
186. Heaton-Jones TG, Ko J, Heaton-Jones DL. Evaluation of medetomidine-ketamine anesthesia with atipamezole reversal in American alligators (*Alligator mississippiensis*). *J Zoo Wildl Med.* 2002;33:36–44.
187. Hellebuyck T, Baert K, Pasmans F, et al. Cutaneous hyalohyphomycosis in a girdled lizard (*Cordylus giganteus*) caused by the *Chrysosporium* anamorph of *Nannizziopsis vriesii* and successful treatment with voriconazole. *Vet Derm.* 2010;21:429–433.
188. Hellebuyck T, Pasmans F, Haesebrouck F, et al. Designing a successful antimicrobial treatment against Devriesea agamarum infections in lizards. *Vet Microbiol.* 2009;139:189–192.
189. Helmick KE, Bennett RA, Ginn P, et al. Intestinal volvulus and stricture associated with a leiomyoma in a green turtle (*Chelonia mydas*). *J Zoo Wildl Med.* 2000;31:221–227.
190. Helmick KE, Papich MG, Vliet KA, et al. Pharmacokinetic disposition of a long-acting oxytetracycline formulation after single-dose intravenous and intramuscular administrations in the American alligator (*Alligator mississippiensis*). *J Zoo Wildl Med.* 2004;35:341–346.
191. Helmick KE, Papich MG, Vliet KA, et al. Pharmacokinetics of enrofloxacin after single-dose oral and intravenous administration in the American alligator (*Alligator mississippiensis*). *J Zoo Wildl Med.* 2004;35:333–340.
192. Hernandez-Divers SJ. Pulmonary candidiasis caused by *Candida albicans* in a Greek tortoise (*Testudo graeca*) and treatment with intrapulmonary amphotericin B. *J Zoo Wildl Med.* 2001;32:352–359.
193. Hernandez-Divers SJ. Diagnostic techniques. In: Mader DR, ed. *Reptile Medicine and Surgery.* 2nd ed. St. Louis, MO: Saunders/Elsevier; 2006:490–532.
194. Hernandez-Divers SJ, Cooper JE. Hepatic lipidosis. In: Mader DR, ed. *Reptile Medicine and Surgery.* 2nd ed. St. Louis, MO: Saunders/Elsevier; 2006:806–813.
195. Hernandez-Divers SJ, Knott CD, MacDonald J. Diagnosis and surgical treatment of thyroid adenoma-induced hyperthyroidism in a green iguana (*Iguana iguana*). *J Zoo Wildl Med.* 2001;32:465–475.
196. Hernandez-Divers SJ, Martinez-Jimenez D, Bush S, et al. Effects of allopurinol on plasma uric acid levels in normouricaemic and hyperuricaemic green iguanas (*Iguana iguana*). *Vet Rec.* 2008;162:112–115.
197. Hernandez SM, Schumacher J, Lewis SJ, et al. Selected cardiopulomonolgy values and baroreceptor reflex in conscious green iguanas (*Iguana iguana*). *Am Vet Res.* 2011;72:1519–1526.
198. Hernandez-Divers SM. Reptile critical care. *Exot DVM.* 2003;5(3):81–87.
199. Hess JC, Benson J, Grimm KA, et al. Minimum alveolar concentration of isoflurane and arterial blood gas values in anesthetized green iguanas, *Iguana iguana. J Herpetol Med Surg.* 2008;17:118–124.
200. Hilf M, Swanson D, Wagner R, et al. A new dosing schedule for gentamicin in blood pythons (*Python curtus*): a pharmacokinetic study. *Res Vet Sci.* 1991;50:127–130.
201. Hilf M, Swanson D, Wagner R, et al. Pharmacokinetics of piperacillin in blood pythons (*Python curtus*) and in vitro evaluation of efficacy against aerobic gram-negative bacteria. *J Zoo Wildl Med.* 1991;22:199–203.
202. Hirano LQL. Contenção química e perfil farmacocinético da dextrocetamina, isolada em associação ao midazolam em jacaré-tinga *Caiman crocodilus* Linnaeus (1758) (Crocodylia: Alligatoridade) [Master's dissertation]. http://repositorio.bc.ufg.br/tede/handle/tede/46944,2015.

203. Holz P, Holz RM. Evaluation of ketamine, ketamine/xylazine, and ketamine/midazolam anesthesia in red-eared sliders (*Trachemys scripta elegans*). *J Zoo Wildl Med.* 1994;25:531–537.
204. Holz P, Barker IK, Burger JP, et al. The effect of the renal portal system on pharmacokinetic parameters in the red-eared slider (*Trachemys scripta elegans*). *J Zoo Wildl Med.* 1997;28:386–393.
205. Holz PH, Burger JP, Baker R, et al. Effect of injection site on carbenicillin pharmacokinetics in the carpet python, *Morelia spilota*. *J Herpetol Med Surg.* 2002;12:12–16.
206. Hungerford C, Spelman L, Papich M. Pharmacokinetics of enrofloxacin after oral and intramuscular administration in savannah monitors (*Varanus exanthematicus*). *Proc Annu Conf Am Assoc Zoo Vet.* 1997:89–92.
207. Hunter RP, Koch DE, Coke RL, et al. Azithromycin metabolite identification in plasma, bile, and tissues of the ball python (*Python regius*). *J Vet Pharmacol Ther.* 2003;26:117–121.
208. Innis CJ. Observations on urinalysis of clinically normal captive tortoises. *Proc Annu Conf Assoc Rept Amph Vet.* 1997:109–112.
209. Innis CJ, Boyer TH. Chelonian reproductive disorders. *Vet Clin North Am Exot Anim Pract.* 2002;5:555–578.
210. Innis C, Papich M, Young D. Pharmacokinetics of metronidazole in the red-eared slider turtle (*Trachemys scripta elegans*) after single intracoelomic injection. *J Vet Pharm Therapeut.* 2007;30:168–171.
211. Innis CJ, Ceresia ML, Merigo C, et al. Single-dose pharmacokinetics of ceftazidime and fluconazole during concurrent clinical use in cold-stunned Kemp's ridley turtles (*Lepidochelys kempii*). *J Vet Pharmacol Therap.* 2012;35:82–89.
212. Innis CJ, Feinsod R, Hanlon J, et al. Coelioscopic orchiectomy can be effectively and safely accomplished in chelonians. *Vet Rec.* 2013;172:526–531.
213. Innis C, Kennedy A, Wocial J, et al. Comparison of oxytetracycline pharmacokinetics after multiple subcutaneous injections in three sea turtle species. *J Herp Med Surg.* 2020;30(3):142–147.
214. Innis C, Young D, Wetzlich S, et al. Plasma voriconazole concentrations in four red-eared slider turtles (*Trachemys scripta elegans*) after a single subcutaneous injection. *Proc Annu Conf Assoc Rept Amph Vet.* 2008;72.
215. Innis CJ, Young D, Wetzlich S, et al. Plasma concentrations and safety assessment of voriconazole in red-eared slider turtles (*Trachemys scripta elegans*) after single and multiple subcutaneous injections. *J Herp Med Surg.* 2014;24:28–35.
216. Jacobson ER. Evaluation of the reptile patient. In: Jacobson ER, Kollias GV Jr., eds. *Exotic Animals.* New York, NY: Churchill Livingstone; 1988:1–18.
217. Jacobson ER. Antimicrobial drug use in reptiles. In: Prescott JF, Baggot JD, eds. *Antimicrobial Therapy in Veterinary Medicine.* Ames, IA: Iowa State University Press; 1993:543–552.
218. Jacobson ER, Brown MP, Chung M, et al. Serum concentration and disposition kinetics of gentamicin and amikacin in juvenile American alligators. *J Zoo Anim Med.* 1988;19:188–194.
219. Jacobson E, Gronwall R, Maxwell L, et al. Plasma concentrations of enrofloxacin after single-dose oral administration in loggerhead sea turtles (*Caretta caretta*). *J Zoo Wildl Med.* 2005;36:628–634.
219a. Jacobson E, Harmon G, Laille E, et al. Plasma concentrations of praziquantel in loggerhead sea turtles (*Caretta caretta*) following administration of single and multiple doses. *Proc Annu Conf Assoc Rept Amph Vet.* 2002:37–39.
220. James LE, Williams CJA, Bertelsen MF, et al. Anaesthetic induction with alfaxalone in the ball python (*Python regius*): dose response and effect of injection site. *Vet Anaesth Analg.* 2018;45:329–337.
221. Jepson L. *Snakes. Exotic Animal Medicine: A Quick Reference Guide.* Philadelphia, PA: Saunders/Elsevier; 2009:315–357.
222. Jepson L. Turtles and tortoises. In: *Exotic Animal Medicine: A Quick Reference Guide.* Philadelphia, PA: Saunders/Elsevier; 2009:358–411.

223. Johnson JG, Naples LM, Chu C, et al. Cutaneous squamous cell carcinoma in a panther chameleon (*Furcifer pardalis*) and treatment with carboplatin implantable beads. *J Zoo Wildl Med*. 2016;47:931–934.
224. Johnson JH, Benson PA. Laboratory reference values for a group of captive ball pythons (*Python regius*). *Am J Vet Res*. 1996;57:1304–1307.
225. Johnson JH, Jensen JM, Brumbaugh GW, et al. Amikacin pharmacokinetics and the effects of ambient temperature on the dosage regimen in ball pythons (*Python regius*). *J Zoo Wildl Med*. 1997;28:80–88.
226. Judd HL, Laughlin GA, Bacon JP, et al. Circulating androgen and estrogen concentrations in lizards (*Iguana iguana*). *Gen Comp Endocrinol*. 1976;30:391–395.
227. Kaminishi APS, de Freitas AC, Henderson R, et al. Antinociceptive and physiological effects of subcutaneously administration of fentanyl in *Trachemys* sp. (Testudines: Emydidae). *Intl J Advanced Engineer Res Sci*. 2019;6:311–316.
228. Kane LP, Allender MC, Archer G, et al. Pharmacokinetics of nebulized and subcutaneously implanted terbinafine in cottonmouths (*Agkistrodon piscivorus*). *J Vet Pharmacol Therap*. 2017;40:575–579.
229. Kanui TI, Hole K. Morphine and pethidine antinociception in the crocodile. *J Vet Pharmacol Ther*. 1992;15:101–103.
230. Karklus AA, Sladky KK, Johnson SM. Respiratory and antinociceptive effects of dexmedetomidine and doxapram in ball pythons (*Python regius*). *Am J Vet Res*. 2021;82:11–21.
231. Kaufman GE, Seymour RE, Bonner BB, et al. Use of rocuronium for endotracheal intubation of North American Gulf Coast box turtles. *J Am Vet Med Assoc*. 2003;222:1111–1115.
232. Kehoe S, Divers S, Mayer J, et al. Efficacy of single-dose oxfendazole to treat oxyurid nematodiasis in the green iguana (*Iguana iguana*). *J Herp Med Surg*. 2020;30(3):137–141.
233. Keller K. Terbinafine. *J Exot Pet Med*. 2012;2:181–185.
234. Kennedy A, Innis C, Rumbeiha W. Determination of glomerular filtration rate in juvenile Kemp's ridley turtles (*Lepidochelys kempii*) using iohexol clearance, with preliminary comparison of clinically healthy turtles vs. those with renal disease. *J Herp Med Surg*. 2012;22:25–29.
235. Kharbush R, Gutwillig A, Hartzler K, et al. Transdermal fentanyl in ball pythons (*Python regius*) does not provide antinociception and decreases breathing frequency despite high plasma fentanyl levels and brain mu-opioid receptor expression similar to opioid-responsive turtles. *Am J Vet Res*. 2017;78:785–795.
236. Kimble SJA, Williams RN. Temporal variance in hematologic and plasma biochemical reference intervals for free ranging Eastern box turtles (*Terrapene carolina carolina*). *J Wildl Dis*. 2012:799–802.
237. Kinney ME, Johnson SM, Sladky KK. Behavioral evaluation of red-eared slider turtles (*Trachemys scripta elegans*) administered either morphine or butorphanol following unilateral gonadectomy. *J Herp Med Surg*. 2011;21:54–62.
238. Kirchgessner M, Mitchell MA. Chelonians. In: Mitchell MA, Tully TN Jr., eds. *Manual of Exotic Pet Practice*. St. Louis, MO: Saunders/Elsevier; 2009:207–249.
239. Kirchgessner M, Mitchell M, Domenzain L, et al. Evaluating the effect of leuprolide acetate on testosterone levels in captive male green iguanas (*Iguana iguana*). *J Herpetol Med Surg*. 2009;19:128–131.
240. Kischinovsky M, Duse A, Wang T, et al. Intramuscular administration of alfaxalone in red-eared slider turtles (*Trachemys scripta elegans*) - effects of dose and body temperature. *Vet Anaesth Analg*. 2013;40:13–20.
241. Klaphake E. A fresh look at metabolic bone diseases in reptiles and amphibians. *Vet Clin North Am Exot Anim Pract*. 2010;13:375–392.
242. Klaphake E. Personal observation; 2016.
243. Klaphake E, Gibbons PM, Sladky KK, et al. Reptiles. In: Carpenter JW, ed. *Exotic Animal Formulary*. 5th ed. St. Louis, MO: Elsevier; 2018:81–166.

244. Klingenberg RJ. A comparison of fenbendazole and ivermectin for the treatment of nematode parasites in ball pythons, *Python regius. Bull Assoc Rept Amph Vet.* 1992;2:5–6.
245. Klingenberg RJ. Management of the anorectic ball python. *Proc North Am Vet Conf.* 1996:830.
246. Klingenberg RJ. *Understanding Reptile Parasites.* Irvine, CA: Advanced Vivarium Systems; 2007:1–200.
247. Knafo SE, Divers SJ, Rivera S, et al. Sterilisation of hybrid Galapagos tortoises (*Geochelone nigra*) for island restoration. Part 1: endoscopic oophorectomy of females under ketamine-medetomidine anaesthesia. *Vet Rec.* 2011;168:78–82.
248. Knotek Z. Alfaxalone as an induction agent for anaesthesia in terrapins and tortoises. *Vet Rec.* 2014;175:327–329.
249. Knotkova Z, Doubek J, Knotek Z, et al. Blood cell morphology and plasma biochemistry in Russian tortoises (*Agrionemys horsfieldi*). *Acta Vet Brno.* 2002;71:191–198.
250. Koelle P. Urinalysis in tortoises. *Proc Annu Conf Assoc Rept Amph Vet.* 2000:111–113.
251. Koelle P. Efficacy of allopurinol in European tortoises with hyperuricemia. *Proc Annu Conf Assoc Rept Amph Vet.* 2001:185–186.
252. Koelle P, Hoffmann R. Urinalysis in European tortoises - part II. *Proc Annu Conf Assoc Rept Amph Vet.* 2002:117.
253. Kojimoto A, Uchida K, Horii Y, et al. Amebiasis in four ball pythons, *Python regius. J Vet Med Sci.* 2001;63(12):1365–1368.
254. Kolmstetter CM, Cox S, Ramsay EC. Pharmacokinetics of metronidazole in the yellow rat snake, *Elaphe obsoleta quadrivitatta. J Herpetol Med Surg.* 2001;11(2):4–8.
255. Kolmstetter CM, Frazier D, Cox S, et al. Pharmacokinetics of metronidazole in the green iguana, *Iguana iguana. Bull Assoc Rept Amph Vet.* 1998;8:4–7.
256. Konda ME. The therapeutic effects of mebendazole and piperazine on certain helminth parasites of the garden lizard, *Calotes versicolor. Int J Parasitol.* 1992;22:843–845.
257. Lai OR, Di Bello A, Soloperto S, et al. Pharmacokinetic behavior of meloxicam in loggerhead sea turtles (*Caretta caretta*) after intramuscular and intravenous administration. *J Wildl Dis.* 2015;51:509–512.
258. Lai OR, Marín P, Laricchiuta P, et al. Pharmacokinetics of marbofloxacin in loggerhead sea turtles (*Caretta caretta*) after single intravenous and intramuscular doses. *J Zoo Wildl Med.* 2009;40:501–507.
259. Lai OR, Marín P, Laricchiuta P, et al. Pharmacokinetics of injectable marbofloxacin after intravenous and intramuscular administration in red-eared sliders (*Trachemys scripta elegans*). *J Vet Pharmacol Ther.* 2020;43:129–134.
260. Lane T. Crocodilians. In: Mader DR, ed. *Reptile Medicine and Surgery.* 2nd ed. St. Louis, MO: Saunders Elsevier; 2006:100–117.
261. Lanza A, Baldi A, Spugnini EP. Surgery and electrochemotherapy for the treatment of cutaneous squamous cell carcinoma in a yellow-bellied slider (*Trachemys scripta scripta*). *J Am Vet Med Assoc.* 2015;246:455–457.
262. Larouche CB, Beaufrère H, Mosley C, et al. Evaluation of the effects of midazolam and flumazenil in the ball python (*Python regius*). *J Zoo Wildl Med.* 2019;50:579–588.
263. Larouche CB, Mosley C, Beaufrère H, et al. Effects of midazolam and nitrous oxide on the minimum anesthetic concentration of isoflurane in the ball python (*Python regius*). *Vet Anaesth Analg.* 2019;46:807–814.
264. Latney LV, McDermott C, Scott G, et al. Surgical management of maxillary and premaxillary osteomyelitis in a reticulated python (*Python reticulatus*). *J Am Vet Med Assoc.* 2016;248(9):1027–1033.
265. Lawrence K, Muggleton PW, Needham JR. Preliminary study on the use of ceftazidime, a broad spectrum cephalosporin antibiotic, in snakes. *Res Vet Sci.* 1984;36:16–20.
266. Lawrence K, Palmer GH, Needham JR. Use of carbenicillin in 2 species of tortoise (*Testudo graeca* and *Testudo hermanni*). *Res Vet Sci.* 1986;40:413–415.
267. Lawrence K, Needham JR, Palmer GH, et al. A preliminary study on the use of carbenicillin in snakes. *J Vet Pharmacol Therapeut.* 1984;7:119–124.

268. Lawton MPC. Anaesthesia. In: Benyon PH, Lawton MPC, Cooper JE, eds. *Manual of Reptiles*. Ames, IA: Iowa State University Press; 1992:170–183.
269. Lawton MPC. Pain management after surgery. *Proc North Am Vet Conf.* 1999:782.
270. Leal WP, Carregaro AB, Bressan TF, et al. Antinociceptive efficacy of intramuscular administration of morphine sulfate and butorphanol tartrate in tegus (*Salvator merianae*). *Am J Vet Res.* 2016;78:1019–1024.
271. Lindemann DM, Allender MC, Rzadkowska M, et al. Pharmacokinetics, efficacy, and safety of voriconazole and itraconazole in healthy cottonmouths (*Agkistrodon piscivorus*) and massasauga rattlesnakes (*Sistrurus catenatus*) with snake fungal disease. *J Zoo Wild Med.* 2017;48:757–766.
272. Lloyd ML. Crocodilia. In: Fowler ME, Miller RE, eds. *Zoo and Wild Animal Medicine*. 5th ed. Philadelphia, PA: Elsevier Saunders; 2003:59–70.
273. Lloyd ML. Crocodilian anesthesia. In: Fowler ME, Miller RE, eds. *Zoo & Wild Animal Medicine: Current Therapy 4*. Philadelphia, PA: WB Saunders; 1999:205–216.
274. Lloyd ML. Reptilian dystocias review - causes, prevention, management, and comments on the synthetic hormone vasotocin. *Proc Annu Conf Am Assoc Zoo Vet.* 1990:290–296.
275. Lloyd ML, Reichard T, Odum RA. Gallamine reversal in Cuban crocodiles (*Crocodilus rhombifer*) using neostigmine alone vs. neostigmine with hyaluronidase. *Proc Annu Conf Assoc Rept Amph Vet.* 1994:117–120.
276. Lock BA, Heard DJ, Dennis P. Preliminary evaluation of medetomidine/ketamine combinations for immobilization and reversal with atipamezole in three tortoise species. *Bull Assoc Rept Amph Vet.* 1998;8:6–9.
277. López J, Waters M, Routh A, et al. Hematology and plasma chemistry of the ploughshare tortoise (*Astrochelys yniphora*) in a captive breeding program. *J Zoo Wildl Med.* 2017;48(1):102–115.
278. Luppi M, Costa M, Malta M, et al. Treatment of *Rhabdias labiata* with levamisole and ivermectin in boa constrictor (*Boa constrictor amarali*). *Veterinaria Noticias.* 2007;13:61–65.
279. Machado CC, Silva LFN, Ramos PRR, et al. Seasonal influence on hematologic values and hemoglobin electrophoresis in Brazilian *Boa constrictor amarali*. *J Zoo Wildl Med.* 2006;37:487–491.
280. MacLean RA, Harms CA, Braun-McNeill J. Propofol anesthesia in loggerhead (*Caretta caretta*) sea turtles. *J Wildl Dis.* 2008;44:143–150.
281. Mader DR. IME - Use of calcitonin in green iguanas, *Iguana iguana*, with metabolic bone disease. *Bull Assoc Rept Amph Vet.* 1993;3:5.
282. Mader DR. Gout. In: Mader DR, ed. *Reptile Medicine and Surgery*. Philadelphia, PA: WB Saunders; 1996:374–379.
283. Mader DR. Understanding local analgesics: practical use in the green iguana, *Iguana iguana*. *Proc Annu Conf Assoc Rept Amph Vet.* 1998:143–147.
284. Mader DR. Metabolic bone diseases. In: Mader DR, ed. *Reptile Medicine and Surgery*. 2nd ed. St. Louis, MO: Saunders/Elsevier; 2006:841–851.
285. Mader DR. Thermal burns. In: Mader DR, ed. *Reptile Medicine and Surgery*. 2nd ed. St. Louis, MO: Saunders/Elsevier; 2006:916–923.
286. Mader DR, Conzelman GM, Baggot JD. Effects of ambient temperature on half life and dosage regimen of amikacin in the gopher snake. *J Am Vet Med Assoc.* 1985;187:1134–1136.
287. Mader DR, Horvath CC, Paul-Murphy J. The hematocrit and serum profile of the gopher snake (*Pituophis melanoleucas catenifer*). *J Zoo Anim Med.* 1985;16:139–140.
288. Makau CM, Towett PK, Abelson KSP, et al. Modulation of nociception by amitriptyline hydrochloride in the Speke's hinge-back tortoise (*Kiniskys spekii*). *Vet Med Sci.* 2021;7:1034–1041.
289. Mallo KM, Harms CA, Lewbart GA, et al. Pharmacokinetics of fluconazole in loggerhead sea turtles (*Caretta caretta*) after single intravenous and subcutaneous injections, and multiple subcutaneous injections. *J Zoo Wildl Med.* 2002;33:29–35.
290. Manire CA, Anderson ET, Byrd L, et al. Dehydration as an effective treatment for brevetoxicosis in loggerhead sea turtles (*Caretta caretta*). *J Zoo Wildl Med.* 2013;44:447–452.

291. Manire CA, Hunter RP, Koch DE, et al. Pharmacokinetics of ticarcillin in the loggerhead sea turtle (*Caretta caretta*) after single intravenous and intramuscular injections. *J Zoo Wildl Med.* 2005;36:44–53.
292. Manire CA, Rhinehart HL, Pennick GJ, et al. Steady-state plasma concentrations of itraconazole after oral administration in Kemp's ridley sea turtles, *Lepidochelys kempi. J Zoo Wildl Med.* 2003;34:171–178.
293. Mans C. Clinical update on diagnosis and management of disorders of the digestive system of reptiles. *J Exot Pet Med.* 2013;22:141–162.
294. Mans C. Clinical technique: intrathecal drug administration in turtles and tortoises. *J Exot Pet Med.* 2014;23:67–70.
295. Mans C. Sedation of pet birds. *J Exot Pet Med.* 2014;23:152–157.
296. Mans C, Braun J. Update on common nutritional disorders of captive reptiles. *Vet Clin North Am Exot Anim Pract.* 2014;17:369–395.
297. Mans C, Foster JD. Endoscopy-guided ectopic egg removal from the urinary bladder in a leopard tortoise (*Stigmochelys pardalis*). *Can Vet J.* 2014;58:569–572.
298. Mans C, Sladky KK. Endoscopically guided removal of cloacal calculi in three African spurred tortoises (*Geochelone sulcate*). *J Am Vet Med Assoc.* 2012;240:869–875.
299. Mans C, Drees R, Sladky KK, et al. Effects of body position and extension of the neck and extremities on lung volume measured via computed tomography in red-eared slider turtles (*Trachemys scripta elegans*). *J Am Vet Med Assoc.* 2013;243:1190–1196.
300. Mans C, Lahner LL, Baker BB, et al. Antinociceptive efficacy of buprenorphine and hydromorphone in red-eared slider turtles (*Trachemys scripta elegans*). *J Zoo Wildl Med.* 2012;43:662–665.
301. Mans C, Sladky KK, Schumacher J. General anesthesia. In: Divers SJ, Stahl SJ, eds. *Mader's Reptile and Amphibian Medicine and Surgery.* 3rd ed. St. Louis, MO: Elsevier; 2019:447–464.
302. Marin P, Bayon A, Fernandez-Varon E, et al. Pharmacokinetics of danofloxacin after single dose intravenous, intramuscular, and subcutaneous administration to loggerhead turtles *Caretta caretta. Dis Aquat Organ.* 2008;82:231–236.
303. Marín P, Lai OR, Laricchiuta P, et al. Pharmacokinetics of marbofloxacin after a single oral dose to loggerhead sea turtles (*Caretta caretta*). *Res Vet Sci.* 2009;87:284–286.
304. Marks SK, Citino SB. Hematology and serum chemistry of the radiated tortoise (*Testudo radiata*). *J Zoo Wildl Med.* 1990;21:342–344.
305. Martel A, Hellebuyck T, Van Waeyenberghe L. Treatment of infections with *Nannizziopsis vriesii*, an emergent reptilian dermatophyte. *Proc Annu Conf Assoc Rept Amph Vet.* 2009:69–70.
306. Martelli P, Lai OR, Krishnasamy K, et al. Pharmacokinetic behavior of enrofloxacin in estuarine crocodile (*Crocodylus porosus*) after single intravenous, intramuscular, and oral doses. *J Zoo Wildl Med.* 2009;40:696–704.
307. Martinez-Jimenez D, Hernandez-Divers SJ. Emergency care of reptiles. *Vet Clin North Am Exot Anim Pract.* 2007;10:557–585.
308. Mathes KA, Holz A, Fehr M. Blood reference values of terrestrial tortoises (*Testudo* spp.) kept in Germany. *Tierarztl Prax Ausg K Klientiere Heimtiere.* 2006;34:268–274.
309. Matt CL, Nagamori Y, Stayton E, et al. *Kalicephalus* hookworm infection in four corn snakes (*Pantherophis guttatus*). *J Exot Pet Med.* 2020;34:62–66.
310. Mauldin GN, Done LB. Oncology. In: Mader DR, ed. *Reptile Medicine and Surgery.* 2nd ed. St. Louis, MO: Saunders/Elsevier; 2006:299–322.
311. Mautino M, Page CD. Biology and medicine of turtles and tortoises. *Vet Clin North Am Small Anim Pract.* 1993;23:1251–1270.
312. Maxwell LK, Jacobson ER. Preliminary single-dose pharmacokinetics of enrofloxacin after oral and intramuscular administration in green iguanas (*Iguana iguana*). *Proc Annu Conf Am Assoc Zoo Vet.* 1997;25.
313. Mayer J. Characterizing the hematologic and plasma chemistry profiles of captive Chinese water dragons, *Physignathus cocincinus. J Herpetol Med Surg.* 2005;15:45–52.

314. Mayer J, Knoll J, Wrubel KM, et al. Characterizing the hematologic and plasma chemistry profiles of captive crested geckos (*Rhacodactylus ciliatus*). *J Herpetol Med Surg.* 2011;21:68–75.
315. McArthur S. Problem solving approach to common diseases of terrestrial and semi-aquatic chelonians. In: McArthur S, Wilkinson R, Meyer J, eds. *Medicine and Surgery of Tortoises and Turtles*. Oxford, UK: Blackwell Publishing; 2004:309–377.
316. McArthur SDJ, Wilkinson RJ, Barrows MG. Tortoises and turtles. In: Meredith A, Redrobe S, eds. *BSAVA Manual of Exotic Pets*. 4th ed. Gloucestershire, GB: British Small Animal Veterinary Association; 2002:208–222.
317. McBride M, Hernandez-Divers SJ, Koch T, et al. Preliminary evaluation of pre- and postprandial 3[alpha]-hydroxy bile acids in the green iguana, *Iguana iguana*. *J Herpetol Med Surg*. 2006;16:129–134.
318. McBride MP, Wojick KB, Georoff TA, et al. *Ophidiomyces ophiodiicola* dermatitis in eight free-ranging timber rattlesnakes (*Crotalus horridus*) from Massachusetts. *J Zoo Wildl Med.* 2015;46:86–94.
319. McEntire MS, Reinhart JM, Allender MC, et al. Antifungal susceptibility patterns of *Nannizziopsis guarroi* and the single-dose pharmacokinetics of orally administered terbinafine in the bearded dragon (*Pogona vitticeps*). *Proc Annu Conf Am Assoc Zoo Vet.* 2020:25.
320. McFadden MS, Bennett RA, Reavill DR, et al. Clinical and histologic effects of intracardiac administration of propofol for induction of anesthesia in ball pythons (*Python regius*). *J Am Assoc Vet Med.* 2011;239:803–807.
321. McGuire JL, Hernandez SM, Smith LL, et al. Safety and utility of an anesthetic protocol for the collection of biological samples from gopher tortoises. *Wildl Soc Bull.* 2014;38:43–50.
322. Mehlhorn H, Schmahl G, Mevissen I. Efficacy of a combination of imidacloprid and moxidectin against parasites of reptiles and rodents: case reports. *Parasitol Res.* 2005;97(Suppl 1):S97–S101.
323. Mehlhorn H, Schmahl G, Frese M, et al. Effects of a combinations of emodepside and praziquantel on parasites of reptiles and rodents. *Parasitol Res.* 2005;97(Suppl 1):S65–S69.
324. Messonnier S. Formulary for exotic pets. *Vet Forum.* 1996;Aug:46–49.
325. Meyer J. Gastrographin as a gastrointestinal contrast agent in the Greek tortoise (*Testudo hermanni*). *J Zoo Wildl Med.* 1998;29:183–189.
326. Miller HA, Brandt PJ, Frye FL, et al. *Trichomonas* associated with ocular and subcutaneous lesions in geckos. *Proc Annu Conf Assoc Rept Amph Vet.* 1994:102–107.
327. Miller LJ, Fetterer DP, Garza NL, et al. A fixed moderate-dose combination of tiletamine+zolazepam outperforms midazolam in induction of short-term immobilization of ball pythons (*Python regius*). *PLoS ONE.* 2018;13:1–15.
328. Millichamp NJ. Surgical techniques in reptiles. In: Jacobson ER, Kollias GV Jr., eds. *Exotic Animals*. New York, NY: Churchill Livingstone; 1988:49–74.
329. Millichamp NJ. Ophthalmology. In: Girling SJ, Raiti P, eds. *BSAVA Manual of Reptiles*. 2nd ed. Quedgeley, UK: British Small Animal Veterinary Association; 2004:199–209.
330. Mitchell M. Ophidia. In: Fowler ME, Miller RE, eds. *Zoo and Wild Animal Medicine*. 5th ed. Philadelphia, PA: Saunders/Elsevier; 2003:82–91.
331. Mitchell MA. Therapeutics. In: Mader DR, ed. *Reptile Medicine and Surgery*. 2nd ed. St. Louis, MO: Saunders/Elsevier; 2006:631–664.
332. Mitchell MA. Managing the reptile patient in the veterinary hospital: establishing a standards of care model for nontraditional species. *J Exot Pet Med.* 2010;19:56–72.
333. Montali RJ, Bush M, Smeller JM. Pathology of nephrotoxicity of gentamicin in snakes - model for reptilian gout. *Vet Pathol.* 1979;16:108–115.
334. Monticelli P, Ronaldson HL, Hutchinson JR, et al. Medetomidine-ketamine-sevoflurane anaesthesia in juvenile Nile crocodiles (*Crocodylus niloticus*). *Vet Anaesth Analg.* 2019;46:84–89.
335. Morgan-Davies AM. Immobilization of the Nile crocodile (*Crocodilus niloticus*) with gallamine triethiodide. *J Zoo Anim Med.* 1980;11:85–87.

336. Morici M, DiGiuseppe M, Spadola F, et al. Intravenous alfaxalone anaesthesia in leopard geckos (*Eublepharis macularius*). *J Exot Pet Med.* 2018;27:11–14.
337. Morici M, Interlandi C, Costa GL, et al. Sedation with intracloacal administration of dexmedetomidine and ketamine in yellow-bellied sliders (*Trachemys scripta scripta*). *J Exot Pet Med.* 2017;26:188–191.
338. Morici M, Lubian E, Costa GL, et al. Difference between cranial and caudal intravenous alfaxalone administration in yellow-bellied sliders (*Trachemys scripta scripta*). *Acta Vet Eurasia.* 2021;47:88–92.
339. Naldo JL, Libanan NL, Samour JH. Health assessment of a spiny-tailed lizard (*Uromastyx* spp.) population in Abu Dhabi, United Arab Emirates. *J Zoo Wildl Med.* 2009;40:445–452.
340. Naples LM, Langan JN, Mylniczenko ND, et al. Islet cell tumor in a Savannah monitor (*Varanus exanthematicus*). *J Herpetol Med Surg.* 2009;19:97–105.
341. Nardini G, Barbarossa A, Dall'Occo A, et al. Pharmacokinetics of cefovecin sodium after subcutaneous administration to Hermann's tortoises (*Testudo hermanni*). *Am J Vet Res.* 2014;75:918–923.
342. Nardini G, Di Girolamo N, Leopardi S, et al. Evaluation of liver parenchyma and perfusion using dynamic contrast-enhanced computed tomography and contrast-enhanced ultrasonography in captive green iguanas (*Iguana iguana*) under general anesthesia. *BMC Vet Res.* 2014;10:112–120.
343. Nathan R. Treatment with ovicentesis, prostaglandin E2 then prostaglandin F2á to aid oviposition in a spotted python, *Antaresia maculosa. Bull Assoc Rept Amph Vet.* 1996;6:4.
344. Necas P. *Chameleons, Nature's Hidden Jewels.* Malabar, FL: Krieger Publishing; 1999:113–119.
345. Neiffer DL, Lydick D, Burks K, et al. Hematologic and plasma biochemical changes associated with fenbendazole administration in Hermann's tortoises (*Testudo hermanni*). *J Zoo Wildl Med.* 2005;36:661–672.
346. Nevarez JG, Mitchell MA, Le Blanc C, et al. Determination of plasma biochemistries, ionized calcium, vitamin D_3, and hematocrit values in captive green iguanas (*Iguana iguana*) from El Salvador. *Proc Annu Conf Assoc Rept Amph Vet.* 2002:87–91.
347. Nichols DK, Lamirande EW. Use of methohexital sodium as an anesthetic in two species of colubrid snakes. *Proc Joint Conf Am Assoc Zoo Vet/Assoc Rept Amph Vet.* 1994:161–162.
348. Norton TM. Chelonian emergency and critical care. *Semin Avian Exot Pet Med.* 2005;14:106–130.
349. Norton TM, Clauss T, Sommer R, et al. Pharmacokinetic behavior of meloxicam in loggerhead (*Caretta caretta*), Kemp's ridley (*Lepidochelys kempii*), and green (*Chelonia mydas*) sea turtles after subcutaneous administration. *J Zoo Wildl Med.* 2021;52(1):295–299.
350. Norton TM, Cox S, Nelson SE, et al. Pharmacokinetics of tramadol and O-desmethyltramadol in loggerhead sea turtles (*Caretta caretta*). *J Zoo Wildl Med.* 2015;46:262–265.
351. Norton TM, Jacobson ER, Caligiuri R, et al. Medical management of a Galapagos tortoise (*Geochelone elephantopus*) with hypothyroidism. *J Zoo Wildl Med.* 1989;20:212–216.
352. Norton TM, Spratt J, Behler J, et al. Medetomidine and ketamine anesthesia with atipamezole reversal in free-ranging gopher tortoises, Gopherus polyphemus. *Proc Annu Conf Assoc Rept Amph Vet.* 1998:25–27.
353. Odette O, Churgin SM, Sladky KK, et al. Anesthetic induction and recovery parameters in bearded dragons (*Pogona vitticeps*): comparison of isoflurane delivered in 100% oxygen versus 21% oxygen. *J Zoo Wildl Med.* 2015;46:534–539.
354. Olesen MG, Bertelsen MF, Perry SF, et al. Effects of preoperative administration of butorphanol or meloxicam on physiologic responses to surgery in ball pythons. *J Am Vet Med Assoc.* 2008;233:1883–1888.
355. Olsson A, Phalen D. Medetomidine immobilization and atipamazole reversal in large estuarine crocodiles (*Crocodylus porosus*) using metabolically scaled dosages. *Aust Vet J.* 2012;90:240–244.

356. Olsson A, Phalen D. Preliminary studies of chemical immobilization of captive juvenile estuarine (*Crocodylus porosus*) and Australian freshwater crocodiles (*Crocodylus johnstoni*) with medetomidine and reversal with atipamazole. *Vet Anaesth Analg.* 2012;39:345–356.
357. Olsson A, Phalen D, Dart C. Preliminary studies of alfaxalone for intravenous immobilization of juvenile captive estuarine crocodiles (*Crocodylus porosus*) and Australian freshwater crocodiles (*Crocodylus johnstoni*) at optimal and selected suboptimal thermal zones. *Vet Anaesth Analg.* 2013;40:494–502.
358. Oonincx DGAB, Stevens Y, van den Borne JJGC, et al. Effects of vitamin D-3 supplementation and UVB exposure on the growth and plasma concentration of vitamin D-3 metabolites in juvenile bearded dragons (*Pogona vitticeps*). *Comp Biochem Physiol B Biochem Mol Biol.* 2010;156:122–128.
359. Oppenheim YC, Moon PF. Sedative effects of midazolam in red-eared sliders (*Trachemys scripta elegans*). *J Zoo Wildl Med.* 1995;26:409–413.
360. Origgi FC. Testudinid herpesviruses: a review. *J Herp Med Surg.* 2012;22:42–54.
361. O'Shea R, Ball RL. Use of bovine tendon collagen for wound repair in *Varanus komodoensis*. *Proc Annu Conf Assoc Rept Amph Vet.* 2010:66–69.
362. Page CD. Current reptilian anesthesia procedures. In: Fowler ME, ed. *Zoo & Wild Animal Medicine: Current Therapy 3*. Philadelphia, PA: WB Saunders; 1993:140–143.
363. Page CD, Mautino M, Derendorf H, et al. Multiple dose pharmacokinetics of ketoconazole administered orally to gopher tortoises (*Gopherus polyphemus*). *J Zoo Wildl Med.* 1991;22:191–198.
364. Paré JA, Crawshaw GJ, Barta JR. Treatment of cryptosporidiosis in Gila monsters (*Heloderma suspectum*) with paromomycin. *Proc Annu Conf Assoc Rept Amph Vet.* 1997;23.
365. Patson C, Doss G. Mans C. Evaluation of tiletamine-zolazepam sedation in inland bearded dragons (*Pogona vitticeps*) following intramuscular and subcutaneous administration. *J Herp Med Surg.* 2021;31(3):204–210.
366. Perrin KL, Bertelsen MF. Intravenous alfaxalone and propofol anesthesia in the bearded dragon (*Pogona vitticeps*). *J Herp Med Surg.* 2017:123–126.
367. Petersen NT. Terbutaline. *J Exot Pet Med.* 2012;21:260–263.
368. Petritz O, Son TT. Emergency and critical care. In: Divers SJ, Stahl SJ, eds. *Mader's Reptile and Amphibian Medicine and Surgery*. 3rd ed. St. Louis, MO: Elsevier; 2019:967–976.
369. Phillips BE, Posner LP, Lewbart GA, et al. Effects of alfaxalone administered intravenously to healthy yearling loggerhead sea turtles (*Caretta caretta*) at three different doses. *J Am Vet Med Assoc.* 2017;250:909–917.
370. Plumb DC. Probenecid. In: *Plumb's Veterinary Drug Handbook*. 8th ed. Ames, IA: Wiley-Blackwell; 2015:1214–1216.
371. Poapolathep S, Giorgi M, Chaiyabutr N, et al. Pharmacokinetics of ceftriaxone in freshwater crocodiles (*Crocodylus siamensis*) after intramuscular administration at two dosages. *J Vet Pharmacol Ther.* 2020;43(2):141–146.
372. Poapolathep S, Giorgi M, Chaiyabutr N, et al. Pharmacokinetics of enrofloxacin and its metabolite ciprofloxacin in freshwater crocodiles (*Crocodylus siamensis*) after intravenous and intramuscular administration. *J Vet Pharmacol Ther.* 2020;43:19–25.
373. Poapolathep S, Giorgi M, Hantrakul S, et al. Pharmacokinetics of marbofloxacin in freshwater crocodiles (*Crocodylus siamensis*) after intravenous and intramuscular administration. *J Vet Pharmacol Ther.* 2017;40:57–61.
374. Poapolathep S, Giorgi M, Klangkaew N, et al. Pharmacokinetic profiles of amoxicillin trihydrate in freshwater crocodiles (*Crocodylus siamensis*) after intramuscular administration at two doses. *J Vet Pharmacol Ther.* 2020;43(4):307–312.
375. Preston DL, Mosley CAE, Mason RT. Sources of variability in recovery time from methohexital sodium anesthesia in snakes. *Copeia.* 2010;3:496–501.
376. Prezant RM, Isaza R, Jacobson ER. Plasma concentrations and disposition kinetics of enrofloxacin in gopher tortoises (*Gopherus polyphemus*). *J Zoo Wildl Med.* 1994;25:82–87.

377. Proneca LM, Fowler S, Kleine S, et al. Coelioscopic-assisted sterilization of female Mojave desert tortoises (*Gopherus agassizii*). *J Herp Med Surg*. 2014;24:95–100.
378. Proneca LM, Fowler S, Kleine S, et al. Single surgeon coelioscopic orchiectomy of desert tortoises (*Gopherus agassizii*) for population management. *Vet Rec*. 2014;175:404–409.
379. Pye GW, Carpenter JW. Ketamine sedation followed by propofol anesthesia in a slider, *Trachemys scripta*, to facilitate removal of an esophageal foreign body. *Bull Assoc Rept Amph Vet*. 1998;8:16–17.
380. Quesada RJ, Aitken-Palmer C, Conley K, et al. Accidental submeningeal injection of propofol in gopher tortoises (*Gopherus polyphemus*). *Vet Rec*. 2010;167:494–495.
381. Raiti P. Veterinary care of the common kingsnake, *Lampropeltis getula*. *Bull Assoc Rept Amph Vet*. 1995;5:11–18.
382. Raiti P. Administration of aerosolized antibiotics in reptiles. *Exot DVM*. 2002;4(3):87–90.
383. Raj R, Mukherjee P, Chaudhuri S, et al. Surgical removal of necrosed venom gland in Indian spectacled cobra (*Naja naja*)- a case report. *Bull UASVM Vet Med*. 2017;74:126–128.
384. Ramsay EC, Dotson TK. Tissue and serum enzyme activities in the yellow rat snake (*Elaphe obsoleta quadrivitatta*). *Am J Vet Res*. 1995;56:423–428.
385. Raphael B, Clark CH, Hudson Jr R. Plasma concentration of gentamicin in turtles. *J Zoo Anim Med*. 1985;16:136–139.
386. Raphael BL. Chelonians. In: Fowler ME, Miller RE, eds. *Zoo and Wild Animal Medicine*. 5th ed. Philadelphia, PA: Saunders/Elsevier; 2003:48–58.
387. Raphael BL, Papich M, Cook RA. Pharmacokinetics of enrofloxacin after a single intramuscular injection in Indian star tortoises (*Geochelone elegans*). *J Zoo Wildl Med*. 1994;25:88–94.
388. Rasys AM, Divers SJ, Lauderdale JD, et al. A systematic study of injectable anesthetic agents in the brown anole lizard (*Anolis sagrei*). *Lab Anim*. 2020;54:281–292.
389. Redrobe S, MacDonald J. Sample collection and clinical pathology of reptiles. *Vet Clin North Am Exot Anim Pract*. 1999;2:709–730.
390. Reptile Care Sheets. Reptiles Magazine. https://www.reptilesmagazine.com/care-sheets. Accessed December 13, 2020.
391. Rettenmund CL, Boyer DM, Orrico WJ, et al. Long-term oral clarithromycin administration in chelonians with subclinical *Mycoplasma* spp. infection. *J Herp Med Surg*. 2017;27:58–61.
392. Rivas AE, Boyer DM, Torregrosa K, et al. Treatment of *Cryptosporidium serpentis* infection in a king cobra (*Ophiophagus hannah*) with paromomycin. *J Zoo Wildl Med*. 2018; 49(4):1061–1063.
393. Rivera S. Health assessment of the reptilian reproductive tract. *J Exot Pet Med*. 2008; 17:259–266.
394. Rivera S, Divers SJ, Knafo SE, et al. Sterilisation of hybrid Galapagos tortoises (*Geochelone nigra*) for island restoration. Part 2: phallectomy of males under intrathecal anaesthesia with lidocaine. *Vet Rec*. 2011;168:78–81.
395. Rockwell K, Mitchell MM. Antiinflammatory therapy. In: Divers SJ, Stahl SJ, eds. *Mader's Reptile and Amphibian Medicine and Surgery*. 3rd ed. St. Louis, MO: Elsevier; 2019:1162–1164.
396. Rockwell K, Mitchell MM. Antiparasitic therapy. In: Divers SJ, Stahl SJ, eds. *Mader's Reptile and Amphibian Medicine and Surgery*. 3rd ed. St. Louis, MO: Elsevier; 2019:1165–1170.
397. Rockwell K, Boykin K, Padlo J, et al. Evaluating the efficacy of alfaxalone in corn snakes (*Pantherophis guttatus*). *Vet Anaesth Analg*. 2021;48(3):364–371.
398. Rojo-Solís C, Ros-Rodriguez JM, Valls M. Pharmakokinetics of meloxicam (Metacam) after intravenous, intramuscular, and oral administration in red-eared slider turtles (*Trachemys scripta elegans*). *Proc Joint Conf Am Assoc Zoo Vet/Am Assoc Wildl Vet*. 2009:228.
399. Rooney MB, Levine G, Gaynor J, et al. Sevoflurane anesthesia in desert tortoises (*Gopherus agassizii*). *J Zoo Wildl Med*. 1999;30:64–69.
400. Rooney TA, Eshar D, Gardhouse S, et al. Evaluation of dexmedetomidine-midazolam-ketamine combination administered intramuscularly in captive ornate box turtles (*Terrapene ornata ornata*). *Vet Anaesth Analg*. 2021 online 13 August 2021.

401. Rosenthal K. Chemotherapeutic treatment of a sarcoma in a corn snake. *Proc Joint Conf Am Assoc Zoo Vet/Assoc Rept Amph Vet.* 1994;46.
402. Rossi J. Practical reptile dermatology. *Proc North Am Vet Conf.* 1995:648–649.
403. Rossi JV. Emergency medicine of reptiles. *Proc North Am Vet Conf.* 1998:799–801.
404. Rowland MN. Use of a deslorelin implant to control aggression in a male bearded dragon (*Pogona vitticeps*). *Vet Rec.* 2011;169:127.
405. Ruiz T, Campos WNS, Peres TPS, et al. Intraocular pressure, ultrasonographic and echobiometric findings of juvenile Yacare caiman (*Caiman yacare*) eye. *Vet Ophthalmol.* 2015;18:40–45.
406. Sadar M, Ambros B. Use of alfaxalone or midazolam-dexmedetomidine-ketamine for implantation of radiotransmitters in bullsnakes (*Pituophis catenifer sayi*). *J Herp Med Surg.* 2018;28:93–98.
407. Sadar MJ, Hawkins MG, Taylor IT, et al. Pharmacokinetics of ceftiofur crystalline free acid sterile suspension in green iguanas (*Iguana iguana*) after single intramuscular administration. *J Zoo Wildl Med.* 2018;49:86–91.
408. Salvadori M, DeVito V, Owen H, et al. Pharmacokinetics of enrofloxacin and its metabolite ciprofloxacin after intracoelomic administration in tortoises (*Testudo hermanni*). *Israel J Vet Med.* 2015;70:45–48.
409. Salvadori M, Vercelli C, De Vito V, et al. Pharmacokinetic and pharmacodynamic evaluations of a 10 mg/kg enrofloxacin intramuscular administration in bearded dragons (*Pogona vitticeps*): a preliminary assessment. *J Vet Pharm Ther.* 2017;40:62–69.
410. Sanches L. Anestesia espinhal no lagarto *Iguana iguana* (Linnaeus, 1758). [Master's dissertation]. http://hdl.handle.net/11449/1157077,2014.
411. Scheelings TF, Gatto C, Reina RD. Anaesthesia of hatchling green sea turtles (*Chelonia mydas*) with intramuscular ketamine-medetomidine-tramadol. *Aust Vet J.* 2020;98:511–516.
412. Scheelings TF, Dobson EC, Hooper C, et al. Cutaneous and systemic mycoses from infection with *Lecanicillium* spp. in captive Guthega skinks (*Liopholis guthega*). *Aust Vet J.* 2015;93:248–251.
413. Scheelings TF, Holz P, Haynes L, et al. A preliminary study of the chemical restraint of selected squamate reptiles with alfaxalone. *Proc Annu Conf Assoc Rept Amph Vet.* 2010:114–115.
414. Schillinger L, Girling S. Cardiology. In: Divers SJ, Stahl SJ, eds. *Mader's Reptile and Amphibian Medicine and Surgery.* 3rd ed. St. Louis, MO: Elsevier; 2019:669–698.
415. Schilliger L, Betremieux O, Rochet J, et al. Absorption and efficacy of a spot-on combination containing emodepside plus praziquantel in reptiles. *Rev Med Vet (Toulouse).* 2009;160:557–561.
416. Schnellbacher R. Butorphanol. *J Exot Pet Med.* 2010;19:192–195.
417. Schobert E. Telazol use in wild and exotic animals. *Vet Med.* 1987;82:1080–1088.
418. Schroeder CA, Johnson RA. The efficacy of intracoelomic fospropofol in red-eared sliders (*Trachemys scripta elegans*). *J Zoo Wildl Med.* 2013;44:941–950.
419. Schumacher J. Lacertilia. In: Fowler ME, Miller RE, eds. *Zoo and Wild Animal Medicine.* 5th ed. Philadelphia, PA: Saunders/Elsevier; 2003:73–81.
420. Schumacher J, Yelen T. Anesthesia and analgesia. In: Mader DR, ed. *Reptile Medicine and Surgery.* 2nd ed. St. Louis, MO: Saunders/Elsevier; 2006:442–452.
421. Schuster EJ, Strueve J, Fehr MJ, et al. Measurement of intraocular pressure in healthy unanesthetized inland bearded dragons (*Pogona vitticeps*). *Am J Vet Res.* 2015;76:494–499.
422. Schuszler L, Popovic D, Zaha C, et al. Observations on xylazine-ketamine-isoflurane anesthesia in constrictor snakes. *Sciendo.* 2018;74:474–478.
423. Shan Q, Zheng G, Liu S, et al. Pharmacokinetic/pharmacodynamic relationship of marbofloxacin against *Aeromonas hydrophila* in Chinese soft-shelled turtles (*Trionyx sinensis*). *J Vet Pharmacol Ther.* 2015;38(6):537–542.
424. Sharun K, Satheesh A, Alexander J. Diagnosis and therapeutic management of gastrointestinal parasitism among the captive population of Indian star tortoise (*Geochelone elegans* Schoepff, 1795) at Zoological Garden, Thiruvananthapuram, Kerala, India. *J Parasit Dis.* 2020;44(2):453–456.

425. Shepard MK, Divers S, Braun C, et al. Pharmacodynamics of alfaxalone after single-dose intramuscular administration in red-eared sliders (*Trachemys scripta elegans*): a comparison of two different doses at two different ambient temperatures. *Vet Anaesth Analg.* 2013;40:590–598.
426. Siddle MR, Hanak E, Parker DL, et al. Cholecystectomy for the treatment of enterococcal cholecystitis and cholelithiasis in an inland bearded dragon (*Pogona vitticeps*): a case report. *J Exot Pet Med.* 2020:64–68.
427. Sim RR. Voriconazole. *J Exot Pet Med.* 2016;25:342–347.
428. Sim RR, Allender MC, Crawford LK, et al. Ranavirus epizootic in captive Eastern box turtles (*Terrapene carolina carolina*) with concurrent herpesvirus and *Mycoplasma* infection: management and monitoring. *J Zoo Wildl Med.* 2016;47:256–270.
429. Skovgaard N, Crossley DA, Wang T. Low cost of pulmonary ventilation in American alligators (*Alligator mississippiensis*) stimulated with doxapram. *J Exp Biol.* 2016;219:933–936.
430. Sladky KK. *Unpublished data.* 2017.
431. Sladky KK, Mans C. Clinical analgesia in reptiles. *J Exot Pet Med.* 2012;21:17–32.
432. Sladky KK, Kinney ME, Johnson SM. Analgesic efficacy of butorphanol and morphine in bearded dragons and corn snakes. *J Am Vet Med Assoc.* 2008;233:267–273.
433. Sladky KK, Kinney ME, Johnson SM. Effects of opioid receptor activation on thermal antinociception in red-eared slider turtles (*Trachemys scripta*). *Am J Vet Res.* 2009;70:1072–1078.
434. Sladky KK, Miletic V, Paul-Murphy J, et al. Analgesic efficacy and respiratory effects of butorphanol and morphine in turtles. *J Am Vet Med Assoc.* 2007;230:1356–1362.
435. Sleeman JM, Gaynor J. Sedative and cardiopulmonary effects of medetomidine and reversal with atipamezole in desert tortoises (*Gopherus agassizii*). *J Zoo Wildl Med.* 2000;31:28–35.
436. Smith JA, McGuire NC, Mitchell MA. Cardiopulmonary physiology and anesthesia in crocodilians. *Proc Annu Conf Assoc Rept Amph Vet.* 1998:17–21.
437. Spadola F, Morici M, Knotek Z. Combination of lidocaine/prilocaine with tramadol for short time anaesthesia-analgesia in chelonians: 18 cases. *Acta Vet Brno.* 2015;84:71–75.
438. Spörle H, Gobel T, Schildger B. Blood levels of some anti-infectives in the spur-thighed tortoise (*Testudo hermanni*). *Proc 4th Intl Colloq Path Med Rept Amph.* 1991:120–128.
439. Stahl SJ. Captive management, breeding, and common medical problems of the veiled chameleon (*Chamaeleo calyptratus*). *Proc Annu Conf Assoc Rept Amph Vet.* 1997:29–40.
440. Stahl SJ. Common diseases of the green iguana. *Proc North Am Vet Conf.* 1998:806–809.
441. Stahl SJ. Reproductive disorders of the green iguana. *Proc North Am Vet Conf.* 1998:810–813.
442. Stahl SJ. Medical management of bearded dragons. *Proc North Am Vet Conf.* 1999:789–792.
443. Stahl SJ. Diseases of the reptile pancreas. *Vet Clin North Am Exot Anim Pract.* 2003;6:191–212.
444. Stahl SJ. Pet lizard conditions and syndromes. *Semin Avian Exot Pet Med.* 2003;12:162–182.
445. Stahl SJ. Clinician's approach to the chameleon patient. *Proc North Am Vet Conf.* 2006:1667–1670.
446. Stahl S, Donoghue S. Pharyngostomy tube placement, management and use for nutritional support in chelonian patients. *Proc Annu Conf Assoc Rept Amph Vet.* 1997:93–97.
447. Stamper MA, Papich MG, Lewbart GA, et al. Pharmacokinetics of ceftazidime in loggerhead sea turtles (*Caretta caretta*) after single intravenous and intramuscular injections. *J Zoo Wildl Med.* 1999;30:32–35.
448. Stegman N, Heatley JJ. The use of haloperidol in mitigation of human-directed aggression in boid snakes. *Proc Annu Conf Assoc Rept Amph Vet.* 2010:113.
449. Stilwell JM, Stilwell NK, Stacy NI, et al. Extension of the known host range of intranuclear coccidiosis: infection in three captive red-footed tortoises (*Chelonoidis carbonaria*). *J Zoo Wildl Med.* 2017;48(4):1165–1171.
450. Stirl R, Krug P, Bonath KH. Tiletamine/zolazepam sedation in boa constrictors and its influence on respiration, circulation, and metabolism. *Proc Conf Euro Assoc Zoo Wildl Vet.* 1996:115–119.
451. Stöhr AC, Globokar-Vrhovec M, Pantchev N. *Choleoeimeria* spp. prevalence in captive reptiles in Germany and a new treatment option in a Lawson's dragon (*Pogona henrylawsoni*). *J Herp Med Surg.* 2021;30(4):261–269.

452. Strahl-Heldreth DE, Clark-Price SC, Keating SCJ, et al. Effect of intracoelomic administration of alfaxalone on the righting reflex and tactile stimulus response of common garter snakes (*Thamnophis sirtalis*). *J Am Vet Med Assoc.* 2019;80:144–151.
453. Stringer EM, Garner MM, Proudfoot JS, et al. Phaeohyphomycosis of the carapace in an Aldabra tortoise (*Geochelone gigantea*). *J Zoo Wildl Med.* 2009;40:160–167.
454. Suarez-Yana T, Montes D, Zuniga R, et al. Hematologic, morphometric, and biochemical analytes of clinically healthy green sea turtles (*Chelonia mydas*) in Peru. *Chelonian Conserv Biol.* 2016;15:153–157.
455. Suedmeyer WK. Iron deficiency in a group of American alligators: diagnosis and treatment. *J Small Exot Anim Med.* 1991;1:69–72.
456. Sykes JM. Updates and practical approaches to reproductive disorders in reptiles. *Vet Clin North Am Exot Anim Pract.* 2010;13:349–373.
457. Sykes JM, Klaphake E. Reptile hematology. *Vet Clin North Am Exot Anim Pract.* 2015;18:63–82.
458. Sykes JM, Ramsay EC, Schumacher J, et al. Evaluation of an implanted osmotic pump for delivery of amikacin to corn snakes (*Elaphe guttata guttata*). *J Zoo Wildl Med.* 2006;37:373–380.
459. Széll Z, Sréter T, Varga I. Ivermectin toxicosis in a chameleon (*Chamaeleo senegalensis*) infected with *Foleyella furcata*. *J Zoo Wildl Med.* 2001;32(1):115–117.
460. Talent LG. Effect of temperature on toxicity of a natural pyrethrin pesticide to green anole lizards (*Anolis carolinensis*). *Environ Toxicol Chem.* 2005;24(12):3113–3116.
461. Tang PK, Divers SJ, Sanchez S. Antimicrobial susceptibility patterns for aerobic bacteria isolated from reptilian samples submitted to a veterinary diagnostic laboratory: 129 cases (2005-2016). *J Am Vet Med Assoc.* 2020;257(3):305–312.
462. Tang PK, Blake D, Hedley J, et al. Efficacy of a topical formulation containing emodepside and praziquantel (Profender®, Bayer) against nematodes in captive tortoises. *J Herp Med Surg.* 2017;27:116–122.
463. Taylor Jr RW, Jacobson ER. Hematology and serum chemistry of the gopher tortoise, *Gopherus polyphemus*. *Comp Biochem Physiol A.* 1982;72:425–428.
464. Teare JA. Species360 physiological reference intervals for captive wildlife. *Species360*: Bloomington, MN; 2013. https://zims.species360.org/Main.aspx . Accessed November 5, 2016.
465. Teare JA, Bush M. Toxicity and efficacy of ivermectin in chelonians. *J Am Vet Med Assoc.* 1983;183:1195–1197.
466. Theusen LR, Bertelsen MF, Brimer L, et al. Selected pharmacokinetic parameters for cefovecin in hens and green iguanas. *J Vet Pharmacol Therap.* 2009;32:613–617.
467. Thompson KA, Papich MG, Higgins B, et al. Ketoprofen pharmacokinetics of R-and S-isomers in juvenile loggerhead sea turtles (*Caretta caretta*) after single intravenous and single- and multidose intramuscular administration. *J Vet Pharmacol Therap.* 2018;41:340–348.
468. Thompson PE. Effects of quinine on saurian malarial parasites. *J Infect Dis.* 1946;78:160–166.
469. Tothill A, Johnson J, Branvold H, et al. Effect of cisapride, erythromycin, and metoclopramide on gastrointestinal transit time in the desert tortoise, *Gopherus agassizii*. *J Herpetol Med Surg.* 2000;10:16–20.
470. Troiano J, Gould E, Gould I. Hematological reference intervals in Argentine lizard *Tupinambis merianae*. *Comp Clin Path.* 2008;17:169–174.
471. Tuttle AD, Papich M, Lewbart GA, et al. Pharmacokinetics of ketoprofen in the green iguana (*Iguana iguana*) following single intravenous and intramuscular injections. *J Zoo Wildl Med.* 2006;37:567–570.
472. Uney K, Altan F, Aboubakr M, et al. Pharmacokinetics of meloxicam in red-eared slider turtles (*Trachemys scripta scripta*) after single intravenous and intramuscular injections. *Am J Vet Res.* 2016;77:439–444.
473. Uney K, Altan F, Cetin G, et al. Pharmacokinetics of cefquinome in red-eared slider turtles (*Trachemys scripta elegans*) after single intravenous and intramuscular injections. *J Vet Pharmacol Ther.* 2018;41:e40–e44.

474. Van Waeyenberghe L, Baert K, Pasmans F, et al. Voriconazole, a safe alternative for treating infections caused by the *Chrysosporium* anamorph of *Nannizziopsis vriesii* in bearded dragons (*Pogona vitticeps*). *Med Mycol.* 2010;48:880–885.
475. Vercelli C, De Vito V, Salvadori M, et al. Blood concentrations of marbofloxacin and its in vivo effect in yellow-bellied slider turtles (*Trachemys scripta scripta*) after a single intracoelomic injection at 3 dose rates. *J Exot Pet Med.* 2016;25:295–304.
475a. Vigneault A, Lair S, Gara-Boivin C, et al. Evaluation of the safety of multiple intramuscular doses of ketoprofen in bearded dragons (*Pogona vitticeps*). *J Herp Med Surg.* 2022;32:123–129.
476. Vree TB, Vree JB, Kolmer EB, et al. N-oxidation, O-demethylation, and excretion of trimethoprim by the turtle *Pseudemys scripta elegans. Vet Quart.* 1989;11(2):125–128.
477. Walden M. *The Epidemiology of Coccidia in Bearded Dragons (Pogona vitticeps).* Baton Rouge, LA: Louisiana State University, Dissertation; 2008:1–145.
478. Walden M, Mitchell MA. Evaluation of three treatment modalities against *Isospora amphiboluri*) in inland bearded dragons (*Pogona vitticeps*). *J Exot Pet Med.* 2012;21:213–218.
479. Wallace BP, George RH. Alternative techniques for obtaining blood samples from leatherback turtles. *Chelonian Conser Biol.* 2007;6:147–149.
480. Wambugu SN, Towett PK, Kiama SG, et al. Effects of opioids in the formalin test in the Speke's hinged tortoise (*Kinixys spekii*). *J Vet Pharmacol Ther.* 2010;33:347–351.
481. Wangen K. Cisapride. *J Exot Pet Med.* 2013;22:301–304.
482. Waxman S, Prados AP, de Lucas JJ, et al. Pharmacokinetic behavior of enrofloxacin and its metabolite ciprofloxacin in Urutu pit vipers (*Bothrops alternatus*) after intramuscular administration. *J Zoo Wildl Med.* 2014;45:78–85.
483. Waxman S, Prados AP, de Lucas JJ, et al. Pharmacokinetics of enrofloxacin and its metabolite ciprofloxacin after single intramuscular administration in South American rattlesnake (*Crotalus durissus terrificus*). *Pakistan Vet J.* 2015;35:494–498.
484. Wellehan JFX, Gunkel CI. Emergent diseases in reptiles. *Semin Avian Exot Pet Med.* 2004;13:160–174.
485. White SD, Bourdeau P, Bruet V, et al. Reptiles with dermatological lesions: a retrospective study of 301 cases at two university veterinary teaching hospitals (1992-2008). *Vet Dermatol.* 2010;22:150–161.
486. Whitehead M. Permethrin toxicity in exotic pets. *Vet Rec.* 2010;166(10):306–307.
487. Whiting SD, Guinea ML, Fomiatti K, et al. Plasma biochemical and PCV ranges for healthy, wild, immature hawksbill sea turtles (*Eretmochelys imbricata*). *Vet Rec.* 2014;174:608.
488. Williams CJ, James LE, Bertelsen MF, et al. Tachycardia in response to remote capsaicin injections as a model for nociception in the ball python (*Python regius*). *Vet Anaesth Analg.* 2015;43:429–434.
489. Williams SR, Sims MA, Roth-Johnson L, et al. Surgical removal of an abscess associated with *Fusarium solani* from a Kemp's ridley sea turtle (*Lepidochelys kempii*). *J Zoo Wildl Med.* 2012;43:402–406.
490. Wills S, Beaufrère H, Watrous G, et al. Proximal duodenoileal anastomosis for treatment of small intestinal obstruction and volvulus in a green iguana (*Iguana iguana*). *J Am Vet Med Assoc.* 2016;249:1061–1066.
491. Wimsatt JH, Johnson J, Mangone BA, et al. Clarithromycin pharmacokinetics in the desert tortoise (*Gopherus agassizii*). *J Zoo Wildl Med.* 1999;30:36–43.
492. Wimsatt J, Tothill A, Offermann CF, et al. Long-term and per-rectum disposition of clarithromycin in the desert tortoise (*Gopherus agassizii*). *J Am Assoc Lab Anim Sci.* 2008:41–45.
493. Wissman MA, Parsons B. Dermatophytosis of green iguanas (*Iguana iguana*). *J Small Exot Anim Med.* 1993;2:133–136.
494. Wood FE, Critchley KH, Wood JR. Anesthesia in green the sea turtle, *Chelonia mydas. Am J Vet Res.* 1982;43:1882.
495. Wright K. Omphalectomy of reptiles. *Exot DVM.* 2001;3(1):11–15.
496. Wright KM. Common medical problems of tortoises. *Proc North Am Vet Conf.* 1997:769–771.

497. Wright KM, Skeba S. Hematology and plasma chemistries of captive prehensile-tailed skinks (*Corucia zebrata*). *J Zoo Wildl Med.* 1992;23:429–432.

498. Wright TL, Gjeltema J, Wack RF, et al. Plasma voriconazole concentrations following single- and multiple dose subcutaneous injections in Western pond turtles (*Actinemys marmorata*). *J Zoo Wildl Med.* 2021;5(2):538–547.

499. Yaw TJ, Mans C, Johnson SM, et al. Effect of injection site on alfaxalone-induced sedation in ball pythons (*Python regius*). *J Sm Anim Pract.* 2018;59:747–751.

500. Young LA, Schumacher J, Papich MG, et al. Disposition of enrofloxacin and its metabolite ciprofloxacin after intravascular injection in juvenile Burmese pythons (*Python molurus bivittatus*). *J Zoo Wildl Med.* 1997;28:71–79.

501. Zaias J, Norton T, Fickel A, et al. Biochemical and hematologic values for 18 clinically healthy radiated tortoises (*Geochelone radiata*) on St Catherines Island, Georgia. *Vet Clin Pathol.* 2006;35:321–325.

502. Ziolo M, Bertelsen M. Effects of propofol administered via the supravertebral sinus in red-eared sliders. *J Am Vet Med Assoc.* 2009;234:390–393.

Chapter 5 **Birds**

David Sanchez-Migallon Guzman | Hugues Beaufrère | Kenneth R. Welle | Jill Heatley | Marike Visser | Craig A. Harms

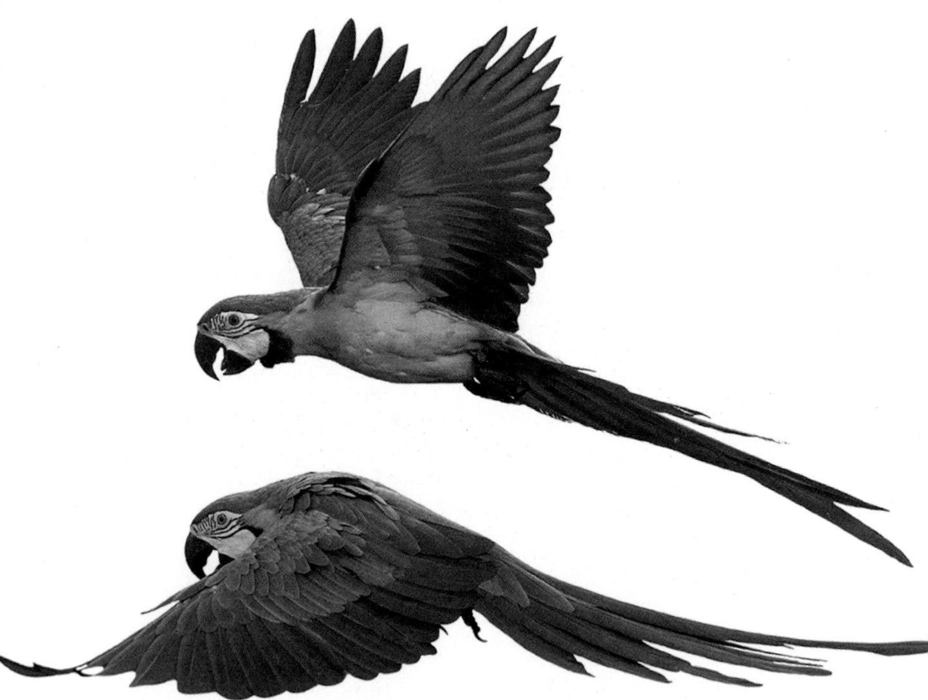

For ease of use of the Birds chapter, water and feed dosages are generally listed last.

TABLE 5-1 Antimicrobial Agents Used in Birds.[a]

Agent	Dosage	Species/Comments
Amikacin	—	Aminoglycoside antibiotic; poorly absorbed from gastrointestinal tract; potentially nephrotoxic and ototoxic; maintain hydration and avoid concurrent use of other nephroactive drugs[106]
	7 mg/kg IV q24h[401]	Emus/PK; mean serum levels declined below a target trough of 4 µg/mL at 24 hr
	7.6 mg/kg IM q8h[441]	Ostriches/PK; causes myositis; painful injection
	10 mg/kg IM q12h[658]	Cranes
	10-20 mg/kg IM, IV q8-12h[360,555,736,840]	African grey parrots, Amazon parrots, cockatiels, cockatoos/PK; blue-fronted Amazon parrots peak IV and IM concentrations 100 µg/mL and 38 µg/mL; cockatiels IM peak and trough concentrations 27.3 µg/mL and 0.9 µg/mL
	15-20 mg/kg SC, IM, IV q8-12h[241]	Passerines, pigeons/5 days maximum[790]
	15-20 mg/kg IM q24h[99]	Raptors/PK; peak 65 µg/mL; trough at 12 hr: 2.3 µg/mL; use low end of dose range for smaller hawks
	15-30 mg/kg IM q12-24h[240,959]	Most species, including passerines/ use in combination with other agents for *Mycobacterium*; see Table 5-45
	528 mg/L drinking water[939]	Ratites/egg dip
	3 g/40 packet bone cement[943]	PMMA bead formation (1:14 ratio); same dose for all aminoglycoside beads; consider absorbable calcium sulfate beads as alternative to PMMA
Amoxicillin sodium	—	Amoxicillin sodium is the sodium salt form of a semisynthetic aminopenicillin antibiotic with bactericidal activity; broad-spectrum β-lactamase-sensitive penicillin[106]
	50 mg/kg IM q12-24h[236,240]	Pigeons/PK; gram-positive bacteria
	100 mg/kg IM, IV q4-8h[802]	Bustards/PK; administer q4h IM or q8h IV to maintain blood levels >2 mg/mL
	150 mg/kg IM q8h[793]	Passerines, softbills
	250 mg/kg IM q12-24h[236,240]	Pigeons/PK; gram-positive and gram-negative bacteria
Amoxicillin trihydrate	—	
	15-22 mg/kg PO q8h[939]	Ratites
	20 mg/kg PO q12-24h[238]	Pigeons/PK; mean half-life 66 min
	30 mg/kg IM q12h × 5 days[134]	Pigeons
	40-80 mg/kg PO q12h × 5 days[134]	Pigeons
	100 mg/kg PO q12-24h[245]	Pigeons/PK
	100 mg/kg PO q8h[60]	Most species, including raptors

Continued

TABLE 5-1 Antimicrobial Agents Used in Birds. (cont'd)

Agent	Dosage	Species/Comments
Amoxicillin trihydrate (cont'd)	100-150 mg/kg PO q12h[178]	Raptors
	100-200 mg/kg IM q4-8h[245]	Pigeons/57% bioavailability compared to IV, double the IM dose when comparing to IV; Cmax 28 μg/mL at 0.5 hr
	150 mg/kg SC, IM q24h × 5 days (administer q48h with long-acting preparation)[802]	Pigeons
	150 mg/kg PO, IV[879]	Pigeons/PK, PD; *Streptococcus bovis*
	150-175 mg/kg PO q12h[177]	Passerines (towhees), psittacines
	150-175 mg/kg PO q4-8h[793]	Pigeons, psittacines
	65 mg/L drinking water[939]	Ratites
	200-400 mg/L drinking water[369]	Canaries/aviary use
	500-800 mg/L drinking water[376]	Pigeons
	1500 mg/L drinking water × 5 days[879]	Pigeons/PK, PD; *Streptococcus bovis*
	1500-4500 mg/L drinking water[177]	Psittacines
	300-500 mg/kg soft feed[369]	Canaries/aviary use
	600 mg/kg soft feed[177]	Psittacines
Amoxicillin/ clavulanate (Clavamox, Zoetis)	—	β-lactamase inhibitor[106]
	7-14 mg/kg IM q24h[134]	Ostriches
	10-15 mg/kg PO q12h[939]	Ratites
	105 mg/kg IM q12h[263]	Pigeon/MIC ≤0.5 mg/L
	125 mg/kg PO q12h[702]	Most species, including pigeons, psittacines, raptors
	125 mg/kg PO q8h[668]	Blue-fronted Amazon parrots/PK
	125 mg/kg PO q6h[177]	Psittacines
	125-250 mg/kg PO q8-12h[242]	Collared doves/PK
Ampicillin sodium	—	Broad-spectrum β-lactamase-sensitive penicillin[106]
	50 mg/kg IM q6-8h[260]	Amazon parrots/PK; localized infections
	100 mg/kg IM q4h[260]	Amazon parrots/PK
	150 mg/kg IM q12-24h[239]	Passerines, softbills
	150 mg/kg IM q12-24h[260]	Pigeons/PK
	150-200 mg/kg PO q8-12h[260]	Amazon parrots/PK; therapeutic levels not achieved in blue-naped Amazons at this dosage
	174 mg/kg PO q24h[207]	Pigeons/PK, PD; *Streptococcus bovis*
	528 mg/L drinking water[207]	Pigeons/PK, PD; *Streptococcus bovis*

TABLE 5-1 Antimicrobial Agents Used in Birds. (cont'd)

Agent	Dosage	Species/Comments
Ampicillin trihydrate	—	Broad-spectrum β-lacatamase-sensitive penicillin; minimal activity for common gram-negative infections of birds; poor gastrointestinal absorption[793]
	4-7 mg/kg SC, IM q8h[939]	Ratites (excluding emus)
	11-15 mg/kg PO q8h[939]	Ratites
	15 mg/kg IM q12h[131]	Raptors/PK
	15-20 mg/kg SC, IM q12h[131]	Emus, cranes/PK
	25 mg/kg PO q12-24h[240]	Pigeons/PK
	100 mg/kg PO q12-24h[240]	Pigeons/PK
	100 mg/kg IM q12h[658]	Cranes
	100 mg/kg IM q4h[391]	Most species, including psittacines
	100-200 mg/kg PO q6-8h[391]	Psittacines
	155 mg/kg IM q12-24h[245]	Pigeons/PK; amoxicillin preferred over ampicillin for IM use in pigeons
	500 mg powder/L drinking water[391]	Psittacines/*Pseudomonas*
	1000-2000 mg/L drinking water[369]	Canaries/aviary use
	2000-3000 mg/kg soft feed[369]	Canaries/aviary use
Azithromycin (Zithromax, Pfizer)	—	Macrolide antibiotic; effective against most aerobic and anaerobic gram-positive bacteria, may be effective against gram-negative organisms; active against *Mycobacterium* (including atypical species), *Chlamydia*, and *Mycoplasma*[106]
	10 mg/kg PO q48h × 5 treatments 124[147]	Blue and gold macaws/PK; nonintracellular infections
	40 mg/kg PO q24h × 30 days[147]	Blue and gold macaws/PK; intracellular infections (i.e., *Chlamydia*)
	40 mg/kg PO q48h × 21 days[814]	Cockatiels/PK, PD; treatment course for *Chlamydia*
	43-45 mg/kg PO q24h[391]	Most species including psittacines, passerines/ intracellular infections including *Mycobacterium* spp.; used with ethambutol and rifabutin (see Table 5-45)
	50-80 mg/kg PO q24h × 3 days on, off 4 days, repeat up to 3 wk[768]	Most species/*Mycobacterium* spp.; do not use if hepatic or renal disease; can mix with lactulose (stable refrigerated for 3-4 wk)
	50-400 mg/L drinking water[391]	Ratites/*Clostridium perfringens*; prepare daily
	100-500 mg/kg feed[134]	Ostriches <3 mo of age

Continued

TABLE 5-1 Antimicrobial Agents Used in Birds. (cont'd)

Agent	Dosage	Species/Comments
Azithromycin - sustained release granules	35mg/kg PO, then 25 mg/kg q24h[1006]	Pigeons/PK, PD; MIC ≤0.03 mg/mL
	1058 mg/L drinking water[594]	Most species
Carbenicillin	—	Broad-spectrum β-lactamase-sensitive penicillin; no longer commercially available
	100 mg/kg IM q8h[56]	Most species
Cefadroxil	—	First-generation cephalosporin; limited activity against gram-negative pathogens[106]
	20 mg/kg PO q12h[980]	Ratites
	100 mg/kg PO q12h × 7 days[379]	Most psittacines, pigeons/14-21 day therapy may be indicated for severe or deep pyodermas
Cefazolin	—	First-generation cephalosporin; limited activity against gram-negative pathogens[106]
	25-30 mg/kg IM, IV q8h[140]	Cranes
	25-50 mg/kg IM, IV q12h[768]	Most species
	50-75 mg/kg IM q12h[789]	Most species
	50-100 mg/kg PO, IM q12h[716]	Raptors
Cefotaxime	—	Third-generation cephalosporin with broad-spectrum activity for many gram-positive and gram-negative pathogens[106]
	25 mg/kg IM q8h[942]	Ratites/young birds
	50-100 mg/kg IM q8-12h[658]	Cranes
	75-100 mg/kg IM, IV q4-8h[391]	Most species, including softbills, psittacines, passerines
	75-100 mg/kg IM q12h[420]	Raptors
	100 mg/kg IM q8-12h[376]	Pigeons
Cefovecin (Convenia, Zoetis)	—	Third-generation cephalosporin; not recommended for use in birds due to short half-life[833]
Cefoxitin	—	Second-generation cephalosporin with a wide range of activity against many gram-positive and gram-negative bacteria
	50-75 mg/kg IM, IV q6-8h[391]	Most species, including softbills
	50-100 mg/kg IM, IV q6-12h[391]	Psittacines
Ceftazidime	—	Third-generation cephalosporin; extensive activity against gram-negative bacteria[106]
	50-100 mg/kg IM, IV q4-8h[391]	Most species
Ceftiofur (Naxcel, Zoetis)	—	Third-generation cephalosporin with activity against *Pasteurella*[106]
	10 mg/kg IM q8-12h[926]	Orange-winged Amazon parrots/PK
	10 mg/kg IM q4h[926]	Cockatiels/PK; higher doses may be required for resistant infections
	10-20 mg/kg IM q12h[391]	Ratites

TABLE 5-1 Antimicrobial Agents Used in Birds. (cont'd)

Agent	Dosage	Species/Comments
Ceftiofur (Naxcel, Zoetis) (cont'd)	50 mg/kg IM q12h[391]	Ostrich chicks
	50-100 mg/kg q4-8h[391]	Most species, including psittacines and passerines
Ceftiofur extended release formulation (Excede, Zoetis)	—	
	10 mg/kg IM[476]	Flamingos/PK; 10 mg/kg reached levels above MIC through 96 hr in 9/11 birds
	10 mg/kg IM[798]	Red-tailed hawks/PK; 10 mg/kg may allow targeted plasma levels for 36-45 hr
	10 mg/kg IM[797a]	Bald eagles/PK; may provide target plasma levels of 1 µg/mL for 110 hr or 4 µg/mL for 60 hr
	20 mg/kg IM[975a]	Cattle egrets/PK; may provide target plasma levels for 72 hr
	20 mg/kg IM[798]	Red-tailed hawks/PK; may provide target plasma levels for 96 hr
	20 mg/kg IM[979a]	Bald eagles/PK; may provide target plasma levels of 4 µg/mL for 160 hr or 4 µg/mL for 80 hr
	50 mg/kg IM[947a]	Ring-necked doves/PK; may provide target plasma levels for 108 hr
Ceftriaxone	—	Third-generation cephalosporin; effective against gram-positive and gram-negative bacteria, including some activity against *Pseudomonas*[106]
	75-100 mg/kg IM q4-8h[391]	Most species
Cephalexin	—	First-generation cephalosporin; active against many gram-positive and some gram-negative bacteria[106]
	15-22 mg/kg PO q8h[939]	Ratites (excluding emus)
	35-50 mg/kg IM q2-3h[133]	Psittacines <500 g/PK
	35-50 mg/kg PO, IM q6-8h[133]	Pigeons, emus, cranes, raptors, psittacines >500 g/PK; dose psittacines q6h
	40-100 mg/kg PO, IM q6-8h[391]	Most species, including raptors, psittacines, passerines
	50 mg/kg PO q6h × 3-5 days[391]	Raptors, pigeons
	100 mg/kg PO q8-12h[376]	Pigeons/14-21-day therapy may be indicated for severe or deep pyodermas
	100 mg/kg PO q4-6h[133]	Pigeons, emus, cranes/PK
Cephalothin	—	First-generation cephalosporin; active against many gram-positive and some gram-negative bacteria[106]
	30-40 mg/kg IM, IV q6h[939]	Ratites (excluding emus)
	100 mg/kg IM q8-12h[420]	Raptors
	100 mg/kg IM, IV q6-8h[391]	Most species, including psittacines, ratites
	100 mg/kg IM q6h[133]	Pigeons, emus, cranes/PK
	100 mg/kg IM, IV q2-6h[241]	Passerines

Continued

TABLE 5-1 Antimicrobial Agents Used in Birds. (cont'd)

Agent	Dosage	Species/Comments
Cephradine	—	First-generation cephalosporin; active against many gram-positive and some gram-negative bacteria[106]
	35-50 mg/kg PO q4-6h[767]	Most species/14-21-day therapy may be indicated for severe or deep pyodermas
	100 mg/kg PO q4-6h[767]	Pigeons, emus, cranes
Chloramphenicol palmitate (oral suspension)	—	Phenicol; broad spectrum, including anaerobes but can cause blood dyscrasias in humans;[106] because large differences in pharmacokinetics exist between birds and mammals and even among avian species, extrapolation between species is not recommended;[243] not commercially available in the United States but can be compounded
	25 mg/kg PO q8h × 5 days[134]	Pigeons
	30-50 mg/kg PO q6-8h[391]	Psittacines, including budgerigars
	35-50 mg/kg PO q8h × 3 days[939]	Ratites
	50 mg/kg PO q6-12h[391]	Raptors
	50-100 mg/kg PO q6-12h[391]	Most species, including passerines
	250 mg/kg PO q6h[376]	Pigeons
	100-200 mg/L drinking water[768]	Canaries
Chloramphenicol succinate	30 mg/kg IM q8h × 3-5 days[305]	Raptors
	35-50 mg/kg SC, IM, IV q8h × 3 days[939]	Ratites
	50 mg/kg IM q24h[162]	Eagles/PK
	50 mg/kg IM q8-12h[241]	Passerines
	50 mg/kg IM, IV q6-12h[162,391]	Most species, including budgerigars, passerines, pigeons, raptors
	50 mg/kg IM q6h[162]	Macaws, conures/PK
	50-80 mg/kg IM q12-24h[241]	Passerines
	60-100 mg/kg IM q8h[376]	Pigeons
	100 mg/kg SC q8h[658]	Cranes
	100 mg/kg IM q6h[241]	Passerines
	200 mg/kg IM q12h × 5 days[430]	Budgerigars/PK
Chlorhexidine	—	Biguanides; antiseptic activity against most gram-positive and some gram-negative bacteria; not bacterial spores[987]
	2.6-7.9 mL of 2% solution/L drinking water[768]	Most species/bacterial infection; topical application may be fatal to nun (mannikin) and parrot finches[768]
	7.9 mL/L water[939]	Ratites/egg disinfectant spray at 40-42°C (104-108°F)

TABLE 5-1 Antimicrobial Agents Used in Birds. (cont'd)

Agent	Dosage	Species/Comments
Chlorine (Na hypochlorite)	5 mg/L drinking water[789]	Water disinfectant; 0.1 mL of 5.25% bleach/L approximates this concentration
Chlortetracycline (Aureomycin Soluble Powder, Cyanamid)	—	Broad-spectrum tetracycline with activity against a wide range of gram-positive and gram-negative bacteria including *Chlamydia* and *Mycoplasma*[106]
	6-10 mg/kg IM q24h[399]	Raptors
	15-20 mg/kg PO q8h[939]	Ratites
	40-50 mg/kg PO q8h (w/grit), or q12h (w/o grit)[391]	Pigeons/PK
	100 mg/kg PO q6h[177]	Psittacines
	250 mg/kg PO q24h[399]	Raptors
	130-400 mg/L drinking water[376]	Pigeons
	500 mg/L drinking water or nectar[391]	Most species/prepare fresh q8-12h
	1000-1500 mg/L drinking water[391]	Canaries, psittacines/prophylaxis against *Chlamydia*
	5000 mg/L drinking water × 45 days[177]	Psittacines/*Chlamydia*
	100 mg/kg of feed[938]	Pigeons/*Salmonella*
	500 mg/kg of feed[240]	Budgerigars/*Chlamydia*
	5000 mg/kg soft feed × 45 days[177]	Psittacines/*Chlamydia*
	0.5% pellets × 30-45 days[237]	Small psittacines/reduce calcium content of diet to 0.7%
	1% pellets × 30-45 days[237]	Large psittacines/reduce calcium content of diet to 0.7%
	1000-2000 mg/kg soft mixed feed × 45 days[239]	Most psittacines, canaries
Ciprofloxacin	—	Fluoroquinolone with wide spectrum against gram-negative and some gram-positive bacteria; activity against *Chlamydia* and *Mycoplasma*[106]
	3-6 mg/kg PO q12h[939]	Ratites
	5-20 mg/kg PO q12h × 5-7 days[790]	Pigeons
	10 mg/kg PO q12h × 7 days[2]	Ostrich chicks
	10-20 mg/kg PO q12h[307]	Raptors
	15-20 mg/kg PO, IM q12h[241,391,940]	Most species, including psittacines, passerines
	20-40 mg/kg PO, IV q12h[391]	Most species, including psittacines, canaries, raptors

Continued

TABLE 5-1 Antimicrobial Agents Used in Birds. (cont'd)

Agent	Dosage	Species/Comments
Ciprofloxacin (cont'd)	50 mg/kg PO q12h[429]	Raptors/PK
	80 mg/kg PO q24h[959]	Most species/*Mycobacterium*; use in combination with other agents (see Table 5-46)
	250 mg/L drinking water × 5-10 days[790]	Pigeons
Clarithromycin	—	Macrolide; effective against most aerobic and anaerobic gram-positive bacteria; may be effective against gram-negative organisms; active against *Mycobacterium* (including atypical species), *Chlamydia*, and *Mycoplasma*;[106] see Table 5-46
	10 mg/kg PO q24h[639]	Penguins
	60 mg/kg PO q24h[524]	Psittacines
	85 mg/kg PO q24h[792]	Most species/*Mycobacterium* spp.; allometrically scaled
Clindamycin	—	Lincosamide; broad spectrum against anaerobic bacteria; limited against aerobic pathogens; widely distributed to tissues including bone[106]
	5.5 mg/kg PO q8h[616]	Ostriches
	12.5 mg/kg PO q12h[370]	Great horned owls/skin grafts; given in combination with enrofloxacin
	25 mg/kg PO q8h[289]	Psittacines, raptors
	50 mg/kg PO q8-12h[291]	Most species/7-10 day course recommended for raptors with osteomyelitis
	100 mg/kg PO q24h × 3-5 days[391]	Most species, including psittacines, passerines, raptors, pigeons/*Clostridium*
	100 mg/kg PO q12h × 7 days[702]	Psittacines
	150 mg/kg PO q24h[358]	Pigeons, raptors/osteomyelitis
	200 mg/L drinking water[190]	Pigeons
Clofazimine (Lamprene, Novartis)	—	Antimycobacterial agent; active against both slow- and fast-growing mycobacteria; use in combination with amikacin
	1-5 mg/kg PO q24h × 3-12 mo[391]	Psittacines, raptors/*Mycobacterium*; use in combination with other agents (see Table 5-46)
	6-12 mg/kg PO q12h[391]	Most species/*Mycobacterium*; use in combination with other agents (see Table 5-46)
Cloxacillin	—	Narrow-spectrum β-lactamase-resistant penicillin; inactive against many gram-positive organisms[106]
	100-250 mg/kg PO, IM q24h[391]	Most species
	250 mg/kg PO q12h × 7-10 days[89]	Raptors

TABLE 5-1 Antimicrobial Agents Used in Birds. (cont'd)

Agent	Dosage	Species/Comments
Cycloserine (Seromycin, Lilly)	5 mg/kg PO q12-24h × 3-12 mo[391]	Raptors/*Mycobacterium*; use in combination with other agents (see Table 5-45)
Danofloxacin mesylate (A180, Zoetis)	—	Fluoroquinolone with wide spectrum against gram-negative and some gram-positive bacteria; active against *Chlamydia* and *Mycoplasma*[106]
	5 mg/kg PO, IM, IV[601]	Hyacinth macaws
	10 mg/kg IM, SC q24h[183]	Chukar partridge (*Alectoris chukar*)/Cmax 8.05 µg/mL (IV), 9.58 µg/mL (IM)
	15 mg/kg IM q24h[835]	Brown pelicans (*Pelecanus occidentalis*)/Cmax 2.5 µg/mL; AUC 13.75 µg/h/mL
	20 mg/kg PO q24h[183]	Chukar partridge (*Alectoris chukar*)/Cmax 3.39 µg/mL
Doxycycline	—	Broad-spectrum tetracycline with activity against a wide range of gram-positive and gram-negative bacteria; drug of choice for *Chlamydia* and *Mycoplasma*; products or foods containing Al, Ca, Mg, and Fe reduce or alter absorption;[106] 12.5-25 mg/kg PO q12-24h resulted in elevations in AST and serum bile acids as well as hepatocellular damage in lorikeets[1018]
	2-3.5 mg/kg PO q12h[939]	Ratites
	7.5-8 mg/kg PO q12-24h[768]	Passerines, nectar feeders, pigeons/PK; administer without grit[238]
	10-20 mg/kg PO q24h × 3-5 days[134]	Pigeons
	25 mg/kg PO q12h[455]	Psittacines, raptors/some gram-negative bacterial infections and possibly *Leucocytozoon*
	25 mg/kg (w/grit) PO q12h[1019]	Pigeons/PK
	25-50 mg/kg PO q12-24h[391]	Most species, including parrots (African grey parrots, Amazon parrots, cockatoos, macaws) and pigeons/may cause regurgitation; use low end of dose range for macaws and cockatoos
	35 mg/kg PO q24h × 21 days[814]	Cockatiels/PK, PD; *Chlamydia*
	40 mg/kg PO q24h[207]	Pigeons/PK, PD
	130 mg/L drinking water[177]	Parrots
	200 mg/L drinking water[265]	Pigeons
	250 mg/L drinking water[238]	Canaries
	280 mg/L drinking water[718]	Cockatiels/PK; see Table 5-42 for recipe
	400 mg/L drinking water[268]	Cockatiels/PK, PD; spiral bacteria
	500 mg/L drinking water × 45 days[670]	Fruit doves/PK, PD

Continued

TABLE 5-1 Antimicrobial Agents Used in Birds. (cont'd)

Agent	Dosage	Species/Comments
Doxycycline (cont'd)	500 mg/L drinking water[207]	Psittacines, pigeons/*Streptococcus bovis* in pigeons
	800 mg/L drinking water (mix the contents of 16 × 100 mg capsules with 2 L water)[297]	African grey parrots, Goffin's cockatoos/PK; protect solution from exposure to light; make fresh daily
	250-300 mg/kg seed[90]	Budgerigars
	500 mg/kg wet weight seeds[718]	Cockatiels/PK; see Table 5-42 for recipe
	1000 mg/kg feed[391,723]	Large psittacines on dehulled seed (PK), macaws on corn (PK), canaries, large psittacines on soft feed (10 mg/mL syrup mixed into 29% kidney beans, 29% canned corn, 29% cooked rice, 13% dry oatmeal cereal)
Doxycycline (Doxirobe gel, Zoetis)	Topical[888]	Most species/apply to beak or pododermatitis lesions; use in conjunction with debridement; antibiotic is released for 28 days
Doxycycline (pharmacist-compounded micronized doxycycline hyclate)	75-100 mg/kg IM q7d[793]	Cockatoos/anecdotal reports of sudden death with compounded product; inadequate drug levels achieved in cockatiels at 100 mg/kg IM q10d[718]; adequate drug levels achieved with 100 mg/kg given IM in cockatoos, Amazon parrots and SC in African grey parrots, but severe soft-tissue reactions seen[293]
Doxycycline (Vibravenös, Pfizer)	—	Broad-spectrum tetracycline with activity against a wide range of gram-positive and gram-negative bacteria; drug of choice for *Chlamydia* and *Mycoplasma*;[106] not available in the United States
	25-50 mg/kg IM q5-7d × 5-7 treatments[391]	Psittacines
	60-100 mg/kg SC, IM q5-7d[238]	Psittacines, pigeons
	75 mg/kg IM q7d × 4-6 wk[59]	Macaws
	75-100 mg/kg IM q5-7d × 4-6 wk[391]	Psittacines, including macaws, budgerigars
	100 mg/kg SC, IM q5-7d × 7 doses[354]	Houbara bustards/PK; *Chlamydia*
Doxycycline hyclate (injection)	—	Cardiovascular collapse associated with the propylene glycol carrier can occur after rapid IV injection[316]
	15 mg/kg IV q24h[9]	Ostrich/extremely poor oral and IM bioavailability; only administer IV; Cmax 80 µg/mL
	25-50 mg/kg slow bolus IV q24h × 3 days[793]	Psittacines
	75-100 mg/kg SC, IM q5-7d[236]	Pigeons/PK

TABLE 5-1 Antimicrobial Agents Used in Birds. (cont'd)

Agent	Dosage	Species/Comments
Doxycyline hyclate capsule	300 mg doxycycline mixed in soybean oil/kg low-fat psittacine pellets[301]	Cockatiels/*Chlamydia* and spiral bacterial infections; feed as sole diet for 47 days
Enrofloxacin	—	Fluoroquinolone with wide spectrum against gram-negative and some gram-positive bacteria; active against *Chlamydia* and *Mycoplasma*;[106] administration may be associated with emesis;[802] given PO, the IM formulation produces therapeutic plasma concentration;[420] best to avoid IM administration; IM administration is believed to be painful and may result in tissue necrosis and sterile abscesses; in parenteral administration, best to dilute with sterile NaCl and give SC; best to avoid IV use in raptors;[282] some fluoroquinolones have been used in PMMA beads with success;[256] joint deformities reported in squab chondrocytes with 200-800 mg/L drinking water;[501] however, enrofloxacin has been commonly used at the recommended dosages without reports of adverse effects;[298,768] no detected effect on cartilage in day-old poultry chicks[696]
	1.5-2.5 mg/kg PO, SC q12h[507]	Ratites
	2.2 mg/kg IV q12h[402]	Emus/PK
	5 mg/kg IM q12h × 2 days[939]	Ratites
	5 mg/kg PO, IM q12-24h[940]	African grey parrots
	5 mg/kg SC, IM q12h[940]	Cockatiels
	5-10 mg/kg SC, IM q24h[240]	African grey parrots
	5-10 mg/kg PO q8h[391]	Passerines, pigeons/PK
	5-15 mg/kg PO, SC, IM q12h[391]	Raptors, psittacines, pigeons/drug of choice for *Salmonella typhimurium*
	5-20 mg/kg PO q12-24h × 5-10 days[391]	Pigeons
	10 mg/kg PO, IV q24h[507]	Emus/PK
	10 mg/kg PO q12h[142]	Cockatiels
	10 mg/kg PO, IM, IV q12h[44]	Houbara bustard (*Chlamydotis undulata macqueenii*); 97% IM bioavailabiity; 62% PO bioavailability
	10-15 mg/kg PO, IM q12h × 5-7 days[391]	Raptors
	10-20 mg/kg PO q24h[238]	Passerines, psittacines, pigeons (PK)
	15 mg/kg PO, IM q24h[44]	Houbara bustard (*Chlamydotis undulata macqueenii*); 97% IM bioavailabiity; 62% PO bioavailability
	15 mg/kg PO, SC q24h[642]	Caribbean flamingos/Cmax 5.25- 5.77 µg/mL

Continued

TABLE 5-1 Antimicrobial Agents Used in Birds. (cont'd)

Agent	Dosage	Species/Comments
Enrofloxacin (cont'd)	15 mg/kg PO, IV q24h[974a]	African penguins/PK
	15 mg/kg PO q24h[702]	Psittacines
	15 mg/kg PO, SC q12h[291]	Most species
	15 mg/kg PO q12h[551]	Ostrich chicks, pigeons (administration to adult birds led to therapeutic levels in crop milk)
	15 mg/kg PO, IM, IV q12h[382]	Raptors/PK; IV administration in owls may result in weakness, tachycardia, vasoconstriction[282,382]
	15-30 mg/kg PO, IM q12h[296]	African grey parrots/PK
	20 mg/kg PO, SC, IM q12h[391]	Pigeons/administer parenterally, followed by oral treatment
	20-30 mg/kg PO q12-24h[265]	Pigeons
	30 mg/kg PO, IM q24h[941]	Psittacines
	45 mg/kg PO q24h[378]	Pigeons
	0.2 mg/mL saline, flush q24h × 10 days[89]	Raptors/nasal flush
	25-50 mg/L drinking water[114]	Cranes (sandhill)/did not provide sufficient plasma levels
	100-200 mg/L drinking water[232,790,802]	Psittacines, pigeons/PK; may need up to 300 mg/L to prevent recurrence of infection in pigeons[802]
	190-750 mg/L drinking water[296]	African grey parrots/PK
	200 mg/L drinking water[295]	Psittacines/PK; maintains plasma concentrations adequate only for highly susceptible bacteria
	200 mg/L drinking water[239]	Canaries
	500 mg/L drinking water[540]	Psittacines
	200 mg/kg soft feed[239]	Canaries
	250 mg/kg feed[238]	Budgerigars/PK
	250-1000 mg/kg feed q24h[391]	Psittacines, passerines
	500 mg/kg feed[540]	Psittacines, including Patagonian conures/PK; mix into steamed corn diet
	1000 mg/kg feed[540]	Senegal parrots/PK; mix into steamed corn diet
Erythromycin	—	Macrolide antibiotic; effective against most aerobic and anaerobic gram-positive bacteria; may be effective against gram-negative organisms; active against *Mycobacterium* (including atypical species), *Chlamydia*, and *Mycoplasma*;[106] IM injection may cause severe muscle necrosis[389]
	5-10 mg/kg PO q8h[939]	Ratites
	10-20 mg/kg IM q24h[240]	Passerines
	10-20 mg/kg PO q12h[802]	Psittacines

TABLE 5-1 Antimicrobial Agents Used in Birds. (cont'd)

Agent	Dosage	Species/Comments
Erythromycin (cont'd)	50-100 mg/kg PO q8-12h[240]	Passerines
	60 mg/kg PO q12h[409]	Most species
	71 mg/kg PO q24h[207]	Pigeons/PK, PD; *Streptococcus bovis*
	100 mg/kg PO[960]	Pigeons/PK, PD; low plasma levels but higher lung and trachea levels
	125 mg/kg PO q8h[376]	Pigeons
	125 mg/L drinking water[239]	Canaries
	132 mg/L drinking water (10 days on, 5 days off, 10 days on)[391]	Most species, including canaries
	250-500 mg/L drinking water × 3-5 days[177]	Psittacines
	525-800 mg/L drinking water[376]	Pigeons
	1000 mg/L drinking water[207,960]	Pigeons/PK, PD; *Streptococcus bovis*; plasma levels low; one study reported that lung and trachea levels were subtherapeutic
	1500 mg/L drinking water[802]	Most species
	200 mg/kg soft feed[239]	Canaries, psittacines
Ethambutol	—	Antimycobacterial agent; use in combination with other agents (see Table 5-45)
	10 mg/kg PO q12h[59]	Most species
	15-20 mg/kg PO q12h × 3-12 mo[391]	Psittacines, raptors/*Mycobacterium*
	15-30 mg/kg PO q12-24h[241]	Passerines/*Mycobacterium*
	30 mg/kg PO q24h[792]	Most species/*Mycobacterium*
Flumequine (Biocik, Amacol)	—	Fluoroquinolone antibiotic with wide spectrum against gram-negative and some gram-positive bacteria; active against *Chlamydia* and *Mycoplasma*;[106] not available in the United States
	30 mg/kg PO, IM q8-12h[236]	Passerines, pigeons (PK)
Furazolidone (NF180, Hess and Clark)	—	Nitrofuran antibiotic, wide spectrum but potency is relatively low;[106] linked with cardiomyopathy in birds; therapeutic action is confined to the gastrointestinal tract
	15-20 mg/kg PO q24h[241]	Passerines
	100-200 mg/L drinking water[768]	Canaries
	200 mg/kg soft food[768]	Canaries
	908 mg/kg feed[938]	Pigeons/*Salmonella*

Continued

TABLE 5-1 Antimicrobial Agents Used in Birds. (cont'd)

Agent	Dosage	Species/Comments
Gentamicin	—	Extended spectrum aminoglycoside; potentially nephrotoxic; maintain hydration and avoid concurrent use of other nephroactive drugs;[94,95,106] avoid doses higher than 2.5-5 mg/kg q8-12h[95,300]
	1-2 mg/kg IM q8h[939]	Ratites (excluding emus)/use only as last resort
	2.5 mg/kg IM q8h[95]	Raptors/PK
	3-10 mg/kg IM q6-12h[241]	Passerines
	5 mg/kg IM q12h[736]	Cockatiels/PK; peak 4.6 µg/mL; trough 0.17 µg/mL
	5 mg/kg IM q8h[132,196]	Emus, cranes/PK
	5-10 mg/kg IM q4h[132,196,796]	Pigeons/PK; *Salmonella*
	7 mg/kg q8h[442]	Ostriches/PK; use with caution
	40 mg/kg PO q8-24h[241]	Passerines/15-25 g
	2-3 drops ophthalmic solution intranasal q8h[940]	Most species
Isoniazid	—	Antimycobacterial agent; should be used in combination with other drugs (see Table 5-45)
	5-15 mg/kg PO q12h[240]	Most species, including passerines
	30 mg/kg PO q24h[959]	Most species
Kanamycin	—	Extended spectrum aminoglycoside; potentially nephrotoxic; maintain hydration and avoid concurrent use of other nephroactive drugs[106]
	10-20 mg/kg IM q12h[391]	Most species, including passerines/enteric infections
	13-65 mg/L drinking water × 3-5 days[391]	Most species/make fresh daily
Lincomycin	—	Lincosamide antibiotic; broad spectrum against anaerobic bacteria; limited activity against aerobic organisms; wide distribution, including bone[106]
	0.25-0.5 mL intraarticular q24h × 7-10 days[793]	Raptors
	25-50 mg/kg PO q12h[373]	Raptors/musculoskeletal surgical repair
	35-50 mg/kg PO q12-24h[241]	Passerines
	35-50 mg/pigeon PO q24h × 7-14 days[584]	Pigeons
	50-75 mg/kg PO, IM q12h × 7-10 days[391]	Psittacines, raptors/pododermatitis, osteomyelitis
	100 mg/kg PO q24h[768]	Raptors
	100 mg/kg IM q12h[90]	Psittacines
	100-200 mg/L drinking water[239]	Canaries

TABLE 5-1 Antimicrobial Agents Used in Birds. (cont'd)

Agent	Dosage	Species/Comments
Lincomycin (cont'd)	Topical[373]	Raptors/mixture of 50 mg/mL lincomycin and 10 mg/mL tobramycin was used to flush the flexor tendon sheath
Lincomycin/ spectinomycin (LS-50 Water Soluble, Zoetis; Linco-Spectin 100 Soluble Powder, Zoetis)	—	Lincosamide in combination with an aminoglycoside; combination is effective against *Mycoplasma*[106]
	50 mg/kg PO q24h[391]	Most species
	¼-½ tsp/L drinking water × 10-14 days[166]	Most species/using soluble powder 16.7 g lincomycin and 33.3 g spectinomycin per 2.55 oz packet of powder
Marbofloxacin (Zeniquin, Zoetis)		Fluoroquinolone with wide-spectrum against gram-negative and some gram-positive bacteria; active against *Chlamydia* and *Mycoplasma*[106]
	2 mg/kg IV[829]	Bilgorajska geese (*Anser anser domesticus*)/MIC ≤0.125 µg/mL
	2-3 mg/kg IO q24h[330]	Buzzard (*Buteo buteo*)/PK; IO: Cmax 1.92µg/mL; AUC 8.53 µg*h/mL
	2.5 mg/kg IV q24h[331]	Vulture/PK; targets MIC 0.2 µg/mL
	2.5-5 mg/kg PO q24h[146]	Blue and gold macaws/PK
	5 mg/kg IM, IV[208]	Ostriches/PK
	9-15 mg/kg IV q24h[328]	Mallard duck/PK; Cmax 1.34 µg/mL; targets MICs of 0.125-0.2 µg/mL
	10 mg/kg PO[829]	Bilgorajska geese (*Anser anser domesticus*)/MIC ≤0.125 µg/mL
	10-15 mg/kg PO, IM q12-24h[802,329]	Raptors, bustards (PO dosage is PK)[329]
Meropenem	—	Broad-spectrum β-lactamase-sensitive penicillin with extended spectra, including *Pseudomonas* and many anaerobes[106]
	175 mg/kg IM q24h[841]	Pigeons/PK
Metronidazole	—	Nitroimidazole antibiotic and antiprotozoal agent active against most anaerobes; penetrates blood-brain barrier;[106] see Table 5-4
	10 mg/kg IM q24h × 2 days[391]	Psittacines
	10-30 mg/kg PO q12h × 10 days[941]	Psittacines
	50 mg/kg PO q24h × 5-7 days[391]	Most species, including raptors, psittacines/ anaerobes
	50 mg/kg PO q12h × 30 days[789]	Amazon parrots, cockatoos/anaerobic and hemorrhagic enteritis

Continued

TABLE 5-1 Antimicrobial Agents Used in Birds. (cont'd)

Agent	Dosage	Species/Comments
Minocycline	—	Broad-spectrum tetracycline with active against a wide range of gram-positive and gram-negative bacteria; drug of choice for *Chlamydia* and *Mycoplasma*; readily penetrates blood-brain barrier[106]
	10 mg/kg PO q12h[639]	Penguins
	15 mg/kg PO q12h[399]	Raptors
	5000 mg/kg feed[15]	Parakeets/use as antibiotic-impregnated millet
Neomycin	—	Aminoglycoside antibiotic; poorly absorbed from gastrointestinal tract; potentially nephrotoxic and ototoxic[106]
	5-10 mg/kg IM q12h[399]	Raptors/toxic if overdosed
	10 mg/kg PO q8-12h[129]	Most species
	80-100 mg/L drinking water[768]	Canaries
	10 mg/kg PO q24h[241]	Passerines
	Topical q6-12h[798]	Most species/superficial wounds; cover with bandage; may be absorbed systemically and may cause ototoxicity and nephrotoxicity
Nitrofurazone	—	Nitrofuran antibiotic; wide spectrum but potency is relatively low;[106] high risk of neurotoxicity and toxicosis; do not use on open wounds associated with pneumatic bones[768]
Norfloxacin	—	Fluoroquinolone with wide spectrum against gram-negative and some gram-positive bacteria; active against *Chlamydia* and *Mycoplasma*[106]
	3-5 mg/kg PO q12h[939]	Ratites
Oleandomycin	—	Macrolide antibiotic; not available in the United States
	25 mg/kg IM q24h[241]	Passerines
	50 mg/kg PO q24h[241]	Passerines
Ormetoprim-sulfadimethoxine (Primor, Zoetis)	—	Potentiated sulfonamide combination antibiotic; broad spectrum[106]
	60 mg/kg PO q12h[378]	Pigeons
	475-951 mg/L drinking water × 7-10 days[378]	Pigeons
Oxytetracycline	—	Broad-spectrum tetracycline with activity against a wide range of gram-positive and gram-negative bacteria; drug of choice for *Chlamydia* and *Mycoplasma*; IM administration may cause muscle irritation or necrosis[106]

TABLE 5-1 Antimicrobial Agents Used in Birds. (cont'd)

Agent	Dosage	Species/Comments
Oxytetracycline (cont'd)	2 mg/mL nebulization q4-6h[253]	Parakeets/PK; requires ultrasonic nebulizer; therapeutic concentrations of antibiotic were present in lung and trachea; not effective in treating systemic infections outside the respiratory tract
	5 mg/kg IM q12h[980]	Ratites
	10 mg/kg IM q3d[939]	Ratites
	16 mg/kg IM q24h[923]	Great horned owls/PK
	25-50 mg/kg PO, IM q8h × 5-7 days[89]	Raptors
	48 mg/kg IM q48h[420]	Owls
	50 mg/kg IM q24h × 5-7 days[802]	Psittacines
	50 mg/kg PO q6-8h[376]	Pigeons
	50-75 mg/kg SC[289]	Goffin's cockatoos, blue and gold macaws
	50-100 mg/kg SC, IM q2-3d[241,299]	Passerines, cockatoos/PK
	50-200 mg/kg IM q3-5d[802]	Raptors
	58 mg/kg IM q24h[923]	Amazon parrots/PK
	80 mg/kg IM q48h[802]	Pigeons <400 g
	200 mg/kg IM q24h[59,89]	Most species, including waterfowl/*Pasteurella*
	130-400 mg/L drinking water[376]	Pigeons
	650-2000 mg/L drinking water × 5-14 days[177]	Psittacines
	300 mg/kg soft feed × 5-14 days[177]	Psittacines
	8 g/40 g packet bone cement[134]	PMMA beads (ratio 1:5); consider absorbable calcium sulfate beads as alternative to PMMA
Penicillin benzathine/Procaine	—	Anecdotal reports suggest procaine penicillin should not be used in birds <1 kg BW because of possible toxic effects[940]
	200 mg/kg IM q24h[59]	Most species
Penicillin G	6 mg/kg IV[163]	Ostriches, emus/PD; rapidly eliminated; small volume of distribution
Penicillin procaine	—	Anecdotal reports suggest procaine penicillin should not be used in birds <1 kg BW; adverse reactions (possible toxic effects) described in finches, canaries, budgerigars, cockatiels[286,940]
Piperacillin	—	Broad-spectrum β-lactamase-sensitive penicillin with extended spectra including *Pseudomonas*, *Proteus*, and others;[106] is only available in combination with tazobactam; see piperacillin/tazobactam

Continued

TABLE 5-1 Antimicrobial Agents Used in Birds. (cont'd)

Agent	Dosage	Species/Comments
Piperacillin (cont'd)	25 mg/kg IM[940]	Ratites (chicks <6 mo of age)
	87 mg/kg IM q4h[148]	Amazon parrots/PK; MIC ≤4 μg/mL
	100 mg/kg IM q12h[238]	Psittacines/PK
	100 mg/kg IM q12h[1]	Ostrich chicks/administer concurrent with amikacin (20 mg/kg IM q12h)
	100 mg/kg IM, IV q8-12h[658,744,802]	Pigeons, raptors, cranes
	100 mg/kg IM q4-6h[775]	Red-tailed hawks, great horned owls/PK
	100-200 mg/kg IM, IV q6-12h[793,802]	Most species, including psittacines
	200 mg/kg IM q8h[761]	Raptors
	200 mg/kg IM, IV q4-8h[291,793,940]	Most species, including passerines
	0.02 mL (4 mg) in macaw eggs; 0.01 mL (2 mg) in small eggs[593]	Eggs/inject 200 mg/mL solution into air cell on days 14, 18, and 22
	500 mg/mL topical[213]	Raptors/pododermatitis; 8 mL DMSO, 2mL dexamethasone (2 mg/mL), and 2 mL piperacillin (500 mg/mL)
Piperacillin/ tazobactam	—	β-lactamase-protected penicillin combination; synergistic effect allows activity against organisms resistant to piperacillin alone; broad-spectrum activity[106]
	100 mg/kg IM, IV q8-12h[646]	Most species, including psittacines/reports of good clinical response; recommended at 100 mg/kg IV q6h for severe polymicrobic bacteremia
	100 mg/kg IM q3-4h[148]	Hispaniolan Amazon parrots/PK; to control infections attributed to susceptible bacteria with an MIC of ≤4 μg/mL
Polymyxin B	—	Polypeptide antibiotic; toxicity limits use to topical preparations or PO for gastrointestinal infections; narrow spectrum against some gram-negative bacteria[106]
	10-15 mg/kg IM q24h[399]	Raptors/not absorbed if given PO
	50,000 U/L drinking water[445]	Canaries
	50,000 U/kg soft feed[454]	Canaries
Povidone-iodine	Topical to lesions, then rinse off[89]	Raptors/wound cleansing; antibacterial, antifungal activity
Rifabutin (Mycobutin, Pfizer)	15-45 mg/kg PO q24h[391]	Antimycobacterial agent; use in combination with other agents (see Table 5-45)
Rifampicin	—	See rifampin
Rifampin	—	Most species/*Mycobacterium*; use with other agents (see Table 5-45); may cause/ be associated with hepatitis, CNS signs, depression, and vomiting; yellow-orange urates observed in bustards[793]

TABLE 5-1 Antimicrobial Agents Used in Birds. (cont'd)

Agent	Dosage	Species/Comments
Rifampin (cont'd)	10-20 mg/kg PO q12-24h[240,789,938]	Most species, including passerines, psittacines/*Mycobacterium*
	45 mg/kg PO q24h[241,878,959]	Most species, including Amazon parrots, cranes
Silver sulfadiazine	Topical q12-24h[270]	Most species/topical sulfonamide, specifically for burn wounds;[106] ulcers; Amazon foot necrosis; bandage application preferred
Spectinomycin	—	Aminoglycoside antibiotic[106]
	10-30 mg/kg IM q8-12h[90]	Psittacines
	25-35 mg/kg IM q8-12h[377]	Pigeons
	165-275 mg/L drinking water[378]	Pigeons
	200-400 mg/L drinking water[239]	Canaries
	400 mg/kg soft feed[239]	Canaries
Spiramycin	—	Macrolide antibiotic; effective against most aerobic and anaerobic gram-positive bacteria; may be effective against gram-negative organisms; active against *Mycobacterium* (including atypical species), *Chlamydia*, and *Mycoplasma*;[106] not available in the United States
	20 mg/kg IM q24h[399]	Raptors
	250 mg/kg PO q24h[585]	Most species, including raptors/poorly absorbed
	200-400 mg/L drinking water[239]	Canaries
	400 mg/kg soft feed[239]	Canaries
Streptomycin	—	Narrow-spectrum aminoglycoside; activity against gram-negative aerobic bacteria[106] and *Mycobacterium*; use in combination with other agents (see Table 5-45); there is reported ototoxicity in chickens resulting in vestibular disease; once medication stopped, clinical signs slowly resolved[343]
	30 mg/kg IM q12h[59]	Most species
Sulfachlorpyridazine	—	Potentiated sulfonamide combination broad-spectrum antibiotic and antiprotozoal[106]
	150-300 mg/L drinking water[768]	Canaries
	400 mg/L drinking water × 7-10 days[788]	Pigeons
Sulfadimethoxine	—	Potentiated sulfonamide combination broad-spectrum antibiotic and antiprotozoal[106]
	50 mg/kg PO q24h[141]	Cranes
	25-55 mg/kg PO q24h × 3-7 days[450,760]	Raptors/loading dose at higher end × 1 day

Continued

TABLE 5-1 Antimicrobial Agents Used in Birds. (cont'd)

Agent	Dosage	Species/Comments
Sulfadimethoxine (cont'd)	190-250 mg/L drinking water[585]	Pigeons/loading dose 375 mg/L drinking water
	330-400 mg/L drinking water on day 1 followed by 200-265 mg/L × 4 days[378]	Pigeons
Tetracycline	—	Broad-spectrum tetracycline with activity against a wide range of gram-positive and gram-negative bacteria; drug of choice for *Chlamydia* and *Mycoplasma*[106]
	50 mg/kg PO q8[241,768]	Most species, including passerines
	200-250 mg/kg PO q12-24h[767]	Most species/gavage
	40-200 mg/L drinking water[391]	Most species, including game birds
	100 mg/L drinking water[738]	Rheas
	200 mg/L drinking water[789]	Pigeons
	666 mg/L drinking water[802]	Pigeons
Tiamulin (Denagard; Elanco)	—	Tiamulin fumarate antibiotic; active against gram-positive organisms including anaerobes[106]
	25-50 mg/kg PO q24h[212]	Most species
Ticarcillin (Ticar, SmithKline Beecham)	—	Broad-spectrum β-lactamase-sensitive penicillin with extended spectra including *Pseudomonas* and many anaerobes[106]
	75-100 mg/kg IM q4-6h[793]	Amazon parrots
	150-200 mg/kg IV q2-4h[241]	Passerines, softbills
	200 mg/kg IM q2-4h[840]	Blue-fronted Amazon parrots/IV peak 1160 μg/mL; IM peak 15 μg/mL
	200 mg/kg IM, IV q6-12h[391]	Most species, including pigeons, raptors/*Pseudomonas*[289]
Ticarcillin/ clavulanate (Timentin, Glaxo SmithKline)	100 mg/kg IM, IV[176]	Most species/frequency not reported
	200 mg/kg IM, IV q12h[789]	Most species
Tilmicosin (Micotil 300 Injection, Provitil-powder and Pulmotil AC-liquid, Elanco)	—	Macrolide antibiotic; effective against most aerobic and anaerobic gram-positive bacteria; may be effective against gram-negative organisms; active against *Mycobacterium* (including atypical species), *Chlamydia*, and *Mycoplasma*;[106] handle with caution; potentially fatal to humans;[710] see Table 6-1 for poultry dosages
Tobramycin	—	Extended spectrum; potentially nephrotoxic; maintain hydration and avoid concurrent use of other nephroactive drugs[106]

TABLE 5-1 Antimicrobial Agents Used in Birds. (cont'd)

Agent	Dosage	Species/Comments
	2.5-5 mg/kg IM, IV q8-12h[177]	Psittacine, passerines, raptors
	10 mg/kg IM q12h × 5-7 days[391]	Raptors
	0.25-0.5 mL intra-articular irrigation q24h × 7-10 days[89]	Raptors/septic arthritis
	Irrigation	A mixture of lincomycin (50 mg/mL) and tobramycin (10 mg/mL) was used to irrigate the flexor tendon sheath[373]
Trimethoprim	—	Bacteriostatic activity against some gram-positive and gram-negative bacteria
	10-20 mg/kg PO q8h[236,240,585]	Psittacines, passerines, pigeons/PK
Trimethoprim/ sulfadiazine	—	Potentiated sulfonamide combination antibiotic; broad spectrum[106]
	8 mg/kg SC, IM q12h[658]	Cranes
	12-60 mg/kg PO q12h × 5-7 days[89]	Raptors/useful for sensitive infections in neonates
	16-24 mg/kg PO q8-12h[658]	Cranes
	20 mg/kg SC, IM q12h[177]	Psittacines
	30 mg/kg PO, IM, IV q12h[372]	Ostriches/PK; Cmax 35.5 (sulfa) and 37.5 (trimethoprim) µg/mL regardless of route
	30 mg/kg PO q8h[372]	Psittacines/combine with pyrimethamine for treatment of sarcocystosis
	60 mg/kg PO q12h[378]	Pigeons
	107 mg/L drinking water[98]	Galliformes
	475-950 mg/L drinking water × 7-10 days[378]	Pigeons
Trimethoprim/ sulfamethoxazole	—	Potentiated sulfonamide combination antibiotic; broad spectrum[106]
	8 mg/kg IM q12h[802]	Psittacines
	10-50 mg/kg PO q24h[241]	Passerines
	20 mg/kg PO q8-12h[802]	Psittacines
	21 mg/kg PO q12h[1]	Ostriches
	40-50 mg/kg PO q12h[291]	Psittacines
	48 mg/kg PO, IM q12h[455]	Raptors
	60 mg/kg PO q24h[236]	Pigeons/PK
	60-72 mg/kg PO q12h[140]	Cranes
	75 mg/kg IM q12h[59]	Most species/reduce dose if regurgitation occurs[289]

Continued

TABLE 5-1 Antimicrobial Agents Used in Birds. (cont'd)

Agent	Dosage	Species/Comments
Trimethoprim/ sulfamethoxazole (cont'd)	100 mg/kg PO q12h[59]	Most species, including psittacines
	144 mg/kg PO q8-12h[793]	Most species
	360-400 mg/L drinking water × 10-14 days[788]	Most species, including pigeons
Trimethoprim/ sulfatroxazole	—	Potentiated sulfonamide combination antibiotic; broad spectrum[106]
	10-50 mg/kg PO q12h[241]	Passerines
Tylosin	—	Macrolide antibiotic; effective against most aerobic and anaerobic gram-positive bacteria, may be effective against gram-negative organisms; active against *Mycobacterium* (including atypical species), *Chlamydia*, and *Mycoplasma*; potentially irritating to muscle when administered IM[106]
	3-5 mg/kg IM, IV q12h[939]	Ratites
	5-10 mg/kg PO q8h[939]	Ratites
	15 mg/kg IM q8h[543]	Cranes/PK
	15-30 mg/kg IM q12h × 3 days[391]	Raptors
	17 mg/kg IM q24h × 7 days[610]	Emus/*Mycoplasma*
	20-40 mg/kg IM q8h[802]	Psittacines
	25 mg/kg IM q8h[543]	Emus/PK
	25 mg/kg IM q6h[543]	Pigeons, quail/PK
	30 mg/kg IM q12h[89]	Most species/*Mycoplasma*
	50 mg/kg PO q24h[391]	Passerines, pigeons
	50 mg/L drinking water[789]	Most species
	250-400 mg/L drinking water[239]	Canaries
	300 mg/L drinking water × 6 wk[651]	House finches/*Mycoplasma*
	500 mg/L drinking water × 3-28 days[391]	Pigeons, emus/*Mycoplasma*
	800 mg/L drinking water[378]	Pigeons
	1000 mg/L drinking water × 21 days[586]	House finches/*Mycoplasma*; give in conjunction with ophthalmic ciprofloxacin
	2000 mg/L drinking water[391]	Pigeons/*Mycoplasma*, *Haemophilus*

[a]Many drug doses used in birds are empirical. Patients should be monitored for adverse effects and treatment failure.[289]

TABLE 5-2 Antifungal Agents Used in Birds.

Agent	Dosage	Species/Comments
Amphotericin B	—	Polyene macrolide antifungal agent; broad activity against various types of fungi, but susceptibility varies as to species; ineffective against dermatophytes: primary use is for systemic fungal infections[107]
	1 mg/kg intratracheal q8-12h, dilute to 1 mL with sterile water[745,768]	Psittacines, raptors/aspergillosis
	1 mg/kg intratracheal q12h × 12 days, then q48h × 5 wk[89]	Raptors/syringeal aspergilloma
	1.5 mg/kg IV q8h × 3-7 days[391,745]	Most species
	100-109 mg/kg PO by gavage q12h × 10-30 days[617]	Budgerigars/*Macrorhabdus*; compound in simple syrup; resistance reported in budgerigars in Australia[702]
	0.05 mg/mL sterile water[60]	Most species/nasal flush
	0.2 mL PO q12h × 10 days[177]	Budgerigars/*Macrorhabdus*; use IV formulation (5 mg/mL)
	0.25-1 mL PO q24h × 4-5 days[89]	Raptor neonates/candidiasis
	1 mg/kg intralesionally[722]	Conures/pulmonary lesions; administered endoscopically with injection needle along with systemic therapy
	1000 mg/L drinking water × 28 days[702,713]	Budgerigars/*Macrorhabdus*
	Topical[177]	Apply 10% solution to oropharynx
	1.35 mg/kg topical q24h of liposomally encapsulated formulation in sterile, water-soluble lubricating gel[100]	Herons
	7 mg/mL saline q12h[943]	Most species/nebulization × 15 min
Amphotericin B (3% cream)	Topical to affected area q12h[768]	Most species/mycoses
Clotrimazole	—	Imidazole antifungal agent; variable sensitivity between yeasts and fungi; superficial mycoses and candidiasis[107]
	2 mg/kg intratracheal q24h × 5 days[789]	Psittacines/syringeal aspergilloma; apply with catheter directly into syrinx during anesthesia
	Inject 10 mg/kg into air sacs[789]	Psittacines/dilute in propylene glycol to 2.5 mg/mL; divide total dose between the four most accessible air sacs; toxic and may result in death in African grey parrots and other birds if injected into the viscera or IM[789]
	10 mg/mL saline flush[702]	Most species/effective against *Aspergillus* at sites that can be flushed; nasal flush using 1% solution
	1% solution[943]	Nebulization × 30-60 min

Continued

TABLE 5-2 Antifungal Agents Used in Birds. (cont'd)

Agent	Dosage	Species/Comments
Enilconazole emulsion	—	Imidazole antifungal agent; variable sensitivity between yeasts and fungi; superficial mycoses and candidiasis;[107] used topically and for nasal flush
	1 mg (0.5 mL)/kg intratracheal of a 1:10 dilution q24h × 7-14 days[812]	Falcons/aspergillosis
	6 mg/kg PO q12h[15]	Eclectus parrots/glossal candidiasis; increased AST activity after 7 days of treatment
	200 mg/L drinking water[15]	Canaries/cutaneous dermatophytosis
	Topical or intratracheal 1:10-1:100 dilution[90]	Psittacines/aspergillosis, candidiasis
	Topical 1:10 dilution q12h × 21-28 days[89]	Raptors/cutaneous aspergillosis, candidiasis
	3 topical soakings q3d[745]	Raptors, ostriches/dermatophytosis
	0.1 mL/kg in 5 mL sterile water, nebulize × 30 min, 5 days on, 2 off, up to 90 days[397]	Raptors/aspergillosis
Fluconazole	—	Imidazole antifungal agent; variable sensitivity between yeasts and fungi; systemic mycoses and candidiasis; relatively good penetration into CSF;[107] death observed in budgerigars at 10 mg/kg PO q12h (this dose was also ineffective against avian gastric yeast)[702]
	2-5 mg/kg PO q24h × 7-10 days[89,665]	Most species, including raptors/gastrointestinal, systemic candidiasis; CNS, ocular mycoses
	4-6 mg/kg PO q12h[287]	Juvenile psittacines/candidiasis
	5 mg/kg PO q24h[741]	Cockatiels/PK; candidiasis
	5-10 mg/kg PO q24h[58,59]	Gouldian finches/candidiasis
	8 mg/kg PO q24h × 30 days[941]	Psittacines/cryptococcosis
	10 mg/kg PO q48h[741]	Cockatiels/PK; candidiasis
	10 or 20 mg/kg PO q48h[294]	African grey parrot/PK; common yeast species; mucosal, systemic yeast infections; 2-3 treatments for resistant candidiasis; death of budgerigars at 10 mg/kg PO q12h; this latter dose ineffective against avian gastric yeast
	10-20 mg/kg PO q24-48h × 30 days[445]	Red-tailed hawks, gyrfalcons/aspergillosis
	15 mg/kg PO q12h × ≥28 days[788,791]	Pigeons/aspergillosis
	15 mg/kg PO q12h × 30 days following cessation of clinical signs[11]	Psittacines/chronic nasal aspergillosis

TABLE 5-2 Antifungal Agents Used in Birds. (cont'd)

Agent	Dosage	Species/Comments
Fluconazole (cont'd)	25 mg/L nectar[387,669]	Hummingbirds/aspergillosis
	50 mg/L drinking water × 14-60 days[789]	Most species/systemic mycoses; candidiasis
	100 mg/L drinking water × 8 days[741]	Cockatiels/ PK candidiasis
	150 mg/L drinking water[78,59]	Gouldian finches/candidiasis
	100 mg/kg soft food[58,59]	Gouldian finches/candidiasis
Flucytosine	—	Fluorinated pyrimidine antifungal agent; not used as sole agent because resistance develops rapidly; effective against *Cryptococcocus*, *Candida*, and *Aspergillus*; excellent CSF, aqueous humor peneteration;[107] use prophylactically in raptors (especially falcons) to prevent aspergillosis[a]
	20-30 mg/kg PO q6h × 20-90 days[420]	Raptors/aspergillosis
	20-75 mg/kg PO q12h × 21 days[802]	Psittacines/generalized yeast or fungal infections
	50 mg/kg PO q12h × 14-28 days[665]	Psittacines, passerines, raptors
	50-75 mg/kg PO q8h[745] 75 mg/kg q12h × 5-7 days, then q24h × 14 days[745]	Raptors/aspergillosis prophylaxis; treat 1 wk prior to and 2 wk after move for domestically raised gyrfalcons and gyrfalcon hybrids from age 45 days
	75-120 mg/kg PO q6h[665]	Most species
	80-100 mg/kg PO q12h[939]	Ratites
	100-250 mg/kg PO q12h[457,458]	Psittacine neonates
	250 mg/kg PO q12h × 14-17 days[908]	Finches/endoventricular mycoses; can use with chlorhexidine in drinking water
	50-250 mg/kg feed[767]	Psittacines, mynah birds
Griseofulvin	—	Systemic antifungal agent; effective against common dermatophytes[107]
	10 mg/kg PO q12h × 21 days[802]	Pigeons/dermatophytosis; gavage
	30-50 mg/kg in drinking water q24h[938]	Ostriches/mycotic dermatitis
Iodine, 1% solution	Topical[745]	Most species/oral or cutaneous candidiasis
Itraconazole	—	Imidazole antifungal agent; variable sensitivity between yeasts and fungi; systemic mycoses and candidiasis; relatively good penetration into CSF;[107] commercially available suspension is recommended as a first choice; use caution using compounded formulations because bulk drug may not be bioavailable or stable[127,202]

Continued

TABLE 5-2 Antifungal Agents Used in Birds. (cont'd)

Agent	Dosage	Species/Comments
Itraconazole (cont'd)	5-10 mg/kg PO q24h[667]	Blue-fronted Amazon parrots/PK; aspergillosis; 10 mg/kg required [therapeutic] for poorly perfused tissues; anorexia, depression, toxicity at higher doses in African grey parrots[288,702]
	5-10 mg/kg PO q12-24h × 10-14 days, then q48h[420]	Raptors/aspergillosis prophylaxis[a]
	5-10 mg/kg PO q12h × 5 days, followed by q24h for a total of 14 days[745]	Raptors/suggested for Class I aspergillosis (mild, vague signs, inconclusive diagnostics, without histologic confirmation)
	5-10 mg/kg PO q12h × 5 days, followed by q24h × 60-90 days[745]	Raptors/Class II-IV aspergillosis
	5-10 mg/kg PO q12h[466,767,896]	Passerines (towhees), penguins/aspergillosis prophylaxis in passerines; aspergillosis, candidiasis, and cryptococcosis in others
	6 mg/kg PO q12h[557]	Pigeons/PK; dosage achieved fungicidal [plasma]
	6-8 mg/kg PO q12h × 5-7 days then q24h × 14 days[745]	Raptors/aspergillosis prevention; treat 1 wk prior and 2 wk after move for domestically raised gyrfalcons and gyrfalcon hybrids from age 45 days
	6-10 mg/kg PO[442]	Ratites
	10 mg/kg PO q24h[391,453]	Gentoo penguins, red-tailed hawks/PK
	10 mg/kg PO q24h × 14-90 days with food[665,666,702]	Psittacines/use in combination with nonazoles
	10 mg/kg PO q12h × 21-60 days[177,908]	Finches/endoventricular mycoses; can use with chlorhexidine in drinking water
	15 mg/kg PO q12h up to 4-6 wk[420]	Raptors/aspergillosis
	20 mg/kg PO q24h[127,925]	Mallard ducks, penguins/PK
	26 mg/kg PO q12h[557]	Pigeons/PK; fungicidal levels in respiratory tissue; further toxicologic studies required
	200 mg/kg feed up to 100 days[758]	Gouldian finches/PK; dermatomycoses; beads from capsules were mixed with small amount of oil and seed
Ketoconazole	—	Imidazole antifungal agent; fungistatic; variable sensitivity between yeasts and fungi; systemic fungal infections[107]
	5-10 mg/kg PO q24h[939]	Ratites
	8 mg/kg PO q12h × 30 days[84,442]	Ostriches
	10-20 mg/kg PO q24h[84,442]	Ostriches
	15 mg/kg PO q12h[450,455]	Raptors/candidiasis
	20 mg/kg PO q24h × 14 days[177,490]	Psittacines, passerines, raptors

TABLE 5-2 Antifungal Agents Used in Birds. (cont'd)

Agent	Dosage	Species/Comments
Ketoconazole (cont'd)	20 mg/kg PO q8h × 7-14 days[702]	Psittacines/refractory candidiasis
	20-30 mg/kg PO q8h[665]	Cockatoos
	20-40 mg/kg PO q12h × 15-60 days[784,791]	Pigeons
	25 mg/kg PO q12h × 14 days[802]	Ratites, raptors/aspergillosis
	30 mg/kg PO q12h × 7-14 days[490]	Amazon parrots/PK
	50 mg/kg/day PO[180]	Toucans
	60 mg/kg PO q12h[975]	Raptors, common buzzards (PK)/aspergillosis
	200 mg/L drinking water, nectar, or soft feed × 7-14 days[58,285,286,387]	Canaries, hummingbirds, Gouldian finches/ dissolve crushed tablet in ½-1 tsp vinegar
Miconazole	—	Imidazole antifungal agent; topical preparations for local dermatophytosis;[107] injectable product not available in the United States
	5 mg/kg intratracheal q12h × 5 days[391]	Psittacines/10 mg/mL solution diluted with saline; syringeal mycoses; use with flucytosine; clotrimazole may be an alternative
	10 mg/kg IM q24h × 6-12 days[802]	Raptors/generalized aspergillosis
	20 mg/kg IV q8h[802]	Psittacines/candidiasis, cryptococcosis
	Topical to affected areas q12h[745]	Most species/cutaneous fungal infections; used in conjunction with oral itraconazole; dermatophytosis
Nystatin	—	Polyene macrolide antifungal agent; used topically or orally to treat gastrointestinal candidiasis; can be effective against other yeast and fungi; it is not (or is not appreciably) absorbed from the gastrointestinal tract[107]
	5000 U/bird PO q12h × 10 days[275,276]	Goldfinches/*Macrorhabdus*; ineffective in budgerigars
	20,000-100,000 U/bird PO q24h × 7 days[98,802]	Pigeons/candidiasis
	100,000 U/kg PO q12h[377,450,455]	Pigeons, raptors
	250,000-430,000 U/kg PO q12h[387]	Hummingbirds
	250,000-500,000 U/kg PO q12h[939]	Ratites
	300,000 U/kg PO q12h × 7-14 days[89,285,664]	Most species
	300,000-600,000 U/kg PO q8-12h × 7-14 days[175-177]	Psittacines

Continued

TABLE 5-2 Antifungal Agents Used in Birds. (cont'd)

Agent	Dosage	Species/Comments
Nystatin (cont'd)	500,000 U/kg PO q8h × 5 days[191]	Toucanetes (saffron)/candidiasis
	Topical q6h[428]	Hummingbirds/candidiasis; direct application using a cotton swab
	25,000 U/L nectar[428]	Hummingbirds
	100,000 U/L drinking water[57,58,239]	Canaries, finches
	200,000 U/kg soft feed[57,58]	Canaries, finches
Povidone-iodine	Topical to lesions, then rinse[59,89]	Raptors/wound cleansing; antibacterial, antifungal activity
Sodium benzoate	1 tsp/L water × 5 wk[409,412]	Cleared infection in nonbreeding budgerigars; 0.5 tsp/L caused neurologic signs, death in breeding budgies[412]
Silver sulfadiazine	Topical to affected areas q12-24h[272,768]	Most species, bandage application preferred
STA solution (salicyclic acid 3 g, tannic acid 3 g, ethyl alcohol to 100 mL)	Topical[768,793]	Fungal dermatitis
Terbinafine	—	Allylamine antifungal used topically for dermatophytes; fungicidal; systemic fungal infections;[107] questionable therapeutic potential for treatment of aspergillosis in avian species; higer dose or use in combination with itraconazole may be more effective[292]
	10-15 mg/kg PO q12-24h[201]	Most species/PK
	15 mg/kg PO q24h[79]	Penguins/PK
	15-30 mg/kg PO q12h[292]	Most species
	22 mg/kg PO q24h[80]	Raptors/PK
	60 mg/kg PO q24h[269]	Hispaniolan Amazon parrots/PK
	60 mg/kg PO q8h[778]	Common shelduck/PK
	1 mg/mL solution via nebulization[259]	Hispaniolan Amazon parrots/PK raw powder maintained MIC concentrations for 4 hr vs. 1 hr for crushed tablets
Voriconazole	—	Imidazole antifungal agent[107] used in avian species for the treatment of aspergillosis;[844] some pigeon strains resistant;[84] difficult to extrapolate drug doses between species; voriconazole toxicity reported for multiple penguin species;[424] compounded suspensions stable up to 30 days at room temperature[649]
	5 mg/kg PO q24h[423a]	African penguins/PK
	10 mg/kg PO q12h or 20 mg/kg q24h[82,83,84]	Pigeons/PK and PD

TABLE 5-2 Antifungal Agents Used in Birds. (cont'd)

Agent	Dosage	Species/Comments
Voriconazole (cont'd)	10-15 mg/kg PO q8h, food delays absorption [335,678,846]	Red-tailed hawks/PK
	12-18 mg/kg PO q12h[302]	African grey parrots/PK
	12.5 mg/kg PO q12h[225,834]	Falcons/PK
	18 mg/kg PO q8h[819]	Amazon parrots/PK
	20 mg/kg PO q24h × 21 days[128,677,924]	Many species

[a]Prophylactic use of antifungal agents may be indicated in newly captured or admitted birds of susceptible species and in birds undergoing change of management or transfer of enclosure.[745]

TABLE 5-3 Antiviral and Immunomodulating Agents Used in Birds.

Agent	Dosage	Species/Comments
Acyclovir	—	Antiviral agent for herpesviruses cytomegalovirus; IM injection of IV water-soluble sodium salt may cause severe muscle necrosis; phlebitis; neurologic signs may occur with IV administration; best administered prior to clinical signs; treat birds a minimum of 7 days; unstable reconstituted solution may be frozen in aliquots[15,793]
	80 mg/kg PO q8h x 7 days[653]	Quaker parrot/PD; psittacine herpesvirus prophylaxis or treatment
	120 mg/kg PO q12h[794]	Tragopans/PK
	330 mg/kg PO q12h × 4-7 days[458]	Psittacine neonates/psittacine herpesvirus
	330 mg/kg PO q12h × 7-14 days[420]	Raptors/falcon and owl herpesvirus; may cause vomiting
	1000 mg/L drinking water, gavage[189,766]	Quaker parrot/herpesvirus
	≤400 mg/kg feed[189]	Quaker parrot/herpesvirus
Amantadine	1 mg/kg PO q24h × 3 wk[349]	African grey parrots/no effect on avian bornavirus infection
Cyclosporine	~ 2 mg/kg PO q24h suspended in sesame oil[366]	Cockatiel/blocks proventricular dilatation and cell infiltrative diseases of birds infected with parrot bornavirus; may alleviate clinical signs of affected birds;[487] CBC monitoring and prophylactic concurrent treatment with itraconazole recommended
	3.5 mg/kg PO q12h[448]	Eclectus parrots/immune-mediated hemolytic anemia; efficacy unproven
Famciclovir	25 mg/kg PO q12h[936]	Ducklings/PD; antiviral for duck hepatitis; no toxic effects reported
Imiquimod cream	Topically 3x/wk[521,523]	Parrots/cloacal papillomatosis; may boost host cell-mediated immunity; masses may decrease in size; lack of complete remission

Continued

TABLE 5-3 Antiviral and Immunomodulating Agents Used in Birds. (cont'd)

Agent	Dosage	Species/Comments
Interferon α2	—	Glycoprotein with immunomodulating, antiproliferative, and antiviral activity
	30 U q24h x 5 days; 30 U 2x/wk × 2 wk; 30 U q7d × 2 wk (route not specified)[353]	May cause temporary improvement of proventricular dilatation disease
	60-240 U/kg SC, IM q12h[853] or 300-1200 U/kg PO q12h[789]	Most species/stock solution: mix 1 mL (3,000,000 U/mL) with 100 mL sterile water (30,000 U/mL); freeze as 2 mL vials up to 1 yr; mix 2 mL of stock into 1 L LRS (= 60 U/mL); refrigerate up to 3 mo
	1500 U/kg PO q24h[15]	Psittacines
	1,000,000 U IM q48h to q7d × 3 treatments[889]	African grey parrots/circovirus; omega alpha-2 interferon
	1000 U/L drinking water × 14-28 days[788]	Pigeons/circovirus
Levamisole	2 mg/kg SC, IM q14d x 3 treatments[119,768]	Most species including macaws/immunostimulation; low therapeutic index with mortality reported
	11 mg/L drinking water × 3-5 wk[165]	Most species/25 mg/mL oral solutions can be prepared from tablets or powder with sterile water for irrigation and refrigerated for up to 90 days of storage[156]
Penciclovir (Denavir, Novartis)	10 mg/kg IP q24h × 12-24 wk[536]	Ducks/PD antiviral of herpesviruses; duck hepatitis B virus; reduction in viral levels without observed toxicity; dissolve in 2 mL of 1% DMSO
Propionibacterium acnes Immunostimulant (ImmunoRegulin, Neogen)	0.13 mg/kg (up to 0.08 mg [0.2 mL] max) SC, IM days 1, 3, 7, 14, 28, 42, then q30d[45]	Psittacines/immune therapy for chronic feather picking; do not use with corticosteroids; enhances cell-mediated immunity, natural killer cells activity, and macrophage and lymphokine production

TABLE 5-4 Antiparasitic Agents Used in Birds.

Agent	Dosage	Species/Comments
Albendazole (11.36%) (Valbazen, Zoetis)	—	Broad-spectrum anthelmintic; may be toxic in keas, some Columbiformes and other spp. at 50-100 mg/kg[418,887]
	5 mg/kg PO q12h × 3 days, repeat in 14 days[43]	Ratites/protozoal infections
	5.2 mg/kg PO q12h × 3 days, repeat in 14 days[939]	Ratites/flagellates, cestodes
	6 mg/kg PO once[210]	Ostriches/100% effective against *Libyostrongylus dentatus* and *L. douglassii*
	15-20 mg/kg PO once[391]	Toucans
	20 mg/kg PO, repeat in 7 days[564]	Cranes/effective against some trematodes

TABLE 5-4 Antiparasitic Agents Used in Birds. (cont'd)

Agent	Dosage	Species/Comments
Albendazole (11.36%) (Valbazen, Zoetis) (cont'd)	25 mg/kg PO q24h × 90 days, then repeat × 120 days when signs returned[705]	Cockatoos/*Encephalitozoon hellem* keratoconjunctivitis
	25-50 mg/kg PO q24h × 3-4 days[887]	Doves, rock partridges/*Capillaria;* toxicity occurred in some birds, use with caution
	50 mg/kg PO q24h × 5 days[137]	Amazon parrots/microsporidian keratoconjunctivitis
Amprolium	—	Pyridimine derivative coccidiostat; although rarely encountered, efficacy can be reduced by high doses of thiamine;[886] resistance common; some coccidial organisms of mynahs, toucans have shown resistance[43]
	2.2 mg/kg PO[145]	Sandhill cranes/ineffective in preventing experimentally induced disseminated visceral coccidiosis
	15-30 mg/kg PO q24h × 1-5 days[232]	Most species/treatment should be repeated after 5 days due to coccidial prepatent period[232]
	30 mg/kg PO q24h[510]	Merlins/may cause thiamine deficiency
	30 mg/kg PO q24h × 5 days[43,510]	Raptors
	5-100 mg/L drinking water × 5-7 days[43,873]	Most species/flock treatment
	50-100 mg/L drinking water × 5-7 days[203,232,391]	Most species, including passerines, parakeets
	60 mg/L drinking water[391]	Cranes
	200 mg/L drinking water[379]	Pigeons/flock treatment
	250 mg/L drinking water × 7 days[391]	Psittacines (keas)/*Sarcocystis;* use in combination with pyrimethamine and primaquine
	¼ tsp/L drinking water × 3-5 days[391]	Pigeons/20% soluble powder
	0.0125 mg/kg feed[564]	Cranes/coccidiosis prophylaxis
	0.025 mg/kg feed × 14 days[564]	Cranes/coccidiosis treatment
	115-235 mg/kg feed [391]	Poultry/coccidia; *Sarcocystis;* lower dose is prophylactic; higher dose is therapeutic
Cambendazole (Equiben, Merial)	60-100 mg/kg PO q24h × 3-7 days[232,391]	Most species
	75 mg/kg PO q24h × 2 day[43,381]	Pigeons
Carbaryl 5% (Sevin Dust, Garden Tech)	Topical; light dusting of plumage or nest box litter (1-2 tsp)[43,564]	Most species/ants, ectoparasites; remove treated litter after 24 hr

Continued

TABLE 5-4 Antiparasitic Agents Used in Birds. (cont'd)

Agent	Dosage	Species/Comments
Carnidazole (Spartrix, Wildlife Pharma-ceuticals)	—	Treatment for *Trichomonas, Hexamita, Histomonas*[43]
	5 mg/bird PO[391]	Doves (adults), pigeons (squabs)
	10 mg/bird PO[915]	Pink pigeons (adults)/*Trichomonas;* squabs ≤18 days old administer 5 mg
	12.5-25 mg/kg PO once[43,159]	Pigeons, raptors/*Trichomonas*, use lower dose with juvenile birds; combine with dimetridazole to treat flock
	20 mg/kg PO once[391]	Pigeons
	20 mg/kg q24h PO × 2 days[391]	Raptors
	20-25 mg/kg PO once[43,232,510]	Raptors/single dose not always effective in falcons, bustards with advanced infections; use lower dose for juveniles
	20-30 mg/kg PO q24h × 1-2 days[43,159]	Most species, including pigeons, psittacines
	20-30 mg/kg PO q24h × 5 days[22,873]	Passerines/*Trichomonas;* house finches reliably cleared *Trichomonas gallinae* if caught prior to clinical signs
	30 mg/kg PO once[306]	Raptors/*Trichomonas*
	30 mg/kg PO q12-24h × 3 days[450,754]	Raptors/*Trichomonas*
	30-50 mg/kg PO, repeat in 10-14 days[768]	Cockatiels/*Giardia*
	33 mg/kg PO, repeat in 14 and 28 days[58]	Society finches, Gouldian finches/flagellates; 0.5 mg/adult (based on 15 g); 0.25 mg/nestling (based on 7.5 g)
	50 mg/kg PO once[420]	Raptors
	120 mg/kg PO as single dose or divided over 2-5 days[945]	American kestrels, screech owls/*Trichomonas* infections resistant to treatment with lower doses
Chloroquine phosphate[a]	—	Generally used with primaquine for *Plasmodium, Haemoproteus,* and *Leucocytozoon;* overdose can result in death[43]
	10 mg/kg PO q7d[391]	Most species/preventive treatment for *Plasmodium* once bird is stable; use with primaquine (1 mg/kg PO q7d)
	10 mg/kg PO, then 5 mg/kg at 6, 12, 18 hr, then q24h × 10 days[43,963]	Magellanic penguins/upon diagnosis of *Plasmodium;* if still positive on blood smear after this regimen, continue with sulfadiazine-trimethoprim 40 mg/kg PO × 10 days
	10 mg/kg PO, then 5 mg/kg at 6, 24, 48 hr[142]	Raptors/use with 0.3 mg/kg primaquine (at 24 hr following the initial chloroquine dose) q24h × 7 days

TABLE 5-4 Antiparasitic Agents Used in Birds. (cont'd)

Agent	Dosage	Species/Comments
Chloroquine phosphate (cont'd)	10-15 mg/kg PO q12h × 2 doses, then q24h[510]	Raptors/*Plasmodium;* use with primaquine
	10-25 mg/kg PO, then 5-15 mg/kg at 6, 18, 24 hr[232]	Use in conjunction with primaquine
	20 mg/kg PO or IV, then 10 mg/kg at 6, 18, 24 hr; repeat q7d × 3-5 treatments[391]	Raptors/*Plasmodium;* IV is recommended for initial dose in acute cases; use with 1 mg/kg primaquine q24h × 2 days
	25 mg/kg PO, then 15 mg/kg PO at 12, 24, 48 hr[43,391,830]	Most species, including raptors/use with 0.75-1.3 mg/kg primaquine at 0 hr
	60 mg/kg PO q24h × 7 days[391]	Raptors/*Haemoproteus;* use in conjunction with mefloquine and primaquine
	2000 mg/L drinking water q24h × 14 days[159]	Passerines/juice covers bitter taste of drug
Chlorsulon (Curatrem, Merial)	—	Benzenesulfonamide anthelmintic and flukicide
	20 mg/kg PO q2wk × 3 treatments[510]	Raptors
Clazuril (Appertex, Janssen)	—	Benzene-acetonitrile anticoccidial; drug detected in eggs after multiple dosing[143]
	2.5 mg/bird PO once; can repeat monthly[964]	Pigeons/oocyst shedding commences 20 days post treatment
	5 mg/kg PO once[159]	Pigeons
	5-10 mg/kg PO q24h × 2 days[399,510]	Raptors
	5-10 mg/kg PO q72h × 3 treatments[43,178,510]	Raptors
	6.25 mg/kg PO once[45]	Pigeons
	7 mg/kg PO × 3 days, off 2 days, on 3 days[43,232]	Most species
	30 mg/kg PO once[159]	Raptors
	1.1 or 5.5 mg/kg feed[145]	Sandhill cranes/ineffective in preventing experimentally induced disseminated visceral coccidiosis
Coumaphos (powder containing 3% w/v coumaphos 2% w/v propoxur 5% w/v sulphanilamide; Negasunt, Bayer)	Topical dust onto feathers[43]	Most species/ectoparasites; useful for fly-blown wounds; contains carbamate propoxur
	20 mg/kg PO q14d × 3 treatments[43,510,767]	Psitacines, raptors/trematodes, cestodes
Crotamiton (Eurax, Westwood-Squibb)	Topical to affected areas[43]	Most species/mites (i.e., *Knemidokoptes*); use in combination with ivermectin
Cypermethrin (5%) (Max Con, Y-Tex)	Spray or dip with 2% solution[43]	Pigeons, ostriches/lice, mites; treatment of premises infested with *Dermanyssus* spp.

Continued

TABLE 5-4 Antiparasitic Agents Used in Birds. (cont'd)

Agent	Dosage	Species/Comments
Deltamethrin	50 mg/L topical spray[391]	Ostriches/lice; spray until runoff
Dichlorophene (tapeworm tablets, Happy Jack)	100 mg PO q10d × 2 treatments, repeat in 10 days prn[475]	Pigeons/cestodes; administer after a 12-hr fast
Diclazuril (Protazil, Merck)	—	Benzene-acetonitrile anticoccidial; some *Eimeria* resistance in poultry documented;[4,739] rotation suggested for long-term prevention
	10 mg/kg PO q12h on days 0, 1, 2, 4, 6, 8, 10[232,587]	Passerines, including Hawaiian crows/*Toxoplasma*
	5 mg/L drinking water[232]	Passerines/*Toxoplasma*
Dimetridazole (Emtryl 40% powder, MedPet)	—	*Trichomonas, Giardia, Hexamita, Spironucleus, Histomonas;* low therapeutic index; hepatotoxic to lories, some passerines (e.g., robins), and fledgling birds;[43] not recommended for finches; highly toxic to geese, ducks, and pigeons;[886] not available in many countries (United States, European Union) because of human health risks; Canada has banned use in food-producing animals;[640] do not give during breeding season
	50 mg/kg PO q24h × 10 days[626]	Falcons/*Enterocytozoon bieneusi*
	50 mg/kg PO or in drinking water q24h × 6 days[159]	Pigeons
	100 mg/L drinking water[239]	Canaries, finches
	200-400 mg/L drinking water × 5 days[232,391]	Psittacines/caution, toxic if overdosed; do not use in finches and Pekin robins; use lower dose in lorikeets and mynahs[232]
	250 mg/L drinking water × 4-6 days[391]	Gouldian finches/*Cochlostoma, Trichomonas*
	265 mg/L drinking water[391]	Pigeons
	300 mg/L drinking water × 10 days[45]	Bustards/prevention of *Trichomonas*
	400 mg/L drinking water × 3 days[427]	Pigeons/PK and PD; bioavailability reduced with feed
	666 mg/L drinking water × 7-12 days[43]	Pigeons/*Trichomonas, Giardia, Hexamita*
	900 mg/L drinking water × 5 days, followed by 700 mg/L × 10 days[43]	Bustards/treatment of choice for *Trichomonas*
	¼-½ tsp/gal drinking water × 3-5 days[378]	Pigeons/CNS symptoms if overdosed; because of variable water consumption, use lower dose in hot weather and higher dose in cool weather
	200-500 mg/kg feed[134]	Ostriches (≤3 mo of age)/*Trichomonas*
Doramectin (Dectomax, Zoetis)	1 mg/kg SC, IM,[43,510] repeat in 2 wk[159]	Raptors, bustards/used to treat gastrointestinal nematodes, lungworms, eyeworms, mites[43]

TABLE 5-4 Antiparasitic Agents Used in Birds. (cont'd)

Agent	Dosage	Species/Comments
Doxycycline	20 mg/kg PO q12h × 10 days[357]	Humboldt penguins/*Plasmodium*
Febantel (Vercom, Bayer)	5 mg/kg PO[585]	Ostriches
	20 mg/kg PO[585]	Ostriches
	30 mg/kg PO once[38,232]	Pigeons/PK and PD; ascarids; repeated doses required to eliminate *Capillaria obsignata*
	37.5 mg/kg PO once[43]	Pigeons
Fenbendazole (Panacur, Merck)	—	Most species/anthelmintic effective against cestodes, nematodes, trematodes, *Giardia*, acanthocephalans; toxicity documented in pigeons and doves;[345,418,675,772] may be toxic for other species, including raptors,[789] vultures,[101,420] lories,[675] storks,[101,977] pelicans;[539] can cause feather abnormalities if administered during molting;[43] ineffective against finch ventricular worms;[43] can be toxic to bone marrow, causing leukopenia[232]
	8-10 mg/kg q24h × 3-4 days[232]	Most species
	10-20 mg/kg PO q24h × 3 days[159]	Pigeons/nematodes
	10-50 mg/kg PO, repeat in 14 days[420,455]	Raptors/nematodes, trematodes
	15 mg/kg PO[179,391]	Ostriches/"wire worms," nematodes, cestodes
	15 mg/kg PO q24h × 5 days[43]	Psittacines
	15 mg/kg PO × 5 days, then off 5 days × 4 treatments[599]	Umbrella cockatoos/proventricular Spiruroidea (nematodes)
	15 mg/kg PO q3wk[179]	Ratite chicks/nematodes; administer at this frequency until 4 mo old, then at adult prophylaxis dosing intervals
	15-25 mg/kg PO × 4-5 days[864]	Tinamous
	15-45 mg/kg PO[391]	Ostriches
	20 mg/kg PO q24h × 10-14 days[178]	Raptors/filarids
	20-25 mg/kg PO q24h × 5 days[178,306,510,751]	Raptors/*Capillaria*
	20-50 mg/kg PO q24h[43,391]	Psittacines, pigeons/ascarids in psittacines, treat once and repeat in 10 days; trematodes and microfilaria, treat for 3 days; *Capillaria*, treat for 5 days
	20-50 mg/kg PO q24h × 3 days, repeat in 2 wk[976]	Penguins[a]
	20-50 mg/kg PO q24h × 3 days, repeat in 21 days[420]	Raptors

Continued

TABLE 5-4 Antiparasitic Agents Used in Birds. (cont'd)

Agent	Dosage	Species/Comments
Fenbendazole (Panacur, Merck) (cont'd)	25 mg/kg PO, repeat in 14 days[172,875]	Most species, including owls/ascarids
	25 mg/kg PO q24h × 5 days,[159] repeat in 10-14 days[420]	Raptors/*Capillaria*, spirurids
	25 mg/kg PO q6wk[179]	Ratites/cestode prophylaxis
	25-50 mg/kg PO once[232]	Most species
	30 mg/kg PO once[43]	Bustards
	30 mg/kg PO q24h × 5-8 days[18]	Falcons/eliminated *Serratospiculoides* fecal eggs and larvae
	33 mg/kg PO q24h × 3 days[177]	Psittacines, passerines, raptors/microfilaria, trematodes
	50 mg/kg PO q24h × 3-5 days[232,391,652,873]	Most species, including pigeons, Bali mynahs/ nematodes, trematodes, *Giardia*
	50 mg/kg PO q24h × 5 days[564]	Cranes/*Capillaria*, gapeworms
	50 mg/kg PO q12h × 5 days[391]	Cockatoos/filarid adulticide treatment; use with ivermectin (0.2 mg/kg once)
	50 mg/kg q24h × 5 days[264]	Scops owls (fledglings)/treatment of *Gongylonema pulchrum* oral plaques
	50-100 mg/kg PO, repeat in 14 days[564]	Cranes/intestinal strongyles, ascarids
	100 mg/kg PO once, repeat in 10-14 days[510]	Raptors/*Capillaria*, spirurids
	100 mg/kg PO q24h × 5 days[140]	Cranes/*Capillaria*
	50 mg/L drinking water × 5 days[391]	Finches
	125 mg/L drinking water × 5 days[391]	Most species/nematodes
Fipronil	—	Do not use spot-on preparation; use with caution in raptors, pigeons, passerines/ectoparasites; apply via pad to base of neck, tail base, and under each wing; avoid plumage during application; alcohol may create dry, brittle feathers; do not soak bird; do not exceed 7.5 mg/kg in zebra finches[481] and wild[337] species; significant toxicity reported from mortality to sublethal effects such as cytotoxic effects,[223] impaired immune function,[546] and reduced growth and reproductive success,[499] often at concentrations well below those associated with mortality;[337,482] environmental contamination and secondary intoxication are of concern[337,480]
	3 mg/kg; spray on skin once[232]	
	7.5 mg/kg; spray on skin once, repeat in 30 days prn[43,159,306,873]	

TABLE 5-4 Antiparasitic Agents Used in Birds. (cont'd)

Agent	Dosage	Species/Comments
Flubendazole (Flutelmium 7.5%, Janssen-Cilag)	30-60 mg/kg feed × 7 days[391]	Tinamous/follow Veterinary Feed Directive (VFD) guidelines
Hydroxychloroquine sulfate	—	Antimalarial
	830 mg/L drinking water × 6 wk[391]	Pigeons/*Plasmodium*
Hygromycin B (Hygromix 8, Elanco)	—	Aminoglycoside antibiotic used as anthelmintic feed additive; follow VFD guidelines
Imidocarb dipropionate (Imizol, Merck)	—	Antiprotozoal effective against *Babesia*
	5-7 mg/kg IM once, repeat in 7 days[809,988]	Raptors/*Babesia;* some cases require a total of 3 treatments
Ipronidazole (Ipropran, Roche)	—	*Giardia, Trichomonas, Histomonas;* not available in the United States; 61 g/2.65 oz
	130 mg/L drinking water × 7 days[391]	Most species, including pigeons
	250 mg/L drinking water × 3-7 days[391]	Psittacines, pigeons
Ivermectin	—	All species/most nematodes, acanthocephalans, leeches, most ectoparasites (including *Knemidokoptes, Dermanyssus*); can dilute with water or saline for immediate use; dilute with propylene glycol for extended use; parenteral ivermectin may be toxic to finches and budgerigars;[391] brain inflammation detected as an adverse effect in king pigeons;[155] suspected toxicity reported in a nanday conure at 0.2 mg/kg[695]
	0.2 mg/kg PO, SC, IM once, can repeat in 10-14 days[43,159,378,442,564,663,873]	Most species, including psittacines, passerines, pigeons, raptors, guinea fowl, ratites, cranes/ use in combination with fenbendazole at 50 mg/kg PO q12h × 5 days for microfilaria in cockatoos[391]
	0.2 mg/kg IM once[205,210]	Ostriches/only 60% effective against *Libyostrongylus dentatus* and *L. douglassii*
	0.2-0.4 mg/kg PO, SC, repeat 7-14 days[976]	Penguins
	0.2-1 mg/kg PO, SC, IM q14d × 2-3 treatments[510]	Raptors
	0.2 mg/kg SC, topical on skin; can repeat 1-2 wk for 3-4 applications[159,203,244,861]	Canaries, finches/quill mites, *Knemidokoptes;* dilute to 0.02% solution with propylene glycol, can apply directly to lesions on cere, legs; also effective against the tracheal mite *Ptilonyssus morofskyi*[27]
	0.4 mg/kg SC once[391]	Raptors, passerines/*Capillaria* in towhees

Continued

TABLE 5-4 Antiparasitic Agents Used in Birds. (cont'd)

Agent	Dosage	Species/Comments
Ivermectin (cont'd)	0.4 mg/kg IM q7d × 7 treatments[799]	Golden eagles/required additional treatment with selamectin to achieve eradication of a novel *Micknemidokoptes* spp. mite
	0.5-1 mg/kg PO, IM once[378]	Pigeons
	1 mg/kg SC, repeat in 7 days[805]	Falcons/*Serratospiculum*
	2 mg/kg IM once[920]	Falcons/*Capillaria;* no adverse effects observed at this dose
	0.8-1 mg/L drinking water[239]	Canaries
	1 drop (0.05 mL) to skin q7d × 3 treatments[43]	Pigeons, Passerines/*Knemidokoptes, Dermanyssus*
Levamisole (Tramisol, Schering-Plough)	—	Many species/nematodes; immunostimulant; low therapeutic index (toxic reactions, deaths reported); do not use in debilitated birds;[43] IM administration may cause severe toxicity; limb paralysis, vomiting, dyspnea reported in a parakeet; do not use in white-faced ibis or in lories; withhold food before treatment to prevent regurgitation[391]
	1.5 mg/kg split into 2 doses and administered topically in eyes[624]	Ostriches/PD; effective against *Philophthalmus gralli*
	2-5 mg/kg SC, IM, repeat in 10-14 days × 3 treatments[43]	Psittacines/immunostimulant
	7.5 mg/kg PO, SC[134]	Ostriches
	7.5 mg/kg IM once; can repeat in 7 days[43]	Pigeons
	10-20 mg/kg PO, SC q24h × 2 days[178,420]	Raptors
	10-20 mg/kg SC once[43,391,510]	Most species
	15-20 mg/bird PO once, repeat in 10 days[159]	Pigeons
	20 mg/kg PO once[43]	Psittacines, pigeons, raptors
	20-40 mg/kg IM once[232,510]	Raptors
	20-50 mg/kg PO × 1-3 days[43]	Psittacines/low therapeutic index
	25 mg/kg PO once[564]	Crane chicks/*Capillaria*, intestinal strongyles, ascarids
	30 mg/kg PO q3wk[179]	Ratite chicks/administer at this dosage until 4 mo of age, then reduce to adult prophylaxis interval thereafter
	30 mg/kg PO q10d[179]	Ratites/cestodes, nematodes
	40 mg/kg PO once[43,510,564]	Psittacines, pigeons, raptors, cranes/*Capillaria*, intestinal strongyles, ascarids

TABLE 5-4 Antiparasitic Agents Used in Birds. (cont'd)

Agent	Dosage	Species/Comments
Levamisole (Tramisol, Schering-Plough) (cont'd)	100-200 mg/L drinking water × 3 days, repeat in 2 wk[159,232]	Psittacines, passerines, raptors
	264-396 mg/L drinking water × 1-3 days[391]	Most species, including pigeons
	300-400 mg/L drinking water for 24 hr, repeat in 7 days[43]	Pigeons/loft treatment for capillariasis, ascaridiasis
	375 mg/L drinking water as sole water source for 24 hr, repeat in 7 days[43]	Pigeons
Mebendazole (Telmin Suspension, Telmintic Powder, Schering-Plough)	5-6 mg/kg PO q24h × 3-5 days, repeat in 21 days[391]	Pigeons
	5-7 mg/kg PO[939]	Ostriches
	10 mg/kg PO q12h × 5 days[391]	Canaries/avoid use during breeding season
	10-25 mg/kg q12h × 5 days[232]	Most species
	20 mg/kg PO q24h × 10-14 days[43,178,510]	Raptors/filarids
	25 mg/kg PO q12h × 5 days[191]	Psittacines, ramphastids (toucans)/nematodes; may not be effective for proventricular and ventricular parasites
	25 mg/kg PO q12h × 5 days, repeat q30d[420]	Raptors/intestinal nematodiasis
	50 mg/kg PO, repeat in 10-14 days[420]	Raptors/intestinal nematodiasis
	10-20 mg/L drinking water × 3-5 days[232,391]	Pigeons
Mefloquine HCl (Lariam, Hoffman-LaRoche)	—	Antimalarial; active against erythrocytic and tissue schizonts of some *Plasmodium*[760,921]
	30 mg/kg PO q12h × 1 day, then q24h × 1-2 days[456,510,921,988]	Raptors
	30 mg/kg PO q12h × 1 day, then q24h × 2 days, then q7d[510]	Raptors/long-term administration up to 6 mo reported
	30 mg/kg PO q7d[357]	Penguins/*Plasmodium* routine prevention during insect season
	50 mg/kg PO q24h[633]	Raptors/*Haemoproteus;* used in conjunction with chloroquine at doses up to 60 mg/kg
	50 mg/kg PO q24h × 7 days[159]	Raptors/*Plasmodium*

Continued

TABLE 5-4 Antiparasitic Agents Used in Birds. (cont'd)

Agent	Dosage	Species/Comments
Melarsomine dihydrochloride (Immiticide, Merial)	—	Organic arsenical
	0.25 mg/kg IM q24h × 4 days[159]	Raptors/*Leucocytozoon*
Melarsomine dihydrochloride (M)/ ivermectin (I)	(M) 0.25 mg/kg IM q24h × 2 days followed 10 days later with (I) 1 mg/kg IM[918]	Falcons/*Serratospiculum;* reduced clinical signs and eliminated shedding of embryonated eggs
Mepacrine HCl	—	Nonsteroidal antiinflammatory used as an antiprotozoal for *Giardia* in humans
	0.24 mg/kg PO q12h[232]	Canaries/*Plasmodium*
Metronidazole	—	Most species/antiprotozoal, including alimentary tract protozoa (especially flagellates such as *Giardia, Histomonas, Spironucleus, Trichomonas*); resistance identified in racing pigeons[785]
	10-20 mg/kg IM q12-24h × 2 days[391]	Pigeons, psittacines
	10-30 mg/kg PO, IM q12h × 10 days [43,941]	Psittacines
	20-25 mg/kg PO q12h[939]	Ratites
	25 mg/kg PO q12h × 2-10 days[389]	Psittacine neonates
	25-50 mg/kg PO q12-24h × 5-10 days[391]	Companion birds/treatment, control, or prevention of *Giardia, Trichomonas*, and *Hexamita*
	25-50 mg/kg PO q12-24h[291]	Pigeons/use lower dose with twice-daily dosing
	30 mg/kg PO via gavage once[274,873]	Passerines, including finches/*Cochlosoma*
	30 mg/kg PO q12h × 5-10 days[58]	Raptors, Gouldian finches, psittacines/*Trichomonas*
	30-50 mg/kg PO q24h × 3-5 days[755]	Raptors/*Trichomonas*
	40 mg/kg PO q24h[391]	Rheas
	40 mg/kg PO q24h × 7 days[391]	Budgerigars/*Trichomonas*
	40-50 mg/kg PO q24h × 5-7 days[159]	Pigeons
	50 mg/kg PO q12-24h[232]	Most species/*Trichomonas, Giardia, Cochlosoma*
	50 mg/kg PO q24h × 5-7 days[43,178,306,420]	Raptors/*Trichomonas, Giardia*
	50 mg/kg PO q12h × 5 days[159,473]	Pigeons, passerines, raptors
	50-100 mg/kg PO q24h[510]	Raptors

TABLE 5-4 Antiparasitic Agents Used in Birds. (cont'd)

Agent	Dosage	Species/Comments
Metronidazole (cont'd)	100 mg/kg PO q24h × 3 days[807]	Falcons/*Trichomonas*
	100-150 mg PO total dose divided over 5 days[43]	Pigeons
	40 mg/L drinking water[274]	Finches/*Cochlosoma*
	40-80 mg/L drinking water × 3 days[232]	Most species/*Trichomonas*, *Giardia*, *Cochlosoma*
	100 mg/L drinking water[291]	Canaries
	200 mg/L drinking water × 7 days[159]	Passerines
	370 mg/L drinking water[391]	Passerines/protozoal sinusitis
	400 mg/L drinking water × 5-15 days[391]	Passerines/protozoal sinusitis
	1057 mg/L drinking water[391]	Pigeons
	1250 mg/L drinking water × 7-10 days[391]	Ratites
	100 mg/kg soft feed[391]	Canaries
Milbemycin oxime	2 mg/kg PO once[232]	Budgerigars, African finches, and European finches may be more sensitive
Monensin (Coban 45, Elanco)	—	Ionophore antibiotic; anticoccidial feed additive
	94 mg/kg feed[144]	Cranes/coccidia (including disseminated visceral coccidiosis)
	99 mg/kg feed[145,564]	Sandhill cranes/prevented experimentally induced disseminated visceral coccidiosis
Moxidectin (ProHeart, Zoetis)	—	Falcons/*Serratospiculum*, *Capillaria*, acanthocephalans, *Paraspiralatus sakeri,* and *Physaloptera alata*[43]
	0.2 mg/kg PO[159,805]	Raptors/nematodes
	0.2 mg/kg IM once[191]	Ramphastids (toucans)/repeat if necessary
	0.2 mg/kg IM once[210]	Ostriches/100% effective against *Libyostrongylus dentatus*, *L. douglassii*
	0.2-0.4 mg/kg PO, IM once[232]	
	0.5 mg/kg PO[43,510]	Raptors
	0.5-1 mg/kg PO[158]	Raptors/*Capillaria*
	1 mg/bird topically once, or can repeat q10d × 2 treatments[391]	Budgerigars/*Knemidokoptes;* no adverse effects seen at this dose in this species
Niclosamide (Yomesan, Bayer)	—	Cestodes, trematodes; rarely used since praziquantel is more efficacious; may be toxic for geese and some anseriformes; not available in the United States
	50-100 mg/kg PO, repeat in 10-14 days[232,391]	Ostriches

Continued

TABLE 5-4 Antiparasitic Agents Used in Birds. (cont'd)

Agent	Dosage	Species/Comments
Niclosamide (Yomesan, Bayer) (cont'd)	100 mg/kg PO q6wk[179]	Ostriches/cestode prophylaxis
	220 mg/kg PO, repeat in 10-14 days[391]	Most species
	250 mg/kg PO q14d prn[139]	Cranes
	500 mg/kg PO q7d × 4 wk[391]	Finches
Ormetoprim-sulfadimethoxine (Primor, Zoetis)	0.015% ormetoprim and 0.026% sulfadimethoxine in food × 3 wk[564]	Cranes/coccidiosis
Oxfendazole (Benzelmin, Syntex)	5 mg/kg PO once[391]	Ostriches/nematodes
	5 mg/kg PO q6wk[179]	Ratites/cestode, nematode prophylaxis
	5 mg/kg PO q3wk[179]	Ratite chicks/nematodes; administer at this frequency until 4 mo of age, then reduce to adult prophylactic dosing interval
	10-40 mg/kg PO once[232,578,895]	Most species, including finches/nematodes
	15-25 mg/kg PO once[191]	Ramphastids (toucans)/repeat in 15 days prn
	20 mg/kg PO once[399]	Raptors
Paromomycin	—	Highest efficacy of all drugs tested thus far against *Cryptosporidium;* oocyst output decreased by 67%-82% in chickens;[885] may result in secondary bacterial or mycotic infections; use with caution if ulcerative bowel lesions are suspected because renal toxicity may occur;[291] ineffective against *Histomonas*[419]
	100 mg/kg PO q12h × 7 days[1,232,396]	Most species, including macaw chicks, falcons/ mix a 250 mg capsule with 10 mL water to facilitate dosing; poorly absorbed
	1000 mg/kg soft food or hulled millet[391]	Gouldian finches/*Cryptosporidium;* may predispose to fungal infections
Permethrin	Dust plumage lightly[43]	Pigeons/lice, fleas
Permethrin, high-cis (Harker's Louse Powder, Harkers)	Topical application[43]	Raptors, psittacines/ectoparasites
Piperazine (Wazine, Fleming Laboratories)	—	Most species/ascarids, oxyurids; less efficacious than fenbendazole; seldom used in companion birds
	35 mg/kg PO q24h × 2 days[391]	Pigeons/ascarids
	50-100 mg/kg PO once[391,886]	Emus, ostriches
	100 mg/kg PO, repeat in 14 days[391,578]	Raptors
	100-250 mg/kg PO once[232]	Ascarids; resistance common
	250 mg/kg PO once[391]	Psittacines, pigeons

TABLE 5-4 Antiparasitic Agents Used in Birds. (cont'd)

Agent	Dosage	Species/Comments
Piperazine (Wazine, Fleming Laboratories) (cont'd)	79 mg/L drinking water × 2 days[391]	Pigeons/ascarids
	1000 mg/L drinking water × 3 days[391,578]	Raptors, pigeons
	1000-2000 mg/L drinking water × 1-2 days[159,391]	Game birds, pigeons
	3700 mg/L drinking water × 12 hr, repeat in 14-21 days[159]	Passerines
Piperonyl butoxide/ pyrethrin (Ridmite Powder, Johnson)	Dust plumage, repeat in 10 days[43,232]	Psittacines
	Dust plumage, repeat in 21 days[43]	Raptors
Piperonyl butoxide/ pyrethrin/methoprene (Avian Insect Liquidator, Vetafarm)	Apply to plumage, spray cages, aviaries, bird rooms, and surroundings[43]	Most species/fleas, lice, mosquitoes, moths, and some mites
Ponazuril (Marquis 5% paste; Bayer)	—	Triazine coccidiocidal drug; metabolite of toltrazuril
	10-20 mg/kg PO, repeat in 10-14 days	Most species, including pigeons, waterfowl[143]
	20 mg/kg q24h × 7 days[961]	Falcons/respiratory *Cryptosporidium baileyi*
Praziquantel (Droncit, Bayer)	—	Most species/cestodes, trematodes; injectable form toxic in finches and associated with depression, death in some species[43,391]
	1 mg/kg PO[43]	Bustards/well tolerated
	5-10 mg/kg PO, repeat after 2-4 wk[43,178,510]	Psittacines, passerines, raptors
	5-10 mg/kg PO, SC q24h × 14 days[391,420]	Raptors/trematodes
	6 mg/kg PO, IM, repeat in 10-14 days[564]	Cranes/cestodes, trematodes
	7.5 mg/kg PO[616]	Ostriches
	7.5 mg/kg SC, IM, repeat in 2-4 wk[159,177]	Most species except finches
	9 mg/kg IM, repeat in 10 days[43,391]	Psittacines/cestodes
	10 mg/kg PO, SC, IM once; repeat in 7 days[306]	Raptors/cestodes, trematodes
	10 mg/kg SC, IM q24h × 3 days, then PO × 11 days[420,941]	Psittacines, raptors/trematodes
	10 mg/kg IM q24h × 3 days, then PO q24h × 11 days[338]	Toucans/trematodes

Continued

TABLE 5-4 Antiparasitic Agents Used in Birds. (cont'd)

Agent	Dosage	Species/Comments
Praziquantel (Droncit, Bayer) (cont'd)	10 mg/kg PO, SC, IM q24h × 14 days[191]	Toucans/trematodes; follow with 6 mg/kg PO q24h × 14 days[391]
	10-20 mg/kg PO, repeat in 10-14 days[43,159,232,379]	Most species
	15-20 mg/kg PO, SC, IM, repeat in 2 wk prn[976]	Penguins/use higher dose PO
	25 mg/kg PO, IM, repeat in 10-14 days[654,873]	Passerines, including Bali mynahs/cestodes
	30-50 mg/kg PO, SC, IM, repeat in 14 days[455,873]	Passerines, raptors/cestodes; use lower dose in passerines
	12 mg crushed and baked into 9″ × 9″ × 2″ cake[391]	Finches/withhold regular feed
	57-85 mg nebulized in 100% oxygen for 15 min q24 × 3 treatments[218]	Blue-crowned motmot, fairy-bluebirds/air sac trematodes *Szidatitrema* spp. reduced shedding; no adverse effects[218]
Primaquine[a]	—	Pigeons, raptors, game birds, penguins[a]/hematozoa (i.e., *Plasmodium, Haemoproteus, Leucocytozoon*); use in conjunction with chloroquine; dosage based on amount of active base rather than total tablet weight
	0.3 mg/kg PO (at 24 hr following the initial chloroquine dose) q24h × 7 days[391]	Raptors/use with chloroquine (10 mg/kg at 0 hr, then 5 mg/kg at 6, 24, 48 hr)
	0.3 mg/kg PO q24h × 10 days[357,976]	Penguins[a]/*Plasmodium;* use with chloroquine (10 mg/kg at 0 hr, then 5 mg/kg at 6, 18, 24 hr)
	0.3-1 mg/kg PO q24h × 3-10 days[232]	Most species/*Atoxoplasma, Sarcocystis;* use with chloroquine
	0.75 mg/kg PO q3-7days[357]	African and Humboldt penguins[a]/during vector season, depending on institution
	0.75 mg/kg PO q24h × 5 days[919]	Falcons/*Haemoproteus tinnunculi*
	0.75-1 mg/kg PO once[876]	Raptors/*Plasmodium;* use with chloroquine (25 mg/kg at 0 hr, then 15 mg/kg at 12, 24, and 48 hr); palliative therapy
	1 mg/kg PO on day 2, then q24h × 3 days[126]	Magellanic penguins[a]/*Plasmodium*, use with chloroquine (10 mg/kg at 0, 6, 12, 18, 24 hr on day 1, then 5 mg/kg q24h × 3 days)
	1 mg/kg PO q7d[756]	Most species/use with chloroquine (10 mg/kg q7d) as a preventive regimen for birds recovering from *Plasmodium* infection
	1 mg/kg PO q24h × 2 days, repeat q7d × 3-5 treatments to prevent relapse[756]	Raptors/*Plasmodium;* use with chloroquine (20 mg/kg IV initially, followed by 10 mg/kg PO at 6, 18, 24 hr)
	1 mg/kg PO q24h X 10 treatments[962]	Seabirds/babesiosis
	1 mg/kg at 0, 24 hr then q24h × 10-14 days[357,988]	African penguins,[a] raptors/upon diagnosis of *Plasmodium*, administer with mefloquine 30 mg/kg PO at 0, 12, 24, 48 hr

TABLE 5-4 Antiparasitic Agents Used in Birds. (cont'd)

Agent	Dosage	Species/Comments
Primaquine (cont'd)	1 mg/kg PO q24h × 45 days[982]	Psittacines (keas)/*Sarcocystis;* use in combination with amprolium, enrofloxacin, and pyrimethamine
	1.25 mg/kg PO q24h × 10-14 days[693]	Medium-sized (3-5 kg) penguins[a]/upon diagnosis of *Plasmodium*, administer with chloroquine 10 mg/kg PO q24h × 10-14 days; then 5 mg/kg PO q12h × 3 days; some institutions stop here, others continue primaquine and chloroquine 5 mg/kg PO q24h
	1.25 mg/kg PO q24h (March until October; Northern hemisphere)[357,976]	African and Humboldt penguins[a]/prophylactic therapy against *Plasmodium*
	3.75 mg/kg PO q3-7days (March until October; Northern hemisphere)[357]	African and Humboldt penguins[a]/prophylactic therapy against *Plasmodium*
	4 mg PO q48h[976]	Medium-sized (3-5 kg) penguins[a]/during vector season (or year-round, depending on location of institution) in capsule with sulfadiazine 125 mg and folic acid 0.4 mg
Pyrantel pamoate	—	Intestinal nematodes; poorly absorbed, so increased safety margin[232]
	4.5 mg/kg PO, repeat in 10-14 days[43,564,994]	Cranes, psittacines, including cockatoo chicks[994]
	5-7 mg/kg PO[939]	Ostriches
	7 mg/kg PO, repeat in 14 days[172]	Most species
	7-20 mg/kg PO, repeat in 14 days[420]	Raptors
	7-25 mg/kg PO once[232]	Nematodes
	20 mg/kg PO once[43,178,510]	Raptors
	20-25 mg/kg PO[379]	Pigeons
	70 mg/kg PO once[191]	Ramphastids (toucans)/repeat if necessary
	148 mg/L drinking water[391]	Psittacines, pigeons/medication floats
Pyrethrins (0.15%) (Adams, Pfizer)	Dust plumage lightly to moderately prn[232,391,564]	Most species, including psittacines, pigeons/ ectoparasites
Pyrimethamine	—	*Toxoplasma, Atoxoplasma, Sarcocystis;* may be effective for *Leucocytozoon;* supplement with folic or folinic acid
	0.25-0.5 mg/kg PO q12h[510]	Raptors
	0.25-0.5 mg/kg PO q12h × 30 days[43,178]	Raptors/*Sarcocystis, Toxoplasma*
	0.5 mg/kg PO q12h × 14-28 days[159,232]	Most species/use for 28 days for *Leucocytozoon* in raptors
	0.5 mg/kg PO q12h × 45 days[982]	Psittacines (keas)/*Sarcocystis;* use in combination with amprolium and primaquine

Continued

TABLE 5-4 Antiparasitic Agents Used in Birds. (cont'd)

Agent	Dosage	Species/Comments
Pyrimethamine (cont'd)	0.5-1 mg/kg PO q12h × 2-4 days, then 0.25 mg/kg PO q12h × 30 days[291]	Companion birds/*Sarcocystis;* use in combination with trimethoprim-sulfa 5 mg/kg IM q12h or 30-100 mg/kg PO q12h × 7 days
	0.5-1 mg/kg PO q12h × 30 days[673]	Eclectus, Amazon parrots/use with trimethoprim-sulfadiazine (30 mg/kg)
	100 mg/kg feed[291]	Most species
Quinacrine HCl[a] (Atabrine, Sanofi)	—	Most species/*Atoxoplasma, Plasmodium;* chloroquine and primaquine are preferred; overdosage may cause hepatoxicity
	5-10 mg/kg PO, IM q24h[510]	Raptors/*Plasmodium*
	5-10 mg/kg PO q24h × 7-10 days[43,232,450]	Most species/use higher doses for *Lankesterella, Plasmodium*
	7.5 mg/kg PO q24h × 10 days[43,391]	Most species/*Atoxoplasma*
	26-79 mg/L drinking water × 10-21 days[43,379]	Pigeons
Rafoxanide (Flukex, Univet; Ranide, MSD)	10 mg/kg PO[232]	Raptors/trematodes, cestodes; not available in the United States
Resorantel (Terenol-S, Intervet)	130 mg/kg PO[179,391]	Ostriches/highly effective against the cestrode *Houttuynia struthionis* when administered with or without fenbendazole
Ronidazole (Ronivet-S, Vetafarm)	—	Antiprotozoal used against trichomoniasis; toxicity documented with overdose in drinking water in society finches[999]
	2.5 mg/kg PO × 6 days[379]	Pigeons
	6-10 mg/kg PO q24h × 6-10 days[391]	Most species
	10-20 mg/kg PO q24h × 7 days[159]	Pigeons
	12.5 mg/kg PO q24h × 6 days[43]	Pigeons
	50-400 mg/L drinking water × 5 days[159]	Passerines
	60 mg/L drinking water[272]	Finches/*Cochlosoma*
	100-200 mg/L drinking water × 7 days[391]	Cockatiels, pigeons/higher dosage required for resistant strains in pigeons
	100-600 mg/L drinking water × 3-5 days[379]	Pigeons
	400 mg/L drinking water × 5-7 days[43,239]	Canaries, pigeons/flock treatment; *Trichomonas;* preventive dose[43]
	600 mg/L drinking water × 5-7 days[43]	Pigeons/*Trichomonas;* flock treatment
	1000 mg/L drinking water q24h[159]	Pigeons/equivalent to 12.5 mg/kg/day
	400 mg/kg soft feed[238]	Canaries

TABLE 5-4 Antiparasitic Agents Used in Birds. (cont'd)

Agent	Dosage	Species/Comments
Selamectin (Revolution, Zoetis)	—	No adverse effects, including neurologic signs, were seen in healthy zebra finches with doses up to 92 mg/kg[97]
	20 mg/kg topically[742]	Lorikeets/PK; maintained therapeutic levels for 14 days.
	23 mg/kg topically, repeat in 3-4 wk[96]	Budgerigars/*Knemidokoptes*; improvement in 13/14 birds at 4 wk, with no neurologic signs identified but monitor for weight loss
	23 mg/kg topically, repeat in 4 wk[799]	Golden eagles/treatment for *Micnemidocoptes* spp.; no evidence of toxicity at this dosage
Sulfachlorpyrazine (ESB3, Novartis)	—	Coccidiostat; affects the intestinal stages of *Atoxoplasma*;[239] not available in the United States but can be obtained through the Bali mynah Species Survival Plan[564]
	1 g of 30% powder/L drinking water × 5 days, off 3 days, on 5 days, then repeat cycle × 4 treatments; administer treatment 3× annually[654]	Bali mynahs/*Atoxoplasma;* significantly reduced or totally cleared oocyst shedding for extended time; it is uncertain if the drug is safe to use when parents are feeding chicks; supplement with vitamin B_6
Sulfachlorpyridazine (Vetisulid, Boehringer-Ingelheim)	—	Coccidiostat; used as replacement for sulfachlorpyrazine in the United States; contraindicated with dehydration, liver disease, renal disease;[232] treatment >2 wk may require folic acid supplementation[232]
	100-400 mg/L drinking water × 3-5 days/wk; repeat[232]	Passerines/repeat after 5 days to allow for prepatent period of coccidia
	150-300 mg/L drinking water;[239] 5 days/wk × 2-3 wk[203]	Passerines, including canaries/may need to treat for months for systemic coccidiosis
	300 mg/L drinking water × 5 days, off 3 days, on 5 days, then repeat cycle × 4 treatments; administer treatment 3 × annually[654,873]	Passerines, including Bali mynahs/*Atoxoplasma*
	300 mg/L drinking water × 7-10 days[379]	Pigeons
	300-1000 mg/L drinking water × 3 days, off 2 days, then repeat course[159]	Pigeons
	400 mg/L drinking water × 30 days[391]	Cockatiels, budgerigars/mixture is stable for up to 5 days if refrigerated; change daily; mix well
	400-500 mg/L drinking water × 5 days, off 2 days, on 5 days[391]	Most species

Continued

TABLE 5-4 Antiparasitic Agents Used in Birds. (cont'd)

Agent	Dosage	Species/Comments
Sulfadimethoxine (12.5%)	20 mg/kg PO q12h[391]	Most species/prevention and treatment of coccidiosis; contraindicated with dehydration, liver disease, renal disease;[232] treatment >2 wk may require folic acid supplementation[232]
	20-50 mg/kg PO q12h × 3-5 days/wk; repeat treatment[232]	Passerines/repeat after 5 days to allow for prepatent period of coccidia[232]
	25 mg/kg PO q12h × 5 days[379]	Most species
	25-50 mg/kg PO q24h × 3 days[291]	Raptors
	25-50 mg/kg PO q24h × 3 days, off 2 days, then q24h × 3 days[420]	Raptors
	25-55 mg/kg PO q24h × 3-7 days[753]	Raptors/*Eimeria, Sarcocystis*
	50 mg/kg PO once, then 25 mg/kg PO q24h × 7-10 days[420]	Raptors
	50 mg/kg PO q24h × 5 days, off 3 days, on 5 days[941]	Psittacines
	50 mg/kg PO q24h × 14 days[564]	Cranes/coccidiosis
	250 mg/kg IM q24h × 3 days, off 2 days, on 3 days[125]	Pigeons/PK and PD; close to toxic level
	250-500 mg/L drinking water × 5-7 days/wk; repeat treatment[232]	Passerines/repeat after 5 days to allow for coccidial prepatent period[232]
	330-400 mg/L drinking water × 1 day, then 200 mg/L × 4 days[379]	Pigeons/supplement with vitamin B for 5 days
Sulfadimidine sodium (33.3%)	—	Contraindicated with dehydration, liver disease, renal disease;[232] treatment >2 wk may require folic acid supplementation[232]
	40-50 mg/kg PO q24h × 7 days or 3 days on, 2 days off[159]	Pigeons
	50-150 mg/kg PO, IM q12h × 3-5 days/wk; repeat treatment[232]	Passerines/repeat after 5 days to allow for coccidial prepatent period[232]
	50-150 mg/kg PO, IM q24h × 5-7 days[391]	Raptors/coccidia; lack of efficacy reported in merlins[391]
	3300-6600 mg/L drinking water × 5 days[232]	Passerines/repeat after 5 days to allow for coccidial prepatent period[232]
	3330-6660 mg/L drinking water × 3-5 days on, 2 days off; repeated twice[43]	Pigeons/coccidia; may be effective against *Toxoplasma*

TABLE 5-4 Antiparasitic Agents Used in Birds. (cont'd)

Agent	Dosage	Species/Comments
Sulfamethazine (Sulmet, Boehringer-Ingelheim)	—	See sulfonamides; coccidiostat; contraindicated with dehydration, liver disease, renal disease;[232] treatment >2 wk may require folic acid supplementation[232]
	50-65 mg/pigeon PO × 3 days, off 2-3 days; repeat × 2-3 days[500]	Pigeons
	50-65 mg/pigeon PO × 5 days[379,500]	Pigeons/supplement vitamin B for 5 days[379]
	75 mg/kg PO q24h × 3 days, off 2 days, on 3 days[391]	Parakeets
	75-185 mg/kg PO q24h × 3 days[232]	Passerines/repeat after 5 days to allow for prepatent period[232]
	125 mg/L drinking water × 3 days, off 2 days, on 3 days[391]	Most species
	400 mg/L drinking water once, then 200-270 mg/L × 4 days[379]	Pigeons
Sulfaquinoxaline (Sulquin 6-50, Zoetis)	—	Sulfonamide used for prevention and treatment of coccidiosis; contraindicated with dehydration, liver disease, renal disease;[232] treatment >2 wk may require folic acid supplementation[232]
	100 mg/kg PO q24h × 3 days, off 2 days, on 3 days[232,391]	Lories, pigeons, passerines
	250 mg/L drinking water × 5-7 days[232]	Passerines/repeat after 5 days to allow for prepatent period of coccidia
	500 mg/L (1.8 mL/L) drinking water × 6 days, off 2 days, on 6 days[790]	Pigeons
Sulfonamides	—	Competitvely inhibit paraaminobenzoic acid, required by schizonts for folic acid synthesis;[500] contraindicated with dehydration, liver disease, or bone marrow suppression; gastrointestinal upset, regurgitation are common, especially in macaws; use for longer than 2 wk may require vitamin B (folic acid) supplementation
Tetracycline (T)/ furaltadone (F)	(T) 400 mg + (F) 400 mg/L drinking water for 7 days[802]	Pigeons/indicated for trichomoniasis, hexamitiasis; avoid in adults feeding young less than 10 days of age
Thiabendazole	—	Most species/nematodes (especially *Syngamus trachea*), acanthocephalans; generally less efficacious than fenbendazole; may be toxic to cranes and ratites[43]
	40-100 mg/kg PO q24h × 7 days[43,232,391]	Most species
	50 mg/kg PO, repeat in 14 days[391]	Ostriches

Continued

TABLE 5-4 Antiparasitic Agents Used in Birds. (cont'd)

Agent	Dosage	Species/Comments
Thiabendazole (cont'd)	100 mg/kg PO once, repeat in 10-14 days[43,391,564]	Raptors, cranes/intestinal strongyles, ascarids
	100 mg/kg PO q24h × 7-10 days[391]	Most species/gapeworms, ascarids
	100-200 mg/kg PO q12h × 10 days[178]	Raptors/nematodes; may interfere with egg laying
	100-500 mg/kg PO once[43,232,391]	Most species
	250-500 mg/kg PO, repeat in 10-14 days[43,941]	Most species, including psittacines/ascarids
	425 mg/kg feed × 14 days[142]	Cranes
Toltrazuril (Baycox, Bayer)	—	Coccidiocidal;[500] efficacious for refractory coccidiosis; has been successful in reducing mortality from *Atoxoplasma* in canaries and other passerines and may affect systemic stages of the disease;[654] not very effective against *Atoxoplasma* when given in water; bitter taste, mixing with soft drinks (i.e., cola) increases palatability;[43] 2.5% solution is very alkaline and should not be gavaged directly into the crop[500]
	50 mg/kg PO once[143]	Most species/*Giardia, Trichomonas, Entamoeba*
	7 mg/kg PO q24h × 2-3 days[411,455]	Budgerigars, raptors
	7-15 mg/kg PO q24h × 3 days[232]	Passerines/*Atoxoplasmosis*
	10 mg/kg PO q24h × 2 days[753]	Raptors/preferred treatment for *Caryospora*
	10 mg/kg PO q48h × 3 treatments[43]	Raptors/treatment of choice for coccidiosis in falcons
	12.5 mg/kg PO q24h × 14 days[654,873]	Passerines, including Bali mynahs/*Atoxoplasma;* dosage is based on a limited number of clinical cases
	12.5 mg/kg PO q24h × 2 days, off 5 days, repeat prn[435]	Blue-crowned laughing thrush/PD; reduced clinical signs and all intestinal stages of *Isospora* spp. within 7 days, white blood cell effects within 3 mo
	12.5 mg/kg PO q24h × 2 days in hand-feeding, then 45 mg/L drinking water × 2 days, repeat prn[596]	Cirl buntings/PD; reduced intestinal stages of *Isospora* spp., 72/75 affected birds released
	15-25 mg/kg PO q24h × 2 days[43,510]	Raptors
	15-25 mg/kg PO q48h × 3 treatments[510]	Raptors
	20-35 mg/kg PO once[232,964]	Pigeons/higher dose prevents shedding up to 4 wk; lower dose is minimum dose required to suppress oocyst shedding

TABLE 5-4 Antiparasitic Agents Used in Birds. (cont'd)

Agent	Dosage	Species/Comments
Toltrazuril (Baycox, Bayer) (cont'd)	25 mg/kg q24h × 2 days[568]	Pigeons/PD; not effective against *S. chalchasi* when administered on day 0, 10, or 40 postinoculation
	25 mg/kg PO q7d × 3 treatments[159,306]	Raptors/*Caryospora*, coccidiosis
	2 mg/L drinking water × 2 consecutive days/wk [143,177]	Psittacines
	5 mg/L drinking water × 2 days; repeat in 14-21 days[545]	Lories/10 mg/L administered during second course of treatment
	20 mg/kg in drinking water × 2 days[500]	Pigeons
	25 mg/L drinking water × 2 days; repeat in 14-21 days[545]	Cockatiels, passerines, including goldfinches, manikins, siskins/coccidia
	25-75 mg/L drinking water × 5 days[232]	Canaries/*Atoxoplasma* spp.
	75 mg/L drinking water × 2 days/wk × 4 wk[203]	Passerines
	75 mg/L drinking water × 5 days[381]	Pigeons
	125 mg/L drinking water × 5 days[43]	Pigeons
	200-400 mg/kg feed[143]	Chickens/*Histomonas;* depressed weight gain on higher dosage
Trimethoprim/ sulfadiazine	—	See sulfonamides
	5 mg/kg IM q12h[391]	Companion birds/*Sarcocystis;* use in conjunction with pyrimethamine (0.5-1 mg/kg PO q12h × 2 days, then 0.25 mg/kg PO q12h × 30 days)
	30 mg/kg PO q8-12h[91,420]	Most species, including psittacines, raptors/*Sarcocystis* (treat for at least 6 wk); coccidia
	30-100 mg/kg PO q12h × 7 days[391]	Companion birds/*Sarcocystis;* use in conjunction with pyrimethamine (0.5-1 mg/kg PO q12h × 2 days, then 0.25 mg/kg PO q12h × 30 days)
	60 mg/kg PO, SC q12h × 3 days, off 2 days, on 3 days[43]	Raptors/coccidia
	80 mg (trimethoprim) + 40 mg (sulfadiazine)/mL drinking water[991]	Canaries/*Toxoplasma gondii*
Trimethoprim/ sulfamethoxazole	10-50 mg/kg q24h[873]	Passerines
	16-24 mg/kg (based on trimethoprim) PO q12-24h[564]	Cranes/coccidiosis
	25 mg/kg PO q24h[391]	Toucans, mynahs/coccidia

Continued

TABLE 5-4 Antiparasitic Agents Used in Birds. (cont'd)

Agent	Dosage	Species/Comments
Trimethoprim/ sulfamethoxazole (cont'd)	30 mg/kg PO q12-24h[159]	Passerines/antiprotozoal
	480 mg/L drinking water q24h[159]	Pigeons/antiprotozoal

[a]Because adult penguins regurgitate food to chicks, use of this regimen must be considered carefully during chick rearing.

TABLE 5-5 Chemical Restraint/Anesthetic/Sedative/Analgesic Agents Used in Birds.[a,b]

Agent	Dosage	Species/Comments
Acepromazine	—	Phenothiazine tranquilizer; see etorphine and ketamine for combinations
	0.1-0.2 mg/kg IV[391]	Ratites/most commonly used in combination with other anesthetics; rarely used in other bird species
	0.25-0.5 mg/kg IM[391]	
Acetaminophen	5 mg/L drinking water[391]	Most species/antipyretic, analgesic; overdosage may be associated with hepatotoxicity
Alfaxalone (Alfaxan, Jurox)	—	Not to be confused with dosing information for alfaxalone/alfadalone (Saffan, Schering-Plough); this is a completely new formulation, so doses cannot be extrapolated from older literature using alfaxalone/alfadalone; see dexmedetomidine for combination
	2 mg/kg IV[969]	Flamingos/induction; induction significantly shorter and quality smoother than with isoflurane alone; decreased isoflurane maintenance requirements but produced moderate cardiorespiratory effects not seen in isoflurane-only group; recovery times similar with both groups, without significant differences in quality or length
	10 mg/kg IM[984] 25 mg/kg IM[984]	Quaker parrots/lower dose significantly longer induction time (13.5 ± 4.5 min) compared to higher dose (6.0 ± 1.3 min), while recovery time significantly longer in the high-dose group (86.2 ± 13.4 min) than the low-dose group (44.4 ± 10.8 min); muscle tremors and hyperexcitation evident in both groups
	20 mg/kg IM[672]	Yellow-legged gulls/loss of righting reflex achieved in only 1/6 birds after 20 min; could not intubate; some birds manifested adverse effects like muscle twitches, wing and tail flapping, and opisthotonus
Alfaxalone (A)/ fentanyl (F)	(A) 20 mg/kg + (F) 20 µg/kg IM[672]	Yellow-legged gulls/loss of righting reflex achieved in only 2/6 birds after 12.5 min; could not intubate; significant reduction in respiratory rate; some birds manifested adverse effects like muscle twitches, wing and tail flapping, and opisthotonus

TABLE 5-5 Chemical Restraint/Anesthetic/Sedative/Analgesic Agents Used in Birds. (cont'd)

Agent	Dosage	Species/Comments
Alfaxalone (A)/ fentanyl (F)/ midazolam (Mi)	(A) 20 mg/kg + (F) 20 µg/kg + (Mi) 1 mg/kg IM[672]	Yellow-legged gulls/loss of righting reflex achieved in 6/6 birds after 20 min; could not intubate; significant heart rate and respiratory rate reduction; a number of birds manifested adverse effects like muscle twitches, wings and tail flapping, and opisthotonus
Alfaxalone (A)/ midazolam (Mi)	(A) 10 mg/kg + (Mi) 1 mg/kg IM[984]	Quaker parrots/lower induction time than same dose (A) alone (6.5 ± 2.9 min) but significantly longer recovery time (103.5 ± 15.1 min); reduced muscle tremors and hyperexcitability
	(A) 20 mg/kg + (Mi) 1 mg/kg IM[672]	Yellow-legged gulls/loss of righting reflex in 5/6 birds after 8 min; a number of birds manifested adverse effects like muscle twitches, wings and tail flapping, and opisthotonus
Alphachloralose (Fisher Scientific)	—	Chloral derivative of glucose which depresses cortical centers of the brain; induces hypothermia; low therapeutic index in chickens suggests only marginally safe in domestic species or for field applications where dosage difficult to control[391]
	250-430 mg/cup of bait[291]	Cranes, American crows/immobilization; 160-210 mg/4.5 kg sandhill crane; cranes could generally be approached within 1-2 hr of feeding and releasable 8-22 hr later
Atipamezole (Antisedan, Zoetis)	—	α_2-adrenergic antagonist; 1:1 volume reversal of dexmedetomidine is general rule; although the same effect is expected as with medetomidine (no longer available except via compounding pharmacy)[931]
	2.5-5 × medetomidine dose IM, IV[826,828]	Psittacines, pigeons, raptors/righting reflex regained 2-10 min after administration
	0.25-0.5 mg/kg IM[291,416,715,826,828]	Most species, including psittacines, pigeons
	0.4 mg/kg ½ IV, ½ SC[513]	Ostriches
	6 mg/kg intranasally[967]	Ring-necked parakeets/dose divided evenly between nares and given slowly; significantly reduced recumbency time after detomidine administration
Atropine sulfate	—	Anticholinergic agent
	0.01-0.02 mg/kg SC, IM, IV[391]	Most species/preanesthetic
	0.04-0.1 mg/kg SC, IM, IV, IO, intratracheal[391]	Most species/bradycardia; higher doses with CPR
Azaperone (Stresnil, Elanco)	—	Butyrophenone neuroleptic agent; see metomidate for combination; not available in the United States
	0.73 mg/kg IM[939]	Ratites/sedation
	1-4 mg/kg IM, IV[391]	Ostriches/premedication, sedation

Continued

TABLE 5-5 Chemical Restraint/Anesthetic/Sedative/Analgesic Agents Used in Birds. (cont'd)

Agent	Dosage	Species/Comments
Benzocaine	Topical anesthesia[391]	Small birds/minor wound repair
Bupivacaine HCl	—	Local anesthetic agent; 4-6 hr duration of action in mammals;[182] may be shorter acting in some birds;[562] recommend minimizing dose to limit potential toxic effects;[226] see bupivacaine combination[391]
	2 mg/kg infused SC[391]	
	2-8 mg/kg perineurally	Mallard ducks/variable efficacy for brachial plexus block[120]
Buprenorphine HCl	—	Partial μ-opioid agonist[c]
	0.1 mg/kg IM[683,684]	African grey parrots/PK and PD; reached human analgesic plasma concentrations but ineffective for analgesia
	0.1-0.6 mg/kg IM[151,362]	American kestrels/PK and PD; resulted in thermal antinociception for ≥6 hr
	0.25 mg/kg IM[590]	Red-tailed hawks/PD; did not change any scored pain behaviors significantly in cross-over study
	0.25-0.5 mg/kg IM[321]	Pigeons/PD; dose-dependent increased withdrawal time from noxious stimulus for 2-5 hr
	0.6, 1.2 and 1.8 mg/kg IM[820a]	Cockatiels/PK and PD; did not change thermal foot withdrawal time or aggitation-sedation scores significantly
Buprenorphine (Simbadol, Zoetis)	—	Concentrated formulation; not to be confused with compounded sustained-release product, as dosing may differ
	0.3 mg/kg SC q24h[342] 1.8 mg/kg SC q48h[342]	Red-tailed hawks/PK; plasma concentrations of >1 ng/mL were maintained for these time periods
Buprenorphine sustained release (Bup-SR, ZooPharm)	—	Compounded sustained-release product; not to be confused with concentrated formulation, as dosing may differ
	1.8 mg/kg SC, IM q24h[821]	American kestrels/PK and PD; thermal antinociceptive response for 12-24 hr
Butorphanol tartrate	—	Opioid agonist-antagonist;[c] PO bioavailability <10% in Hispaniolan Amazon parrots; PO route not recommended;[820] butorphanol combination follows; see dexmedetomidine, ketamine, and xylazine for combinations
	0.05-0.25 mg/kg IV[939]	Ratites
	0.5 mg/kg IM, IV q1-4h[764]	Great horned owls, red-tailed hawks/PK: $t_{1/2}$ IM, IV very short (approx. 1-2 hr); more rapid clearance and shorter $t_{1/2}$ when given IV medial metatarsal vein than IV median ulnar vein

TABLE 5-5 Chemical Restraint/Anesthetic/Sedative/Analgesic Agents Used in Birds. (cont'd)

Agent	Dosage	Species/Comments
Butorphanol tartrate (cont'd)	0.5-4 mg/kg IM, IV q1-4h[193,32 1,485,683,764,820,872]	Most species, including psittacines/no isoflurane-sparing effects detected in harlequin ducks when administered IM 15 min prior to induction[625]
	1-2 mg/kg IM[192,193]	African grey parrots, cockatoos, blue-fronted Amazon parrots/PD; significantly reduced ED_{50} of isoflurane for African greys and cockatoos but not for Amazon parrots; African grey parrots had more significant reduction of withdrawal response to electrical stimulus at 2 mg/kg
	1-6 mg/kg IM[816]	American kestrels/PD; did not cause thermal antinociception suggestive of analgesia; hyperalgesia in males at higher doses
	2-5 mg/kg IM, IV q2-3h[485,820,872]	Hispaniolan Amazon parrots/PK; low mean plasma concentrations at 2 hr postinjection; PD: withdrawal from electrical stimuli reduced after 2 mg/kg IM; effective preemptive analgesia with sevoflurane anesthesia for endoscopy[485]
	3 mg/kg (premedication) + 75 µg/kg/min IV CRI (maintenance)[532]	Psittacines/PD; significantly reduced isoflurane MAC
Butorphanol (B)/ midazolam (Mi)	(B) 1 mg/kg IM + (Mi) 0.5 mg/kg IM[505]	Psittacines/induction time and isoflurane concentration were reduced in the B + Mi group; induction quality scores were improved in the B + Mi group and no adverse effects on anesthesia and cardiovascular stability were observed
Carfentanil (Wildnil, Wildlife Pharmaceuticals)	—	Super-potent opioid agonist;[c] carfentanil combination follows; not generally recommended for use in birds; no longer commercially available in the United States
	0.024 mg/kg IM[391]	Ostriches (free-ranging)/darted from helicopter
	0.03 mg/kg IM[391]	Ratites
Carfentanil (C)/ xylazine (X)	(C) 3 mg + (X) 150 mg IM per ostrich[728]	Ostriches (free-ranging)/darted from helicopter
Desflurane (Suprane, Baxter)	—	Fluorine halogenated ether; fast induction, rapid recovery;[396] no significant differences from isoflurane and sevoflurane in a red-tailed hawk[348]
Detomidine (Dormosedan, Zoetis)	—	α_2-adrenergic agonist
	12 mg/kg intranasally[967]	Ring-necked parakeets/dose divided into each naris and given slowly; sedation <3 min but did not allow dorsal recumbency or manipulation; reversal with atipamezole significantly reduced time to recovery

Continued

TABLE 5-5 Chemical Restraint/Anesthetic/Sedative/Analgesic Agents Used in Birds. (cont'd)

Agent	Dosage	Species/Comments
Detomidine (Dormosedan, Zoetis) (cont'd)	12-15 mg intranasally[968]	Canaries/dose divided into each naris and given slowly; higher dose prolonged sedation but could not place in dorsal recumbency; prolonged duration of effect (257 ± 1.5 min); completely reversed with yohimbine intranasally
Dexmedetomidine HCl (Dexdomitor, Zoetis)	—	α_2 agonist; active optical enantiomer of racemic compound medetomidine; ½ the dose of medetomidine but same volume due to concentration has been used as a general guideline;[d] although the same effects would be expected as with medetomidine (not commercially available, but can be compounded); limited data on the efficacy and safety of dexmedetomidine in birds to date; dexmedetomidine combinations follow
	25 µg/kg IM[828]	Common buzzards/adequate restraint to prevent reaction to handling but did not allow for intubation; loss of righting reflex = 3.5 ± 1 min; no arrhythmias, excitement, or major adverse effects noted; complete reversal with atipamezole
	75 µg/kg IM[828]	Common kestrels/adequate restraint to prevent reaction to handling but did not allow for intubation; loss of righting reflex = 7 ± 1.2 min; no arrhythmias, excitement, or major adverse effects noted; complete reversal with atipamezole
Dexmedetomidine (D)/alfaxalone (A)	(D) 0.4 mg/kg + (A) 20 mg/kg IM[1014]	Domestic doves/time to loss of consciousness = 102 ± 48 sec, loss of righting reflex = 240 ± 135 sec; two birds could not undergo endoscopic procedure; one bird died due to prolonged recovery; significant variability in heart rate and respiratory rate; not recommended at these doses for minimally invasive procedures
Dexmedetomidine (D)/ketamine (K)/ butorphanol (B)	(D) 0.4 mg/kg + (K) 40 mg/kg + (B) 1 mg/kg IM[1014]	Domestic doves/mean time to loss of consciousness and loss of righting reflex was 80 ± 44 sec and 162 ± 102 sec, respectively; all birds experienced a prolonged recovery period (>1 hr); significant variability in heart rate and respiratory rate; not recommended at these doses for minimally invasive procedures
Dexmedetomidine (D)/midazolam (Mi)	(D) 80 µg/kg + (Mi) 5 mg/kg intranasally[416]	Pigeons/PD; effective immobilization 20 to 30 min after intranasal administration; birds tolerated postural changes without resistance; significant decreases in heart rate and respiratory rate that persisted until the end of sedation; atipamezole antagonized sedation and cardiorespiratory side effects within 10 min

TABLE 5-5 Chemical Restraint/Anesthetic/Sedative/Analgesic Agents Used in Birds. (cont'd)

Agent	Dosage	Species/Comments
Dexmedetomidine (D)/thiafentanil oxalate (Th)/ tiletamine-zolazepam (Tz)	—	Ultra-short-acting opioid agonist (Th); not currently available in the United States; α_2 agonist (D); dissociative anesthetic (Tz)
	(D) 0.2 mg + (Th) 7 mg + (Tz) 100 mg IM per bird[930]	Greater rheas/anesthesia administered via remote injection; smooth induction/recovery; respiratory depression in 1/8 birds but recovered with reversal
Diazepam	—	Benzodiazepine; used alone for sedation, seizure control, tranquilization, and/or appetite stimulation; IM administration may cause severe muscle irritation and absorption may be delayed; reversal with flumazenil; see ketamine for combinations
	0.05-0.5 mg/kg IV[391]	Most species
	0.1-0.3 mg/kg IV[391,442]	Ratites/tranquilization; smooth anesthetic recovery
	0.2-0.5 mg/kg IM[233]	Most species/premedication; onset in 15-20 min
	0.25-0.5 mg/kg IM, IV q24h × 2-3 days[906]	Raptors/appetite stimulant
	0.5 mg/kg PO[391]	Passerines/calms fractious species while improving acceptance to a novel captive diet; oral solution (1 mg/mL, Roxane Laboratories) works best
	0.5-1 mg/kg IM, IV q8-12h[43]	Raptors/sedation; anticonvulsant
	0.8 mg/kg intranasally[28]	Ostriches (juvenile)/slower onset (4.3 ± 0.4 min) than midazolam (2.9 ± 1.2 min); moderate sedation was achieved for standing chemical restraint with the maximum duration effect of 9.2 ± 2.5 min
	1-2 mg/kg IV[391]	Ostriches/administer just prior to recovery from teletamine/zolazepam to counter its undesirable effects
	2.5-4 mg/kg PO[391]	Most species/sedation
	5 mg/kg PO[391]	Ostriches/standing sedation
	5 mg/kg IV[313,391]	Emus, rheas/sedation
	6 mg/kg IM[946]	Rock partridges/decrease in cloacal temperature; prolonged recoveries (149 ± 8.3 min)
	10 mg/kg IM[720]	Zebra finches/deep sedation, dorsal recumbency achieved in minutes and lasted for several hours; reversed completely with flumazenil

Continued

TABLE 5-5 Chemical Restraint/Anesthetic/Sedative/Analgesic Agents Used in Birds. (cont'd)

Agent	Dosage	Species/Comments
Diazepam (cont'd)	12 mg/kg intranasally[967]	Ring-necked parakeets/dose divided into each naris and given slowly; time to onset 3.5 ± 1.2 min, dorsal recumbency 11.0 ± 6.4 min; not sedate enough for any manipulation; flumazenil intranasally significantly reduced recumbency time
	12.5-15.6 mg/kg intranasally[968]	Canaries/dose divided into each naris and given slowly; dorsal recumbency for approx. 35 min; flumazenil intranasally significantly reduced recumbency time
	13 ± 1 mg/kg intranasally[93]	Finches/onset of sedation significantly slower (1.8 ± 0.2 min) compared with midazolam (1.0 ± 0.3 min); longer duration of dorsal recumbency observed after diazepam (68 ± 13 min) than with midazolam (32 ± 8 min); diazepam produced significantly longer duration of sedation (182 ± 18.) than midazolam (74 ± 9)
	13.6 ± 1.1 mg/kg intranasally[800]	Budgerigars/onset of sedation significantly longer after diazepam (2.8 ± 0.9 min) than midazolam (1.3 ± 0.4 min); diazepam produced significantly longer duration of sedation (165 ± 19 min) than midazolam (72 ± 9 min); adequate sedation for diagnostic, minor therapeutic procedures
Diprenorphine	0.04-0.06 mg/kg IV[808]	Ostriches/opioid antagonist
Dobutamine	—	β_1-adrenergic agonist with weak β_2 activity and selective α_1 activity; used to treat anesthetic-induced hypotension
	15 µg/kg/min IV[837]	Hispaniolan Amazon parrots/PD; significant increase in direct arterial pressure within 4-7 min
Dopamine HCl	—	Catecholamine neurotransmitter activating dopamine receptors; inotropic vasopressor used to treat anesthetic-induced hypotension
	7-10 µg/kg/min IV[837]	Hispaniolan Amazon parrots/PD; significant increase in direct arterial pressure within 4-7 min; greater effects on direct arterial pressures than dobutamine
Etorphine HCl (M-99, Wildlife Pharmaceuticals)	—	Super-potent opioid agonist;[c] may be inadequate when used as sole agent;[442] see etorphine combinations
	0.025 mg/kg IM[391]	Ostriches
Etorphine (E)/ acepromazine (A)	(E) 0.04-0.07 mg/kg + (A) 0.19 mg/kg IM[808]	Ostriches (10-12 mo of age)
	(E) 3.6 mg/bird + (A) 15 mg/ bird IM[808]	Ostriches

TABLE 5-5 Chemical Restraint/Anesthetic/Sedative/Analgesic Agents Used in Birds. (cont'd)

Agent	Dosage	Species/Comments
Etorphine (E)/ acepromazine (A)/ xylazine (X)	(E) 0.04 mg/kg + (A) 0.16 mg/kg + (X) 0.66 mg/kg IM[808]	Ostriches/sedation for simple procedures lasting 10-20 min
Etorphine (E)/ ketamine (K)	(E) 6-12 mg/bird IM + (K) 200-300 mg/bird IM[391]	Ostriches (adults)
Fentanyl citrate	—	Short-acting μ-opioid agonist[c]
	20 μg bolus + 0.2-0.5 μg/kg/min IV CRI[679,688]	Red-tailed hawks/PK and PD; reduced isoflurane MAC 31%-55% in a dose-related manner, without significant effects on heart rate, blood pressure, $paCO_2$, or paO_2
	20 μg bolus + 1.5-6 μg/kg/min IV CRI[679]	Hispaniolan Amazon parrots/PK and PD; reduced isoflurane in a dose-related manner similar to red-tailed hawks but with much higher dosages; significant decreases in heart rate, indirect blood pressure; monitor closely
	0.02 mg/kg IM[413]	Cockatoos/PK and PD; rapid absorption, elimination; no effect withdrawal to thermal, electrical stimulus
	0.2 mg/kg SC[413]	Cockatoos/PK and PD; some analgesia; large dose and volume; hyperactivity first 15-30 min in some birds
Fentanyl (F)/ midazolam (M)	(F) 30 μg bolus + (M) 1-2 mg/kg IM, then (F) 30 μg/kg/h IV CRI + (M) 1 mg/kg/h IV CRI[671]	Wild birds/partial IV anesthesia (PIVA) with isoflurane anesthesia for orthopedic surgery; recovery = 63.2 ± 24.0 min with excellent quality; no significant change in HR detected
Flumazenil	—	Benzodiazepene antagonist
	0.02-0.1 mg/kg IM, IV[6,391]	Most species
	0.05 mg/kg intranasally[574]	Hispaniolan Amazon parrots
	0.13 mg/kg intranasally[967]	Ring-necked parakeets/dose divided evenly between nares and given slowly; significantly reduced recumbency time
	0.25-0.31 mg/kg intranasally[968]	Canaries/dose divided evenly between nares and given slowly; significantly reduced recumbency time
	0.3 mg/kg IM[720]	Zebra finches/smooth, complete recovery after deep sedation with diazepam
Gabapentin	—	GABA analogue; used to treat human neuropathic pain
	3 mg/kg PO q24h[871]	Senegal parrots/analgesia; used with fluoxetine so difficult to determine efficacy alone; bird appeared sedated 3 days after initiation of administration
	10 mg/kg PO q12h[231,232]	Little corella/long-term (>90 days) analgesia; sole analgesic for self-mutilation; no adverse effects noted

Continued

TABLE 5-5 Chemical Restraint/Anesthetic/Sedative/Analgesic Agents Used in Birds. (cont'd)

Agent	Dosage	Species/Comments
Gabapentin (cont'd)	11 mg/kg PO q12h[857]	Prairie falcons/long-term (>90 days) analgesia; adjunct to multimodal therapy for self-mutilation; bird exhibited neurologic signs, diarrhea when dosed at 110 mg/kg but no adverse effects at 82 mg/kg
	11 mg/kg PO q8h[1003]	Great horned owls/PK; maintained plasma concentrations >2 μg/mL ≈ 8 hr
	15 mg/kg PO q8h[47]	Hispaniolan Amazon parrots/PK; maintained plasma concentrations ≥ human analgesic concentration ≈ 8 hr
	25 mg/kg q12h[124]	Flamingos/PK; maintained plasma concentrations ≥ human analgesic concentration ≈ 12 hr[124]
Glycopyrrolate	—	Anticholinergic agent; slower onset than atropine
	0.01-0.02 mg/kg IM, IV[391]	Most species/preanesthetic; rarely indicated
	0.04 mg/kg IV[939]	Ratites
Hydromorphone	0.1-0.6 mg/kg IM q3-6h[817,822]	American kestrels/PK and PD: doses of 0.1, 0.3, and 0.6 mg/kg IM significantly increased thermal foot withdrawal responses; appreciable sedation with 0.6 mg/kg
	0.1, 0.3, and 0.6 mg/kg IM[417]	Cockatiels/PK and PD; doses did not significantly increase thermal foot withdrawal responses; 0.3 and 0.6 mg/kg produced mild sedation[417]
	1-2 mg/kg[815]	Orange-winged Amazon/PK and PD; this dosage had thermal antinociceptive activity through 6 hr, but caused agitation[815]
Isoflurane	—	Inhalant anesthetic agent of choice in birds; dose-dependent hypotension with all inhalants; raptors, macaws may be more likely to exhibit isoflurane-induced arrhythmias;[11,391] no significant differences in ventilation or O_2 transport between dorsal and lateral recumbency in red-tailed hawks[392]
	0.5%-4% (usually 1.5%-2%)[391]	Ostriches/use following preanesthetic medication
	1%-3%[854]	Cinereous vultures/dose-dependent increases in heart rate and $ETCO_2$ and decreases in direct blood pressure and respiratory acidosis during spontaneous ventilation
	1.115%[874]	Emus/PD; minimum anesthetic concentration
	1.3%[552,553]	Cranes, ducks/minimum anesthetic concentration
	1.44 ± 0.07%[193]	Cockatoos/PD; ED_{50}

TABLE 5-5 Chemical Restraint/Anesthetic/Sedative/Analgesic Agents Used in Birds. (cont'd)

Agent	Dosage	Species/Comments
Isoflurane (cont'd)	1.46 ± 0.30%[153]	Crested serpent eagles/minimum anesthetic concentration; time-related increase in $ETCO_2$ and decreases in body temperature and respiratory rates
	1.8 ± 0.4%[108]	Pigeons/PD; minimum anesthetic concentration; dose-dependent hypercapnia, hypotension, mild hypothermia and 2nd- and 3rd-degree atrioventricular blocks
	2.05 ± 0.45%[688]	Red-tailed hawks/PD; minimum anesthetic concentration
	3%-5%[391]	Ostriches/when used without preanesthetic medication
	3%-5% induction, 1.5%-2.5% maintenance[391]	Most species
Ketamine HCl	—	Dissociative anesthetic; seldom used as sole agent because of poor muscle relaxation and prolonged (up to 3 hr), violent recovery; may produce excitation or convulsions in pigeons, gallinules, water rails, golden pheasants, Hartlaub's turacoes, ratites, and vultures;[442,810] may fail to produce general anesthesia in some species including great horned owls, snowy owls, Cooper's hawks, sharp-shinned hawks; see dexmedetomidine and etorphine for combinations; ketamine combinations follow
	5 mg/kg IV q10min prn[442]	Ratites/maintenance
	5-30 mg/kg IM, IV[42,391]	Raptors/sedation
	10-50 mg/kg SC, IM, IV[233,391]	Psittacines, pigeons, ratites, waterfowl/restraint 30-60 min; smaller species require a higher dose; large birds tend to recover more slowly
	25 mg/kg IM[391]	Emus/may need to supplement 5-9 mg/kg IV q10min
	50 mg/kg IO[465]	Pigeons/provided effective anesthesia
	50-100 mg/kg PO in bait[89,178,793]	Raptors/sedation to catch an escaped bird; place in a 30 g piece of meat
Ketamine (K)/ acepromazine (A)	(K) 10-25 mg/kg + (A) 0.5-1 mg/kg IM[983]	Most species/high dose for birds <250 g
Ketamine (K)/ diazepam (D)	(K) 2-5 mg/kg IV + (D) 0.25 mg/kg IV[391]	Ostriches/ketamine may be given 15-30 min after diazepam
	(K) 3-8 mg/kg + (D) 0.5-1 mg/kg IM[399]	Eagles, vultures
	(K) 5-30 mg/kg + (D) 0.5-2 mg/kg IV[391]	Most species/psittacines and pigeons lower end of range is preferred
	(K) 8-15 mg/kg + (D) 0.5-1 mg/kg IM[399]	Falcons

Continued

TABLE 5-5 Chemical Restraint/Anesthetic/Sedative/Analgesic Agents Used in Birds. (cont'd)

Agent	Dosage	Species/Comments
Ketamine (K)/ diazepam (D) (cont'd)	(K) 10 mg/kg + (D) 0.2 mg/kg IM[35]	Pigeons/rapid induction with an increase in anesthesia duration; good muscle relaxation and a smooth, slow recovery
	(K) 10 mg/kg + (D) 0.5 mg/kg IM[681]	Amazon parrots/PD; significantly reduced sevoflurane MAC
	(K) 10-40 mg/kg IV + (D) 1-1.5 mg/kg IM, IV[754]	Raptors, waterfowl/induction or surgical anesthesia (rapid bolus may produce apnea, arrhythmia, and increased risk of death)
	(K) 20 mg/kg + (D) 1 mg/kg IV[191]	Toucans/short procedures (15-20 min)
	(K) 20-40 mg/kg IM + (D) 1-1.5 mg/kg IM[623]	Birds >250 g
Ketamine (K)/ butorphanol (B)/ medetomidine (Me)	—	Medetomidine no longer available but can be compounded; see dexmedetomidine
	(K) 3 mg/kg + (B) 1 mg/kg + (Me) 40 µg/kg IM[1007]	Psittacines/premedication or supplement to isoflurane; reduces isoflurane requirement and improves ventilation
	(K) 50 mg + (B) 50 µg + (Me) 50 µg IM per pigeon[32]	Pigeons/PD; satisfactory anesthesia in 7/8 pigeons; heart rate, respiratory rate decreased within 10 min following Me + B injection; arrhythmias in 3/8 pigeons; cloacal temperature decreased gradually during anesthesia
Ketamine (K)/ medetomidine (Me)	—	Unreliable level of sedation in pigeons at (K) 5 mg/kg + (Me) 80 µg/kg IM;[715] medetomidine not currently available but can be compounded
	(K) 1.5-2 mg/kg + (Me) 60-85 µg/kg IM, IV[391]	Pigeons/sedation
	(K) 2 mg/kg + (Me) 80 µg/kg IM[513]	Ostriches/sedation
	(K) 2-4 mg/kg + (Me) 25-75 µg/kg IV[433]	Raptors
	(K) 2.5-7 mg/kg + (Me) 50-100 µg/kg IV[434]	Large psittacines
	(K) 3-5 mg/kg + (Me) 50-100 µg/kg IM[433]	Raptors
	(K) 3-7 mg/kg + (Me) 75-150 µg/kg IM[434]	Large psittacines
	(K) 25 mg/kg + (Me) 100 µg/kg IM[759]	Psittacines/anesthesia
Ketamine (K)/ midazolam (Mi)	(K) 10-40 mg/kg + (Mi) 0.2-4 mg/kg SC, IM[232,391,623]	Most species, including psittacines
	(K) 40-50 mg/kg + (Mi) 3.65 mg/kg intranasally[967]	Ring-necked parakeets/dose divided into each naris and given slowly; onset of action <3 min, dorsal recumbency for 71 ± 47 min; recovery times reduced with flumazenil intranasally

TABLE 5-5 Chemical Restraint/Anesthetic/Sedative/Analgesic Agents Used in Birds. (cont'd)

Agent	Dosage	Species/Comments
Ketamine (K)/ midazolam (Mi)/ butorphanol (B)	(Mi) 0.2 mg/kg + (B) 0.4 mg/kg IM followed by (K) 8.7 ± 0.5 mg/kg IV[40]	Ostriches/PD; anesthesia; followed by intubation and isoflurane anesthesia
Ketamine (K)/ tiletamine/ zolazepam (Tz)	(K) 15 mg/kg + (Tz) 10 mg/kg IM[503]	Raptors/anesthesia
Ketamine (K)/ xylazine (X)	—	Often associated with cardiac depressive effects and rough recoveries
	(K) 0.45 mg/kg + (X) 25 mg/kg IM[585]	Ostriches
	(K) 2-3 mg/kg IV + (X) 5-10 mg/kg IM[134]	Ostriches
	(K) 2-5 mg/kg IV + (X) 0.25 mg/kg IV[134]	Ostriches
	(K) 2.2-3.3 mg/kg + (X) 2.2 mg/kg IM[442]	Ratites/administer xylazine 10-15 min before ketamine
	(K) 4.4 mg/kg + (X) 2.2 mg/kg IV[420,518]	Psittacines, raptors
	(K) 5 mg/kg + (X) 1 mg/kg IM[98]	Ostriches
	(K) 8 mg/kg IV + (X) 4 mg/kg IM[17]	Ostriches/ketamine administered 20 min after xylazine; produced sufficient surgical plane of anesthesia as an adjunct to isoflurane anesthesia
	(K) 10 mg/kg + (X) 0.5-1 mg/kg IM[16,588]	Ratites, turkey vultures
	(K) 10-15 mg/kg + (X) 2 mg/kg IM[623]	Owls
	(K) 10-30 mg/kg + (X) 2-6 mg/kg IM[623]	Psittacines/birds <250 g require dose at higher end of range
	(K) 20 mg/kg + (X) 1-2 mg/kg IV slow bolus[191]	Toucans
	(K) 25 mg/kg + (X) 2.5 mg/kg IM[623]	Cockatiels
	(K) 25-30 mg/kg + (X) 2 mg/kg IM[623]	Falcons, hawks
	(K) 30 mg/kg + (X) 6.5 mg/kg IM[623]	Budgerigars
	(K) 40-50 mg/kg + (X) 10 mg/kg intranasally[967]	Ring-necked parakeets/dose divided evenly between nares and given slowly; time to sedation, 7.7 ± 1.4 min; dorsal recumbency, 12.2 ± 14.1 min; yohimbine IM shortened recovery

Continued

TABLE 5-5 Chemical Restraint/Anesthetic/Sedative/Analgesic Agents Used in Birds. (cont'd)

Agent	Dosage	Species/Comments
Ketamine (K)/ xylazine (X)/ acepromazine (A)	(K) 34 mg/kg + (X) 0.2 mg/kg + (A) 0.1 mg/kg IM[442]	Ostriches
Lidocaine	—	Local anesthetic agent with a duration of action in mammals of 90-200 min;[182] previous reports state that the dose of lidocaine used in birds should be ≤3.3 mg kg;[391] a recent study in chickens showed 6 mg/kg IV was not associated with adverse cardiovascular effects[116]
	1 mg/kg perineurally each nerve[249]	Raptors/sciatic-femoral nerve block under inhalant anesthesia
	1-3 mg/kg[391]	Most species
	2 mg/kg perineurally[199]	Hispaniolan Amazon parrots/brachial plexus block via palpation or ultrasound guidance; onset of block tended to be faster when ultrasonography was used but neither technique produced an effective block
Medetomidine[d] (Domitor, Pfizer)	—	Not commercially available; can be compounded; dosages listed here as a general guide for possible dexmedetomidine dosing; α_2-adrenergic agonist; 80-2000 µg/kg IM was associated with inadequate sedation in the pigeon;[715,826] 100 µg/kg IM did not immobilize ostrich chicks;[951] see ketamine and thiafentanil for combinations; see dexmedetomidine for more details
	60-85 µg/kg IM[42]	Psittacines
	150-350 µg/kg IM[42]	Raptors
Meperidine HCl	—	Short-acting opioid agonist[c]
	1-4 mg/kg IM[768,939]	Most species, including ratites (at 1 mg/kg)/ sedation; analgesia
Midazolam HCl	—	Benzodiazepine; shorter acting than diazepam, water soluble; see butorphanol, dexmedetomidine, and ketamine for combinations
	0.1-2 mg/kg IM, IV[6]	Most species/premedication at lower doses; onset ≈ 15 min when administered IM
	0.15 mg/kg IV[442]	Ostriches/rapid sternal recumbency in adults
	0.2 mg/kg SC, IM[43]	Psittacines/for use in combination with ketamine
	0.3-0.4 mg/kg IM[442,588]	Ostriches, emus/premedication; sedation of adult emus

TABLE 5-5 Chemical Restraint/Anesthetic/Sedative/Analgesic Agents Used in Birds. (cont'd)

Agent	Dosage	Species/Comments
Midazolam HCl (cont'd)	0.4 mg/kg intranasally[28]	Ostrich (juvenile)/significantly shorter onset time (2.9 ± 1.2 min) compared with diazepam (4.3 ± 0.4 min) with longer duration of sedation; moderate sedation for standing chemical restraint, with maximum duration effects of 7.0 ± 1.4 min; deep sedation achieved with 0.8 mg/kg intranasally with sternal recumbency for 22 ± 5 min
	0.4 mg/kg IV[442]	Emus
	0.5-1 mg/kg IM, IV q8h[43]	Raptors/anticonvulsant
	2 mg/kg intranasally[575]	Hispaniolan Amazon parrots/mild to moderate sedation in 3 min; reduced vocalizations, struggling and defensive behaviors for 15 min; reversed with flumazenil intranasally
	2 mg/kg IM[948]	Canada geese/sedation for 15-20 min
	5 mg/kg intranasally[416]	Pigeons/PD; minimal side effects on vital functions but caused inadequate immobilization of pigeons for restraint in dorsal recumbency
	2 mg/kg intranasally[832]	Wild macaws/PD; provided approximately 20 min of sedation in 80% of macaws
	7.3-8.8 mg/kg intranasally[967]	Ring-necked parakeets/dose divided into each naris and given slowly; time to onset, 3 min; dorsal recumbency, 58 ± 24 min; flumazenil intranasally significantly reduced recovery time
	12.5-15.6 mg/kg intranasally[968]	Canaries/dose divided into each naris and given slowly; time to onset, <3 min; dorsal recumbency, 17 ± 5 min; flumazenil intranasally significantly reduced recovery time
	13 ± 1 mg/kg intranasally[93]	Finches/time to onset of sedation significantly faster (1.0 ± 0.3 min) than xylazine or diazepam; shorter duration of dorsal recumbency observed (32 ± 8 min) compared with diazepam (68 ± 13 min); significantly shorter duration of sedation (74 ± 9 min) than diazepam (182 ± 18 min) and xylazine (360 ± 41 min); no complications noted
	13.2 ± 1.3 mg/kg intranasally[800]	Budgerigars/time to onset of sedation significantly shorter (1.3 ± 0.4 min) than xylazine (2.6 ± 0.9 min) and diazepam (2.8 ± 0.8 min); sedation significantly shorter (72 ± 9 min) than with xylazine and diazepam; adequate sedation for diagnostic and minor therapeutic procedures
Morphine sulfate	—	Opioid agonist;[c] early work in chickens demonstrated confusing clinical dosage results

Continued

TABLE 5-5 Chemical Restraint/Anesthetic/Sedative/Analgesic Agents Used in Birds. (cont'd)

Agent	Dosage	Species/Comments
Nalbuphine HCl	—	Opioid partial κ-agonist and partial μ-antagonist;[c] due to its low abuse potential, this opioid is currently not a DEA scheduled substance at the time of writing
	12.5 mg/kg IM q2-3h[470,823]	Hispaniolan Amazon parrots/PK and PD; excellent IM bioavailability; little sedation and no adverse effects; rapidly cleared after IM and IV dosing; thermal foot withdrawal threshold values increased ≥3 hr; higher dosages (25, 50 mg/kg IM) did not significantly increase withdrawal values
Naloxone HCl	—	Opioid antagonist; shorter-acting than naltrexone
	0.01 mg/kg IV[40]	Ostriches
	2 mg IV q14-21h[391]	Most species, including psittacines
Naltrexone HCl	—	Opioid antagonist; longer-acting than naloxone
	300-330 mg IM, IV[468,585,728]	Ostriches/opioid antagonist
Nitrous oxide	—	Sufficient oxygen must be provided to avoid hypoxic mixtures; may cause some cardiovascular depression;[396] do not use in birds with normal subcutaneous air pockets (e.g., pelicans, hornbills) or in birds with marginal respiratory reserves[6,396]
Nitrous oxide (N)/ isoflurane (I)/ vecuronium (V)	(N) 0.3 L/kg/min of O_2 and (1:1, min 33% O_2) + (I) 1-2.4% + (V) 0.2 mg/kg IV[491,493]	Most species/mydriasis and anesthesia; gases are administered via air sac cannulation; vecuronium effective up to 256 min in pigeons
Pentobarbital sodium	—	Short-acting barbiturate; see Table 5-17 for other indications
	13.3 mg/kg IV[585]	Emus/premedicate with diazepam
Propofol	—	IV sedative-hypnotic agent; intubation, ventilation, and supplemental oxygen is strongly recommended[561,842]
	1-5 mg/kg IV[233]	Many species/give slowly for induction to minimize apnea; intubation and IPPV required
	1.33 mg/kg IV[43,420]	Psittacines, raptors
	2.9-4.7 mg/kg IV (induction); 0.4-0.55 mg/kg/min IV (maintenance)[393]	Red-tailed hawks, great horned owls/PK and PD; minimal blood pressure effects, but ventilation significantly reduced; prolonged recoveries with moderate-to-severe excitatory CNS signs may occur in these species at these doses
	3 mg/kg IV (induction); 0.2 mg/kg/min IV (maintenance)[513]	Ostriches/PD; anesthesia

TABLE 5-5 Chemical Restraint/Anesthetic/Sedative/Analgesic Agents Used in Birds. (cont'd)

Agent	Dosage	Species/Comments
Propofol (cont'd)	3.7 mg/kg IV (induction); 0.3 mg/kg/min IV (maintenance)[92]	King penguins/rapid and smooth induction and calm recovery
	4 mg/kg IV (induction); 0.5 mg/kg/min IV (maintenance)[571]	Barn owls/anesthesia
	5 mg/kg IV (induction); 0.5 mg/kg/min IV (maintenance)[832]	Wild turkeys/PD; anesthesia
	5 mg/kg IV (induction); 1 mg/kg/min IV (maintenance)[515]	Hispaniolan Amazon parrots/PD; recovery times (15.4 ± 15.2 min) were prolonged and variable when compared with isoflurane; 6/10 birds had agitated recoveries; light anesthetic plane in 8/10 birds
	14 mg/kg IV[284,420]	Pigeons, raptors/anesthesia; 2-7 min duration; severe respiratory depression and apnea documented in pigeons
Sevoflurane	2.35%[700]	Thick-billed parrots/PD; minimum anesthetic concentration when using mechanical stimulation; minimum anesthetic concentration was much higher (4.24%) when using electrical stimulus
	3 ± 0.6%[109]	Pigeons/PD; minimum anesthetic concentration; SAP decreased significantly, $PECO_2$ increased significantly despite an increase in respiratory rate; sinus arrhythmias were detected in two birds; time to tracheal intubation and recovery were 2.5 ± 0.7 and 6.4 ± 1.7 min, respectively; recovery was rapid and uneventful in all birds
	6% induction; 3.5% maintenance[262]	Crested caracara/PD; smooth induction/recovery; reduced respiratory rate and arterial blood pressures
	Incremental increases up to 7% prn (induction)[485,724]	Psittacines/anesthesia; similar to isoflurane; provides more rapid recovery; less incidence of ataxia during recovery[396,491,724]
Tapentadol	30 mg/kg PO[252]	Hispaniolan Amazons/PK; oral mu agonist noradrenaline reuptake inhibitor, similar to tramadol
		Poor bioavailability; only 2/7 birds achieved detectable concentrations[252]
Thiafentanil oxalate (T)/medetomidine (Me)	—	Ultra-short-acting opioid agonist[c] (T); α_2 agonist (Me); neither drug currently available in the United States
	(T) 0.175 mg/kg + (Me) 0.092 mg/kg IM[195]	Emus (adults)/anesthesia via remote injection; rapid induction (6.8 min) and recovery (3.2 min)

Continued

TABLE 5-5 Chemical Restraint/Anesthetic/Sedative/Analgesic Agents Used in Birds. (cont'd)

Agent	Dosage	Species/Comments
Tiletamine/zolazepam (Telazol, Zoetis)	—	Dissociative anesthetic associated with prolonged, rough recoveries; see dexmedetomidine and ketamine for combinations; tiletamine/zolazepam combinations follow
	1-8 mg/kg IV[442,623]	Ratites (adults)/induction and/or short procedures
	2-12 mg/kg IM[537,897]	Ratites (adults)/induction and/or short procedures;[314] recommend 3-5 mg/kg IM for captive birds and 5 mg/kg IM for free-ranging birds
	4-25 mg/kg IM[178,838,951]	Most species, including psittacines, raptors, ostriches, flamingos/sedation
	5-10 mg/kg IM[43,89,420,468,503,518,519]	Ostrich (chicks), raptors, psittacines/good immobilization
	9-30 mg/kg IM[838]	Owls, wood partridges/restraint
	10 mg/kg IM[503,838]	Raptors
	15-22 mg/kg IM[623,838]	Budgerigars, emus
	40-80 mg/kg PO[178]	Raptors
	80 mg/kg in feed[437,1012]	Eurasian buzzards/sufficient in most birds to allow safe handling after 30-60 min; birds receiving drug in powder form reached a deeper plane of anesthesia more quickly
Tiletamine-zolazepam (Tz)/ thiafentanil oxalate (Th)/ dexmedetomidine (D	—	Ultra-short-acting opioid agonist[c] (Th), not currently available in the United States; α_2 agonist (D); dissociative anesthetic (Tz)
	(Tz) 100 mg + (Th) 7 mg + (D) 0.2 mg IM per bird[931]	Greater rheas/anesthesia administered via remote injection; smooth induction/recovery; respiratory depression in 1/8 birds but recovered when reversed
Tolazoline HCl (Tolazine, Akorn)	—	α_2-adrenergic antagonist
	1 mg/kg IV[468]	Ostriches
	15 mg/kg IV[16]	Turkey vultures
Tramadol HCl	—	Synthetic analog of codeine with opioid, α-adrenergic, and serotonergic receptor activity; O-desmethyltramadol (M1) metabolite is more potent μ-opiate agonist in mammals
	5 mg/kg PO, IV q12h[881,883]	Bald eagles/PK; similar plasma concentrations to humans for analgesia but analgesia not evaluated; PO bioavailability in bald eagles higher than in humans, dogs;[883] sedation evident after multiple dosing; monitor for sedation and reduce dose and/or frequency prn

TABLE 5-5 Chemical Restraint/Anesthetic/Sedative/Analgesic Agents Used in Birds. (cont'd)

Agent	Dosage	Species/Comments
Tramadol HCl (cont'd)	5 mg/kg PO q2-9h[818]	American kestrels/PD
	8-11 mg/kg PO q12h[881,884]	Red-tailed hawks/PK; only three birds; 15 mg/kg PO q12h data model suggested more frequent dosing to achieve human analgesic plasma tramadol concentrations; analgesia not evaluated;[881] birds sedated after multiple dosing; monitor for sedation and reduce dose and/or frequency prn[881]
	10 mg/kg PO q24h[477]	African penguins/PK: maintained plasma concentrations for 24 hr
	30 mg/kg PO q6h[824,882]	Hispaniolan Amazon parrots/PK and PD; similar plasma concentrations to humans for analgesia; effectively reduced thermal withdrawal response for 6 hr
Xylazine	—	α_2-adrenergic agonist; not recommended by itself for tranquilization and seldom used in pet birds due to adverse effects—excitement, convulsions, bradycardia, arrhythmias, bradypnea, hypoxemia, hypercarbia, and death when used alone; reversible with yohimbine, atipamezole; most useful in ratites;[810] see carfentanil, etorphine, and ketamine for combinations
	0.2-1 mg/kg IM[442,728]	Ratites/calming sedation
	1-2.2 mg/kg IM, IV[43]	Raptors, psittacines/in combination with ketamine (1:3 or 1:5); still widely used in raptors in some countries
	1-20 mg/kg IM, IV[420]	Raptors/sedation
	20 mg/kg divided intranasally[967]	Ring-necked parakeets/time to onset, 7.9 ± 2.8 min but sedation not adequate for manipulation; reversed with yohimbine intranasally
	24-30 mg/kg divided intranasally[968]	Canaries/heavy sedation; prolonged sedation but could not place in dorsal recumbency at either dose; reversed with yohimbine intranasally
	25.6 ± 2.2 mg/kg intranasally[800]	Budgerigars/time to onset 2.6 ± 0.9 min; significantly longer sedation that midazolam or diazepam; quality of sedation insufficient to perform clinical procedures
Xylazine (X)/ butorphanol (B)	(X) 1.06-2.75 mg/kg + (B) 0.1-0.55 mg/kg IM[537]	Ratites, including rheas/sedation, premedication; higher doses were needed in rheas
Yohimbine HCl (Yobine, Akorn)	—	α_2-adrenergic antagonist; excitement and mortality observed at doses >1 mg/kg[396]
	0.1-0.2 mg/kg IV[43]	Psittacines, raptors
	0.1-0.2 mg/kg IM, IV[420]	Raptors
	0.1-1 mg/kg[391]	Most species

Continued

TABLE 5-5 Chemical Restraint/Anesthetic/Sedative/Analgesic Agents Used in Birds. (cont'd)

Agent	Dosage	Species/Comments
Yohimbine HCl (Yobine, Akorn) (cont'd)	0.11-0.275 mg/kg IM, IV once[398]	Budgerigars
	0.125 mg/kg IV[442,468,728]	Ratites
	12 mg/kg intranasally[967]	Ring-necked parakeets/dose divided evenly between nares and administered slowly; successful reversal of xylazine intranasally
	12-15 mg/kg intranasally[968]	Canaries/dose divided evenly between nares and administered slowly; successful reversal of xylazine and detomidine

[a]For other analgesic recommendations, refer to Table 5-6 Nonsteroidal Anti-inflammatory Agents Used in Birds.

[b]The anesthetic agents of choice in most avian species are the inhalant agents, isoflurane and sevoflurane.

[c]All opioid agonists and agonist-antagonists may cause respiratory depression; profound bradypnea may occur with potent opioid agonists.

[d]The effects of the volume:volume use of the dexmedetomidine and medetomidine may not be equivalent, so the dose of dexmedetomidine may need to be adjusted based on clinical response.

TABLE 5-6 Nonsteroidal Antiinflammatory Agents Used in Birds.

Agent	Dosage	Species/Comments
Aspirin (acetylsalicylic acid)	—	Contraindicated with tetracycline, insulin, or allopurinol therapy[5]
	5 mg/kg PO q8h[391]	Most species
	25 mg/kg IV[36,37]	Ostriches, pigeons/PK; rapid clearance except longer $t_{1/2}$ in pigeon
	50 mg/kg PO q8h[255]	Psittacines
	150 mg/kg PO[391]	Psittacines
	325 mg/250 mL drinking water[391]	Most species/make fresh q8-12h; alters taste of water (may not be well accepted)
Carprofen	—	Caution should be used when administering to *Gyps* vultures[197,311] and pigeons[1016]
	1-2 mg/kg PO, IM, IV q12-24h[178,420]	Most species, including raptors
	2-10 mg/kg SC, IM[43,255,391]	Psittacines, passerines, raptors
	2-10 mg/kg IM q24h up to 7 days[1016]	Pigeons/PD; 2, 5, and 10 mg/kg associated with increases in plasma AST, ALT, mottled yellow livers, pale muscle injection sites, and histologic changes in the kidney, liver (lipidosis, necrosis, portal hepatitis), and muscle injection sites
	3 mg/kg IM q12h[687]	Hispaniolan Amazon parrots/PD; markedly reduced arthritis pain 2 hr postadministration, but short-term effect thus more frequent dosing recommended

TABLE 5-6 Nonsteroidal Antiinflammatory Agents Used in Birds. (cont'd)

Agent	Dosage	Species/Comments
Carprofen (cont'd)	5-10 mg/kg PO, IM[391]	Raptors/postoperative analgesia
	30 mg/kg IM[143]	Chickens/PD; arthritis painful behaviors reduced for only 1 hr post-treatment with this dose[143]
Celecoxib (Celebrex, Pfizer)	10-20 mg/kg PO q24h × 6-24 wk[167,200]	Psittacines/clinical proventricular dilatation disease; clinical improvement may be seen within 7-14 days; compounded formulation of 10 mg/mL stable for approximately 90 days at room temperature[234]
		Cockatiels/PK; high to complete oral absorption[224]
Diclofenac	—	Recent massive mortalities in 3 vulture species lead to banning of diclofenac in India, Pakistan, and Nepal; severe renal lesions suggested toxicity of the kidneys or the renal supportive vascular system;[197,603,635,656,913] diclofenac toxicity has also been reported in Steppe eagles in India[855] and is suspected in other species; aceclofenac is rapidly metabolized to diclofenac in cattle, thus should also be avoided for its potential toxicity[323]
	12.5 mg PO once[43]	Pigeons/arthritis
	Topical opththalmic drops	Chickens/PK; ophthalmic administration yielded plasma levels of diclofenac, but no toxicity[356]
Dimethylsulfoxide (DMSO) (90%) (Domoso, Zoetis)	1 mL/kg topical to affected area q4-7d[391]	Most species/anti-inflammatory, analgesic; systemic absorption; use gloves during application
Dipyrone	20-25 mg/kg SC, IM, IV q8-12h[939]	Ratites/analgesic for intestinal disorders; antipyretic
Flunixin meglumine	—	Potential nephrotoxicity; hydration is essential; use only for short duration (<5 days);[179] 5 mg/kg led to renal ischemia and necrosis in Siberian cranes;[682] histologic lesions occurred in budgerigars administered 5.5 mg/kg and severity increased with duration of therapy;[694] histologic glomerular changes were demonstrated in bobwhite quail given doses as low as 0.1 mg/kg (severity of lesions was directly correlated to dose);[486] avoid in *Gyps* vultures;[197,311] IM administration caused muscle necrosis in ducks;[563] regurgitation may occur after administration[456]
	0.2 mg/kg IM[939]	Ratites
	0.5 mg/kg IM[396]	Most species, including psittacines
	1-10 mg/kg IM, IV q24h[389,420,438,750]	Most species, including raptors, psittacines
	1.1 mg/kg IV[36,37]	Ostriches, pigeons/PK; ostrich $t_{1/2}$ = 10 min
	1.1 mg/kg IM q12h[1,3]	Ostriches/myositis[3]

Continued

TABLE 5-6 Nonsteroidal Antiinflammatory Agents Used in Birds. (cont'd)

Agent	Dosage	Species/Comments
Flunixin meglumine (cont'd)	1.5 mg/kg IM q24h × 3 days[134]	Ostriches
	5 mg/kg IV[632]	Budgerigars, Patagonian conures/PK: elimination half-life and mean residence time rapid and similar in both spp.
	5.5 mg/kg IM q24h × 3 or 7 days[694]	Budgerigars/some renal changes at 3 days; 6/8 birds had tubular necrosis at 7 days
Ibuprofen	—	Avoid in *Gyps* vultures[197]
	5-10 mg/kg PO q8-12h[255]	Psittacines/use pediatric suspension for small birds
Ketoprofen	—	Avoid in *Gyps* vultures, mortalities reported at clinical doses;[311,636] 7/11 Cape Griffon vultures administered 5 mg/kg PO died within 48 hr[638]
	1 mg/kg IM q24h × 1-10 days[43,89]	Raptors
	1-5 mg/kg IM q12h[745]	Raptors
	2.5 mg/kg IM q24h × 3 or 7 days[694]	Budgerigars/low frequency of glomerular congestion, degeneration/dilation of tubules occurred at 3-7 days of treatment
Mavacoxib	4 mg/kg PO[224,334]	Cockatiels/PK[224] and PD[334]; COX-2 selective NSAID; high oral bioavailability and long elimination half-life (135 hr); safety studies needed;[224] inhibited signs of illness in LPS injection model of inflammation[334]
	6 mg/kg PO[421]	Caribbean flamingos/PK; reached canine therapeutic levels, $t_{1/2}$ about 74 hr[421]
Meloxicam	—	No reported mortalities in over 700 cases of 60 species of birds, including *Gyps* vultures,[197,913,914] but few studies to date evaluating renal effects of higher doses;[227,615,869] the combination of avian bornavirus challenge and meloxicam treatment resulted in severe disease and death in cockatiels, whereas challenge alone or meloxicam treatment alone were not lethal within the duration of this study[414,415]
	0.1 mg/kg IM q24h × 3 or 7 days[694]	Budgerigars/mild glomerular congestion and tubular degeneration at 3 and 7 days
	0.5 mg/kg PO q12h × 14 days[615]	African grey parrots/PD; mild to no hematological or biochemical changes, and no histologic lesions in 9 of 10 birds after 14 days of treatment
	0.5 mg/kg IV[36]	Ostriches, pigeons/PK; variable distribution; ostrich had more rapid $t_{1/2}$ (0.5 hr) than other species studied

TABLE 5-6 Nonsteroidal Antiinflammatory Agents Used in Birds. (cont'd)

Agent	Dosage	Species/Comments
Meloxicam (cont'd)	0.5 mg/kg PO, IV[511]	Red-tailed hawks, great horned owls/PK; significant differences in pharmacokinetics between species strongly discourages extrapolation between species; hawks had shortest half-life (0.49 hr) of any species recorded to date; once daily dosing not applicable at this dose in these species
	0.5 mg/kg PO, IM q8-12h[1017]	Lesser flamingos/PK; PO had higher bioavailability and longer elimination half-life than IM, but the plasma concentrations may be insufficient to provide analgesia; IM administration achieved the desired plasma concentration but would require more frequent administration
	0.5-1 mg/kg PO q12h[995]	Ring-necked parakeets/PK; no analgesic evaluation
	0.5 mg/kg IM q24h - 1 mg/kg PO q48h[622]	African penguins/PK
	0.5 mg/kg IM q6-8h[103]-1.5 mg/kg SC q8-12h[538]	Caribbean (American) flamingos/PK
	0.5-2 mg/kg PO, IM q12h × 9 days[222]	Pigeons/PD; 0.5 mg/kg dose ineffective in minimizing postoperative orthopedic pain; 2 mg/kg provided quantifiable analgesia that appeared safe under experimental conditions
	0.5-3 mg/kg PO q8-12h[103,538]	Caribbean (American) flamingos/PK; oral bioavailability only 45% when compared with SC administration; fasting status may change absorption;[538] results in these 2 studies differ significantly (possibly associated with fasting vs. nonfasting or other differences in the population); higher dose than 0.5 mg/kg may be required for PO administration;[103] selecting a dose midway between the 2 extremes may be the most reasonable
	1 mg/kg PO, IM, IV[614]	African grey parrots/PK; slower absorption and lower bioavailability than IM (40%)
	1 mg/kg PO[224]	Cockatiels/PK; low oral absorption (11%)[224]
	1 mg/kg PO, IM, IV q12h[174,611]	Hispaniolan Amazon parrots/PK and PD; improved weight-bearing on arthritic limb compared with lower doses; PO lower bioavailability than parenteral; PO did not attain plasma concentrations similar to humans for analgesia; concentrations similar to humans for analgesia for IM, IV for 6 hr
	1-2 mg/kg q12h[608]	Zebra finches/PK; both doses reached low plasma levels; dosing at 12 hr intervals or less probably needed; safe for 4 days[608]

Continued

TABLE 5-6 Nonsteroidal Antiinflammatory Agents Used in Birds. (cont'd)

Agent	Dosage	Species/Comments
Meloxicam (cont'd)	1.6 mg/kg PO q12h × 15 days[227]	Hispaniolan Amazon parrots/PD; no apparent negative changes in several renal, gastrointestinal, or hemostatic variables in healthy birds
	2 mg/kg PO, IM[637]	Cape Griffon vultures/PK; rapid metabolism and short elimination $t_{1/2}$ (<45 min) suggests low potential for drug accumulation
	2, 10, 20 mg/kg PO q12h × 7 days[911]	American kestrels; histologic evaluation showed a significant correlation between hepatic lipidosis and meloxicam dose; 2/9 birds developed gastric ulcers at highest dose
	5 mg/kg transdermally[130]	Red-tailed hawks/PK; compounded meloxicam in pluronic lecithin organogel (PLO); no detectable levels at 1.5 or 3 mg/kg; inconsistent levels at 5 mg/kg below levels for PO, IM[130]
Meloxicam SR (sustained-release meloxicam formulation	3 mg/kg SC[813]	Hispaniolan Amazon parrots/PK; highly variable results; use of this formulation in this species cannot be recommended without further study[813]
Wildlife Pharmaceuticals, Windsor, CO, USA)	3 mg/kg SC[865]	American flamingos/PK; did not extend interval of dosing; not recommended[865]
Phenylbutazone	—	Caution with use in *Gyps* vultures; mortalities associated with use[197,311]
	3.5-7 mg/kg PO q8-12h[255]	Psittacines
	10-14 mg/kg PO q12h[939]	Ratites
	20 mg/kg PO q8h[391]	Raptors
Piroxicam	—	Indicated for chronic osteoarthritis; has been used to treat pain associated with chronic degenerative joint disease in cranes and other species
	0.5 mg/kg PO q12h[391]	Psittacines
	0.5-0.8 mg/kg PO q12h[391]	Whooping cranes/acute myopathy; chronic degenerative joint disease
	0.5-1 mg/kg[469]	Brolga cranes/PK; no adverse effects; achieved concentrations known to be analgesic in humans[469]

TABLE 5-7 Hormones and Steroids Used in Birds.

Agent	Dosage	Species/Comments
Adrenocorticotropic hormone (ACTH)	1-2 U/kg IM[391]	Psittacines/ACTH stimulation test
	16-26 U/bird IM[548,1013]	Psittacines/obtain baseline sample, administer ACTH, then sample in 1-2 hr; stress of handling and venipuncture may invalidate results
	50-125 µg/bird IM[391]	Pigeons
Boldenone undecylenate (Equipoise, Zoetis)	1.1 mg/kg IM q21d[939]	Ratites/anabolic steroid
Buserelin (Receptal, Intervet India)	0.5-1 µg/kg q48h up to 3 treatments[43]	Psittacines/used to suppress chronic egg laying
	8 µg/kg IM[549]	Cockatiels, sulfur-crested cockatoos/ increased circulating testosterone after single injection
Buserelin acetate depot (Suprefact, Sanofi Aventis Canada)	10 µg/kg SC implant[184]	Budgerigars/when administered in inguinal region, increased reproductive activity and egg laying
Cabergoline	10-50 µg/kg q12-24h[43]	Psittacines/egg laying
Calcitonin	4 U/kg IM q12h × 14 days[391]	Most species/reduce hypercalcemia (caused by cholecalciferol rodenticide toxicity)
	10 µg/kg IM[1002]	Pigeons/significant reduction in plasma calcium over 5 days
Chorionic gonadotropin (hCG)	500-1000 U/kg IM on day 1, 3, 7 q3-6wk prn[391]	Most species/inhibits egg laying; administer on days 3 and 7 if hen lays after day 1
Delmadinone	1 mg/kg[43]	Antiandrogen sometimes effective for neurotic regurgitation in budgerigars
Deslorelin (Suprelorin, Virbac)	—	GnRH agonist available as 4.7 mg and 9.4 mg long-term implants; also used for long-term management of ovarian neoplasia in cockatiels[471,644] and Sertoli cell tumors in budgerigars;[901] anecdotal evidence of decreased efficacy over time with repeated administration;[30] to date, only approved for use in adrenocortical disease in ferrets in the United States
	4.7 mg implant placed SC intrascapularly[912]	Cockatiels/suppressed egg laying for ≥180 days; 5/13 implanted birds laid first egg between 192 and 230 days following implant placement; no difference in egg shape, color, shell quality, or number of eggs per clutch was observed between treated and control groups
	4.7 mg implant placed IM[185]	Domestic pigeons/effectively controlled egg laying for at least 49 days; significantly reduced serum LH concentrations in males and females compared to pretreatment levels for 56 and 84 days, respectively

Continued

TABLE 5-7 Hormones and Steroids Used in Birds. (cont'd)

Agent	Dosage	Species/Comments
Deslorelin (Suprelorin, Virbac) (cont'd)	5 mg/kg implant SC[629]	Male zebra finches/transiently suppressed testosterone concentrations, reversible when implant removed
Desmopressin	4.6 µg/kg IM q12h[893]	African grey parrots/long-term treatment of central diabetes insipidus; dosage adjusted as needed up to 24 µg/kg 16 mo after initial diagnosis
Dexamethasone[a]	0.2-1 mg/kg IM, IV once or q12-24h × 2-7 days, then q48h × 5 days[43,391]	Most species
	2-4 mg/kg IM, IV q12-24h[43,391]	Most species, including ratites/shock, trauma
	2-8 mg/kg SC, IM, IV q12-24h[658]	Cranes/reduce doses for long-term therapy
Dexamethasone sodium phosphate[a]	2-4 mg/kg SC, IM, IV q6-24h[43,391]	Most species, including raptors/head trauma, shock, hyperthermia; higher dose for shock, head trauma, and endotoxemia
Diethylstilbestrol diphosphate (Stilphostrol, Bayer)	0.025-0.075 mg/kg IM[391]	Most species/narrow therapeutic index
	0.4 mg/L drinking water[391]	Most species
Dinoprost tromethamine	—	See prostaglandin $F_2\alpha$
Dinoprostone	—	See prostaglandin E_2
Estradiol benzoate	—	Estrogens have been associated with severe adverse reactions in small mammals;[710] anemia, hypercholesterolemia, and hyperlipidemia were observed in penguins[406]
	0.3-0.5 mg/kg PO q24h × 1 mo[406]	Penguins/induces molt
	10-15 mg/kg IM q7d × 4 treatments[406]	Penguins/induces molt
Flumethasone (Flucort, Glenmark)[a]	1-1.5 mg/kg PO, SC, IM, IV[939]	Ratites/glucocorticoid; antiinflammatory
Glipizide	1 mg/kg PO q12h[422]	Most species
Hydrocortisone[a]	3-4.5 mg/kg PO q12h[939]	Ratites
	10 mg/kg IM, IV[391]	Psittacines, passerines, raptors
	40-50 mg/kg IV q24h[939]	Ratites
Insulin	0.002 U/bird IM q12-48h[391]	Budgerigars/NPH insulin
	0.01-0.1 U/bird IM q12-48h[391]	Amazon parrots/NPH insulin
	0.1-0.5 U/bird IM q24h or prn[391]	Toco toucans

TABLE 5-7 Hormones and Steroids Used in Birds. (cont'd)

Agent	Dosage	Species/Comments
Insulin (cont'd)	0.2-10.7 U/kg SC, IM q12h[55]	Bali mynah/PZI insulin: commercial and compounded products used with differing results, so increase/change dose/product with caution
	0.5-3 U/kg IM[391]	Psittacines/NPH insulin
	1.4 U/kg IM q12-24h[391,445]	Cockatiels, toco toucans/NPH insulin
	2 U/bird IM[391]	Toco toucans/ultralente or PZI insulin; adjust dose or frequency based on glucose curves
Lecirelin (Dalmarelin; Selecta, Germany; Vetcare, Finland; Fatro, Ireland, Israel, Italy, Netherlands; Ufamed, Switzerland; Reprorelin: Vetoquinol, France)	5-21 µg/kg transcutaneous (combined with cream vehicle) administered to skin over right jugular[774]	Canaries/time from start of treatment to onset of egg laying was significantly shorter for treated birds than controls, irrespective of photoperiod given
Leuprolide acetate (Lupron Depot, TAP Pharmaceuticals; Lupron Kit, Florida Infusion Pharmacy [a single-dose leuprolide acetate compounded formulation is available from Professional Arts Pharmacy, Baltimore, MD])	—	Synthetic GnRH agonist depot drug; prevents ovulation; may be indicated in some cases of sexually related feather picking or mutilation;[341] variable results obtained; in treating reproductive diseases, administration before onset of egg laying may be more successful than treatment during breeding; single report of anaphylaxis following chronic administration in two elf owls;[904] rarely seen in humans unless impurities in formulation
	(No. of days for desired effect) × (52 or 156 µg/kg) = dosage IM[605]	Cockatiels/PD
	100 µg/kg q14d × 3 treatments[391,439]	Most species/feather-damaging behavior
	200-800 µg/kg IM q2-6wk[391,446]	Most species
	375 µg/bird IM[42,606]	Cockatiels/inhibits ovulation
	400-1000 µg/kg IM q2-3 wk[573]	Psittacines
	500 µg/kg IM q14d[1009]	Psittacines (>300 g)/for most problems, begin with three treatments
	750 µg/kg IM q14d[1009]	Psittacines (≤300 g)/for most problems, begin with three treatments
	800 µg/kg IM[484]	Hispaniolan Amazon parrots/hormonal effects may taper off between 7 and 21 days after administration
	1250 µg/kg IM once[406]	Penguins/induced molt in 1 of 2 birds dosed
	1500 µg/kg IM q2-4wk[471]	Long-term management of ovarian neoplasia[471]

Continued

TABLE 5-7 Hormones and Steroids Used in Birds. (cont'd)

Agent	Dosage	Species/Comments
Levothyroxine (l-thyroxine)	—	May induce molt; monitor blood levels and body weight
	5-200 µg/kg PO q12h[781]	Amazon parrots
	20 µg/kg PO q12-24h[43,159,391]	Most species, including psittacines, pigeons, and raptors
	25 µg q24h × 7 days, then 50 µg q24h × 7 days, then 75 µg q24h × 7 days, then 50 µg q24h × 7 days, then 25 µg q24h × 7 days[420]	Raptors (750-1000 g)/induces molt; scale dose up or down by up to 50% for larger or smaller birds
Medroxyprogesterone acetate	—	This agent is not recommended; previously used for sexually related feather picking or chronic egg laying; high incidence of adverse effects, including lethargy, polydipsia, polyphagia, polyuria, immunosuppression, weight gain, liver disease, thromboembolism, diabetes mellitus, salpingitis, sudden death[341]
	5-25 mg/kg SC, IM, repeat q4-6wk prn[374,391]	Psittacines/suppresses ovulation; antipruritic (feather picking in male parrots)
	5-50 mg/kg SC, IM q4-6wk[43]	Psittacines/higher dosages recommended for smaller birds (e.g., 50 mg/kg for 150 g bird)[585]
	15-30 mg/kg IM q7d × 4-5 treatments[757]	Penguins/induces molt 60-90 days postinjection
	30 mg/kg SC, repeat in 90 days prn[391]	Most species
	1000 mg/kg feed[391]	Pigeons/inhibits ovulation
Megestrol acetate	—	Progestin; adverse effects can be severe (diabetic-like); not generally recommended, so dosages are not provided
Methylprednisolone acetate[a]	0.5-1 mg/kg PO, IM[391]	Most species/allergies (Amazon foot necrosis);[767] use orally once weekly, then taper to once monthly, then stop
	200 mg/bird IM, repeat prn[939]	Ratites (adults)
Nandrolene laurate (Laurabolin, Intervet)	—	Testosterone derivative; used in the treatment of chronic, debilitating disease; may be hepatotoxic
	0.2-2 mg/kg IM once[391]	Most species
	0.4 mg/kg SC, IM q21d[43]	Psittcines, raptors, bustards
Oxytocin	—	Use of oxytocin should be preceded by calcium administration for egg binding; contraindicated unless uterovaginal sphincter is well dilated and uterus is free of adhesions; used alone to stop uterine bleeding[391]

TABLE 5-7 Hormones and Steroids Used in Birds. (cont'd)

Agent	Dosage	Species/Comments
Oxytocin (cont'd)	0.5-5 U/kg, may repeat q30min[391]	Most species, including raptors
	5-10 U/kg IM once[391]	Psittacines/in some cases, multiple injections are recommended
	20-30 U/bird IM q24h × 2 treatments[939]	Ratites (adults)/egg binding
Prednisolone (prednisone)[a]	0.5-1 mg/kg IM, IV[391]	Most species
	1-1.25 mg/kg PO q48h[939]	Ratites
	2 mg/kg IM, IV q12-24h[658]	Cranes/shock, trauma, chronic lameness
	2-4 mg/kg IM, IV[420]	Raptors/shock
	0.5-1 mg/kg PO q24h[248]	Harpy eagle/inflammatory bowel disease; prednisone; initial treatment with lower dose ineffective but at 1 mg/kg resolved clinical disease; treatment was 5 wk with 5 more wk tapering to zero[248]
Prednisolone sodium succinate (Solu-Delta-Cortef, Zoetis)[a]	0.5-1 mg/kg IM, IV[391]	Psittacines/antiinflammatory
	1.5-2 mg/kg IM q12h[939]	Ratites/immunosuppression (see prednisolone for prolonged therapy)
	2-4 mg/kg IM, IV once[391]	Psittacines/shock; trauma; endotoxemia; immunosuppression
	5-8.5 mg/kg IV q1h[939]	Ratites/shock
	10-20 mg/kg IM, IV q15min prn[391]	Most species/head trauma; cardiopulmonary resuscitation
Prednisone	—	See prednisolone
Prostaglandin E_2 (dinoprostone) (Prepidil Gel, Pfizer)	0.02-0.1 mg/kg applied topically to uterovaginal sphincter[391]	Most species, including psittacines, raptors/dystocia; relaxes uterovaginal sphincter; lower dosage may be effective; freeze into aliquots
Prostaglandin $F_{2\alpha}$ (dinoprost tromethamine) (Lutalyse, Zoetis)	0.02-0.1 mg/kg IM, or intracloacal once[802]	Most species, including psittacines, raptors, and waterfowl/dystocia; may be helpful when the egg is located distally and the uterovaginal sphincter is dilated; can result in uterine rupture, bronchoconstriction, hypertension, death
Somatostatin	0.003 mg/kg SC q12h[463]	Toucans (sulfur-breasted)/diabetes mellitus; some clinical improvement observed; hyperglycemia and elevated glucagon levels persisted
Tamoxifen citrate	—	Nonsteroidal antiestrogen
	2 mg/kg PO q24h given on 2 consecutive days per wk for 38-46 wk[560]	Budgerigars/effects suggested by change in cere color from white/brown to blue; leukopenia was the most significant adverse effect
	40 mg/kg IM[406]	Penguins/induces molt

Continued

TABLE 5-7 Hormones and Steroids Used in Birds. (cont'd)

Agent	Dosage	Species/Comments
Testosterone	—	Anabolic steroid; may adversely affect spermatogenesis; contraindicated with hepatic or renal disease[165]
	2-8 mg/kg SC, IM once[43]	Most species/stimulates sexual behavior in the male; baldness in canaries
	8-8.5 mg/kg IM q7d prn[15]	Most species, including psittacines/anemia due to debilitation; increases libido; use with caution
	10-15 mL stock solution/L drinking water × 5 days-2 mo[391]	Canaries/finish molt or regain singing; stock solution: 100 mg parenteral suspension/30 mL drinking water (3333 mg/L); mix fresh daily
Thyroid-releasing hormone	15 µg/kg IM once[391]	Most species
Thyroid-stimulating hormone (thyrotropin; TSH)	0.1 U/bird IM (bovine)[380]	Cockatiels/3-24-fold higher T_4 6 hr after receiving TSH
	0.2 U/kg IM (human)[351]	Macaws/PD; T_4 doubled in 6/11 birds 4 hr after receiving TSH
	1 U/kg IM (human)[350,351,1013]	Hispaniolan parrots, blue-fronted Amazon parrots, African grey parrots, pigeons/PD; T_4 doubled in Hispaniolan and blue-fronted parrots 6 hr after receiving TSH
	1-2 U/kg IM (human)[547]	Psittacines/obtain blood at 0 hr, then 4-6 hr after TSH stimulation

[a]Steroid administration may predispose birds to aspergillosis and other mycoses.[420] Administration may also be associated with the development of polyuria/polydypsia/polyphagia, increased protein catabolism, glucosuria, and diabetes mellitus. Toxic levels may be attained even with topical application.[404] Administration should ideally not exceed 5 days. Rapid onset, shorter-acting drugs are generally less likely to cause serious adverse effects.

TABLE 5-8 Nebulization Agents Used in Birds.[a]

Agent	Dosage	Species/Comments
N-acetyl-L-cysteine 10%-20% (Mucomyst, Bristol)	—	See other antimicrobials and drugs for combinations
	22 mg/mL sterile water until dissipated[62]	Most species/mucolytic agent; tracheal irritation and reflex bronchoconstriction reported in mammals; use is preceded by bronchodilators in mammals[763]
Amikacin	5-6 mg/mL sterile water or saline × 15 min q8-12h[62]	Most species/discontinue if polyuria develops
Aminophylline	3 mg/mL sterile water or saline × 15 min[62]	Most species/bronchial and pulmonary vasculature smooth muscle relaxation; incompatible with amikacin, cephalothin, clindamycin, erythromycin, oxytetracycline, methylprednisone, penicillin G, tetracycline; consult with specialized references for more information[710]

TABLE 5-8 Nebulization Agents Used in Birds. (cont'd)

Agent	Dosage	Species/Comments
Amphotericin B (Fungizone, Squibb)	—	May lead to hypokalemia; corticosteroids may exacerbate this effect;[710] minor systemic absorption with aerosol administration; can be nebulized long term;[710] mix with sterile water; may precipitate with saline and other electrolytic solutions
	0.1-1 mg/mL sterile water × 15-60 min q12-24h[41,62,976]	Most species including birds of prey, penguins, and parrots (0.5-1 mg/mL q30-40 min is usually used)
	0.25 mg/mL saline × 15 min q12h[387]	Hummingbirds/low efficacy; may cause weight loss
Amphotericin B liposome (AmBisome, Astellas Pharma)	—	Most species/do not mix with saline or other drugs; nebulization does not alter the liposome formulation[14]
	1-4 mg/kg diluted in sterile water x 15-60 min[65]	Most species
	3 mg/kg intratracheal aerosol administration[707]	Mallard ducks/PK; concentrations above MIC of 1 µg/g for up to 9 days; drug distribution is uneven in the lung parenchyma
Cefotaxime	10 mg/mL saline × 10-30 min q6-12h[62]	Most species
Ceftriaxone	40 mg/mL sterile water × 1 hr[461]	Bantam chickens/PK; 1 g ceftriaxone without or with 10-15 mL DMSO; no significant serum levels measured.
Chloramphenicol	13 mg/mL saline[164]	Most species/human health concerns; the development of aplastic anemia reported in humans; prohibited by the FDA for use in food animals
Clotrimazole (1%) (Lotrimin, Schering)	10 mg/mL propylene glycol or polyethylene glycol × 30-45 min q24h × 3 days, off 2 days, repeat prn for up to 4 mo[62]	Most species/treatment of aspergillosis; can be toxic to psittacines at this dose
	10 mg/mL polyethylene glycol × 30-60 min164	Raptors, psittacines/used in combination with systemic antifungals
	5-10% clotrimazole in propyethylene glycol with 5% DMSO x 1h[746]	Raptors
Dexamethasone sodium phosphate	0.16 mg/mL in saline[600]	Eclectus parrot with tracheal stent placement
Doxycycline hyclate (Vibramycin injection, Pfizer)	13 mg/mL saline[62]	Psittacines
Enilconazole (Imaverol, Janssen; Clinafarm, Schering)	0.2 mg/5 mL saline q12h × 21 days[534]	Most species, including raptors, psittacines
	10 mg/mL sterile water[62]	Most species/antifungal

Continued

TABLE 5-8 Nebulization Agents Used in Birds. (cont'd)

Agent	Dosage	Species/Comments
Enilconazole (Imaverol, Janssen; Clinafarm, Schering) (cont'd)	50 mg in 25 mL saline x 30-45 min q12h[41]	Raptors
	29 mg in a 1-2 g smoke pellet x 30 min[950]	Chickens/PD; fumigation (not nebulization); successfully prevented mortality in experimental infection and decreased morbidity
Enrofloxacin (Baytril, Bayer)	10 mg/mL saline[41,62]	Most species
Erythromycin	5-20 mg/mL saline × 15 min q8h[164,793]	Most species
F10	1:250 dilution[41]	Raptors/prevention and treatment of aspergillosis
	0.2% superconcentrate[966]	Falcons/using a fogging system; prevention and treatment of aspergillosis
Gentamicin	3-6 mg/mL saline or sterile water and 1-2 mL acetylcysteine (20%) × 20 min q8h[41,62,793]	Most species, including cranes and raptors
Itraconazole	1-10% nanoparticulate suspension x 30 min[786]	Japanese quail/PK; reached high lung levels
	4% nanoparticulate suspension x 30 min q24h[998]	Japanese quail/PD; less effective than 10% in experimental aspergillosis
	10% nanoparticulate suspension x 30 min q24h[998]	Japanese quail/PD; experimental aspergillosis, blocked lethality in low spore load group and delayed disease progression in high spore load group
	Nanoparticulate suspension x 30 min (unreported concentration)[502]	Pigeons/PD; tissue therapeutic dose
Lincomycin	250 mg/mL water[164]	Most species
	250 mg aerosolized drug/m^3 chamber × 15-30 min[152]	Chickens/PK; antibiotic; therapeutic concentrations in blood, lungs, and trachea for up to 24 hr
Oxytetracycline	2 mg/mL × 60 min q4-6h[253]	Parakeets/PK; therapeutic concentrations in lungs and trachea, low plasma concentrations
	1 g/m^3 of air using a Devilbiss ultrasonic nebulizer, or 0.075 g/m^3 of air using a Fogmaster fogger[949]	Turkey poults
Piperacillin	10 mg/mL saline × 10-30 min q6-12h[41,62]	Most species/available only in combination with tazobactam in the United States
Polymyxin B sulfate	66,000 U/mL saline[304]	Psittacines/poorly absorbed from respiratory epithelium
Praziquantel	56.8-85.2 mg in 100% oxygen x 5-15 min q24h[218]	Blue-crowned motmots, fairy-bluebirds/ treatment of air sac flukes, decreased parasite burden
Sodium chloride	0.9 % or 3% (hypertonic)[62]	Viscosity of respiratory secretions may be decreased by hydration, mucolytic properties[104]

TABLE 5-8 Nebulization Agents Used in Birds. (cont'd)

Agent	Dosage	Species/Comments
Spectinomycin (Spectam, Ceva)	13 mg/mL saline[164,304]	Most species
Sterile water	—	Viscosity of respiratory secretions may be decreased by hydration[104]
Sulfadimethoxine (Albon, SmithKline)	13 mg/mL saline[164,304]	Most species
Terbinafine	1 mg/mL crushed pills in sterile water x 15min[259]	Hispaniolan Amazon parrots/PK; plasma levels above MIC for 1 hr; solution concentration was lower than expected at 0.9 mg/mL
	1 mg/mL raw powder in sterile water x15 min[259]	Hispaniolan Amazon parrots/PK; plasma levels above MIC for 4 hr
	1 mg/mL q8-12h, 10-15 mg/kg[16]	Raptors
Terbutaline	0.01 mg/kg with 9 mL saline[62]	Psittacines/bronchodilation
Tylosin (Tylan, Elanco)	10 mg/mL saline × 10-60 min q12h[304,793]	Most species
	20 mg/mL DMSO or distilled water × 1 hr[542,543]	Most species, pigeons, quail/PK
Voriconazole	10 mg/mL of NaCl 0.9% x 15 min[82]	Pigeons/PK; low plasma concentrations; no measurable drug in the lungs 1 hr after nebulization; plasma and lung levels below MIC for *Aspergillus*
	10-15 mg/kg saline x 15-30 min q12-8h[16,62]	Most species, raptors

[a]Nebulization is an adjunctive therapy indicated for: rhinitis, sinusitis, tracheitis, pneumonia, airsacculitis, and syringeal aspergilloma, where there is air movement occurring in the patient's disease state; optimal particle size for deposition in the trachea is 2-10 μm; optimal particle size for peripheral airways and air sacs is 0.5-5 μm; treatments of 30-45 min repeated q4-12h are recommended (longer nebulization periods of 1 to several hours may be required[839,927]); caution: do not overhydrate airways. Saline or propylene glycol can be used as a carrier.[839] A variety of nebulizers exist: air jet nebulizers (most commonly used), ultrasonic nebulizers. Air jet nebulizers are better to nebulize viscous liquid.[63] Pressurized metered-dose inhalers are air jet nebulizers and should be used with a holding chamber (e.g., Aerokat).[62]

TABLE 5-9 Agents Used in the Treatment of Toxicologic Conditions of Birds.

Agent	Dosage	Species/Comments
Atropine sulfate	—	Antidote for muscarinic effects of organophosphate/carbamate (acetylcholinesterase inhibitors) toxicosis; does not treat nicotinic effects[752]
	0.01-0.02 mg/kg SC, IM[104]	Most species/facilitates bronchodilation in acutely dyspneic animals; treatment of choice for anticholinesterase-induced respiratory distress
	0.03-0.05 mg/kg SC, IM, IV q8h[939]	Ratites

Continued

TABLE 5-9 Agents Used in the Treatment of Toxicologic Conditions of Birds. (cont'd)

Agent	Dosage	Species/Comments
Atropine sulfate (cont'd)	0.04-0.1 mg/kg IM[104]	Psittacines/bronchodilation in acutely dyspneic animals; treatment of choice for anticholinesterase-induced respiratory distress
	0.1 mg/kg IM, IV q3-4h[43]	Waterfowl, raptors
	0.2-0.5 mg/kg IM, IV q3-4h[251]	Most species, including pigeons, raptors/ cholinesterase inhibitors toxicosis
	0.5 mg/kg IV, IM q6-8h[748]	Raptors/cholinesterase inhibitors toxicosis
Bismuth sulfate 1.75% (Bismusal, Bimeda)	2 mL/kg PO[43]	Most species/weak adsorbent, demulcent; gastrointestinal irritation; may be useful for toxin removal
Botulinum type C antitoxin (100 U/mL) (National Wildlife Health Center, Madison, WI, USA)	1 mL IP[583] once	Waterfowl/not commercially available; produced for experimental use in migratory birds
Botulinum antitoxin	0.05-1 mL/day IP[804]	Most species
Calcium EDTA (edetate calcium disodium)	—	Preferred initial chelator for lead and zinc toxicosis; may cause renal tubular necrosis in mammals; maintain hydration and monitor patient for PU/PD; SC, IM absorbed well;[710] poorly effective at removing lead in soft tissues; combine with DMSA in severe cases[752]
	10-40 mg/kg IM q12h × 5-10 days[804]	Raptors, most species
	20-70 mg/kg IV[206]	Most species/empirical diagnosis; signs should resolve for up to 48 hr; diluted 1:4 in saline
	25-50 mg/kg IV q12h[627]	Geese
	30 mg/kg SC q24h x 5 days[709]	Egyptian, cinereous vultures
	35-100 mg/kg SC, IM, IV diluted with saline q12h for 5 days[270,752]	Raptors
	40 mg/kg IM q12h[220]	Cockatiels/PD; reduces lead levels when used alone or with DMSA
	50 mg/kg IM q12h × up to 23 days[806]	Raptors/no deleterious effects observed
	100 mg/kg IM q12h x 5-25 days[804]	Falcons/no observed deleterious effects
Charcoal, activated	—	Adsorbs toxins from the intestinal tract; may be mixed with hemicellulose to act as a bulk laxative to aid in the passage of ingested toxins; administration prior to cathartic use may help bind small particles of heavy metal;[206] see magnesium hydroxide (Table 5-18) for combination

TABLE 5-9 Agents Used in the Treatment of Toxicologic Conditions of Birds. (cont'd)

Agent	Dosage	Species/Comments
Charcoal, activated (cont'd)	52 mg/kg PO once[607]	A component of oiled bird treatment; alternatively, may use bismuth
	1-3 g/kg[997]	Most species
	2-8 g/kg PO[43,251]	Most species
Deferasirox (Jadenu, Novartis)	Not specified	Oropendolas/induced white discoloration of feathers[917]
Deferiprone (Ferriprox, Apotex, Ontario, Canada)	50 mg/kg PO q12h × 30 days[917,986]	Toucans, pigeons, chickens/iron chelation; may produce rust-colored urates
	50 mg/kg PO q12h[985]	Pigeons/PK
	75 mg/kg PO q24h x 90 days[827]	Hornbills/PD; n = 3
Deferoxamine mesylate (Desferal, Novartis)	—	Preferred iron chelator for hemochromatosis; may take 3 mo to see response; may cause reddish discoloration of urine; avoid in birds with renal disease; combine with a low iron diet;[516,917] poorly absorbed from the gastrointestinal tract[710]
	40 mg/kg IM q24h × 7 days[652]	Bali mynahs
	50 mg/kg IM q12h × 14 days[325]	Macaws
	100 mg/kg SC, IM q24h up to 3.5 mo[181,516,917]	Most species, including toucans
	100 mg/kg SC q24h × 16 wk[661]	European starlings/PD
Dimercaprol (BAL in oil, Becton Dickinson)	2.5-5 mg/kg IM q4h × 2 days, then q12h × 10 days or until recovery[941]	Most species/heavy metal toxicosis; arsenical compound toxicosis; occasionally used for lead, mercury, and gold intoxication (if ingestion <2 hr);[710] cross blood-brain barrier, nephrotoxic, and painful upon injection[752,997]
	25-35 mg/kg PO q12h × 3-5 wk[43]	Most species/give 5 days/wk
Dimercaptosuccinic acid (DMSA or succimer) (DMSA, Aldrich; Chemet, Bock Pharmacal)	—	Oral chelator for lead or zinc; may be effective for mercury toxicity; does not chelate lead from bones; combine with Ca-EDTA in severe cases[752,997]
	25-35 mg/kg PO q12h × 5 day/wk × 3-5 wk[251]	Most species, including raptors/lead toxicosis
	30 mg/kg PO q12h × ≥7 days[410,752]	Most species, raptors/lead toxicosis
	35 mg/kg PO q12h × 34 wk[559]	Budgerigars/PD; prevented experimental lead toxicosis

Continued

TABLE 5-9 Agents Used in the Treatment of Toxicologic Conditions of Birds. (cont'd)

Agent	Dosage	Species/Comments
Dimercaptosuccinic acid (DMSA or succimer) (DMSA, Aldrich; Chemet, Bock Pharmacal) (cont'd)	40 mg/kg PO q12h × 21 days[220]	Cockatiels/PD; lead toxicosis; reduces lead levels when used alone or in combination with CaEDTA; 80 mg/kg resulted in death in >60% of cockatiels
Diphenhydramine	2 mg/kg PO, IM q12h[48,892]	Macaws/used to treat extrapyramidal effects of clomipramine/haloperidol/amitriptyline
Grit	80 particles of fine grit (silica 0.2 mm) or 20 particles of coarse grit (silica, 1-2 mm)[559]	Budgerigar/PD; experimental lead particles administration; faster elimination time than controls but not statistically significant
	3-5 pieces[251]	Most species/reduce size of metal particles
Lipid emulsion 20% (Intralipid)	2 mL/kg IV over 15 min, then 0.25 mL/kg/min over 60 min, repeat 3 times[49]	Double-crested cormorants/ brevetoxicosis
Magnesium hydroxide (M)/ activated charcoal (C) (Milk of Magnesia, Roxane)	(M) 10-12 mL + (C) 1 tsp powder[509]	Most species/cathartic;[a] adsorbent
Magnesium sulfate (Epsom salts)	500-1000 mg/kg PO q12-24h × 1-3 days[43]	Raptors, waterfowl/cathartic used in lead toxicosis to reduce lead absorption[a]
Peanut butter	1 mL combined with mineral oil (2:1)[559]	Budgerigar/cathartic;[a] experimental lead particles administration; faster elimination time than controls but not statistically significant
Penicillamine (Cuprimine, Merck)	—	Preferred chelator for copper toxicosis; may be used for lead, zinc, and mercury toxicosis; significant gastrointestinal side effects (emesis)[710]
	30 mg/kg PO q12h × ≥7 days[410]	Most species/initially supplemented with CaEDTA once in severe neurologic disease
	30-55 mg/kg PO q12h × 7-14 days[509]	Most species, including raptors, waterfowl
	50-55 mg/kg PO q24h × 1-6 wk[206]	Most species, including psittacines, raptors/use in combination with CaEDTA for several days followed by penicillamine × 3-6 wk[206]
	55 mg/kg PO q12h x 10 days[804]	Most species
Phytonadione	—	See vitamin K
Pralidoxime (2-PAM) (Protopam, Wyeth-Ayerst)	—	Administer within 24-36 hr of organophosphate intoxication; use lower dose in combination with atropine;[941] contraindicated for some carbamate poisoning[752]
	10-100 mg/kg IM q24-48h or repeat once q6h[43,509]	Psittacines, raptors, waterfowl
	100 mg/kg IM once[858]	Raptors/monocrotophos toxicosis

TABLE 5-9 Agents Used in the Treatment of Toxicologic Conditions of Birds. (cont'd)

Agent	Dosage	Species/Comments
Pralidoxime (2-PAM) (Protopam, Wyeth-Ayerst) (cont'd)	100 mg/kg IM once[859]	Goslings/PD; experimental diazinon toxicosis; lower dosages (25-50 mg/kg) were less effective
Psyllium (Metamucil)	1 mL of a solution made of 1/2 tsp diluted in 60 mL of water[559]	Budgerigar/PD; cathartic;[a] experimental lead particles administration, similar elimination time than controls
Sodium sulfate (Glauber's salt) (GoLytely, Braintree; anydrous sodium sulfate, ACS grade, Fisher Scientific)	—	Cathartic;[a] contraindicated with impaired gastrointestinal function; maintain hydration
	500 mg/kg PO q48h[220]	Cockatiels/PD; did not result in further decreases in lead concentrations when given to birds receiving CaEDTA alone or in combination with DMSA
	2000 mg/kg PO q24h × 2 days[585]	Most species
Succimer (Chemet, Bock Pharmacal)	—	See dimercaptosuccinic acid (DMSA)
Tea (black tea leaves) (Ceylon CO_2-decaffeinated tea leaves, Frontier Natural)	8 g/kg diet[849]	Starlings/hepatic iron concentrations did not increase significantly in starlings on an iron-enriched diet when supplemented with tea leaves; tea containing approximately 20% (by weight) condensed tannins were blended directly into the food mixture (8 g/kg diet)
Tetanus antitoxin (equine)	50 IU IV over 15 min[72]	Falcon/tetanus
Vitamin K1 (Veda-K1, Vedco)	0.2-2.2 mg/kg IM q4-8h until stable, then q24h PO, IM × 14-28 days[509,752]	Most species, including raptors/rodenticide anticoagulant toxicosis
	2.5 mg/kg SC q12h[630]	Red-tailed hawks/secondary brodifacoum toxicosis

[a]Cathartics increase gastrointestinal motility and are used to evacuate the gut and prevent absorption of toxins.

TABLE 5-10 Psychotropic and Antiepileptic Agents Used in Birds.[a,b]

Agent	Dosage	Species/Comments
Amitriptyline (Flavil, Stuart)	—	Tricyclic antidepressant; inhibits serotonin and norepinephrine reuptake; mild antihistamine effect;[582,954] feather damaging behavior, anxiety, phobia;[582] severe extrapyramidal side effects encountered in a blue and gold macaw at 5 mg/kg PO;[48] as for all antidepressants, start at low dose and titrate up to effect
	1-5 mg/kg PO q12-24h[43,221]	Most species
	2 mg/kg PO q24h[267]	Psittacines/minimum of 30 days

Continued

TABLE 5-10 Psychotropic and Antiepileptic Agents Used in Birds. (cont'd)

Agent	Dosage	Species/Comments
Amitriptyline (Flavil, Stuart) (cont'd)	1.5-4.5 mg/kg PO[973]	Grey parrots, cockatoos/PK; erratic plasma concentrations generally below therapeutic levels
	9 mg/kg PO[973]	Grey parrots, cockatoos/PK; good levels but unpredictable half-life, toxicity in 1/3 African grey parrots
Buspirone HCl (Buspar, Bristol-Myers Squibb)	0.5 mg/kg PO q12h[460]	Anxiolytic; used in one case to control behavior interpreted as paradoxical anxiety caused by clomipramine
Carbamazepine (Tegretol, Novartis)	3-10 mg/kg PO q24h[954] 166 mg/L drinking water[954]	Most species/anticonvulsant, analgesic; may cause bone marrow suppression (including aplastic anemia and agranulocytosis) and hepatotoxicity
Chlorpromazine	—	Phenothiazine; dopamine antagonist[710] used in some cases of feather picking; no antianxiety effects; correct underlying problems and discontinue within 30 days; efficacy diminishes in 14-30 days when given PO; may cause ataxia, regurgitation, drowsiness;[954] rarely recommended in avian behavioral disorders
	0.1-0.2 mg/kg IM once[954]	Cockatoos, ring-necked parakeets/use with carbamazepine following removal of elizabethan collar; mild sedation and decreases obsessive behaviors
	Mix 1 mL stock solution/120 mL drinking water or 0.2-1 mL/kg stock PO q12-24h prn[954]	Most species/stock solution: crush five 25 mg tablets and mix with 31 mL simple syrup; start at low dose initially; mild sedation
Clomipramine (Anafranil, Novartis; Clomicalm, Novartis)	—	Most selective for serotonin reuptake inhibition among tricyclic antidepressants; weak antihistamine; may cause regurgitation, drowsiness; adverse effects in mammals include cardiac conduction abnormalities, tachyarrhythmias, postural hypotension, dry mucous membranes, urinary retention, constipation, and lowering of the seizure threshold;[460,954] as for other psychoactive molecules, wait 2 wk before adjusting dose;[221] reported adverse reactions in psittacines (macaws, cockatoos, grey parrots) include general illness, extrapyramidal signs, increased anxiety, serotonine overload, and death;[221,460,892,954] indicated for compulsive disorders, feather-damaging behavior, fear, phobia, and anxiety in combination with appropriate environmental changes and behavior modifications[221,582,954]
	1 mg/kg PO q12h starting dose; 1-5 mg/kg PO q12h therapeutic range[221]	Psittacines, most birds/anxiety, fear, feather damaging behavior, self-mutilation[221]

TABLE 5-10 Psychotropic and Antiepileptic Agents Used in Birds. (cont'd)

Agent	Dosage	Species/Comments
Clomipramine (Anafranil, Novartis; Clomicalm, Novartis) (cont'd)	1 mg/kg PO q24h or divided q12h × 6 wk[735]	Psittacines/feather-damaging behavior; occasional regurgitation and drowsiness observed; 2 of 11 birds decreased feather picking[735]
	3 mg/kg PO q12h[852]	Cockatoos/PD; placebo-controlled clinical trial; no appreciable deleterious side effects; no significant differences between baseline and posttreatment bloodwork or body weight; significant decrease in feather damaging behavior at 3 and 6 wk
Clonazepam	0.5 mg/kg PO q12h[73]	Grey parrot; antiepileptic; developed tolerance after 7 months
Deslorelin 4.7 mg implant (Suprelorin, Virbac)	4.7 mg and 9.4 mg implant q3-6 months[952]	Most birds/decrease reproduction-related behavior
Diazepam	—	Benzodiazepine sedative; anxiolytic/stress-associated feather picking; useful for acute seizure management; IM diazepam has a delayed absorption and causes muscle irritation
	0.2-2 mg/kg PO q6-8h[572]	Psittacines/sedation
	0.25-0.5 mg/kg IM, IV q24h × 2-3 days[906]	Raptors/appetite stimulant
	0.5 mg/kg PO[333]	Amakihi/calm fractious species while improving acceptance to a novel captive diet; oral solution (1 mg/mL; Roxane Laboratories) worked best
	0.5-1.5 mg/kg IM, IV, intracloacal q8-12h[219]	Most species/control of seizures
	1 mg/kg/h IV, CRI, decrease after 12-24h without seizures[219]	Most species/acute seizure
	10-15 mg/kg IM[720,968]	Small passerines/sedation
	10-20 mg/L drinking water[344]	Most species
Diphenhydramine	—	Antihistamine; mild hypnotic effects; suspected allergic feather picking
	2-4 mg/kg PO q12h[582,952]	Most species
	2 mg/L drinking water[582,952]	Most species
	2 mg/kg IM, PO q12h[892]	Blue and gold macaw/treatment of extrapyramidal side effects of a haloperidol/clomipramine combination
Doxepin	—	Tricyclic antidepressant; antihistamine; may be useful to treat pruritus
	0.5-5 mg/kg PO q12h[952]	Most species/feather picking, anxiety, pruritus
Fluoxetine (Prozac, Dista)	—	Selective serotonin reuptake inhibitor; antidepressant; adjunctive treatment for depression-induced feather picking, compulsive disorders, anxiety disorders, phobia, aggression[582]

Continued

TABLE 5-10 Psychotropic and Antiepileptic Agents Used in Birds. (cont'd)

Agent	Dosage	Species/Comments
Fluoxetine (Prozac, Dista) (cont'd)	0.5-1 mg/kg PO q24h starting dose; 1-5 mg/kg PO q12-24h therapeutic range[221]	Psittacines/feather-damaging behavior
	1 mg/kg PO q24h[850]	Cockatiel/toe-chewing behavior
	1-4 mg/kg PO q24h, up to 20 mg/kg[582]	Parrots
Gabapentin	11 mg/kg PO q8h[1003]	Great horned owl/PK
	15 mg/kg PO q8h[47]	Hispaniolan Amazon parrots/PK
	20 mg/kg PO q12h[73]	African grey parrot/seizures
	25 mg/kg PO q12h[124]	Caribbean flamingo/PK
Haloperidol (Haldol, McNeil)	—	Butyrophenone dopamine antagonist tranquilizer; may cause anorexia, depression, hypotension, bradycardia, ataxia, sedation;[954] no antianxiety effects;[221] efficacy may be mainly based on inhibition of movement and sedation;[221] use is controversial;[221] extrapyramidal signs and/or death reported in various species of macaw;[526,892] Quaker parrots and cockatoos may be more sensitive to side effects[954]
	0.1-0.9 mg/kg PO q24h[582,952]	Most species
	1-2 mg/kg IM q14-21d[952]	Most species, including psittacines
	6.4 mg/L drinking water × 7 mo[425]	Grey parrots/feather picking
Hydroxyzine (Atarax, Roerig)	—	Antihistamine with mild sedative effects
	2-2.2 mg/kg PO q8h[504,582,952]	Most species/feather picking/pruritis
	30-40 mg/L drinking water[952]	Most species
Leuprolide acetate	750 µg/kg IM; BW ≤300g[582]	Parrots/sexual behaviors
	500 µg/kg IM; BW >300g[582]	
	100-1000 µg/kg q2-3 wk (for 3 treatments)[582,952]	Parrots/hormonal feather-damaging behavior/reproductive behaviors
Levetiracetam	50-100 mg/kg PO q8h[73]	African grey parrot/long-term seizure management; therapeutic drug monitoring was performed
	100-150 mg/kg PO q8h[462]	Pionus parrot/long-term seizure management
	5.4-190 mg/kg PO q8-12h[972]	African grey parrots/PK; population pharmacokinetics; short half-life (2.3 hr); no dose recommendation but q8h recommended
	50 mg/kg PO q8h[836]	Hispaniolan Amazon parrots/PK
	100 mg/kg PO q12h[836]	
Lorazepam (Ativran, Wyeth Ayerst)	—	Benzodiazepine with anxiolytic and sedative effects
	0.05-0.1 mg/kg PO q12h[221]	Anxiety, sedation

TABLE 5-10 Psychotropic and Antiepileptic Agents Used in Birds. (cont'd)

Agent	Dosage	Species/Comments
Naloxone HCl (Narcan, DuPont)	2 mg/kg IV[952]	Psittacines/opioid antagonist; may be used to determine the response of stereotypic behavior to antagonist therapy; reduction of the behavior should be observed within 20 min
Naltrexone HCl	1.5 mg/kg PO q8-12h × 1-18 mo[952]	Most species/opioid antagonist; feather-damaging behavior; self-mutilation; contraindicated in patients with liver disease; may need to increase dosage 2-6 × to be effective; dissolve tablet in 10 mL sterile water; preservative does not go into solution
Nortriptyline (Pamelor, Sandoz)	16 mg/L drinking water (2 mg/120 mL)[582,952]	Most species/tricyclic antidepressant; feather-damaging behavior; seldom used; decrease dose or discontinue if hyperactivity develops; taper dose to discontinue
Paroxetine (Paxil, SmithKline Beecham)	1-2 mg/kg PO q24h[467,582]	Macaws, ibises/selective serotonin reuptake inhibitor (SSRI); feather damaging behavior; self-mutilation; generally requires long-term therapy; fewer side effects than tricyclic antidepressants and other SSRIs[954]
	1 mg kg PO q24h starting dose; 1-4 mg/kg PO q12-24h therapeutic range[221]	Most birds
	3 mg/kg PO q24h[467]	Waldrapp ibis
	4 mg/kg PO q12h, bulk chemical compounded in water[957]	Grey parrots/PK; slow absorption and low oral bioavailability; bioavailability increased with repeated dosing; commercial oral suspension (Seroxat) resulted in nondetectable plasma levels; large individual differences
Phenobarbital sodium	—	Barbiturate anticonvulsant; mild sedative effect; long-term seizure management; adjust dosage based on blood levels; may cause deep sedation and inability to perch; hepatotoxic; oral formulations may not reach therapeutic plasma levels in parrots[73,717]
	1-7 mg/kg PO q12-24h[952]	Most species/feather picking; mild sedative effect
	2 mg/kg PO q12h[73]	Grey parrot/antiseizure; therapeutic drug monitoring did not show detectable plasma level
	2-10 mg/kg/h CRI[219]	Most species
	17 mg/kg PO[717]	Grey parrots/PK; used diluted commercial intravenous solution and compounded suspension; plasma levels below therapeutic levels
	50-80 mg/L drinking water[725]	Most species, including Amazon parrots/idiopathic epilepsy
Potassium bromide	—	Long-term seizure management; use as sole agent or in conjunction with phenobarbital; monitor blood levels which may take up to several weeks to establish steady state

Continued

TABLE 5-10 Psychotropic and Antiepileptic Agents Used in Birds. (cont'd)

Agent	Dosage	Species/Comments
Potassium bromide (cont'd)	20-200 mg/kg PO q12h with loading dose of additional 80 mg/kg PO q12h x3 days[73]	Grey parrot/antiseizure; therapeutic drug monitoring showed low plasma level below therapeutic levels (<0.7 mg/mL)
	25-75 mg/kg PO[952]	Most species
	80 mg/kg PO q24h[111]	Umbrella cockatoo/serum drug levels ranged from 1.7-2.2 mg/mL
Zonisamide	19.8-80 mg/kg PO q8-12h[972]	African grey parrots/PK; population pharmacokinetics; half-life was highly variable (10.9 ± 18 hr); no dose recommendation but q8-12h recommended
	20 mg/kg PO q8-12h[73,462]	Grey parrots, white-crowned pionus/anti-seizures; therapeutic drug monitoring performed in one case
	20 mg/kg PO[811]	Chickens/PK; 2/8 birds of multiple escalating dose study developed immune-mediated anemia
	20 mg/kg PO q12h[472]	Hispaniolan Amazon parrots/PK

[a]The use of psychotropic agents in birds is controversial because safety, efficacy, and pharmacologic effects are poorly documented;[954] anxiolytics or tricyclic antidepressants may be useful for stereotypic behaviors or mutilation; selective serotonin reuptake inhibitors may prove helpful for compulsive behaviors; consider metabolic scaling when calculating dosages; psychotropic agents should always be part of a global treatment plan including behavior modifications and environmental changes. It is recommended to start these medications at the lowest end of the reported range, then assess effects after 10-14 days, then increase the dose (typically doubled) and re-evaluate in 2 weeks.[221] We thank Marion Desmarchelier, DVM, Dipl. ACZM, Dipl. ACVB, for commenting on this section.

[b]See also Table 5-55 Guidelines for Selection of Psychotherapeutic Agents for Birds.

TABLE 5-11 Nutritional/Mineral Support and Supplementation Used in Birds.

Agent	Dosage	Species/Comments
Biotin	0.05 mg/kg PO q24h × 30-60 days[43]	Raptors/beak and nail regrowth
Brewer's yeast	30 mg/bird in feed[43]	Pigeons/brittle plumage
Calcium	—	Recommended dietary levels;[a] higher dietary levels than in commercial food were found in wild macaw chicks (1.4%)[121]
	3-7 mg/kg feed (0.3-0.7%)[209]	Maintenance diet for most birds
	3-10 mg/kg feed (0.3-1%)[447]	Laying parrots
	3.5 mg/kg feed (0.35 %)[497]	Egg-laying cockatiel
	4-8 mg/kg feed (0.4-0.8%)[641]	Growing Muscovy ducks
	8.5 mg/kg feed (0.85%)[497]	Egg-laying budgerigars

TABLE 5-11 Nutritional/Mineral Support and Supplementation Used in Birds. (cont'd)

Agent	Dosage	Species/Comments
Calcium borogluconate (10%)	10 mg/kg PO q24h[891]	African grey parrots/hypocalcemia; in addition to UVb supplementation and diet correction
	50-100 mg/kg IM, IV[90]	Psittacines/20% solution
	100-500 mg/kg SC, IV (slow) once[43]	Raptors/hypocalcemia
Calcium glubionate	—	Most species/hypocalcemia, calcium supplementation
	25 mg/kg PO[57,420]	Most species, including raptors, psittacines
	150 mg/kg PO q12h[423,941]	Most species
	750 mg/L drinking water[423]	Most species
Calcium gluconate (10%)	—	Hypocalcemia; dilute 1:1 with saline or sterile water for IM or IV injections; use NaCl 0.9% as IV fluid or precipitation may occur
	25-50 mg/kg SC, IV (slow)[43]	Pigeons
	50-100 mg/kg IM, SC (diluted), IV (slow)[420,423,767]	Most species, including psittacines, pigeons, raptors
	50-150 mg/kg IV over 15-20 min[63]	Most birds/ionized hypocalcemia, hyperkalemia
	100-300 mg/kg SC diluted 1:1-2 with saline[922]	Most species
	100-500 mg/kg SC, IV (slow) once[802]	Raptors/hypocalcemia
	1 mL/30 mL (3300 mg/L) drinking water[941]	Psittacines/calcium supplementation
Calcium lactate/calcium glycerophosphate (Calphosan, Glenwood)	5-10 mg/kg IM q7d prn[57,420,423]	Most species, including raptors/hypocalcemia
	50-100 mg/kg IV (slow bolus) once[730]	Grey parrots
Calcium levulinate	75-100 mg/kg IM, IV[423]	Most species/hypocalcemia
L-carnitine	1000 mg/kg feed[211]	Budgerigars/PD; lipomas; average lipoma size decreased significantly
Dextrose (50%)	50-100 mg/kg IV (slow bolus) to effect[793,941]	Psittacines/hypoglycemia; can dilute with fluids
	500-1000 mg/kg IV (slow bolus)[726]	Hypoglycemia; can dilute with fluids
	0.5 mL/kg IV over 15 min[63]	Most species/hypoglycemia
Diatrizoate meglumine sodium (37% iodine) (Renografin-76, Solvay)	—	Parenteral treatment of goiter is generally reserved for emergency situations
	122 mg/kg IM[767]	Budgerigars/thyroid hyperplasia

Continued

TABLE 5-11 Nutritional/Mineral Support and Supplementation Used in Birds. (cont'd)

Agent	Dosage	Species/Comments
Essential fatty acids	0.5 mL/kg PO q24h × 50 days or indefinitely[43]	Raptors/pruritic dermatitis (atopy)
Fatty acids (omega-3, omega-6)	0.1-0.2 mL/kg of flaxseed oil to corn oil mixed at a ratio of 1:4 PO or added to food; ratio of omega-6:omega-3 is 4-5:1[254]	Psittacines, pigeons/glomerular disease; used to reduce thromboxane A2 synthesis in platelets and glomerular cells; adjunct therapy for arthritis, feather picking, mutilators, and neoplasia; 2-4 wk of therapy are required to recognize effects; may increase dietary vitamin E requirements; consider supplementation with chronic use
	0.11 mL/kg q24h in a 5:1 ratio of omega-6:omega-3[229]	Psittacines/glomerulonephritis, pancreatitis
	10% flaxseeds[699]	Quaker parrots/PD; shift in HDL subgroups; higher plasma phospholipid omega-3 fatty acids
	A-linolenic acid, 0.2-4% of daily energy[698]	Quaker parrots/PD; no change in blood cholesterol compared to control group; changes in polyunsaturated fatty acid blood profile
	Fish oil, 3% dietary supplementation[400]	Cockatiels/PD; decrease in blood cholesterol; more effective than flaxseed oil
	Flaxseed oil, 3.5% dietary supplementation[400]	Cockatiels/PD; decrease in blood lipid; less effective than fish oil
Hemicellulose (Metamucil, Searle)	—	For bulk in diet; facilitates defecation in bowel deficit disorders and other conditions
	0.5 tsp/60 mL hand-feeding formula or baby food gruel[509]	Psittacines/bulk diet to delay absorption of an ingested toxin
	1 Tbs/60 mL water q24h[939]	Ostrich chicks/impaction
	1 mL of solution of ½ tsp diluted in 60 mL of water[559]	Budgerigars/no difference from controls in elimination rate of ventricular lead particles
Inositol	20 g/kg of food[661,662]	Starling/PD; not effective to decrease liver stored iron but prevented an increase in stored iron concentration
Iodine (Lugol's iodine)	0.2 mL/L drinking water daily[423]	Most species/thyroid hyperplasia
	2 parts iodine + 28 parts water; 3 drops into 100 mL drinking water[43]	Budgerigars/thyroid hyperplasia
Iodine (sodium iodide 20%)	—	Parenteral treatment of goiter is generally reserved for emergency situations or initial treatment of severe thyroid dysplasia; continue with oral therapy when improvement is noted
	2 mg (0.01 mL)/bird IM prn[57]	Budgerigars
	60 mg (0.3 mL)/kg IM[423]	Most species/thyroid hyperplasia
Iron	20-60 mg/kg feed[516,550,661]	Species susceptible to iron storage disease/levels recommended for a low-iron diet

TABLE 5-11 Nutritional/Mineral Support and Supplementation Used in Birds. (cont'd)

Agent	Dosage	Species/Comments
Iron dextran	10 mg/kg IM, repeat in 7-10 days prn[767]	Most species, including raptors, waterfowl/iron deficiency anemia; use cautiously in species in which iron storage disease is common (e.g., toucans, mynahs, starlings, birds of paradise, other passerines)
Lactobacillus (Bene-Bac, Pet-Ag)	1 pinch/day/bird in food[941]	Psittacines/stimulation of normal gastrointestinal flora regrowth
Lactobacillus acidophilus	0.25 g/dose mixed with diet, 2.5-6 × 10^6 CFU/dose[944]	Neonatal cockatiel/PD; increased growth rate in birds receiving the gel form; no effect in birds receiving the powder form; no overall benefit noted
	1 tsp/L hand-feeding formula[391]	Most species
Magnesium sulfate	20 mg/kg IM[478]	Grey parrot/dietary hypomagnesemia and seizures
Niacin (nicotinic acid)	50 mg/kg PO q8h[725]	Psittacines/yolk emboli; give with gemfibrozil (30 mg/kg PO)
Pancreatic enzyme powder (Viokase-V Powder, Fort Dodge)	—	Most species/exocrine pancreatic insufficiency; maldigestion; mix with food and let stand 30 min[941]
	2-5 g/kg feed[391]	Most species
	1/8 tsp/kg feed[391]	Most species
	1/8 tsp/60-120 g lightly oil-coated seed[391]	Most species
	1/8 tsp/30-120 mL hand-feeding formula prn[391]	Psittacine neonates
Pancreatic enzyme powder (Pancrezyme, Virbac)	1 pinch in food[110]	May be beneficial to hatchlings of species fed regurgitant, such as woodpeckers and some others; emaciated birds
Phytonadione	—	See vitamin K1
Potassium chloride (KCl)	0.5 mmol/kg PO q12h[65]	Most species/hypokalemia
Selenium (Seletoc, Schering)	0.05-0.1 mg Se/kg IM q14d[767]	Most species/neuromuscular diseases (capture myopathy, white muscle disease, some cardiomyopathies); may be useful in some cockatiels with jaw, eyelid, and tongue paralysis
	0.06 mg Se/kg IM q3-14d[423]	
Sodium chloride (buffered salt tablet)	450 mg PO daily[312]	Penguins/prevents atrophy of salt gland; may not be needed[976]
Tannic acid	20 g/kg of food[661,662]	Starling/PD; not effective to decrease liver stored iron but prevented an increase in stored iron concentration
Tea (black)	8g/kg of food (black Ceylon decaffeinated)[849]	Starling/PD; effectively limited iron absorption

Continued

TABLE 5-11 Nutritional/Mineral Support and Supplementation Used in Birds. (cont'd)

Agent	Dosage	Species/Comments
Vitamin A (Aquasol A Parenteral, Astra)	—	1 µg = 14 IU; 1 µg retinol = 3.3 IU; 1 µg beta-carotene = 1.7 IU; 3000 µg/kg dietary vitamin A after 269 days induced increased plasma retinol, splenic hemosiderosis, and altered vocalization patterns in cockatiels;[498] toxicosis may follow oversupplementation[498,676]
	200 U/kg IM[454]	Raptor juveniles/supplemental therapy for pox infection
	2000 U/kg PO, IM[34]	Psittacines/adjunctive therapy for pox infection
	5000 U/kg IM q24h × 14 days, then 250-1000 U/kg q24h PO[177]	Psittacines/adjunctive therapy for respiratory or epithelial disease
	20,000 U/kg IM[929]	Most species/hypovitaminosis A; maximum dose; improves skin healing
	33,000 U/kg (10,000 U/300 g) IM q7d[423]	Most species/hypovitaminosis A
	50,000 U/kg IM q7d[457]	Psittacine neonates
	1 mL/135 kg IM[2]	Ostriches/hypovitaminosis A
Vitamin B1 (thiamine)	—	Thiamine deficiency; requirements may be higher if thiaminase is present in diet[b]
	1-3 mg/kg PO q24h[420,767]	Most species including raptors, penguins, cranes/daily supplement for CNS signs
	1-50 mg/kg PO q24h × 7 days or indefinitely[43]	Raptors
	2 mg/kg IM[939]	Ratites/curly toe paralysis
	4 mg/kg IM followed by 2 mg/kg PO q12h × 5 days[138]	Juvenile goshawks/hypovitaminosis B_1 with neurological signs
	10-50 mg/kg PO q24h[510]	Raptors
	25-30 mg/kg fish (wet basis)[87]	Piscivorous species/recommended level of supplementation
	2850 mg/L drinking water q7d[802]	Pigeons
Vitamin B_{12} (cyanocobalamin)	0.25-0.5 mg/kg IM q7d[420,767,802]	Most species, including psittacines, raptors/anemia
	2-5 mg/bird SC[938]	Pigeons/vitamin B12 deficiency
Vitamin B complex	—	Usually dosed based on thiamine (see vitamin B1); deaths have been reported in falcons following injections, which was attributed to an overdose of vitamin B_6 (pyridoxine);[804] has been used to treat folate and cobalamine dietary deficiency in a hyacinth macaw[361]

TABLE 5-11 Nutritional/Mineral Support and Supplementation Used in Birds. (cont'd)

Agent	Dosage	Species/Comments
Vitamin C (ascorbic acid)	20-50 mg/kg IM q1-7d[454,767]	Most species, including raptors/nutritional support; supplemental therapy for pox infection
	150 mg/kg PO q24h[371]	Willow ptarmigan chicks/PD; supplemental daily requirements over 265 mg/kg diet
Vitamin D3 (Vital E-A + D, Schering)	—	1 µg = 40 IU; macaws are more susceptible to toxic side effects; vitamin D_2 is poorly effective in birds[209]
	3300 U/kg (1000 U/300 g) IM q7d prn[423]	Most species/hypovitaminosis D3; hypervitaminosis D may occur with excessive use
	5000 U IM once, then 200 U PO q24h x 88d[499]	Red-legged seriema chicks/hypovitaminosis D; in combination with UVb supplementation
	6600 U/kg IM once[1001]	Most species
Vitamin E (Vitamin E20, Horse Health Products; Bo-SE, Schering Plough)	—	1 mg d α-tocopherol acetate = 1.5 IU; 1 mg dL α-tocopherol acetate = 1.1 IU; injectable vitamin E may have lower efficacy than oral[579]
	0.06 mg/kg IM q7d[802]	Psittacines/hypovitaminosis E
	0.06 mg/kg IM[939]	Ratites/prevention or treatment of capture myopathy
	15 mg/kg PO once[569]	Swainson's hawk/PD; administer without food
	70 mg/kg IM q24h for up to 5 days[1015]	Pelicans/hypovitaminosis E; steatitis
	200-300 mg/kg IM[585]	Ostrich chicks
	200-400 mg/bird PO q24h[7]	Great blue herons
	73.5 mg/kg fish (wet basis)[1015]	Pelicans/supplementation; excessive supplementation (550-10560 IU/kg) has been associated with coagulopathy in pink-backed pelicans[650]
	100 mg/kg fish (wet basis)[87,1015]	Piscivorous species/recommended level of supplementation
	4400-8800 mg/kg feed[16]	Ostrich chicks/hypovitaminosis E
Vitamin E/γ-linolenic acid (2%), linoleic acid (71%) (Derm Caps, DVM Pharmaceuticals)	0.1 mL/kg PO q24h[767]	Most species/feather picking; use liquid from gel caps
Vitamin K1 (phytonadione)	0.2-2.2 mg/kg IM q4-8h until stable, then q24h × 14 days[509]	Most species/rodenticide toxicity
	2.5 mg/kg SC q12h[630]	Red-tailed hawk/treatment of brodifacoum toxicosis
	5 mg/kg IM q24h for several days[939]	Ratites/coagulopathy

Continued

TABLE 5-11 Nutritional/Mineral Support and Supplementation Used in Birds. (cont'd)

Agent	Dosage	Species/Comments
Vitamin K1 (phytonadione) (cont'd)	10-12.5 mg/kg SC q12h × 4 days[1015]	Pelicans/coagulopathy
	10-20 mg/kg IM q12-24h[15]	Psittacines
	0.1 mg/kg feed[444]	Turkeys/PD; as effective as 1-2 mg/kg in reducing plasma prothrombin time

[a]Grains and seeds commonly fed to parrots contain calcium levels of approximately 0.02-0.1% DM.
[b]Food items known to contain appreciable amounts of thiaminase include clams, herring, smelt, and mackerel.[87]

TABLE 5-12 Ophthalmologic Agents Used in Birds.[a]

Agent	Dosage	Species/Comments
Amphotericin B	125 µg/5 mL sterile water subconjunctival[188]	Ducks (ornamental)/candidiasis of third eyelid
Amphotericin B ointment (4%) (formulated)	Topical q24h[188]	Ducks (ornamental)/candidiasis of third eyelid; administered in conjunction with systemic antifungal therapy
Atracurium	0.05 µL intracameral[150]	Great horned owl/mydriasis for cataract surgery
	0.01 mg intracameral[65]	Parrots/mydriasis for cataract surgery
	1:5 dilution of 10 mg/mL solution, intracameral, maximum 1 mL injection[161]	Penguins/mydriasis for cataract surgery; out of 14 penguins, 71% had moderate mydriasis, 7% had minimal mydriasis, 21% showed no effect
Atropine (0.4-0.5%)	0.6 mg/bird topical[733]	Cockatoos/PD; partial mydriasis; some birds have iridal smooth muscle; may cause ocular irritation, weakness, shallow breathing; dilute with 0.9% saline[a]
	Topical[122]	Ratites/partial mydriasis; use in combination with curariform drugs; some ratites have iridal smooth muscle[a]
	1 drop of 1% atropine[544]	Double-crested cormorants/PD; no mydriasis when used alone
Bacitracin/neomycin/polymyxin B sulfate	Topical q6-8h[67]	Most species/antibiotics; corneal ulcers, conjunctivitis
Chloramphenicol ophthalmic drops	1 drop topical q6-8h[445]	Pigeons/antibiotic
Ciprofloxacin HCl (0.3%) (Ciloxan, Alcon)	1 drop topical q4-8h[7,67]	Most species/antibiotic; corneal ulcers, conjunctivitis (e.g., *Chlamydia, Mycoplasma*)
	One drop topical q12h; use in conjunction with tylosin 1 mg/mL drinking water × 21-77 days[586]	House finches/PD; *Mycoplasma gallisepticum* conjunctivitis

TABLE 5-12 Ophthalmologic Agents Used in Birds. (cont'd)

Agent	Dosage	Species/Comments
Demercarium bromide (0.125%) (Humorsol, Merck)	1 drop topical[7]	Most species/topical anesthetic; allows removal of *Thelazia*
Dexamethasone	—	Pigeons/PD; ophthalmic administration results in significant adrenocortical suppression for 24 hr at 4 µg/drop[981]
Dexamethasone (0.1%) ophthalmic drops	1 drop topical q4-8h[420]	Raptors/traumatic anterior uveitis without corneal ulceration
Diclofenac	1 drop topical q12h[65]	Most species/caution in species susceptible to toxicosis (*Gyps* vultures, pigeons)[655]
Edetate disodium ophthalmic drops	1 drop several times daily[710]	Most species/used to treat calcific keratopathy
Flurbiprofen 0.03%	Topical[67,863]	Most birds, raptors/uveitis
Fumagillin (Fumidil B; Mid-Continent Agrimarketing)	1 drop topical q2h[137]	Amazon parrots/fungal and microsporidial keratoconjunctivitis in combination with oral albendazole
	0.114 mg/mL drops q2-3h until 1 wk post clinical signs[877]	Lovebirds/*Encephalitozoon hellem* conjunctivitis; used in combination with albendazole
	60 mg in sterile water topical[877]	Most species/filter solution to remove bacteria before applying
Gentamicin sulfate	1 drop topical q12 × 21 days[979]	House finches/PD; mycoplasmosis treatment in combination with oral enrofloxacin; was not effective
Isoflurane	1-3% maintenance[67]	Most species/mydriasis[a]
	1-2.4% maintenance by air sac perfusion[193,494]	Most species/mydriasis; ocular surgery
Miconazole (Monistat IV, Janssen)	1 drop topical q2h[137]	Amazon parrots/microsporidian keratitis
Miconazole vaginal cream (2%) (Monistat, Ortho-McNeal)	Topical[7]	Most species/antifungal
	Topical q24h × 7 days[474]	Ring-billed gull/third eyelid candidiasis
Natamycin (Natacyn, Alcon)	1 drop topical q6h[767]	Most species/antifungal; gradually taper off
Neomycin/polymixin/ dexamethasone (0.1%)	1 drop topical q8-24h[150]	Great horned owl/post cataract surgery
Oxybuprocaine (0.45%)	Topical[496]	Pigeons, buzzards/topical anesthetic of choice due to reliable effect with minimal side effects
Phenylephrine (2.5%)	Topical[122]	Ratites/partial mydriasis; use in combination with curariform drugs; some ratites have iridal smooth muscle[a]

Continued

TABLE 5-12 Ophthalmologic Agents Used in Birds. (cont'd)

Agent	Dosage	Species/Comments
Phenylephrine (4-5%)	—	4-5% ophthalmic solution is not available in the United States
	6 mg/bird topical[733]	Cockatoos/PD; partial mydriasis; some birds have iridal smooth muscle; may cause ocular irritation, weakness, shallow breathing; dilute with 0.9% saline
	Topical[544]	Cormorants/PD; mydriasis; used in combination with vecuronium bromide and atropine
Phenylephrine (10%)	2 drops topical, diluted to 1%[326,327,989]	Various species/diagnosis of Horner's syndrome
Pimaricin (Natacyn, Alcon)	1 drop topical q6h, taper after 14-21 days[767]	Most species/polyene antifungal
Prednisolone acetate	—	Pigeons/PD; ophthalmic administration results in significant adrenocortical suppression for 4 hr at 35 µg /drop[981]
Prednisolone acetate (1%)	1 drop topical q4-8h[420]	Raptors/traumatic anterior uveitis without corneal ulceration
Prednisolone acetate (0.12%)	1 drop topical q4h[388]	Macaw/uveitis and hyphema secondary to lymphoma
Proparacaine (0.5%) (Proxymetacaine)	Topical[496]	Topical anesthetic
	1 drop/eye[897]	Hispaniolan Amazon parrots/PD; at 10 min: no difference in phenol red thread test values, lower Schirmer tear test values
Rocuronium bromide (1%)	0.12 mg/eye[54]	European kestrels/PD; maximal mydriasis at 90 min, onset of action at 20 min, duration of action of 250 min; decreases IOP[51]
	0.15 mg/eye[46]	Hispaniolan Amazon parrots/PD; mydriasis starting at 5-10 min and lasting for 360 min
	0.2 mg/eye[52]	Little owls/PD; maximal mydriasis at 40 min, onset of action at 20 min, duration of action of 290 min; decreases IOP[51]
	0.35-0.70 mg/eye[53]	Tawny owls/PD; maximal mydriasis at 60-80 min (depending on dose), onset of action at 20 min, duration of action of 240 min
	0.4 mg/eye[52]	Common buzzards/PD; maximal mydriasis at 90 min, onset of action at 20 min, duration of action of 240 min
	20 µL/eye[697]	Hispaniolan Amazon parrots/PD; mydriasis from 20 to 360 min; some birds had transient palpebral paresis
Tetracaine (6%)	Topical[496]	Topical anesthetic

TABLE 5-12 Ophthalmologic Agents Used in Birds. (cont'd)

Agent	Dosage	Species/Comments
Tissue plasminogen activator (rTPA) (TNKase Tenecteplase, Genetech)	50 µg via injection[495]	Raptors/hyphema (use paracentesis into the anterior eye chamber); intraocular hemorrhage (use intravitreous injection)
Tissue plasminogen activator (rTPA) (Activase)	400 µL via injection[24]	Great horned owl/hyphema
	25 µg intracameral[33]	Prevention of hyphema post cataract surgery
Tobramycin	1 drop q6-12h[65]	Most species
Triamcinolone (Vetalog, Fort Dodge)	0.1-0.25 mL subconjunctival[420]	Raptors/traumatic anterior uveitis without corneal ulceration in patients where restraint is a concern
	0.075 mg/kg subconjunctival[150]	Great horned owls/cataract surgery
Trypan blue 0.06%	Intracameral injection[863]	Raptors/injection in anterior chamber to stain the lens capsule.
d-tubocurarine (Curarin-Asta, Asta-Werke, Bielefeld, Germany)	—	Mydriatic agent;[a] recommended for therapeutic use only; administer into anterior chamber; high risk of intraocular injury; topical application has no effect[493]
	0.01-0.03 mL of 0.3% solution, intracameral[67,492,494,628]	Most species, including pigeons, raptors/dilation within 15 min; duration 4-12 hr
Tylosin	Topical (mix powder 1:10 with sterile water)[7]	Cockatiels/conjunctivitis; use in conjunction with systemic treatment
Vecuronium bromide (Norcuron, Organon)	—	Mydriatic agent; may cause respiratory paralysis or shallow breathing, ataxia, death (especially when applied bilaterally);[604] neostigmine may counteract systemic effects[a]
	0.096 mg/bird of 0.08% solution topical[733]	Cockatoos, blue-fronted Amazon parrots, African grey parrots/PD
	0.16 mg/eye (0.4% solution)[544]	Double-crested cormorants/PD; mydriasis; combination with atropine and phenylephrine provided more consistent and longer mydriasis
	0.18-0.22 mg/kg topical[733]	African grey parrots/PD
	0.18-0.29 mg/kg topical[733]	Cockatoos/PD
	0.24-0.28 mg/kg topical[733]	Blue-fronted Amazon parrots/PD
	0.96 mg/bird topical[733]	Cockatoos/use caution with bilateral application
	1 drop of 0.4% solution topical[990]	Cormorants, loons/dilation at 30-45 min; duration >2 hr
	2 drops of 0.4% solution topical q15min × 3 treatments[604]	Kestrels/PD; maximal effect in 65 ± 12 min
	0.5% solution topical[604]	Raptors/duration 1 hr

Continued

TABLE 5-12 Ophthalmologic Agents Used in Birds. (cont'd)

Agent	Dosage	Species/Comments
Vecuronium (V)/ nitrous oxide (N)/ isoflurane (I)	(V) 0.2 mg/kg IV + 1:1 ratio of oxygen to 33% (N) at 0.3 L/kg/min + (I) 1-2.4%[491,493]	Most species/mydriasis and anesthesia; gases are administered via air sac cannulation; vecuronium effective up to 256 min in pigeons[a]

[a]Variable amounts of skeletal muscle are present in the avian iris, giving birds voluntary control over pupil dilation. In many avian patients, the pupils are best dilated by restraining the animal in a dark room. Consensual pupillary light reflex is generally absent in birds.

TABLE 5-13 Oncologic Agents and Radiation Therapy Used in Birds.

Agent	Dosage	Species/Comments
Acemannan (Carravet, Carrington Laboratories)	1 mg/kg SC q7d × 4 treatments[993]	Cockatoos/chemotherapeutic adjunct therapy
	2 mg/kg intralesional q7d × 4 treatments[993]	Cockatoos/use prior to surgical debulking in fibrosarcoma
Asparaginase (Elspar, Merck)	400 U/kg IM q7d[315]	Cockatoos/lymphosarcoma; premedicate with diphenhydramine
	400 IU/kg SC, 3000 IU total dose[870]	Black swan/lymphocytic leukemia, in combination with lomustine, poor response
	1650 U/kg SC once[797]	Great horned owls/sarcoma; associated with severe bone marrow suppression
Bleomycin	0.5 mg/kg intralesional with electrochemotherapy[729]	Cockatiel/uropygial squamous cell carcinoma; curative
Carboplatin	5 mg/kg IV, IO over 3 min[279,566]	Sulphur-crested cockatoos/PD; mix with 5% dextrose to 400 mg/L
		Budgerigar/renal adenocarcinoma; diluted in sterile water; leg paresis showed improvement over 2 mo; mass continued to grow
	5 mg/kg intralesional[993]	Amazon parrots/squamous cell carcinoma; mix with sesame oil or plasma at a concentration of 10 mg/mL
	5 mg/kg IO q4wk × 3 doses[1010]	Green-winged macaw/pancreatic adenocarcinoma
	15 mg/kg IV q5wk × 4 doses[157]	Mallard duck/Sertoli cell tumor; 13 mo survival
	17.2 mg/kg × 4 doses 3-10 wk apart[1010]	Amazon parrot/choanal squamous cell carcinoma; 9 mo survival
	27 mg/kg q4wk × 4 doses[1010]	Cockatiel/cutaneous squamous cell carcinoma; 3 mo survival
	24 mg/kg q4wk × 4 doses[1010]	Amazon parrot/cutaneous squamous cell carcinoma; 1 yr survival
	125 mg/m^2 IV (slow bolus) q14-21d[1008]	Amazon parrots/bile duct carcinoma; dilute with 5% dextrose[a]
	Impregnated calcium-based matrix beads (4.6 mg/bead), intralesional[825]	Kori bustard/myxosarcoma

TABLE 5-13 Oncologic Agents and Radiation Therapy Used in Bird. (cont'd)

Agent	Dosage	Species/Comments
Chlorambucil (Leukeran, GlaxoSmithKline)	1 mg/bird PO 2×/wk[648]	Pekin ducks/lymphocytic leukemia or lymphosarcoma; responded to treatment initially but euthanized 1 mo after presentation because of respiratory distress and hemorrhages
	1 mg/kg PO 2×/wk[368]	Green-winged macaw/chronic lymphocytic leukemia; developed thrombocytopenia and discontinued; died after 29 wk
	1.5 mg/kg PO q72h[322]	Starling/chronic lymphocytic leukemia; followup of 6 mo
	2 mg/kg PO 2×/wk[773]	Umbrella cockatoos/cutaneous lymphosarcoma
	2 mg total dose PO q48h[870]	Black swan/lymphocytic leukemia; minimal response
	2 mg/kg PO twice weekly[1004]	Java sparrow/thymic lymphoma; reduction in mass; treatment discontinued after bird became anorexic at 19 wk
	2 mg tablet twice weekly[570]	Great horned owl/lymphoma; no response
Cisplatin	0.2 mg/kg intralesional[273]	Black-footed penguin/choanal squamous cell carcinoma; 13 mo remission
	1 mg/kg IV over 1 hr[277,278]	Cockatoos/PK and PD; may cause nephrotoxicity; administer IV fluids 1 hr before and 2 hr after infusion
	17.5 mg/m² q7d for 4 treatments, intralesional[483]	African grey parrot/multiple integumentary squamous cell carcinomas; did not seem effective
	Intralesional (undisclosed dose)[737]	Blue and gold macaw/facial fibrosarcoma; in combination with radiation therapy; 29 mo remission
	Intralesional (undisclosed dose)[432]	Goose/lipoblastomatosis-xanthomatosis; unsuccessful
Cyclophosphamide	200 mg/m² IO q7d[391]	Cockatoos/lymphosarcoma[a]
	300 mg/m² PO once[797]	Great horned owls/histiocytic sarcoma;[a] dose associated with severe bone marrow suppression
	5 mg/kg 4 days/wk[368]	Green-winged macaw/lymphocytic leukemia; good response
	10 mg/m² PO q24h[825]	Kori bustard/myxosarcoma; metronomic therapy in combination with meloxicam
Deslorelin implant	4.6 mg SC q4-6mo[471]	Cockatiels/ovarian adenocarcinoma
Diphenhydramine	2 mg/kg IO once[315]	Cockatoos/before chemotherapy
Doxorubicin	2 mg/kg IV[339,340]	Cockatoos/PD; may produce mild transient inappetence; frequency was not determined; PK of metabolite doxorubicinol showed no toxicity[340]
	30 mg/m² IO q2d[315]	Cockatoos/lymphosarcoma;[a] premedicate with diphenhydramine

Continued

TABLE 5-13 Oncologic Agents and Radiation Therapy Used in Bird. (cont'd)

Agent	Dosage	Species/Comments
Doxorubicin (cont'd)	60 mg/m^2 IV q30d[235]	Blue-fronted Amazon parrots/osteosarcoma;[a] premedicate with diphenhydramine 30 min before; dilute with saline and give over 30 min (anesthesia recommended); 20 mo remission
Hexyl ether pyropheophorbide-a (Photochlor, Roswell Park Cancer Institute)	0.3 mg/kg IV[909,910]	African rose-ringed parakeet, hornbill/ photosensitizing agent; use 24 hr prior to photodynamic therapy
L-carnitine	1000 mg/kg of food[211]	Budgerigars/PD; lipoma size decrease
Leuprolide acetate	1500-3000 µg/kg IM q2-3 wk[471]	Cockatiels/ovarian adenocarcinoma
Lomustine	60 mg/m^2 PO q3wk[870]	Black swan/lymphocytic leukemia, in combination with L-asparaginase; minimal response
Methylprednisolone	2 mg/bird IM once[23]	African grey parrot/bronchial carcinoma
Porfimer sodium (Photofrin, QLT PhotoTherapeutics)	3 mg/kg IV[783]	Cockatiels/photodynamic therapy
Prednisolone	2.2 mg/kg q12h[1004]	Java sparrow/thymic lymphoma; 61 wk survival
Prednisone	0.5-1 mg/kg q24h[368,870]	Adjunctive treatment in chemotherapeutic protocols; palliative care; multiple case reports
	1 mg/kg PO q24h[368]	Green-winged macaw/chronic lymphocytic leukemia; combination therapy; discontinued after 6 wk because of thrombocytopenia
	1.6 mg/kg PO q24h[797]	Great horned owls/sarcoma
Radiation therapy	20 cGy fractions for 10 treatments, total dose of 2 Gy[870]	Black swan/lymphocytic leukemia; total body radiation; partial response
	1 Gy at 2.5 Gy/min × 3-4 doses[198]	Military macaws/PD; radiation of normal choana; delivered dose was slightly lower (0.94-0.97 G) than calculated
	2.5 Gy fractions, total dose of 50 Gy[363]	Thick-billed parrot/beak melanoma; 2.5 mo survival
	4 Gy fractions q48h over 22 days, total dose of 40 Gy[512]	Blue and gold macaw/wing fibrosarcoma, in combination with cisplatin chemotherapy; remission observed over 2 mo and until 15 mo
	4 Gy fractions 3 days/wk for a total dose of 40 Gy[685]	African grey parrot/periocular lymphoma; 2 mo survival
	4 Gy fractions 4 d/wk, total dose of 40 Gy[317]	Budgerigar/metacarpal hemangiosarcoma; complete tumor regression observed; death 8 wk later from metastasis
	4 Gy fractions 3 d/wk × 4 wk, total dose of 48 Gy; then booster dose of 8 Gy 5 wk later[576]	Buffon's macaw/squamous cell carcinoma of the beak; no evidence of tissue or tumor damage

TABLE 5-13 Oncologic Agents and Radiation Therapy Used in Bird. (cont'd)

Agent	Dosage	Species/Comments
Radiation therapy (cont'd)	4 Gy fractions 3 days/wk, total dose of 44 Gy[737]	Blue and gold macaw/facial fibrosarcoma in combination with intralesional cisplatin; erythema over the tumor site; 29 mo remission
	4 Gy fractions, total doses of 48, 60, or 72 Gy[50]	Ring-necked parakeets/PD; radiation of normal skin and crop; no adverse radiation effects detected
	4 Gy fractions 3 days/wk × 6 wk, total dose of 68 Gy[309]	Umbrella cockatoo/intraocular osteosarcoma; 2 mo survival
	6 Gy fractions, total dose of 24 Gy[525]	Grey parrot/thymoma; curative at 9 mo in combination with surgery
	8 Gy fractions, total dose of 24 Gy[856]	Green-winged macaw/carcinoma, initial mass reduction but recurred
	8 Gy fractions q1wk, total dose 32 Gy[916]	Grey parrot/squamous cell carcinoma, palliative
	10 Gy fractions at 0, 7, and 21 days, 2 additional doses 1 mo later, total dose of 50 Gy[8]	American flamingo/cutaneous squamous cell carcinoma; no tumor reduction
Silymarin (milk thistle)	100-150 mg/kg PO divided q8-12h[26]	Hepatic antioxidant/protectant; use in patients with liver disease and as ancillary to chemotherapy; use a low-alcohol or alcohol-free liquid formulation
Strontium (Sr-90 ophthalmic applicator)	100 Gy/area x 1-3 areas[645]	Budgerigars, cockatiels/uropygial squamous cell carcinoma; good response at 2-9 mo
	4 areas irradiated with 100 Gy, repeated 1 wk later[708]	Grey parrot/uropygial squamous cell carcinoma; good response at 6 mo
Vincristine sulfate	0.1 mg/kg IV q7-14d[773]	Cockatoos/monitor CBC weekly; complete remission
	0.5 mg/m² IV, then 0.75 mg/m² q7d × 3 treatments[648]	Ducks/lymphoma; lymphocytic leukemia[a]
	0.75 mg/m² IO q7d × 3 treatments[315]	Cockatoos/lymphosarcoma[a]

[a]Body weight (kg) = surface area (m²); 0.5 kg = 0.06 m²; 1 kg = 0.1 m²; 2 kg = 0.15 m²; 3 kg = 0.2 m²; 4 kg = 0.25 m²; 5 kg = 0.29 m²

TABLE 5-14 Antimicrobial-Impregnated Polymethylmethacrylate (PMMA) Agents Used in Birds.[a,266,391,567,932]

Agent	Dosage	Species/Comments
Amikacin	1.25-2.5 g/20 g polymer powder[266]	PD/elution of amikacin from PMMA beads was greater when the powdered form was used compared with liquid amikacin
Bone cement (various manufacturers)	—	Polymer powder and liquid monomer for use in making antibiotic-impregnated beads; some bone cements may lead to higher rate of drug elution than others[598]

Continued

TABLE 5-14 Antimicrobial-Impregnated Polymethylmethacrylate (PMMA) Agents Used in Birds. (cont'd)

Agent	Dosage	Species/Comments
Calcium sulfate beads (Kerrier, info@kerrier.com)	—	Absorbable alternative to PMMA
Cefazolin	1-2 g/20 g polymer powder[446]	
Cefotaxime	2 g/20 g polymer powder[446]	Mix antibiotic powder with bone cement powder, then add liquid for mixing
Ceftazidime	2 g/20 g polymer powder[446]	Mix antibiotic powder with bone cement powder, then add liquid for mixing
Ceftiofur (Naxcel, Pfizer)	2 g/20 g polymer powder[266]	Studies show elution for approximately 7 days only[173]
Ciprofloxacin	—	Release for 360 days[937]
Clindamycin	—	PMMA beads with clindamycin had adequate drug levels for more than 90 days[567,761]
Enrofloxacin (Baytril, Bayer)	—	Raptors/pododermatitis[761]
Gentamicin	1 g powder or solution/20 g polymer powder[266]	PD/elution concentration remained greater than MIC for common pathogens for 30 days; powder and liquid forms of gentamicin had similar elution rates from PMMA
	1 mL of 50 mg/mL solution/20 g polymer powder[761]	Raptors/pododermatitis
	Ratio PMMA:gentamicin of 20:1[734]	Good elution for at least 21 days
Gentamicin (Septopal, Merck)	Premade beads	Commercially available in Europe; not available in the United States
Hydroxyapatite cement (BoneSource, Osteogenics)	—	Polymer powder used as an alternative to bone cement; absorbs into muscle and tissue; osteoconductive in bone; fabricates with water which aids in formulation with liquid antibiotics[266]
Itraconazole	16% intraconazole-impregnated PMMA fed as grit stones[896]	Indian peafowl/PD; antifungal agent; when used as grit, therapeutic levels achieved in 2 days and decreased over 7 days; beads from capsules mix into PMMA uniformly before hardening; PMMA cut into 1-g size pieces (grit stone size) after hardening
Meropenem	Ratio PMMA:meropenem of 5:1[39]	Elution for 15 days
Metronidazole	Ratio PMMA:metronidazole of 20-40:1[734]	Good elution for at least 21 days
Oxytetracycline	4.5 mL of 200 mg/mL solution/20 g polymer powder[761]	Raptors/pododermatitis
(R) Rifampin/(P) pefloxacin (Pelwin, 5% soluble powder, Wockhardt)	1 part (R) + 1 part (P) is finely ground in equal volumes in a mortar and pestle; thoroughly mix with 5 parts PMMA powder[761]	Rifampin powder taken from oral capsules; pefloxacin powder obtained from the preparation intended for oral use in poultry

TABLE 5-14 Antimicrobial-Impregnated Polymethylmethacrylate (PMMA) Agents Used in Birds. (cont'd)

Agent	Dosage	Species/Comments
(R) Rifampin/(P) piperacillin	1 part (R) + 1 part (P) is combined and finely ground in a mortar and pestle; thoroughly mix with 5 parts PMMA powder[761]	Rifampin powder taken from oral capsules; piperacillin powder taken from parenteral preparation prior to reconstitution (piperacillin is available only in combination with tazobactam in the United States)
Tobramycin	—	Release for 220 days[567]

[a]Antimicrobial-impregnated polymethylmethacrylate (PMMA) is used to elute antimicrobial agents for long-term treatment of infected lesions. Following are guidelines for its use and preparation:

- Choose antibiotic based on culture and sensitivity.
- Mix 1-2 g of sterile antibiotic powder with 40-60 g of PMMA powder. Add approximately 2 Tbs to antibiotic at a time. The use of liquid antibiotic reduces the mechanical strength of the bead.
- Shake mixture well (for at least 2 min) to make it homogeneous.
- Add liquid monomer as usual.
- The dough is placed in a catheter tip syringe and extruded, rolled into beads, and placed onto steel surgical wire. Dough may also be injected into a red rubber catheter and cut into variable sizes after setting. The smaller the bead, the greater the elution of antibiotic.[932]
- Gas sterilization or UV radiation is recommended; beads are aerated for at least 24 hr at room temperature.
- The wound is aggressively debrided and beads are placed within it; the wound is then closed and the beads are left within the site until the wound is no longer infected.
- In human medicine, beads are removed after 2-6 wk. Despite their antibiotic release, beads act as a surface to which bacteria preferentially adhere, grow, and potentially develop antibiotic resistance. [647] Beads are difficult to remove if left in place for more than 14 days.[674]

TABLE 5-15 Agents Used in the Treatment of Oiled Birds.

Agent	Dosage	Species/Comments
Bismuth subsalicylate	2-5 mg/kg PO once[607]	Adsorbent; gavage; alternatively can use activated charcoal
Charcoal, activated (Toxiban, Vet-A-Mix)	52 mg/kg PO once[607]	Adsorbent; gavage; alternatively can use bismuth subsalicylate
Charcoal, activated/ electrolyte slurry (Toxiban, Vet-A-Mix)	50 mL/kg by gavage[934]	3 bottles of charcoal slurry (3.75 g/kg) added to 250 mL of electrolyte solution
Detergent (Dawn, Procter & Gamble)	1-2% bath[935] 1-5% bath[607]	Submerse bird up to mid-neck region; rinse with water; use water at 39-41°C (103-105°F) and 40-60 psi (pounds per square inch; 1.9-2.9 kPa); water should be soft(ened);[607,618] sea water may also be used[281,591]
Fluid therapy	—	See Table 5-38 for guidelines
Iron dextran	10 mg/kg IM q5-7d[607]	If PCV +25%
Lactulose	0.3 mL/kg PO q12h[589]	Prophylactic laxative
Margarine	Topical application[740]	Anhinga, great blue heron; removal of polyisobutylene on plumage; dish soap was unsuccessful

Continued

TABLE 5-15 Agents Used in the Treatment of Oiled Birds. (cont'd)

Agent	Dosage	Species/Comments
Oral electrolyte solutions (Pedialyte; Ross Labs)	30 mL/kg by gavage[934]	Most species/at field stabilization site
Papaya enzyme	1 tablet PO q12h[589]	Prophylactic laxative
Thiamine/vitamin B1	25-30 mg/kg fish[607]	Piscivorous species

TABLE 5-16 Agents Used in Bird Emergencies.[a]

Agent	Dosage	Species/Comments
Aminophylline	4 mg/kg PO q6-12h[941]	Can give orally after initial response
	4 mg/kg IM q12h[867]	Amazon parrot/smoke inhalation injury
	10 mg/kg IV q3h[941]	Use for pulmonary edema
Atropine sulfate	0.5 mg/kg IM, IV, IO, intratracheal[793]	CPR
	0.02 mg/kg IM, IV, IO[531]	CPR, bradycardia
Blood homologous transfusion	—	Administer over 1-4 hr; use filter;[436] half-life of 8-10 days; heterologous blood transfusion may not be effective[214,217]
Calcium gluconate	1-5 mg elemental calcium/kg/h[63]	CRI for ionized hypocalcemia
	50-150 mg/kg IM, IV (slow bolus)[63,531]	Hypocalcemia; dilute 50 mg/mL; hyperkalemia; facilitates potassium movement across cell membranes
Dextran 70	10-20 mL/kg IV[177]	Most species/hypovolemic shock
Dextrose (50%)	50-100 mg/kg IV (slow bolus to effect) [793,941]	Hypoglycemia; can dilute with fluids
	0.25 mL/kg (125 mg/kg) IV after 1:1 dilution with saline[531]	Hypoglycemia
	0.5 mL/kg (250 mg/kg) IV over 15 min[63]	Hypoglycemia
	500-1000 mg/kg IV (slow bolus)[726]	Hypoglycemia; can dilute with fluids
Dobutamine	5-15 µg/kg/min[837]	Hispaniolan Amazon parrots/PD; less effective than dopamine
Dopamine	5-10 µg/kg/min[837]	Hispaniolan Amazon parrots/PD; more effective than dobutamine
Doxapram	2 mg/kg IV, IO[531]	CPR; respiratory arrest
	5-10 mg/kg IM, IV once[420]	Raptors/respiratory depression or arrest
Epinephrine (1:1000)	0.5-1 mL/kg IM, IV, IO, intratracheal[793]	CPR; bradycardia
	0.01 mg/kg[531]	CPR

TABLE 5-16 Agents Used in Bird Emergencies. (cont'd)

Agent	Dosage	Species/Comments
Hemoglobin glutamer-200 (Oxyglobin, OPK Biotech)	—	Hemoglobin polymer; hemoglobin replacement product; anemia treatment; currently unavailable
	3-10 mL/kg IV (slow)[6]	Most species
	5 mL/kg IV[531]	Mallard duck/PD; no difference in mortality rate from crystalloid fluids in a hemorrhagic shock model (but a trend of decreased mortality)
	10 mL/kg IV[418]	Raptors
Hetastarch	5 mL/kg IV[533]	Mallard duck/PD; no difference in mortality rate from crystalloid fluids in a hemorrhagic shock model
	10-15 mL/kg IV (slow) q8h× 1-4 treatments[420]	Most species, including raptors/ hypoproteinemia; hypovolemia
	20 mL/kg/day; 5 mL/kg bolus may be repeated twice[63]	Hypovolemia, half-life: 25 hr
Insulin/dextrose 50%	0.5 IU/kg + 2 g dextrose/ insulin unit[63]	Hyperkalemia
Mannitol	0.2-2 g/kg IV (slow) q24h[391]	Raptors/cerebral edema; anuric renal failure
Norepinephrine	0.1-0.5 µg/kg/min CRI[65]	Hypotension
Oxyglobin	—	See Hemoglobin glutamer-200
Pentastarch	20 mL/kg/day; 5 mL/kg IV bolus[63]	Hypovolemia, half-life: 2.5 hr
Potassium chloride (KCl)	Maintenance: 15-20 mmol/L Moderate hypoK: 40 mmol/L Severe hypoK: 60 mmol/L[63]	Supplement IV/IO fluids; hypokalemia; do not exceed 0.5 mmol/kg/h
Sodium bicarbonate	1 mmol/kg IV q15-30min to maximum of 4 mmol/kg total dose[165]	Metabolic acidosis
	0.3*BW(kg)*base excess, IV bolus[63]	Most species/metabolic acidosis; give over 30-60 min
Terbutaline	0.01 mg/kg PO, IM q6h[529]	Psittacines/α2-selective smooth muscle bronchodilator
Vasopressin	0.8 U/kg[531]	CPR

[a]Because of the presence of peripheral vasoconstriction, subcutaneous administration is not adequate for patients in shock.[749]

TABLE 5-17 Euthanasia Agents Used in Birds.[a]

Agent	Dosage	Species/Comments
Carbon dioxide (CO_2)	20-80%[847]	Zebra finches/PD; 80% CO_2 was recommended to minimize duration
	>40%[520]	Most species/danger to person administering gas; compressed gas is the only recommended source; higher concentrations are required for newly hatched chicks (80-90%)[520]

Continued

TABLE 5-17 Euthanasia Agents Used in Birds. (cont'd)

Agent	Dosage	Species/Comments
Carbon monoxide (CO)	Minimum 6% concentration in a closed container[520]	Most species/unconsciousness occurs rapidly; inexpensive; danger to person administering gas; compressed gas recommended[520]
Euthanasia solution (pentobarbital sodium 390 mg/mL, phenytoin sodium 50 mg/mL)	0.2-1 mL/kg IV, ICe[391]	Most species/birds may react unpredictably with IV administration; ICe administration is smooth, quiet; proper carcass disposal is necessary because secondary poisoning of wild scavenging birds may occur;[395,795,970] induces significant histopathologic changes that may impair interpretation (especially for lungs)[355,731]
	19.5 mg/bird ICe[847]	Zebra finches/PD; with or without isoflurane anesthesia
	220 mg/kg IO[686]	Starlings/PD
	430-602 mg/kg oral transmucosal[332]	Most birds died within 5 min, followed by IV pentobarbital in some birds
	693-754 mg/kg IO[686]	Sparrows/PD
Isoflurane	Saturated cotton ball in closed container or face mask[831]	Most species/very rapid induction; wing flapping and vocalizing may occur
Methoxyflurane	Saturated cotton ball in closed container or face mask[831]	Most species/induction may be slower than with isoflurane
Pentobarbital	—	See Euthanasia solution above
Potassium chloride	1-2 mmol/kg IV[520]	Most species/must be provided in conjunction with prior general anesthesia
	3-10 mmol/kg[732]	Parrots/PD; no histologic artifacts; death in 0.5-1.1 min, performed under isoflurane anesthesia

[a]The American Veterinary Medical Association accepts inhalant anesthetic overdose, carbon monoxide, carbon dioxide, KCl (after anesthesia), and barbiturate overdose as humane euthanasia methods.[520] Cervical dislocation and decapitation are conditionally acceptable for research and poultry. Thoracic compression is commonly used for wild passerine birds.[686]

TABLE 5-18 Miscellaneous Agents Used in Birds.

Agent	Dosage	Species/Comments
Acemannan (Carravet, Veterinary Products Labs)	Topical[272]	Most species/hydrogel wound dressing; wound healing; increases cytokine production, fibroblast proliferation, and epidermal growth[a]
Acetylsalicylic acid (aspirin)	5 mg/kg PO q48h[73]	Most species, grey parrot/antithrombotic agent
Allopurinol	—	Xanthine oxidase inhibitor/use in treatment of gout is controversial: 50 mg/kg given to red-tailed hawks was toxic, leading to marked elevations in plasma oxypurinol, xanthine, and hypoxanthine with secondary renal dysfunction[558]

TABLE 5-18 Miscellaneous Agents Used in Birds. (cont'd)

Agent	Dosage	Species/Comments
Allopurinol (cont'd)	10-30 mg/kg PO q12-24h[46,787]	Most species/gout
	25 mg/kg PO q24h[558,712]	Red-tailed hawks/PD; no significant effect on plasma uric acid levels
	1 mL stock solution/30 mL drinking water mixed fresh several times daily (300 mg/L)[43,767]	Budgerigars/decrease initial dose to 25% recommended dose in severe cases and gradually increase over several days; use with colchicine in severe cases; stock solution: 100 mg tablet/10 mL sterile water
Aloe vera	Topical[272,445]	Most species/antiinflammatory; antithromboxane activity; beneficial in treating burns, electrical injury, or dying skin flaps;[a] see heparin for combination
Amantadine	5 mg/kg PO q24h[86]	Orange-winged Amazon parrots/PK
Aminoloid (Aminoloid, Schering)	0.25-0.75 mg/kg IM, repeat in 10-14 days[43]	Raptors/induction of molt
Aminopentamide hydrogen sulfate (Centrine, Fort Dodge)	0.05 mg/kg SC, IM q12h up to 5 doses[288]	Most species/regurgitation
	0.11 mg/kg SC, IM q8-12h × 1 day, then q12h × 1 day, then q24h × 1 day[102]	Most species/regurgitation
Aminophylline	5 mg/kg PO, IV q12h[529]	Psittacines
	8-10 mg/kg PO, IM, IV q6-8h[420,939]	Most species, ratites/may be diluted prior to injection; initial doses may be given IV; subsequent doses given oral once response is observed
Amlodipine	0.1-0.4 mg/kg PO q12-24h[278]	Parrots/hypertension
	0.8 mg/kg PO q24h[280]	Parrots/hypertension
Ammonium solution	Topical prn[767]	Most species/analgesic; antipruritic; anti-inflammatory; can use on fresh wounds; avoid overusage[a]
Arginine vasopressin	24 µg/kg IM q12h[893]	African grey parrot/central diabetes insipidus; oral administration was not effective
Arginine vasotocin	0.5-4 µg/kg intranasal q12h[517]	African grey parrot/central diabetes insipidus
Armor All Protectant (Armor All Protectant Corp)	Topical to affected plumage[85]	Most species/soften sticky-trap glue-covered plumage; use detergent (Dawn) to remove Armor All
Atenolol	5-10 mg/kg PO q12-24h[69]	Most species
Atorvastatin (Lipitor)	10 mg/kg PO q24h[777]	Hispaniolan Amazon parrots/PK, PD; no significant changes to plasma lipid profiles over a 30-day period
	10-20 mg/kg PO q12h[64]	Parrots/hypercholesterolemia; needs to be compounded from tablets; should not be taken while feeding grapefruit or concurrently with azole antifungals[61]

Continued

TABLE 5-18 Miscellaneous Agents Used in Birds. (cont'd)

Agent	Dosage	Species/Comments
Barium sulfate	—	Dilute 72% suspension 1:1 with water; dilute 92% suspension 1:2 with water; 60% suspension effective in Amazon parrots;[74,261] more dilute concentrations (20-25%) can also be used[971]
	15 mL/kg PO of 1:1 barium 60% and hand-feeding formula[74]	Amazon parrots/PD; contrast fluoroscopy
	20 mL/kg PO of barium 25%[971]	Amazon parrots/PD; contrast fluoroscopy, radiography
	20-25 mL/kg PO via gavage[336,971]	Most species
	25 mL/kg PO[246,247]	Barred owls, red-tailed hawks/PD; contrast fluoroscopy
	25-50 mL/kg PO[336]	Most species/smaller species require relatively more contrast media; African grey parrots, 25 mL/kg; Quaker parakeets and budgerigars, 50 mL/kg
Benazepril	0.5 mg/kg PO q24h[69,283,848]	Parrots
Bismuth subsalicylate (Pepto-Bismol, Procter & Gamble)	1-2 mL/kg PO q12h[43,509]	Most species/weak adsorbent; gastrointestinal irritation
Bromhexine HCl	1.5 mg/kg IM q12-24h[165]	Most species/expectorant
	3-6 mg/kg IM[104,177]	Most species, including psittacines, passerines, raptors
	6.5 mg/L drinking water[104]	Psittacines
	1200 mg/L drinking water[177]	Most species
Carvedilol	1-9 mg/kg PO q12-24h[283]	Parrots
Cimetidine	—	Prototype histamine-2 blocker used to reduce gastrointestinal acid production
	3-5 mg/kg PO, IV q8h[939]	Ratites
	5 mg/kg PO, IM q8-12h[789]	Psittacines/proventriculitis; gastric ulceration
	5-10 mg/kg IM q12h[939]	Ratites
Cisapride (Propulsid, Janssen)	—	Gastrointestinal prokinetic agent; stimulates motility in mammals[710]
	0.5-1.5 mg/kg PO q8-12h[445]	Most species
Citrate phosphate dextrose adenine solution (CPDA)	1 part CPDA:5-6 parts whole blood[347,621]	Most species/anticoagulant for blood collection for transfusion; not for extended storage of whole blood;[621] a cryopreservation study has also been published[347]
Citric acid	5000 mg/L drinking water[177]	Most species/reduces the effect of calcium and magnesium on the absorption of tetracyclines

TABLE 5-18 Miscellaneous Agents Used in Birds. (cont'd)

Agent	Dosage	Species/Comments
Colchicine	—	Unique antiinflammatory used in the treatment of gout or hepatic fibrosis/ cirrhosis;[710] may potentiate gout formation in some cases[767]
	0.01 mg/kg PO q12h[171]	Juvenile macaws/gout
	0.04 mg/kg PO q12-24h[408]	Most species/gradually increase to q12h
	0.2 mg/kg PO q12h[767]	Psittacines
Copper sulfate (Cu-7, Searle)	Topical[43]	Most species/ulcerative dermatitis
Cyclosporine	10-20 mg/kg PO q24h[65]	Most species/no detectable plasma level in a single African grey parrot case
	10 mg/kg PO q12h[415]	Cockatiels/PD; effective at preventing avian bornaviral clinical signs; most birds still had histopathological lesions and multiple PCR positive organs
	0.2 mg/bird[366]	Cockatiels/PD; compounded in sesame oil; effective at preventing avian bornaviral clinical signs[366]
	10 mg/kg IV[947]	Pekin ducks/PD; low plasma levels and high clearance
2-deoxy-2-fluoro-d-glucose	37 MBq (1 mCi)[880]	Amazon parrots/PD; PET-scan
	128.5 ± 20.2 MBq (3.5 ± 0.5 mCi)[452]	Bald eagles/PD; PET-scan
Digoxin	—	Toxic reactions include depression, ataxia, vomiting, diarrhea; contraindicated with renal or liver disease; monitoring of serum digoxin, potassium, magnesium, calcium, and ECG is recommended; induced arrhythmias in pigeons at 0.2 mg/kg/day[609]
	0.01-0.02 mg/kg PO q12h[177]	Psittacines, passerines, raptors/congestive heart disease
	0.02 mg/kg PO q24h × 5 days[367]	Budgerigars, sparrows (PD)/produces a plasma concentration of 1.6 µg/mL (within mammalian therapeutic range); this dose led to signs of toxicity in a mynah[782]
	0.05 mg/kg PO q24h[996]	Quaker parakeets/PD; congestive heart failure; cardiomyopathy
	0.066 mg/kg IV q12h[689]	Pekin ducks/PD; short half-life
	0.13 mg/L drinking water[177]	Psittacines, passerines, raptors/congestive heart disease
Dimethylsulfoxide (90%)	1 mL/kg topical to affected area q4-7d[445,767]	Most species/antiinflammatory, analgesic; systemic absorption; use gloves during application
Dioctyl sodium sulfosuccinate	33 mL/L drinking water[457]	Psittacine chicks/constipation; use only if chick is drinking

Continued

TABLE 5-18 Miscellaneous Agents Used in Birds. (cont'd)

Agent	Dosage	Species/Comments
Diphenhydramine	1-4 mg/kg PO q8-12h[789,952]	Most species/hypersensitivity, pruritus, anxiety; may cause hypotension
	2 mg/kg IV, IO once[315]	Cockatoos/use prior to chemotherapy
	20-40 mg/L drinking water[177]	Most species
Diphenoxylate with atropine (Lomotil, Searle)	2-2.5 mg/kg PO q8h[939]	Ratites/opiate; gastrointestinal motility modifier
EDTA-tromethamine or EDTA-Tris	IT, intranasal, or wound lavage[43]	Most species/potentiates the effect of antibiotics on resistant bacteria;[271] lysozyme solution mix: 3.07 g Trizma HCl, 3.17 g Trizma base, 1.12 g disodium EDTA in 100 mL water; Tris-EDTA may also be added to chlorhexidine solution[31]
Enalapril	0.8 mg/kg PO q12h[194]	African penguin/heart failure
	0.25 mg/kg PO q24h[597]	
	1.25 mg/kg PO q8-12h[691]	Pigeons, Amazon parrots/PD; a dose of 10 mg/kg PO q24h for 21 days did not result in side effects in pigeons
	2.5-5 mg/kg PO q12h[692]	Amazon parrot/right-sided heart failure; long-term therapy
	5 mg/kg PO q24h[903]	Lovebirds
Ferric subsulfate	Topical[767]	Most species/hemostasis of bleeding nail or beak tip; will cause necrosis if used on open skin lesions
Furosemide	—	Diuretic; overdose can cause dehydration and electrolyte abnormalities
	0.1-2.2 mg/kg PO, IM, SC, IV q6-24h[69,283,690,969]	Most species, including psittacines, raptors, pigeons, mynahs, ratites, penguins; lories are extremely sensitive[767,941]
	0.15 mg/kg IM[457]	Psittacine neonates/pulmonary congestion
	1-5 mg/kg IM q2-12h[282,283]	Parrots/acute treatment of congestive heart failure
	1-13 mg/kg PO q8-12h[282,283]	Parrots/maintenance treatment of congestive heart failure
	2-6 mg/kg PO, IM[420]	Raptors
Gadopentate dimeglumine (Magnevist, Berlex)	0.25 mmol/kg IV[780]	Pigeons/PD; contrast agent for magnetic resonance imaging
Gallium-67 citrate (Ga-67)	0.5 mCi (microcuries)/bird IV[464]	Green-winged macaws/radiopharmaceutical used for detection of infection and inflammatory lesions; requires a gamma camera for imaging
Gemfibrozil	30 mg/kg PO q8h[725]	Psittacines/lipid regulating agent; yolk emboli; sometimes effective in controlling signs; gradual improvement may be seen over weeks to months; give with niacin

TABLE 5-18 Miscellaneous Agents Used in Birds. (cont'd)

Agent	Dosage	Species/Comments
Glipizide	—	Sulfonylurea antidiabetic; contraindicated in ketotic patients
	0.5 mg/kg PO q12h[714]	Cockatiels/diabetes mellitus; did not reduce blood glucose in a Bali mynah at that dose[55]
	1.25 mg/kg PO q24h[445]	Most species/diabetes mellitus; did not reduce blood glucose in a macaw at that dose[325]
	2 mg/kg PO q8-12h[65]	Cockatiels/diabetes mellitus; reduced blood glucose and fructosamine in one case
Glycosaminoglycan	—	See polysulfated glycosaminoglycan
Guaifenesin	0.8 mg/kg PO q12h[706]	Severe macaws/expectorant, bronchodilation
Heparin	2 U/mL whole blood[214]	Cockatiels, conures/anticoagulant for blood transfusions
Heparin/aloe vera	Topical to affected area[445]	Most species/antiinflammatory; dilute 1000 U heparin/150 mg aloe vera[a]
Hyaluronidase	5 U/kg IV q12h × 1-3 days then 2×/wk prn[533]	Psittacines/egg yolk-related disease; egg yolk visually apparent in blood or serum; dilute with an equal or greater quantity of isotonic NaCl
	75-150 U/L fluids[535]	Most species/increases absorption rate of fluids
	Few drops to the lumen of feather shaft at the base[399]	Raptors/flight feather pulling
Hydroxyzine (Atarax, Roerig)	2 mg/kg PO q8-12h[952]	Most species/allergic pruritus; feather picking; self-mutilation
	34-40 mg/L drinking water[952]	Most species/respiratory allergy; feather picking
Iohexol (Omnipaque, Sanofi Winthrop)	2-3 mL/kg IV over 3-5 sec[76,78]	Most parrots/PD; angiography; CT contrast; distribution of contrast is extremely fast in vascular system; deaths have been observed in small birds (<150 g)[592]
	20 mL/kg PO[579]	Cockatiels/PD; fluoroscopy for evaluating gastrointestinal motility.
	25-30 mL/kg PO[261]	Cockatoos, Amazon parrots/gavage; radiographic gastrointestinal iodinated contrast media; 1:1 dilution with water can also be used
	50 mL/kg PO[336]	Quaker parrots, budgerigars
Iopamidol	2 mL/kg IV over 3-5 sec[65]	Most parrots/CT contrast; deaths have been observed in small birds (<150 g)[592]
	2 mL/bird IV[1005]	Grey parrots/PD; CT angiography; most reliable protocol achieved with post contrast medium infusion with 0.4 mL saline
	4-5.3 mL IV over 2 min[479]	Parrots, anseriformes, charadriiformes/CT angiography; CT scan started 30 sec into the contrast delivery

Continued

TABLE 5-18 Miscellaneous Agents Used in Birds. (cont'd)

Agent	Dosage	Species/Comments
Isoxsuprine	5-10 mg/kg PO q24h × 20-40 days[43]	Raptors/peripheral vasodilator; wingtip edema
	10 mg/kg PO q24h[866]	Amazon parrot/single case report of presumed atherosclerosis
	10 mg/kg PO q12-24h[283]	Parrots
Kaolin/pectin	2 mL/kg PO q6-12h[391]	Psittacine neonates/intestinal protectant; antidiarrheal
	≤15 mL/kg PO q8-12h, repeat prn[43]	Raptors/nonspecific diarrhea
Lactulose	—	Does not treat liver disease; reduces blood ammonia levels; exerts osmotic effect in birds with caeca through fermentation to acetic and lactic acid[710]
	150-650 mg/kg (0.2-1 mL/kg) PO q8-12h[43]	Most species, including psittacines/hepatic encephalopathy
	200 mg/kg (0.3 mL/kg) PO q8-12h[458]	Psittacine neonates
Magnesium hydroxide (M)/ activated charcoal (C)	(M) 10-12 mL + (C) 1 tsp powder PO[509]	Most species/cathartic; adsorbent
Magnesium sulfate (Epsom salts)	—	Purgative, cathartic; may cause lethargy;[509] see peanut butter for combination
	0.25-1 g/kg PO q24h × 1-2 days[43,509]	Most species, including raptors
	1⁄4 tsp/bird PO[939]	Ratite juveniles/obstipation
	2 Tbs/bird PO[939]	Ratite adults/obstipation
Mannitol	—	Osmotic diuretic used to treat cerebral edema, especially after head trauma; may be used with furosemide; also used to treat glaucoma
	0.25-2 g/kg q24h IV (slow bolus)[391]	Most species, including raptors
	1500 mg/kg IV q6h[939]	Ratites
Maropitant	1 mg/kg SC, IM[65]	Parrots
Methocarbamol	10 mg/kg PO q24h[595]	Lesser flamingo/capture myopathy
	32.5 mg/kg PO q12[767]	Swans, cranes (demoiselle)/capture myopathy
	50 mg/kg IV (slow bolus)[767]	Most species, including swans, demoiselle cranes/muscle relaxation; capture myopathy; may be given q12h for muscle relaxation
Metoclopramide	—	Gastrointestinal motility disorders; regurgitation; slow crop motility; extrapyramidal signs may be seen as an adverse effect[65]
	0.1 mg/kg IV[939]	Ostriches

TABLE 5-18 Miscellaneous Agents Used in Birds. (cont'd)

Agent	Dosage	Species/Comments
Metoclopramide (cont'd)	0.5-1 mg/kg PO, IM, IV q8-12h[767]	Most species, including psittacines/ gastrointestinal ileus; regurgitation
	1 mg/kg IM[113]	Amazon parrots/PD; no alterations in motility observed at that dose
	2 mg/kg IM, IV q8-12h[43]	Raptors, waterfowl/crop stasis; ileus
	12.5 mg/kg PO[939]	Ratites/gastrointestinal disorders
Mexiletine	4-8 mg/kg PO q12-24h[65]	Parrots
Mineral oil	—	Cathartic; used to aid passage of grit and other foreign bodies; administer directly into the crop because oral administration may result in aspiration pneumonia; see peanut butter for combination
	5-10 mL/kg PO via gavage[509,941]	Most species, including psittacines/cathartic
	15 mL/kg PO via gavage[939]	Ratite adults/impaction
Nicarbazin (Ovocontrol, Innolytics)	—	Inhibits sperm receptor sites on the vitelline membrane to prevent fertilization of eggs; check federal and state permit requirements prior to use
	Formulated pellets provided at baiting stations (www.ovocontrol.com)	Pigeons, waterfowl/egg hatch control
Peanut butter	Peanut butter and mineral oil (2:1)[391]	Most species/add to diet; cathartic
	Dilute peanut butter and magnesium sulfate[391]	Most species/add to diet; cathartic; dilute with water
	1 mL combined with mineral oil (2:1)[559]	Budgerigar/cathartic;[a] experimental lead particles administration; faster elimination time than controls but not statistically significant
Pentoxifylline	15 mg/kg PO q24h[953]	Parrots/peripheral arterial disease due to atherosclerosis; combined with atorvastatin and/or enalapril
	15-25 mg/kg PO q8-12h[580,978]	Most species/frostbite
	30 mg/kg PO q12h x 5 days[65,71]	Most species; improve peripheral perfusion; peripheral arterial disease; raptor wingtip edema
Perflutren lipid microspheres (Definity, Lantheus medical)	0.1 mL/bird IV[76]	Most birds/ultrasound contrast agent; necessitate a mechanical activating device
	0.1 mL/bird IV diluted with 0.9 mL NaCl[77]	Red-tailed hawks/PD; lasted several min in cardiac chambers
Pimobendan	0.25 mg/kg PO q12h[117]	Harris's hawk/congestive heart failure; therapeutic drug monitoring performed
	0.25 mg/kg PO q12h[597]	African penguins/heart failure

Continued

TABLE 5-18 Miscellaneous Agents Used in Birds. (cont'd)

Agent	Dosage	Species/Comments
Pimobendan (cont'd)	0.25 mg/kg PO q12h[68,848,955]	Parrots
	6-10 mg/kg PO q12h[282,283]	Parrots
	6 mg/kg PO q12h[194]	African penguins/heart failure
	10 mg/kg PO q12h[812]	Hispaniolan Amazon parrots/PD
Policosanol	0.3-2 mg PO q25h[303]	Psittacines/hyperlipidemia; use was reported in two birds
Polysulfated glycosaminoglycan (PSGAG) (Adequan, Luitpold)	—	Used for osteoarthritis in a variety of birds; coagulopathies including three deaths reported in four birds following IM injection[21]
	10 mg/kg IM, IA q7d × 3 mo[907]	Most species, including pheasants, vultures, cranes/noninfectious or traumatic joint dysfunction; 250 mg/mL for intraarticular use; 500 mg/mL for IM use
	500 mg/bird IM q4d × 7 treatments[939]	Ratites
Probenecid	—	Not currently recommended for the treatment of gout; may exacerbate the condition[5]
	125 mg/kg PO q6h[171]	Macaw chicks/antigout
Probucol (Lorelco, Marion Merrell Dow)	1 drop stock/300 g PO q12h × 2-4 mo[445,767]	Most species/low-density lipoprotein cholesterolemia; contains iron: use cautiously in species susceptible to hemochromatosis; may increase bile acids; use with low-fat diet; prepare stock: crush 250 mg tablet/7.5 mL lactulose
Propentofylline (Vivitonin, Hoechst)	5 mg/kg PO q12h × 20-40 days[43]	Raptors/wingtip edema; dry gangrene syndrome
Propranolol	0.04 mg/kg IV (slow)[767]	Most species/supraventricular arrhythmia, atrial flutter, fibrillation
	0.2 mg/kg IM[767]	
Proprantheline	0.1-0.3 mg/kg PO q8h[955]	Parrots/antiarrhythmic
Psyllium (Metamucil, Procter & Gamble)	0.5 tsp/60 mL hand-feeding formula[509]	Most species/bulk diet; can use mineral oil as alternative or in addition to psyllium
	1 Tbs/60 mL water/bird PO, up to 120 mL/day[939]	Ratite chicks/impaction
	1 mL of a solution made of 1/2 tsp diluted in 60 mL of water[559]	Budgerigar/cathartic;[a] experimental lead particles administration; similar elimination time than controls
Rosuvastatin	10-25 mg/kg PO[75]	Hispaniolan Amazon parrots/PD; low plasma levels
Sildenafil	1 mg/kg PO q12h[194]	African penguin/distention of pulmonary vasculature
	1-5 mg/kg PO q8-12h[283]	Parrots
	2.5 mg/kg PO q8h[115]	Amazon parrot/pulmonary hypertension treatment

TABLE 5-18 Miscellaneous Agents Used in Birds. (cont'd)

Agent	Dosage	Species/Comments
Silymarin (milk thistle)	10-100 mg/kg PO q24h x21 days[359]	Pigeons/PD; no demonstrable hepatoprotective effect in experimental hepatitis
	35 mg/kg PO q12h[426]	Pigeons/PD; decreased mortality and liver enzymes elevation in acetaminophen-induced acute hepatic toxicity
	100-150 mg/kg PO divided q8-12h[26]	Most species/hepatic antioxidant; use in patients with liver disease and as ancillary to chemotherapy; use a low-alcohol or alcohol-free liquid formulation
Skin-So-Soft (Avon)	Topical to affected plumage[85]	Most species/softens and removes sticky-trap glue from plumage; use Dawn dish detergent to remove Skin-So-Soft product[a]
Sodium tetradecyl sulfate	2 mg/kg diluted at 5% topical[70]	Most species/fibrotic agent; topical administration in cervicocephalic diverticulum in case of hyperinflation
Spironolactone	1 mg/kg PO q12h[69,283,848]	Parrots/diuretic
Sucralfate	25 mg/kg PO q8h[767]	Most species, including raptors/oral, esophageal, gastric, duodenal ulcers; give 1 hr before food or other drugs[391]
^{99m}Technetium-diethylene-triaminepenta-acetic acid (DTPA)	42 ± 0.16 MBq (1.158 ± 0.164 mCi [microcuries])/bird IV[577]	Pigeons/PD; radiopharmaceutical agent of choice for the assessment of renal function
^{99m}Technetium-disofenin	1 mCi (microcuries) in a commercial liquid or solid diet PO[216]	Grey parrots/radionucleotide used for gastrointestinal scintigraphy in birds
^{99m}Technetium-mebrofenin	1.5-2.0 mCi[359,364]	Pigeons/PD; liver scintigraphy
Terbutaline	0.01 mg/kg PO, IM q6h[529]	Psittacines/α2-selective smooth muscle bronchodilator
	0.1 mg/kg PO q12-24h[789]	Macaws, Amazon parrots/bronchodilator; obstructive pulmonary disease; pneumonitis
Theophylline	2 mg/kg PO q12h[706]	Severe macaws/bronchodilation
	5-10 mg/kg PO q12h[65]	Blue and gold macaws/chronic obstructive pulmonary disease
	10 mg/kg PO q12h[65]	Amazon parrot/syringeal mass in a single case
Trilostane	1 mg/kg PO q24h[956]	Senegal parrot/Cushing's disease
Trypsin-balsam Peru-castor oil (Granulex, Pfizer)	Topical[272]	Most species/digests necrotic tissue (may have debriding action); may have analgesic effects; may cause local inflammation and pyogenic reaction; do not use for long-term management[a]
Tyrode's solution	Offer in place of drinking water[767]	Cockatiels/restores renal-medullary gradient; add 8 g NaCl, 0.13 g CaCl2, 0.2 g KCl, 0.1 g MgCl2, 0.05 g Na2HPO4, 1 g NaHCO3, 1 g glucose to 1 L water

Continued

TABLE 5-18 Miscellaneous Agents Used in Birds. (cont'd)

Agent	Dosage	Species/Comments
Urate oxidase (Uricozyme, Sanofi Winthrop)	100-200 U/kg IM q24[711,712]	Red-tailed hawks, pigeons/PD; significantly lowered plasma uric acid, including postprandial plasma uric acid
Ursodeoxycholic acid	15 mg/kg PO q24h[65]	Most species
Vegetable oil	15 mL/kg PO[939]	Ratites/impaction
Yeast cell derivatives (Preparation H, WhiteHall)	Topical q24h[941]	Most species/pododermatitis; stimulation of epithelialization; one of the commercial products contains 1% hydrocortisone[a]

[a]Many topical agents contain oils that adhere to plumage. These agents should be used sparingly and generally in non-feathered regions to prevent losing the insulative properties of the plumage.

TABLE 5-19 Hematologic and Biochemical Values of Select Psittaciformes.

Measurement	African Grey Parrot (*Psittacus* spp.)[186,320]	Amazon Parrots (*Amazona* spp.)[186,320]	Amazon Parrot, Orange-winged (*Amazona amazonica*)[965]
Hematology			
PCV (%)	45-53	41-53	51 (42-60)
RBC (10^6/μL)	2.84-3.62	2.45-3.18	2.47 (2.40-3.67)
Hgb (g/dL)	12.7-15.9	12.2-15.9	—
MCV (fL)	144-155	160-175	166 (138-193)
MCH (pg)	36.4-43.9	47.2-56.8	—
MCHC (g/dL)	25.4-28.1	29.1-31.9	—
WBC (10^3/μL)	6-13	6-17	8 (0.7-16)
Heterophils 10^3/μL (%)	4.64-7.52	3.81-8.73	3.07 (0.71-7.24)
	45-73	31-71	—
Lymphocytes 10^3/μL (%)	1.96-5.15	2.40-6.48	4.55 (0-10.8)
	19-50	20-54	—
Monocytes 10^3/μL (%)	0-0.21	0.12-0.36	0.38 (0.09-0.86)
	0-2	1-3	—
Eosinophils 10^3/μL (%)	0-0.10	0.12-0.24	0.05
	0-1	1-2	—
Basophils 10^3/μL (%)	0-0.1	0-0.12	—
	0-1	0-1	—
H:L ratio	—	—	—

TABLE 5-19 Hematologic and Biochemical Values of Select Psittaciformes. (cont'd)

Measurement	African Grey Parrot (*Psittacus* spp.)	Amazon Parrots (*Amazona* spp.)	Amazon Parrot, Orange-winged (*Amazona amazonica*)
Chemistries			
ALP (U/L)	20-160	15-150	46 (18-120)
ALT (U/L)	5-12	5-11	—
Amylase (U/L)	210-530	205-510	—
AST (U/L)	109-305	141-437	168 (125-375)
Bile acid (μmol/L)			
RIA	13.7-73.6	10.3-79.3	—
Colorimetric	12-96	33-154	20 (8-88)
BUN (mg/dL)	3-5.4	—	1 (0-2)
Calcium (mg/dL)	7.7-11.3	8.2-10.9	9.1 (7.7-10.4)
Chloride (mmol/L)	—	—	110 (105-114)
Cholesterol (mg/dL)	160-425	180-305	237 (110-363)
CK (U/L)	228-322	125-345	341 (182-1459)
Creatinine (mg/dL)	0.1-0.4	0.1-0.4	—
GGT (U/L)	1-10	—	—
Glucose (mg/dL)	206-275	221-302	266 (213-371)
LDH (U/L)	145-465	155-425	—
Lipase (U/L)	35-350	35-225	—
Phosphorus (mg/dL)	3.2-5.4	3.1-5.5	3.1 (1.2-5.0)
Potassium (mmol/L)	2.9-4.6	3-4.5	3.2 (1.3-5.0)
Protein, total (g/dL)	3.2-5.2	3-5.2	4.2 (3.4-4.9)
Albumin (g/dL)	1.22-2.52	1.79-2.81	—
Globulin (g/dL)	—	—	—
A:G ratio	1.02-2.59	1.21-2.29	—
Prealbumin (g/dL)	0.30-0.92	0.6-1.23	—
α-globulin (g/dL)	0.06-0.20 (α_1)	0.09-0.23 (α_1)	—
	0.10-0.28 (α_2)	0.20-0.42 (α_2)	—
β-globulin (g/dL)	0.49-0.88	0.33-0.89	—
γ-globulin (g/dL)	0.21-0.81	0.21-0.72	—
Sodium (mmol/L)	157-165	125-155	150 (146-154)
Triglycerides (mg/dL)	45-145	49-190	14 (69-234)
Uric acid (mg/dL)	2.7-8.8	2.1-8.7	1.6 (1.9-12.7)

Continued

TABLE 5-19 Hematologic and Biochemical Values of Select Psittaciformes. (cont'd)

Measurement	Budgerigar Parakeet (*Melopsittacus undulatus*)[320,407]	Caique (*Pionites* spp.)[186,320]	Cockatiel (*Nymphicus hollandicus*)[186,320]
Hematology			
PCV (%)	44-58	47-55	43-57
RBC (10^6/µL)	3.77-4.6	—	3.1-4.4
Hgb (g/dL)	12.4-16.9	—	10.2-14.7
MCV (fL)	116-127	—	126-142
MCH (pg)	23.1-30.9	—	26.4-35.8
MCHC (g/dL)	19.8-23.9	—	20.4-25.2
WBC (10^3/µL)	3-10	8-15	5-11
Heterophils 10^3/µL (%)	2.68-4.55 (40-75)	4.68-8.64 (39-72)	3.68-5.76 (46-72)
Lymphocytes 10^3/µL (%)	1.47-4.02 (20-45)	2.4-7.32 (20-61)	2.08-4.8 (26-60)
Monocytes 10^3/µL (%)	0-0.13 (0-2)	0-0.24 (0-2)	0-0.08 (0-1)
Eosinophils 10^3/µL (%)	0 (0)	0-0.12 (0-1)	0-0.16 (0-2)
Basophils 10^3/µL (%)	0-0.13 (0-1)	0-0.12 (0-1)	0-0.08 (0-1)
H:L ratio	—	—	—
Chemistries			
ALP (U/L)	10-80	—	20-250
ALT (U/L)	—	—	5-11
Amylase (U/L)	302-560	244-290	205-490
AST (U/L)	55-154	193-399	160-383
Bile acid (µmol/L)			
RIA	20-65	11.8-56.7	11.7-80.7
Colorimetric	32-117	12-112	44-108
BUN (mg/dL)	3-5.2	—	2.9-5
Calcium (mg/dL)	6.4-11.2	7.1-11.5	7.3-10.7
Chloride (mmol/L)	—	—	—
Cholesterol (mg/dL)	145-275	—	140-360
CK (U/L)	54-252	134-427	58-245
Creatinine (mg/dL)	0.1-0.4	—	0.1-0.4
GGT (U/L)	1-10	—	1-30
Glucose (mg/dL)	254-399	167-366	249-363
LDH (U/L)	154-271	—	120-455
Lipase (U/L)	—	—	30-280

TABLE 5-19 Hematologic and Biochemical Values of Select Psittaciformes. (cont'd)

Measurement	Budgerigar Parakeet (*Melopsittacus undulatus*)	Caique (*Pionites* spp.)	Cockatiel (*Nymphicus hollandicus*)
Phosphorus (mg/dL)	3-5.2	—	3.2-4.8
Potassium (mmol/L)	2.2-3.7	—	2.4-4.6
Protein, total (g/dL)	2-3	2.4-4.6	2.4-4.8
Albumin (g/dL)	—	0.96-2.04	0.78-1.75
Globulin (g/dL)	—	—	—
A:G ratio	—	1.09-2.76	1.01-2.19
Prealbumin (g/dL)	—	0.33-0.89	0.59-1.24
α-globulin (g/dL)	—	0.05-0.17 (α_1)	0.05-0.32 (α_1)
	—	0.13-0.38 (α_2)	0.07-0.39 (α_2)
β-globulin (g/dL)	—	0.34-0.99	0.34-0.81
γ-globulin (g/dL)	—	0.13-0.50	0.15-0.60
Sodium (mmol/L)	139-159	—	130-153
Triglycerides (mg/dL)	—	—	45-200
Uric acid (mg/dL)	3-8.6	3.4-12.2	3.5-11

Measurement	Cockatoos (*Cacatuidae*)[320,431]	Conures (*Aratinga* and *Pyrrhura* spp.)[186,320]	Eclectus Parrot (*Eclectus roratus*)[186,320]
Hematology			
PCV (%)	40-54	42-54	45-55
RBC (10^6/μL)	2.44-3.34	2.9-4.5	2.5-3.7
Hgb (g/dL)	11.1-16.0	12-16	11.1-13.9
MCV (fL)	158-175	90-190	157-170
MCH (pg)	40.4-53.7	28-55	37.5-44.6
MCHC (g/dL)	25.8-31.5	—	22.69-27.53
WBC (10^3/μL)	5-13	5-13	9-15
Heterophils 10^3/μL (%)	4.68-7.49 (45-72)	4.22-6.91 (44-72)	5.75-8.75 (46-70)
Lymphocytes 10^3/μL (%)	2.08-5.20 (20-50)	2.11-4.89 (22-51)	2.87-7.12 (23-57)
Monocytes 10^3/μL (%)	0-0.2 (0-2)	0-0.09 (0-1)	0-0.12 (0-1)
Eosinophils 10^3/μL (%)	0-0.2 (0-2)	0-0.09 (0-1)	0-0.12 (0-1)

Continued

TABLE 5-19 Hematologic and Biochemical Values of Select Psittaciformes. (cont'd)

Measurement	Cockatoos (*Cacatuidae*)	Conures (*Aratinga* and *Pyrrhura* spp.)	Eclectus Parrot (*Eclectus roratus*)
Basophils $10^3/\mu L$ (%)	0-0.1 (0-1)	0-0.09 (0-1)	0-0.12 (0-1)
H:L ratio	—	—	1-2
Chemistries			
ALP (U/L)	15-255	80-250	—
ALT (U/L)	6-12	5-13	5-11
Amylase (U/L)	200-510	100-450	200-645
AST (U/L)	117-314	178-307	148-378
Bile acid (µmol/L)			
RIA	10.3-79.1	8.3-85.2	9.7-87.5
Colorimetric	34-112	32-105	30-110
BUN (mg/dL)	3-5.1	2.5-5.4	3.5-5
Calcium (mg/dL)	8.3-10.8	7.9-10.8	7.9-11.4
Chloride (mmol/L)	—	—	—
Cholesterol (mg/dL)	135-355	120-400	130-350
CK (U/L)	106-305	154-355	118-345
Creatinine (mg/dL)	0.1-0.4	0.1-0.4	0.1-0.4
GGT (U/L)	1-45	1-15	1-20
Glucose (mg/dL)	214-302	217-323	220-294
LDH (U/L)	220-550	120-390	200-425
Phosphorus (mg/dL)	2.5-5.5	2-10	2.9-6.5
Potassium (mmol/L)	2.5-4.5	3.4-5	3.5-4.3
Protein, total (g/dL)	3-5	2.8-4.6	3-5
Albumin (g/dL)	1.11-2.28	1.01-1.94	1.23-2.26
Globulin (g/dL)	—	—	—
A:G ratio	1.06-2.54	1.08-2.73	1.09-2.50
Prealbumin (g/dL)	0.29-0.83	0.39-1.12	0.31-1.18
α-globulin (g/dL)	0.07-0.16 (α_1) 0.09-0.26 (α_2)	0.07-0.17 (α_1) 0.18-0.43 (α_2)	0.08-0.19 (α_1) 0.10-0.30 (α_2)
β-globulin (g/dL)	0.39-0.89	0.30-0.81	0.46-0.89
γ-globulin (g/dL)	0.18-0.61	0.12-0.55	0.17-0.63
Sodium (mmol/L)	130-155	135-149	130-145
Triglycerides (mg/dL)	45-200	50-300	—
Uric acid (mg/dL)	2.9-11.0	3.0-11.4	2.5-8.7

TABLE 5-19 Hematologic and Biochemical Values of Select Psittaciformes. (cont'd)

Measurement	Grey-Cheeked Parakeet (*Brotogeris pyrrhoptera*)[320]	Jardine's Parrot (*Poicephalus gulielmi*)[186]	Lories and Lorikeets[186,320,394]
Hematology			
PCV (%)	45-56	41-53	47-55
RBC (10^6/µL)	—	3.03-4.47	3.3-4
Hgb (g/dL)	—	—	10.8-14.8
MCV (fL)	—	—	128-140
MCH (pg)	—	—	27.5-31.4
MCHC (g/dL)	—	—	20.3-23.1
WBC (10^3/µL)	4-12	4.1-12.6	8-13
Heterophils 10^3/µL (%)	3.74-5.64 (45-68)	— (55-75)	4.21-6.48 (39-60)
Lymphocytes 10^3/µL (%)	1.83-3.98 (22-48)	— (25-45)	2.38-7.45 (22-69)
Monocytes 10^3/µL (%)	0-0.08 (0-1)	— (0-2)	0-0.22 (0-2)
Eosinophils 10^3/µL (%)	0-0.08 (0-1)	— (0-1)	0-0.11 (0-1)
Basophils 10^3/µL (%)	0-0.08 (0-1)	— (0-1)	— (0-1)
H:L ratio	—	—	—
Chemistries			
ALP (U/L)	—	80-156	—
ALT (U/L)	—	5-12	—
Amylase (U/L)	—	100-425	20-65
AST (U/L)	189-388	150-278	141-369
Bile acid (µmol/L)			
RIA	—	10.2-61.7	20-65
Colorimetric	15-81	—	20-97
BUN (mg/dL)	—	2.8-5.6	—
Calcium (mg/dL)	8.0-11.6	7.0-12.8	8-12
Chloride (mmol/L)	—	—	—
Cholesterol (mg/dL)	96-249	100-300	100-257
CK (U/L)	164-378	110-310	178-396
Creatinine (mg/dL)	—	—	—
GGT (U/L)	—	1-15	—

Continued

TABLE 5-19 Hematologic and Biochemical Values of Select Psittaciformes. (cont'd)

Measurement	Grey-Cheeked Parakeet (*Brotogeris pyrrhoptera*)	Jardine's Parrot (*Poicephalus gulielmi*)	Lories and Lorikeets
Glucose (mg/dL)	210-385	199-348	200-400
LDH (U/L)	154-356	119-335	124-302
Phosphorus (mg/dL)	—	2-6.8	—
Potassium (mmol/L)	—	3-4.5	—
Protein, total (g/dL)	2.5-4.5	2.8-4	1.9-4.1
Albumin (g/dL)	—	1.17-1.92	1.3-2.1
Globulin (g/dL)	—	—	0.9-2.4
A:G ratio	—	1.32-2.56	1-2.3
Prealbumin (g/dL)	—	0.12-0.42	—
α-globulin (g/dL)	—	0.07-0.16 (α_1)	—
	—	0.08-0.22 (α_2)	—
β-globulin (g/dL)	—	0.38-0.84	—
γ-globulin (g/dL)	—	0.12-0.47	—
Sodium (mmol/L)	—	133-153	—
Tryglycerides (mg/dL)	—	60-130	—
Uric acid (mg/dL)	0.3-12	2.5-12	2-11.9

Measurement	Lovebirds (*Agapornis* spp.)[186,320]	Macaws (*Ara* and *Anodorhynchus* spp.)[186,320]	Parrotlets (*Forpus* spp.)[320]
Hematology			
PCV (%)	44-55	42-56	48-55
RBC (10^6/μL)	3.25-3.95	2.7-4.5	—
Hgb (g/dL)	10.8-14.8	15-17	—
MCV (fL)	128-140	125-170	—
MCH (pg)	27.5-31.4	36-55	—
MCHC (g/dL)	20.3-23.1	29-35	—
WBC (10^3/μL)	7-16	10-20	5-13
Heterophils 10^3/μL (%)	3.33-9.21 (40-75)	7.6-11.4 (50-75)	4.84-6.51 (55-74)
Lymphocytes 10^3/μL (%)	3.34-6.20 (20-53)	3.50-8.06 (23-53)	2.11-4.4 (19-70)
Monocytes 10^3/μL (%)	0-0.12 (0-1)	0-0.15 (0-1)	0-0.09 (0-1)

TABLE 5-19 Hematologic and Biochemical Values of Select Psittaciformes. (cont'd)

Measurement	Lovebirds (*Agapornis* spp.)	Macaws (*Ara* and *Anodorhynchus* spp.)	Parrotlets (*Forpus* spp.)
Eosinophils $10^3/\mu L$ (%)	0-0.23 (0-2)	0 (0)	0-0.09 (0-1)
Basophils $10^3/\mu L$ (%)	0-0.23 (0-6)	0-0.15 (0-1)	0-0.09 (0-1)
H:L ratio	—	—	—
Chemistries			
ALP (U/L)	10-90	20-230	—
ALT (U/L)	5-13	5-12	—
Amylase (U/L)	90-400	150-550	—
AST (U/L)	125-377	105-324	110-224
Bile acid (μmol/L)			
RIA	8.5-77.1	7.6-60	—
Colorimetric	12-90	7-100	—
BUN (mg/dL)	2.8-5.5	3-5.6	—
Calcium (mg/dL)	7.2-10.6	8.2-10.9	—
Chloride (mmol/L)	—	—	—
Cholesterol (mg/dL)	95-335	100-390	—
CK (U/L)	58-337	101-300	—
Creatinine (mg/dL)	0.1-0.4	0.5-0.6	—
GGT (U/L)	2.5-18	1-30	—
Glucose (mg/dL)	246-381	228-325	252-384
LDH (U/L)	105-355	70-350	—
Lipase (U/L)	30-320	30-250	—
Phosphorus (mg/dL)	2.8-4.9	—	—
Potassium (mmol/L)	2.1-4.8	2-5	—
Protein, total (g/dL)	2.4-3.6	2.6-5.0	—
Albumin (g/dL)	0.98-1.68	1.12-2.43	—
Globulin (g/dL)	—	—	—
A:G ratio	1.06-2.09	1.08-2.55	
Prealbumin (g/dL)	0.37-0.68	0.24-0.80	—
α-globulin (g/dL)	0.08-0.17 (α_1)	0.07-0.18 (α_1)	—
	0.12-0.37 (α_2)	0.15-0.45 (α_2)	—
β-globulin (g/dL)	0.33-0.78	0.34-0.85	—
γ-globulin (g/dL)	0.12-0.38	0.15-0.58	—

Continued

TABLE 5-19 Hematologic and Biochemical Values of Select Psittaciformes. (cont'd)

Measurement	Lovebirds (*Agapornis* spp.)	Macaws (*Ara* and *Anodorhynchus* spp.)	Parrotlets (*Forpus* spp.)
Sodium (mmol/L)	125-155	140-165	—
Triglycerides (g/L)	45-200	—	—
Uric acid (mg/dL)	2.5-12	2.9-10.6	4.1-12

Measurement	Pionus Parrots (*Pionus* spp.)[186,320]	Quaker Parakeet (*Myopsitta monachus*)[186,320]	Senegal Parrot (*Poicephalus senegalus*)[186,320]
Hematology			
PCV (%)	44-54	30-58	45-60
RBC (10^6/μL)	2.4-4	—	2.4-4
Hgb (g/dL)	11-16	—	12.3-14.0
MCV (fL)	85-210	—	139-151
MCH (pg)	26-54	—	33.1-39.4
MCHC (g/dL)	24-31	—	23.4-27.4
WBC (10^3/μL)	5-13	8-17	6-14
Heterophils 10^3/μL (%)	0.48-7.10 (55-74)	— (0-24)	4.70-7.81 (44-73)
Lymphocytes 10^3/μL (%)	1.82-6.72 (19-70)	— (74-90)	2.35-7.49 (22-70)
Monocytes 10^3/μL (%)	0-0.10 (0-1)	— (1-4)	0-0.11 (0-1)
Eosinophils 10^3/μL (%)	0-0.10 (0-1)	— (0-2)	0-0.21 (0-2)
Basophils 10^3/μL (%)	0-0.10 (0-1)	— (0-6)	0-0.11 (0-1)
H:L ratio	—	—	—
Chemistries			
ALP (U/L)	80-290	70-300	70-300
ALT (U/L)	5-12	5-11	5-11
Amylase (U/L)	200-500	100-400	190-550
AST (U/L)	140-359	225-375	183-352
Bile acid (μmol/L)			
RIA	6.1-62.7	9.6-83.2	13.8-87.4
Colorimetric	15-92	21-90	20-94
BUN (mg/dL)	3-5.4	2.9-5.4	2.9-5.4

TABLE 5-19 Hematologic and Biochemical Values of Select Psittaciformes. (cont'd)

Measurement	Pionus Parrots (*Pionus* spp.)	Quaker Parakeet (*Myopsitta monachus*)	Senegal Parrot (*Poicephalus senegalus*)
Calcium (mg/dL)	7.8-10.8	7-10.0	7.6-10.7
Chloride (mmol/L)	—	—	—
Cholesterol (mg/dL)	130-295	110-295	130-340
CK (U/L)	169-354	110-311	100-330
Creatinine (mg/dL)	0.1-0.4	0.1-0.4	0.1-0.4
GGT (U/L)	1-18	1-15	1-15
Glucose (mg/dL)	228-312	229-318	220-284
LDH (U/L)	125-380	120-300	150-350
Lipase (U/L)	30-250	25-225	32-250
Phosphorus (mg/dL)	2.9-6.6	2.9-6.5	—
Potassium (mmol/L)	3.5-4.6	2.8-4.6	3-5
Protein, total (g/dL)	3.6-5.2	3.0-4.8	2.8-4.2
Albumin (g/dL)	—	0.92-2.48	1.19-1.81
Globulin (g/dL)	—	—	—
A:G ratio	0.6-1.9	1.07-2.38	1.41-2.66
Prealbumin (g/dL)	1.52-2.37	0.91-2.46	0.55-0.99
α-globulin (g/dL)	0.08-0.23 (α_1) 0.11-0.36 (α_2)	0.08-0.21 (α_1) 0.22-0.45 (α_2)	0.08-0.15 (α_1) 0.11-0.25 (α_2)
β-globulin (g/dL)	0.40-0.95	0.37-0.79	0.32-0.87
γ-globulin (g/dL)	0.23-0.69	0.19-0.77	0.15-0.45
Sodium (mmol/L)	145-155	140-155	130-155
Triglycerides (mg/dL)	60-225	50-200	45-145
Uric acid (mg/dL)	2.0-7.9	3.5-11.5	2.5-7.8

TABLE 5-20 Hematologic and Biochemical Values for Juveniles of Select Psittaciformes.

Measurement	Mean ± SD (Range)				
	Cockatoos (*Cacatua* spp.)[169] (9 species) (*n* = 152)[a]	Lorikeet, Green-naped (*Trichoglossus haematodus haematodus*)[392] (n=102)[b]	Macaws (*Ara* spp.)[170] (7 species) (*n* = 113)[a]	Macaw, Blue and Gold (*Ara ararauna*)[170] (*n* = 43)[a]	Parrot, Eclectus (*Eclectus roratus*)[168] (*n* = 111)[a]
Hematology					
PCV (%)	39.7 ± 9 (25-59)	52 ± 3.8 (44.2–59.0)	41.7 ± 8.4 (25-55)	40 ± 7.7	43.8 ± 8.4 (26-58)
RBC (10^6/μL)	2.53 ± 0.63 (1.5-4)	—	2.9 ± 0.8 (1.5-4.5)	2.7 ± 0.7	2.69 ± 0.67 (1.5-4)
Hgb (g/dL)	11.4 ± 2.9 (6.5-17)	—	12.3 ± 3.3 (7-17)	11 ± 2.9	12.5 ± 3 (6.5-18)
WBC (10^3/μL)	12.9 ± 6.3 (5.5-25)	7.4 ± 2.4 (4.0-13.7)	19.2 ± 6.9 (7-30)	18.9 ± 5.6	13.7 ± 6.3 (5.5-25)
Heterophils (%)	50.8 ± 11.7 (27-74)	31.0 ± 15.0 (8.7-70.0)	55.3 ± 10 (37-75)	52 ± 10 —	53.9 ± 11.4 (35-75)
Bands (%)	1.3 ± 2.3 (0-7)	—	0.6 ± 1.7 (0-5)	0.1 ± 0.7 —	0.5 ± 1.5 (0-5)
Lymphocytes (%)	41.2 ± 11.9 (17-65)	66.2 ± 15.1 (30.0-90.3)	39 ± 10 (20-60)	42 ± 10 —	39.5 ± 11.5 (20-65)
Monocytes (%)	5.8 ± 3.4 (0-12)	2.1 ± 1.8 (0.0-6.0)	4.4 ± 2.9 (1-10)	4.3 ± 2.7 —	5 ± 2.7 (1-11)
Eosinophils (%)	0	0.2 ± 0.6 (0-2.4)	0 ± 0.2 (0-1)	0 —	0.1 ± 0.3 (0-1)
Basophils (%)	0.9 ± 1.1 (0-4)	—	0.5 ± 1 (0-3)	0.9 ± 1.3 —	1.1 ± 1 (0-3)

TABLE 5-20 Hematologic and Biochemical Values for Juveniles of Select Psittaciformes. (cont'd)

	Mean ± SD (Range)				
Measurement	Cockatoos (*Cacatua* spp.) (9 species) (n = 152)	Lorikeet, Green-naped (*Trichoglossus haematodus haematodus*) (n=102)	Macaws (*Ara* spp.) (7 species) (n = 113)	Macaw, Blue and Gold (*Ara ararauna*) (n = 43)	Parrot, Eclectus (*Eclectus roratus*) (n = 111)
Chemistries					
ALP (U/L)	579 ± 239 (200-1000)	—	970 ± 397 (290-1600)	1200 ± 390	489 ± 159 (200-900)
ALT (U/L)	2 ± 3 (0-13)	—	3 ± 2 (0-9)	4 ± 3	4 ± 3 (0-10)
AST (U/L)	143 ± 79 (50-400)	215 ± 42.4 (159-349)	104 ± 31 (60-180)	101 ± 24	140 ± 58 (65-260)
BUN (mg/dL)	2 ± 2.2 (0-6)		2.4 ± 2.3 (0-6)	1.9 ± 2.2	1.7 ± 2.4 (0-6)
Calcium (mg/dL)	9.6 ± 0.7 (8-11)	8.7 ± 0.6 (6.9-9.7)	9.9 ± 0.5 (8.5-10.8)	10 ± 0.5	9.3 ± 0.4 (8.5-10.2)
Chloride (mmol/L)	110 ± 6 (97-120)	114 ± 4.7 (101-122)	106 ± 6 (96-118)	104 ± 5	111 ± 5 (100-120)
Cholesterol (mg/dL)	251 ± 105 (100-500)	186 ± 28.9 (134-250)	165 ± 62 (75-300)	164 ± 67	268 ± 80 (125-450)
CK (U/L)	510 ± 235 (140-1000)	774 ± 277 (373-1533)	550 ± 312 (180-1100)	540 ± 267	616 ± 472 (200-1600)
Creatinine (mg/dL)	0.4 ± 0.1 (0.2-0.7)	—	0.4 ± 0.1 (0.3-0.6)	0.4 ± 0.1	0.4 ± 0.1 (0.2-0.5)
GGT (U/L)	2.6 ± 1.7 (0-6)	—	1.8 ± 1.2 (0-4)	1.7 ± 1.2	4 ± 2 (0-7)
Glucose (mg/dL)	253 ± 24 (200-300)	236 ± 37.5 (152-317)	281 ± 30 (225-330)	288 ± 31	258 ± 18 (220-300)

Continued

TABLE 5-20 Hematologic and Biochemical Values for Juveniles of Select Psittaciformes. (cont'd)

	Mean ± SD (Range)				
Measurement	Cockatoos (*Cacatua* spp.) (9 species) (n = 152)	Lorikeet, Green-naped (*Trichoglossus haematodus haematodus*) (n=102)	Macaws (*Ara* spp.) (7 species) (n = 113)	Macaw, Blue and Gold (*Ara ararauna*) (n = 43)	Parrot, Eclectus (*Eclectus roratus*) (n = 111)
LDH (U/L)	371 ± 285 (150-1000)	—	138 ± 84 (35-275)	144 ± 98	228 ± 101 (100-400)
Phosphorus (mg/dL)	6.1 ± 1.1 (3.5-8)	4.0 ± 1.7 (1.14-8.6)	6.5 ± 1 (4.6-6.9)	6.6 ± 0.9	6.8 ± 1.2 (4.5-9)
Potassium (mmol/L)	3.6 ± 0.7 (2.5-5.5)	2.4 ± 0.6 (1.4-3.7)	2.9 ± 0.8 (2-4.2)	2.7 ± 0.6	2.8 ± 0.7 (2-4.6)
Protein, total (g/dL)	2.8 ± 0.7 (1.5-4)	—	2.6 ± 0.6 (1.5-3.5)	2.5 ± 0.7	2.9 ± 0.5 (1.8-3.8)
Albumin (g/dL)	1.1 ± 0.3 (0.3-1.6)	1.2 ± 0.2 (0.8-1.6)	1.2 ± 0.3 (0.6-1.7)	1.2 ± 0.3	1.3 ± 0.3 (0.8-1.8)
Globulin (g/dL)	1.7 ± 0.5 (0.8-2.5)	1.6 ± 0.3 (1.2-2.0)	1.3 ± 0.6 (0.8-1.9)	1.3 ± 0.6	1.5 ± 0.3 (0.8-2.2)
A:G ratio	0.6 ± 0.2 (0.4-1)	—	0.8 ± 0.3 (0.5-1)	0.8 ± 0.2	0.9 ± 0.2 (0.6-1.1)
Sodium (mmol/L)	145 ± 6 (135-155)	152 ± 5.1 (143-163)	145 ± 6 (135-156)	142 ± 6	148 ± 6 (138-158)
Uric acid (mg/dL)	2.9 ± 2.3 (0.2-8.5)	5.7 ± 3.2 (1.8-12)	2.3 ± 2.1 (0.2-6)	1.9 ± 2.5	2 ± 1.6 (0.2-6.5)

[a]*n* = Number of blood samples (multiple blood samples were obtained from some individuals over time).
[b]Mean and SD (reference interval); reference intervals were determined by nonparametric method with 90% confidence interval using the bootstrap method.

TABLE 5-21 Hematologic and Biochemical Values of Select Passeriformes.

Measurement	Canary (*Serinus canaria*)[318]	Common Hill Mynah[a] (*Gracula religiosa*)[29]
PCV (%)	45-56	47.6 ± 4.9
RBC ($10^6/\mu L$)	2.5-3.8	3.8 ± 0.4
Hgb (g/dL)	12-16	14.3 ± 1.2
MCV (fL)	90-210	126 ± 11.7
MCH (pg)	26-55	38.4 ± 3.6
MCHC (g/dL)	22-32	30.1 ± 1.5
WBC ($10^3/\mu L$)	3-10	20.8 ± 5.8
Heterophils $10^3/\mu L$	—	—
(%)	(50-80)	(43.8 ± 8)
Lymphocytes $10^3/\mu L$	—	—
(%)	(20-45)	(48.7 ± 7.5)
Monocytes $10^3/\mu L$	—	—
(%)	(0-1)	(4.6 ± 4.1)
Eosinophils $10^3/\mu L$	—	—
(%)	(0-2)	(4.1 ± 2.5)
Basophils $10^3/\mu L$	—	—
(%)	(0-1)	(0.8 ± 0.7)
H:L ratio	—	—
ALP (U/L)	20-135	—
ALT (U/L)	—	—
AST (U/L)	14-345	130-350
Bile acid (μmol/L)		
RIA	23-90	—
Colorimetric	—	—
Calcium (mg/dL)	5.5-13.5	9-13
Chloride (mmol/L)	—	—
Cholesterol (mg/dL)	150-400	—
CK (U/L)	55-350	—
Creatinine (mg/dL)	0.1-0.4	0.1-0.6
GGT (U/L)	1-14	—
Glucose (mg/dL)	205-435	190-350
LDH (U/L)	120-450	600-1000
Phosphorus (mg/dL)	2.9-4.9	—
Potassium (mmol/L)	2.2-4.5	0.3-5.1
Protein, total (g/dL)	2.8-4.5	2.3-4.5
Albumin (g/dL)	—	—
Globulin (g/dL)	—	—
A:G ratio	—	—
Sodium (mmol/L)	135-165	136-152
Uric acid (mg/dL)	4-12	4-10

[a]Values reported in captive adult males.

TABLE 5-22 Hematologic and Biochemical Values of Select Ratites.

Measurement	Emu (*Dromaius novaehollandiae*)[442,769]	Ostrich (*Struthio camelus*)[527,528]	Rhea, Greater (*Rhea americana*)[a,230,324]
Hematology			
PCV (%)	40-60	32 ± 3	40.8 ± 4.5
RBC (10^6/µL)	2.5-4.5	1.7 ± 0.4	1.21 ± 0.80
Hgb (g/dL)	—	12.2 ± 2.0	10.4 ± 1.4
MCV (fL)	—	174 ± 42	44.7 ± 20.1
MCH (pg)	—	—	113.5 ± 52.9
MCHC (g/dL)	—	33 ± 5	25.6 ± 2.5
WBC (10^3/µL)	8-25	5.5 ± 1.9	12.1 ± 4.1
Heterophils 10^3/µL (%)	— (45-75)	— (63 ± 8)	— (64.1 ± 9.9)
Lymphocytes 10^3/µL (%)	— (20-40)	— (34 ± 7)	— (26.9 ± 9.6)
Monocytes 10^3/µL (%)	— (0-2)	— (3 ± 1)	— (6.4 ± 3.0)
Eosinophils 10^3/µL (%)	— (0-1)	— (0.3 ± 0.5)	— (2.1 ± 2.1)
Basophils 10^3/µL (%)	— (0-1)	— (0.2 ± 0.5)	— (0.5 ± 1.3)
H:L ratio	—	—	—
Chemistries			
ALP (U/L)	—	575 ± 248	—
AST (U/L)	80-380	131 ± 31	20-192
Bile acid (µmol/L)			
RIA	6-45	—	—
Colorimetric	—	—	—
Calcium (mg/dL)	8.8-12.5	9.2	2.6-8.2
Chloride (mmol/L)	—	100 ± 16	—
Cholesterol (mg/dL)	68-170	108	—
CK (U/L)	100-750	688 ± 208	0-2640
Creatinine (mg/dL)	0.22	0.32	—
GGT (U/L)	—	1.5 ± 2.9	—
Glucose (mg/dL)	100-290	250	37.8-158.6
LDH (U/L)	310-1200	1565 ± 660	269-1640
Phosphorus (mg/dL)	3.8-7.2	3.7	—
Potassium (mmol/L)	3.5-6.5	3 ± 0.8	—
Protein, total (g/dL)	3.4-5.6	3.7 ± 0.7	3.4-6.2
Albumin (g/dL)	1-2.5	—	—
Sodium (mmol/L)	—	147 ± 34	—
Uric acid (mg/dL)	4.5-14	8.2	—

TABLE 5-23 Hematologic and Biochemical Values of Select Piciformes and Columbiformes.

Measurement	Toucan (*Ramphastos* spp.)[a,320]	Pigeon (*Columba livia*)[556,845]
Hematology		
PCV (%)	42-60 (49.8)	49 ± 3.8
RBC (10^6/µL)		—
Hgb (g/dL)		—
MCV (fL)		—
MCH (pg)		—
MCHC (g/dL)		—
WBC (10^3/µL)	8-18 (13.5)	8348 ± 4813
Heterophils 10^3/µL	—	1369 ± 1031
[%]	[41-62 (51.9)]	—
Lymphocytes 10^3/µL	—	5877 ± 4099
[%]	[35-70 (50.5)]	—
Monocytes 10^3/µL	—	225 ± 232
[%]	[0-2 (0)]	—
Eosinophils 10^3/µL	—	9 ± 25
[%]	[0-3 (0)]	—
Basophils 10^3/µL	—	120 ± 130
[%]	[0-1 (0)]	—
H:L ratio	—	—
Chemistries		
ALP (U/L)	14-88 (43.4)	160-780
ALT (U/L)	—	19-48
AST (U/L)	141-340 (243.3)	45-123
Bile acid (µmol/L)		
RIA	—	—
Colorimetric	16-86 (54.4)	22-60
BUN (mg/dL)	—	2.4-4.2
Calcium (mg/dL)	8.8-11.8 (10.2)	7.6-10.4
Chloride (mmol/L)	—	101-113
Cholesterol (mg/dL)	104-254 (175.1)	—
CK (U/L)	—	110-480
Creatinine (mg/dL)	—	0.3-0.4
GGT (U/L)	—	0-2.9
Glucose (mg/dL)	222-363 (297.9)	232-369
LDH (U/L)	180-319 (257)	30-205
Phosphorus (mg/dL)	—	1.8-4.1

Continued

TABLE 5-23 Hematologic and Biochemical Values of Select Piciformes and Columbiformes. (cont'd)

Measurement	Toucan (*Ramphastos* spp.)	Pigeon (*Columba livia*)
Potassium (mmol/L)	—	3.9-4.7
Protein, total (g/dL)	2.8-4.4 (3.5)	2.1-3.3
Albumin (g/dL)	1.4-2.4 (2.1)	1.3-2.2
Globulin (g/dL)	1.4-2.2 (1.8)	0.6-1.2
A:G ratio	—	1.5-3.6
Sodium (mmol/L)	—	141-149
Uric acid (mg/dL)	2.4-14 (7.9)	2.5-12.9

[a]Numbers in parentheses represent the mean.

TABLE 5-24 Hematologic and Biochemical Values of Select Raptors. Accipitriformes

Measurement	Bald Eagle (*Haliaeetus leucocephalus*)[451]	Golden Eagle (*Aquila chrysaetos*)[a,390,643]
Hematology		
PCV (%)	35-57	35-47 (41)
RBC ($10^6/\mu L$)	2.60-4.05	1.9-2.7 (2.4)
Hgb (g/dL)	—	12.1-15.2 (13.8)
MCV (fL)	—	160-184 (174)
MCH (pg)	—	56.3-62.7 (58.9)
MCHC (g/dL)	—	32.3-35.9 (34)
WBC ($10^3/\mu L$)	4.1-27.3	5.9-24 (12.3)
Heterophils $10^3/\mu L$	—	—
(%)	(50-93)	(49-86)
Lymphocytes $10^3/\mu L$	—	—
(%)	(4-38)	(14-38)
Monocytes $10^3/\mu L$	—	—
(%)	(0-4)	(0-9)
Eosinophils $10^3/\mu L$	—	—
(%)	(0-9)	(1-5)
Basophils $10^3/\mu L$	—	—
(%)	(0-1)	(0-1)
H:L ratio	—	—
Fibrinogen (g/L)	—	2-4.1 (2.9)
Chemistries		
ALP (U/L)	—	15-36
ALT (U/L)	—	—

TABLE 5-24 Hematologic and Biochemical Values of Select Raptors. Accipitriformes (cont'd)

Measurement	Bald Eagle (*Haliaeetus leucocephalus*)	Golden Eagle (*Aquila chrysaetos*)
AST (U/L)	131-956	95-210
Bile acid (µmol/L)		
RIA	—	—
Calcium (mg/dL)	8.2-10.4	7.4-9.5
Chloride (mmol/L)	—	—
Cholesterol (mg/dL)	—	—
CK (U/L)	190-1797	—
GGT (U/L)	—	—
Glucose (mg/dL)	246-431	250-408
LDH (U/L)	—	320-690
Phosphorus (mg/dL)	—	1.9-3.6
Potassium (mmol/L)	—	—
Protein, total (g/dL)	2.2-4.6	2.5-3.9
Albumin (g/dL)	1.09-2.05	1-1.4
Globulin (g/dL)	0.19-0.59	—
A:G ratio	0.57-1.59	—
Sodium (mmol/L)	—	—
Uric acid (mg/dL)	1.8-15.3	4.4-12

[a]Numbers in parentheses represent the mean.

Measurement	Red-tailed Hawk (*Buteo jamaicensis*)[803]	Common Buzzard (*Buteo buteo*)[403]	Harris's hawk (*Parabuteo unicinctus*)[b,136,440,803]
PCV (%)	31-43	40.8 ± 4.4	32-44
RBC (10^6/µL)	2.4-3.6	2.94 ± 0.82	2.13-2.76
Hgb (g/dL)	10.7-16.6	—	10.1-16.7
MCV (fL)	150-178	145 ± 25	147-163
MCH (pg)	46-57.4	48.3 ± 10.2	45.4-51.1
MCHC (g/dL)	297-345	32.4 ± 6.7	30.1-33.0
WBC (10^3/µL)	19.1-33.4	8.04 ± 1.77	4.8-10
Heterophils 10^3/µL	—	4.58 ± 1.2	—
(%)	35 ± 11	63 ± 13.1	2.3-6.7
Lymphocytes 10^3/µL	—	1.4 ± 0.73	—
(%)	44 ± 9	20 ± 9.5	0.6-2.4

Continued

TABLE 5-24 Hematologic and Biochemical Values of Select Raptors. Accipitriformes (cont'd)

Measurement	Red-tailed Hawk (*Buteo jamaicensis*)	Common Buzzard (*Buteo buteo*)	Harris's hawk (*Parabuteo unicinctus*)
Monocytes $10^3/\mu L$	—	0.05 ± 0.08	—
(%)	6 ± 3	0 ± 1	0.2-1.5
Eosinophils $10^3/\mu L$	—	1.2 ± 1.1	—
(%)	13 ± 4	16 ± 13.8	0-0.8
Basophils $10^3/\mu L$	—	0.6 ± 0.1	—
(%)	Rare	0 ± 0.7	0-1.6
H:L ratio	—	—	—
Fibrinogen (g/L)	—	—	—
Chemistries			
ALP (U/L)	22-138	—	15-36
ALT (U/L)	3-50	13.1 ± 5.9	—
AST (U/L)	76-492	227.7 ± 155.5	95-210
Bile acid (µmol/L)			
RIA	8.4-10.2	—	—
Calcium (mg/dL)	10-12.8	11.2 ± 2.5	8.4-10.6
Chloride (mmol/L)	118-129	—	113-119
Cholesterol (mg/dL)	—	—	—
CK (U/L)	—	393.2 ± 187.8	224-650
GGT (U/L)	0-20	3.5 ± 0.7	2-6.9
Glucose (mg/dL)	292-390	301.1 ± 53.1	220-283
LDH (U/L)	0-2640	631.5 ± 153.0	160-563
Phosphorus (mg/dL)	1.9-4	4.6 ± 3.3	3-4.4
Potassium (mmol/L)	2.6-4.3	—	0.8-2.3
Protein, total (g/dL)	3.9-6.7	3.1 ± 1.5	3.1-4.6
Albumin (g/dL)	—	—	1.4-1.7
Globulin (g/dL)	—	—	2.1-2.9
A:G ratio	—	—	0.45-0.55
Sodium (mmol/L)	143-162	—	155-171
Uric acid (mg/dL)	8.1-16.8	6.0 ± 1.5	9-13.2

Measurement	Sharp-shinned Hawk (*Accipiter striatus*)[719]	Northern Goshawk (*Accipiter gentilis*)[160]	Turkey Vulture (*Cathartes aura*)[a,803]
Hematology			
PCV (%)	44-52	43–53	51-58 (54)

TABLE 5-24 Hematologic and Biochemical Values of Select Raptors. Accipitriformes (cont'd)

Measurement	Sharp-shinned Hawk *(Accipiter striatus)*	Northern Goshawk *(Accipiter gentilis)*	Turkey Vulture *(Cathartes aura)*
RBC (10^6/μL)	—	2.6–3.48	2.4-2.9 (2.7)
Hgb (g/dL)	—	12.1–17.7	15.7-17.3 (16.3)
MCV (fL)	—	141–156	194-224 (204)
MCH (pg)	—	—	58.6-65 (61.7)
MCHC (g/dL)	—	—	28.6-32 (30.2)
WBC (10^3/μL)	7.7-16.8	4–11	10.5-31.9 (20.1)
Heterophils 10^3/μL	—	3.5–6.97	—
(%)	(16-24)	—	(59-64)
Lymphocytes 10^3/μL	—	0.3–3.1	—
(%)	(54-75)	—	(8-18)
Monocytes 10^3/μL	—	0–0.1	—
(%)	(0-3)	—	(0-1)
Eosinophils 10^3/μL	—	0–0.65	—
(%)	(5-11)	—	(3-4)
Basophils 10^3/μL	—	0–0.35	—
(%)	(0-1)	—	(0)
H:L ratio	—	—	—
Chemistries			
ALP (U/L)	—	15.6–87.5	—
ALT (U/L)	—	0–44	—
AST (U/L)	—	176–409	—
Bile acid (μmol/L)			
RIA	—	—	—
Calcium (mg/dL)	—	8.6–10.7	—
Chloride (mmol/L)	—	—	—
Cholesterol (mg/dL)	—	154-444	—
CK (U/L)	—	218–775	—
GGT (U/L)	—	—	—
Glucose (mg/dL)	—	207–286	—
LDH (U/L)	—	—	—
Phosphorus (mg/dL)	—	2.4-13.7	—
Potassium (mmol/L)	—	—	—
Protein, total (g/dL)	2.4-3.2	2.63–4.2	—

Continued

TABLE 5-24 Hematologic and Biochemical Values of Select Raptors. Accipitriformes (cont'd)

Measurement	Sharp-shinned Hawk *(Accipiter striatus)*	Northern Goshawk *(Accipiter gentilis)*	Turkey Vulture *(Cathartes aura)*
Albumin (g/dL)	—	0.88-1.24	—
Globulin (g/dL)	—	1.8–2.92	—
A:G ratio	—	0.4-0.57	—
Sodium (mmol/L)	—	155–171	—
Uric acid (mg/dL)	—	—	—

Falconiformes

Measurement	American Kestrel (*Falco sparverius*)[250]	Gyrfalcon (*Falco rusticolus*)[803]	Peregrine Falcon (*Falco peregrinus*)[440,727,803]
Hematology			
PCV (%)	43 ± 3.2	49 ± 2	37-53
RBC (10^6/µL)	—	—	3-4
Hgb (g/dL)	—	—	118-188
MCV (fL)	14.5-57	—	118-176
MCH (pg)	11-33	—	40-48.4
MCHC (g/dL)	24-58	—	319-352
WBC (10^3/µL)	9.8 ± 4.9	4.6 ± 1.7	3.3-21 (13 ± 3)
Heterophils 10^3/µL	—	—	—
(%)	(47 ± 3	51 ± 5	65 ± 12
Lymphocytes 10^3/µL	—	—	—
(%)			
	(46 ± 3)	(45 ± 5)	35 ± 13
Monocytes 10^3/µL	—	—	—
(%)	(2 ± 0.2)	(1 ± 1)	(0)
Eosinophils 10^3/µL	—	—	—
(%)	(1 ± 0.2)	(1 ± 1)	(0)
Basophils 10^3/µL	—	—	—
(%)	(2 ± 0.2)	(Rare)	(0)
Chemistries			
ALP (U/L)	232 ± 72	257	97-350
ALT (U/L)	41 ± 33	—	19-54
AST (U/L)	77 ± 29	97	20-52

TABLE 5-24 Hematologic and Biochemical Values of Select Raptors. Accipitriformes (cont'd)

Measurement	American Kestrel (*Falco sparverius*)	Gyrfalcon (*Falco rusticolus*)	Peregrine Falcon (*Falco peregrinus*)
Bile acid (μmol/L)			
RIA	—	—	20-118
Calcium (mg/dL)	7.1 ± 0.8	9.6	8.4-10.2
Chloride (mmol/L)	108 ± 33	125	121-134
Cholesterol (mg/dL)	—	—	175-401
CK (U/L)	1739 ± 734	402	357-850
GGT (U/L)	—	—	0-7
Glucose (mg/dL)	305 ± 40	318	11-16
LDH (U/L)	—	—	625-1210
Phosphorus (mg/dL)	3 ± 0.9	—	3.4
Potassium (mmol/L)	2.2 ± 0.7	—	1.6-3.2
Protein, total (g/dL)	3.2 ± 0.5	2.89	2.5-4
Albumin (g/dL)	1 ± 0.2	—	0.8-1.3
Globulin (g/dL)	1.2 ± 0.4	—	1.6-2.8
A:G ratio	0.9 ± 0.4	—	0.4-0.6
Sodium (mmol/L)	158 ± 3	160	152-168
Uric acid (mg/dL)	9 ± 6	13.9	4.4-22

Strigiformes

Measurement	Barn Owl (*Tyto alba*)[c,19,20]	Barred Owl (*Strix varia*)[c,19,20]	Eastern Screech Owl (*Megascops asio*)[c,19,20]
Hematology			
PCV (%)	48 ± 4 (41-57)	44 ± 4 (38-52)	47 ± 3 (40-54)
RBC (10^6/μL)	2.4 ± 0.4 (1.6-3.3)	3.0 ± 0.9 (1.0-4.7)	3.4 ± 7 (1.7-4.8)
Hgb (g/dL)	—	—	—
MCV (fL)	202 ± 29 (135-270)	156 ± 38 (77-236)	145 ± 26 (89-200)
MCH (pg)	—	—	—
MCHC (g/dL)	—	—	—
WBC (10^3/μL) PBT	13.1 ± 5.9 (5.0-28.8)	18.9 ± 7.4 (2.6-33.7)	15.4 ± 6.3 (1.2-28.1)
NHT	8.3 ± 5.0 (2.5-22.1)	6.6 ± 2.9 (2.3-13.9)	8.4 ± 3.9 (3.1-19.8)
EST	12.4 ± 6.1 (3.8-28.6)	16.5 ± 3.6 (8.8-23.0)	15.2 ± 6.3 (1.8-28.5)
Heterophils 10^3/μL (%)	6.9 ± 2.8 (3.2-15.0) 56 ± 15 (26-85)	4.7 ± 1.8 (0.5-8.6) 28 ± 12.5 (10-52)	4.0 ± 1.6 (0.4-7.3) 27 ± 10 (6-47)
Lymphocytes 10^3/μL (%)	3.1 ± 2.1 (0.3-8.6) 23 ± 10 (2-41)	9.6 ± 5.5 (0.9-22.7) 48 ± 15 (18-80)	6.0 ± 3.6 (0.9-15.9) 38 ± 13 (12-65)

Continued

TABLE 5-24 Hematologic and Biochemical Values of Select Raptors. Accipitriformes (cont'd)

Measurement	Barn Owl (*Tyto alba*)	Barred Owl (*Strix varia*)	Eastern Screech Owl (*Megascops asio*)
Monocytes $10^3/\mu L$ (%)	1.0 (0.1-1.3) 7 ± 5 (0-17)	2.5 ± 1.8 (0.2-7.6) 12 ± 6 (3-29)	2.3 ± 1.1 (0.5-5.0) 15 ± 6 (3-27)
Eosinophils $10^3/\mu L$ (%)	1.6 ± 1.5 (0.2-7.4) 12 ± 7 (2-34)	2.1 ± 2.2 (0.4-4.3) 11 ± 4 (1-20)	2.8 ± 1.8 (0.4-7.9) 18 ± 8 (5-39)
Basophils $10^3/\mu L$ (%)	0.3 ± 0.3 (0.0-1.1) 2 ± 2 (2-34)	0.2 ± 0.2 (0.0-4.4) 1 ± 1 (1-3)	0.3 ± 0.4 (0.0-1.3) 2 ± 2 (0-6)
H:L ratio	38 ± 4.5 (0.8-22.2)	0.7 ± 0.7 (0.1-2.7)	0.9 ± 0.8 (0.8-15.8)
Fibrinogen (g/L)	—	—	—
Chemistries			
ALP (U/L)	—	—	—
ALT (U/L)	—	—	—
AST (U/L)	151 (93-263)*	88-358†	108-647‡
Bile acid (µmol/L)			
Colorimetric	17.0 (1.0-55.0)*	6.4-54‡	4-59‡
Calcium (mg/dL)	9.16 (4.80-18.8)*	7.44-12.24†	4.9-12.4†
Chloride (mmol/L)	115 (112-120)*	108-122‡	106-119†
Cholesterol (mg/dL)	262 (190-352)*	159-267†	168-336†
CK (U/L)	1243 (158-3415)*	22-3657‡	5-1174‡
GGT (U/L)	0 (0-388)*	0-2 ‡	0-10‡
Glucose (mg/dL)	245 (187-425)*	283-405†	283-455†
LDH (U/L)	173 (76-640)*	63-2103‡	62-2984‡
Phosphorus (mg/dL)	3.12 (1.85-4.39)*	2.78-8.02‡	1.2-8.5‡
Potassium (mmol/L)	4.1 (2.2-6.7)*	1.7-4.9†	1.2-6.2†
Protein, total (g/dL)	3.4 (2.4-4.6)*	2.9-5.0‡	2.5-4.3‡
Albumin (g/dL)	1.9 (1.3-2.3)*	1.2-1.8‡	1.3-2.6†
Globulin (g/dL)	1.5 (1.0-2.4)*	1.7-3.4‡	0.9-2.2†
A:G ratio	1.4 (0.7-1.6)*	0.5-0.8‡	0.6-1.9†
Sodium (mmol/L)	158 (153-166)*	154-169†	152-165†
Uric acid (mg/dL)	11.74 (5.49-18.06)*	1.29-18.05†	2.84-26.30‡

Measurement	Eurasian Eagle Owl (*Bubo bubo*)[c,19,20]	Great Gray Owl (*Strix nebulosa*)[c,19,20]	Great Horned Owl (*Bubo virginianus*)[c,19,20]
Hematology			
PCV (%)	50 ± 9 (NA)	50 ± 5 (39-61)	43 ± 4

TABLE 5-24 Hematologic and Biochemical Values of Select Raptors. Accipitriformes (cont'd)

Measurement	Eurasian Eagle Owl *(Bubo bubo)*	Great Gray Owl *(Strix nebulosa)*	Great Horned Owl *(Bubo virginianus)*
RBC (10^6/µL)	2.0 ± 0.3 (NA)	2.8 ± 0.3 (2.1-3.4)	2.6 ± 0.5
Hgb (g/dL)	—	—	—
MCV (fL)	—	181 ± 26 (127-236)	164 ± 28
MCH (pg)	—	—	—
MCHC (g/dL)	—	—	—
WBC (10^3/µL) PBT	20.9 ± 14.4 (6.6-64.7)	11.1 ± 6.0 (1.8-26)	18.3 ± 9.2 (4.2-42.4)
NHT	17.2 ± 11.6 (3.0-56.6)	4.8 ± 2.5 (1.7-11.4)	17.1 ± 9.6 (4.8-42.6)
EST	20.4 ± 12.6 (6.2-65.8)	13.0 ± 4.6 (2.7-21.7)	20.0 ± 6.2 (7.2-33.0)
Heterophils 10^3/µL (%)	10.9 ± 8.3 (2.3-48.9) 51 ± 12 (24-76)	3.6 ± 2.6 (1.0-12.2) 34 ± 12 (9-58)	9.9 ± 5.8 (2.0-25.5) 54 ± 12 (28-79)
Lymphocytes 10^3/µL (%)	4.0 ± 2.1 (1.5-12.0) 23 ± 11 (5-50)	4.3 ± 3.0 (0.4-12.3) 37 ± 15 (5-69)	3.4 ± 2.3 (0.4-9.7) 18 ± 8 (4-37)
Monocytes 10^3/µL (%)	1.7 ± 1.3 (0.3-5.6) 9 ± 4 (0-17)	1.6 ± 1.0 (0.2-4.7) 14 ± 4 (5-23)	2.1 ± 1.4 (0.2-6.7) 11 ± 4 (2-20)
Eosinophils 10^3/µL (%)	4.0 ± 5.9 (NA) 16 ± 10 (4-46)	1.4 ± 1.6 (0.7-11.9) 12 ± 8 (0-42)	2.6 ± 2.4 (0.4-8.2) 15 ± 8 (2-33)
Basophils 10^3/µL (%)	0.2 ± 0.3 (0.0-0.9) 1 ± 1 (NA)	0.2 ± 0.2 (0.0-0.9) 2 ± 2 (0-7)	0.3 ± 0.4 (0.2-2.9) 2 ± 2 (2-33)
H:L ratio	2.9 ± 1.9 (0.6-9.9)	1.3 ± 1.1 (0.2-5.8)	4.2 ± 4.2 (1.0-19.7)
Fibrinogen (g/L)	—	—	—
Chemistries			
ALP (U/L)	—	—	—
ALT (U/L)	—	—	—
AST (U/L)	—	125-467 ‡	55-277†
Bile acid (µmol/L)	—	—	
Colorometric	—	6-81‡	4.2-48.9‡
Calcium (mg/dL)	—	2.88-11.88†	6.4-12‡
Chloride (mmol/L)	—	107-121†	111-127†
Cholesterol (mg/dL)	—	139-285 †	117-281†
CK (U/L)	—	1-574‡	27-1544‡
GGT (U/L)	—	0-10‡	0-6 ‡
Glucose (mg/dL)	—	245-378†	292-448†
LDH (U/L)	—	65-353‡	106-747‡
Phosphorus (mg/dL)	—	0.50-8.18†	1.76-8.23‡
Potassium (mmol/L)	—	2.1-4.8†	2.3-5.7†

Continued

TABLE 5-24 Hematologic and Biochemical Values of Select Raptors. Accipitriformes (cont'd)

Measurement	Eurasian Eagle Owl (*Bubo bubo*)	Great Gray Owl (*Strix nebulosa*)	Great Horned Owl (*Bubo virginianus*)
Protein, total (g/dL)	—	2.7-4.1‡	3.0-5.1‡
Albumin (g/dL)	—	1.5-2.4†	1.2-1.8‡
Globulin (g/dL)	—	1.0-2.6‡	1.5-3.3‡
A:G ratio	—	0.6-1.9‡	0.4-1.0‡
Sodium (mmol/L)	—	152-168‡	151-172†
Uric acid (mg/dL)	—	3.33-21.37‡	3.09-17.80‡

Measurement	Northern Saw-whet Owl (*Aegolius acadicus*)[c,19,20]	Short-eared Owl (*Asio flammeus*)[c,19,20]	Snowy Owl (*Bubo scandiaca*)[c,19,20]
Hematology			
PCV (%)	48 ± 5 (NA)	48 ± 6 (NA)	49 ± 6 (NA)
RBC (10^6/μL)	2.8 ± 0.5 (NA)	2.6 ± 0.6 (NA)	3.3 ± 0.7 (NA)
Hgb (g/dL)	—	—	—
MCV (fL)	176 ± 29 (NA)	181 ± 29 (NA)	142 ± 23 (NA)
MCH (pg)	—	—	—
MCHC (g/dL)	—	—	—
WBC (10^3/μL) PBT	6.3 ± 3.1 (NA)	11.0 ± 7.3 (NA)	9.6 ± 5.4 (NA)
NHT	5.7 ± 2.5 (NA)	6.0 ± 3.6 (NA)	6.7 ± 6.5 (NA)
EST	11.6 ± 3.6 (NA)	12.4 ± 5.5 (NA)	10.2 ± 5.7 (NA)
Heterophils 10^3/μL (%)	1.8 ± 0.8 (NA) 29 ± 10 (NA)	3.5 ± 2.9 (NA) 30 ± 14 (NA)	4.5 ± 3.4 (NA) 46 ± 19 (NA)
Lymphocytes 10^3/μL (%)	2.4 ± 1.9 (NA) 35 ± 15 (NA)	5.0 ± 3.4 (NA) 47 ± 15 (NA)	3.3 ± 2.8 (NA) 34 ± 17 (NA)
Monocytes 10^3/μL (%)	0.8 ± 0.4 (NA) 13 ± 3 (NA)	1.1 ± 1.1 (NA) 9 ± 5 (NA)	0.9 ± 0.4 (NA) 11 ± 5 (NA)
Eosinophils 10^3/μL (%)	± 0.7 (NA) 22 ± 10 (NA)	1.2 ± 0.8 (NA) 13 ± 8 (NA)	0.8 ± 1.0 (NA) 8 ± 5 (NA)
Basophils 10^3/μL (%)	± 0.1 1 ± 2	0.2 ± 0.3 (NA) 2 ± 2 (NA)	0.0 ± 0.1 (NA) 1 ± 2 (NA)
H:L ratio	1.2 ± 1.2	0.9 ± 1.0 (NA)	2.6 ± 3.6 (NA)
Fibrinogen (g/L)	—	—	—
Chemistries			
ALP (U/L)	—	—	—
ALT (U/L)	—	—	—
AST (U/L)	248 (127-411)*	213 (121-431)*	215 (171-301)*

TABLE 5-24 Hematologic and Biochemical Values of Select Raptors. Accipitriformes (cont'd)

Measurement	Northern Saw-whet Owl *(Aegolius acadicus)*	Short-eared Owl *(Asio flammeus)*	Snowy Owl *(Bubo scandiaca)*
Bile acid (µmol/L)			
Colorometric	50 (21-61)*	19 (4-94)*	27 (8-78)*
Calcium (mg/dL)	9.4 (5.6-10.4)*	6.72 (3.6-9.6)*	8.84 (7.32-11.12)*
Chloride (mmol/L)	113 (92-114)*	114 (104-122)*	113 (109-121)*
Cholesterol (mg/dL)	308 (194-492)*	206 (174-279)*	2612 (152-840)*
CK (U/L)	377(19-4299) *	29 (0-265)*	203 (20-3338)*
GGT (U/L)	0 (0-4)*	0 (0-3)*	0 (0-5)*
Glucose (mg/dL)	319 (272-347)*	319 (261-360)*	338 (218-468)*
LDH (U/L)	140 (6-308)*	180 (92-530)*	209 (132-861)*
Phosphorus (mg/dL)	3.96 (2.79-5.26)*	2.60 (0.93-7.12)*	5.51 (1.64-7.77)*
Potassium (mmol/L)	3.0 (2.6-3.6)*	3.7 (2.9-5.3)*	3.8 (1.5-5.5)*
Protein, total (g/dL)	3.0 (2.7-3.7)*	2.7 (2.1-3.3)*	3.6 (2.6-4.7)*
Albumin (g/dL)	2.1 (1.9-2.7)*	1.4 (1.0-1.7)*	1.4 (0.8-1.9)*
Globulin (g/dL)	0.9 (0.4-1.5)*	1.3 (1.0-1.6)*	1.8 (1.3-3.4)*
A:G ratio	2.3 (1.3-6.5)*	1.1 (0.8-1.4)*	0.8 (0.4-1.3)*
Sodium (mmol/L)	153 (129-155)*	157 (151-161)*	158 (156-170)*
Uric acid (mg/dL)	9 (2.63-12.6)*	7.09 (2.56-25.28)*	11.42 (5.51-22.33)*

[a]Numbers in parentheses represent the mean.
[b]WBC count and differentials for Harris's hawk are absolute values.
[c]Hematology: mean and SD (reference interval); reference intervals were calculated by the robust method or robust method after Box-Cox transformation; NA, insufficient sample size for reference interval calculation (n <20).
Biochemistry: *median (range) (10 < n < 20); reference intervals were not reported when n < 10; †robust technique (n > 20, Gaussian distribution); ‡robust technique with Box-Cox transformation (n > 20, non-Gaussian distribution).

TABLE 5-25 Biologic and Physiologic Values of Select Avian Species.[a,13,33,169,170,228,230,257,310,385,386,445,489,634,776,860,905,974]

Species	Incubation Period (days)[b]	Fledgling Age (days)	Weaning Age (days)		Sexual Maturity	Lifespan in Captivity (Maximum) (yr)	Body Weight (g)[c]
			Parent Raised	Hand Reared			
Psittaciformes							
African grey parrot	26-28[d]	50-65	100-120	75-90	4-6 yr	50-60	454 (370-534)
Amazon parrot	24-29[e]	45-60	90-120	75-90	4-6 yr	>50 (80)	[f]
Budgerigar parakeet	16-18	22-26	30-40	30	6-9 mo	5-10 (18)	30
Cockatiel	18-20	32-38	47-52	42-49	6-12 mo	10-12 (30)	80-90
Cockatoo, galah	22-24	45-55	90-120	80-90	1 yr	40-60	[g]
Cockatoo, large	[h]	60-80	120-150	95-120	5-6 yr	50-60	[g]
Cockatoo, medium	[h]	45-60	90-120	75-100	3-4 yr	40-60	[g]
Conure	[i]	35-40	45-70	60	2-3 yr	25-40	80-100[j]
Eclectus parrot	26-28	72-80	120-150	100-110	4 yr	20-40 (80)	432 (347-512)
Lory/lorikeet	21-27	42-50	62-70	50-60	2 yr	20-30	—
Lovebirds	18-24	30-35	45-55	40-45	6-12 mo	15-30	42-48
Macaw, large	26-28	70-80	120-150	95-120	5-7 yr	75-100	[k]
Macaw, small	23-26	45-60	90-120	75-90	4-6 yr	50-80	[k]
Ring-necked parakeet, Indian	22-23	40-45	55-65	—	3 yr	18-25	115
Passeriformes							
Canary	12-14	14	21	—	<1 yr	6-12	12-30
Mynah	14-15	30	60	—	2-3 yr	12	180-260
Zebra or society finch	12-16	18-20	25-28	—	9-10 mo	4-7	10-16

TABLE 5-25 Biologic and Physiologic Values of Select Avian Species. (cont'd)

Species	Incubation Period (days)[b]	Fledgling Age (days)	Weaning Age (days)		Sexual Maturity	Lifespan in Captivity (Maximum) (yr)	Body Weight (g)[c]
			Parent Raised	Hand Reared			
Columbiformes							
Dove, common ground	12- >14	18	—	—	1 yr	4-8	30
Dove, mourning	13-14	12-14	—	—	—	—	120
Pigeon (rock dove)	16-19	28-35	35	—	1 yr	4-8 (>20)	240-300
Ratites							
Emu	50-57	—	Precocial	—	3-5 yr	30	40-45 kg
Ostrich	41-43	—	Precocial	—	4 yr	80	120-160 kg
Rhea	36-41	—	Precocial	—	1.5-2 yr	—	25 kg

[a]Guidelines only; data vary between references. For raptors, see Table 5-26.

[b]Brotogeris parakeets, 22; Pionus parrot, 25-26; Psittacula parakeets, 23-26; Quaker parakeet, 23; Senegal parrot, 24-25.

[c]Bourke's parakeet, 40 (35-50); kakariki parakeet, 95-100; Princess of Wales parakeet, 108 (100-129); red-rumped parakeet, 65 (60-69).

[d]Congo, 28; Timneh, 26.

[e]Green-cheeked, blue-fronted, 26; spectacled (white-fronted), 24; yellow-naped, yellow-fronted, yellow-crowned, double yellow-headed, 28-29.

[f]Blue-crowned, 740 (618-998); blue-fronted, 432 (361-485); double yellow-headed, 568 (463-694); Mexican red-headed, 360 (343-377); yellow-naped, 596 (476-795).

[g]Bare-eyed, 331; greater sulphur-crested, 806; Leadbeater's (Major Mitchell's), 423 (381-474); lesser sulphur-crested, 303; Moluccan, 808; rose-breasted, 299; triton, 559; umbrella, 552.

[h]Bare-eyed, 23-24; citron-crested, 25-26; greater sulphur-crested, 27-28; Leadbeater's (Major Mitchell's), 26; lesser sulphur-crested, 24-25; Moluccan, 28-29; palm, 28-30; triton, 27-28; umbrella, 28.

[i]Blue-crowned, 23-24; orange-fronted, 30; nanday, 21-23; Patagonian, 24-25; sun, 27-28.

[j]Queen of Bavaria, 262 (252-276).

[k]Blue and gold, 1021; green-winged, 1179; hyacinth, 1355 (1197-1466); military, 788; red-fronted, 458; scarlet, 1103.

TABLE 5-26 Biologic and Physiologic Values of Select Raptors.[88,158,257,307,375,803,860]

Species	Clutch Size	Incubation Period (days)	Interval Between Eggs (days)	Start of Incubation	Fledging (days)	Sexual Maturity (yr)	Longevity (yr)	Body Weight	
								Male	Female
American kestrel	3-7	29-31	—	—	30-31	—	2-7	103-120 g	126-166 g
Bald eagle	1-3	34-36	—	—	70-98	—	—	4.1 kg	5.8 kg
Barn owl	2-9	30-31	2-3	First egg	70-75	7	—	441-470 g	490-570 g
Barred owl	2-4	28-33	—	—	6	—	—	630 g	800 g
Black vulture	1-3	37-48	—	—	80-94	—	—	[a]	[a]
Common kestrel	3-6	27-29	1-2	Second to third egg	—	7	—	136-252 g	154-314 g
Cooper's hawk	3-6	32-36	—	—	27-34	—	—	220-410 g	330-680 g
Eurasian buzzard	2-4	36-38	4	First to second egg	—	2-3	—	0.55-0.85 kg	0.7-1.2 kg
Eurasian eagle owl	2-4	34-36	2-3	First to second egg	6	2-3	50-60	1.5-2.8 kg	1.8-4.2 kg
Golden eagle	1-3	43-45	—	—	6	>5	50-60	2.5-4 kg	3.25-6.35 kg
Gyrfalcon	3-5	34-36	—	—	49-56	—	—	0.96-1.3 kg	1.3-2.1 kg
Harris's hawk	2-5	3	2-3	Penultimate or last egg	43-49	>3	20-30	0.7 kg	1 kg
Merlin	2-7	28-32	—	—	30-35	7	10-14	150-210 g	189-255 g
Northern goshawk	3-5	35-38	2-3	First to second egg	35-42	>3	15-20	0.5-1.2 kg	0.8-1.5 kg
Northern sparrow hawk	4-6	3	2-3	Third to fourth egg	—	1-2	—	—	—
Osprey	2-4	32-43	—	—	48-59	—	—	[b]	[b]
Peregrine falcon	3-4	29-32	2-3	Penultimate or last egg	35-42	>3	15-20	440-750 g	910-1500 g

TABLE 5-26 Biologic and Physiologic Values of Select Raptors. (cont'd)

Species	Clutch Size	Incubation Period (days)	Interval Between Eggs (days)	Start of Incubation	Fledging (days)	Sexual Maturity (yr)	Longevity (yr)	Body Weight	
								Male	Female
Prairie falcon	2-7	29-33	—	—	35-42	—	—	500-650 g	700-975 g
Screech owl, eastern	3-4	—	—	—	—	—	—	158-184 g	180-220 g
Screech owl, western	2-6	21-30	—	—	6	—	—	131-210 g	157-250 g
Sharp-shinned hawk	3-8	32-35	—	—	24-27	—	—	82-125 g	144-208 g
Snowy owl	3-9	30-33	2-3	First egg	6	7	—	1.6 kg	1.1-2 kg
Turkey vulture	1-3	38-41	—	—	66-88	—	—	[c]	[c]

[a]1.7-2.3 kg; weights of males and females were not listed separately.

[b]1-2.1 kg; weights of males and females were not listed separately, but females are generally 25% heavier than males.

[c]0.8-2.3 kg; weights of males and females were not listed separately, but females are slightly heavier than males.

TABLE 5-27 Quick Reference to Abnormalities of the Standard Avian Hematology Profile.[319]

Parameter	Increases	Decreases
PCV/RBC	Dehydration • Increased total protein Erythrocytosis (polycythemia) • Normal or low total protein • Primary rare • Secondary to respiratory or cardiovascular disease	Regenerative anemia • Polychromasia (10%), reticulocytes, immature RBC • Hemorrhagic: trauma, parasites, coagulopathies, ulcerated neoplasms, gastrointestinal ulcers • Hemolytic: septicemia, hemoparasites, toxicities, immune mediated • Presence of Heinz bodies, agglutination of RBC Nonregenerative anemia • Hypoplastic: inflammatory, infectious, myelosuppresive drugs, iron deficiency, food restriction, folic acid deficiency
Heterophils	Inflammatory processes • Bacterial (including *Mycobacterium*) and fungal infections • Excess corticosteroids ○ Endogenous production ○ Exogenous administration Birds with a high heterophil:lymphocyte ratio may mount a greater leukocytic response	Infection • Bacterial and viral (i.e., PBFD) Poor sample preparation, collection, and storage
Lymphocytes	Chronic antigenic stimulation Neoplasia: lymphocytic leukemia Stress response (acute)	Stress response (chronic) Immunosuppresive drugs Viral infection Endotoxemia/septicemia
Monocytes	Granulomatous and/or chronic inflammation (e.g., bacterial, fungal, parasitic) Neoplasia	—
Eosinophils	Gastrointestinal parasitism Type IV hypersensitivity reactions	Corticosteroids Stress response (chronic)
Basophils	Early inflammatory responses Type I hypersensitivity reaction Anaphylactic reaction Induced molting	—
Thrombocytes	—	Vitamin K deficiency Rodenticide toxicity Aflatoxicosis Septicemia-associated DIC (as with polyomavirus and reovirus) Hepatic disease or failure

TABLE 5-28 Quick Reference to Abnormalities of the Standard Avian Biochemical Profile.[a,320]

Parameter	Increases: Nonmedical	Increases: Medical	Decreases: Nonmedical	Decreases: Medical
ALP (U/L)	Juveniles have higher levels	Hyperparathyroidism-induced osteoclastic activity (fractures); egg laying; hepatic disease; enteritis; aflatoxicosis	—	Dietary zinc deficiency
ALT (U/L)	Seasonal variation in raptors; sample hemolysis	—	Seasonal variation in raptors	—
Amylase (U/L)	—	Pancreatitis; gastrointestinal disease; zinc toxicity	—	—
AST (U/L)	Rare; severe lipemia; 300-1000	Liver, muscle, or heart damage; vitamin E/ selenium, methionine deficiency; 300-15,000	—	<50; end-stage liver disease
Blood urea nitrogen (mg/dL)	—	Dehydration; postprandial in high protein diet	—	—
Bile acids (μmol/L)	Lipemia; sample hemolysis, such samples should not be analyzed	Loss of liver function, even with normal enzymes	Lipemic samples that are chemically treated	Response to therapy; liver cirrhosis; microhepatica
Calcium (mg/dL)	Lipemia (or cloudy from other causes); protein elevations; bacterial contamination	Hormonal disorders; egg production; metabolic disease; excess dietary vitamin D; dehydration; osteolytic neoplasia	EDTA; bacterial contamination; young birds have lower levels	<8; metabolic (e.g., renal disease, hypoparathyoidism) and nutritional disorders (hypovitaminosis D and hypomagnesemia); lead poisoning; glucocorticoid administration; low albumin
Cholesterol (mg/dL)	Postprandial;[530] high-fat diet; carnivorous diet; reproductive upregulation females	Metabolic disease; hepatic lipidosis; bile duct obstruction; hypothyroidism; starvation	—	Liver, metabolic disease, maldigestion and malabsorption, starvation
CK (U/L)	>300; healthy birds up to 1000	600-25,000; muscle or heart damage; CNS disease (seizures); vitamin E/selenium deficiency; chlamydiosis; lead toxicity; IM injections	<10; bacterial contamination	Rare
Creatinine (mg/dL)	—	Not useful in birds	—	Not useful in birds

Continued

TABLE 5-28 Quick Reference to Abnormalities of the Standard Avian Biochemical Profile. (cont'd)

Parameter	Increases		Decreases	
	Nonmedical	Medical	Nonmedical	Medical
GGT (U/L)	—	Biliary epithelial and cholestatic disease; low sensitivity but highly specific for liver disease	—	—
GLDH (U/L)	—	Hepatocellular necrosis; low sensitivity for liver disease but highly specific	—	—
Glucose (mg/dL)	Improper dilution; postprandial; posthandling	Stress, 400-600; diabetes, 800-1500; corticosteroids	<100; unseparated blood; bacterial contamination	<100; hepatic dysfunction; septicemia; neoplasia; aspergillosis
LDH (U/L)	Sample hemolysis	300-15,000; liver, heart, or muscle damage; hepatitis; muscle damage	<50	End-stage liver disease
Lipase (U/L)	—	Acute pancreatitis	—	—
Phosphorus (mg/dL)	Postprandial; sample hemolysis	Severe renal disease; nutritional secondary hyperparathyroidism; hypoparathyroidism	EDTA	Hypovitaminosis D; malabsorption; chronic glucocorticoid therapy
Potassium (mmol/L)	Hemolysis; dietary supplementation	Adrenal disease; metabolic disease; severe tissue damage; renal disease; acidosis; dehydration; hemolytic anemia	—	Adrenal disease; metabolic disease; diuretic therapy; alkalosis; overhydration; dietary deficiency
Protein, total (g/dL)	Lipemia; nontemperature-compensated refractometer	Inflammation; dehydration; chronic infection; gamma globulinopathy; lymphoproliferative disease; myelosis	Nontemperature-compensated refractometer	Chronic hepatopathy; malabsorption; renal disease; blood loss; neoplasia; starvation/malnutrition
Sodium (mmol/L)	Dietary supplementation	Dehydration; salt poisoning	—	Renal disease; overhydration
Sorbitol dehydrogenase (U/L)	—	Hepatitis	—	—
Uric acid (mg/dL)	5-15; severe lipemia; dirty nail clip; carnivorous birds have higher levels	Renal disease; gout; dehydration; postprandial; ovulation; tissue damage; starvation; hypervitaminosis D	Overhydration of patient; juvenile levels are lower	End-stage liver disease

[a]The ranges given are not absolute and are to be used as a guide for interpretation of a wide range of avian species.

TABLE 5-29 Blood Gases of Select Avian Species.[a]

Parameter	*Amazona aestiva*[b] (n = 35)[680]	*Falco rusticolus*[c] (n = 30)[731]	*Psittacus* spp.[d] (*n* = 46)[613]
$pH_{37°C}$	7.45 ± 0.05	7.49 ± 0.08	7.32 ± 0.08
PCO_2 (mmHg)	22.1 ± 4	35.5 ± 6.1	29.3 ± 6.1
PO_2 (mmHg)	98.1 ± 7.6	111.8 ± 20.5	37.9 ± 3.8
HCO_3 (mmol/L)	14.8 ± 2.8	22.5 ± 4.0	15 ± 2.4
TCO_2 (mmol/L)	—	23.3 ± 4.0	16.0 ± 2.7
BEecf (mmol/L)	7.9 ± 3.1	0.9 ± 4.9	17-0
Na (mmol/L)	147 ± 2.2	148 ± 1.8	141-159
K (mmol/L)	3.5 ± 0.5	3.3 ± 0.3	3.6 ± 0.5
iCa (mmol/L)	0.8 ± 0.3	1.0 ± 0.1	1.1 ± 0.1
SO_2 (%)	96.2 ± 1.1	98.6 ± 1.0	68.4 ± 10.1
Hct (%)	38.7 ± 6.2	42.1 ± 4.0	—
Hgb (g/dL)	13.2 ± 2.1	14.3 ± 1.4	—
Glu (mg/dL)	—	317 ± 17	247 ± 25
Temperature (°C)	41.8 ± 0.6	41.2 ± 0.5	41.6 ± 0.4
$pH_{Temp°C}$	—	7.4 ± 0.1	7.3 ± 0.1
PCO_2 (mmHg) $_{Temp°C}$	—	35.5 ± 6.1	35.7 ± 7.5
PO_2 (mmHg) $_{Temp°C}$	—	140 ± 21.1	52.5 ± 5.6

[a]*PCO_2*, Partial pressure carbon dioxide; *PO_2*, partial pressure of oxygen; *HCO_3*, bicarbonate concentration; *TCO_2*, total carbon dioxide concentration; *SO_2*, hemoglobin saturated with oxygen.
[b]i-STAT EC7+ cartridges. Mean and SD. Arterial sample under manual restraint.
[c]i-STAT CG8+ cartridges. Mean and SD. Venous sample under isoflurane anesthesia with O_2.
[d]i-STAT EC8+ and CG8+ cartridges. Mean and SD or range. Venous sample under manual restraint.

TABLE 5-30 Lipoprotein Panel of Select Avian Species.

Parameter[a]	*Amazona* spp.[b] (*n* = 29)[743]	African Grey Parrot (*n* = 20)[890]	*Pionus* Parrot (*n* = 29)[890]
Cholesterol (mg/dL)	238 (87-364)	222-297	100-116
Triglycerides (mg/dL)	156 (10-300)	104-190	270-301
HDL (mg/dL)	109 (75-148)	161-176	172-177
LDL (mg/dL)	92 (2-182)	24-100	75-103
VLDL (mg/dL)	31 (2-60)	—	—
LDL:HDL (mg/dL)	0.75 (0.18-1.28)	—	—
Non-HDL-LDL (mg/dL)	1.08 (0.24-1.82)	—	—

[a]*HDL*, High-density lipoprotein; *LDL*, low-density lipoprotein; *VLDL*, very low-density lipoprotein.
[b]Mean and 90% confidence intervals.

TABLE 5-31 Protein Electrophoresis of Select Avian Species.[a,187]

Species	African Grey (*Psittacus erithacus*) (n=139)	Amazon (*Amazona* spp.) (n=58)	Cockatiel (*Nymphicus hollandicus*) (n=62)	Cockatoo (*Cacatua* spp.) (n=83)	Conure (*Aratinga* spp. and *Nandayus nenday*) (n=50)	Eclectus (*Eclectus* spp.) (n=50)	Macaw (*Ara* spp.) (n=80)
Total protein (g/dL)	3.0–4.6	3.0–5.0	2.4–4.2	3.0–5.0	3.0–4.4	2.8–4.6	2.2–4.6
Prealbumin g/dL (%)	0–1.25 (0–13)	0.3–1.15 (11–31)	0.85–1.65 (24–34)	0.21–1.25 (12–28)	0.18–0.95 (14–34)	0.38–0.74 (21–33)	0.25–0.85 (6–24)
Albumin, g/dL (%)	1.48–3.19 (50–69)	1.85–3.24 (37–57)	0.75–1.85 (31–40)	1.75–2.95 (38–56)	1.85–2.68 (32–57)	1.95–2.45 (38–48)	1.25–3.08 (39–59)
α-1-globulins, g/dL (%)	0.03–0.19 (2–7)	0.05–0.32 (2–5)	0.05–0.24 (2–4)	0.05–0.17 (2–5)	0.04–0.21 (2–5)	0.05–0.19 (2–4)	0.04–0.25 (2–4)
α-2-globulins, g/dL (%)	0.05–0.21 (3–7)	0.07–0.32 (3–9)	0.05–0.22 (2–6)	0.05–0.32 (2–7)	0.07–0.25 (2–9)	0.11–0.21 (2–5)	0.04–0.31 (2–7)
β-globulins, g/dL (%)	0.35–0.64 (15–25)	0.38–0.75 (9–21)	0.31–0.68 (12–24)	0.34–0.75 (12–24)	0.38–0.69 (8–17)	0.35–0.65 (11–21)	0.38–0.54 (11–21)
γ-globulins, g/dL (%)	0.12–0.68 (4–13)	0.17–0.60 (4–13)	0.15–0.53 (3–14)	0.21–0.64 (4–14)	0.32–0.62 (4–14)	0.22–0.65 (4–12)	0.21–0.55 (5–15)
A/G ratio[b]	1.3–2.7	1.4–3.2	1.5–2.9	1.3–3.6	1.5–3.1	1.6–3.2	1.2–2.6
A/G ratio[c]	0.6–1.6	1.1–2.1	0.7–1.5	0.8–2.0	0.8–2.2	1.1–1.8	0.8–2.0

[a]95% reference intervals.

[b]A/G ratio calculated as (prealbumin + albumin) ÷ (the sum of all globulins).

[c]A/G ratio calculated as albumin ÷ (the sum of all globulins); prealbumin was not included.

TABLE 5-32 T_4 Values of Select Avian Species.[a,186,547,554,1003]

Species	Baseline T_4 (nmol/L)[b]	Post-TSH (nmol/L)[c,d]
African grey parrot	3.83-27.03[186,445]	—
	1.83 ± 0.57[547]	11.97 ± 3.73[547]
	≤1.93[1013]	23.04 ± 13.26[1013]
Amazon parrot	1.29-14.16[186]	—
	10.54 ± 8.88[547]	35.26 ± 20.5[547]
	5.53 ± 0.36 (red-lored)[1009]	78.64 ± 44.79[1013]
	≤1.93 (blue-fronted)[1009]	98.33 ± 26.38[1013]
Budgerigar	6.44-27.03[186]	—
Canary	9.01-41.18[186]	—
Cockatiel	9.01-30.89[186]	—
	15.24 ± 8.7[547]	50.19 ± 7.28[547]
Cockatoo	17.54 ± 8.4[547]	45.17 ± 16.94[547]
Conure	6.44-25.74[186]	—
	2.27 ± 0.99[547]	17.37 ± 9.92[547]
Eclectus parrot	3.86-25.74[186]	—
Jardine's parrot	2.57-19.31[186]	—
Lory	3.86-15.44[186]	—
Lovebird	2.57-55.34[186,445]	—
Macaw, blue and gold	4.39 ± 2.29[547]	15.91 ± 8.16[547]
Macaw, scarlet	1.72 ± 0.66[547]	8.31 ± 3.99[547]
Pigeon	6.05-35.01[186,445,554]	—
Pionus parrot	6.44-24.45[186]	—
Quaker parrot	5.15-27.03[186]	—
Senegal parrot	6.44-29.6[186]	—

[a]0.5µg/dL = 6.5 nmol/L = 5 ng/mL.[351] To convert thyroxine from µg/dL to nmol/L, multiply by 12.87.[554]

[b]T_4 levels will vary with the time of day and year, with higher levels measured in the winter. Physiologic states such as molting or reproductive activity may also alter the ratio of T_4 to T_3 released. The half-life of thyroid hormones is much shorter in birds than in mammals; therefore, it is difficult to accurately measure single hormone levels.[602]

[c]The canine radioimmunoassay (RIA) kit does not accurately measure total T_4 below 6.5 nmol/L.[351] Results of high-sensitivity total T_4 testing in parrots ranged from 2 to 6 nmol/L. This high sensitivity test is available through the University of Tennessee Clinical Endocrinology Laboratory (865-974-5638).[352]

[d]Low-dose TSH (0.2 U/kg).

TABLE 5-33 Approximate Resting Respiratory Rates of Select Avian Species and by Weight.[178,307,792]

Species	Respiratory Rate (breaths/min)[a]
Amazon parrot	15-45
Budgerigar	60-75
Canary	60-80
Cockatiel	40-50
Cockatoo	15-40
Conure, large	30-45
Conure, small	40-50
Finch	90-110
Lovebird	50-60
Macaw	20-25
Raptor	10-20
Toucan	15-45
Weight (g)	**Respiratory Rate (breaths/min)a**
100	40-52
200	35-50
300	30-45
400	25-30
500	20-30
1000	15-20

[a]Restraint can increase respiratory rate 1.5-2 × the resting rate.

TABLE 5-34 Urinalysis Values Reported in Birds.[118,701]

Parameter	Reference Range	Pigeon[a,365]	Falcon[933]	Ostrich[631]
Specific gravity (g/mL)	1.005-1.020	—	—	—
pH	6.4-8 Laying hens and carnivorous birds may have more acidic urine; cloacal contents may alter urine pH	5.5-6.9	5-7	7.6 ± 1.5
Protein (g/dL)	Negative to trace	0.11-1.99	0.3 ± 0.2	2.6 ± 1.5
Glucose (mg/dL)	Negative to trace	—	24.3 ± 39.6	Negative
Ketones	Negative; ketonuria is sometimes present in migratory birds	—	Negative	Negative
Bilirubin	Negative	—	—	Negative
Urobilinogen	Negative	—	—	Negative

[a]95% confidence interval.

TABLE 5-35 Values Reported for Select Ophthalmic Diagnostic Tests in Avian Species.[a,b,81,443,506,508,612,762,898,900,992]

Species	Tear Production		Intraocular Pressure (mmHg)	
	Phenol Red Thread Test (mm/15 sec)	Schirmer Tear Test (mm/min)	Applanation Tonometry	Rebound Tonometry
Psittacine birds				
Amazon parrots, blue-fronted	21.9 ± 2.3[c]	—	8.3 ± 1.1[c]	—
Amazon parrots, Hispaniolan	12.5 ± 5.0	7.9 ± 2.6	—	—
Amazon parrots, orange-winged	12.6 ± 2.6[c]	—	9.7 ± 1.7[c]	—
Raptors				
Bald eagle	—	14 ± 2	21.5 ± 1.7	—
Barn owl	19.5 ± 7.2	3.6 ± 2.2	18.0 ± 6.6	11.5 ± 4.7
Common buzzard	16.0 ± 7.7	13.7 ± 4.4	19.4 ± 3.9	29.9 ± 6.1
Cooper's hawk	—	—	16.0 ± 1.8	10.7 ± 1.4
Eastern screech owl	—	—	9.3 ± 2.6	6.3 ± 1.3
Eurasian eagle owl	—	—	9.3 ± 1.8	10.5 ± 1.6
Eurasian scops owl	11.8 ± 5	1.0 ± 0.5	14.5 ± 3.9	—
Golden eagle	—	—	21.5 ± 3	—
Great horned owl	—	—	9.9 ± 2.4	9.9 ± 2.4
Kestrel, American	—	—	8.5 ± 4.4	6.8 ± 1.7
Kestrel, common	29.6 ± 4.7	5.8 ± 4	11.9 ± 3.3	11.6 ± 2.7
Northern goshawk	—	—	—	21.2 ± 2.4
Peregrine falcon	—	—	—	15.3 ± 6.1
Red-tailed hawk	—	—	20.3 ± 2.8	19.8 ± 4.9
Snowy owl	—	9.8 ± 2.4	—	9.1 ± 1.9
Swainson's hawk	—	—	20.8 ± 2.3	—
Tawny owl	—	4.3	9.4 ± 1.8	11.1 ± 3.1
Turkey vulture	—	—	15.0 ± 2.1	11.7 ± 1.0

[a]Mean ± SD values reported.

[b]For ultrasonographic ocular measurements, see references.

[c]Median ± S-IQR.

TABLE 5-36 Bone Marrow Differential Cell Counts of 17 Captive, Clinically Healthy Hispaniolan Amazon Parrots in the USA.[843]

Lineage	Cell Type	Mean ± SD (%)	Median (%)	Minimum-Maximum (%)
Erythroid	Rubriblast	± 0.6	2.0	1.0–3.4
	Prorubricyte	5.1 ± 1.0	5.0	2.8–6.8
	Basophilic rubricyte	6.1 ± 1.9	6.6	4.0–11.2
	Early polychromatophilic rubricyte	20.3 ± 6.3	19.7	12.5–31.4
	Late polychromatophilic rubricyte	23.3 ± 5.4	23.0	15.6–33.0
	Polychromatophilic erythrocyte	11.5 ± 5.1	11.6	1.2–18.8
	Total erythroid	**68.9 ± 8.6**	—	—
Granulocytic	Myeloblast	0.8 ± 0.6	0.6	0.2–2.7
	Progranulocyte	2.6 ± 1.7	2.2	0.6–5.4
	Myelocyte			
	Heterophil	2.6 ± 2.0	2.0	0.5–7.9
	Eosinophil	0.3 ± 0.1	0.0	0.0–0.5
	Basophil	0.4 ± 0.1	0.0	0.0–0.6
	Metamyelocyte			
	Heterophil	3.2 ± 2.1	2.7	0.8–7.8
	Eosinophil	Rare[a]	Rare	Rare
	Basophil	Rare	Rare	Rare
	Band			
	Heterophil	6.5 ± 3.4	5.9	2.2–12.0
	Eosinophil	Rare	Rare	Rare
	Basophil	Rare	Rare	Rare
	Mature granulocyte			
	Heterophil	11.9 ± 5.2	10.8	2.4–18.6
	Eosinophil	0.5 ± 0.3	0.4	0.0–1.0
	Basophil	Rare	Rare	Rare
	Total granulocytic	**28.1 ± 3.8**	—	—
Other	Monocyte/macrophage	0.3 ± 0.2	0.2	0–0.8
	Lymphocyte	1.1 ± 0.7	1	0.2–3.0
	Plasma cell	0.5 ± 0.3	0	0–0.6
	Osteoclast	Rare	Rare	Rare

[a]Rare indicates <0.1%.

TABLE 5-37 Checklist of Supportive Care Procedures Used in Companion Birds.[112]

Supportive care is an essential component of companion bird medicine.

1. Minimize handling and other stressors
2. House the bird in a warm, quiet, well-ventilated environment
   - Ensure minimal to no disturbance
   - Debilitated birds are often fluffed and ruffled and require supplemental heat 86°F (30°C)
3. Fluid therapy (see Table 5-38 and Table 5-39)
4. Provide pain management when indicated (see Table 5-5 and Table 5-6)
5. Supplement vitamins as needed
   - Vitamin A, vitamin E/selenium
   - Vitamin B complex in selected cases of injury, anorexia, cachexia, CNS disorders, or blood loss
6. Antibiotics (see Table 5-1)
   - To control primary infections and for injured or debilitated birds where secondary infections may result
7. Iron dextran
   - Iron deficiency or following hemorrhage
8. Normal photoperiod (or subdued lighting, if needed)
9. Oxygen
   - Dyspnea, hypoxia, or severe pneumonia and air sacculitis
10. Maintain body weight
    - Weigh once or twice daily if possible
    - Offer favorite foods and avoid changing diet while ill
11. Gavage or tube feeding[a]
    - Malnourishment, anorexia, cachexia, and dehydration
    - High carbohydrate formula is initially recommended
    - High-protein/high-calorie formulas may be used to increase body weight during recovery

[a]Crop volume may be estimated as 5% BW or 50 mL/kg.

TABLE 5-38 Fluid Therapy Recommendations for Birds.

When evaluating a patient for fluid therapy, the following factors should ideally be considered: hydration status, electrolyte balance, acid-base status, hematologic and biochemical values, and caloric balance.

- Warm fluids to 100-102°F (38-39°C) to help prevent or correct hypothermia
- Use caution when giving dextrose parenterally; 5% dextrose is a good choice for simple dehydration; however, it can exacerbate problems significantly if used concurrent to significant electrolyte loss[581,894]
- When given orally, dextrose is rapidly absorbed from the intestinal tract without creating an influx of fluid into the intestinal lumen and secondary dehydration[581,894]
- Potassium chloride can be diluted in fluids to correct for potassium depletion based on electrolyte analysis (0.1-0.3 mmol/kg)[941]
- Hetastarch at 10-15 mL/kg IV q8h for up to four treatments or dextrans may be effective for hypoproteinemia; synthetic colloids should be used with caution in patients suffering from congestive heart failure or renal failure[620,899]

Total parenteral nutrition may also be considered.[212,215]

Maintenance and Deficit Replacement[420,620,726]

- Determine fluid deficit:
  Fluid deficit (mL) = body weight (g) × % dehydration
- Determine daily maintenance:
  Daily maintenance is estimated at 50 mL (range: 40-60 mL/kg/day in many avian species); the smallest passerines drink 250-300 mL/kg daily[565]
- If possible, replace 50% of the deficit in the first 12-24 hr and the remainder over the next 24-48 hr; some clinicians recommend replacing 20%-25% of the deficit in the first 4-6 hr and the remaining volume during the next 24-72 hr

TABLE 5-39 Routes of Administration and Maximum Suggested Volumes of Fluids That Can Be Administered to Psittacines.[384,747,894]

Route	Maximum Suggested Volume of Fluid[a]
Gavage	• Administer up to 5 mL/100 g bird[b] • Initial volume should be much less in critically ill and anorectic patients (begin with ½ - ⅓ of estimated crop volume) • Crop volume may be up to 10% BW in neonatal birds
Subcutaneous	50 mL/kg[c,d]
Intravenous or intraosseous bolus	Administer up to 10 mL/kg (ideally over a 5-10 min period); in emergencies, could go as high as 25 mL/kg (see Table 5-16)

[a]Combinations of routes (PO, SC, and IV/IO) are recommended if large fluid volumes are administered.
[b]Crop volume may be estimated at 5% of body weight (BW).
[c]Volumes of 10-15 mL/kg may be comfortably given per subcutaneous injection site, although up to 25 mL/kg per site may be given. Overdistension of the area may compromise blood supply to the area and reduce absorption.[894]
[d]Hyaluronidase (Wydase, Wyeth-Ayerst) (1 mL [150 U]/L fluids) may be used in most species to increase the absorption rate of fluids.[455]

TABLE 5-40 Suggested Volumes and Frequency of Gavage Feeding in Anorectic Birds.[726,793]

Species	Volume (mL)[a,b]	Frequency[a]
Finch	0.1-0.5	q4h
Budgerigar	0.5-3	q6h
Lovebird	1-3	q6h
Cockatiel	1-8	q6h
Conure, small	3-12	q6h
Conure, large	7-24	q6-8h
Amazon parrot	5-35	q8h
Cockatoo	10-40	q8-12h
Macaw	20-60	q8-12h

[a]Adjust volume and frequency as crop accommodates larger volumes.
[b]Generally 3%-5% of body weight.[383]

TABLE 5-41 Calculation of Enteral Feeding Requirements for Birds.[721]

When dealing with a debilitated patient that must be tube fed more than once or twice, it is always prudent to make sure you are meeting its caloric requirements.
Basal metabolic rate (BMR) (kcal/day) = $kW^{0.75}$
Maintenance energy requirements (MER) (kcal/day) = (1.5 × BMR)
k = kcal/kg/day constant (nonpasserines = 78, passerines = 129)

- Calculate MER
- Adjust the MER value for debilitated patients, taking their specific clinical condition into account. For instance, an adjustment for sepsis is made by multiplying by 1.5.

Most manufacturers of critical care diets provide information on caloric content (see below);[721] if they do not, call them and ask (see Table 5-43).

Product (Manufacturer)	Protein (%)		Fat (%)		Fiber (%)		CHO (NFE)[a] (%) Dry Matter Basis	Caloric Content (kcal)
	Label Claim (min)	Dry Matter Basis	Label Claim (min)	Dry Matter Basis	Label Claim (max)	Dry Matter Basis		
a/d Canine/Feline Critical Care (Hill's)	8.5	44.2	6.6	30.4	0.5	1.3	15.4	1.3/mL
Carnivore Care (Oxbow)	45	—	32	—	3	—	—	0.8/mL[b]
CliniCare Canine/Feline Liquid Diet (Abbott)	8.2	35.1	5.1	22.2	0.1	0.4	29.5	1/mL
Emeraid Carnivore (Lafeber)	37.8	—	34	—	4.5	—	—	4.98 kcal/g dry weight; 1.60 kcal/mL when prepared as directed
Emeraid Herbivore (Lafeber)[c]	19	—	9.5	—	32	—	—	3.04 kcal/g dry weight; 1 kcal/mL when prepared as directed
Emeraid Omnivore (Lafeber)	20	—	9.5	—	0.5	—	—	4.08 kcal/g dry weight; 1.86 kcal/mL when prepared as directed
Emeraid Nutri-Support (Lafeber)	18.5	—	5	—	1	—	—	2.5/g
Exact Baby Bird Hand Feeding Formula (Kaytee)	22	—	9	—	5	—	—	3.9/g
Exact Macaw Hand Feeding Formula (Kaytee)	19	—	13	—	5	—	—	4.1/g
Formula AA Acute Care (Roudybush)	20	—	10	—	5	—	—	3.5/g DW
Maximum-Calorie Veterinary Formula (Iams)	14	—	12	—	1	—	—	2.1/mL
Recovery Formula (Harrison's)	35	—	19	—	1	—	—	3.9/g

[a]Carbohydrate nitrogen-free extract.
[b]24 kcal/Tbs of powder.
[c]Fed in combination with Emeraid Omnivore to geese and swans.

TABLE 5-42 Doxycycline Recipes Used in Psittacines.[290,718]

Medicated water for cockatiels:

1. Mix doxycycline with tap water to a final concentration of 280 mg/L (0.28 mg/mL) using a magnetic stir bar and plate
2. Prepare daily for 45 days
3. No calcium supplementation should be provided

Medicated seed for cockatiels:

1. Combine 60% hulled millet and 40% hulled sunflower seed with 6.25 mL sunflower oil/kg seed; mix well
2. Mix doxycycline with seeds at 500 mg/kg wet weight using an electric mixer
3. Prepare daily for 45 days
4. No calcium supplementation should be provided

Medicated seed for budgerigars:

1. Create a 1:4 mixture of hulled oat groat and hulled millet
2. Mix well
3. Add approximately 6 mL sunflower oil/kg seed (enough to coat seeds, but not dripping)
4. Mix well
5. Add the contents of doxycycline hyclate capsules aseptically (300 mg drug/kg seed)
6. Prepare daily for 45 days
7. No calcium supplementation should be provided

TABLE 5-43 Select Sources of Formulated and Medicated Diets for Companion and Aviary Birds.

Avi-Sci, Inc[a] 4477 South Williams Road St. Johns, MI 48879, USA www.avi-sci.com	Pretty Bird International, Inc[a] 31008 Fox Hill Ave Stacy, MN 55079, USA www.prettybird.com/
Harrison's Bird Foods 7108 Crossroads Blvd, Suite 325 Brentwood, TN 37027, USA www.harrisonsbirdfoods.com/	Rolf C. Hagen, Inc[a] 50 Hampden Rd Mansfield, MA 02048, USA www.hagen.com/usa/index
Kaytee Products, Inc 521 Clay St, PO Box 230 Chilton, WI 53014, USA www.kaytee.com/	Roudybush Foods[a] 340 Hanson Way Woodland, CA 95776, USA www.roudybush.com/
Lafeber Co 24981 N 1400 East Rd Cornell, IL 61319, USA www.lafebervet.com/	Scenic Bird Food Marion Zoological 2003 E. Center Circle Plymouth, MN 55441, USA www.marionzoological.com/bird/
L'Avian Plus D & D Commodities Ltd. PO Box 359 Stephen, MN 56757, USA www.lavianplus.com	Zeigler Bros, Inc[a] PO Box 95 Gardners, PA 17324, USA www.zeiglerfeed.com
Mazuri Diets PMI Nutrition International LLC PO Box 66812 St. Louis, MO 63166-6812, USA www.mazuri.com/	ZuPreem Diets Premium Nutritional Products, Inc PO Box 2094 Mission, KS 66201, USA www.zupreem.com/

[a]Source of medicated feeds.

TABLE 5-44 Select Nutritional Recommendations for Wild Bird Rehabilitation.[a,123,257,258,308,860]

Aquatic Birds, Including Wading Birds and Seabirds

- Live-prey eating birds like pelicans and herons may not recognize familiar food in an unfamiliar presentation; offer live fish in large tubs, such as a child's wading pool, but be prepared to force feed as needed

Hummingbirds

- It is extremely challenging to meet the nutritional needs of hummingbirds; hummingbirds must constantly replenish energy sources to survive; nectar from plants as well as protein from insects (an estimated 100 mg) are both critical daily dietary requirements
- Nektar-Plus (Nekton) will provide adequate nutritional support, including protein
- Insects, such as *Drosophila* fruit flies, may be released into the enclosure[669]

Raptors

- Rehydrate first (see Table 5-38 and Table 5-39); this is particularly important in birds of prey because the raptor's digestive process requires copious secretions
- For debilitated birds, tube feed a diet rich in protein and fat; offer an enteral tube feeding product (see Table 5-41), ground whole prey (less feet, fur or feathers, gastrointestinal tract), or small amounts of quail breast meat soaked in oral electrolytes
- Feed whole prey after establishing normal gastrointestinal time; offer food the bird will recognize as prey such as eviscerated fish, rats, mice, and/or quail; to increase the chances of self-feeding, offer a variety of foods
- Feed juvenile raptors a whole animal diet of mice or rats supplemented with vitamins; for young nestlings, remove the fur, toenails, and the gastrointestinal tract, then dice the remainder of the body to create a fine "mush"

Songbirds

- Determine if the bird is an omnivore, herbivore, nectarivore, or insectivore and offer a variety of foods; use a good identification book like *The Sibley Guide to Birds*[860] paired with a resource like *The Birder's Handbook*[257] to determine preferred foods
- Offer a variety of foods, such as high-quality birdseed, mealworms, and tiny pieces of fresh fruit and vegetables, in a shallow container or lid
- Presentation of food promotes self-feeding; place earthworms in a pan of soil for thrushes, offer berries still attached to a branch to a mockingbird
- Swifts and swallows may take a live insect on a forcep
- Woodpeckers may eat mealworms trapped in peanut butter spread on bark

[a]See Table 14.1 for more details.

TABLE 5-45 Management of Dystocia or Egg Binding in Birds.[88,391,620]

Definition

- Dystocia or egg binding—obstructive or nonobstructive abnormal oviposition

Etiology—Often Multifactorial

- Environmental stressors
- Nutritional: dehydration, hypocalcemia, low-protein diet, and/or general malnutrition
- Egg-related: abnormal egg size and shape or position
- Hen-related: systemic disease, salpingitis, oviduct perforation, torsion or scarring, and/or neoplasia

Diagnosis

- History/clinical signs/physical findings: nonspecific signs of illness, respiratory distress, persistent tail bobbing, ± blood from vent or in droppings, coelomic distension ± palpable egg
- Complete blood/chemistry panel
- Radiography/ultrasonography

Treatment

- Stabilize the patient
  - Warm, dark, humidified environment
  - Administer warmed fluids, SC, IV, or IO if dehydrated
  - Dextrose: 50% bolus IV or IO; 2.5% in fluids SC if hypoglycemic
  - Calcium gluconate: 50-100 mg/kg IM or SC if hypocalcemic
  - Nutritional support required in most cases
- Medical management
  - Oxytocin: 5 U/kg IM, may repeat q30min
  - Prostaglandin E_2: 0.1 mL/100 g (1 mL/kg) intracloacal on uterovaginal sphincter
- Surgical management
  - Attempt after 12-24 hr unless patient is obstructed and requires faster intervention
  - Sedation with oxygen supplementation or general anesthesia must be used
  - Use caution when manipulating egg; do not press cranially when stabilizing the egg, as this will compromise respiration; instead, use gentle laterolateral digital pressure to direct egg caudally
  - Cloacal ovocentesis
    - 18g-20g needle regardless of patient size
    - Visualize egg/oviductal opening using lubricated speculum or cotton applicators and focal light source
    - Insert needle into egg and aspirate contents while stabilizing egg
    - Gently implode egg with laterolateral digital pressure
    - Extract fragments with curved hemostats
  - Percutaneous ovocentesis
    - 18g-20g needle
    - Stabilize egg against left side of body, then aseptically prepare area
    - Insert needle and aspirate contents
    - Gently implode egg with laterolateral digital pressure if it does not collapse
    - Salpingotomy or salpingohysterectomy

TABLE 5-46 Protocols Used in Treating Mycobacteriosis in Birds.[a,b]

Agent	Drug Combinations and Dosages									
	1[c,958]	2[59]	3[958]	4[958]	5[958]	6[d,89]	7[522]	8[240]	9[949]	10[792]
Azithromycin	—	—	—	—	—	—	—	45 mg/kg PO q24h	—	43 mg/kg PO q24h
Ciprofloxacin	—	—	—	—	80 mg/kg PO q24h	—	—	—	—	15 mg/kg PO q12h[e]
Clarithromycin	—	—	—	—	—	—	55 mg/kg PO q24h	85 mg/kg PO q24h	—	—
Clofazimine	—	—	—	—	—	1.5 mg/kg PO q24h	—	—	6 mg/kg PO q24h	—
Cycloserine	—	—	—	—	—	5 mg/kg PO q12h	—	—	—	—
Enrofloxacin	—	—	30 mg/kg PO q24h	30 mg/kg PO q24h	—	10-15 mg/kg PO, IM q12h	6 mg/kg PO q24h	—	—	—
Ethambutol	30 mg/kg PO q24h	10 mg/kg PO q12h	30 mg/kg PO q24h	30 mg/kg PO q24h	30 mg/kg PO q24h	20 mg/kg PO q24h	30 mg/kg PO q24h	15-30 mg/kg PO q12-24h	30 mg/kg PO q24h	30 mg/kg PO q24h
Isoniazid	30 mg/kg PO q24h	—	—	—	—	—	—	—	—	—
Rifabutin	—	—	15 mg/kg PO q24h	—	—	—	45 mg/kg PO q24h	15-45 mg/kg PO q24h	—	15 mg/kg PO q24h
Rifampin	45 mg/kg PO q24h	15 mg/kg PO q12h	—	45 mg/kg PO q24h	45 mg/kg PO q24h	—	—	—	45 mg/kg PO q24h	—
Streptomycin	—	30 mg/kg IM q12h	—	—	—	—	—	—	—	—

[a]Because of its zoonotic potential, controversy exists concerning whether to treat pet and aviary birds for *Mycobacterium avium*. Because *M. avium* isolates from birds differ from human isolates in antibiotic susceptibility, serovars, and genetic sequencing, pet birds are an unlikely source of *M. avium* in people (except immunosuppressed individuals). Nevertheless, veterinarians who treat birds with this disease do so at their own risk. The veterinarian should be aware that treatment is often lifelong for the bird and that treatment does not necessarily prevent shedding.[59,89,240,522,658,792]

[b]Empirical evaluation of multidrug therapy found that azithromycin (43 mg/kg), rifampin (45 mg/kg), and ethambutol (30 mg/kg) were ineffective in ring-necked doves (*Streptopelia risoria*) naturally infected with avian mycobacteriosis. Culture and sensitivity results indicated resistance to all drugs except for azithromycin.[801]

[c]Mix into dextrose powder, administered with a small amount of food.[958]

[d]Recommended for use in raptors.[89]

[e]Enrofloxacin (15 mg/kg PO q12h), clofazimine (6 mg/kg PO q12h), or amikacin IM, IV can be used in lieu of ciprofloxacin with ethambutol, rifabutin, and azithromycin.[792]

TABLE 5-47 Suggested Chemotherapeutic Protocols Used in Birds.

C.O.P. PROTOCOL FOR LYMPHOMA[315]

- Prednisone 25 mg/m^2 PO q24h
- Cyclophosphamide 200 mg/m^2 IO q7d
- Vincristine 0.75 mg/m^2 IO q7d × 3 treatments
- Doxorubicin 30 mg/m^2 IO q21d
- L-asparaginase 400 U/kg IM q7d
- Interferon α 15,000 U/m^2 SC q2d × 3 treatments
- Diphenhydramine 2 mg/kg IO before doxorubicin and L-asparaginase treatments
- Dexamethasone 1 mg/kg IM before doxorubicin and L-asparaginase treatments

PROTOCOL FOR LYMPHOCYTIC LEUKEMIA OR LYMPHOMA[a,648]

- Vincristine sulfate 0.5 mg/m^2 IV initial dose, then 0.75 mg/m^2 q7d × 3 treatments
- Prednisone 1 mg/454 g PO q12h
- Chlorambucil 1 mg/bird PO 2×/wk

PROTOCOL FOR CUTANEOUS LYMPHOMA[b,773]

- Vincristine 0.1 mg/kg IV q7-14d
- Chlorambucil 2 mg/kg PO 2×/wk

PROTOCOL FOR OSTEOSARCOMA[c,235]

- Diphenhydramine 30 min before doxorubicin treatment (route and dose not given)
- Doxorubicin 60 mg/m^2 is diluted into 6 mL sterile saline and administered IV over 30 min in an anesthetized patient via an angiocatheter in the jugular vein q30d
- Do not extravasate doxorubicin; doxorubicin may cause myelosuppression and cardiac toxicity; monitor the CBC
- Electrocardiography during treatment is recommended

[a]Dosages are for a Pekin duck (*Anas platyrhynchos domesticus*)

[b]Dosages are for an umbrella cockatoo (*Cacatua alba*).

[c]Dosages are for a blue-fronted Amazon parrot (*Amazona aestiva*).

TABLE 5-48 Drug Dosages and Volumes Suggested for Cardiopulmonary Resuscitation (CPR) and in Critical Birds.[a,391,749]

Emergency Drug	Dose	15 g (Canary; Finch)	30 g (Budgerigar)	40-50 g (Lovebird)	100 g (Conure; Cockatiel)	200 g (Mynah)	300 g (Pigeon; Sulphur-crested Cockatoo)	400 g (African Grey Parrot; Eclectus Parrot)	500 g (Umbrella Cockatoo)	750 g (Greater Sulphur-crested Cockatoo)	1 kg (Blue and Gold Macaw)
Atropine (0.2-0.5 mg/mL)	0.5 mg/kg[b]	0.006-0.015 mL	0.012-0.03 mL	0.015-0.05 mL	0.04-0.1 mL	0.08-0.2 mL	0.12-0.3 mL	0.16-0.4 mL	0.2-0.5 mL	0.3-0.75 mL	0.4-1 mL
Calcium gluconate (10%) (100 mg/mL)	50-100 mg/kg	0.007-0.015 mL	0.015-0.03 mL	0.02-0.05 mL	0.05-0.1 mL	0.1-0.2 mL	0.15-0.3 mL	0.2-0.4 mL	0.25-0.5 mL	0.375-0.75 mL	0.5-1 mL
Dexamethasone sodium phosphate (4 mg/mL)	2-4 mg/kg	0.007-0.015 mL	0.015-0.03 mL	0.02-0.05 mL	0.05-0.1 mL	0.1-0.2 mL	0.15-0.3 mL	0.2-0.4 mL	0.25-0.5 mL	0.375-0.75 mL	0.5-1 mL
Dextrose (50%) (diluted with saline)	0.25 mL/kg (slow)	0.004 mL	0.008 mL	0.01-0.125 mL	0.025 mL	0.05 mL	0.075 mL	0.1 mL	0.12 mL	0.18 mL	0.25 mL
Epinephrine (1:1000; 1 mg/mL)	0.1 mg/kg	0.001mL	0.003 mL	0.005 mL	0.01 mL	0.02 mL	0.03 mL	0.04 mL	0.05 mL	0.075 mL	0.1 mL
Isotonic crystalloid fluids (bolus)	10 mL/kg	0.15 mL	0.3 mL	0.4-0.5 mL	1 mL	2 mL	3 mL	4 mL	5 mL	7.5 mL	10 mL
7.5% NaCl	3 mL/kg	0.04 mL	0.09 mL	0.12-0.15 mL	0.3 mL	0.6 mL	0.9 mL	1.2 mL	1.5 mL	2.1 mL	3 mL

Continued

TABLE 5-48 Drug Dosages and Volumes Suggested for Cardiopulmonary Resuscitation (CPR) and in Critical Birds. (cont'd)

Emergency Drug	Dose	15 g (Canary; Finch)	30 g (Budgerigar)	40-50 g (Lovebird)	100 g (Conure; Cockatiel)	200 g (Mynah)	300 g (Pigeon; Sulphur-crested Cockatoo)	400 g (African Grey Parrot; Eclectus Parrot)	500 g (Umbrella Cockatoo)	750 g (Greater Sulphur-crested Cockatoo)	1 kg (Blue and Gold Macaw)
6% Hetastarch	5 mL/kg bolus (20 mL/kg/day)	0.07mL	0.15 mL	0.2-0.25 mL	0.5 mL	1 mL	1.5 mL	2 mL	2.5 mL	3.75 mL	5 mL
Mannitol (20%) (200 mg/mL)	0.5-2 mL/kg	0.0075-0.03 mL	0.015-0.06 mL	0.02-0.1 mL	0.05-0.2 mL	0.1-0.4 mL	0.15-0.6 mL	0.2-0.8 mL	0.25-1 mL	0.375-1.5 mL	0.5-2 mL
Prednisolone sodium succinate (10 mg/mL)	10-20 mg/kg	0.015-0.03 mL	0.03-0.06 mL	0.04-0.1 mL	0.1-0.2 mL	0.2-0.4 mL	0.3-0.6 mL	0.4-0.8 mL	0.5-1 mL	0.75-1.5 mL	1-2 mL
Sodium bicarbonate (1 mmol/mL)	5 mmol/kg	0.075 mL	0.15 mL	0.2-0.25 mL	0.5 mL	1 mL	1.5 mL	2 mL	2.5 mL	3.75 mL	5 mL
Vasopressin (20 U/mL)	0.8 U/kg IV, IO	—	—	—	0.004 mL	0.008 mL	0.012 mL	0.016 mL	0.02 mL	0.03 mL	0.04 mL

[a]Dose in mL/kg body weight, IV, IO, or IM. If weight is not available, base CPR on approximate weight of species closest in size.

[b]Doses published range from 0.02-0.5 mg/kg.

TABLE 5-49 Vaccines Used in Birds (Nonpoultry).[25,135,149,378,449,468,583,619,659,703,765,771,779,941,1000]

Species	Agent	Dosage	Initial	Booster	Comments
See comments	West Nile virus (West Nile-Innovator, Zoetis; equine killed vaccine); (Recombitek-equine rWNV vaccine, Merial; equine recombinant DNA vaccine)	0.5-1 mL IM	Repeat q3-4wk for 2-3 treatments	3 wk	Environmental control is generally considered most important; however, West Nile virus vaccine has been administered to many types of birds, including Ciconiiformes, Columbiformes, Coraciiformes, Passeriformes, Phoenicopteriformes, Psittaciformes, and raptors (including falcons); an antibody response has been documented inconsistently (flamingos, penguins);[154,204,657,660,862] hemolytic anemia reported in lories immunized a year after first set of immunizations[704]
Raptors	Paramyxovirus-1 (V.P. Vaccin Nobilis Lasota, Intervet; poultry vaccine)	Intranasally or added to drinking water	—	Booster in 3-4 wk; protects approximately 6 mo	Hitchner B1 and Lasota strain poultry vaccines in drinking water appear to be effective; may see mild palpebral swelling for a few days[449]
Pigeons, racing	Pigeon paramyxovirus (Nobilis Paramyxo P201, MSD)	0.25 mL SC	4 wk and older pigeons.	—	Killed virus; administer 6 wk before competitions, exhibitions, and coupling season
	Paramyxovirus-1/Pox pigeon (Colombovac, Solvay Animal Health)	0.2 mL SC[a,89]	4 wk of age	—	Killed virus; poor immunologic response to pox
	Pigeon Paramyxovirus) (KM-PMV; ARKO Laboratories)	0.25 mL SC	6 wk of age	2-3 wk, then annually	Killed virus
	Salmonella (Nu-Sal KM-1 Paratyphoid (*Salmonella*);ARKO Laboratories)	0.25 mL SC	5 wk of age	3-4 wk, then every 6 mo	Polyvalent bacterin; avoid vaccinating during breeding season, racing/show, the molt, and pigeons less than 6 wk of age

Continued

TABLE 5-49 Vaccines Used in Birds (Nonpoultry). (cont'd)

Species	Agent	Dosage	Initial	Booster	Comments
	Pigeon poxvirus (Pigeon Pox Vaccine, Hygieia Biologic Laboratories; poultry vaccine)	Through the feather pluck method; feathers removed from the distal aspect of a leg and vaccine is brushed with a sterile cotton-tipped applicator[405]	6 wk of age or older		Live virus; response to vaccine characterized by localized infection characterized by swelling, discoloration, and follicular distension at the site of vaccination; lesions resolved within 1 mo
Psittacines	Polyomavirus (Psittimune APV, Creative Science)	0.25 mL/bird (that will weigh <200 g at maturity) SC[721]	35-50 days of age; chicks may be safely vaccinated as young as 10-20 days of age; degree of protection uncertain[771]	2-3 wk, then annually	May cause discoloration, thickening, or granuloma of skin at vaccination site
	—	0.5 mL/bird (that will weigh >200 g at maturity) SC[721]	—	Last booster should be given at least 2 wk before leaving aviary[770]	May be indicated in the face of an outbreak;[b,771] registered with the United States Department of Agriculture[779]
Emus[928]	Eastern and Western equine encephalitis and tetanus (Equiloid Innovator, Zoetis; equine vaccine)	Same dosage as recommended for the target species (horses) IM	6 wk to 3 mo of age	Repeat 3-4 wk later, then booster annually or biannually before and after breeding season (March/Sept)[928]	Killed virus
Cranes[564]	Eastern and Western equine encephalitis and tetanus (ENCEVAC,Merck/MSD; equine vaccine), (West Nile Innovator + EWT, Zoetis; equine vaccine)	0.25 mL IM	30 days of age	Repeat 3-4 wk later, then booster annually	Killed virus

[a]Vaccinating birds during an outbreak may allow humans to theoretically serve as mechanical vectors.[765]

[b]Choose subcutaneous injection site carefully in pigeons to avoid bleeding; cranial to thigh or lower ⅓ of neck on dorsal midline.

TABLE 5-50 Blood Pressure Values Reported in Birds.

Species	Direct or Indirect	Mean Arterial Pressure (mmHg)	Systolic Arterial Pressure (mmHg)	Diastolic Arterial Pressure (mmHg)
Psittacines	Indirect in conscious birds[530]	—	120-180	—
	Indirect in birds under isoflurane anesthesia[530]	—	90-180	—
Hispaniolan Amazon parrots[a] (*n* = 16)	Direct in birds under isoflurane anesthesia using the wing[10]	155 ± 18 (112-185)	163 ± 18 (119-200)	148 ± 18 (106-171)
	Direct in birds under isoflurane anesthesia using the leg[10]	152 ± 28 (97-190)	159 ± 28 (113-206)	144 ± 30 (83-181)
	Indirect in birds under isoflurane anesthesia using the wing[10]	140 ± 25 (104-197)	—	—
	Indirect in birds under isoflurane anesthesia using the leg[10]	145 ± 28 (96-196)	—	—
Falcons (*n* = 45)	Indirect in birds under isoflurane anesthesia[541]	202 ± 28	—	—
Red-tailed hawks (*n* = 6)	Indirect in birds under sevoflurane anesthesia[b,1011]	155 ± 27	181 ± 25	—
	Indirect in conscious birds[1011]	190 ± 38	236 ± 42	—
	Direct in birds under sevoflurane anesthesia[1011]	159 ± 25 (102-216)	178 ± 27 (124-251)	143 ± 24 (78-198)
	Direct in conscious birds[1011]	201 ± 29 (154-262)	238 ± 39 (161-301)	180 ± 31 (142-254)
Bald eagles (*n* = 17)	Direct in spontaneously breathing birds under general anesthesia[459]	MAP was significantly elevated with isoflurane when compared to sevoflurane	176 ± 14 to 209 ± 14 on isoflurane over 40 min 129 ± 15 to 163 ± 13 on sevoflurane over 40 min	139 ± 14 to 172 ± 14 on isoflurane over 40 min 129 ± 15.2 to 147 ± 14 on sevoflurane over 40 min
	Indirect in conscious birds[12]	124 ± 62	—	—
Pigeons (*n* = 7)	Indirect in conscious birds[108]	—	155 ± 21	—
	Indirect under isoflurane anesthesia	—	87 ± 11	—
Chicken (*n* = 40)	Direct in birds under general anesthesia[488]	136 (114-158)	141 (118-163)	131 (109-153)
Pekin ducks (*n* = 72)	Direct in birds under general anesthesia[514]	143 (111–174)	165 (138–192)	121 (85–157)

[a]There was substantial disagreement between direct systolic arterial blood pressure and indirect blood pressure measurements obtained with the Doppler probe from the wing and from the leg of the Hispaniolan parrot (*Amazona ventralis*); attempts to obtain indirect blood pressure measurements with an oscillometric unit were unsuccessful.[10]

[b]Indirect blood pressure measured using an oscillometric unit was unreliable; indirect blood pressure measurements using a Doppler probe and cuff 3 were closer to direct mean arterial pressure measured from the superficial ulnar artery.

TABLE 5-51 Select Arrhythmias and Some Documented Causes in Birds.[66]

Arrhythmias	ECG Changes	Causes
Excitability Disturbances		
Respiratory sinus arrhythmia	Slowing of HR during expiration	Physiologic
Sinus bradycardia	Low HR, normal sinus rhythm	Vagal stimulation, atropine, anesthesia, hypokalemia, hyperkalemia, vitamin E deficiency, vitamin B_1 deficiency, acetylcholinesterase inhibitors
Sinus tachycardia	High HR, normal sinus rhythm	Sympathetic, catecholamine stimulation
Atrial tachycardia	Series of fast atrial extrasystoles	Atrial distension, ectopic foci
Atrial fibrillation	No normal P waves, irregular SS intervals	Atrial enlargements, cardiac disease
Ventricular premature contraction (VPC)	Wide, bizarre QRS unrelated to P	Ectopic foci, hypokalemia, vitamin B_1 deficiency, vitamin E deficiency, PMV-1, AI, myocardial infarction
Ventricular tachycardia	Series of VPC	Similar causes as for VPCs
Ventricular fibrillation	Chaotic ventricular depolarization	Myocardial hypoxia, shock, severe disorders
Conduction Disturbances		
1st-degree AV block	Long PR intervals	Anesthetics, increased vagal tone
2nd-degree AV block	Long PR intervals, some P without QRS	Anesthetics, increased vagal tone, occasionally normal in pigeons, parrots, raptors
3rd-degree AV block	Escape ventricular rhythm (slow and bizarre QRS), no consistent PR	Severe cardiomegaly
Bundle branch block	Short PR, bizarre and widened QRS	Lead, myopathy, myocarditis, uncommon in birds

TABLE 5-52 ECG Measurements Reference Values on Lead II in Select Avian Species.[a,b,69]

Species	African Grey Parrot	Amazon Parrot	Bald Eagle	Chicken	Cockatoo	Macaw	Pekin Duck	Racing Pigeon	Red-tailed Hawk
n	45	37	20	72	31	41	50	60	11
Heart rate	340-600	340-600	50-160	180-340	259-575	255-555	200-360	160-300	80-220
P amplitude	0.25-0.55	0.25-0.60	0.050-0.325	—	0.13-0.53	0.03-0.47	—	0.4-0.6	-0.1-0.175
P duration	0.012-0.018	0.008-0.017	0.030-0.060	0.035-0.043	0.009-0.025	0.009-0.021	0.015-0.035	0.015-0.020	0.020-0.035
PR interval	0.040-0.055	0.042-0.055	0.070-0.110	0.073-0.089	0.039-0.071	0.040-0.068	0.04-0.08	0.045-0.070	0.050-0.090
S amplitude	0.9-2.2	0.7-2.3	0.150-1.450	0.10-1.0	0.27-1.59	0.27-1.43	0.35-1.03	1.5-2.8	0.300-0.900
QRS duration	0.010-0.016	0.010-0.015	0.020-0.040	0.02-0.028	0.014-0.026	0.002-0.030	0.028-0.044	0.013-0.016	0.020-0.030
T amplitude	0.18-0.6	0.3-0.8	0.050-0.200	0.03-0.28	0.17-0.97	0.12-0.80	0.04-0.40	0.3-0.8	0.000-0.300
QT interval	0.048-0.080	0.050-0.095	0.110-0.165	—	0.065-0.125	0.053-0.109	0.08-0.12	0.060-0.075	0.080-0.165
MEA	–79 to –103	–90 to –107	–30 to –150	–91 to –120	–73 to –89	–76 to –87	–160 to 95	–83 to –99	–50 to –110

[a]Amplitude in mV, Interval/Duration in Sec.

[b]To obtain a 95% reference interval, all published results in the form of mean ± SD were reported as mean ± 2 SD and in the form of mean ± sem were reported as mean ± 2 sem √n; when only the range or a 95% reference interval was published, it was reported as is.

TABLE 5-53 Echocardiographic Reference Intervals (mm) in Select Avian Species Obtained in the Horizontal Four-Chamber View.[a,69]

Parameter	African Grey Parrots	Amazon Parrots	Cockatoos	Diurnal Raptors[b]	Pigeons (Parasternal)
n	60	10	10	100	50
Left ventricle					
Systole length	18.4-26	16.5-25.7	16.4-21.6	9.1-20.3	15.9-19.9
Systole width	4.8-8.8	4.3-9.1	3.0-9.8	4.1-8.5	4.4-6.0
Diastole length	20.2-27.8	17.7-26.5	16.7-23.1	11.0-21.8	17.3-22.9
Diastole width	6.6-10.6	6.4-10.4	5.3-11.3	5.3-10.1	6.2-8.6
FS (%)	13.8-31.4	14.4-31.2	11.6-39.6	—	—
Right ventricle					
Systole length	6.4-12.0	5.8-13.0	7.9-12.7	7.3-18.1	—
Systole width	1.0-4.6	1.7-4.5	7.9-12.7	0.9-3.3	
Diastole length	7.7-15.3	7.7-12.9	6.7-15.9	8.9-18.9	8.3-11.5
Diastole width	2.6-7.0	2.6-7.8	2.5-4.5	0.9-4.1	3.0-5.0
FS (%)	17.0-64.6	26.7-41.5	12.7-53.9	—	—
Aorta					
Systole diameter	2.8-4.4	2.0-4.0	—	—	—
Diastole diameter	2.8-5.2	2.2-4.6	—	2-3.6	2.8-3.2

[a]To obtain a 95% reference interval, all published results in the form of mean ± SD were reported as mean ± 2 SD and in the form of mean ± sem were reported as mean ± 2 sem$\sqrt{n}$; when only the range or a 95% reference interval was published, it was reported as is. FS, fractional shortening. Echocardiographic measurements may not be reliable and clinically useful.
[b]European diurnal raptors included common buzzard, European sparrow hawk, northern goshawk, and black kite.

TABLE 5-54 Spectral Doppler Echocardiographic Reference Intervals (m/s) in Select Avian Species Obtained in the Horizontal Four-Chamber View.[a,69,690,902,903]

Species	*n*	Left Diastolic Inflow	Right Diastolic Inflow	Aortic Systolic Outflow
African grey parrots	—	0.27-0.51	—	0.63-1.15
Amazon parrots	—	0.12-.24	0.12-0.32	0.67-0.99
Barn owls	10	0.14-0.26	0.10-0.34	0.84-1.32
Cockatoos	—	0.02-0.62	—	0.40-1.16
Common buzzard	10	0.16-0.28	0.13-0.25	1.04-1.68
Falcons	15	0.18-0.38	0.17-0.37	1.07-1.43
Harris's hawks	10	0.13-0.25	0.15-0.27	0.75-1.43
Macaws	—	0.40-0.68	—	0.55-1.07

[a]To obtain a 95% reference interval, all published results in the form of mean ± SD were reported as mean ± 2 SD and in the form of mean ± sem were reported as mean ± 2 sem$\sqrt{n}$; when only the range or a 95% reference interval was published, it was reported as is. Parrots were anesthetized; raptors were awake.

TABLE 5-55 Guidelines for Selection of Psychotherapeutic Agents for Birds.[105,582,851,868]

1. Perform a complete medical and behavioral workup:
   - Obtain a detailed medical and behavioral history.
   - Perform a careful physical examination, looking for evidence of feather dysplasia or skin abnormalities.
   - Collect a minimum database that includes complete blood count, plasma biochemistry panel, radiographs, psittacine beak and feather disease testing, as well as paired (affected/nonaffected) skin/feather follicle biopsy when indicated.
2. Once a medical problem has been ruled out or treated, assuming the problem does not abate, form a behavioral diagnosis:
   - It is not enough to determine the bird is feather picking; identify "why" the bird is feather picking; use of "antecedent, behavior, and consequence" data can be particularly helpful.
   - Many behavioral problems are multifactorial in origin.
3. Formulate a treatment plan that incorporates:
   - Environmental modification:
     - Improve the nutritional plane and basic husbandry.
     - Provide environmental enrichment where appropriate.
   - Behavioral modification techniques:
     - Focus on what you want the bird to do and reward the bird for that, and/or engage in stimulating behavior that will accomplish that goal. Do not punish or deprive the bird.
     - Offer behavioral alternatives with emphasis in developing foraging behaviors for treats or food of increasing complexity, and training of basic skills.
   - Behavioral pharmacotherapy can be a useful component of treatment.
   - Whenever possible, consult with a behaviorist, preferably a member of the American College of Veterinary Behaviorists.
4. Behavioral pharmacotherapy, general principles:
   - These drugs may help the bird be more open to change, thereby reducing stress and increasing the chances of success.
     - Most behavioral drugs act by exerting effects on neurotransmitters (NT) in the central nervous system (CNS).
     - Serotonin (5-HT) affects mood, sleep patterns, and appetite; also plays a role in the suppression of impulses; low levels or an imbalance between serotonin and other hormones may be associated with maladaptive behaviors.
     - Norepinephrine (NE) plays an important role in attentiveness, sleeping, dreaming, and learning.
     - Gamma-aminobutyric acid (GABA) is a major inhibitory NT.
   - Behavioral drugs are classified based on their first clinical use in humans or on their structure and effects (tricyclics, selective serotonin reuptake inhibitors); major groups include anxiolytics, antipsychotics, and antidepressants, but their use may be more generalized outside of these broad areas.
   - A number of factors must be considered when selecting a psychotropic agent: the proposed mechanism of action, indications and contraindications, common side effects and the potential for other adverse effects, drug cost, and ease of administration; also consider the bird species, its age and underlying health, as well as reproductive status; see information that follows or consult a veterinary behavior text or a general formulary for more detailed information.

Continued

TABLE 5-55 Guidelines for Selection of Psychotherapeutic Agents for Birds.

- Drugs commonly selected for:
  - Conditions of *fear, phobia, or anxiety* include benzodiazepines and buspirone; antidepressants may also be used for generalized anxiety and separation anxiety.
  - Obsessive-compulsive disorders such as stereotypical behaviors[a] include TCAs and SSRIs.
  - Stereotypy that involves self-injurious behavior includes opioid antagonists (i.e., naltrexone), SSRIs, TCAs, and in select cases, haloperidol.
  - Antipruritic effects include the TCAs; doxepin, followed by amitriptyline, have the most potent antihistaminic activity.[b]
  - Aggression, both hierarchical and anxiety-induced, are the SSRIs.
- Ancillary treatments may include opioid analgesics (Table 5-5), NSAIDs (Table 5-6), hormonal agents (Table 5-7), and/or essential fatty acid supplements when indicated.

5. How much to give, how often, and for how long?
   - Many of the doses in Table 5-10 are based on anecdotal experience or case reports; the few empirical studies referenced use small sample sizes.
   - Warn your client that, in many instances, dosing may be by trial and error; for instance, after giving an antidepressant for 4-8 weeks, it may be necessary to adjust the dose or in some instances, to change drugs.
   - Combination therapy can sometimes enhance drug effectiveness:
     - Benzodiazepines (BZDs) may be combined with antidepressants but reduce the BZD dose to minimize the risk of CNS depression; this combination may be particularly helpful when psychotherapy is first started because it takes weeks for antidepressants to exert an effect.
     - Unless both dosages are decreased, avoid combining drugs where both increase serotonin levels since there is the risk of causing serotonin syndrome.[c]
   - Administer antidepressants for a minimum of 6-8 weeks.
   - Monitor blood work regularly.
   - When and if a beneficial result is achieved, it may be prudent to continue treatment for at least 2-6 months.
   - The process of weaning a bird off of medication may also require trial and error; one technique is to reduce the effective dose by 25% every 3 weeks; if signs recur, return to the lowest effective dose; taper drug dosages over a minimum of 3 weeks.
6. Client education
   - Determine beforehand how you will document treatment response; identify target signs that can be monitored by the owner with respect to intensity, duration, and frequency.
   - Prepare clients for the possibility of trial and error dosing, possible side effects, the duration of treatment that may be necessary, and the length of time before onset of desired effects.
   - Extra-label drug use.

	Anxiolytics			Antidepressants	
Characteristics	Benzodiazepines	Buspirone	Antipsychotics	Tricyclic Compounds (TCAs)	Selective Serotonin Reuptake Inhibitors (SSRIs)
Range of effects	Mild sedation,[d] to anxiolysis, to hypnosis as dose increases	Calming	Reduce motor activity	A variety including potent antihistaminic activity and some sedation	A variety of actions including a mood-stabilizing effect
Specific examples	Diazepam Lorazepam Midazolam High potency: alprazolam Clorazepate	—	Haloperidol	Amitriptyline Clomipramine Imipramine	Fluoxetine Paroxetine Sertraline
Disadvantages	Can interfere with learning and affect behavioral modification	Delayed onset of action (2-4 wk)	See below	Delayed onset of action (2-4 wk)	Delayed onset of action (3-6 wk)
Potential adverse effects	Sedation, ataxia,[d] paradoxical excitation; rare fatal idiopathic hepatic necrosis in cats given diazepam PO	Few to mild; confusion, nausea, anorexia	Extrapyramidal signs: tremors, dystonia, dyskinesia or akathisia; transient anorexia and regurgitation	Anticholinergic signs[e]	Uncommon and transient; anorexia most common[f] and serotonin syndrome is the most serious[c]
Contraindications and precautions	Liver or renal disease; aggression; consider potential for human abuse	Severe renal or hepatic disease	—	Discontinue slowly to prevent withdrawal responses; may lower seizure threshold in humans	—
Taste	Benign, although a bitter aftertaste has been described for diazepam	—	—	Lingering bitter taste	Odorless, tasteless tablets

[a]Stereotypies are repetitive behaviors such as circling or pacing, or in some instances, feather-destructive behavior.

[b]The antihistaminic activity of doxepin is 800 times that of diphenhydramine.

[c]Serotonin syndrome may cause muscle tremors, rigidity, agitation, hyperthermia, vocalization, hypertension or hypotension, tachycardia, seizures, coma, and death.

[d]Mild sedative effects create a risk of bird falling from perch; tolerance to sedation may develop over time.

[e]A variety of anticholinergic signs have been reported in mammals, including dry mouth, fatigue, variable degrees of sedation, constipation, tremor, hypotension, arrhythmias, weight gain, mydriasis, and vomiting; sedation and regurgitation are reported most commonly in birds.[582]

[f]Other possible adverse effects with SSRIs include diarrhea, increased agitation, irritability, insomnia, and in rare instances, vomiting.

REFERENCES

1. Aarons JE. First aid and wound management in the ostrich. *Proc Annu Conf Assoc Avian Vet.* 1995:201–208.
2. Aarons JE. Adverse effects of high environmental temperature on ostrich chicks. *Proc Annu Conf Assoc Avian Vet.* 1996:153–158.
3. Aarons JE. Assessing the down bird. *Proc Annu Conf Assoc Avian Vet.* 1997:175–179.
4. Abbas RZ, Iqbal Z, Khan MN, et al. Prophylactic efficacy of diclazuril in broilers experimentally infected with three field isolates of *Eimeria tenella. Int J Agric Biol.* 2009;11:606–610.
5. Abernathy DR, Arnold GJ, Azarnoff DL et al., eds. *Mosby's Drug Consult.* St. Louis, MO: Mosby; 2003.
6. Abou-Madi N. Avian anesthesia. *Vet Clin North Am Exot Anim Pract.* 2001;4:147–167.
7. Abrams GA, Paul-Murphy J, Murphy CJ. Conjunctivitis in birds. *Vet Clin North Am Exot Anim Pract.* 2002;5:287–309.
8. Abu J, Wünschmann A, Redig PT, et al. Management of a cutaneous squamous cell carcinoma in an American flamingo (*Phoenicopterus ruber*). *J Avian Med Surg.* 2009;23(1):44–48.
9. Abu-Basha EA, Idkaidek NM, Hantash TM. Pharmacokinetics and bioavailability of doxycycline in ostriches (*Struthio camelus*) at two different dose rates. *J Vet Sci.* 2006;7(4):327–332.
10. Acierno MJ, da Cunha A, Smith J, et al. Agreement between direct and indirect blood pressure measurements obtained from anesthetized Hispaniolan Amazon parrots. *J Am Vet Med Assoc.* 2008;233:1587–1590.
11. Aguilar RF, Redig PT. Diagnosis and treatment of avian aspergillosis. In: Bonagura JD, ed. *Kirk's Current Veterinary Therapy XII: Small Animal Practice.* Philadelphia, PA: Saunders; 1995:1294–1299.
12. Aguilar RF, Smith VE, Ogburn P, et al. Arrythmias associated with isoflurane anesthesia in bald eagles (*Haliaeetus leucocephalus*). *J Zoo Wildl Med.* 1995;26:508–516.
13. Alderton D. *A Birdkeeper's Guide to Pet Birds.* Morris Plains, NJ: Tetra Press; 1987.
14. Alexander BD, Winkler TP, Shi S, et al. In vitro characterization of nebulizer delivery of liposomal amphotericin B aerosols. *Pharm Dev Technol.* 2011;16(6):577–582.
15. Allen DG, Pringle JK, Smith DA et al., eds. *Handbook of Veterinary Drugs.* 2nd ed. Philadelphia, PA: JB Lippincott Co; 1998:749–842.
16. Allen JL, Oosterhuis JE. Effect of tolazoline on xylazine-ketamine-induced anesthesia in turkey vultures. *J Am Vet Med Assoc.* 1986;189:1011–1012.
17. Al-Sobayil FA, Ahmed AF, Al-Wabel NA, et al. The use of xylazine, ketamine, and isoflurane for induction and maintenance of anesthesia in ostriches (*Struthio camelus*). *J Avian Med Surg.* 2009;23:101–107.
18. Al-Timimi F, Nolosco P, Al-Timimi B. Incidence and treatment of serratospiculosis in falcons from Saudi Arabia. *Vet Rec.* 2009;165:408–409.
19. Ammersbach M, Beaufrère H, Gionet Rollick A, et al. Laboratory blood analysis in Strigiformes-Part I: hematologic reference intervals and agreement between manual blood cell counting techniques. *Vet Clin Pathol.* 2015;44:94–108.
20. Ammersbach M, Beaufrère H, Gionet Rollick A, et al. Laboratory blood analysis in Strigiformes-Part II: plasma biochemistry reference intervals and agreement between the Abaxis Vetscan V2 and the Roche Cobas c501. *Vet Clin Pathol.* 2015;44:128–140.
21. Anderson K, Garner MM, Reed HH, et al. Hemorrhagic diathesis in avian species following intramuscular administration of polysulfated glycosaminoglycan. *J Zoo Wildl Med.* 2013;44(1):93–99.
22. Anderson NL, Johnson CK, Fender S, et al. Clinical signs and histopathologic findings associated with a newly recognized protozoal disease (*Trichomonas gallinae*) in free-ranging house finches (*Carpodacus mexicanus*). *J Zoo Wildl Med.* 2010;41:249–254.
23. Andre J, Delverdier M. Primary bronchial carcinoma with osseous metastasis in an African grey parrot (*Psittacus erithacus*). *J Avian Med Surg.* 1999;13(3):180–186.
24. Andrew SE, Clippinger TL, Brooks DE, et al. Penetrating keratoplasty for treatment of corneal protrusion in a great horned owl (*Bubo virginianus*). *Vet Ophthalmol.* 2002;5(3):201–205.

25. Angenvoort J, Fischer D, Fast C, et al. Limited efficacy of West Nile virus vaccines in large falcons (*Falco* spp.). *Vet Res*. 2014;45:41.
26. Antinoff N. Improving oncologic diagnostics and therapeutics. *Proc Annu Assoc Avian Med*. 2001:369–381 Published online.
27. Arabkhazaeli F, Madani SA, Ghavami S. Outbreak of an unusual tracheal mite, *Ptilonyssus morofskyi* (Acarina: Rhinonyssidae), in canaries (*Serinus canaria*) with concurrent infection with *Staphylococcus aureus* and *Macrorhabdus ornithogaster*. *J Avian Med Surg*. 2016;30:269–273.
28. Araghi M, Azizi S, Vesal N, et al. Evaluation of the sedative effects of diazepam, midazolam, and xylazine after intranasal administration in juvenile ostriches (*Struthio camelus*). *J Avian Med Surg*. 2016;30:221–226.
29. Archawaranon M. Hematological investigations of captive hill mynah *Gracula religiosa* in Thailand. *Int J Poult Sci*. 2005;4:679–682.
30. Asa C, Boutelle S. Contraception. In: Miller RE, Fowler ME, eds. St. Louis, MO: Elsevier; 2011. *Fowler's Zoo and Wild Animal Medicine Current Therapy*. Vol 7:8–14.
31. Ashworth CD, Nelson DR. Antimicrobial potentiation of irrigation solutions containing tris-[hydroxymethyl] aminomethane-EDTA. *J Am Vet Med Assoc*. 1990;197:1513–1514.
32. Atalan G, Uzun M, Demirkan I, et al. Effect of medetomidine-butorphanol-ketamine anaesthesia and atipamezole on heart and respiratory rate and cloacal temperature of domestic pigeons. *J Vet Med A Physiol Pathol Clin Med*. 2002;49:281–285.
33. Axelson RD. *Caring for Your Pet Bird*. Toronto, ON: Canaviax Publications Ltd; 1981.
34. Axelson RD. Avian dermatology. In: Hoefer HL, ed. *Practical Avian Medicine: The Compendium Collection*. Trenton, NJ: Veterinary Learning Systems; 1997:186–195.
35. Azizpour A, Hassani Y. Clinical evaluation of general anaesthesia in pigeons using a combination of ketamine and diazepam. *J S Afr Vet Assoc*. 2012;83:12.
36. Baert K, de Backer P. Comparative pharmacokinetics of three non-steroidal anti-inflammatory drugs in five bird species. *Comp Biochem Physiol C Toxicol Pharmacol*. 2003;134:25–33.
37. Baert K, Nackaerts J, de Backer P. Disposition of sodium salicylate, flunixin, and meloxicam after intravenous administration in ostriches (*Struthio camelus*). *J Avian Med Surg*. 2002;16:123–128.
38. Baert L, Van Poucke S, Vermeersch H, et al. Pharmacokinetics and anthelmintic efficacy of febantel in the racing pigeon (*Columba livia*). *J Vet Pharmacol Therap*. 1993;16:223–231.
39. Báez LA, Langston C, Givaruangsawat S, et al. Evaluation of in vitro serial antibiotic elution from meropenem-impregnated polymethylmethacrylate beads after ethylene oxide gas and autoclave sterilization. *Vet Comp Orthop Traumatol*. 2011;24(1):39–44.
40. Bailey J, Heard D, Schumacher J, et al. Midazolam, butorphanol, ketamine, and the clinically effective dose of isoflurane anesthesia in ostriches (*Struthio camelus*). *25th Annu Meet Am Coll Vet Anesthesiol*. 38; 2000.
41. Bailey T. Raptors: respiratory problems. In: Chitty J, Lierz M, eds. *BSAVA Manual of Raptors, Pigeons and Passerine Birds*. Gloucester, UK: BSAVA; 2008:223–233.
42. Bailey TA, Apo MM. Pharmaceutics commonly used in avian medicine. In: Samour J, ed. *Avian Medicine*. 2nd ed. Edinburgh, Scotland: Mosby Elsevier; 2008:485–509.
43. Bailey TA, Apo MM. Pharmaceutics commonly used in avian medicine. In: Samour J, ed. *Avian Medicine*. 3rd ed. Edinburgh, Scotland: Mosby Elsevier; 2016:637–678.
44. Bailey TA, Sheen RS, Silvanose C, et al. Pharmacokinetics of enrofloxacin after intravenous, intramuscular and oral administration in houbara bustard (*Chlamydotis undulata macqueenii*). *J Vet Pharm Ther*. 1998;21:288–297.
45. Baillie JW. Alternative therapy ideas for feather picking. *Proc Annu Conf Assoc Avian Vet*. 2001:191–196.
46. Baine K, Hendrix DVH, Kuhn SE, et al. The efficacy and safety of topical rocuronium bromide to induce bilateral mydriasis in Hispaniolan Amazon parrots (*Amazona ventralis*). *J Avian Med Surg*. 2016;30(1):8–13.
47. Baine K, Jones MP, Cox S, et al. Pharmacokinetics of compounded intravenous and oral gabapentin in Hispaniolan Amazon parrots (*Amazona ventralis*). *J Avian Med Surg*. 2015;29:165–173.

48. Barboza T, Beaufrère H. Extrapyramidal side effects in a blue and gold macaw (*Ara ararauna*) treated with amitriptyline. *J Vet Behav*. 2017;22:19–23.
49. Barron H, Kehoe S, Bast R, et al. Use of intravenous lipid emulsion therapy as a novel treatment for brevetoxicosis in double-crested cormorants (*Phalacrocorax auritus*). *Proc ExoticsCon*. 2019:151 Published online.
50. Barron HW, Roberts RE, Latimer KS, et al. Tolerance doses of cutaneous and mucosal tissues in ring-necked parakeets (*Psittacula krameri*) for external beam megavoltage radiation. *J Avian Med Surg*. 2009;23(1):6–9.
51. Barsotti G, Asti M, Giani E, et al. Effect of topical ophthalmic instillation of rocuronium bromide on the intraocular pressure of kestrels (*Falco tinnunculus*) and little owls (*Athene noctuae*). *J Am Vet Med Assoc*. 2019;255:1359–1364.
52. Barsotti G, Briganti A, Spratte JR, et al. Bilateral mydriasis in common buzzards (*Buteo buteo*) and little owls (*Athene noctua*) induced by concurrent topical administration of rocuronium bromide. *Vet Ophthalmol*. 2010;13(Suppl 1):35–40.
53. Barsotti G, Briganti A, Spratte JR, et al. Mydriatic effect of topically applied rocuronium bromide in tawny owls (*Strix aluco*): comparison between two protocols. *Vet Ophthalmol*. 2010;13(Suppl):9–13.
54. Barsotti G, Briganti A, Spratte JR, et al. Safety and efficacy of bilateral topical application of rocuronium bromide for mydriasis in European kestrels (*Falco tinnunculus*). *J Avian Med Surg*. 2012;26(1):1–5.
55. Bartlett SL, Bailey R, Baitchman E. Diagnosis and management of diabetes mellitus in a Bali mynah (*Leucopsar rothschildi*). *J Avian Med Surg*. 2016;30(2):146–151.
56. Bauck L. *A Practitioner's Guide to Avian Medicine*. Lakewood, CO: American Animal Hospital Association; 1993.
57. Bauck L. Nutritional problems in pet birds. *Semin Avian Exot Pet Med*. 1995;4:3–8.
58. Bauck L, Brash M. Survey of diseases of the Lady Gouldian finch. *Proc Annu Conf Assoc Avian Vet*. 1999:204–212.
59. Bauck L, Hoefer HL. Avian antimicrobial therapy. *Semin Avian Exot Pet Med*. 1993;2:17–22.
60. Bauck L, Hillyer E, Hoefer H. Rhinitis: case reports. *Proc Annu Conf Assoc Avian Vet*. 1992:134–139.
61. Beaufrère H. Dyslipidemia/hyperlipidemia. In: Graham J, ed. *5-Minute Veterinary Consult: Avian*. Ames, IA: Blackwell Publishing; 2016:98–100.
62. Beaufrère H. Nebulization in birds. In: Samour J, ed. *Avian Medicine*. 3rd ed. St. Louis, MO: Elsevier; 2016:208–209.
63. Beaufrère H. Parenteral fluid therapy. In: Samour J, ed. *Avian Medicine. 3rd ed*. St. Louis, MO: Elsevier; 2016:209–215.
64. Beaufrère H. Clinical lipidology in psittacine birds. *Proc ExoticsCon*. 2020:10–15 Published online.
65. Beaufrère H. *Personal observation*. 2017/2020.
66. Beaufrère H, Guzman DS-M. Systemic diseases: disorders of the cardiovascular system. In: Samour J, ed. *Avian Medicine*. 3rd ed. St. Louis, MO: Elsevier; 2016:395–407.
67. Beaufrère H, Pinard C. Ocular lesions. In: Mayer J, Donnelly T, eds. *Clinical Veterinary Advisor: Birds and Exotic Pets*. St. Louis, MO: Elsevier; 2013:209–212.
68. Beaufrère H, Aertsens A, Fouquet J. Un cas d'insuffisance cardiaque congestive chez un perroquet gris. *L'Hebdo Vet*. 2007;200:8–10.
69. Beaufrère H, Schilliger L, Pariaut R. Cardiovascular system. In: Mitchell M, Tully T, eds. *Current Therapy in Exotic Pet Practice*. St. Louis, MO: Elsevier; 2016:151–220.
70. Beaufrère H, Summa N, Le K. Respiratory system. In: Mitchell M, Tully T, eds. *Current Therapy in Exotic Pet Practice*. St. Louis, MO: Elsevier; 2016:76–150.
71. Beaufrère H, Holder KA, Bauer R, et al. Intermittent claudication-like syndrome secondary to atherosclerosis in a yellow-naped Amazon parrot (*Amazona ochrocephala auropalliata*). *J Avian Med Surg*. 2011;25(4):266–276.
72. Beaufrère H, Laniesse D, Stickings P, et al. Generalized tetanus in a gyrfalcon (*Falco rusticolus*) with pododermatitis. *Avian Dis*. 2016;60(4):850–855.

73. Beaufrère H, Nevarez J, Gaschen L, et al. Diagnosis of presumed acute ischemic stroke and associated seizure management in a Congo African grey parrot. *J Am Vet Med Assoc.* 2011;239(1):122–128.
74. Beaufrère H, Nevarez J, Taylor WM, et al. Fluoroscopic study of the normal gastrointestinal motility and measurements in the Hispaniolan Amazon parrot (*Amazona ventralis*). *Vet Radiol Ultrasound.* 2010;51(4):441–446.
75. Beaufrère H, Papich MG, Brandão J, et al. Plasma drug concentrations of orally administered rosuvastatin in Hispaniolan Amazon parrots (*Amazona ventralis*). *J Avian Med Surg.* 2015;29(1):18–24.
76. Beaufrère H, Pariaut R, Rodriguez D, et al. Avian vascular imaging: a review. *J Avian Med Surg.* 2010;24(3):174–184.
77. Beaufrère H, Pariaut R, Rodriguez D, et al. Comparison of transcoelomic, contrast transcoelomic, and transesophageal echocardiography in anesthetized red-tailed hawks (*Buteo jamaicensis*). *Am J Vet Res.* 2012;73(10):1560–1568.
78. Beaufrère H, Rodriguez D, Pariaut R, et al. Estimation of intrathoracic arterial diameter by means of computed tomographic angiography in Hispaniolan Amazon parrots. *Am J Vet Res.* 2011;72(2):210–218.
79. Bechert U, Christensen JM, Poppenga R, et al. Pharmacokinetics of orally administered terbinafine in African penguins (*Spheniscus demersus*) for potential treatment of aspergillosis. *J Zoo Wild Med.* 2010;41:263–274.
80. Bechert U, Christensen JM, Poppenga R, et al. Pharmacokinetics of terbinafine after single oral dose administration in red-tailed hawks (*Buteo jamaicensis*). *J Avian Med Surg.* 2010;24:122–230.
81. Beckwith-Cohen B, Horowitz I, Bdolah-Abram T, et al. Differences in ocular parameters between diurnal and nocturnal raptors. *Vet Ophthalmol.* 2015;18(Suppl 1):98–105.
82. Beernaert LA, Baert K, Marin P, et al. Designing voriconazole treatment for racing pigeons: balancing between hepatic enzyme auto induction and toxicity. *Med Mycol.* 2009;47:276–285.
83. Beernaert LA, Pasmans F, Baert K, et al. Designing a treatment protocol with voriconazole to eliminate *Aspergillus fumigatus* from experimentally inoculated pigeons. *Vet Microbiol.* 2009;139:393–397.
84. Beernaert LA, Pasmans F, Van Waeyenberghe L, et al. Avian *Asperigillus fumigatus* strain resistant to both itraconazole and voriconazole. *Antimicrob Agents Chemother.* 2009;53:2199–2201.
85. Bennett R. Common avian emergencies. *Proc 5th Annu Intern Vet Emerg Crit Care Symp*; 1996:698–703.
86. Berg KJ, Guzman DSM, Knych HK, et al. Pharmacokinetics of amantadine after oral administration of single and multiple doses to orange-winged Amazon parrots (*Amazona amazonica*). *Am J Vet Res.* 2020;81(8):651–655.
87. Bernard JB, Allen ME. Feeding captive piscivorous animals: nutritional aspects of fish as food. *Nutritional Advisory Group Handbook.* 1997:1–11.
88. Best R. Breeding problems. In: Beynon PH, Forbes NA, Lawton MPC, eds. *BSAVA Manual of Raptors, Pigeons and Waterfowl.* Ames, IA: Iowa State University Press; 1996:202–215.
89. Beynon PH, Forbes NA, Harcourt-Brown NH. *Manual of Raptors, Pigeons and Waterfowl.* Ames, IA: Iowa State University Press; 1996.
90. Beynon PH, Forbes NA, Lawton MPC. *Manual of Psittacine Birds.* Ames, IA: Iowa State University Press; 1996.
91. Bicknese EJ. Review of avian sarcocystis. *Proc Annu Conf Assoc Avian Vet.* 1993:52–58.
92. Bigby SE, Carter JE, Bauquier S, et al. Use of propofol for induction and maintenance of anesthesia in a king penguin (*Aptenodytes patagonicus*) undergoing magnetic resonance imaging. *J Avian Med Surg.* 2016;30:237–242.
93. Bigham AS, Moghaddam Zamani, Finch AK. (*Taeneopygia guttata*) sedation with intranasal administration of diazepam, midazolam or xylazine. *J Vet Pharmacol Ther.* 2013;36:102–104.
94. Bird JE, Walser MM, Duke GE. Toxicity of gentamicin in red-tailed hawks (*Buteo jamaicensis*). *Am J Vet Res.* 1983;44:1289–1293.

95. Bird JE, Miller KW, Larson AA, et al. Pharmacokinetics of gentamicin in birds of prey. *Am J Vet Res*. 1983;44:1245–1247.
96. Bishop CR, Rorabaugh E. Evaluation of the safety and eficacy of selamectin in budgerigars with *Knemidokoptes* infection. *Proc Annu Conf Assoc Avian Vet*. 2010:79–84.
97. Bishop CR, McCoy B, Peter B. Selamectin tolerance in *Taeniopygia guttata* with *Sternostoma tracheacolum*. *Proc Annu Conf Assoc Avian Vet*. 2007:251–254.
98. Bishop Y, ed. *The Veterinary Formulary*. 5th ed. London, UK: Pharmaceutical Press; 2001.
99. Bloomfield RB, Brooks D, Vulliet R. The pharmacokinetics of a single intramuscular dose of amikacin in red-tailed hawks (*Buteo jamaicensis*). *J Zoo Wildl Med*. 1997;28:55–61.
100. Bonar CJ, Lewandowski AH. Use of a liposomal formulation of amphotericin B for treating wound aspergillosis in a goliath heron (*Ardea goliath*). *J Avian Med Surg*. 2004;18:162–166.
101. Bonar CJ, Lewandowski AH, Schaul J. Suspected fenbendazole toxicosis in 2 vulture species (*Gyps africanus, Torgos tracheliotus*) and marabou storks (*Leptoptilos crumeniferus*). *J Avian Med Surg*. 2003;17:16–19.
102. Bond M. Medication for vomiting psittacines. *J Assoc Avian Vet*. 1993:102 Published online.
103. Boonstra JL, Cox SK, Martin-Jimenez T. Pharmacokinetics of meloxicam after intramuscular and oral administration of a single dose to American flamingos (*Phoenicopterus ruber*). *Am J Vet Res*. 2017;78:267–273.
104. Boothe DM. Drugs affecting the respiratory system. *Vet Clin North Am Exot Anim Pract*. 2000;3:371–394.
105. Boothe DM. Drugs that modify animal behavior. In: Boothe DM, ed. *Small Animal Clinical Pharmacology and Therapeutics*. Philadelphia, PA: Saunders; 2001:457–472.
106. Boothe DM. Antibacterial agents. *The Merck Veterinary Manual*. 11th ed. 2016. Available at: www.merckvetmanual.com/pharmacology/antibacterial-agents. Accessed December 1, 2016.
107. Boothe DM. Antifungal agents. *The Merck Veterinary Manual*. 11th ed. 2016. Available at: www.merckvetmanual.com/pharmacology/antifungal-agents. Accessed December 1, 2016.
108. Botman J, Dugdale A, Gabriel F, et al. Cardiorespiratory parameters in the awake pigeon and during anaesthesia with isoflurane. *Vet Anaesth Analg*. 2016;43:63–71.
109. Botman J, Gabriel F, Dugdale AH, et al. Anaesthesia with sevoflurane in pigeons: minimal anaesthetic concentration (MAC) determination and investigation of cardiorespiratory variables at 1 MAC. *Vet Rec*. 2016;178:560.
110. Bowers V. Small insectivores. In: Duerr R, Gage L, eds. *Hand Rearing Birds*. 2nd ed. Hoboken, NJ: Wiley-Blackwell; 2020:665–682.
111. Bowles HL. Management with potassium bromide of seizures of undetermined origin in an umbrella cockatoo. *Exot DVM*. 2003;4(5):7–8.
112. Bowles H, Lichtenberger M, Lennox A. Emergency and critical care of pet birds. *Vet Clin North Am Exot Anim Pract*. 2007;10:345–394.
113. Bowman MR, Pare JA, Ziegler LE, et al. Effects of metoclopramide on the gastrointestinal tract motility of Hispaniolan parrots (*Amazona ventralis*). *Proc Annu Conf Am Assoc Zoo Vet*. 2002:117–118.
114. Bowman MR, Waldoch J, Pittman JM, et al. Enrofloxacin plasma concentrations in sandhill cranes (*Grus canadensis*) after administration in drinking water: a preliminary study. *Proc Annu Conf Am Assoc Zoo Vet*. 2002:389–390.
115. Brady S, Burgdorf A, Wack R. Treatment of pulmonary hypertension in a mealy Amazon parrot (*Amazona farinosa*) using sildenafil citrate. *J Avian Med Surg*. 2016;30:368–373.
116. Brandão J, da Cunha AF, Pypendop B, et al. Cardiovascular tolerance of intravenous lidocaine in broiler chickens (*Gallus gallus domesticus*) anesthetized with isoflurane. *Vet Anaesth Analg*. 2015;42:442–448.
117. Brandão J, Reynolds CA, Beaufrère H, et al. Cardiomyopathy in a Harris hawk (*Parabuteo unicinctus*). *J Am Vet Med Assoc*. 2016;249(2):221–227.
118. Braun EJ. Comparative renal function in reptiles, birds, and mammals. *Semin Avian Exot Pet Med*. 1998;7:62–71.
119. Breadner S. Chronic *Nocardia* infection in a hyacinth macaw. *Proc Annu Conf Assoc Avian Vet*. 1994:283–285.

120. Brenner DJ, Larsen RS, Dickinson PJ, et al. Development of an avian brachial plexus nerve block technique for perioperative analgesia in mallard ducks (*Anas platyrhynchos*). *J Avian Med Surg*. 2010;24(1):24–34.
121. Brightsmith DJ, McDonald D, Matsafuji D, et al. Nutritional content of the diets of free-living scarlet macaw chicks in southeastern Peru. *J Avian Med Surg*. 2010;24(1):9–23.
122. Brooks DE. Avian cataracts. *Semin Avian Exot Pet Med*. 1997;6:131–137.
123. Brown CS. Wild bird rehabilitation for the practicing veterinarian. *Proc Annu Conf Assoc Avian Vet*. 2003:207–219.
124. Browning GR, Carpenter JW, Magnin GC, et al. Pharmacokinetics of oral gabapentin in Caribbean flamingos (*Phoenicopterus ruber ruber*). *J Zoo Wildl Med*. 2018;49:609–616.
125. von Bruch J, Aufinger P, Jakoby JR. Untersuchungen zur pharmakokinetik und wirkung von intramuskulär, oral und über das trinkwasser verabreichtem sulfadimethoxine an gesunden und kokzidien-infizierten, adulten tauben (*Columba livia* Gmel., 1789, var. dom.). (Pharmacokinetics and efficacy of sulfadimethoxine in healthy and coccidia-infected adult pigeons.). *Vet Bull*. 1986;56:7830.
126. Bueno MG, Lopez RP, de Menezes RM, et al. Identification of *Plasmodium relictum* causing mortality in penguins (*Spheniscus magellanicus*) from São Paulo Zoo, Brazil. *Vet Parasitol*. 2010;173:123–127.
127. Bunting EM, Abou-Madi N, Cox S, et al. Evaluation of oral itraconazole administration in captive Humboldt penguins (*Spheniscus humboldti*). *J Zoo Wildl Med*. 2009;40:508–518.
128. Burhenne J, Haefeli WE, Hess M, et al. Pharmacokinetics, tissue concentrations, and safety of the antifungal agent voriconazole in chickens. *J Avian Med Surg*. 2008;22:199–207.
129. Burke TJ. Antibiotic therapy in pet birds and reptiles. In: Weber AJ, Grey S, Townsend K et al., eds. *Veterinary Pharmaceuticals and Biologicals*. 5th ed. Lenexa, KS: Veterinary Medicine Publishing Co; 1986.
130. Bush KM, Visser M, Boothe DM. Pharmacokinetics of compounded transdermal meloxicam in red-tailed hawks (*Buteo jamaicensis*). *Proc Annu Conf Assoc Avian Vet*. 2017:119.
131. Bush M, Neal LA, Custer RS. Preliminary pharmacokinetic studies of selected antibiotics in birds. *Proc Annu Conf Assoc Avian Vet*. 1979:45–47.
132. Bush M, Locke D, Neal LA, et al. Gentamicin tissue concentration in various avian species following recommended dosage therapy. *Am J Vet Res*. 1981;42:2114–2116.
133. Bush M, Locke D, Neal LA, et al. Pharmacokinetics of cephalothin and cephalexin in selected avian species. *Am J Vet Res*. 1981;42:1014–1017.
134. Byrne RF, Davis C, Lister SA, et al. Prescribing for birds. In: Bishop Y, ed. *The Veterinary Formulary. 5th ed*. London, UK: Pharmaceutical Press; 2001:43–56.
135. Cambre RC, Kenny D. Vaccination of zoo birds against avian botulism with mink botulism vaccine. *Proc Annu Conf Am Assoc Zoo Vet*. 1993:383–385.
136. Campbell TW, Smith SA, Zimmerman KL. Hematology of waterfowl and raptors. In: Weiss DJ, Wardrop KJ, eds. *Schalm's Veterinary Hematology*. 6th ed. Ames, IA: Blackwell Publishing; 2010:978–979.
137. Canny CJ, Ward DA, Patton S, et al. Microsporidian keratoconjunctivitis in a double yellow-headed Amazon parrot (*Amazona ochrocephala oratrix*). *J Avian Med Surg*. 1999;13:279–286.
138. Carnarius M, Hafez HM, Henning A, et al. Clinical signs and diagnosis of thiamine deficiency in juvenile goshawks (*Accipiter gentilis*). *Vet Rec*. 2008;163(7):215–217.
139. Carpenter JW. Cranes (Order Gruiformes). In: Fowler ME, ed. *Zoo and Wild Animal Medicine*. 2nd ed. Philadelphia, PA: Saunders; 1986:315–326.
140. Carpenter JW. Infectious and parasitic diseases of cranes. In: Fowler ME, ed. *Zoo and Wild Animal Medicine: Current Therapy 3*. Philadelphia, PA: Saunders; 1993:229–237.
141. Carpenter JW. Gruiformes (cranes, limpkins, rails, gallinules, coots, bustards). In: Fowler ME, Miller RE, eds. *Zoo and Wild Animal Medicine*. 5th ed. St. Louis, MO: Saunders; 2003:171–180.
142. Carpenter JW. *Personal observation*; 2013.
143. Carpenter JW, Hawkins MG, Barron H. Appendix 1: Table of common drugs and approximate doses. In: Speer B, ed. *Current Therapy in Avian Medicine and Surgery*. St. Louis, MO: Elsevier; 2016:795–824.

144. Carpenter JW, Novilla MN, Hatfield JS. The safety and physiological effects of the anticoccidial drugs monensin and clazuril in sandhill cranes (*Grus canadensis*). *J Zoo Wildl Med.* 1992;23:214–221.
145. Carpenter JW, Novilla MN, Hatfield JS. Efficacy of selected coccidiostats in sandhill cranes (*Grus canadensis*) following challenge. *J Zoo Wildl Med.* 2005;36:391–400.
146. Carpenter JW, Hunter RP, Olsen JH, et al. Pharmacokinetics of marbofloxacin in blue and gold macaws (*Ara ararauna*). *Am J Vet Res.* 2006;67:947–950.
147. Carpenter JW, Olsen JH, Randle-Port M, et al. Pharmacokinetics of azithromycin in the blue and gold macaw (*Ara ararauna*) after intravenous and oral administration. *J Zoo Wildl Med.* 2005;36:606–609.
148. Carpenter JW, Tully Jr TN, Gehring R, et al. Single-dose pharmacokinetics of piperacillin/tazobactam in Hispaniolan Amazon parrots (*Amazona ventralis*). *J Avian Med Surg.* 2017;31(2):95–101.
149. Carpenter NA. Anseriform and galliform therapeutics. *Vet Clin North Am Exot Anim Pract.* 2000;3:1–17.
150. Carter RT, Murphy CJ, Stuhr CM, et al. Bilateral phacoemulsification and intraocular lens implantation in a great horned owl. *J Am Vet Med Assoc.* 2007;230:559–561.
151. Ceulemans SM, Guzman DS, Olsen GH, et al. Evaluation of thermal antinociceptive effects after intramuscular administration of buprenorphine hydrochloride to American kestrels (*Falco sparverius*). *Am J Vet Res.* 2014;75:705–710.
152. Chaleva EI, Vasileva IV, Savova MD. Absorption of lincomycin through the respiratory pathways and its influence on alveolar macrophages after aerosol administration to chickens. *Res Vet Sci.* 1994;57:245–247.
153. Chan FT, Chang GR, Wang HC, et al. Anesthesia with isoflurane and sevoflurane in the crested serpent eagle (*Spilornis cheela hoya*): minimum anesthetic concentration, physiological effects, hematocrit, plasma chemistry and behavioral effects. *J Vet Med Sci.* 2013;75:1591–1600.
154. Chang GJ, Davis BS, Stringfield C, et al. Prospective immunization of the endangered California condors (*Gymnogyps californianus*) protects this species from lethal West Nile virus infection. *Vaccine.* 2007;25:2325–2330.
155. Chen LJ, Sun BH, Qu JP, et al. Avermectin induced inflammation damage in king pigeon brain. *Chemosphere.* 2013;93:2528–2534.
156. Chiadmi F, Lyer A, Cisternino S, et al. Stability of levamisole oral solutions prepared from tablets and powder. *J Pharm Pharm Sci.* 2005;8:322–825.
157. Childs-Sanford SE, Rassnick KM, Alcaraz A. Carboplatin for treatment of a Sertoli cell tumor in a mallard (*Anas platyrhynchos*). *Vet Comp Oncol.* 2006;4(1):51–56.
158. Chitty J. Birds of prey. In: Meredith A, Redrobe S, eds. *BSAVA Manual of Exotic Pets.* Gloucester, UK: British Small Animal Veterinary Association; 2002:179–192.
159. Formulary. In: Chitty J, Lierz M, Chitty J, Lierz M, eds. *BSAVA Manual of Raptors, Pigeons and Passerine Birds.* Gloucester, UK: British Small Animal Veterinary Association; 2008:384–390.
160. Chitty J, Lierz M. Appendix 3-Laboratory reference ranges. In: Chitty J, Lierz M, eds. *BSAVA Manual of Raptors, Pigeons and Passerine Birds.* Gloucester, UK: British Small Animal Veterinary Association; 2008:394–397.
161. Church ML, Priehs DR, Denis H, et al. Technique, postoperative complications, and visual outcomes of phacoemulsification cataract surgery in 21 penguins (27 eyes): 2011-2015. *Vet Ophthalmol.* 2018;21(6):612–621.
162. Clark CH, Thomas JE, Milton JL, et al. Plasma concentrations of chloramphenicol in birds. *Am J Vet Res.* 1982;43:1949.
163. Clarke CR, Kocan AA, Webb AI, et al. Intravenous pharmacokinetics of penicillin G and antipyrine in ostriches and emus. *J Zoo Wildl Med.* 2001;32:74–77.
164. Clippinger TL. Diseases of the lower respiratory tract of companion birds. *Semin Avian Exot Pet Med.* 1997;6:201–208.
165. Clubb SL. Therapeutics. In: Harrison GJ, Harrison LR, eds. *Clinical Avian Medicine and Surgery.* Philadelphia, PA: Saunders; 1986:327–355.

166. Clubb SL. Birds. In: Johnston DE, ed. *The Bristol Veterinary Handbook of Antimicrobial Therapy*. 2nd ed. Trenton, NJ: Veterinary Learning Systems; 1987:188–199.
167. Clubb SL. Clinical management of psittacine birds affected with proventricular dilation disease. *Proc Annu Conf Assoc Avian Vet*. 2006:85–90.
168. Clubb SL, Schubot RM, Joyner K, et al. Hematologic and serum biochemical reference intervals in juvenile eclectus parrots (*Eclectus roratus*). *J Assoc Avian Vet*. 1990;4:218–225.
169. Clubb SL, Schubot RM, Joyner K, et al. Hematologic and serum biochemical reference intervals in juvenile cockatoos. *J Assoc Avian Vet*. 1991;5:16–26.
170. Clubb SL, Schubot RM, Joyner K, et al. Hematologic and serum biochemical reference intervals in juvenile macaws (*Ara sp.* [sic.]). *J Assoc Avian Vet*. 1991;5:154–162.
171. Clyde V, Kollias G. Diet-associated gout in juvenile macaws. *Proc Annu Conf Am Assoc Zoo Vet*. 1989:90.
172. Clyde VL, Patton S. Diagnosis, treatment and control of common parasites in companion and aviary birds. *Semin Avian Exot Pet Med*. 1996;5:75–84.
173. Cockcroft PD, Jones AC, Harris JM. Antibacterial activity of ceftiofur-impregnated polymethylmethacrylate beads following manufacture, storage and sterilisation. *Vet Rec*. 2003;152:21–22.
174. Cole GA, Paul-Murphy J, Krugner-Higby L, et al. Analgesic effects of intramuscular administration of meloxicam in Hispaniolan parrots (*Amazona ventralis*) with experimentally induced arthritis. *Am J Vet Res*. 2009;70:1471–1476.
175. Coles BH. Cage and aviary birds. In: Beynon PH, Cooper JE, eds. *Manual of Exotic Pets*. Worthing, UK: British Small Animal Veterinary Association; 1991:150–179.
176. Coles BH. Appendix 1: An avian formulary. *Avian Medicine and Surgery*. 2nd ed. Oxford, UK: Blackwell Science, Osney Mead; 1997:240–278.
177. Coles BH. Prescribing for exotic birds. In: Bishop Y, ed. *The Veterinary Formulary*. 5th ed. London, UK: Pharmaceutical Press; 2001:99–105.
178. Cooper JE, Appendix IX. Medicines and other agents used in treatment, including emergency anaesthesia kit and avian resuscitation protocol. In: Cooper JE, ed. *Birds of Prey: Health and Disease*. 3rd ed. Ames, IA: Blackwell Publishing, Iowa State Press; 2002:271–277.
179. Cooper RG. Bacterial, fungal and parasitic infections in the ostrich (*Struthio camelus var. domesticus*). *Anim Sci J*. 2005;76:97–106.
180. Cornelissen H. Behavior, anatomy, feeding and medical problems of toucans in captivity. *Proc Eur Conf Avian Med Surg*. 1993:446–453.
181. Cornelissen H, Ducatelle R, Roels S. Successful treatment of a channel-billed toucan (*Ramphastos vitellinus*) with iron storage disease by chelation therapy: sequential monitoring of the iron content of the liver during the treatment period by quantitative chemical and image analyses. *J Avian Med Surg*. 1995;9:131–137.
182. Cornick JL. *Veterinary Anesthesia*. Woburn, MA: Butterworth-Heinemann; 2001:196–198.
183. Corum O, Durna Corum D, Atik O, et al. Pharmacokinetics and bioavailability of danofloxacin in chukar partridge (*Alectoris chukar*) following intravenous, intramuscular, subcutaneous, and oral administrations. *J Vet Pharmacol Ther*. 2019;42(2):207–213.
184. Costantini V, Carraro C, Bucci FA, et al. Influence of a new slow-release GnRH analogue implant on reproduction in the budgerigar (*Melopsittacus undulatus*). *Anim Repro Sci*. 2009;111:289–301.
185. Cowan ML, Martin GB, Monks DJ, et al. Inhibition of the reproductive system by deslorelin in male and female pigeons (*Columba livia*). *J Avian Med Surg*. 2014;28:102–108.
186. Cray C. University of Miami Avian and Wildlife Laboratory avian reference ranges. University of Miami Web site. Available at: http://www.cpl.med.miami.edu/documents/avian_reference_ranges.pdf. Accessed June 15, 2017.
187. Cray C, Rodriguez M, Zaias J. Protein electrophoresis of psittacine plasma. *Vet Clin Pathol*. 2007;36(1):64–72.
188. Crispin SM, Barnett KC. Ocular candidiasis in ornamental ducks. *Avian Pathol*. 1978;7(1):49–59.

189. Cross G. Antiviral therapy. *Semin Avian Exot Pet Med*. 1995;4:96–102.
190. Crosta L, Delli Carri AP. Oral treatment with clindamycin in racing pigeons. *Proc First Conf Eur Comm Assoc Avian Vet*. 1991:293–296.
191. Cubas ZS. Medicine: Family Rhamphastidae (toucans). In: Fowler ME, Cubas ZS, eds. *Biology, Medicine, and Surgery of South American Wild Animals*. Ames, IA: Iowa State University Press; 2001:188–199.
192. Curro TG. Evaluation of the isoflurane-sparing effects of butorphanol and flunixin in psittaciformes. *Proc Annu Conf Assoc Avian Vet*. 1994:17–19.
193. Curro TG, Brunson DB, Paul-Murphy J. Determination of the ED_{50} of isoflurane and evaluation of the isoflurane-sparing effect of butorphanol in cockatoos (*Cacatua* spp.). *Vet Surg*. 1994;23:429–433.
194. Cusack L, Field C, McDermott A, et al. Right heart failure in an African penguin (*Spheniscus demersus*). *J Avian Med Surg*. 2016;30(3):243–249.
195. Cushing A, McClean M. Use of thiafentanil-medetomidine for the induction of anesthesia in emus (*Dromaius novaehollandiae*) within a wild animal park. *J Zoo Wildl Med*. 2010;41:234–241.
196. Custer RS, Bush M, Carpenter JW. Pharmacokinetics of gentamicin in blood plasma of quail, pheasants, and cranes. *Am J Vet Res*. 1979;40:892–895.
197. Cuthbert R, Parry-Jones J, Green RE, et al. NSAIDs and scavenging birds: potential impacts beyond Asia's critically endangered vultures. *Biol Lett*. 2007;3:90–93.
198. Cutler DC, Shiomitsu K, Liu C-C, et al. Comparison of calculated radiation delivery versus actual radiation delivery in military macaws (*Ara militaris*). *J Avian Med Surg*. 2016;30(1):1–7.
199. da Cunha AF, Strain GM, Rademacher N, et al. Palpation- and ultrasound-guided brachial plexus blockade in Hispaniolan Amazon parrots (*Amazona ventralis*). *Vet Anaesth Analg*. 2013;40:96–102.
200. Dahlhausen B, Aldred S, Colaizzi E. Resolution of clinical proventricular dilatation disease by cyclooxygenase 2 inhibition. *Proc Annu Conf Assoc Avian Vet*. 2002:9–12.
201. Dahlhausen B, Lindstrom JG, Radabaugh CS. The use of terbinafine hydrochloride in the treatment of avian fungal disease. *Proc Annu Conf Assoc Avian Vet*. 2000:35–39.
202. Davidson G. Veterinary pharmacy. In: Riviere JE, Papich MG, eds. *Veterinary Pharmacology and Therapeutics*. 9th ed. Hoboken, NJ: Wiley-Blackwell; 2009:1413.
203. Davies RR. Passerine birds: going light. In: Chitty J, Lierz M, eds. *BSAVA Manual of Raptors, Pigeons and Passerine Birds*. Gloucester, UK: British Small Animal Veterinary Association; 2008:365–369.
204. Davis MR, Langan JN, Johnson YJ, et al. West Nile virus seroconversion in penguins after vaccination with a killed virus vaccine or a DNA vaccine. *J Zoo Wildl Med*. 2008;39:582–589.
205. de Andrade JG, Lelis RT, Damatta RA, et al. Occurrence of nematodes and anthelmintic management of ostrich farms from different Brazilian states: *Libyostrongylus douglassii* dominates mixed infections. *Vet Parasitol*. 2011;178:129–133.
206. De Francisco N, Ruiz Troya JD, Agüera EI. Lead and lead toxicity in domestic and free living birds. *Avian Pathol*. 2003;32:3–13.
207. De Herdt P, Devriese LA, De Groote B, et al. Antibiotic treatment of *Streptococcus bovis* infections in pigeons. *Proc Eur Conf Avian Med Surg*. 1993:297–304.
208. de Lucas JJ, Rodríguez C, Waxman S, et al. Pharmacokinetics of marbofloxacin after intravenous and intramuscular administration to ostriches. *Vet J*. 2005;3:364–368.
209. de Matos R. Calcium metabolism in birds. *Vet Clin North Am Exot Anim Pract*. 2008;11(1):59–82.
210. de Souza LP, Lelis RT, Granja IR, et al. Efficacy of albendazole and moxidectin and resistance to ivermectin against *Libyostrongylus douglassii* and *Libyostrongylus dentatus* in ostriches. *Vet Parasitol*. 2012;189:387–389.
211. De Voe RS, Trogdon M, Flammer K. Preliminary assessment of the effect of diet and L-carnitine supplementation on lipoma size and bodyweight in budgerigars (*Melopsittacus undulatus*). *J Avian Med Surg*. 2004;18:12–18.
212. Degernes LA. Topics in emergency medicine: fluid therapy and parenteral nutrition. *Proc Avian Specialty Advanced Prog Small Mam and Rept Med Surg (Annu Conf Assoc Avian Vet)*; 1998:55–60.

213. Degernes LA, Talbot BJ, Mueller LR. Raptor foot care. *J Assoc Avian Vet*. 1990;4(2):93–95.
214. Degernes LA, Crosier ML, Harrison LD, et al. Autologous, homologous, and heterologous red blood cell transfusions in cockatiels (*Nymphicus hollandicus*). *J Avian Med Surg*. 1999;13(1):2–9.
215. Degernes L, Davidson G, Flammer K, et al. Administration of total parenteral nutrition in pigeons. *Am J Vet Res*. 1994;55:660–665.
216. Degernes LA, Fisher PE, Trogdon M, et al. Gastrointestinal scintigraphy in psittacines. *Proc Annu Conf Assoc Avian Vet*. 1999:93–94.
217. Degernes LA, Harrison LD, Smith DW, et al. Autologous, homologous and heterologous red blood cell transfusions in conures of the genus *Aratinga*. *J Avian Med Surg*. 1999;13:10–14.
218. Delaski KM, Nelson S, Dronen NO, et al. Detection and management of air sac trematodes (*Szidatitrema* species) in captive multispecies avian exhibits. *J Avian Med Surg*. 2015;29(4):345–353.
219. Delk K. Clinical management of seizures in avian patients. *J Exot Pet Med*. 2012;21(2):132–139.
220. Denver MC, Tell LA, Galey FD. Comparison of two heavy metal chelators for treatment of lead toxicosis in cockatiels. *Am J Vet Res*. 2000;61:935–940.
221. Desmarchelier MR. Clinical psychopharmacology for the exotic animal practitioner. *Vet Clin North Am Exot Anim Pract*. 2021;24:17–35.
222. Desmarchelier M, Troncy E, Fitzgerald G, et al. Analgesic effects of meloxicam administration on postoperative orthopedic pain in domestic pigeons (*Columba livia*). *Am J Vet Res*. 2012;73:361–367.
223. Dheeraj A, Seema A, Astha C. Effect of fipronil toxicity in haematological parameters in white leghorn cockerels. *Afri J Agricult Res*. 2014;9:2759–2764.
224. Dhondt L, Devreese M, Croubels S, et al. Comparative population pharmacokinetics and absolute oral bioavailability of COX-2 selective inhibitors celecoxib, mavacoxib and meloxicam in cockatiels (*Nymphicus hollandicus*). *Sci Rep*. 2017;7(1):1–12.
225. Di Somma A, Bailey T, Silvanose C, et al. The use of voriconazole for the treatment of aspergillosis in falcons (*Falco* species). *J Avian Med Surg*. 2007;21:307–316.
226. DiGeronimo PM, da Cunha AF, Pypendop B, et al. Cardiovascular tolerance of intravenous bupivacaine in broiler chickens (*Gallus gallus domesticus*) anesthetized with isoflurane. *Vet Anaesth Analg*. 2017;44:287–294.
227. Dijkstra B, Guzman DS, Gustavsen K, et al. Renal, gastrointestinal, and hemostatic effects of oral administration of meloxicam to Hispaniolan Amazon parrots (*Amazona ventralis*). *Am J Vet Res*. 2015;76:308–317.
228. Dodwell GT. *The Complete Book of Canaries*. London, UK: Merehurst Press; 1986.
229. Doneley B. Acute pancreatitis in parrots. *Exot DVM*. 2003;4:13–16.
230. Doneley B. Management of captive ratites. In: Harrison GJ, Lightfoot TL, eds. Palm Beach, FL: Spix Publishing; 2006. *Clinical Avian Medicine*. Vol II:957–989.
231. Doneley B. The use of gabapentin to treat presumed neuralgia in a little corella (*Cacatua sanguinea*). *Proc Austral Assoc Avian Vet*. 2007:169–172.
232. Doneley B. Formulary. In: Doneley B, ed. *Avian Medicine and Surgery in Practice: Companion and Aviary Birds*. London, UK: Manson Publishing; 2011:285–320.
233. Doneley B. *Avian Medicine and Surgery in Practice: Companion and Aviary Birds*. 2nd ed. Boca Raton, FL: CRC Press; 2016.
234. Donnelly RF, Pascuet E, Ma C, et al. Stability of celecoxib oral suspension. *Can J Hosp Pharm*. 2009;62:464–468.
235. Doolen M. Adriamycin® chemotherapy in a blue-front Amazon with osteosarcoma. *Proc Annu Conf Assoc Avian Vet*. 1994:89–91.
236. Dorrestein GM. *Studies on Pharmacokinetics of Some Antibacterial Agents in Homing Pigeons (Columba livia)*: Thesis: Utrecht University; 1986.
237. Dorrestein GM. Formulation and (bio)availability problems of drug formulations in birds. *J Vet Pharmacol Therap*. 1992;15:143–150.
238. Dorrestein GM. Antimicrobial drug use in companion birds. In: Prescott JF, Baggot JD, eds. *Antimicrobial Therapy in Veterinary Medicine*. 2nd ed. Ames, IA: Iowa State University Press; 1993:491–506.

239. Dorrestein GM. Infectious diseases and their therapy in Passeriformes*Antimicrobial Therapy in Caged Birds and Exotic Pets*. Trenton, NJ: Veterinary Learning Systems; 1995:11–27.
240. Dorrestein GM. Antimicrobial drug use in companion birds. In: Prescott JF, Baggot JD, Walker RD, eds. *Antimicrobial Therapy in Veterinary Medicine*. 3rd ed. Ames, IA: Iowa State University Press; 2000:617–636.
241. Dorrestein GM. Passerine and softbill therapeutics. *Vet Clin North Am Exot Anim Pract*. 2000;3:35–57.
242. Dorrestein GM, Kazemi SM, Eksik N, et al. Comparative study of Synulox® and Augmentin after intravenous, intramuscular and oral administration in collared doves (*Streptopelia decaocto*). In: Kösters J et al., ed. *X. Tagung der Fachgruppe "Geflügelkrankheiten." Giessen*. Germany: Deutschen Veterinärmedizinischen Gesellschaft e.V; 1996:42–54.
243. Dorrestein GM, van Gogh H, Rinzema JD. Pharmacokinetic aspects of penicillins, aminoglycosides and chloramphenicol in birds compared to mammals: a review. *Vet Quart*. 1984;6:216–224.
244. Dorrestein GM, van Der Horst HHA, Cremers HJWM, et al. Quill mite (*Dermoglyphus passerinus*) infestation of canaries (*Serinus canaria*): diagnosis and treatment. *Avian Pathol*. 1997;26:195–199.
245. Dorrestein GM, Van Gogh H, Rinzema JD, et al. Comparative study of ampicillin and amoxicillin after intravenous, intramuscular and oral administration in homing pigeons (*Columba livia*). *Res Vet Sci*. 1987;42:343–348.
246. Doss GA, Williams JM, Mans C. Contrast fluoroscopic evaluation of gastrointestinal transit times with and without the use of falconry hoods in red-tailed hawks (*Buteo jamaicensis*). *J Am Vet Med Assoc*. 2017;251(9):1064–1069.
247. Doss GA, Williams JM, Mans C. Determination of gastrointestinal transit times in barred owls (*Strix varia*) by contrast fluoroscopy. *J Avian Med Surg*. 2017;31(2):123–127.
248. Doss GA, Mans C, Johnson L, et al. Diagnosis and management of inflammatory bowel disease in a harpy eagle (*Harpia harpyja*) with suspected fenbendazole toxicosis. *J Am Vet Med Assoc*. 2018;252(3):336–342.
249. d'Ovidio D, Noviello E, Adami C. Nerve stimulator-guided sciatic-femoral nerve block in raptors undergoing surgical treatment of pododermatitis. *Vet Anaesth Analg*. 2015;42:449–453.
250. Dressen PJ, Wimsatt J, Burkhard MJ. The effects of isoflurane anesthesia on hematologic and plasma biochemical values of American kestrels (*Falco sparverius*). *J Avian Med Surg*. 1999;13(3):173–179.
251. Dumonceaux G, Harrison GJ. Toxins. In: Ritchie BW, Harrison GJ, Harrison LR, eds. *Avian Medicine: Principles and Application*. Delray Beach, FL: Wingers Publishing; 1994:1030–1052.
252. Duvall A, Tully TN, Carpenter JW, et al. Pilot study of a single dose of orally administered tapentadol suspension in Hispaniolan Amazon parrots (*Amazona ventralis*). *J Am Med Surg*. 2021;35(1):45–50.
253. Dyer DC, Van Alstine WG. Antibiotic aerosolization: tissue and plasma oxytetracycline concentrations in parakeets. *Avian Dis*. 1987;31:677–679.
254. Echols S, Speer B. Omega-3 fatty acid supplementation: potential uses and limitations. *Proc Annu Assoc Avian Med*. 2000:13–16 Published online.
255. Edling TM. Anaesthesia and analgesia. In: Chitty J, Harcourt-Brown N, eds. *BSAVA Manual of Psittacine Birds*. Gloucester, UK: British Small Animal Veterinary Association; 2005:87–96.
256. Efstathopoulos N, Giamarellos-Bourboulis E, Kanellakopoulou K, et al. Treatment of experimental osteomyelitis by methicillin resistant *Staphylococcus aureus* with bone cement system releasing grepafloxacin. *Injury*. 2008;39:1384–1390.
257. Ehrlich PR, Dobkin DS, Wheye D. *The Birder's Handbook: A Field Guide to the Natural History of North American Birds*. New York, NY: Simon & Schuster; 1988.
258. Elliston E, Perlman J. Meeting the protein requirements of adult hummingbirds in captivity. *J Wildl Rehab*. 2002;25:14–19.
259. Emery LC, Cox SK, Souza MJ. Pharmacokinetics of nebulized terbinafine in Hispaniolan Amazon parrots (*Amazona ventralis*). *J Avian Med Surg*. 2012;26(3):161–166.

260. Ensley PK, Janssen DL. A preliminary study comparing the pharmacokinetics of ampicillin given orally and intramuscularly to psittacines: Amazon parrots (*Amazona* spp.) and blue-naped parrots (*Tanygnathus lucionensis*). *J Zoo Anim Med.* 1981;12:42–47.
261. Ernst S, Goggin JM, Biller DS, et al. Comparison of iohexol and barium sulfate as gastrointestinal contrast media in mid-sized psittacine birds. *J Avian Med Surg.* 1998;12:16–20.
262. Escobar A, Thiesen R, Vitaliano SN, et al. Some cardiopulmonary effects of sevoflurane in crested caracara (*Caracara plancus*). *Vet Anaesth Analg.* 2009;36:436–441.
263. Escudero E, Vicente MS, Carceles CM. Pharmacokinetics of amoxicillin/clavulanic acid combination after intravenous and intramuscular administration to pigeons. *Res Vet Sci.* 1998;65(1):77–81.
264. Esperon F, Martin MP, Lopes F, et al. *Gongylonema* sp. infection in the scops owl (*Otus scops*). *Parasitol Int.* 2013;62:502–504.
265. Esposito JF. Respiratory medicine. *Vet Clin North Am Exot Anim Pract.* 2000;3:395–402.
266. Ethell MT, Bennett RA, Brown MP, et al. In vitro elution of gentamicin, amikacin and ceftiofur from polymethylmethacrylate and hydroxyapatite cement. *Vet Surg.* 2000;29:375–382.
267. Eugenio CT. Amitriptyline HCl: clinical study for treatment of feather picking. *Proc Annu Conf Assoc Avian Vet.* 2003:133–135.
268. Evans EE, Wade LL, Flammer K. Administration of doxycycline in drinking water for treatment of spiral bacterial infection in cockatiels. *J Am Vet Med Assoc.* 2008;232:389–393.
269. Evans EE, Emery LC, Cox SK, et al. Pharmacokinetics of terbinafine after oral administration of a single dose to Hispaniolan Amazon parrots (*Amazona ventralis*). *Am J Vet Res.* 2013;74(6):835–838.
270. Fallon JA, Redig P, Miller TA, et al. Guidelines for evaluation and treatment of lead poisoning of wild raptors. *Wildl Soc Bull.* 2017;41(2):205–211.
271. Farca AM, Piromalli G, Maffei F, et al. Potentiating effect of EDTA-Tris on the activity of antibiotics against resistant bacteria associated with otitis, dermatitis and cystitis. *J Small Anim Pract.* 1997;38:243–245.
272. Ferrell ST, Graham JE, Swaim SF. Avian wound healing and management. *Proc Annu Conf Assoc Avian Vet.* 2002:337–347.
273. Ferrell ST, Marlar AB, Garner M, et al. Intralesional cisplatin chemotherapy and topical cryotherapy for the control of choanal squamous cell carcinoma in an African penguin (*Spensiscus demersus*). *J Zoo Wildl Med.* 2006;37(4):539–541.
274. Filippich LJ, O'Donoghue PJ. *Cochlosoma* infections in finches. *Aust Vet J.* 1997;75:561–563.
275. Filippich LJ, Parker MG. Megabacteria and proventricular/ventricular disease in psittacines and passerines. *Proc Annu Conf Assoc Avian Vet.* 1994:287–293.
276. Filippich LJ, Perry RA. Drug trials against megabacteria in budgerigars (*Melopsittacus undulatus*). *Aust Vet Pract.* 1993;23:184–189.
277. Filippich LJ, Bucher AM, Charles BG. Platinum pharmacokinetics in sulphur-crested cockatoos (*Cacatua galerita*) following single-dose cisplatin infusion. *Aust Vet J.* 2000;78:406–411.
278. Filippich LJ, Bucher AM, Charles BG, et al. Intravenous cisplatin administration in sulphur-crested cockatoos (*Cacatua galerita*): clinical and pathologic observations. *J Avian Med Surg.* 2001;15:23–30.
279. Filippich LJ, Charles BG, Sutton RH, et al. Carboplatin administration in sulphur-crested cockatoos (*Cacatua galerita*): clinical observations. *J Avian Med Surg.* 2005;19:92–97.
280. Fink D, Mans C. Use of amlodipine in psittacine birds: 5 cases (2010-2018). *J Avian Med Surg.* 2021:155–160.
281. Finlayson GR, Chilvers BL, Pearson H, et al. Efficacy of seawater for washing oiled birds during an oil spill response. *Mar Pollut Bull.* 2018;126:137–140.
282. Fitzgerald B, Beaufrère H. Cardiology. In: Speer B, ed. *Current Therapy in Avian Medicine and Surgery.* St. Louis, MO: Elsevier; 2016:252–328.
283. Fitzgerald BC, Dias S, Martorell J. Cardiovascular drugs in avian, small mammal, and reptile medicine. *Vet Clin North Am Exot Anim Pract.* 2018;21(2):399–442.

284. Fitzgerald G, Cooper JE. Preliminary studies on the use of propofol in the domestic pigeon (*Columba livia*). *Vet Sci*. 1990;49:334–338.
285. Flammer K. An overview of antifungal therapy in birds. *Proc Annu Conf Assoc Avian Vet*. 1993:1–4.
286. Flammer K. A review of the pharmacology of antimicrobial drugs in birds. *Proc Avian/Exot Anim Med Symp*. 1994:65–78.
287. Flammer K. Fluconazole in psittacine birds. *Proc Annu Conf Assoc Avian Vet*. 1996:203–204.
288. Flammer K. Approach to the vomiting bird. *Proc 21st Annu Waltham®/OSU Symp*; 1997:19–21.
289. Flammer K. Common bacterial infections and antibiotic use in companion birds. *Antimicrobial Therapy in Exotics; Supplement to Comp Cont Edu Pract Vet*. 1998;20(3A):34–48.
290. Flammer K. Doxycycline-medicated seed for treatment of chlamydiosis. *Proc Annu Conf Assoc Avian Vet*. 2002:7–8.
291. Flammer K. Treatment of bacterial and mycotic diseases of the avian gastrointestinal tract. *Proc North Am Vet Conf*. 2002:851–852.
292. Flammer K. Antifungal drug update. *Proc Annu Conf Assoc of Avian Vet*. 2006;3.
293. Flammer K, Papich M. Assessment of plasma concentration and effects of injectable doxycycline in three psittacine species. *J Avian Med Surg*. 2005;19:216–224.
294. Flammer K, Papich M. Pharmacokinetics of fluconazole after oral administration of single and multiple doses in African grey parrots. *Am J Vet Res*. 2006;67(3):417–422.
295. Flammer K, Whitt-Smith D. Plasma concentrations of enrofloxacin psittacine birds offered water medicated with 200 mg/L of the injectable formulation of enrofloxacin. *J Avian Med Surg*. 2002;16:286–290.
296. Flammer K, Aucoin DP, Whitt DA. Intramuscular and oral disposition of enrofloxacin in African grey parrots following single and multiple doses. *J Vet Pharmacol Therap*. 1991;41:359–366.
297. Flammer K, Whitt-Smith D, Papich M. Plasma concentrations of doxycycline in selected psittacine birds when administered in water for potential treatment of *Chlamydophila psittaci* infection. *J Avian Med Surg*. 2001;15:276–282.
298. Flammer K, Aucoin DP, Whitt DA, et al. Plasma concentrations of enrofloxacin in African grey parrots treated with medicated water. *Avian Dis*. 1990;34:228–234.
299. Flammer K, Aucoin DP, Whitt DA, et al. Potential use of long-acting injectable oxytetracycline for treatment of chlamydiosis in Goffin's cockatoos. *Avian Dis*. 1990;34:1017–1022.
300. Flammer K, Clark CH, Drewes LA, et al. Adverse effects of gentamicin in scarlet macaws and galahs. *Am J Vet Res*. 1990;51:404–407.
301. Flammer K, Massey JG, Roudybush T, et al. Assessment of plasma concentrations and potential adverse effects of doxycycline in cockatiels (*Nymphicus hollandicus*) fed a medicated pelleted diet. *J Avian Med Surg*. 2013;27:187–193.
302. Flammer K, Nettifee-Osborne JA, Webb DJ, et al. Pharmacokinetics of voriconazole after oral administration of single and multiple doses in African grey parrots (*Psittacus erithacus timneh*). *Am J Vet Res*. 2008;69:114–121.
303. Flinchum GB. Potential use of policosanol in the treatment of hyperlipidemia in pet birds. *Exot DVM*. 2003;5:51–55.
304. Forbes N, Beynon PH, Forbes NA, Lawton MPC. Respiratory problems. *Manual of Psittacine Birds*. Ames, IA: Iowa State University Press; 1996:147–157.
305. Forbes NA. Birds of prey. In: Beynon PH, Cooper JE, eds. *BSAVA Manual of Exotic Pets*. Ames, IA: Iowa State University Press; 1991:212–220.
306. Forbes NA. Raptors: parasitic diseases. In: Chitty J, Lierz M, eds. *BSAVA Manual of Raptors, Pigeons and Passerine Birds*. Gloucester, UK: British Small Animal Veterinary Association; 2008:202–211.
307. Forbes NA, Richardson T. Husbandry and nutrition. In: Beynon PH, Forbes NA, Harcourt-Brown NH, eds. *BSAVA Manual of Raptors, Pigeons and Waterfowl*. Ames, IA: Iowa State University Press; 1996:289–298.

308. Ford S, Chitty J, Jones MP. Raptor medicine master class. *Proc Annu Conf Assoc Avian Vet.* 2009:143–162.
309. Fordham M, Rosenthal K, Durham A, et al. Intraocular osteosarcoma in an umbrella cockatoo (*Cacatua alba*). *Vet Ophthalmol.* 2010;13(Suppl):103–108.
310. Forshaw JM, Cooper WT. *Parrots of the World.* 3rd ed. Melbourne, VIC: Lansdowne Editions; 1989.
311. Fourie T, Cromarty D, Duncan N, et al. The safety and pharmacokinetics of carprofen, flunixin and phenylbutazone in the Cape vulture (*Gyps coprotheres*) following oral exposure. *PLoS One.* 2015:10.
312. Fowler GS, Fowler ME. Order Sphenisciformes. In: Fowler ME, Cubas ZS, eds. *Biology, Medicine, and Surgery of South American Wild Animals.* Ames, IA: Iowa State University Press; 2001:53–64.
313. Fowler ME. *Restraint and Handling of Wild and Domestic Animals.* 2nd ed. Ames, IA: Iowa State University Press; 1995.
314. Fowler ME. *Restraint and Handling of Wild and Domestic Animals.* 3rd ed. Ames, IA: Wiley-Blackwell; 2008.
315. France M. Chemotherapy treatment of lymphosarcoma in a Moluccan cockatoo. *Proc Annu Conf Assoc Avian Vet.* 1993:15–19.
316. Frazier DL. Avian toxicology. In: Olsen GH, Orosz SE, eds. *Manual of Avian Medicine.* St. Louis, MO: Mosby; 2000:228–263.
317. Freeman K, Hahn K, Adams W, et al. Radiation therapy for hemangiosarcoma in a budgerigar. *J Avian Med Surg.* 1999;13(1):40–44.
318. Fudge AM. Laboratory reference ranges for selected avian, mammalian, and reptilian species. In: Fudge AM, ed. *Laboratory Medicine: Avian and Exotic Pets.* Philadelphia, PA: Saunders; 2000:375–400.
319. Fudge AM, Joseph V. Disorders of avian leukocytes. In: Fudge AM, ed. *Laboratory Medicine: Avian and Exotic Pets.* Philadelphia, PA: Saunders; 2000:19–25.
320. Fudge AM, Speer BL. Appendix 2: Normal clinical pathologic data. Hematology: laboratory reference ranges for selected species. In: Speer BL, ed. *Current Veterinary Therapy in Avian Medicine and Surgery.* St. Louis, MO: Elsevier; 2016:825–856.
321. Gaggermeier B, Henke J, Schatzmann U. Investigations on analgesia in domestic pigeons (*C. livia*, Gmel., 1789, var. dom.) using buprenorphine and butorphanol. *Proc Eur Assoc Avian Vet.* 2003:70–73.
322. Gaharan S, Gupta A, Boudreaux B, et al. What is your diagnosis? Chronic lymphocytic leukemia. *J Avian Med Surg.* 2012;26(1):45–48.
323. Galligan TH, Taggart MA, Cuthbert RJ, et al. Metabolism of aceclofenac in cattle to vulture-killing diclofenac. *Conserv Biol.* 2016;30:1122–1127.
324. Gallo SS, Ederli NB, Bôa-Morte MO. Hematological, morphological and morphometric characteristics of blood cells from rhea, *Rhea americana* (Struthioniformes: Rheidae): a standard for Brazilian birds. *Brazilian J Biol.* 2015;75:953–962.
325. Gancz A, Wellehan J, Boutette J, et al. Diabetes mellitus concurrent with hepatic haemosiderosis in two macaws (*Ara severa, Ara militaris*). *Avian Pathol.* 2007;36:331–336.
326. Gancz AY, Lee S, Higginson G, et al. Horner's syndrome in an eastern screech owl (*Megascops asio*). *Vet Rec.* 2006;159(10):320–322.
327. Gancz AY, Malka S, Sandmeyer L, et al. Horner's syndrome in a red-bellied parrot (*Poicephalus rufiventris*). *J Avian Med Surg.* 2005;19(1):30–34.
328. Garcia-Montijano M, de Lucas JJ, Rodriguez C, et al. Marbofloxacin disposition after intravenous administration of a single dose in wild mallard ducks (*Anas platyrhynchos*). *J Avian Med Surg.* 2012;26:6–10.
329. García-Montijano M, Gonzáles F, Waxman S, et al. Pharmacokinetics of marbofloxacin after oral administration to Eurasian buzzards (*Buteo buteo*). *J Avian Med Surg.* 2003;17:185–190.

330. Garcia-Montijano M, Waxman S, de Lucas JJ, et al. The pharmacokinetic behaviour of marbofloxacin in Eurasian buzzards (*Buteo buteo*) after intraosseous administration. *Vet J.* 2006;171:551–555.
331. Garcia-Montijano M, Waxman S, de Lucas JJ, et al. Disposition of marbofloxacin in vulture (*Gyps fulvus*) after intravenous administration of a single dose. *Res Vet Sci.* 2010 epub.
332. Gardhouse S, Beaufrère H, Hawkins MG, et al. Evaluation of oral transmucosal administration of pentobarbital for euthanasia of conscious wild birds. *J Appl Anim Welf Sci.* 2021. doi: 10.1080/10888705.2021.1911655 online ahead of print.
333. Gaskins LA, Massey JG, Ziccardi MH. Effect of oral diazepam on feeding behavior and activity of Hawai'i 'amakihi (*Hemignathus virens*). *Appl Anim Behav Sci.* 2008;112:384–394.
334. Gasthuys E, Houben R, Haesendonck R, et al. Development of an in vivo lipopolysaccharide inflammation model to study the pharmacodynamics of COX-2 inhibitors celecoxib, mavacoxib, and meloxicam in cockatiels (*Nymphicus hollandicus*). *J Avian Med Surg.* 2019;33(4):349–360.
335. Gentry J, Montgerard C, Crandall E, et al. Voriconazole disposition after single and multiple oral doses in healthy, adult red-tailed hawks (*Buteo jamaicensis*). *J Avian Med Surg.* 2014;28(3):201–208.
336. Gentz EJ, Dykes NL, Kollias GV. Comparison of barium and iohexol as gastrointestinal contrast media in avian radiography. *Proc Annu Am Assoc Zoo Vet.* 1999:197.
337. Gibbons D, Morrissey C, Mineau P. A review of the direct and indirect effects of neonicotinoids and fipronil on vertebrate wildlife. *Environ Sci Pollution Res.* 2015;22:103–118.
338. Giddings RF. Treatment of flukes in a toucan. *J Am Vet Med Assoc.* 1988;193:1555–1556.
339. Gilbert CM, Filippich LJ, Charles BG. Doxorubicin pharmacokinetics following a single-dose infusion to sulphur-crested cockatoos (*Cacatua galerita*). *Aust Vet J.* 2004;82(12): 769–772.
340. Gilbert CM, Filippich LJ, McGeary RP, et al. Toxicokinetics of the active doxorubicin metabolite, doxorubicinol, in sulphur-crested cockatoos (*Cacatua galerita*). *Res Vet Sci.* 2007;83(1):123–129.
341. Gill JH. Avian skin diseases. *Vet Clin North Am Exot Anim Pract.* 2001;4:463–982.
342. Gleeson MD, Sanchez-Migallon Guzman D, Kynch H, et al. Pharmacokinetics of a concentrated buprenorphine formulation in red-tailed hawks (*Buteo jamaicensis*). *Am J Vet Res.* 2018;69:13–20.
343. Goode CT, Carey JP, Fuchs AF, et al. Recovery of the vestibulocolic reflex after aminoglycoside ototoxicity in domestic chickens. *J Neurophysiol (Bethesda).* 1999;81(3):1025–1035.
344. Gould W. Caring for birds' skin and feathers. *Vet Med.* 1995;90:53–63.
345. Gozalo AS, Schwiebert RS, Lawson GW. Mortality associated with fenbendazole administration in pigeons (*Columba livia*). *J Am Assoc Lab Anim Sci.* 2006;45:63–66.
346. Graham JE, Kollias-Baker C, Craigmill AL, et al. Pharmacokinetics of ketoprofen in Japanese quail (*Coturnix japonica*). *J Vet Pharmacol Ther.* 2005;28:399–402.
347. Graham JE, Meola DM, Kini NR, et al. Comparison of the effects of glycerol, dimethyl sulfoxide, and hydroxyethyl starch solutions for cryopreservation of avian red blood cells. *Am J Vet Res.* 2015;76(6):487–493.
348. Granone TD, de Francisco ON, Killos MB, et al. Comparison of three different anesthetic agents (isoflurane, sevoflurane, desflurane) in red-tailed hawks (*Buteo jamaicensis*). *Vet Anaesth Analg.* 2012;39:29–37.
349. Gray P, Gou J, Shivaprasad HL, et al. Use of antiviral drugs for treatment of avian bornavirus infection. *Proc Annu Conf Assoc Avian Vet.* 2010:19.
350. Greenacre CB. Thyrogen for use in TSH testing of healthy and suspected hypothyroid parrots. *Proc Eur Assoc Avian Vet.* 2009:125–126.
351. Greenacre CB, Olsen J, Wilson GH, et al. The use of synthetic TSH to evaluate the thyroid gland. *Proc Annu Conf Assoc Avian Vet.* 2002;13.
352. Greenacre CB, Young DW, Behrend EN, et al. Validation of a novel high-sensitivity radioimmunoassay procedure for measurement of total thyroxine concentration in psittacine birds and snakes. *Am J Vet Res.* 2001;62:1750–1754.

353. Gregory CR. Proventricular dilatation disease. In: Ritchie BW, ed. *Avian Viruses: Function and Control*. Lake Worth, FL: Wingers Publishing; 1995:439–448.
354. Greth A, Gerlach H, Gerbermann H, et al. Pharmacokinetics of doxycycline after parenteral administration in the houbara bustard (*Chlamydotis undulata*). *Avian Dis*. 1993;37:31–36.
355. Grieves JL, Dick EJ, Schlabritz-Loutsevich NE, et al. Barbiturate euthanasia solution-induced tissue artifact in nonhuman primates. *J Med Primatol*. 2008;37(3):154–161.
356. Griggs AN, Yaw TJ, Haynes JS, et al. Bioavailability and biochemical effects of diclofenac sodium 0.1% ophthalmic solution in the domestic chicken (*Gallus gallus domesticus*). *Vet Ophthalmol*. 2017;20(2):171–176.
357. Grilo ML, Vanstreels RE, Wallace R, et al. Malaria in penguins-current perceptions. *Avian Pathol*. 2016;45:393–407.
358. Grimm F, Serbest E. The therapy of osteomyelitis with clindamycin in patients suffering from fractures. *Proc VIII Tagung über Vogelkrankheiten, München*. 1992:252–254.
359. Grizzle J, Hadley TL, Rotstein DS, et al. Effects of dietary milk thistle on blood parameters, liver pathology, and hepatobiliary scintigraphy in white carneaux pigeons (*Columba livia*) challenged with B1 aflatoxin. *J Avian Med Surg*. 2009;23(2):114–124.
360. Gronwall R, Brown MP, Clubb S. Pharmacokinetics of amikacin in African gray parrots. *Am J Vet Res*. 1989;50:250–252.
361. Gupta A, Tully TN, Beaufrère H, et al. What is your diagnosis? Bone marrow aspirate from a hyacinth macaw (*Anodorhynchus hyacinthinus*). *Vet Clin Pathol*. 2011;40(4):565–566.
362. Gustavsen KA, Guzman DS, Knych HK, et al. Pharmacokinetics of buprenorphine hydrochloride following intramuscular and intravenous administration to American kestrels (*Falco sparverius*). *Am J Vet Res*. 2014;75:711–715.
363. Guthrie AL, Gonzalez-Angulo C, Wigle WL, et al. Radiation therapy of a malignant melanoma in a thick-billed parrot (*Rhynchopsitta pachyrhyncha*). *J Avian Med Surg*. 2010;24(4):299–307.
364. Hadley TL, Daniel GB, Rotstein DS, et al. Evaluation of hepatobiliary scintigraphy as an indicator of hepatic function in domestic pigeons (*Columba livia*) before and after exposure to ethylene glycol. Vet Radiol Ultrasound. 48(2):155-162.
365. Halsema WB, Alberts H, de Bruijne JJ, et al. Collection and analysis of urine from racing pigeons (*Columba livia domestica*). *Avian Pathol*. 1988;17:221–225.
366. Hameed SS, Guo J, Tizard I, et al. Studies on immunity and immunopathogenesis of parrot bornaviral disease in cockatiels. *Virology*. 2018;515:81–91.
367. Hamlin RL, Stalnaker PS. Basis for use of digoxin in small birds. *J Vet Pharmacol Ther*. 1987;10:354–356.
368. Hammond EE, Guzman DS-M, Garner MM, et al. Long-term treatment of chronic lymphocytic leukemia in a green-winged macaw (*Ara chloroptera*). *J Avian Med Surg*. 2010;24(4):330–338.
369. Haneveld-v Laarhoven MA, Dorrestein GM. IME-sudden high mortality in canaries. *J Assoc Avian Vet*. 1990;4:82.
370. Hannon DE, Swaim SF, Milton JL, et al. Full thickness mesh skin grafts in two great horned owls. *J Zoo Wildl Med*. 1993;24:539–542.
371. Hanssen I, Grav HJ, Steen H. Vitamin C deficiency in growing willow ptarmigan (*Lagopus lagopus lagopus*). *J Nutr*. 1979;109:2260–2276.
372. Hantash TM, Abu-Basha EA. Pharmacokinetics and bioavailability of a sulfadiazine/trimethoprim combination following intravenous, intramuscular, and oral administration in ostriches (*Struthio camelus*). *Proc Annu Conf Assoc Avian Vet*. 2008:319–324.
373. Harcourt-Brown NH. Tendon repair in the pelvic limb of birds of prey: part II. Surgical techniques. In: Lumeij JT, Remple JD, Redig PT et al., eds. *Raptor Biomedicine III*. Lake Worth, FL: Zoological Education Network; 2002:217–231.
374. Harcourt-Brown N, Chitty J. Formulary. In: Harcourt-Brown N, Chitty J, eds. *BSAVA Manual of Psittacine Birds*. Gloucester, UK: British Small Animal Veterinary Association; 2005:303–308.
375. Hardey J, Crick H, Wernham C, et al. *Raptors: A Field Guide to Survey and Monitoring*. Edinburgh, SCO: Scottish Natural Heritage; 2006.

376. Harlin RW. Pigeons. *Vet Clin North Am Small Anim Pract.* 1994;24:157–173.
377. Harlin RW. Pigeons. *Proc Annu Conf Assoc Avian Vet.* 1995:361–373.
378. Harlin RW. Pigeon therapeutics. *Vet Clin North Am Exot Anim Pract.* 2000;3:19–34.
379. Harlin RW. Practical pigeon medicine. *Proc Annu Conf Assoc Avian Vet.* 2006:249–262.
380. Harms CA, Hoskinson JJ, Bruyette DS, et al. Development of an experimental model of hypothyroidism in cockatiels (*Nymphicus hollandicus*). *Am J Vet Res.* 1994;55:399–404.
381. Harper FDW. Poor performance and weight loss. In: Beynon PH, Forbes NA, Harcourt-Brown NH, eds. *BSAVA Manual of Raptors, Pigeons and Waterfowl.* Ames, IA: Iowa State University Press; 1996:272–278.
382. Harrenstien LA, Tell LA, Vulliet R, et al. Disposition of enrofloxacin in red-tailed hawks (*Buteo jamaicensis*) and great horned owls (*Bubo virginianus*) after a single oral, intramuscular, or intravenous dose. *J Avian Med Surg.* 2000;14:228–236.
383. Harris D. Therapeutic avian techniques. *Semin Avian Exot Pet Med.* 1997;6:55–62.
384. Harrison GJ. What to do until a diagnosis is made. In: Harrison GJ, Harrison LR, eds. *Clinical Avian Medicine and Surgery.* Philadelphia, PA: Saunders; 1986:356–361.
385. Harrison GJ, Harrison LR, eds. *Clinical Avian Medicine and Surgery.* Philadelphia, PA: Saunders; 1986:662–663.
386. Harvey R. *Practical Incubation.* Suffolk, UK: Payn Essex Printers Ltd, Sudbury; 1990.
387. Harvey-Clark C, Gass CL. IME-Treating aspergillosis in hummingbirds. *J Assoc Avian Vet.* 1993;7:216.
388. Hausmann JC, Mans C, Gosling A, et al. Bilateral uveitis and hyphema in a Catalina macaw (*Ara ararauna* x *Ara macao*) with multicentric lymphoma. *J Avian Med Surg.* 2016;30(2):172–178.
389. Hawk CT, Leary SL. *Formulary for Laboratory Animals.* 2nd ed. Ames, IA: Iowa State University Press; 1999.
390. Hawkey CM, Samour HJ. The value of clinical hematology in exotic birds. In: Jacobson ER, Kollias GV Jr., eds. *Exotic Animals.* New York, NY: Churchill Livingstone; 1988:109–141.
391. Hawkins MG, Barron H, Speer BL, et al. Birds. In: Carpenter JW, ed. *Exotic Animal Formulary.* 4th ed. St. Louis, MO: Elsevier Saunders; 2013:183–437.
392. Hawkins MG, Malka S, Pascoe PJ, et al. Evaluation of the effects of dorsal versus lateral recumbency on the cardiopulmonary system during anesthesia with isoflurane in red-tailed hawks (*Buteo jamaicensis*). *Am J Vet Res.* 2013;74:136–143.
393. Hawkins MG, Wright BD, Pascoe PJ, et al. Pharmacokinetics and anesthetic and cardiopulmonary effects of propofol in red-tailed hawks (*Buteo jamaicensis*) and great horned owls (*Bubo virginianus*). *Am J Vet Res.* 2003;64:677–683.
394. Hawkins S, Adams L, Mans C. Hematologic and plasma biochemical reference values for juvenile green-naped lorikeets (*Trichoglossus haematodus haematodus*). *J Zoo Wildl Med.* 2018;49(4):1032–1035.
395. Hayes B. British Columbia: deaths caused by barbiturate poisoning in bald eagles and other wildlife. *Can Vet J.* 1988;29(2):173–174.
396. Heard D. Anesthesia and analgesia. In: Altman RB, Clubb SL, Dorrestein GM et al., eds. *Avian Medicine and Surgery.* Philadelphia, PA: Saunders; 1997:807–827.
397. Heatley JJ, Gill H, Crandall L, et al. Enilconazole for treatment of raptor aspergillosis. *Proc Annu Conf Assoc Avian.* 2007:287–288.
398. Heaton JT, Brauth SE. Effects of yohimbine as a reversing agent for ketamine-xylazine anesthesia in budgerigars. *Lab Anim Sci.* 1992;42:54–56.
399. Heidenreich M. *Birds of Prey, Medicine and Management.* Malden, MA: Blackwell Science; 1997.
400. Heinze CR, Hawkins MG, Gillies LA, et al. Effect of dietary omega-3 fatty acids on red blood cell lipid composition and plasma metabolites in the cockatiel, *Nymphicus hollandicus. J Anim Sci.* 2012;90(9):3068–3079.

401. Helmick KE, Boothe DM, Jensen JM. Disposition of single-dose intravenously administered amikacin in emus. *J Zoo Wildl Med.* 1997;28:49–54.
402. Helmick KE, Boothe DM, Jensen JM. Disposition of single-dose intravenously administered enrofloxacin in emus. *J Zoo Wildl Med.* 1997;28:43–48.
403. Hernandez M, Martin S, Fores P. Clinical hematology and blood chemistry values for the common buzzard. *J Raptor Res.* 1990;14:113–119.
404. Hess L. Possible complications associated with topical corticosteroid use in birds. *Proc Annu Conf Assoc Avian Vet.* 2001:29–32.
405. Hibl BM, Blackwood RS, Simons BW, et al. Poxvirus infection in a colony of laboratory pigeons (*Columba livia*). *Comp Med.* 2019;69(3):179–183.
406. Hines R, Kolattukuty PE, Sharkey P. Pharmacological induction of molt and gonadal involution in birds. *Proc Annu Conf Assoc Avian Vet.* 1993:127–134.
407. Hochleithner M. Reference values for selected psittacine species using a dry chemistry system. *J Assoc Avian Vet.* 1989;3:207–209.
408. Hoefer H. IME-hepatic fibrosis and colchicine therapy. *J Assoc Avian Vet.* 1991;5:193.
409. Hoefer HL. Antimicrobials in pet birds. In: Bonagura JD, ed. *Kirk's Current Veterinary Therapy XII: Small Animal Practice.* Philadelphia, PA: Saunders; 1995:1278–1283.
410. Hoogesteijn AL, Raphael BL, Calle P, et al. Oral treatment of avian lead intoxication with meso-2,3-dimercaptosuccinic acid. *J Zoo Wildl Med.* 2003;34:82–87.
411. Hooimeijer J. Coccidiosis in lorikeets infectious for budgerigar. *Proc Annu Conf Assoc Avian Vet.* 1993:59–61.
412. Hoppes S. Treatment of *Macrorhabdus ornithogaster* with sodium benzoate in budgerigars (*Melopsittacus undulatus*). *Proc Annu Conf Assoc Avian Vet.* 2011:67.
413. Hoppes S, Flammer K, Hoersch K, et al. Disposition and analgesic effects of fentanyl in white cockatoos (*Cacatua alba*). *J Avian Med Surg.* 2003;17:124–130.
414. Hoppes S, Heatley JJ, Guo JH, et al. Meloxicam treatment in cockatiels (*Nymphicus hollandicus*) infected with avian bornavirus. *J Exot Pet Med.* 2013;22:275–279.
415. Hoppes S, Tizard I, Shivaprasad H, et al. Treatment of avian bornavirus-infected cockatiels (*Nymphicus hollandicus*) with oral meloxicam and cyclosporine. *Proc Annu Conf Assoc Avian Vet.* 2012:27.
416. Hornak S, Liptak T, Ledecky V, et al. A preliminary trial of the sedation induced by intranasal administration of midazolam alone or in combination with dexmedetomidine and reversal by atipamezole for a short-term immobilization in pigeons. *Vet Anaesth Analg.* 2015;42:192–196.
417. Houck EL, Sanchez-Migallon Guzman D, Beaufrère H, et al. Evaluation of the thermal antinociceptive effects and pharmacokinetics of hydromorphone hydrochloride after intramuscular administration to cockatiels (*Nymphicus hollandicus*). *Am J Vet Res.* 2018;79:820–827.
418. Howard LL, Papendick R, Stalis IH, et al. Fenbendazole and albendazole toxicity in pigeons and doves. *J Avian Med Surg.* 2002;16:203–210.
419. Hu J, McDougald LR. The efficacy of some drugs with known antiprotozoal activity against *Histomonas meleagridis* in chickens. *Vet Parasitol.* 2004;121:233–238.
420. Huckabee JR. Raptor therapeutics. *Vet Clin North Am Exot Anim Pract.* 2000;3:91–116.
421. Huckins GL, Carpenter JW, Dias S, et al. Pharmacokinetics of oral mavacoxib in Caribbean flamingos (*Phoenicopterus ruber ruber*). *J Zoo Wildl Med.* 2020;51(1):53–58.
422. Hudelson KS, Hudelson PM. Endocrine considerations. In: Harrison GJ, Lightfoot TL, eds. *Clinical Avian Medicine.* Palm Beach, FL: Spix Publishing; 2006:541–557.
423. Huff DG. Avian fluid therapy and nutritional therapeutics. *Semin Avian Exot Pet Med.* 1993;2:13–16.
423a. Hyatt MW, Wiederhold NP, Hope WW, et al. Pharmacokinetics of orally administered voriconazole in African penguins (*Spheniscus demersus*) after single and multiple doses. *J Zoo Wildl Med.* 2017;48:352–362.
424. Hyatt MW, Georoff TA, Nollens HH, et al. Voriconazole toxicity in multiple penguin species. *J Zoo Wildl Med.* 2015;46:880–888.

425. Iglauer F, Rasim R. Treatment of psychogenic feather picking in psittacine birds with a dopamine antagonist. *J Small Anim Pract.* 1993;34:564–566.
426. Ihedioha JI, Anyogu DC, Ogbonna ME. The effects of silymarin on acetaminophen-induced acute hepatic and renal toxicities in domestic pigeons (*Columba livia*). *J Avian Med Surg.* 2020;34(4):348–357.
427. Inghelbrecht S, Vermeersch H, Ronsmans S, et al. Pharmacokinetics and anti-trichomonal efficacy of a dimetridazole tablet and water-soluble powder in homing pigeons (*Columba livia*). *J Vet Pharmacol Therap.* 1996;19:62–67.
428. Ingram K. Hummingbirds and miscellaneous orders. In: Fowler ME, ed. *Zoo and Wild Animal Medicine.* 2nd ed. Philadelphia, PA: Saunders; 1986:447–456.
429. Isaza R, Budsberg SC, Sundlof SF, et al. Disposition of ciprofloxacin in red-tailed hawks following a single oral dose. *J Zoo Wildl Med.* 1993;24:498–502.
430. Itoh N, Okada H. Pharmacokinetics and tolerability of chloramphenicol in budgerigars (*Melopsittacus undulatus*). *J Vet Med Sci.* 1993;55:439–442.
431. Jaensch SM, Cullen L, Raidal SR. Assessment of liver function in galahs after partial hepatectomy: a comparison of plasma enzyme concentrations, serum bile acid levels, and galactose clearance tests. *J Avian Med Surg.* 2000;14:164–171.
432. Jaensch SM, Butler R, O'Hara A, et al. Atypical multiple, papilliform, xanthomatous, cutaneous neoplasia in a goose (*Anser anser*). *Aust Vet J.* 2002;80(5):277–280.
433. Jalanka HH. Medetomidine-ketamine and atipamezole: a reversible method for chemical restraint of birds. *Proc First Annu Conf Eur Comm Assoc Avian Vet.* 1991:102–104.
434. Jalanka HH. New alpha two adrenoceptor agonists and antagonists. In: Fowler ME, ed. *Zoo and Wild Animal Medicine: Current Therapy.* 3rd ed. Philadelphia, PA: Saunders; 1993:475–476.
435. Jamriska J, Lavilla LA, Thomasson A, et al. Treatment of atoxoplasmosis in the blue-crowned laughing thrush (*Dryonastes courtoisi*). *Avian Pathol.* 2013;42:569–571.
436. Jankowski G, Nevarez J. Evaluation of a pediatric blood filter for whole blood transfusions in domestic chickens (*Gallus gallus*). *J Avian Med Surg.* 2010;24(4):272–278.
437. Janovsky M, Ruf T, Wolfgang Z. Oral administration of tiletamine/zolazepam for the immobilization of the common buzzard (*Buteo buteo*). *J Raptor Res.* 2002;36:188–193.
438. Jenkins JR. Avian critical care and emergency medicine. In: Altman RB, Clubb SL, Dorrestein GM et al., eds. *Avian Medicine and Surgery.* Philadelphia, PA: Saunders; 1997:839–863.
439. Jenkins JR. Feather picking and self-mutilation in psittacine birds. *Vet Clin North Am Exot Anim Pract.* 2001;4:663–667.
440. Jennings IB. Haematology. In: Beynon PH, Forbes NA, Harcourt-Brown NH, eds. *BSAVA Manual of Raptors, Pigeons and Waterfowl.* Ames, IA: Iowa State University Press; 1996:68–78.
441. Jensen J, Westerman E. Amikacin pharmacokinetics in ostrich (*Struthio camelus*). *Proc Annu Conf Am Assoc Zoo Vet.* 1990:238–242.
442. Jensen JM, Johnson JH, Weiner ST. *Husbandry & Medical Management of Ostriches, Emus & Rheas. Wildlife and Exotic Animal TeleConsultants.* TX: College Station; 1992.
443. Jeong MB, Kim YG, Yi NY, et al. Comparison of the rebound tonometer (TonoVet) with the applanation tonometer (TonoPen XL) in normal Eurasian eagle owls (*Bubo bubo*). *Vet Ophthalmol.* 2007;10:376–379.
444. Jin S, Sell JL. Dietary vitamin K1 requirement and comparison of biopotency of different vitamin K sources for young turkeys. *Poult Sci.* 2001;80(5):615–620.
445. Johnson-Delaney CA, Harrison LR, eds. *Exotic Companion Medicine Handbook for Veterinarians.* Lake Worth, FL: Wingers Publishing; 1996.
446. Johnston M. *Personal communication.* 2003.
447. Johnston MS, Ivey ES. Parathyroid and ultimobranchial glands: calcium metabolism in birds. *Semin Avian Exot Pet Med.* 2002;11:84–93.
448. Johnston MS, Son TT, Rosenthal KL. Immune-mediated hemolytic anemia in an eclectus parrot. *J Am Vet Med Assoc.* 2007;230(7):1028–1031.
449. Jones MP. Selected diseases of birds of prey. *Proc Annu Meet Am Board Vet Pract.* 2001:31–39.

450. Jones MP. Selected infectious diseases of birds of prey. *J Exot Pet Med*. 2006;15:5–17.
451. Jones MP, Arheart KL, Cray C. Reference intervals, longitudinal analyses, and index of individuality of commonly measured laboratory variables in captive bald eagles (*Haliaeetus leucocephalus*). *J Avian Med Surg*. 2014;28:118–126.
452. Jones MP, Morandi F, Wall JS, et al. Distribution of 2-deoxy-2-fluoro-d-glucose in the coelom of healthy bald eagles (*Haliaeetus leucocephalus*). *Am J Vet Res*. 2013;74(3):426–432.
453. Jones MP, Orosz SE, Cox SK, et al. Pharmacokinetic disposition of itraconazole in red-tailed hawks (*Buteo jamaicensis*). *J Avian Med Surg*. 2000;14:15–22.
454. Joseph V. Raptor pediatrics. *Semin Avian Exot Pet Med*. 1993;2:142–151.
455. Joseph V. Preventive health programs for falconry birds. *Proc Annu Conf Assoc Avian Vet*. 1995:171–178.
456. Joseph V. Emergency care of raptors. *Vet Clin North Am Exot Anim Pract*. 1998;1:77–98.
457. Joyner KL. Pediatric therapeutics. *Proc Annu Conf Assoc Avian Vet*. 1991:188–199.
458. Joyner KL. Psittacine incubation and pediatrics. In: Fowler ME, ed. *Zoo and Wild Animal Medicine: Current Therapy*. 3rd ed. Philadelphia, PA: Saunders; 1993:247–260.
459. Joyner PH, Jones MP, Ward D, et al. Induction and recovery characteristics and cardiopulmonary effects of sevoflurane and isoflurane in bald eagles. *Am J Vet Res*. 2008;69:13–22.
460. Juarbe-Diaz SJ. Animal behavior case of the month. *J Am Vet Med Assoc*. 2000;216:1562–1564.
461. Junge RE, Naeger LL, LeBeau MA, et al. Pharmacokinetics of intramuscular and nebulized ceftriaxone in chickens. *J Zoo Wildl Med*. 1994;25:224–228.
462. Kabakchiev C, Laniesse D, James F, et al. Diagnosis and long-term management of post-traumatic seizures in a white-crowned pionus (*Pionus senilis*). *J Am Vet Med Assoc*. 2020;256:1145–1152.
463. Kahler J. Somatostatin treatment for diabetes mellitus in a sulfur breasted toucan. *Proc Annu Conf Assoc Avian Vet*. 1994:269–273.
464. Kahler J. The use of gallium scanning in psittacine birds. *Proc Annu Conf Assoc Avian Vet*. 2001:91–93.
465. Kamiloglu A, Atalan G, Kamiloglu NN. Comparison of intraosseous and intramuscular drug administration for induction of anaesthesia in domestic pigeons. *Res Vet Sci*. 2008;85:171–175.
466. Kasper A. Rehabilitation of California towhees. *Proc Annu Conf Assoc Avian Vet*. 1997:83–90.
467. Kearns KS. Paroxetine therapy for feather picking and self-mutilation in the waldrapp ibis (*Genonticus eremita*). *Proc Joint Conf Am Assoc Zoo Vet/Am Assoc Wildl Vet/Wildl Dis Assoc*. 2004:254–255.
468. Keffen R. The ostrich: capture, care, accommodation, and transportation. In: McKenzie A, ed. *Capture and Care Manual*. Pretoria, South Africa: Wildlife Decision Services; 1993:634–652.
469. Keiper NL, Cox SK, Doss GA, et al. Pharmacokinetics of piroxicam in cranes (family Gruidae). *J Zoo Wildl Med*. 2017;48(3):886–890.
470. Keller D, Sanchez-Migallon Guzman D, Kukanich B, et al. Pharmacokinetics of nalbuphine hydrochloride after intravenous and intramuscular administration to Hispaniolan Amazon parrots (*Amazona ventralis*). *Am J Vet Res*. 2011;72:741–745.
471. Keller KA, Beaufrère H, Brandão J, et al. Long-term management of ovarian neoplasia in two cockatiels (*Nymphicus hollandicus*). *J Avian Med Surg*. 2013;27:44–52.
472. Keller KA, Guzman DSM, Boothe DM, et al. Pharmacokinetics and safety of zonisamide after oral administration of single and multiple doses to Hispaniolan amazon parrots (*Amazona ventralis*). *Am J Vet Res*. 2019;80(2):195–200.
473. Kelly-Clarke WK, McBurney S, Forzan MJ, et al. Detection and characterization of a *Trichomonas* isolate from rehabilitated bald eagle (*Haliaeetus leucocephalus*). *J Zoo Wildl Med*. 2013;44:1123–1126.
474. Kern T, Paul-Murphy J, Murphy C, et al. Disorders of the third eyelid in birds: 17 cases. *J Avian Med Surg*. 1996;10(1):12–18.
475. Keymer I. Pigeons. In: Beynon P, Cooper J, eds. *BSAVA Manual of Exotic Pets*. Ames, IA: Iowa State University Press; 1991:180–202.

476. Kilburn JJ, Cox SK, Backues KA. Pharmacokinetics of ceftiofur crystalline free acids, a long-acting cephalosporin, in American flamingos (*Phoenicopterus ruber*). *J Zoo Wildl Med.* 2016;47:457–462.
477. Kilburn JJ, Cox SK, Kottyan J, et al. Pharmacokinetics of tramadol and its primary metabolite O-desmethyltramadol in African penguins (*Spheniscus demersus*). *J Zoo Wildl Med.* 2014;45(1):93–99.
478. Kirchgessner MS, Tully TN, Nevarez J, et al. Magnesium therapy in a hypocalcemic African grey parrot (*Psittacus erithacus*). *J Avian Med Surg.* 2012;26(1):17–21.
479. Kirk N, Echols S, Wilcox C, et al. Comparison of different doses and delivery methods of IsoVue 370 IV for CT contrast study in birds. *Proc ExoticsCon.* 2019:103.
480. Kitulagodage M, Astheimer LB, Buttemer WA. Diacetone alcohol, a dispersant solvent, contributes to acute toxicity of a fipronil-based insecticide in a passerine bird. *Ecotoxicol Environ Saf.* 2008;71:597–600.
481. Kitulagodage M, Buttemer WA, Astheimer LB. Adverse effects of fipronil on avian reproduction and development: maternal transfer of fipronil to eggs in zebra finch *Taeniopygia guttata* and in ovo exposure in chickens *Gallus domesticus*. *Ecotoxicology.* 2011;20:653–660.
482. Kitulagodage M, Isanhart J, Buttemer WA, et al. Fipronil toxicity in northern bobwhite quail *Colinus virginianus*: reduced feeding behaviour and sulfone metabolite formation. *Chemosphere.* 2011;83:524–530.
483. Klaphake E, Beazley-Keane SL, Jones M, et al. Multisite integumentary squamous cell carcinoma in an African grey parrot (*Psittacus erithacus erithacus*). *Vet Rec.* 2006;158(17):593–596.
484. Klaphake E, Fecteau K, DeWit M, et al. Effects of leuprolide acetate on selected blood and fecal sex hormones in Hispaniolan Amazon parrots (*Amazona ventralis*). *J Avian Med Surg.* 2009;23:253–262.
485. Klaphake E, Schumacher J, Greenacre C, et al. Comparative anesthetic and cardiopulmonary effects of pre- versus postoperative butorphanol administration in Hispaniolan Amazon parrots (*Amazona ventralis*) anesthetized with sevoflurane. *J Avian Med Surg.* 2006;20:2–7.
486. Klein PN, Charmatz K, Langenberg J. The effect of flunixin meglumine (Banamine®) on the renal function in northern bobwhite (*Colinus virginianus*): an avian model. *Proc Annu Conf Am Assoc Zoo Vet.* 1994:128–131.
487. Kleinschmidt LM, Hoppes SM, Heatley JJ, et al. Cyclosporine as a palliative treatment for proventricular dilatation disease in psittacines birds. *Proc Annu Conf Assoc Am Zoo Vet.* 2015:47–48.
488. Koch J, Buss EG, Lobaugh B, et al. Blood pressure of chickens selected for leanness or obesity. *Poult Sci.* 1983;62:904–907.
489. Koepff C. *The New Finch Handbook.* 1983.
490. Kollias Jr GV, Palgut J, Rossi J, et al. The use of ketoconazole in birds: preliminary pharmacokinetics and clinical applications. *Proc Annu Conf Assoc Avian Vet.* 1986:103.
491. Korbel R. Inhalation anaesthesia with isoflurane (Forene®) and sevoflurane (SEVOrane) in domestic pigeons (*Columba livia*, Gmel., 1789, var. *domestica*). *Ger Vet Med Soc.* 1998:209–217.
492. Korbel R. Avian ophthalmology—a practically orientated review on recent developments. *Proc Annu Assoc Avian Med.* 2014:139–147.
493. Korbel R. Avian ophthalmology: principles and application. *Proc Annu Conf Assoc Avian Vet: Exot Proc.* 2016:173–180.
494. Korbel RT. Disorders of the posterior eye segment in raptors—examination procedures and findings. In: Lumeij JT, Remple D, Redig PT et al., eds. *Raptor Biomedicine III.* Lake Worth, FL: Zoological Education Network; 2000:179–194.
495. Korbel RT. Investigations into intraocular injection of recombinant tissue plasminogen activator (rTPA) for the treatment of trauma-induced intraocular hemorrhages in birds. *Proc Annu Conf Assoc Avian Vet.* 2003;97.
496. Korbel RT, Goetz B. Investigations on topical anesthesia of the eye in racing pigeons (*Columba livia*) and common buzzards (*Buteo buteo*). *Proc Annu Conf Assoc Avian Vet.* 2001:51–53.

497. Koutsos EA, Matson KD, Klasing KC. Nutrition of birds in the order Psittaciformes: a review. *J Avian Med Surg*. 2001;15(4):257–275.
498. Koutsos EA, Tell LA, Woods LW, et al. Adult cockatiels (*Nymphicus hollandicus*) at maintenance are more sensitive to diets containing excess vitamin A than to vitamin A-deficient diets. *J Nutr*. 2003;133:1898–1902.
499. Kozel CA, Kinney ME, Hanley CS, et al. Medical management of hypovitaminosis D with cholecalciferol and elastic therapeutic taping in red-legged seriema (*Cariama cristata*) chicks. *J Avian Med Surg*. 2016;30(1):53–59.
500. Krautwald-Junghanns ME, Zebisch R, Schmidt V. Relevance and treatment of coccidiosis in domestic pigeons (*Columba livia forma domestica*) with particular emphasis on toltrazuril. *J Avian Med Surg*. 2009;23:1–5.
501. Krautwald-Junghanns ME, Pieper K, Rullof R, et al. Further experiences with the use of Baytril in pet birds. *Proc Annu Conf Assoc Avian Vet*. 1990:226–236.
502. Krautwald-Junghanns ME, Schmidt V, Vorbruggen S, et al. Inhalative nanosuspensions - the future of avian antimycotic therapy? *Proc Int Conf Avian, Herpetol, Exot Mam Med*. 2013:232.
503. Kreeger TJ, Degernes LA, Kreeger JS, et al. Immobilization of raptors with tiletamine and zolazepam (Telazol). In: Redig PT, Cooper JE, Remple DJ et al., eds. *Raptor Biomedicine*. Minneapolis, MN: University of Minnesota Press; 1993:141–144.
504. Krinsley M. IME-use of DermCaps Liquid and hydroxyzine HCl for the treatment of feather picking. *J Assoc Avian Vet*. 1993;7:221.
505. Kubiak M, Roach L, Eatwell K. The influence of a combined butorphanol and midazolam premedication on anesthesia in psittacid species. *J Avian Med Surg*. 2016;30:317–323.
506. Kuhn SE, Jones MP, Hendrix DV, et al. Normal ocular parameters and characterization of ophthalmic lesions in a group of captive bald eagles (*Haliaeetus leucocephalus*). *J Avian Med Surg*. 2013;27:90–98.
507. Kumar PS, Arivuchelvan A, Jagadeeswaran A, et al. Pharmacokinetics of enrofloxacin in emu (*Dromaius novaehollandiae*) birds after intravenous and oral bolus administration. *Proc Nat Acad Sci Indian Sec B-Bio Sci*. 2015;85:845–851.
508. Labelle AL, Whittington JK, Breaux CB, et al. Clinical utility of a complete diagnostic protocol for the ocular evaluation of free-living raptors. *Vet Ophthalmol*. 2012;15:5–17.
509. LaBonde J. Toxicity in pet avian patients. *Semin Avian Exot Pet Med*. 1995;4:23–31.
510. Lacasse C. Falconiformes (falcons, hawks, eagles, kites, harriers, buzzards, ospreys, caracaras, secretary birds, Old World and New World vultures). In: Miller RE, Fowler ME, eds. St. Louis, MO: Elsevier; 2015. *Fowler's Wild Animal Medicine*. Vol 8:127–142.
511. Lacasse C, Gamble KC, Boothe DM. Pharmacokinetics of a single dose of intravenous and oral meloxicam in red-tailed hawks (*Buteo jamaicensis*) and great horned owls (*Bubo virginianus*). *J Avian Med Surg*. 2013;27:204–210.
512. Lamberski N, Théon AP. Concurrent irradiation and intratumoral chemotherapy with cisplatin for treatment of a fibrosarcoma in a blue and gold macaw (*Ara ararauna*). *J Avian Med Surg*. 2002;16(3):234–238.
513. Langan JN, Ramsay EC, Blackford JT, et al. Cardiopulmonary and sedative effects of intramuscular medetomidine-ketamine and intravenous propofol in ostriches (*Struthio camelus*). *J Avian Med Surg*. 2000;14:2–7.
514. Langille BL, Jones DR. Central cardiovascular dynamics of ducks. *Am J Physiol*. 1975;228:1856–1861.
515. Langlois I, Harvey RC, Jones MP, et al. Cardiopulmonary and anesthetic effects of isoflurane and propofol in Hispaniolan Amazon parrots. *J Avian Med Surg*. 2003;17:4–10.
516. Laniesse D, Beaufrère H. Iron storage disease. In: Graham J, ed. *5-Minute Veterinary Consult: Avian*. Ames, IA: Wiley Blackwell; 2016:156–157.
517. Laniesse D, Beaufrère H, Smith D. Diabetes insipidus in a 4 year old Congo African grey parrot (*Psittacus erithacus erithacus*) concurrently infected with avian bornavirus. *Proc Annu Conf Assoc Avian Vet: Exot Proc*. 2016:339.

518. Lawton MPC. Anaesthesia. In: Beynon PH, Forbes NA, Lawton MPC, eds. *BSAVA Manual of Psittacine Birds*. Ames, IA: Iowa State University Press; 1996:49–55.
519. Lawton MPC. Anaesthesia. In: Beynon PH, Forbes NA, Harcourt-Brown NH, eds. *BSAVA Manual of Raptors, Pigeons and Waterfowl*. Ames, IA: Iowa State University Press; 1996:79–88.
520. Leary S, Underwood W, Anthony R, et al. *AVMA Guidelines for the Euthanasia of Animals: 2020 Edition*. Schaumburg, IL: American Veterinary Medical Association; 2020.
521. Legler M, Kothe R, Rautebschlein S, et al. Detection of psittacid herpesvirus 1 in Amazon parrots with cloacal papilloma [internal papillomatosis of parrots, IPP] in an aviary of different psittacine species. *Dtsch Tierarztl Wochenschr*. 2008;115:461–470.
522. Lennox AM. Successful treatment of mycobacteriosis in three psittacine birds. *Proc Annu Conf Assoc Avian Vet*. 2002:111–113.
523. Lennox AM. The use of Aldara™ (imiquimod) for the treatment of cloacal papillomatosis in psittacines. *Exot DVM*. 2002;4:34–35.
524. Lennox AM. Mycobacteriosis in companion psittacine birds: a review. *J Avian Med Surg*. 2007;21:181–187.
525. Lennox A, Rechner K. Radiation therapy for treatment of thymoma in a Congo African grey parrot. *Proc ExoticsCon*. 2019:311–313.
526. Lennox AM, VanDerHeyden N. Haloperidol for use in treatment of psittacine self-mutilation and feather plucking. *Proc Annu Conf Assoc Avian Vet*. 1993:119–120.
527. Levi A, Perelman B, Waner T, et al. Haematological parameters of the ostrich (*Struthio camelus*). *Avian Pathol*. 1989;18:321–327.
528. Levy A, Perelman B, Waner T, et al. Reference blood chemical values in ostriches (*Struthio camelus*). *Am J Vet Res*. 1989;50:1548–1550.
529. Lichtenberger M. Treatment of respiratory inhalant toxins in 4 psittacine birds. *Proc Annu Conf Assoc Avian Vet*. 2003:39–43.
530. Lichtenberger M, Ko J. Critical care monitoring. *Vet Clin North Am Exot Anim Pract*. 2007;10:317–344.
531. Lichtenberger M, Lennox A. Critical care. In: Speer B, ed. *Current Therapy in Avian Medicine and Surgery*. St. Louis, MO: Elsevier; 2016:582–588.
532. Lichtenberger M, Lennox A, Chavez W, et al. The use of butorphanol constant rate infusion in psittacines. *Proc Annu Conf Assoc Avian Vet/Assoc Exot Mam Vet*. 2009:73.
533. Lichtenberger M, Orcutt C, Cray C, et al. Comparison of fluid types for resuscitation after acute blood loss in mallard ducks (*Anas platyrhynchos*). *J Vet Emerg Crit Care*. 2009;19(5):467–472.
534. Lierz M. Use of inhalation chamber for aspergillosis therapy. *Exot DVM*. 2000;2:79–80.
535. Lightfoot TL. Hyaluronidase: therapeutic applications including egg-yolk disease. *Proc Annu Assoc Avian Med*. 2000:17–21.
536. Lin E, Luscombe C, Colledge G, et al. Long-term therapy with the guanine nucleoside analog penciclovir controls chronic duck hepatitis B virus infection in vivo. *Antimicrob Agents Chemother*. 1998;42:2132–2137.
537. Lin HC, Todhunter PG, Power TA, et al. Use of xylazine, butorphanol, tiletamine-zolazepam, and isoflurane for induction and maintenance of anesthesia in ratites. *J Am Vet Med Assoc*. 1997;210:244–248.
538. Lindemann DM, Carpenter JW, KuKanich B. Pharmacokinetics of a single dose of oral and subcutaneous meloxicam in Caribbean flamingos (*Phoenicopterus ruber ruber*). *J Avian Med Surg*. 2016;30:14–22.
539. Lindemann DM, Eshar D, Nietfeld JC, et al. Suspected fenbendazole toxicity in an American white pelican (*Pelecanus erythrorhyncos*). *J Zoo Wildl Med*. 2016;47:681–685.
540. Lindenstruth H, Frost JW. Enrofloxacin (Baytril)—an alternative for psittacosis prevention and therapy in imported psittacines. *DTW Dtsch Tierarztl Wochenschr*. 1993;100:364–368.

541. Lloyd C, Hebel C, Padrtova R. Non-invasive indirect blood pressure measurements in Falconiformes. *Falco*. 2007;30:20–21.
542. Locke D, Bush M. Tylosin aerosol therapy in quail and pigeons. *J Zoo Anim Med.* 1984;15:67–72.
543. Locke D, Bush M, Carpenter JW. Pharmacokinetics and tissue concentrations of tylosin in selected avian species. *Am J Vet Res*. 1982;43:1807–1810.
544. Loerzel SM, Smith PJ, Howe A, et al. Vecuronium bromide, phenylephrine and atropine combinations as mydriatics in juvenile double-crested cormorants (*Phalacrocorax auritus*). *Vet Ophthalmol*. 2002;5:149–154.
545. Lohr JE, Haberkorn A. Efficacy of toltrazuril against natural infections with intestinal coccidia in aviary birds. *Praktische-Tierarzt*. 1998;79:419–422.
546. Lopez-Antia A, Ortiz-Santaliestra ME, Camarero PR, et al. Assessing the risk of fipronil-treated seed ingestion and associated adverse effects in the red-legged partridge. *Environ Sci Technol*. 2015;49:13649–13657.
547. Lothrop CD, Loomis MR, Olsen JH. Thyrotropin stimulation test for evaluation of thyroid function in psittacine birds. *J Am Vet Med Assoc*. 1985;186:47–48.
548. Lothrop CD, Olsen JH, Loomis MR, et al. Evaluation of adrenal function in psittacine birds using ACTH. *J Am Vet Med Assoc*. 1985;187:1113–1115.
549. Lovas EM, Johnston SD, Filippich LJ. Using a GnRH agonist to obtain an index of testosterone secretory capacity in the cockatiel (*Nymphicus hollandicus*) and sulphur-crested cockatoo (*Cacatua galerita*). *Aust Vet J*. 2010;88:52–56.
550. Lowenstine L, Stasiak I. Update on iron overload in zoological species. In: Miller RE, Fowler ME, eds. St. Louis, MO: Elsevier; 2015. *Fowler's Zoo and Wild Animal Medicine*. Vol 8:674–681.
551. Lublin A, Raz C, Weisman Y. Excretion of Baytril (enrofloxacin) in pigeon milk as an approach to treat squabs. *Israel J Vet Med*. 1996;51:125–128.
552. Ludders JW, Mitchell GS, Rode J. Minimal anesthetic concentration and cardiopulmonary dose response of isoflurane in ducks. *Vet Surg*. 1990;19:304–307.
553. Ludders JW, Rode J, Mitchell GS. Isoflurane anesthesia in sandhill cranes (*Grus canadensis*): minimal anesthetic concentration and cardiopulmonary dose-response during spontaneous and controlled breathing. *Anesth Analg*. 1989;68:511–516.
554. Lumeij JT. Appendix: hematology and biochemistry: Columbiformes. In: Ritchie BW, Harrison GJ, Harrison LR, eds. *Avian Medicine: Principles and Application*. Lake Worth, FL: Wingers Publishing; 1994:1339–1340.
555. Lumeij JT. Psittacine antimicrobial therapy*Antimicrobial Therapy in Caged Birds and Exotic Pets*. Trenton, NJ: Veterinary Learning Systems; 1995:38–48.
556. Lumeij JT, de Bruijne JJ. Blood chemistry reference values in racing pigeons (*Columba livia* domestica). *Avian Pathol*. 1985;14:401–408.
557. Lumeij JT, Gorgevska D, Woestenborghs R. Plasma and tissue concentrations of itraconazole in racing pigeons (*Columba livia domestica*). *J Avian Med Surg*. 1995;9(1):32–35.
558. Lumeij JT, Sprang EPM, Redig PT. Further studies on allopurinol induced hyperuricaemia and visceral gout in red-tailed hawks. *Avian Path*. 1998;27:390–393.
559. Lupu C, Robins S. Comparison of treatment protocols for removing metallic foreign objects from the ventriculus of budgerigars (*Melopsittacus undulatus*). *J Avian Med Surg.* 2009;23(3):186–193.
560. Lupu CA. Evaluation of side effects of tamoxifen in budgerigars. *J Avian Med Surg.* 2000;14:237–242.
561. Machin KL, Caulkett NA. Evaluation of isoflurane and propofol anesthesia for intraabdominal transmitter placement in nesting female canvasback ducks. *J Wildl Dis*. 2000;36:324–334.
562. Machin KL, Livingston A. Plasma bupivacaine levels in mallard ducks (*Anas platyrhynchos*) following a single subcutaneous dose. *Proc Annu Conf Am Assoc Zoo Vet/Am Assoc Wildl Vet/Assoc Rept Amph Vet/Nat Assoc Zoo Wildl Vet*. 2001:159–163.

563. Machin KL, Tellier LA, Lair S, et al. Pharmacodynamics of flunixin and ketoprofen in mallard ducks (*Anas platyrhynchos*). *J Zoo Wildl Med.* 2001;32:222–229.
564. MacLean RA, Beaufrère H. Gruiformes (cranes, limpkins, rails, gallinules, coots, bustards). In: Miller RE, Fowler ME, eds. St. Louis, MO: Elsevier; 2015. *Fowler's Zoo and Wildlife Medicine.* Vol 8:155–163.
565. Macwhirter P. Passeriformes. In: Ritchie RW, Harrison GJ, Harrison LR, eds. *Avian Medicine: Principles and Application.* Lake Worth, FL: Wingers Publishing; 1994:1172–1199.
566. Macwhirter P, Pyke D, Wayne J. Use of carboplatin in the treatment of renal adenocarcinoma in a budgerigar. *Exot DVM.* 2002;4.2:11–12.
567. Mader JT, Calhoun J, Cobos J. In vitro evaluation of antibiotic diffusion from antibiotic-impregnated biodegradable beads and polymethylmethacrylate beads. *Antimicrob Agents Chemother.* 1997;41:415–418.
568. Maier K, Olias P, Gruber AD, et al. Toltrazuril does not show an effect against pigeon protozoal encephalitis. *Parasitol Res.* 2015;114:1603–1606.
569. Mainka SA, Dierenfeld ES, Cooper RM, et al. Circulating α-tocopherol following intramuscular or oral vitamin E administration in Swainson's hawks (*Buteo swainsonii*). *J Zoo Wildl Med.* 1994;25:229–232.
570. Malka S, Crabbs T, Mitchell EB, et al. Disseminated lymphoma of presumptive T-cell origin in a great horned owl (*Bubo virginianus*). *J Avian Med Surg.* 2008;22:226–233.
571. Mama KR, Phillips LG, Pascoe PJ. Use of propofol for induction and maintenance of anesthesia in a barn owl (*Tyto alba*) undergoing tracheal resection. *J Zoo Wildl Med.* 1996;27:397–401.
572. Mans C. Sedation of pet birds. *J Exot Pet Med.* 2014;23:152–157.
573. Mans C, Pilny A. Use of GnRH-agonists for medical management of reproductive disorders in birds. *Vet Clin North Am Exot Anim Pract.* 2014;17:23–33.
574. Mans C, Guzman DS, Lahner LL, et al. Sedation and physiologic response to manual restraint after intranasal administration of midazolam in Hispaniolan Amazon parrots (*Amazona ventralis*). *J Avian Med Surg.* 2012;26:130–139.
575. Mans C, Sanchez-Migallon Guzman D, Lahner LL, et al. Intranasal midazolam for conscious sedation in Hispaniolan Amazon parrots (*Amazona ventralis*). *Proc Annu Conf Am Assoc Zoo Vet.* 2010:160.
576. Manucy T, Bennett R, Greenacre C, et al. Squamous cell carcinoma of the mandibular beak in a Buffon's macaw (*Ara ambigua*). *J Avian Med Surg.* 1998;12(3):158–166.
577. Marshall KL, Craig LE, Jones MP, et al. Quantitative renal scintigraphy in domestic pigeons (*Columba livia domestica*) exposed to toxic doses of gentamicin. *Am J Vet Res.* 2003;64:453–462.
578. Marshall R. Avian anthelmintics and antiprotozoals. *Semin Avian Exot Pet Med.* 1993;2:33–41.
579. Martel A, Mans C, Doss GA, et al. Effects of midazolam and midazolam-butorphanol on gastrointestinal transit time and motility in cockatiels (*Nymphicus hollandicus*). *J Avian Med Surg.* 2018;32(4):286–293.
580. Martel-Arquette A, Mans C, Sladky K. Management of severe frostbite in a grey-headed parrot *(Poicephalus fuscicollis suahelicus*). *J Avian Med Surg.* 2016;30(1):39–45.
581. Martin HD, Kollias GV. Evaluation of water deprivation and fluid therapy in pigeons. *J Zoo Wildl Med.* 1989;20:173–177.
582. Martin KM. Psittacine behavioral pharmacotherapy. In: Leuscher AU, ed. *Manual of Parrot Behavior.* Ames, IA: Blackwell Publishing; 2006:267–280.
583. Martinez R, Wobeser G. Immunization of ducks for type C botulism. *J Wildl Dis.* 1999;35:710–715.
584. Marx D. Preventive health care with diagnostics. *AAV Today.* 1988;2:92–94.
585. Marx KL, Roston MA. *The Exotic Animal Drug Compendium: An International Formulary.* Trenton, NJ: Veterinary Learning Systems; 1996.
586. Mashima TY, Ley DH, Stoskopf MK, et al. Evaluation of treatment of conjunctivitis associated with *Mycoplasma gallisepticum* in house finches (*Carpodacus mexicanus*). *J Avian Med Surg.* 1997;11:20–24.

587. Massey JG, Work TM. Diclazuril therapy for clinical toxoplasmosis. *Proc Annu Conf Assoc Avian Vet*. 2000:29–39.
588. Matthews NS. Anesthesia for big birds (ostriches and emus). *Proc North Am Vet Conf*. 1993:705.
589. Mazet JAK, Newman SH, Gilardi KVK, et al. Advances in oiled bird emergency medicine and management. *J Avian Med Surg*. 2002;16:146–149.
590. Mazor-Thomas JE, Mann PE, Karas AZ, et al. Pain-suppressed behaviors in the red-tailed hawk (*Buteo jamaicensis*). *Appl Anim Behav Sci*. 2014;152:83–91.
591. McConnell HM, Morgan KJ, Sine A, et al. Using sea water for cleaning oil from seabird feathers. *Meth Ecol Evol*. 2015;6(10):1235–1238.
592. McCready JE, Gardhouse SM, Beaufrère H, et al. Mortality rate of birds following intravenous administration iodinated contrast medium for computed tomography. *J Am Vet Med Assoc*. 2021;259:77–83.
593. McDonald SE. IME-injecting eggs with antibiotics. *J Assoc Avian Vet*. 1989;1:9.
594. McDonald SE. IME-summary of medications for use in psittacine birds. *J Assoc Avian Vet*. 1989;3:120–127.
595. McEntire MS, Sanchez CR. Multimodal drug therapy and physical rehabilitation in the successful treatment of capture myopathy in a lesser flamingo (*Phoeniconaias minor*). *J Avian Med Surg*. 2017;31(3):232–238.
596. McGill I, Feltrer Y, Jeffs C, et al. Isosporoid coccidiosis in translocated cirl buntings (*Emberiza cirlus*). *Vet Rec*. 2010;167:656–660.
597. McNaughton A, Frasca S, Mishra N, et al. Valvular dysplasia and congestive heart failure in a juvenile African penguin (*Spheniscus demersus*). *J Zoo Wildl Med*. 2014;45(4):987–990.
598. Meeker DG, Cooper KB, Renard RL, et al. Comparative study of antibiotic elution profiles from alternative formulations of polymethylmethacrylate bone cement. *J Arthroplasty*. 2019;34(7):1458–1461.
599. Mejia-Fava J, Divers SJ, Jimenez DA, et al. Diagnosis and treatment of proventricular nematodiasis in an umbrella cockatoo (*Cacatua alba*). *J Am Vet Med Assoc*. 2013;242:1122–1126.
600. Mejia-Fava J, Holmes SP, Radlinsky M, et al. Use of a nitinol wire stent for management of severe tracheal stenosis in an eclectus parrot (*Eclectus roratus*). *J Avian Med Surg*. 2015;29(3):238–249.
601. Menao MC, Bottino JA, Biasia I, et al. *Salmonella typhimurium* infection in hyacinth macaw (*Anodorhynchus hyacinthinus*). *Arquivos-do-Instituto-Biologico-Sao-Paulo*. 2000;67:43–47.
602. Merryman JI, Buckles EL. The avian thyroid gland. *J Avian Med Surg*. 1998;12:234–242.
603. Meteyer CU, Rideout BA, Gilbert M, et al. Pathology and proposed pathophysiology of diclofenac poisoning in free-living and experimentally exposed oriental white-backed vultures (*Gyps bengalensis*). *J Wildl Dis*. 2005;41:707–716.
604. Mikaelian I, Paillet I, Williams D. Comparative use of various mydriatic drugs in kestrels (*Falco tinnunculus*). *Am J Vet Res*. 1994;55:270–272.
605. Millam JR. Leuprolide acetate can reversibly prevent egg laying in cockatiels. *Proc Annu Conf Assoc Avian Vet*. 1993;46.
606. Millam JR, Finney HL. Leuprolide acetate can reversibly prevent egg laying in cockatiels (*Nymphicus hollandicus*). *Zoo Biol*. 1994;13:149–155.
607. Miller EA, Welte SC. Caring for oiled birds. In: Fowler ME, Miller RE, eds. *Zoo and Wild Animal Medicine: Current Therapy 4*. Philadelphia, PA: Saunders; 1998:300–309.
608. Miller KA, Hill NJ, Carrasco SE, et al. Pharmacokinetics and safety of intramuscular meloxicam in zebra finches (*Taeniopygia guttata*). *J Am Assoc Lab Anim Sci*. 2019;58(5):589–593.
609. Miller MS. Electrocardiography. In: Harrison G, Harrison L, eds. *Clinical Avian Medicine and Surgery*. Philadelphia, PA: Saunders; 1986:286–292.
610. Mohan R. *Mycoplasma* in ratites. *Proc Annu Conf Assoc Avian Vet*. 1993:294–296.
611. Molter CM, Court MH, Hazarika S, et al. Pharmacokinetics of parenteral and oral meloxicam in Hispaniolan parrots (*Amazona ventralis*). *Proc Annu Conf Assoc Avian Vet/Assoc Exot Mam Vet*. 2009:317–318.

612. Monção-Silva R, Ofri R, Raposo AC, et al. Ophthalmic diagnostic tests in parrots (*Amazona amazonica*) and (*Amazona aestiva*). *J Exot Pet Med.* 2016;25:186–193.
613. Montesinos A, Ardiaca M. Acid-base status in the avian patient using a portable point-of-care analyzer. *Vet Clin North Am Exot Anim Pract.* 2013;16:47–69.
614. Montesinos A, Ardiaca M, Gilabert JA, et al. Pharmacokinetics of meloxicam after intravenous, intramuscular and oral administration of a single dose to African grey parrots (*Psittacus erithacus*). *J Vet Pharmacol Ther.* 2017;40:279–284.
615. Montesinos A, Ardiaca M, Juan-Salles C, et al. Effects of meloxicam on hematologic and plasma biochemical analyte values and results of histologic examination of kidney biopsy specimens of African grey parrots (*Psittacus erithacus*). *J Avian Med Surg.* 2015;29:1–8.
616. Moore DM, Rice RL. Exotic animal formulary. In: Holt KM, Boothe DM, Gaumnitz J et al., eds. *Veterinary Values.* 5th ed. Lenexa, KS: Veterinary Medicine Publishing Group; 1998:159–245.
617. Moore RP, Snowden KF, Phalen DN, et al. Diagnosis, treatment, and prevention of megabacteriosis in the budgerigar (*Melopsittacus undulatus*). *Proc Annu Conf Assoc Avian Vet.* 2001:161–163.
618. Morgan K, Ziccardi M. Veterinary care of oiled birds. In: Samour J, ed. *Avian Medicine.* 3rd ed. St. Louis, MO: Elsevier; 2016:286–293.
619. Morishita TY. Clinical assessment of gallinaceous birds and waterfowl in backyard flocks. *Vet Clin North Am Exot Anim Pract.* 1999;2:383–404.
620. Morrisey JK. Avian emergency medicine and critical care. In: Hoefer HL, ed. *Practical Avian Medicine: The Compendium Collection.* Trenton, NJ: Veterinary Learning Systems; 1997:53–57.
621. Morrisey JK, Hohenhaus AE, Rosenthal K, et al. Comparison of three media for the storage of avian whole blood. *Proc Annu Conf Am Assoc Zoo Vet.* 1998:149–150.
622. Morrison J, Greenacre CB, George R, et al. Pharmacokinetics of a single dose of oral and intramuscular meloxicam in African penguins (*Spheniscus demersus*). *J Avian Med Surg.* 2018;32(2):102–108.
623. Muir III WW, Hubbell JA, Bednarski RA, et al. Anesthetic procedures in exotic animals. In: Muir WW III., Hubbell JA, Bednarski RA, et al., eds. *Handbook of Veterinary Anesthesia.* St. Louis, MO: Elsevier Mosby; 2013:450–489.
624. Mukaratirwa S, Chimbwanda M, Matekwe N, et al. A comparison of the efficacy of doramectin, closantel and levamisole in the treatment of the "oriental eye fluke," *Philophthalmus gralli*, in commercially reared ostriches (*Struthio camelus*). *J S Afr Vet Assoc.* 2008;79:101–103.
625. Mulcahy DM, Stoskopf MK, Esler D. Lack of isoflurane-sparing effect of butorphanol in field anesthesia of harlequin ducks (*Histrionicus histrionicus*). *Proc Annu Conf Am Assoc Zoo Vet/Intl Assoc Aquat Anim Med.* 2000:532–533.
626. Muller MG, Kinne J, Schuster RK, et al. Outbreak of microsporidiosis caused by *Enterocytozoon bieneusi* in falcons. *Vet Parasitol.* 2008;152:67–78.
627. Murase T, Ikeda T, Goto I, et al. Treatment of lead poisoning in wild geese. *J Am Vet Med Assoc.* 1992;200:1726–1729.
628. Murphy CJ. Raptor ophthalmology. *Compend Contin Educ Pract Vet.* 1987;9:241–260.
629. Murphy K, Wilson DA, Burton M, et al. Effectiveness of the GnRH agonist deslorelin as a tool to decrease levels of circulating testosterone in zebra finches. *Gen Comp Endocrinol.* 2015;222:150–157.
630. Murray M, Tseng F. Diagnosis and treatment of secondary anticoagulant rodenticide toxicosis in a red-tailed hawk (*Buteo jamaicensis*). *J Avian Med Surg.* 2008;22:41–46.
631. Mushi EZ, Binta MG, Isa JW. Biochemical composition of urine from farmed ostriches (*Struthio camelus*) in Botswana. *J South Afr Vet Assoc.* 2001;72:46–48.
632. Musser JMB, Heatley JJ, Phalen DN. Pharmacokinetics after intravenous administration of flunixin meglumine in budgerigars (*Melopsittacus undulatus*) and Patagonian conures (*Cyanoliseus patagonus*). *J Am Vet Med Assoc.* 2013;242:205–208.

633. Mutlow A, Forbes N. *Haemoproteus* in raptors: pathogenicity, treatment, and control. *Proc Annu Conf Assoc Avian Vet.* 2000:157–163.
634. Naether CA. *Raising Pigeons and Doves.* New York, NY: David McKay Co; 1979.
635. Naidoo V, Swan GE. Diclofenac toxicity in *Gyps vulture* is associated with decreased uric acid excretion and not renal portal vasoconstriction. *Comp Biochem Physiol C Toxicol Pharmacol.* 2008;149:269–274.
636. Naidoo V, Venter L, Wolter K, et al. The toxicokinetics of ketoprofen in *Gyps coprotheres*: toxicity due to zero-order metabolism. *Arch Toxicol.* 2010;84:761–766.
637. Naidoo V, Wolter K, Cromarty AD, et al. The pharmacokinetics of meloxicam in vultures. *J Vet Pharmacol Ther.* 2008;31:128–134.
638. Naidoo V, Wolter K, Cromarty D, et al. Toxicity of non-steroidal anti-inflammatory drugs to *Gyps* vultures: a new threat from ketoprofen. *Biol Lett.* 2010;6:339–341.
639. Napier JE, Hinrichs SH, Lampen F, et al. An outbreak of avian mycobacteriosis caused by *Mycobacterium intracellulare* in little blue penguins (*Eudyptula minor*). *J Zoo Wildl Med.* 2009;40:680–686.
640. National Registration Authority for Agricultural and Veterinary Chemicals. *Dimetridazole* Scope Document. Canberra, Australia. 2002. Available at: http://www.apvma.gov.au/chemrev/dimetridazole_scope.pdf. Accessed June 16, 2017.
641. National Research Council. *Nutrient Requirements of Poultry.* Washington, DC: National Academy Press; 1994.
642. Nau MR, Carpenter JW, KuKanich B, et al. Pharmacokinetics of a single dose of oral and subcutaneous enrofloxacin in Caribbean flamingos (*Phoenicopterus ruber ruber*). *J Zoo Wildl Med.* 2017;48(1):72–79.
643. Nazifi S, Nabinejad A, Sepehrimanesh M, et al. Haematology and serum biochemistry of golden eagle (*Aquila chrysaetos*) in Iran. *Comp Clin Pathol.* 2008;17:197–201.
644. Nemetz L. Deslorelin acetate long-term suppression of ovarian carcinoma in a cockatiel (*Nymphicus hollandicus*). *Proc Annu Conf Assoc Avian Vet.* 2012:37–42.
645. Nemetz L, Broome M. Strontium-90 therapy for uropygial neoplasia. *Proc Annu Conf Assoc Avian Vet.* 2004:15–20.
646. Nemetz LP, Lennox AM. Zosyn: a replacement for Pipracil in the avian patient. *Proc Annu Conf Assoc Avian Vet.* 2004:11–13.
647. Neut D, van de Belt H, van Horn JR, et al. Residual gentamicin-release from antibiotic-loaded polymethylmethacrylate beads after 5 years of implantation. *Biomaterials.* 2003;24:1829–1831.
648. Newell SM. Diagnosis and treatment of lymphocytic leukemia and malignant lymphoma in a Pekin duck (*Anas platyrhyncos domesticus*). *J Assoc Avian Vet.* 1991;5:83–86.
649. Nguyen KQ, Hawkins MG, Taylor IT, et al. Stability and uniformity of extemporaneous preparations of voriconazole in two liquid suspension vehicles at two storage temperatures. *Am J Vet Res.* 2009;7:908–914.
650. Nichols D, Wolff M, Phillips L, et al. Coagulopathy in pink-backed pelicans (*Pelecanus rufescens*) associated with hypervitaminosis E. *J Zoo Wildl Med.* 1989;20(1):57–61.
651. Nolan PM, Duckworth RA, Hill GE, et al. Maintenance of a captive flock of house finches free of infection by *Mycoplasma gallisepticum*. *Avian Dis.* 2000;44:948–952.
652. Norton TM. *Medical protocols recommended by the US Bali mynah SSP.* Available at: http://www.aazv.org/page/547/Bali-Mynah-Medical-Protocols.htm. 2001. Accessed August 8, 2021.
653. Norton TM, Gaskin J, Kollias GV, et al. Efficacy of acyclovir against herpesvirus infection in Quaker parakeets. *Am J Vet Res.* 1991;52:2007–2009.
654. Norton TM, Neiffer DL, Seibels B, et al. *Atoxoplasma medical protocols recommended by the passerine Atoxoplasma working group.* Available at: https://www.aazv.org/page/545; 2007. Accessed August 8, 2021.
655. Oaks J, Meteyer C. Nonsteroidal anti-inflammatory drugs in raptors. In: Miller RE, Fowler ME, eds. St. Louis, MO: Elsevier; 2011. *Fowler's Zoo and Wild Animal Medicine: Current Therapy.* Vol 7:349–355.

656. Oaks JL, Gilbert M, Virani MZ, et al. Diclofenac residues as the cause of vulture population decline in Pakistan. *Nature*. 2004;427:630–633.
657. Okeson DM, Llizo SY, Miller CL, et al. Antibody response of five bird species after vaccination with a killed West Nile virus vaccine. *J Zoo Wildl Med*. 2007;38:240–244.
658. Olsen GH, Carpenter JW, Langenberg JA. Medicine and surgery. In: Ellis DH, Gee GF, Mirande CM, eds. *Cranes: Their Biology, Husbandry, and Conservation*. Washington, DC: National Biological Service/International Crane Foundation; 1996:142–143.
659. Olsen GH, Turell MJ, Pagac BB. Efficacy of eastern equine encephalitis immunization in whooping cranes. *J Wildl Dis*. 1997;33:312–315.
660. Olsen GH, Miller KJ, Docherty DE, et al. Pathogenicity of West Nile virus and response to vaccination in sandhill cranes (*Grus canadensis*) using a killed vaccine. *J Zoo Wildl Med*. 2009;40:263–271.
661. Olsen GP, Russell KE, Dierenfeld E, et al. A comparison of four regimens for treatment of iron storage disease using the European starling (*Sturnus vulgaris*) as a model. *J Avian Med Surg*. 2006;20:74–79.
662. Olsen GP, Russell KE, Dierenfeld E, et al. Impact of supplements on iron absorption from diets containing high and low iron concentrations in the European starling (*Sturnus vulgaris*). *J Avian Med Surg*. 2009;20(2):67–73.
663. Onderka D, Doornenbal E. Mycotic dermatitis in ostriches. *Can Vet J*. 1992;33:547–548.
664. Orosz SE. Antifungal drug therapy in avian species. *Vet Clin North Am Exot Anim Pract*. 2003;6(2):337–350.
665. Orosz SE, Frazier DL. Antifungal agents: a review of their pharmacology and therapeutic indications. *J Avian Med Surg*. 1995;9:8–18.
666. Orosz SE, Schroeder EC, Frazier DL. Itraconazole: a new antifungal drug for birds. *Proc Annu Conf Assoc Avian Vet*. 1994:13–19.
667. Orosz SE, Schroeder EC, Frazier DL. Pharmacokinetic properties of itraconazole in blue-fronted Amazon parrots (*Amazona aestiva aestiva*). *J Avian Med Surg*. 1996;10:168–173.
668. Orosz SE, Jones MP, Cox SK, et al. Pharmacokinetics of amoxicillin plus clavulanic acid in blue-fronted Amazon parrots (*Amazona aestiva aestiva*). *J Avian Med Surg*. 2000;14:107–112.
669. Orr KA, Fowler ME. Order Trochiliiformes (hummingbirds). In: Fowler ME, Cubas ZS, eds. *Biology, Medicine, and Surgery of South American Wild Animals*. Ames, IA: Iowa State University Press; 2001:174–179.
670. Padilla LR, Flammer K, Miller RE. Doxycycline-medicated drinking water for treatment of *Chlamydophila psittaci* in exotic doves. *J Avian Med Surg*. 2005;19:88–91.
671. Paesano F, Ceccherelli R, Briganti A. Partial intravenous anaesthesia (PIVA) with infusion of fentanyl and midazolam during orthopedic surgery in wild birds. *Intl Conf Avian Herp Exot Mam Med*. 2015:332.
672. Paesano F, Ceccherelli R, Di Chiara G, et al. Clinical effects of alfaxalone based protocols in the yellow legged gull (*Larus michahellis*). *Intl Conf Avian Herp Exot Mam Med*. 2015;334.
673. Page DC, Schmidt RE, English JH, et al. Antemortem diagnosis and treatment of sarcocystosis in two species of psittacines. *J Zoo Wildl Med*. 1992;23:77–85.
674. Paley D, Herzenberg JE. Intramedullary infections treated with antibiotic cement rods: preliminary results in nine cases. *J Orthoped Trauma*. 2002;16:723–729.
675. Papendick R, Stalis I, Harvey C, et al. Suspected fenbendazole toxicity in birds. *Proc Annu Conf Am Assoc Zoo Vet/Am Assoc Wildl Vet*. 1998:144–146.
676. Park F. Vitamin A, toxicosis in a lorikeet flock. *Vet Clin North Am Exot Anim Pract*. 2006;9(3):495–502.
677. Parrot TY, Cray C, Martin S. Daily dosing of voriconazole and correlation with serological testing. *Proc Annu Conf Assoc Avian Vet*. 2010:69–70.
678. Parsley RA, Tell LA, Gehring R. Pharmacokinetics of a single dose of voriconazole administered orally with and without food to red-tailed hawks (*Buteo jamaicensus*). *Am J Vet Res*. 2017;78(4):433–439.

679. Pascoe PJ, Pypendop BH, Phillips JCP, et al. Pharmacokinetics of fentanyl after intravenous administration in isoflurane-anesthetized red-tailed hawks (*Buteo jamaicensis*) and Hispaniolan Amazon parrots (*Amazona ventralis*). *Am J Vet Res*. 2018;79:606–613.
680. Paula VV, Fantoni DT, Otsuki DA, et al. *Blood-gas and electrolyte values for Amazon parrots (Amazona aestiva). Pesquisa Vet Brasil.* 2008;28:108–112.
681. Paula VV, Otsuki DA, Auler Junior JO, et al. The effect of premedication with ketamine, alone or with diazepam, on anaesthesia with sevoflurane in parrots (*Amazona aestiva*). *BMC Vet Res*. 2013;9:142.
682. Paul-Murphy J, Ludders JW. Avian analgesia. *Vet Clin North Am Exot Anim Pract*. 2001;4:35–45.
683. Paul-Murphy JR, Brunson DB, Miletic V. Analgesic effects of butorphanol and buprenorphine in conscious African grey parrots. *Am J Vet Res*. 1999;60:1218–1221.
684. Paul-Murphy J, Hess JC, Fialkowski JP. Pharmacokinetic properties of a single intramuscular dose of buprenorphine in African grey parrots (*Psittacus erithacus erithacus*). *J Avian Med Surg*. 2004;18:224–228.
685. Paul-Murphy J, Lowenstine L, Turrel J. Malignant lymphoreticular neoplasm in an African gray parrot. *J Am Vet Med Assoc*. 1985;187(11):1216–1217.
686. Paul-Murphy J, Engilis A, Pascoe P, et al. Comparison of pentobarbital and thoracic (cardiac) compression to euthanize anesthetized sparrows (*Passer domesticus*) and starlings (*Sturnus vulgaris*). *Proc Annu Conf Assoc Avian Vet: Exot Proc*. 2016:69–70.
687. Paul-Murphy JR, Sladky KK, Krugner-Higby LA, et al. Analgesic effects of carprofen and liposome-encapsulated butorphanol tartrate in Hispaniolan parrots (*Amazona ventralis*) with experimentally induced arthritis. *Am J Vet Res*. 2009;70:1201–1210.
688. Pavez JC, Hawkins MG, Pascoe PJ, et al. Effect of fentanyl target-controlled infusions on isoflurane minimum anaesthetic concentration and cardiovascular function in red-tailed hawks (*Buteo jamaicensis*). *Vet Anaesth Analg*. 2011;38:344–351.
689. Pedersoli WM, Ravis WR, Lee HS, et al. Pharmacokinetics of single doses of digoxin administered intravenously to ducks, roosters, and turkeys. *Am J Vet Res*. 1990;51(11):1751–1755.
690. Pees M, Krautwald-Junghanns M-E, Straub J. Evaluating and treating the cardiovascular system. In: Harrison GJ, Lightfoot TL, eds. Evaluating and treating the cardiovascular system. *Clinical Avian Medicine*. 2006;Vol I:379–394.
691. Pees M, Kuhring K, Demiraij F, et al. Bioavailability and compatibility of enalapril in birds. *Proc Annu Conf Assoc Avian Vet*. 2006:7–11.
692. Pees M, Schmidt V, Coles B, et al. Diagnosis and long-term therapy of right-sided heart failure in a yellow-crowned Amazon (*Amazona ochrocephala*). *Vet Rec*. 2006;158:445–447.
693. Penguin Taxon Advisory Group. *Penguin (Spheniscidae) Care Manual*. Silver Springs, FL: Association of Zoos and Aquariums; 2014.
694. Pereira ME, Werther K. Evaluation of the renal effects of flunixin meglumine, ketoprofen and meloxicam in budgerigars (*Melopsittacus undulatus*). *Vet Rec*. 2007;160:844–846.
695. Perpinan D, Melero R. Suspected ivermectin toxicity in a nanday parakeet (*Nandayus nenday*). *Proc Annu Conf Am Assoc Zoo Vet*. 2003:298–299.
696. Peters TL, Fulton RM, Roberson KD, et al. Effect of antibiotics on in vitro and in vivo avian cartilage degradation. *Avian Dis*. 2002;46:75–86.
697. Petritz OA, Sanchez-Migallon Guzman D, Gustavsen K, et al. Evaluation of the mydriatic effects of topical administration of rocuronium bromide in Hispaniolan Amazon parrots (*Amazona ventralis*). *J Am Vet Med Assoc*. 2016;248(1):67–71.
698. Petzinger C, Heatley JJ, Bailey CA, et al. Lipid metabolic dose response to dietary alpha-linolenic acid in monk parrot (*Myiopsitta monachus*). *Lipids*. 2014;49(3):235–245.
699. Petzinger C, Larner C, Heatley JJ, et al. Conversion of α-linolenic acid to long-chain omega-3 fatty acid derivatives and alterations of HDL density subfractions and plasma lipids with dietary polyunsaturated fatty acids in Monk parrots (*Myiopsitta monachus*). *J Anim Physiol Anim Nutr (Berl)*. 2014;98(2):262–270.

700. Phair KA, Larsen RS, Wack RF, et al. Determination of the minimum anesthetic concentration of sevoflurane in thick-billed parrots (*Rhynchopsitta pachyrhyncha*). *Am J Vet Res.* 2012;73:1350–1355.
701. Phalen DN. Avian renal disorders. In: Fudge AM, ed. *Laboratory Medicine: Avian and Exotic Pets.* Philadelphia, PA: Saunders; 2000:61–68.
702. Phalen DN. Common bacterial and fungal infectious diseases in pet birds. *Suppl Compend Contin Educ Pract Vet.* 2003;25:43–48.
703. Phalen DN. Implications of viruses in clinical disorders. In: Harrison GJ, Lightfoot TL, eds. Palm Beach, FL: Spix Publishing; 2006. *Clinical Avian Medicine.* Vol II:721–745.
704. Phalen DN. Preventive medicine and screening. In: Harrison GJ, Lightfoot TL, eds. Palm Beach, FL: Spix Publishing; 2006. *Clinical Avian Medicine.* Vol II:573–585.
705. Phalen DN, Logan KS, Snowden KF. *Encephalitozoon hellem* infection as the cause of a unilateral chronic keratoconjunctivitis in an umbrella cockatoo (*Cacatua alba*). *Vet Ophthalmol.* 2006;9:59–63.
706. Phalen DN, Hays HB, Filippich LJ, et al. Heart failure in a macaw with atherosclerosis of the aorta and brachiocephalic arteries. *J Am Vet Med Assoc.* 1996;209:1435–1440.
707. Phillips A, Fiorello CV, Baden RM, et al. Amphotericin B concentrations in healthy mallard ducks (*Anas platyrhynchos*) following a single intratracheal dose of liposomal amphotericin B using an atomizer. *Med Mycol.* 2018;56(3):322–331.
708. Pignon C, Mayer J. Radiation therapy of uropygial gland carcinoma in psittacine species. *Proc Annu Conf Assoc Avian Vet.* 2011;263.
709. Pikula J, Hajkova P, Bandouchova H, et al. Lead toxicosis of captive vultures: case description and responses to chelation therapy. *BMC Vet Res.* 2013;9(1):11.
710. Plumb DC. *Plumb's Veterinary Drug Handbook.* 9th ed. Ames, IA: Wiley-Blackwell; 2018.
711. Poffers J, Lumeij JT, Redig PT. Investigations into the uricolytic properties of urate oxidase in a granivorous (*Columba livia domestica*) and in a carnivorous (*Buteo jamaicensis*) avian species. *Avian Pathol.* 2002;31:573–579.
712. Poffers J, Lumeij JT, Timmermans-Sprang EPM, et al. Further studies on the use of allopurinol to reduce plasma uric acid concentrations in the red-tailed hawk (*Buteo jamaicensis*) hyperuricaemic model. *Avian Pathol.* 2002;31:567–572.
713. Poleschinski JM, Straub JU, Schmidt V. Comparison of two treatment modalities and PCR to assess treatment effectiveness in macrorhabdosis. *J Avian Med Surg.* 2019;33(3):245–250.
714. Pollock C, Pledger T, Renner M. Diabetes mellitus in avian species. *Proc Annu Assoc Avian Med.* 2001:151–155.
715. Pollock CG, Schumacher J, Orosz SE, et al. Sedative effects of medetomidine in pigeons. *J Avian Med Surg.* 2001;15:95–100.
716. Porter SL. Vehicular trauma in owls. *Proc Annu Conf Assoc Avian Vet.* 1990:164–170.
717. Powers LV, Papich MG. Pharmacokinetics of orally administered phenobarbital in African grey parrots (*Psittacus erithacus erithacus*). *J Vet Pharmacol Ther.* 2011;34(6):615–617.
718. Powers LV, Flammer K, Papich M. Preliminary investigation of doxycycline plasma concentrations in cockatiels (*Nymphicus hollandicus*) after administration by injection or in water or feed. *J Avian Med Surg.* 2000;14:23–30.
719. Powers LV, Pokras M, Rio K, et al. Hematology and occurrence of hemoparasites in migrating sharp-shinned hawks (*Accipiter striatus*) during fall migration. *J Raptor Res.* 1994;28:178–185.
720. Prather JF. Rapid and reliable sedation induced by diazepam and antagonized by flumazenil in zebra finches (*Taeniopygia guttata*). *J Avian Med Surg.* 2012;26:76–84.
721. Product insert.
722. Proenca LM, Mayer J, Schnellbacher R, et al. Antemortem diagnosis and successful treatment of pulmonary candidiasis in a sun conure (*Aratinga solstitialis*). *J Avian Med Surg.* 2014;28:316–321.
723. Prus SE, Clubb SL, Flammer K. Doxycycline plasma concentrations in macaws fed a medicated corn diet. *Avian Dis.* 1992;36:480–483.

724. Quandt JE, Greenacre CB. Sevoflurane anesthesia in psittacines. *J Zoo Wildl Med.* 1999;30:308–309.
725. Quesenberry K. Avian neurologic disorders. In: Birchard S, Sherding R, eds. *Manual of Small Animal Practice.* 2nd ed. Philadelphia, PA: Saunders; 2000:1459–1463.
726. Quesenberry KE, Hillyer EV. Supportive care and emergency therapy. In: Ritchie BW, Harrison GJ, Harrison LR, eds. *Avian Medicine: Principles and Application.* Lake Worth, FL: Wingers Publishing; 1994:382–416.
727. Quintavalla F, Zucca P. Birds of prey: blood chemistry profile for peregrine falcons (*Falco peregrinus*) and eagle owls (*Bubo bubo*) in a raptor centre in north Italy. *Proc Eur Conf Assoc Avian Vet.* 1993:544–551.
728. Raath JP, Quandt SKF, Malan JH. Ostrich (*Struthio camelus*) immobilisation using carfentanil and xylazine and reversal with yohimbine and naltrexone. *J South Afr Vet Assoc.* 1992;63(4):138–140.
729. Racnik J, Zadravec M, Svara T, et al. Electrochemotherapy with bleomycin in the treatment of squamous cell carcinoma of uropygial gland in a cockatiel (*Nymphicus hollandicus*). *Int Conf Avian, Herpetol Exot Mam Med.* 2017:356 Published online.
730. Rae M. Endocrine disease in pet birds. *Semin Avian Exot Pet Med.* 1995;4:32–38.
731. Raghav R, Middleton R, Ahamad R, et al. Analysis of arterial and venous blood gases in healthy gyrfalcons (*Falco rusticolus*) under anesthesia. *J Avian Med Surg.* 2015;29:290–297.
732. Raghav R, Taylor M, Guincho M, et al. Potassium chloride as a euthanasia agent in psittacine birds: clinical aspects and consequences for histopathologic assessment. *Can Vet J.* 2011;52(3):303–306.
733. Ramer JC, Paul-Murphy J, Brunson D, et al. Effects of mydriatic agents in cockatoos, African gray parrots, and blue-fronted Amazon parrots. *J Am Vet Med Assoc.* 1996;208:227–230.
734. Ramos JR, Howard RD, Pleasant RS, et al. Elution of metronidazole and gentamicin from polymethylmethacrylate beads. *Vet Surg.* 2003;32(3):251–261.
735. Ramsay EC, Grindlinger H. Use of clomipramine in the treatment of obsessive behavior in psittacine birds. *J Assoc Avian Vet.* 1994;8:9.
736. Ramsay EC, Vulliet R. Pharmacokinetic properties of gentamicin and amikacin in the cockatiel. *Avian Dis.* 1993;37:628–634.
737. Ramsay E, Bos J, McFadden C. Use of intratumoral cisplatin and orthovoltage radiotherapy in treatment of a fibrosarcoma in a macaw. *J Assoc Avian Vet.* 1993;7(2):87–90.
738. Randolph K. Equine encephalitis virus in ratites. *Proc Annu Conf Assoc Avian Vet.* 1995:249–252.
739. Rathinam T, Chapman HD. Sensitivity of isolates of *Eimeria* from turkey flocks to the anticoccidial drugs amprolium, clopidol, diclazuril, and monensin. *Avian Dis.* 2009;53:405–408.
740. Ratliff CM, Hernandez A, Watson CB, et al. Use of margarine for the successful removal of polyisobutylene in an anhinga (*Anhinga anhinga*) and great blue heron (*Ardea herodias*). *J Avian Med Surg.* 2020;34(1):70–77.
741. Ratzlaff K, Papich MG, Flammer K. Plasma concentrations of fluconazole after a single oral dose and administration in drinking water in cockatiels (*Nymphicus hollandicus*). *J Avian Med Surg.* 2011;25:23–31.
742. Raulic J, Couture E, Baudry F, et al. Pharmacokinetics of selamectin after a single transcutaneous dose in lorikeets (*Trichoglossus* spp.). *Proc ExoticsCon.* 2019.
743. Ravich M, Cray C, Hess L, et al. Lipid panel reference intervals for Amazon parrots (*Amazona* species). *J Avian Med Surg.* 2014;28:209–215.
744. Redig P. *Medical Management of Birds of Prey: A Collection of Notes on Selected Topics.* St. Paul, MN: The Raptor Center; 1993.
745. Redig P. Infectious diseases; fungal diseases. In: Samour J, ed. *Avian Medicine.* London, UK: Harcourt Publishers; 2000:275–291.
746. Redig P. Aspergillosis. In: Samour J, ed. Aspergillosis. *Avian Medicine.* 2016:460–472.

747. Redig PT. Fluid therapy and acid-base balance in the critically ill avian patient. *Proc Annu Conf Assoc Avian Vet*. 1984:59–73.
748. Redig PT. Treatment protocol for bumblefoot types 1 and 2. *AAV Today*. 1987;1:207–208.
749. Redig PT. Avian emergencies. In: Beynon PH, Forbes NA, Harcourt-Brown NH, eds. *BSAVA Manual of Raptors, Pigeons and Waterfowl*. Ames, IA: Iowa State University Press; 1996:30–41.
750. Redig PT. Nursing avian patients. In: Beynon PH, Forbes NA, Harcourt-Brown NH, eds. *Manual of Raptors, Pigeons and Waterfowl*. Ames, IA: Iowa State University Press; 1996:42–46.
751. Redig PT. Falconiformes (vultures, hawks, falcons, secretary bird). In: Fowler ME, Miller RE, eds. *Zoo and Wild Animal Medicine*. 5th ed. Philadelphia, PA: Saunders; 2005:150–161.
752. Redig P, Arent L. Raptor toxicology. *Vet Clin North Am Exot Anim Pract*. 2008;11:261–282.
753. Redig PT, Cruz-Martinez L. Raptors. In: Tully TN, Dorrestein GM, Jones AK, eds. *Avian Medicine*. Edinburgh, SCO: Saunders Elsevier; 2009:209–242.
754. Redig PT, Duke GE. Intravenously administered ketamine HCl and diazepam for anesthesia of raptors. *J Am Vet Med Assoc*. 1976;169:886–888.
755. Redig PT, Ponder J. Raptors: practical information every avian practitioner can use. *Proc Annu Conf Assoc Avian Vet*. 2010:171–180.
756. Redig PT, Talbot B, Guarnera T. Avian malaria. *Proc Annu Conf Assoc Avian Vet*. 1993:173–181.
757. Reidarson TH, McBain JF, Denton D. The use of medroxyprogesterone acetate to induce molting in chinstrap penguins. *J Zoo Wildl Med*. 1999;30:278–280.
758. Reiss AE, Badcock NR. Itraconazole levels in serum, skin and feathers of Gouldian finches (*Chloebia gouldiae*) following in-seed medication. *Proc Joint Conf Am Assoc Zoo Vet/Am Assoc Wildl Vet*. 1998:142–143.
759. Reither NP. Medetomidine and atipamezole in avian practice. *Proc Eur Conf Avian Med Surg*. 1993:43–48.
760. Remple JD. Intracellular hematozoa of raptors: a review and update. *J Avian Med Surg*. 2004;18:75–88.
761. Remple JD, Forbes NA. Antibiotic-impregnated polymethyl methacrylate beads in the treatment of bumblefoot in raptors. In: Lumeij JT, Remple JD, Redig PT et al., eds. *Raptor Biomedicine III*. Lake Worth, FL: Zoological Education Network; 2002:255–263.
762. Reuter A, Muller K, Arndt G, et al. Reference intervals for intraocular pressure measured by rebound tonometry in ten raptor species and factors affecting the intraocular pressure. *J Avian Med Surg*. 2011;25:165–172.
763. Riedesel D. Respiratory pharmacology. In: Hsu W, ed. *Handbook of Veterinary Pharmacology*. Ames, IA: Wiley-Blackwell; 2008:221–233.
764. Riggs SM, Hawkins MG, Craigmill AL, et al. Pharmacokinetics of butorphanol tartrate in red-tailed hawks (*Buteo jamaicensis*) and great horned owls (*Bubo virginianus*). *Am J Vet Res*. 2008;69:596–603.
765. Ritchie BW. *Avian Viruses: Function and Control*. Lake Worth, FL: Wingers Publishing; 1995.
766. Ritchie BW. Diagnosing and preventing common viral infections in companion birds. *Proc 21st Annu Waltham/OSU Symp*; 1997:7–13.
767. Ritchie BW, Harrison GJ. Formulary. In: Ritchie BW, Harrison GJ, Harrison LR, eds. *Avian Medicine: Principles and Application*. Lake Worth, FL: Wingers Publishing; 1994:457–478.
768. Ritchie BW, Harrison GJ. Formulary. In: Ritchie BW, Harrison GJ, Harrison LR, Abridged, eds. *Avian Medicine: Principles and Application*. Lake Worth, FL: Wingers Publishing; 1997:227–253.
769. Ritchie BW, Harrison GJ, Harrison LR. Hematology and biochemistry. In: Ritchie BW, Harrison GJ, Harrison LR, eds. *Avian Medicine: Principles and Application*. Lake Worth, FL: Wingers Publishing; 1994:1331–1347.
770. Ritchie BW, Latimer KS, Leonard J, et al. Safety, immunogenicity and efficacy of an inactivated avian polyomavirus vaccine. *Am J Vet Res*. 1998;59:143–148.
771. Ritchie BW, Vaughn SB, St. Leger J, et al. Use of an inactivated virus vaccine to control polyomavirus outbreaks in nine flocks of psittacine birds. *J Am Vet Med Assoc*. 1998;212:685–690.

772. Rivera S, McClearen J, Reavill DR. Suspected fenbendazole toxicity in pigeons (*Columba livia*). *Proc Annu Conf Assoc Avian Vet*. 2000:207–209.
773. Rivera S, McClearen JR, Reavill DR. Treatment of nonepitheliotropic cutaneous B-cell lymphoma in an umbrella cockatoo (*Cacatua alba*). *J Avian Med Surg*. 2009;23:294–302.
774. Robbe D, Todisco G, Giammarino A, et al. Use of a synthetic GnRH analog to induce reproductive activity in canaries (*Serinus canaria*). *J Avian Med Surg*. 2008;22:123–126.
775. Robbins PK, Tell LA, Needham ML, et al. Pharmacokinetics of piperacillin after intramuscular injection in red-tailed hawks and great horned owls. *J Zoo Wildl Med*. 2000;31:47–51.
776. Roberts MF. *Pigeons*. Jersey City, NJ: TFH Publications; 1962.
777. Robertson JA, Guzman DSM, Graham JL, et al. Evaluation of orally administered atorvastatin on plasma lipid and biochemistry profiles in hypercholesterolemic Hispaniolan Amazon parrots (*Amazona ventralis*). *J Avian Med Surg*. 2020;34(1):32–40.
778. Rojo-Solís C, García-Párraga D, Montesinos A, et al. Pharmacokinetics of single dose oral terbinafine in common shelducks (*Tadorna tadorna*). *J Vet Pharmacol Ther*. 2021;44:510–515.
779. Romagnano A. Examination and preventive medicine protocols in psittacines. *Vet Clin North Am Exot Anim Pract*. 1999;2(2):333–355.
780. Romagnano A, Shiroma JT, Heard DJ, et al. Magnetic resonance imaging of the brain and coelomic cavity of the domestic pigeon (*Columba livia domestica*). *Vet Radiol Ultrasound*. 1996;37(6):431–440.
781. Rosenthal KL, Johnston M. Hypothyroidism in a red-lored Amazon (*Amazona autumnalis*). *Proc Annu Conf Assoc Avian Vet*. 2003:33–36.
782. Rosenthal K, Stamoulis M. Diagnosis of congestive heart failure in an Indian hill mynah bird (*Gracula religiosa*). *J Assoc Avian Vet*. 1993;7:27–30.
783. Rosenthal K, Duda L, Ivey ES, et al. A report of photodynamic therapy for squamous cell carcinoma in a cockatiel. *Proc Annu Conf Assoc Avian Vet*. 2001:175–176.
784. Rosskopf WJ, Woerpel RW. Practical avian therapeutics with dosages of commonly used medications. *Proc Basics Avian Med (Sydney, Australia)*. 1996:75–81.
785. Rouffaer LO, Adriaensen C, De Boeck C, et al. Racing pigeons: a reservoir for nitro-imidazole-resistant *Trichomonas gallinae*. *J Parasitol*. 2014;100:360–363.
786. Rundfeldt C, Wyska E, Steckel H, et al. A model for treating avian aspergillosis: serum and lung tissue kinetics for Japanese quail (*Coturnix japonica*) following single and multiple aerosol exposures of a nanoparticulate itraconazole suspension. *Med Mycol*. 2013;51(8):800–810.
787. Rupiper D. Allopurinol in simple syrup for gout. *J Assoc Avian Vet*. 1993:217–219 Published online.
788. Rupiper DJ. Diseases that affect race performance of homing pigeons. Part 1: Husbandry, diagnostic strategies, and viral diseases. *J Avian Med Surg*. 1998;12:70–77.
789. Rupiper DJ.*Personal communication*. 2004.
790. Rupiper DJ, Ehrenberg M. Introduction to pigeon practice. *Proc Annu Conf Assoc Avian Vet*. 1994:203–211.
791. Rupiper DJ, Ehrenberg M. Practical pigeon medicine. *Proc Annu Conf Assoc Avian Vet*. 1997:479–497.
792. Rupley AE. Respiratory bacterial, fungal and parasitic diseases. *Proc Avian Specialty Advanced Prog Small Mam Rept Med Surg (Annu Conf Assoc Avian Vet)*. 1997:23–44.
793. Rupley AE. Critical care of pet birds. *Vet Clin North Am Exot Anim Pract*. 1998;1:11–41.
794. Rush EM, Hunter RP, Papich M, et al. Pharmacokinetics and safety of acyclovir in tragopans (*Tragopan* species). *J Avian Med Surg*. 2005;19(4):271–276.
795. Russell RE, Franson JC. Causes of mortality in eagles submitted to the National Wildlife Health Center 1975-2013. *Wildl Soc Bull*. 2014;38(4):697–704.
796. Sabrautzki S. The course of gentamicin concentrations in serum and tissues of pigeons. Inaugural dissertation Tierärztliche Fakultät der Ludwig-Maximilians-Universität München. *Vet Bull*. 1983;54:5915.
797. Sacre B, Oppenheim Y, Steinberg H, et al. Presumptive histiocytic sarcoma in a great horned owl. *J Zoo Wildl Med*. 1992;23:113–121.

797a. Sadar MJ, Cox SK, Duvall A, et al. Pharmacokinetics of a single intramuscular injection of ceftiofur crystalline free acid in bald eagles (*Haliaeetus leucocephalus*). *J Avian Med Surg.* 2021;35:290–294.
798. Sadar MJ, Hawkins MG, Drazenovich T, et al. Pharmacokinetic-pharmacodynamic integration of an extended-release ceftiofur formulation administered to red-tailed hawks (*Buteo jamaicensis*). *Proc Annu Conf Assoc Avian Vet.* 2014:11.
799. Sadar MJ, Sanchez-Migallon Guzman D, Mete A, et al. Mange caused by a novel *Micnemidocoptes* mite in a golden eagle (*Aquila chrysaetos*). *J Avian Med Surg.* 2015;29:231–237.
800. Sadegh AB. Comparison of intranasal administration of xylazine, diazepam, and midazolam in budgerigars (*Melopsittacus undulatus*): clinical evaluation. *J Zoo Wildl Med.* 2013;44:241–244.
801. Saggese MD, Tizard I, Phalen DN. Efficacy of multi-drug therapy with azithromycin, rifampin, and ethambutol for the treatment of ring-necked doves (*Streptopelia risoria*) naturally infected with avian mycobacteriosis. *Proc Annu Conf Assoc Avian Vet.* 2007:27–29.
802. Samour J. Pharmaceutics commonly used in avian medicine. In: Samour J, ed. *Avian Medicine.* Philadelphia, PA: Mosby; 2000:388–418.
803. Samour J. Management of raptors. In: Harrison GJ, Lightfoot TL, eds. Palm Beach, FL: Spix Publishing; 2006. *Clinical Avian Medicine.* Vol II:948–954.
804. Samour J. Toxicology. In: Samour J, ed. *Avian Medicine.* 3rd ed. St. Louis, MO: Elsevier; 2016:275–286.
805. Samour JH, Naldo J. Serratospiculiasis in captive falcons in the Middle East: a review. *J Avian Med Surg.* 2001;15:2–9.
806. Samour JH, Naldo J. Diagnosis and therapeutic management of lead toxicosis in falcons in Saudi Arabia. *J Avian Med Surg.* 2002;16:16–20.
807. Samour JH, Naldo J. Diagnosis and therapeutic management of trichomoniasis in falcons in Saudi Arabia. *J Avian Med Surg.* 2003;17:135–143.
808. Samour JH, Irwin-Davies J, Faraj E. Chemical immobilisation in ostriches using etorphine hydrochloride. *Vet Rec.* 1990;127:575–576.
809. Samour JH, Naldo JL, John SK. Therapeutic management of *Babesia shortii* infection in a peregrine falcon (*Falco peregrinus*). *J Avian Med Surg.* 2005;19:294–296.
810. Samour JH, Jones DM, Knight JA, et al. Comparative studies of the use of some injectable anesthetic agents in birds. *Vet Rec.* 1984;115:6–11.
811. Sanchez-Migallon Guzman D. Advances in avian clinical therapeutics. *J Exot Pet Med.* 2014;23(1):6–20.
812. Sanchez-Migallon Guzman D, Beaufrère H, Kukanich B, et al. Pharmacokinetics of a single oral dose of pimobendan in Hispaniolan Amazon parrot (*Amazona ventralis*). *J Avian Med Surg.* 2014;28(2):95–101.
813. Sanchez-Migallon Guzman D, Court MH, Zhu Z, et al. Pharmacokinetics of a sustained-release formulation of meloxicam after subcutaneous administration to Hispaniolan Amazon parrots (*Amazona ventralis*). *J Avian Med Surg.* 2017;31(3):219–224.
814. Sanchez-Migallon Guzman D, Diaz-Figueroa O, Tully Jr T, et al. Evaluating 21-day doxycycline and azithromycin treatments for experimental *Chlamydophila psittaci* infection in cockatiels (*Nymphicus hollandicus*). *J Avian Med Surg.* 2010;24:35–45.
815. Sanchez-Migallon Guzman D, Douglas JM, Beaufrère H, et al. Evaluation of the thermal antinociceptive effects and pharmacokinetics of hydromorphone hydrochloride in orange-winged Amazon parrots (*Amazona amazonica*). *Am J Vet Res.* 2020;81:775–782.
816. Sanchez-Migallon Guzman D, Drazenovich TL, KuKanich B, et al. Evaluation of thermal antinociceptive effects and pharmacokinetics after intramuscular administration of butorphanol tartrate to American kestrels (*Falco sparverius*). *Am J Vet Res.* 2014;75:11–18.
817. Sanchez-Migallon Guzman D, Drazenovich TL, Olsen GH, et al. Evaluation of thermal antinociceptive effects after intramuscular administration of hydromorphone hydrochloride to American kestrels (*Falco sparverius*). *Am J Vet Res.* 2013;74:817–822.

818. Sanchez-Migallon Guzman D, Drazenovich TL, Olsen GH, et al. Evaluation of thermal antinociceptive effects after oral administration of tramadol hydrochloride to American kestrels (*Falco sparverius*). *Am J Vet Res.* 2014;75(2):117–127.
819. Sanchez-Migallon Guzman D, Flammer K, Papich MG, et al. Pharmacokinetics of voriconazole after oral administration of single and multiple doses in Hispaniolan Amazon parrots (*Amazona ventralis*). *Am J Vet Res.* 2010;71:460–467.
820. Sanchez-Migallon Guzman D, Flammer K, Paul-Murphy J, et al. Pharmacokinetics of butorphanol after oral, intravenous and intramuscular administration in Hispaniolan Amazon parrots (*Amazona ventralis*). *J Avian Med Surg.* 2011;25:185–191.
820a. Sanchez-MIgallon Guzman D, Houck EL, Knych HKD, et al. Evaluation of the thermal antinociceptive effects and pharmacokinetics after intramuscular administration of buprenorphine hydrochloride to cockatiels (*Nymphicus hollandicus*). *Am J Vet Res.* 2018;79:1239–1245.
821. Sanchez-Migallon Guzman D, Knych H, Olsen G, et al. Evaluation of the thermal antinociceptive effects and pharmacokinetics of a sustained-release buprenorphine formulation in American kestrels (*Falco sparverius*). *Proc 36th Annu Conf Assoc Avian Vet ExoticsCon.* 2015:13.
822. Sanchez-Migallon Guzman D, KuKanich B, Drazenovich TL, et al. Pharmacokinetics of hydromorphone hydrochloride after intravenous and intramuscular administration of a single dose to American kestrels (*Falco sparverius*). *Am J Vet Res.* 2014;75:527–531.
823. Sanchez-Migallon Guzman D, Kukanich B, Keuler NS, et al. Antinociceptive effects of nalbuphine hydrochloride in Hispaniolan Amazon parrots (*Amazona ventralis*). *Am J Vet Res.* 2011;72:736–740.
824. Sanchez-Migallon Guzman D, Souza MJ, Braun JM, et al. Antinociceptive effects after oral administration of tramadol hydrochloride in Hispaniolan Amazon parrots (*Amazona ventralis*). *Am J Vet Res.* 2012;73(8):1148–1152.
825. Sander SJ, Hope KL, McNeill CJ, et al. Metronomic chemotherapy for myxosarcoma treatment in a kori bustard (*Ardeotis kori*). *J Avian Med Surg.* 2015;29(3):210–215.
826. Sandmeier P. Evaluation of medetomidine for short-term immobilization of domestic pigeons (*Columba livia*) and Amazon parrots (*Amazona* species). *J Avian Med Surg.* 2000;14:8–14.
827. Sandmeier P, Clauss M, Donati OF, et al. Use of deferiprone for the treatment of hepatic iron storage disease in three hornbills. *J Am Vet Med Assoc.* 2012;240(1):75–81.
828. Santangelo B, Ferrari D, Di Martino I, et al. Dexmedetomidine chemical restraint in two raptor species undergoing inhalation anaesthesia. *Vet Res Commun.* 2009;33:S209–S211.
829. Sartini I, Łebkowska-Wieruszewska B, Lisowski A, et al. Concentrations in plasma and selected tissues of marbofloxacin after oral and intravenous administration in Bilgorajska geese (*Anser anser domesticus*). *N Z Vet J.* 2020;68(1):31–37.
830. Scaglione FE, Cannizzo FT, Chiappino L, et al. *Plasmodium* spp. in a captive raptor collection of a safaripark in northwest Italy. *Res Vet Sci.* 2016;104:123–125.
831. Schaeffer D. Avian euthanasia. *Proc Annu Assoc Avian Med.* 1996:287–288.
832. Schäffer DP, Raposo AC, Libório FA, et al. Intranasal administration of midazolam in blue-and-yellow macaws (*Ara araruana*): evaluation of sedative effects. *Vet Anaesth Analg.* 2016;43(4):459–460.
833. Schink B, Korbel RT. Investigations on pharmacokinetics and pharmacodynamics of cefovecin in domestic pigeons. *Proc Annu Conf Assoc Avian Vet.* 2010:301–302.
834. Schmidt V, Demiraj F, Di Somma A, et al. Plasma concentrations of voriconazole in falcons. *Vet Rec.* 2007;161:265–268.
835. Schmitt TL, Nollens HH, Simeone CA, et al. Population pharmacokinetics of danofloxacin after single intramuscular dose administration in California brown pelicans (*Pelecanus occidentalis californicus*). *J Avian Med Surg.* 2019;33(4):361–368.
836. Schnellbacher R, Beaufrère H, Arnold RD, et al. Pharmacokinetics of levetiracetam in healthy Hispaniolan Amazon parrots (*Amazona ventralis*) after oral administration of a single dose. *J Avian Med Surg.* 2014;28(3):193–200.

837. Schnellbacher RW, da Cunha AF, Beaufrère H, et al. Effects of dopamine and dobutamine on isoflurane-induced hypotension in Hispaniolan Amazon parrots (*Amazona ventralis*). *Am J Vet Res*. 2012;73(7):952–958.
838. Schobert E. Telazol use in wild and exotic animals. *Vet Med*. 1987(Oct):1080–1088.
839. Schoemaker N, Schottert M, Mesu S, et al. Distribution of nebulized fluorescein-labeled propylene glycol or saline in pigeons. *Proc ExoticsCon*. 2015:3–4.
840. Schroeder EC, Frazier DL, Morris PJ, et al. Pharmacokinetics of ticarcillin and amikacin in blue-fronted Amazon parrots (*Amazona aestiva aestiva*). *J Avian Med Surg*. 1997;11:260–267.
841. Schuetz S, Krautwald-Junghanns ME, Lutz F, et al. Pharmacokinetic and clinical studies of the carbapenem antibiotic, meropenem, in birds. *Proc Annu Conf Assoc Avian Vet*. 2001:183–190.
842. Schumacher J, Citino SB, Hernandez K, et al. Cardiopulmonary and anesthetic effects of propofol in wild turkeys. *Am J Vet Res*. 1997;58:1014–1017.
843. Schwartz D, Sanchez-Migallon Guzman D, Beaufrère H, et al. Morphologic and quantitative evaluation of bone marrow aspirates from Hispaniolan Amazon parrots (*Amazona ventralis*). *Vet Clin Path*. 2019;48(4):645–651.
844. Scope A, Burhenne J, Haefeli WE, et al. Pharmacokinetics and pharmacodynamics of the new antifungal agent voriconazole in birds. *Proc Eur Assoc Avian Vet*. 2005:217–221.
845. Scope A, Filip T, Gabler C, et al. The influence of stress from transport and handling on hematologic and clinical chemistry blood parameters of racing pigeons (*Columba livia domestica*). *Avian Dis*. 2002;46:224–229.
846. Scott DE. Successful treatment of aspergillosis with voriconazole in a red-tailed hawk (*Buteo jamaicensis*). *Proc Annu Conf Assoc Avian Vet*. 2011:53–57.
847. Scott KE, Bracchi LA, Lieberman MT, et al. Evaluation of best practices for the euthanasia of zebra finches (*Taeniopygia guttata*). *J Am Assoc Lab Anim Sci*. 2017;56(6):802–806.
848. Sedacca CD, Campbell TW, Bright JM, et al. Chronic cor pulmonale secondary to pulmonary atherosclerosis in an African grey parrot. *J Am Vet Med Assoc*. 2009;234(8):1055–1059.
849. Seibels B, Lamberski N, Gregory CR, et al. Effective use of tea to limit dietary iron available to starlings (*Sturnus vulgaris*). *J Zoo Wildl Med*. 2003;34:314–316.
850. Seibert LM. Animal behavior case of the month. A cockatiel was examined because of repetitive chewing of the third digit of the right foot. *J Am Vet Med Assoc*. 2004;224(9):1433–1435.
851. Seibert LM, Tobias K, Sequin B. Understanding behavior: husbandry considerations for better behavioral health in psittacine species. *Compend Contin Educ Vet*. 2007;29:303–306.
852. Seibert LM, Crowell-Davis SL, Wilson GH, et al. Placebo-controlled clomipramine trial for the treatment of feather picking disorder in cockatoos. *J Am Anim Hosp Assoc*. 2004;40:261–269.
853. Sellers C.*Personal communication*. 2003.
854. Seok SH, Jeong DH, Hong IH, et al. Cardiorespiratory dose-response relationship of isoflurane in cinereous vulture (*Aegypius monachus*) during spontaneous ventilation. *J Vet Med Sci*. 2017;79(1):160–165.
855. Sharma AK, Saini M, Singh SD, et al. Diclofenac is toxic to the Steppe eagle (*Aquila nipalensis*): widening the diversity of raptors threatened by NSAID misuse in South Asia. *Bird Conserv Intl*. 2014;24:282–286.
856. Shashy P. Carcinoma in a green-winged macaw (*Ara chloropterus*). *Proc ExoticsCon*. 2019:306–309.
857. Shaver SL, Robinson NG, Wright BD, et al. A multimodal approach to management of suspected neuropathic pain in a prairie falcon (*Falco mexicanus*). *J Avian Med Surg*. 2009;23:209–213.
858. Shlosberg A. Treatment of monocrotophos-poisoned birds of prey with pralidoxime iodide. *J Am Vet Med Assoc*. 1976;169(9):989–990.
859. Shlosberg A, Egyed MN, Eilat A, et al. Efficacy of pralidoxime iodide and obidoxime dichloride as antidotes in diazinon-poisoned goslings. *Avian Dis*. 1976;20(1):162–166.
860. Sibley DA. *The Sibley Guide to Birds*. New York, NY: Knopf; 2000.

861. Siddalls M, Currier TA, Pang J, et al. Infestation of research zebra finch colony with 2 novel mite species. *Comp Med.* 2015;65:51–53.
862. Siegal-Willot JL, Carpenter JW, Glaser AL. Lack of detectable antibody response in greater flamingos (*Phoeniopterus ruber ruber*) after vaccination against West Nile virus with a killed equine vaccine. *J Avian Med Surg.* 2006;20:89–93.
863. Sigmund AB, Jones MP, Ward DA, et al. Long-term outcome of phacoemulsification in raptors - a retrospective study (1999-2014). *Vet Ophthalmol.* 2019;22(3):360–367.
864. Silveira LF, Hofling E, Moro MEG, et al. Order Tinamiformes (tinamous). In: Fowler ME, Cubas ZS, eds. *Biology, Medicine, and Surgery of South American Wild Animals.* Ames, IA: Iowa State University Press; 2001:72–80.
865. Sim RR, Cox SK. Pharmacokinetics of a sustained-release formulation of meloxicam after subcutaneous administration to American flamingos (*Phoenicopterus ruber*). *J Zoo Wildl Med.* 2018;49(4):839–843.
866. Simone-Freilicher E. Use of isoxsuprine for treatment of clinical signs associated with presumptive atherosclerosis in a yellow-naped Amazon parrot (*Amazona ochrocephala auropalliata*). *J Avian Med Surg.* 2007;21:215–219.
867. Simone-Freilicher E. Recurrent smoke-induced respiratory infections in a ruby blue-headed pionus parrot *(Pionus menstruus rubrigularis)*. *J Avian Med Surg.* 2008;22(2):138–145.
868. Simpson BS, Papich MG. Pharmacologic management in veterinary behavioral medicine. *Vet Clin North Am Small Anim Pract.* 2003;33:365–404.
869. Sinclair KM, Church ME, Farver TB, et al. Effects of meloxicam on hematologic and plasma biochemical analysis variables and results of histologic examination of tissue specimens of Japanese quail (*Coturnix japonica*). *Am J Vet Res.* 2012;73:1720–1727.
870. Sinclair KM, Hawkins MG, Wright L, et al. Chronic T-cell lymphocytic leukemia in a black swan (*Cygnus atratus*): diagnosis, treatment, and pathology. *J Avian Med Surg.* 2015;29(4):326–335.
871. Siperstein LJ. Use of neurontin (gabapentin) to treat leg twitching/foot mutilation in a Senegal parrot. *Proc Annu Conf Assoc Avian Vet/Assoc Exot Mam Vet.* 2007:335.
872. Sladky KK, Krugner-Higby L, Meek-Walker E, et al. Serum concentrations and analgesic effects of liposome-encapsulated and standard butorphanol tartrate in parrots. *Am J Vet Res.* 2006;67:775–781.
873. Smith JA. Passeriformes (songbirds, perching birds). In: Miller RE, Fowler ME, eds. St. Louis, MO: Elsevier; 2015. *Fowler's Zoo and Wildlife Medicine.* Vol 8:236–246.
874. Smith JA, Tully TN, Cornick JL. Determination of isoflurane minimum anesthetic concentration in emus. *Proc Annu Conf Assoc Avian Vet.* 1997:181–182.
875. Smith SA. Diagnosis and treatment of helminths in birds of prey. In: Redig PT, Cooper JE, Remple JD et al., eds. *Raptor Biomedicine.* Minneapolis, MN: University of Minnesota Press; 1993:21–27.
876. Smith SA. Parasites of birds of prey: their diagnosis and treatment. *Semin Avian Exot Pet Med.* 1996;5:97–105.
877. Snowden K, Phalen DN. *Encephalitozoon* infection in birds. *Semin Avian Exot Pet Med.* 2004;13:94–99.
878. Snyder SB, Richard MJ. Treatment of avian tuberculosis in a whooping crane (*Grus americana). Proc Annu Conf Am Assoc Zoo Vet.* 1994:167–170.
879. Soenens J, Vermeersch H, Baert K, et al. Pharmacokinetics and efficacy of amoxycillin in the treatment of an experimental *Streptococcus bovis* infection in racing pigeons (*Columba livia*). *Vet J.* 1998;156:59–65.
880. Souza M, Wall J, Stuckey A, et al. Static and dynamic (18) FDG-PET in normal Hispaniolan Amazon parrots (*Amazona ventralis*). *Vet Radiol Ultrasound.* 2011;52(3):340–344.
881. Souza MJ, Cox SK. Tramadol use in zoologic medicine. *Vet Clin North Am Exot Anim Pract.* 2011;14:117–130.
882. Souza MJ, Gerhardt L, Cox S. Pharmacokinetics of repeated oral administration of tramadol hydrochloride in Hispaniolan Amazon parrots (*Amazona ventralis*). *Am J Vet Res.* 2013;74(7):957–962.

883. Souza MJ, Martin-Jimenez T, Jones MP, et al. Pharmacokinetics of intravenous and oral tramadol in the bald eagle (*Haliaeetus leucocephalus*). *J Avian Med Surg*. 2009;23:247–252.
884. Souza MJ, Martin-Jimenez T, Jones MP, et al. Pharmacokinetics of oral tramadol in red-tailed hawks (*Buteo jamaicensis*). *J Vet Pharmacol Ther*. 2010;34:86–88.
885. Sreter T, Szell Z, Varga I. Anticryptosporidial prophylactic efficacy of enrofloxacin and paromomycin in chickens. *J Parasitol*. 2002;88:209–211.
886. Stadler C, Carpenter JW. Parasites of backyard game birds. *Semin Avian Exot Pet Med*. 1996;5:85–96.
887. Stalis IH, Rideout BA, Allen JL, et al. Possible albendazole toxicity in birds. *Proc Joint Conf Am Assoc Zoo Vet/Wildl Dis Assoc/Am Assoc Wildl Vet*. 1995:190–191.
888. Stanford M. Use of Doxirobe Gel®. *Exot DVM*. 2002;4:11.
889. Stanford M. Interferon treatment of circovirus infection in grey parrots (*Psittacus erithacus*). *Vet Rec*. 2004;154:435–436.
890. Stanford M. Significance of cholesterol assays in the investigation of hepatic lipidosis and atherosclerosis in psittacine birds. *Exot DVM*. 2005;7(3):28–34.
891. Stanford M. Clinical pathology of hypocalcaemia in adult grey parrots (*Psittacus erithacus*). *Vet Rec*. 2007;161:456–457.
892. Starkey SR, Morrisey JK, Hickam JD, et al. Extrapyramidal side effects in a blue and gold macaw (*Ara ararauna*) treated with haloperidol and clomipramine. *J Avian Med Surg*. 2008;22:234–239.
893. Starkey SR, Wood C, de Matos R, et al. Central diabetes insipidus in an African grey parrot. *J Am Vet Med Assoc*. 2010;237:415–419.
894. Steinhort LA. Avian fluid therapy. *J Avian Med Surg*. 1999;13:83–91.
895. Steinhort LA. Diagnosis and treatment of common diseases of finches. In: Bongaura JD, ed. *Kirk's Current Veterinary Therapy XIII*. Philadelphia, PA: Saunders; 2000:1119–1123.
896. Stetter MD, Sheppard C, Cook RA. Itraconazole-impregnated synthetic grit for sustained release dosing in avian species. *Proc Annu Conf Am Assoc Zoo Vet*. 1996:181–185.
897. Stewart JS. IME-restraint and anesthesia of ratites. *J Assoc Avian Vet*. 1990;4:90.
898. Stiles J, Buyukmihci NC, Farver TB. Tonometry of normal eyes in raptors. *Am J Vet Res*. 1994;55:477–479.
899. Stone EG. Preliminary evaluation of hetastarch for the management of hypoproteinemia and hypovolemia. *Proc Annu Conf Assoc Avian Vet*. 1994:197–199.
900. Storey ES, Carboni DA, Kearney MT, et al. Use of phenol red thread tests to evaluate tear production in clinically normal Amazon parrots and comparison with Schirmer tear test findings. *J Am Vet Med Assoc*. 2009;235:1181–1187.
901. Straub J, Zenker I. First experience with hormonal treatment of Sertoli cell tumors in budgerigars (*Melopsittacus undulatus*) with absorbable, extended-release GnRH chips (Suprelorelin®). *Proc 1st Intl Conf Avian Herpetol Exot Mam Med*. 2013:299–300.
902. Straub J, Forbes NA, Pees M, et al. Pulsed-wave Doppler-derived velocity of diastolic ventricular inflow and systolic aortic outflow in raptors. *Vet Rec*. 2004;154:145–147.
903. Straub J, Pees M, Enders F, et al. Pericardiocentesis and the use of enalapril in a Fischer's lovebird (*Agapornis fischeri*). *Vet Rec*. 2003;152:24–26.
904. Stringer EM, De Voe RS, Loomis MR. Suspected anaphylaxis to leuprolide acetate depot in two elf owls (*Micrathene whitneyi*). *J Zoo Wildl Med*. 2011;42:166–168.
905. Stunkard JA. *Diagnostics, Treatment and Husbandry of Pet Birds*. Edgewater: Stunkard; 1984.
906. Suarez DL. Appetite stimulation in raptors. In: Redig PT, Cooper JE, Remple DJ et al., eds. *Raptor Biomedicine*. Minneapolis, MN: University of Minnesota Press; 1993:225–228.
907. Suedmeyer WK. IME-use of Adequan in articular diseases of avian species. *J Assoc Avian Vet*. 1993;7:105.
908. Suedmeyer WK, Haynes N, Roberts D. Clinical management of endoventricular mycoses in a group of African finches. *Proc Annu Conf Assoc Avian Vet*. 1997:225–227.
909. Suedmeyer WK, McCaw D, Turnquist S. Attempted photodynamic therapy of squamous cell carcinoma in the casque of a great hornbill (*Buceros bicornis*). *J Avian Med Surg*. 2001;15(1):44–49.

910. Suedmeyer WK, Henry C, McCaw D, et al. Attempted photodynamic therapy against patagial squamous cell carcinoma in an African rose-ringed parakeet (*Psittacula kremeri*). *J Zoo Wildl Med.* 2007;38(4):597–600.
911. Summa NM, Sanchez-Migallon Guzman D, Larrat S, et al. Evaluation of high dosages of oral meloxicam in American kestrels (*Falco sparverius*). *J Avian Med Surg.* 2017;31(2):108–116.
912. Summa NM, Sanchez-Migallon Guzman D, Wils-Plotz EL, et al. Evaluation of the effects of a 4.7-mg deslorelin acetate implant on egg laying in cockatiels (*Nymphicus hollandicus*). *Am J Vet Res.* 2017;78:745–751.
913. Swan GE, Cuthbert R, Quevedo M, et al. Toxicity of diclofenac to *Gyps* vultures. *Biol Lett.* 2006;2:279–282.
914. Swarup D, Patra RC, Prakash V, et al. Safety of meloxicam to critically endangered *Gyps* vultures and other scavenging birds in India. *Anim Cons.* 2007;10:192–198.
915. Swinnerton KJ, Greenwood AG, Chapman RE, et al. The incidence of the parasitic disease trichomoniasis and its treatment in reintroduced and wild pink pigeons *Columba mayeri*. *Ibis.* 2005;147:772–782.
916. Swisher SD, Phillips KL, Tobias JR, et al. External beam radiation therapy of squamous cell carcinoma in the beak of an African grey parrot (*Psittacus timneh*). *J Avian Med Surg.* 2016;30:250–256.
917. Sykes IV J. Piciformes (honeyguides, barbets, woodpeckers, toucans). In: Miller RE, Fowler ME, eds. St. Louis, MO: Elsevier; 2015. *Fowler's Zoo and Wild Animal Medicine.* Vol 8:230–235.
918. Tarello W. Serratospiculosis in falcons from Kuwait: incidence, pathogenicity and treatment with melarsomine and ivermectin. *Parasite.* 2006;13:59–63.
919. Tarello W. Clinical signs and response to primaquine in falcons with *Haemoproteus tinnunculi* infection. *Vet Rec.* 2007;161:204–206.
920. Tarello W. Efficacy of ivermectin (Ivomec) against intestinal capillariosis in falcons. *Parasite.* 2008;15:171–174.
921. Tavernier P, Saggese M, Van Wettere A, et al. Malaria in an eastern screech owl (*Megascops asio*). *Avian Dis.* 2005;9:433–435.
922. Taylor W, Smith D, Beaufrère H. Birds. In: Mathews K, ed. *Veterinary Emergency + Critical Care Manual.* 3rd ed. Guelph, Canada: Lifelearn Animal Health; 2017:981–1002.
923. Teare JA, Schwark WS, Shin SJ, et al. Pharmacokinetics of a long-acting oxytetracycline preparation in ring-necked pheasants, great horned owls and Amazon parrots. *Am J Vet Res.* 1985;46:2639–2643.
924. Tell LA, Clemons KV, Kline Y, et al. Efficacy of voriconazole in Japanese quail (*Coturnix japonica*) experimentally infected with *Aspergillus fumigatus*. *Med Mycol.* 2010;48:234–244.
925. Tell LA, Craigmill AL, Clemons KV, et al. Studies on itraconazole delivery and pharmacokinetics in mallard ducks (*Anas platyrhynchos*). *J Vet Pharmacol Ther.* 2005;28:267–274.
926. Tell L, Harrenstien L, Wetzlich S, et al. Pharmacokinetics of ceftiofur sodium in exotic and domestic avian species. *J Vet Pharmacol Ther.* 1998;21:85–91.
927. Tell LA, Stephens K, Teague SV, et al. Study of nebulization delivery of aerosolized fluorescent microspheres to the avian respiratory tract. *Avian Dis.* 2012;56(2):381–386.
928. Tengelsen LA, Bowen RA, Royals MA, et al. Response to and efficacy of vaccination against eastern equine encephalomyelitis virus in emus. *J Am Vet Med Assoc.* 2001;218:1469–1473.
929. Tennant B. *Small Animal Formulary.* Mid Glamorgan, Wales: Stephens & Geroge Ltd; 1994.
930. Ter Beest J, McClean M, Cushing A, et al. Efficacy of thiofentanil-dexmedetomidine-Telazol for greater rhea (*Rhea americana*) immobilizations. *Proc Joint Conf Am Assoc Zoo Vet/Am Assoc Wildl Vet.* 2010:202.
931. Ter Beest J, McClean M, Cushing A, et al. Thiafentanil-dexmedetomidine-Telazol anesthesia in greater rheas (*Rhea americana*). *J Zoo Wildl Med.* 2012;43(4):802–807.
932. Tobias K, Schneider R, Besser T. Use of antimicrobial-impregnated polymethyl methacrylate. *J Am Vet Med Assoc.* 1996;208(6):841–845.

933. Tschopp R, Bailey T, Di Somma A, et al. Urinalysis as a noninvasive health screening procedure in Falconidae. *J Avian Med Surg.* 2007;21:8–12.
934. Tseng FS. Considerations in care for birds affected by oil spills. *Semin Avian Exot Pet Med.* 1999;8:21–31.
935. Tseng FS, Ziccardi M, Hernandez SM, Barron HW, Miller EA, et al. Care of oiled wildlife-*Medical Management of Wildlife Species: a Guide for Practitioners.* Hoboken, NJ: Wiley; 2020:75–84.
936. Tsiquaye KN, Slomka MJ, Maung M. Oral famciclovir against duck hepatitis B virus replication in hepatic and nonhepatic tissues of ducklings infected in ovo. *J Med Virol.* 1994;42:306–310.
937. Tsourvakas S, Alexandropoulos C, Karatzios C, et al. Elution of ciprofloxacin from acrylic bone cement and fibrin clot: an in vitro study. *Acta Orthop Belg.* 2009;75(4):537–542.
938. Tudor DC. *Pigeon Health and Disease.* Ames, IA: Iowa State University Press; 1991.
939. Tully TN. Therapeutics. In: Tully TN, Shane SM, eds. *Ratite Management, Medicine, and Surgery.* Malabar, FL: Krieger Publishing; 1996:155–163.
940. Tully TN. Formulary. In: Altman RB, Clubb SL, Dorrestein GM et al., eds. *Avian Medicine and Surgery.* Philadelphia, PA: Saunders; 1997:671–688.
941. Tully TN. Psittacine therapeutics. *Vet Clin North Am Exot Anim Pract.* 2000;3:59–90.
942. Tully TN.*Personal communication.* 2003.
943. Tully Jr TN. Birds. In: Mitchell MA, Tully TN Jr., eds. *Manual of Exotic Pet Practice.* St. Louis, MO: Saunders/Elsevier; 2009:250–298.
944. Tully TN, Shane SM, Kearney MY. Evaluation of two *Lactobacillus acidophilus* formulations as dietary supplements in neonatal cockatiels (*Nymphicus hollandicus*). *J Avian Med Surg.* 1998;12(1):25–29.
945. Ueblacker SN. Trichomoniasis in American kestrels (*Falco sparverius*) and Eastern screech-owls (*Otus asio*). In: Lumeij JT, Remple JD, Redig PT et al., eds. *Raptor Biomedicine III.* Lake Worth, FL: Zoological Education Network; 2000:59–63.
946. Uzun M, Onder F, Atalan G, et al. Effects of xylazine, medetomidine, detomidine, and diazepam on sedation, heart and respiratory rates, and cloacal temperature in rock partridges (*Alectoris graeca*). *J Zoo Wildl Med.* 2006;37:135–140.
947. Vaden SL, Cullen JM, Riviere JE. Pharmacokinetics of cyclosporine in woodchucks and Pekin ducks. *J Vet Pharmacol Ther.* 1995;18(1):30–33.
947a. Valitutto MT, Newton AL, Wetzlich S, et al. Pharmacokinetics and clinical safety of a sustained-release formulation of ceftiofur crystalline free acid in ringneck doves (*Streptopelia risoria*) after a single intramuscular injection. *J Zoo Wildl Med.* 2021;52:81–89.
948. Valverde A, Honeyman VL, Dyson DH, et al. Determination of a sedative dose and influence of midazolam on cardiopulmonary function in Canada geese. *Am J Vet Res.* 1990;51:1071–1074.
949. Van Alstine WG, Dyer DC. Antibiotic aerosolization: tissue and plasma oxytetracycline concentrations in turkey poults. *Avian Dis.* 1985;29:430–436.
950. Van Cutsem J. Antifungal activity of enilconazole on experimental aspergillosis in chickens. *Avian Dis.* 1983;27(1):36–42.
951. van Heerden J, Keffen R. Preliminary investigation into the immobilizing of ostriches. *J South Afr Vet Assoc.* 1991;62:114–117.
952. van Zeeland Y. Medication for behavior modification in birds. *Vet Clin North Am Exot Anim Pract.* 2018;21(1):115–149.
953. van Zeeland Y, Schoemaker N. The use of pentoxifylline in birds. *Proc ExoticsCon.* 2018:195–196.
954. van Zeeland Y, Friedman S, Bergman L. Behavior. In: Speer B, ed. *Current Therapy in Avian Medicine and Surgery.* St. Louis, MO: Elsevier; 2016:177–251.
955. van Zeeland Y, Schoemaker N, Lumeij J. Syncopes associated with second degree atrioventricular block in a cockatoo. *Proc Annu Conf Assoc Avian Vet.* 2010:345–346.
956. van Zeeland Y, Bastiaansen P, Kooistra H, et al. Diagnosis and treatment of Cushing's syndrome in a Senegal parrot. *Proc ExoticsCon.* 2015:119.

957. van Zeeland YRA, Schoemaker NJ, Haritova A, et al. Pharmacokinetics of paroxetine, a selective serotonin reuptake inhibitor, in grey parrots (*Psittacus erithacus erithacus*): influence of pharmaceutical formulation and length of dosing. *J Vet Pharmacol Ther*. 2013;36(1):51–58.
958. VanDerHeyden N. Update on avian mycobacteriosis. *Proc Annu Conf Assoc Avian Vet*. 1994:53–61.
959. VanDerHeyden N. New strategies in the treatment of avian mycobacteriosis. *Semin Avian Exot Pet Med*. 1997;6:25–33.
960. Vanhaecke E, De Backer P, Remon JP, et al. Pharmacokinetics and bioavailability of erythromycin in pigeons (*Columba livia*). *J Vet Pharmacol Ther*. 1990;13:356–360.
961. Van Sant F, Stewart GR. Ponazuril used as a treatment for suspected *Cryptosporidium* infection in 2 hybrid falcons. *Proc Annu Conf Assoc Avian Vet*. 2009:368–371.
962. Vanstreels RET, Hurtado R, Snyman A, et al. Empirical primaquine treatment of avian babesiosis in seabirds. *J Avian Med Surg*. 2019;33:258–264.
963. Vanstreels RET, Kolesnikovas CKM, Sandri S, et al. Outbreak of avian malaria associated to multiple species of *Plasmodium* in Magellanic penguins undergoing rehabilitation in southern Brazil. *PLoS One*. 2014;9.
964. Vercruysse J. Efficacy of toltrazuril and clazuril against experimental infections with *Eimeria labbeana* and *E. columbarum* in racing pigeons. *Avian Dis*. 1990;34:73–79.
965. Vergneau-Grosset C, Polley T, Holt DC, et al. Hematologic, plasma biochemical, and lipid panel reference intervals in orange-winged Amazon parrots (*Amazona amazonica*). *J Avian Med Surg*. 2016;30:335–344.
966. Verwoerd D. Aerosol use of a novel disinfectant as part of an integrated approach to preventing and treating aspergillosis in falcons in the UAE. *Falco*. 2002;17:15–18.
967. Vesal N, Eskandari MH. Sedative effects of midazolam and xylazine with or without ketamine and detomidine alone following intranasal administration in ring-necked parakeets. *J Am Vet Med Assoc*. 2006;228:383–388.
968. Vesal N, Zare P. Clinical evaluation of intranasal benzodiazepines, alpha-agonists and their antagonists in canaries. *Vet Anaesth Analg*. 2006;33:143–148.
969. Villaverde-Morcillo S, Benito J, Garcia-Sanchez R, et al. Comparison of isoflurane and alfaxalone (Alfaxan) for the induction of anesthesia in flamingos (*Phoenicopterus roseus*) undergoing orthopedic surgery. *J Zoo Wildl Med*. 2014;45:361–366.
970. Viner TC, Hamlin BC, McClure PJ, et al. Integrating the forensic sciences in wildlife case investigations: a case report of pentobarbital and phenytoin toxicosis in a bald eagle (*Haliaeetus leucocephalus*). *Vet Pathol*. 2016;53(5):1103–1106.
971. Vink-Nooteboom M, Lumeij JT, Wolvekamp WT. Radiography and image-intensified fluoroscopy of barium passage through the gastrointestinal tract in six healthy Amazon parrots (*Amazona aestiva*). *Vet Radiol Ultrasound*. 2003;44:43–48.
972. Visser M, Boothe DM. Population pharmacokinetics of levetiracetam and zonisamide in the African grey parrot (*Psittacus erithacus*). *Proc ExoticsCon*. 2015:7–10.
973. Visser M, Ragsdale MM, Boothe DM. Pharmacokinetics of amitriptyline HCl and its metabolites in healthy African grey parrots (*Psittacus erithacus*) and cockatoos (*Cacatua* species). *J Avian Med Surg*. 2015;29(4):275–281.
974. Vriends MM. *Simon & Schuster's Guide to Pet Birds*. New York, NY: Simon & Schuster; 1984.

974a. Wack AN, KuKanich B, Bronson B, et al. Pharmacokinetics of enrofloxacin after single dose oral and intravenous administration in the African penguin (*Spheniscus demersus*). *J Zoo Wildl Med*. 2012;43:309–316.

975. Wagner CH, Hochleitner M, Rausch W-D. Ketoconazole plasma levels in buzzards. *Proc First Conf Eur Comm Assoc Avian Vet*. 1991:333–340.

975a. Waldoch JA, Cox SK, Armstrong DL. Pharmacokinetics of a single intramuscular injection of long-acting ceftiofur crystaliline-free acid in cattle egrets (*Bubulcus ibis*). *J Avian Med Surg*. 2017;31:314–318.

976. Wallace RS. Sphenisciformes (penguins). In: Miller RE, Fowler ME, eds. St. Louis, MO: Elsevier; 2015. *Fowler's Zoo and Wild Animal Medicine*. Vol 8:82–88.

977. Weber MA, Terrell SP, Neiffer DL, et al. Bone marrow hypoplasia and intestinal crypt cell necrosis associated with fenbendazole administration in five painted storks. *J Am Vet Med Assoc*. 2002;221:417–419.
978. Wellehan J. Frostbite in birds: pathophysiology and treatment. *Comp Contin Educ Pract Vet*. 2003;25(10):776–781.
979. Wellehan JFX, Zens MS, Calsamiglia M, et al. Diagnosis and treatment of conjunctivitis in house finches associated with mycoplasmosis in Minnesota. *J Wildl Dis*. 2001;37(2):245–251.
980. Welsh RD, Nieman RW, Vanhooser SL, et al. Bacterial infections in ratites. *Vet Med*. 1997;92:992–998.
981. Westerhof I, Pellicaan C. Effects of different application routes of glucocorticoids on the pituitary-adrenocortical axis in pigeons (*Columba livia domestica*). *J Avian Med Surg*. 1995;9(3):175–181.
982. Weston HS. The successful treatment of sarcocystosis in two keas (*Nestor nobilis*) at the Franklin Park Zoo. *Proc Annu Conf Am Assoc Zoo Vet*. 1996:186–191.
983. Wheler C. Avian anesthetics, analgesics, tranquilizers. *Semin Avian Exot Pet Med*. 1993;2:7–12.
984. Whitehead MC, Hoppes SM, Musser JMB, et al. The use of alfaxalone in Quaker parrots (*Myiopsitta monachus*). *J Avian Med Surg*. 2019;33:340–348.
985. Whiteside DP, Barker IK, Conlon PD, et al. Pharmacokinetic disposition of the oral iron chelator deferiprone in the domestic pigeon (*Columba livia*). *J Avian Med Surg*. 2007;21(2):121–129.
986. Whiteside DP, Barker IK, Mehren KG, et al. Clinical evaluation of the oral iron chelator deferiprone for the potential treatment of iron overload in bird species. *J Zoo Wildl Med*. 2004;35(1):40–49.
987. Wickstrom ML. Antiseptics and disinfectants. *The Merck Veterinary Manual*. 11th ed. Available at: www.merckvetmanual.com/pharmacology/antiseptics-and-disinfectants. Accessed August 9, 2021.
988. Willette M, Ponder J, Cruz-Martinez L, et al. Management of select bacterial and parasitic conditions of raptors. *Vet Clin North Am Exot Anim Pract*. 2009;12:491–517.
989. Williams DL, Cooper JE. Horner's syndrome in an African spotted eagle owl (*Bubo africanus*). *Vet Rec*. 1994;134(3):64–66.
990. Williams M, Smith PJ, Loerzel SM, et al. Evaluation of the efficacy of vecuronium bromide as a mydriatic in several different species of aquatic birds. *Proc Annu Conf Assoc Avian Vet*. 1996:113–117.
991. Williams SM, Fulton RM, Render JA, et al. Ocular and encephalic toxoplasmosis in canaries. *Avian Dis*. 2001;45:262–267.
992. Wills S, Pinard C, Nykamp S, et al. Ophthalmic reference values and lesions in two captive populations of northern owls: great grey owls (*Strix nebulosa*) and snowy owls (*Bubo scandiacus*). *J Zoo Wildl Med*. 2016;47:244–255.
993. Wilson GH, Graham J, Roberts R, et al. Integumentary neoplasms in psittacine birds: treatment strategies. *Proc Annu Conf Assoc Avian Vet*. 2000:211–214.
994. Wilson GH, Greenacre CB, Howerth EW, et al. Ascaridosis in a group of psittacine birds. *J Avian Med Surg*. 1999;13:32–39.
995. Wilson GH, Hernandez-Divers S, Budsberg SC, et al. Pharmacokinetics and use of meloxicam in psittacine birds. *Proc Annu Conf Assoc Avian Vet*. 2004:7–9.
996. Wilson RC, Zenoble RD, Horton Jr CR, et al. Single dose digoxin pharmacokinetics in the Quaker conure (*Myiopsitta monachus*). *J Zoo Wildl Med*. 1989;20:432–434.
997. Wismer T. Advancements in diagnosis and management of toxicologic problems. In: Speer B, ed. *Current Therapy in Avian Medicine and Surgery*. St. Louis, MO: Elsevier; 2016:589–599.
998. Wlaź P, Knaga S, Kasperek K, et al. Activity and safety of inhaled itraconazole nanosuspension in a model pulmonary *Aspergillus fumigatus* infection in inoculated young quails. *Mycopathologia*. 2015;180(1-2):35–42.
999. Woods LW, Higgins RJ, Joseph VJ, et al. Ronidazole toxicosis in 3 society finches (*Lonchura striata*). *Vet Pathol*. 2010;47:231–235.

1000. Woolcock PR. Duck hepatitis virus type I: studies with inactivated vaccines in breeder ducks. *Avian Pathol.* 1991;20:509–522.
1001. Worell AB. Therapy of noninfectious avian disorders. *Semin Avian Exot Pet Med.* 1993;2:42–47.
1002. Yadav S, Srivastav AK. Influence of calcitonin administration on ultimobranchial and parathyroid glands of pigeon, *Columba livia. Microsc Res Tech.* 2009;72:380–384.
1003. Yaw TJ, Zaffarano BA, Gall A, et al. Pharmacokinetic properties of a single administration of oral gabapentin in the great horned owl (*Bubo virginianus*). *J Zoo Wildl Med.* 2015;46(3):547–552.
1004. Yu PH, Chi CH. Long-term management of thymic lymphoma in a Java sparrow (*Lonchura oryzivora*). *J Avian Med Surg.* 2015;29(1):51–54.
1005. Yu PH, Lee YL, Chen CL, et al. Comparison of three computed tomographic angiography protocols to assess diameters of major arteries in African grey parrots (*Psittacus erithacus*). *Am J Vet Res.* 2018;79(1):42–53.
1006. Zań R, Burmańczuk A, Stępień-Pyśniak D, et al. Pharmacokinetics and pharmacodynamics of a single dose of sustained-release azithromycin formulation in pigeons. *Pol J Vet Sci.* 2020;23(1):43–50.
1007. Zantop D. Medetomidine in birds. *Exot DVM.* 1999;1:34.
1008. Zantop DW. Treatment of bile duct carcinoma in birds with carboplatin. *Exot DVM.* 2000;2:76–78.
1009. Zantop DW. Using leuprolide acetate to manage common avian reproductive problems. *Exot DVM.* 2000;2:70.
1010. Zehnder A, Graham J, Reavill D, Speer B, et al. Neoplastic diseases in avian species*Current Therapy in Avian Medicine and Surgery*. St. Louis, MO: Elsevier; 2016:107–141.
1011. Zehnder AM, Hawkins MG, Pascoe PJ, et al. Evaluation of indirect blood pressure monitoring in awake and anesthetized red-tailed hawks (*Buteo jamaicensis*): effects of cuff size, cuff placement, and monitoring equipment. *Vet Anaesth Analg.* 2009;36:464–479.
1012. Zenker W, Janovsky M, Kurzwell J, et al. Immobilisation of the Eurasian buzzard (*Buteo buteo*) with oral tiletamine/zolazepam. In: Lumeij JT, Remple JD, Redig PT et al., eds. *Raptor Biomedicine III*. Lake Worth, FL: Zoological Education Network; 2002:295–300.
1013. Zenoble RD, Kemppainen RJ, Young DW, et al. Endocrine responses of healthy parrots to ACTH and thyroid stimulating hormone. *J Am Vet Med Assoc.* 1985;187:1116–1118.
1014. Zoller G, Chassang L, Loos P, et al. Evaluation of dexmedetomidine-alfaxalone- butorphanol and dexmedetomidine-ketamine-butorphanol anesthesia in domestic doves (*Streptotelia risoria*). *Proc Annu Assoc Avian Vet ExoticsCon.* 2016:49.
1015. Zollinger TJ, Gamble KC, Alvarado TP, et al. Rhabdomyolysis, steatitis, and coagulopathy in East African white pelicans (*Pelecanus onocrotalus*) and pink-backed pelicans (*Pelecanus rufescens*). *Proc Annu Conf Am Assoc Zoo Vet.* 2002:111–113.
1016. Zollinger TJ, Hoover JP, Payton ME, et al. Clinicopathologic, gross necropsy, and histologic findings after intramuscular injection of carprofen in a pigeon (*Columba livia*) model. *J Avian Med Surg.* 2011;25:173–184.
1017. Zordan MA, Papich MG, Pich AA, et al. Population pharmacokinetics of a single dose of meloxicam after oral and intramuscular administration to captive lesser flamingos (*Phoeniconaias minor*). *Am J Vet Res.* 2016;77:1311–1318.
1018. Zuba JR, Singleton C, Papendick R. Avian chlamydiosis and doxycycline toxicity in a flock of free-contact rainbow lorikeets (*Trichoglossus haematodus haematodus*): considerations, concerns, and quandaries. *Proc Annu Conf Am Assoc Zoo Vet.* 2002:105–107.
1019. Zwijnenberg RJG, Vulto AG, Van Miert AS, et al. Evaluation of antibiotics for racing pigeons (*Columba livia var. domestica*) available in the Netherlands. *J Vet Pharmacol Therap.* 1992;15:364–378.

Chapter 6 Backyard Poultry, Gamebirds, and Waterfowl

Rocio Crespo | Olivia A. Petritz

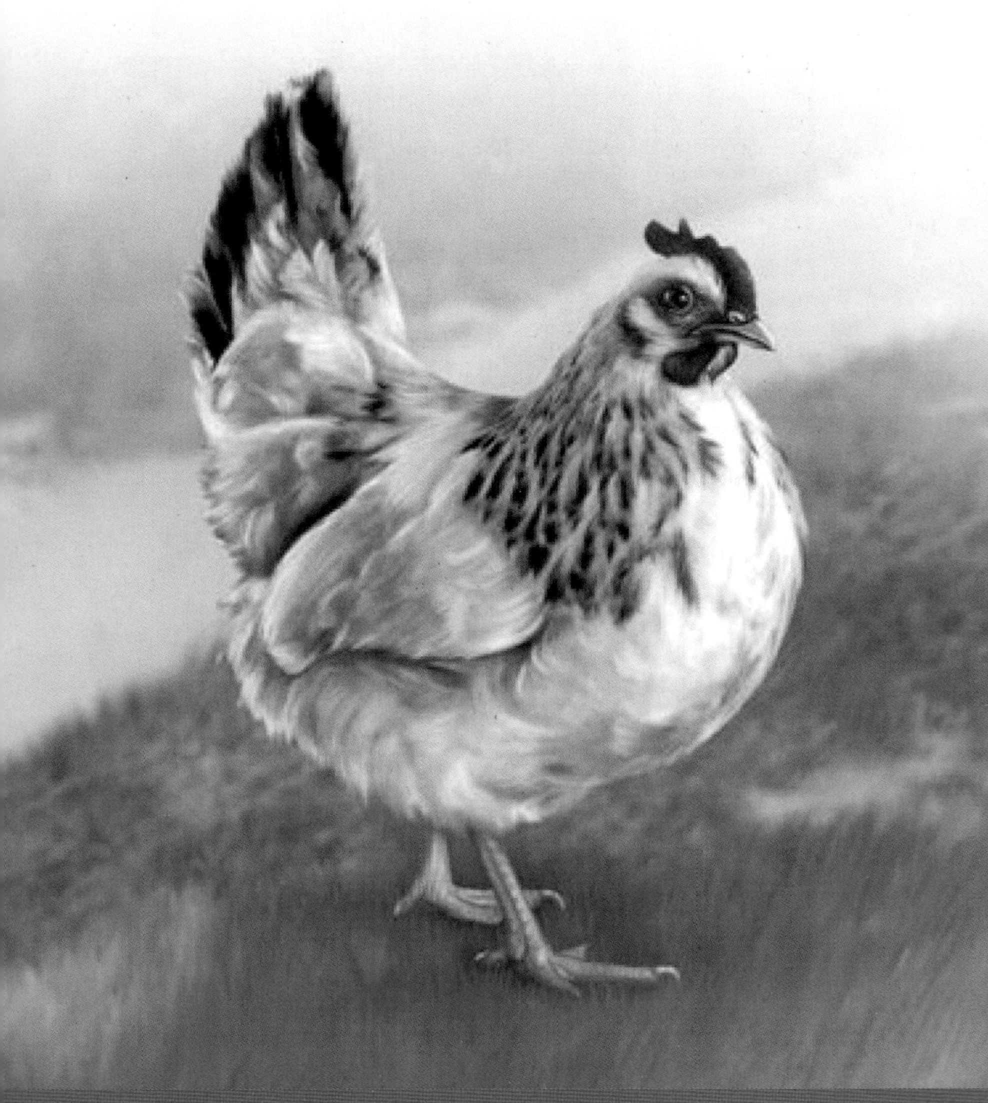

INTRODUCTION

The U.S. Department of Agriculture (USDA) defines poultry to include chickens, doves, ducks, geese, grouse, guinea fowl, partridges, pea fowl, pheasants, pigeons, quail, swans, and turkeys.[18] Many of these poultry species are considered food-producing animal species and, as such, these species are regulated by the U.S. Food and Drug Administration (FDA).[226] Even if the individual animal of any of these species is never used for food, it is still regulated by the FDA. The FDA prohibits the use of certain drugs with no allowable extralabel drug use in any food-producing animal species. These prohibited drugs are clearly identified in the tables (i.e., Tables 6.1 to 6.13), and the doses are provided in case they are needed for a similar but non-food-producing animal species (e.g., Attwater's prairie chicken), and listings should in no way be misconstrued as an endorsement of using FDA-prohibited drugs in any food-producing animal species. Please refer to the appropriate tables at the end of this chapter regarding the definitions of prohibited drugs, extralabel drugs, labeled drugs, and drugs needing a Veterinary Feed Directive prior to choosing a drug and dose. Please refer to the Food Animal Residue Avoidance Databank at www.farad.org and other sources listed in Table 6.26 for meat and egg withdrawal times.[77]

Be aware that most drug dosages are listed in standard international units (SI), such as mg/kg, but some dosages may be in conventional units, such as mg/lb, mg/gallon, or grams/ton to match the dose on the label.

TABLE 6-1 Antimicrobial Agents Used in Backyard Poultry, Gamebirds, and Waterfowl.[a,b]

Agent	Dosage	Species/Comments
Amikacin	5.3 mg/kg IV RLP once[186]	Chickens/pododermatitis; regional limb perfusion (RLP) into medial metatarsal vein with a tourniquet placed proximal to hock joint for 15 min[186]
	10 mg/kg SC, IM q8h × 14 days[120]	Ring-necked pheasants/PK; renal toxicosis appeared at 11 days; uric acid levels abnormal up to 7 days after cessation
	20 mg/kg IM q8h[64]	Chickens/PK
Amoxicillin/ clavulanate (Clavamox, Zoetis)	125 mg/kg PO q8h[1]	Poultry
	125 mg/kg PO q12h[199]	Chickens/PK; tablets PO did not reach therapeutic plasma concentrations at this route and dose
	500 mg/L drinking water[247]	Chickens/PK
Amoxicillin trihydrate	15 mg/kg/day PO × 3 days[68]	Chickens, turkeys
	15 mg/kg PO × 3-5 days; if in drinking water, concentration should be such that the bird consumes the recommended dose[167]	Chickens/not laying eggs for human consumption[167]

Continued

TABLE 6-1 Antimicrobial Agents Used in Backyard Poultry, Gamebirds, and Waterfowl. (cont'd)

Agent	Dosage	Species/Comments
Amoxicillin trihydrate (cont'd)	15-20 mg/kg PO × 3-5 days; if in drinking water, concentration should be such that the bird consumes the recommended dose[167]	Turkeys/not laying eggs for human consumption[167]
	20 mg/kg PO[129]	Chickens, turkeys/no frequency listed
	20 mg/kg PO × 3 days; if in drinking water, concentration should be such that the bird consumes the recommended dose[167]	Ducks/not laying eggs for human consumption[167]
	330 mg/L (1 g/3 L) drinking water q2d × 3 treatments[25,41]	Waterfowl
Ampicillin trihydrate	170 mg/L drinking water[25,37]	Gamebirds
	250 mg/8 oz drinking water[25]	Galliformes
	1000 mg/L drinking water[25,188]	Galliformes/flock use
Ampicillin/sulbactam	300 mg/kg IM q8h[73]	Turkeys/PK
Apramycin (Apralan, Elanco)	—	Therapeutic levels not achieved in Japanese quail at 50 mg/kg IV;[125] not available in the United States
	250-500 mg/L drinking water[37]	Gamebirds, poultry/primarily used against *Salmonella* spp.
Bacitracin methylene disalicylate (Solu-Tracin 200, Solu-Tracin 50, BMD Soluble 50%, Zoetis)	27.5-158 mg/L drinking water[170]	Chickens
	220 mg/L drinking water[41]	Quail/*Clostridium perfringens;* prepare daily
	400 mg/gal drinking water[170]	Turkeys
	55-220 mg/kg feed[148]	Quail
Cefovecin (Convenia, Zoetis)	10 mg/kg SC, IM, IV q1h[221]	Chickens/PK; not recommended for use in birds due to short half-life Poultry/restricted drug[a]
Cefquinome	2 mg/kg IM, IV single dose[244]	Black swans/PK; recommended splitting dose to 1 mg/kg q12h to treat susceptible *E. coli* infections effectively Poultry/restricted drug
	2 mg/kg IM, IV q4h[238]	Chickens/PK Poultry/restricted drug
	5 mg/kg IM q24h[243]	Ducks/no effect PO Poultry/restricted drug[a]

TABLE 6-1 Antimicrobial Agents Used in Backyard Poultry, Gamebirds, and Waterfowl. (cont'd)

Agent	Dosage	Species/Comments
Ceftiofur (Naxcel, Zoetis)	0.08-0.2 mg/chick SC once[170,171]	Chickens (1- to 3-day-old chicks)/as a single SC injection in the neck for the control of early mortality associated with *E. coli* organisms;[171] restricted drug[a]
	0.16 mg/chick SC q24h[219]	Chickens (chicks)/PK; treatment of early mortality associated with *E. coli* Poultry/restricted drug[a]
	0.17-0.5 mg/poult SC once[170,171]	Turkeys (1- to 3-day-old poults)/as a single SC injection in the neck for the control of early mortality associated with *E. coli* organisms; restricted drug[a]
	0.17-0.5 mg/poult SC q24h[219]	Turkeys, poultry/restricted drug[a]
	2-4 mg/kg SC q24h[45]	Ducks, poultry/restricted drug[a]
	2.8-5.8 mg/kg SC q24h[219]	Turkeys (poults)/PK; treatment of early mortality associated with *E. coli* Poultry/restricted drug[a]
	2 mg/kg IV regional limb perfusion q24h[116]	Chickens; plasma and synovial fluid exceeded therapeutic threshold Poultry/restricted drug
Ceftiofur crystalline-free acid (Excede, Zoetis)	10 mg/kg IM q72h[102]	American black ducks/PK Major poultry species/restricted drug
	10 mg/kg IM q72h[237]	Helmeted guinea fowl/PK Major poultry species/restricted drug
Ceftriaxone	100 mg/kg IM q4h[111]	Chickens/PK Poultry/restricted drug[a]
Cephalexin	35-50 mg/kg IM q2-3h[36]	Quail, ducks/PK Major poultry species/restricted drug[a]
Cephalothin	100 mg/kg IM q2-3h[36]	Quail, ducks/PK Major poultry species/restricted drug[a]
Chloramphenicol palmitate (oral suspension)	50 mg/kg PO q6-12h[12]	Chickens/PK Poultry/restricted drug[a]
Chloramphenicol succinate	22 mg/kg IM, IV q3h[55]	Ducks/PK Major poultry species/restricted drug[a]
	50 mg/kg IM q24h[47]	Peafowl Major poultry species/restricted drug[a]
	50 mg/kg IM, IV q6-12h[47]	Chickens (PK), turkeys (PK), geese (PK), ducks Poultry/restricted drug[a]
	79 mg/kg IM q12h[47]	Turkeys/PK Poultry/restricted drug[a]

Continued

TABLE 6-1 Antimicrobial Agents Used in Backyard Poultry, Gamebirds, and Waterfowl. (cont'd)

Agent	Dosage	Species/Comments
Chlortetracycline bisulfate (Aureomycin Soluble Powder, Zoetis)	55 mg/kg PO × 7-14 days[226]	Turkeys/control of complicating bacterial organisms associated with bluecomb (transmissible enteritis, coronaviral enteritis); prepare fresh solution daily as a sole source of chlortetracycline; do not slaughter animals for food within 24 hr of treatment; do not use for more than 14 days[226]
	40-120 mg/L drinking water[37]	Galliformes (gamebirds)
	100-400 mg/gal drinking water[170]	Turkeys
	100-1000 mg/gal drinking water[170]	Chickens
	200-400 mg/gal drinking water[226]	Chickens/control of infectious synovitis caused by *Mycoplasma synoviae*; prepare fresh solution daily as sole source of chlortetracycline; do not slaughter animals for food within 24 hr of treatment; do not use for more than 14 days; do not use in laying chickens[226]
	400 mg/gal drinking water[226]	Turkeys (growing)/control of infectious synovitis caused by *Mycoplasma synoviae*; prepare fresh solution daily as sole source of chlortetracycline; do not slaughter animals for food within 24 hr of treatment; do not use for more than 14 days[226]
	400-800 mg/gal drinking water[226]	Chickens/control of chronic respiratory disease (CRD) and air sac infections caused by *Mycoplasma gallisepticum* and *E. coli*; prepare fresh solution daily as sole source of chlortetracycline; do not slaughter animals for food within 24 hr of treatment; do not use for more than 14 days; do not use in laying chickens[226]
	1000 mg/gal drinking water[226]	Chickens/control of mortality due to fowl cholera caused by *Pasteurella multocida;* prepare fresh solution daily as sole source of chlortetracycline; do not slaughter animals for food within 24 hr of treatment; do not use for more than 14 days; do not use in laying chickens[226]
	2500 mg/L drinking water[43,248] and 2500 mg/kg feed[248]	Chickens, turkeys/PK; simultaneous medication of water and feed required to reach therapeutic level
Ciprofloxacin	2 mg/kg IV[165]	Chicks/no toxic effects observed; prohibited drug[b]
	10-20 mg/kg PO q12h[65]	Chickens/prohibited drug[b]

TABLE 6-1 Antimicrobial Agents Used in Backyard Poultry, Gamebirds, and Waterfowl. (cont'd)

Agent	Dosage	Species/Comments
Danofloxacin mesylate (A180, Zoetis)	5 mg/kg PO, IM, IV[65,210]	Chickens/PK, PD; higher therapeutic efficacy of water medication for enrofloxacin compared to danofloxacin can be expected when given at 5 mg/kg;[118] prohibited drug[b]
	50 mg/L drinking water × 3 days[151,210]	Chicks/*Mycoplasma;* prohibited drug[b]
Doxycycline (Vibramycin, Zoetis)	8-25 mg/kg PO q12h[41]	Waterfowl
	20 mg/kg PO q24h × 3 days[240]	Laying chickens/PK
	20 mg/kg PO q24h × 4 days[14]	Broiler chickens/PK
	20 mg/kg IM, IV q12h[241]	Muscovy ducks/PK; single dose; PO route not recommended at this dose/formulation due to poor oral bioavailability
	20 mg/kg PO × 5 days, or IV single dose[214]	Japanese quail/PK; egg and meat residues reported for this dose and route
	50 mg/kg PO q12h × 3-5 days[27]	Waterfowl/45 days for chlamydiosis
	100 mg/L drinking water[71]	Chickens/PK
Enrofloxacin	—	IM formulation has an extremely alkaline pH and should not be given repeatedly; best to avoid IV use in birds; fluoroquinolones may be used in PMMA beads with success;[62] prohibited drug[b]
	5 mg/kg/day PO × 5 days[85]	Chickens/PK; accumulates in eggs; prohibited drug[b]
	10 mg/kg PO q12h × 4 days[15,17]	Chickens/PK; high efficacy for intestinal salmonellosis; prohibited drug[b]
	10-15 mg/kg PO, IM q12h × 5-7 days[25]	Waterfowl/prohibited drug[b]
	50 mg/kg via nebulization × 4 hr (day 1, AM), then 25 mg/kg × 4 hr/day × 4 days[222]	Muscovy, Pekin ducklings/*Riemerella* (*Pasteurella*); prohibited drug[b]
	50 mg/L drinking water[97,117]	Chickens, turkeys/PK; prohibited drug[b]
	50-100 mg/L drinking water[37]	Gamebirds/prohibited drug[b]
Erythromycin	30 mg/kg PO, SC, IM, IV[84]	Broiler chickens/PK; single dose
	102 mg/L drinking water[57]	Chicks/PK
Erythromycin phosphate (Gallimycin, Cross Vetpharm Group)	500 mg/gal drinking water × 5-7 days[171]	Chickens (broilers, replacements)/aid control of chronic respiratory disease (5 days) and aid control of infectious coryza due to *Avibacterium paragallinarum;* do not use in replacement pullets over 16 wk of age; do not use in chickens producing eggs for human consumption; solutions older than 3 days should not be used

Continued

TABLE 6-1 Antimicrobial Agents Used in Backyard Poultry, Gamebirds, and Waterfowl. (cont'd)

Agent	Dosage	Species/Comments
Gamithromycin	6 mg/kg SC, IV[233]	Broiler chickens/PK
Gentamicin sulfate (Garasol, Intervet)	0.2 mg SC[170]	Chickens/35-day meat withdrawal time
		Turkeys/65-day meat withdrawal time
	3 mg/kg IM q12h[175]	Turkeys/PK
	5 mg/kg IM q8h[51,93]	Pheasants/PK
	5 mg/kg PO, SC, IM, IV[3,4]	Laying hens/PK; oral route not recommended due to poor oral bioavailability
	10 mg/kg IM q6h[51,93]	Quail/PK
Lincomycin HCl (Lincocin, Upjohn)	64 mg/gal drinking water[170]	Chickens
	2 g/L drinking water × 5-7 days[25]	Waterfowl
Lincomycin hydrochloride monohydrate (Lincomix, Zoetis)	2 g/L drinking water × 5-7 days[27]	Waterfowl/*Pasteurella; Mycoplasma* tenosynovitis
Lincomycin/spectinomycin (LS-50 Water Soluble, Upjohn; Linco-Spectin 100 Soluble Powder, Upjohn)	2.5-5 mg/chick IM once[89]	Chickens (chicks)/PD; may prevent *E. coli* and *Staphylococcus aureus* infections; injectable form not available in the United States
	528 mg/L drinking water for first 5 days of age[90]	Turkey poults/PD; *Mycoplasma* airsacculitis
	750 mg/L drinking water × 3-7 days[25]	Waterfowl/*Mycoplasma* synovitis, sinusitis
Lincomycin hydrochloride monohydrate/spectinomycin sulfate tetrahydrate (LS 50 Water Soluble Powder, Zoetis)	2 g/gal drinking water for first 5-7 days of age[170]	Chicken (up to 7 days old)/aid in control of airsacculitis
	750 mg/L drinking water × 3-7 days[41]	Waterfowl
Marbofloxacin (Zeniquin, Zoetis)	2 mg/kg PO q24h[16]	Chickens (broilers)/PK; prohibited drug[b]
	3-12 mg/kg PO q24h[92]	Turkeys/PK; prohibited drug[b]
Neomycin	80-264 mg/L drinking water[41]	Waterfowl
	126 mg/L drinking water[37]	Galliformes
	70-220 mg/kg feed × 14-21 days[41]	Waterfowl, galliformes/*Clostridium*, necrotizing enteritis
Neomycin sulfate (Neomycin 325 Soluble Powder, Zoetis)	10 mg/lb (22 mg/kg) body weight in drinking water × 2-5 days[226]	Turkeys (growing)/for the control of mortality associated with *E. coli*

TABLE 6-1 Antimicrobial Agents Used in Backyard Poultry, Gamebirds, and Waterfowl. (cont'd)

Agent	Dosage	Species/Comments
Nitrofuran	26 mg/L drinking water × 5-7 days[41]	Galliformes/prohibited drug[b,224]
	50-200 mg/kg feed × 5-7 days[41]	Galliformes/*Clostridium; Salmonella;* prohibited drug[b,224]
Norfloxacin (Noroxin, Merck; Vetriflox 20% Oral Solution, Lavet)	8 mg/kg PO q24h[17]	Chickens/PK; prohibited drug[b,224]
	10 mg/kg PO q24h[25,123]	Chickens, geese/PK; prohibited drug[b,224]
	10 mg/kg PO q6-8h[25,123]	Turkeys/PK; prohibited drug[b,224]
	15 mg/kg in water × 2-4 hr[193]	Turkeys/PD; once-per-day pulse dosing was more efficacious than continuous dosing in the water; prohibited drug[b,224]
	20-40 mg/kg PO q24h × 5 days[133]	Chickens/prohibited drug[b,224]
	100 mg/L drinking water × 5 days[193]	Chickens/PK; prohibited drug[b,224]
	175 mg/L drinking water × 5 days[25,190]	Chickens/prohibited drug[b,224]
Novobiocin (Albamix Feed Medication, Zoetis)	4-5 mg/lb body weight/day in feed[226]	Turkeys/aid in the treatment of breast blisters associated with susceptible staphylococcal infections
	5-8 mg/lb body weight/day in feed[226]	Turkeys/aid in the control of recurring outbreaks of fowl cholera caused by susceptible strains of *Pasteurella multocida* following initial treatment with 7-8 mg/lb body weight/day
	6-7 mg/lb body weight/day in feed × 5-7 days[226]	Chickens/aid in the treatment of breast blisters associated with susceptible staphylococcal infections; administer as sole ration feed that contains not less than 200 g/ton of feed; not for laying chickens
	10-14 mg/lb body weight/day in feed × 5-7 days[226]	Chickens/treatment of susceptible staphylococcal infections; administer as sole ration in feed that contains not less than 350 g/ton of feed; not for laying chickens
Novobiocin sodium	15-30 mg/kg PO q24h[209]	Poultry/effective against some gram-positive cocci
	220-385 mg/kg feed[93]	Poultry, waterfowl
Orbifloxacin (Orbax, Intervet)	15-20 mg/kg PO q24h[94]	Japanese quail/PK
		Poultry/prohibited drug[b,226]
Ormetoprim-sulfadimethoxine (Primor, Zoetis)	200-800 mg/kg feed[41]	Waterfowl/colibacillosis

Continued

TABLE 6-1 Antimicrobial Agents Used in Backyard Poultry, Gamebirds, and Waterfowl. (cont'd)

Agent	Dosage	Species/Comments
Oxytetracycline	5 mg/kg SC, IM q12-24h[30]	Chickens (chicks)/PD
	10 mg/kg IM q24h × 3-4 days[78]	Broiler chickens/PK; short-acting formulation (50 mg/mL)
	20 mg/kg IM q72h[78]	Broiler chickens/PK; long-acting formulation (200 mg/mL)
	23 mg/kg IV q6-8h[213]	Pheasants/PK
	43 mg/kg IM q24h[213]	Pheasants/PK
Oxytetracycline (Liquamycin injectable, LA 200, Zoetis)	—	Chickens (broilers, breeders), turkeys/*Mycoplasma gallisepticum*; *M. synoviae*; *E. coli*; *Pasteurella multocida*; treatment must be discontinued at least 5 days prior to slaughter; do not administer to laying hens unless the eggs are used for hatching only; in light turkey breeds, no more than 55 mg/kg of body weight is administered; treatment not to exceed a total of 4 consecutive days[223]
	6.25 mg/chick or poult/day SC diluted 1 part drug to 3 parts sterile water[223]	Chickens, turkeys (1 day to 2 wk of age)
	12.5 mg/pullet or poult/day SC diluted 1 part drug to 3 parts sterile water[223]	Chickens, turkeys (2-4 wk of age)
	15 mg/kg PO, SC, IM, IV[245]	Broiler chickens/PK; PO route not recommended due to poor oral bioavailability
	25 mg/chicken/day SC[223]	Chickens (4-8 wk of age)
	50 mg/chicken or poult/day SC[223]	Chickens (8 wk of age), turkeys (4-6 wk of age)
	100 mg/chicken or poult/day SC[223]	Chickens (adult), turkeys (6-12 wk of age)
	200 mg/poult/day SC undiluted[223]	Turkeys (12 wk of age and older)
Oxytetracycline (Terramycin Soluble Powder, Zoetis)	25 mg/lb body weight × 7-14 days[226]	Turkeys (growing)
	200-400 mg/gal drinking water × 7-14 days[226]	Turkeys (not laying eggs for human consumption)
	200-800 mg/gal drinking water × 7-14 days[226]	Chickens
	37 g/15 L drinking water × 5-7 days[25]	Waterfowl/pasteurellosis and other sensitive bacterial infections
	2500 mg/L drinking water and 2500 mg/kg feed[93,248]	Chickens (PK), turkeys (PK), waterfowl/simultaneous medication of water and feed required to reach therapeutic concentration

TABLE 6-1 Antimicrobial Agents Used in Backyard Poultry, Gamebirds, and Waterfowl. (cont'd)

Agent	Dosage	Species/Comments
Penicillin	50,000 U/kg IM[41]	Waterfowl/*Erysipelas*; new duck disease
Penicillin G (Penicillin G Potassium, Zoetis)	1,500,000 U/gal drinking water × 5 days[226]	Turkeys/not laying eggs for human consumption
Penicillin procaine	100 mg/kg IM q24-48h[99]	Turkeys/PK
Sarafloxacin (Saraflox, Abbott)	10 mg/kg PO q8h[25]	Chickens/prohibited drug[b,226]
	20-40 mg/L drinking water × 5 days[25]	Chickens/colibacillosis; prohibited drug[b,226]
	30-50 mg/L drinking water × 5 days[25]	Turkeys/colibacillosis; prohibited drug[b,226]
Spectinomycin	0.5 g/gal drinking water[226]	Chickens (floor-raised broilers)/use first 3 days of life × 3 days; 1 day following each vaccination[226]
	1 g/gal drinking water[226]	Chickens (broilers)/use first 3-5 days of life[226]
	2 g/gal drinking water[226]	Chickens (growing)/use first 3 days of life × 3 days; use 1 day following each vaccination[226]
Streptomycin	30 mg/kg IM q12h[25]	Chickens
	50 mg/kg x 5 days (may be given via drinking water; make sure to adjust for BW; for standard size chicken = 0.5 g/L)[82]	Chickens/PK; not laying eggs for human consumption
	0.6-0.9 g/gal drinking water x ≤ 5 days[223]	Chickens/not laying eggs for human consumption
Sulfachloropyridazine/ trimethoprim (Cosumix Plus, Ciba)	400 mg/kg feed[25]	Geese
Sulfadimethoxine	0.938 g/gal (0.025%) × 6 days[226]	Turkeys (meat)/fowl cholera; do not administer to turkeys over 24 wk of age; withdraw 5 days prior to slaughter[223]
	1.875 g/gal (0.05%) × 6 days[226]	Chickens (broilers and replacements)/fowl cholera and infectious coryza; do not administer to chickens over 16 wk of age; withdraw 5 days prior to slaughter[226]
Sulfamethazine (SMZ, Cross Vetpharm Group)	110 to 273 mg/kg body weight/day in drinking water[226]	Turkeys/not laying eggs for human consumption[226]
	128-187 mg/kg body weight/day in drinking water[223]	Chickens/not laying eggs for human consumption[223]
Sulfaquinoxaline (Sulquin 6-50, Zoetis; Sul-Q-Nox, Huvepharma)	0.04% in drinking water × 2-3 days[226]	Chickens, turkeys/acute fowl cholera (*Pasteurella multocida*); fowl typhoid (*Salmonella gallinarum*)
	250-500 mg/kg feed[41]	Waterfowl/avian cholera; new duck disease

Continued

TABLE 6-1 Antimicrobial Agents Used in Backyard Poultry, Gamebirds, and Waterfowl. (cont'd)

Agent	Dosage	Species/Comments
Tetracycline	10 mg/kg PO, IV[246]	Broiler chicks/PK
	65 mg/kg IV[13]	Chickens/PK
	40-200 mg/L drinking water[41]	Gamebirds
Tiamulin (Denagard; Elanco)	12.5 mg/kg PO q24h × 3 days[105]	Poultry/intestinal spirochetosis; adverse effects, including death, if administered with ionophores
	25 mg/kg PO q24h × 5 days[105]	Layer hens/intestinal spirochetosis, not to be administered with ionophores
	300-400 mg/kg feed × 7 days[28]	Gamebirds
Tiamulin/ chlortetracycline (Tetramutin, Elanco)	1-1.5 mg/kg feed × 7 days[208]	Chickens/*Mycoplasma*; *Brachyspira*-related diseases; may be used with salinomycin at low doses of 60 mg/kg without signs of incompatibility[93]
Tilmicosin (Micotil 300 Injection, Provitil-powder and Pulmotil AC-liquid, Elanco)	30 mg/kg PO q24h[4]	Poultry/PK; not labeled for use in poultry[93]
	100-500 mg/L drinking water × 5 days[110,113]	Poultry chicks/*Mycoplasma*
Tobramycin	5 mg/kg IM, IV[124]	Broiler chickens/PK; dose not recommended due to extremely low plasma concentrations
	5 mg/kg IM, IV[59]	Ducks/PK; rate of drug elimination slower than other avian species
	20 mg/kg PO[124]	Broiler chickens/PK; dose not recommended due to extremely low plasma concentrations
Trimethoprim/ sulfadiazine	107 mg/L drinking water[28]	Galliformes
Trimethoprim/ sulfamethoxazole	20-50 mg/kg PO q12h[1]	Ducks
	50 mg/kg PO q12h[1]	Chickens
Tylosin (Tylan, Elanco)	10-40 mg/kg IM q6-8h[188]	Poultry
	20-30 mg/kg IM q8h × 3-7 days[25,27]	Waterfowl/*Mycoplasma*
	25 mg/kg IM q6h[131]	Quail/PK
	50 mg/kg PO q24h × 5 days[203]	Broiler chicken/PK
	100 mg/10 mL saline nasal flush × 10 days[25]	Waterfowl/*Mycoplasma*
	500 mg/L drinking water × 3-28 days[93,110,210]	Galliformes, waterfowl/*Mycoplasma*
	851-1419 mg/gal (225-375 ppm) in drinking water × 5 days[226]	Chickens/control mortality caused by necrotic enteritis[226]
	2000 mg/gal (528 ppm) in drinking water × 1-5 days[226]	Chickens (broiler and replacement chicks)/ chronic respiratory disease[226]

TABLE 6-1 Antimicrobial Agents Used in Backyard Poultry, Gamebirds, and Waterfowl. (cont'd)

Agent	Dosage	Species/Comments
Tylosin (Tylan, Elanco) (cont'd)	2000 mg/gal (528 ppm) in drinking water × 2-5 days[226]	Turkeys/infectious sinusitis associated with *Mycoplasma gallisepticum*[226]
	2.5 g/5 L drinking water × 3 days[25]	Waterfowl
Virginiamycin (Stafac, Phibro)	22 mg/kg feed[209]	Poultry

[a]The FDA restricts the extralabel use of the cephalosporin class of antibiotics, except for cephapirin, in food-producing animal species, such as chickens and turkeys.[77,93,226]

[b]The FDA prohibits the use of chloramphenicol, clenbuterol, diethylstilbestrol (DES), fluoroquinolone-class antibiotics, glycopeptides (all agents, including vancomycin), medicated feeds, nitroimidazoles (all agents, including dimetridazole, ipronidazole, metronidazole, and others), and nitrofurans (all agents, including furazolidone, nitrofurazone, and others), with no allowable extralabel drug use, in any food-producing animal species.[77,226]

TABLE 6-2 Antifungal Agents Used in Backyard Poultry, Gamebirds, and Waterfowl.

Agent	Dosage	Species/Comments
Amphotericin B (Liposomal amphotericin B suspension; AmBisome, Astellas)	3 mg/kg intratracheal via atomizer[179]	Mallard ducks/tissue concentrations
Copper sulfate ("bluestone")	Dissolve 0.5 lb copper sulfate and 0.5 cup vinegar in 1 gal of water for a "stock" solution; dispense stock solution at the rate of 1 oz per gal for the final drinking solution[152]; alternate method of preparing the solution: dissolve 1 oz copper sulfate and 1 Tbs of vinegar in 15 gal water[152]	Poultry/mycosis (thrush) in the crop; "followup" treatment after flushing crop with Epsom salt solution[152]
Epsom salts	1 tsp Epsom salt in 1 oz water to flush crop[152]	Chicken/mycotic ingluvitis; individual dose
	1 lb Epsom salt per 15 lb feed[152]	Poultry/laxative or flush prior to copper sulfate treatment; give the Epsom salt feed mixture as the sole feed source for a 1-day period
Fluconazole	100 mg/kg PO q24h[178]	Chickens/avian gastric yeast
Flucytosine (Ancobon, Roche)	60 mg/kg PO q12h[5]	Galliformes, swans/birds >500 g; syringeal aspergilloma
	150 mg/kg PO q12h[5]	Galliformes, swans/birds <500 g; syringeal aspergilloma
Itraconazole	—	Study using SC controlled-release gel formulation in ducks showed unacceptable tissue and plasma levels of the drug[218]
	5 mg/kg PO q24h[5]	Galliformes, swans/aspergillosis

Continued

TABLE 6-2 Antifungal Agents Used in Backyard Poultry, Gamebirds, and Waterfowl. (cont'd)

Agent	Dosage	Species/Comments
Itraconazole (cont'd)	5-10 mg/kg PO q12h[188]	Waterfowl
	10 mg/kg PO q24h × 7-10 days[25]	Waterfowl/prophylactic dose
	10 mg/kg PO q12h 4-6 wk[25]	Waterfowl/therapeutic dose
Ketoconazole	12.5 mg/kg PO q24h × 30 days[188]	Swans/candidiasis
Nystatin	300,000 U/kg PO q12h × 7-14 days[25]	Waterfowl
Voriconazole	10 mg/kg PO, IV q12h[35]	Chickens/PK
	20 mg/kg PO q8-12h[115]	Mallard ducks/PK
	40 mg/kg PO q24h[217]	Quail/PD

TABLE 6-3 Antiparasitic Agents Used in Backyard Poultry, Gamebirds, and Waterfowl.[a]

Parasite	Agent	Dosage	Species/Comments
Protozoa[b]	Amprolium (Amprol, Huvepharma; Corid, Merial)	Follow label of approved preparation; orally via drinking water or feed	Coccidiosis caused by *Eimeria* spp.; coccidiostat
		13-26 mg/kg PO[88]	Chickens/PK, PD; bioavailability almost 4 times greater in fasted birds
		1.2 mL/L (1 tsp/gal) drinking water × 3-5 days and continue with 0.3 mL/L (1/4 tsp/gal) drinking water × 1 to 2 wk[171]	Poultry/20% soluble powder (at 0.024% level, followed by 0.006%)
		3 mL/L (2 tsp/gal) drinking water × 3-5 days and continue with 0.6 mL/L (1/2 tsp/gal) drinking water × 1-2 wk[171]	Poultry/using a 9.6% solution (at 0.024% level, followed by 0.006%)
	Chloroquine phosphate	5 mg/kg PO q24h or in feed[206]	Gamebirds/generally used with primaquine for *Plasmodium*, *Haemoproteus*, and *Leucocytozoon*; overdose can result in death[25]
		2000 mg/L drinking water q24h × 14 days[206]	Gamebirds/juice covers bitter taste of drug
	Clazuril (Appertex, Janssen)	5-10 mg/kg PO q24h × 3 days, off 2 days, on 3 days[144]	Poultry
		125-250 mg/kg feed[206]	Gamebirds/coccidiosis; *Leucocytozoon; Plasmodium*

TABLE 6-3 Antiparasitic Agents Used in Backyard Poultry, Gamebirds, and Waterfowl. (cont'd)

Parasite	Agent	Dosage	Species/Comments
Protozoa (cont'd)	Diclazuril (Clinicox 0.5%, Huvepharma AD; DiClosol 1%, Pharmaswede)	5 mg/L drinking water × 6 days[19]	Chickens/reduced oocyst viability and virulence
		5-10 mg/L drinking water × 2 days[63]	Chickens/effective in preventing disease and reducing total oocysts, lesions, and mortality in infected birds with mixed *Eimeria* infections
	Oregano essential oil (Orego-Stim 5%, Meriden AnimalHealth Ltd)	500 ppm in feed[154]	Chickens (growing)/PD; coccidiostat; (not statistically significant) lower oocysts per gram of feces and lower coccidiosis lesion scores compared to the untreated group
	Primaquine	0.03 mg/kg PO q24h × 3 days[206]	Gamebirds/hematozoa (i.e., *Plasmodium*, *Haemoproteus*, *Leucocytozoon*); use in conjunction with chloroquine; dosage based on amount of active base rather than total tablet weight
	Pyrimethamine (Fansidar, Roche)	0.25-0.5 mg/kg PO q12h × 30 days[93]	Waterfowl/*Sarcocystis*; *Toxoplasma*
		0.5 mg/kg PO q12h × 30 days[27]	Waterfowl/*Sarcocystis*
		1 mg/kg feed[206]	Gamebirds
	Pyrimethamine/ sulfaquinoxaline (Microquinox, C-Vet Livestock Products)	60 mg/L drinking water, 3 days on, 2 days off, 3 days on[25]	Waterfowl/coccidiosis
	Sulfadiazine/ trimethoprim (DiTrim, Zoetis)	60 mg/kg PO q12h × 3 days[25]	Waterfowl/coccidiosis
	Sulfadimethoxine (12.5%)	0.938 g/gal or 250 mg/L (0.025%) × 6 days[206,226]	Turkeys (meat)/coccidiosis; withdraw 5 days before slaughter; do not administer to turkeys over 24 wk (168 days) of age
		1.875 g/gal or 500 mg/L (0.05%) × 6 days[206,226]	Chickens (broilers and replacements)/coccidiosis; withdraw 5 days before slaughter; do not administer to chickens over 16 wk (112 days) of age
	Sulfadimethoxine/ ormetoprim (Rofenaid 40, Zoetis)	10 mg/kg feed[206]	Gamebirds/coccidiosis; *Leucocytozoon*; *Sarcocystis*
	Sulfamethazine (Sulmet, Huvepharma; Sulmet, Boehringer Ingelheim)	125-185 mg/kg PO q24h × 2 days, then 64-94 mg/kg × 4 days[109]	Chickens

Continued

TABLE 6-3 Antiparasitic Agents Used in Backyard Poultry, Gamebirds, and Waterfowl. (cont'd)

Parasite	Agent	Dosage	Species/Comments
Protozoa (cont'd)		2 Tbs (1 fl oz)/gal to provide 58-85 mg/lb/day (128-187 mg/kg/day) body weight in chickens and 50-124 mg/lb/day (110-273 mg/kg/day) body weight in turkeys × 2 days, then reduce medication by 50% × 4 days[171]	Chickens, turkeys/coccidiosis
	Sulfaquinoxaline (20% solution, Huvepharma)	0.04% in drinking water × 2-3 days, off 3 days, then use 0.025% × 2 days (repeat 0.025% × 2 days if needed)[226]	Chickens/coccidiosis caused by *Eimeria tenella*, *E. necatrix*, *E. acervulina*, *E. maxima*, and *E. brunetti*; do not change litter unless absolutely necessary; do not give flushing mashes; medicated chickens must actually consume enough medicated water to provide a recommended dosage of approximately 22-99 mg/kg/day depending on the age, class of animal, ambient temperature, and other factors; do not give to chickens within 10 days of slaughter for food; do not medicate chickens producing eggs for human consumption; make fresh drinking water daily[226]
		0.025% in drinking water × 2 days, off 3 days, on 2 days, off 3 days, and on 2 days; repeat if necessary[226]	Turkeys/coccidiosis caused by *Eimeria meleagridis* and *E. adenoides*;[226] must consume enough medicated water to provide approximately 77-121 mg/kg/day depending on age, class of animal, ambient temperature; do not give to turkeys within 10 days of slaughter for food; do not use in turkeys producing eggs for human consumption
	Tinidazole (Fasigyn, Pfizer)	—	*Giardia*; *Trichomonas*; *Entamoeba*
		200-400 mg/kg feed[104]	Chickens/*Histomonas*; depressed weight gain on higher dosage
	Toltrazuril (Baycox, Bayer)	—	Coccidiocidal; efficacious for refractory coccidiosis; 2.5% solution is very alkaline and should not be gavaged directly into the crop[121]
		1 ml of 2.5% solution/2 L drinking water × 2 days[75]	Waterfowl

TABLE 6-3 Antiparasitic Agents Used in Backyard Poultry, Gamebirds, and Waterfowl. (cont'd)

Parasite	Agent	Dosage	Species/Comments
Protozoa (cont'd)		12.5 mg/L drinking water × 2 days[25]	Waterfowl
		25 mg/L drinking water × 2 days[63]	Chickens
	Trimethoprim/ sulfachlorpyridazine (1:5 ratio; Cosumix Plus, Novartis)	400 mg/kg feed[109]	Geese
	Trimethoprim/ sulfadiazine	60 mg/kg PO, SC q12h × 3 days, off 2 days, on 3 days[25]	Waterfowl/coccidiosis
	Trimethoprim/ sulfamethoxazole	320-525 mg/L drinking water[25]	Poultry/coccidiosis
Helminths	Albendazole (11.36%) (Valbazen, Zoetis)	Not listed for poultry in US	General dewormer (nematodes, cestodes, and flukes)
		10 mg/kg PO once[157]	Poultry/PK; dose 40 mg/kg or higher reduce egg hatchability
	Clorsulon (Curatrem, Merial)	20 mg/kg PO × 3 treatments q2wk[25]	Waterfowl/trematodes; cestodes
	Fenbendazole (Safeguard, Ralston Purina; Panacur, Intervet)	—	Effective against cestodes, nematodes, trematodes, *Giardia*, acanthocephalans; can cause feather abnormalities if administered during molting[25]
		1.5-3.9 mg/kg PO q24h × 3 days[25,211]	Chickens/PK, PD; *Capillaria*
		5-15 mg/kg q24h × 5 days[25]	Waterfowl
		10-50 mg/kg PO once; repeat in 10 days[142]	Chickens/*Ascaris* spp.
		10-50 mg/kg PO q24h × 5 days[142]	Chickens/*Capillaria* and other nematodes
		20 mg/kg PO once[25]	Waterfowl
		125 mg/L of drinking water × 5 days[142]	Chickens/nematodes other than *Capillaria*
		16 mg/kg feed × 6 days[142]	Turkeys (growing)/*Ascaridia dissimilis*; *Heterakis gallinarium*
		20 mg/kg PO once[232]	Pheasants/cestodes; nematodes; acanthocephalans; reduced *Heterakis* and *Eimeria* in pheasants
		20-100 mg/kg PO once[142]	Chickens/nematodes other than *Capillaria*

Continued

TABLE 6-3 Antiparasitic Agents Used in Backyard Poultry, Gamebirds, and Waterfowl. (cont'd)

Parasite	Agent	Dosage	Species/Comments
Helminths (cont'd)		53-500 mg/kg feed × 5-7 days[87,206]	Gamebirds (pheasant, partridges, quail)/*Syngamus*; nematodes; trematodes
		80 mg/kg feed[211]	Chickens/PK, PD; *Capillaria*
	Flubendazole (Flubenol, Elanco)	20 mg/kg feed × 7 days[67]	Turkeys/broad-spectrum anthelmintic
		30 mg/kg feed × 7 days[25]	Chickens/nematodes
		60 mg/kg feed × 7 days[67]	Partridges, pheasants/broad-spectrum anthelmintic Chickens/tapeworms
	Hygromycin B (Hygromix 8, Elanco)	—	Aminoglycoside antibiotic used as anthelmintic feed additive
		8-12 g/ton feed[142]	Chickens/*Ascaridia; Heterakis; Capillaria*
		9-13 mg/kg feed[206]	Gamebirds/ascarids; cecal worms; some efficacy against *Capillaria*
		18-26 mg/kg feed × 2 mo[206]	Gamebirds/cecal worms
	Ivermectin	—	Most nematodes, acanthocephalans, leeches, most ectoparasites (including *Knemidokoptes, Dermanyssus*); can dilute with water or saline for immediate use; dilute with propylene glycol for extended use
		0.2 mg/kg PO, SC, IM once, can repeat in 10-14 days[25]	Not approved in poultry; PK data in eggs not available
	Levamisole	—	Nematodes; immunostimulant; low therapeutic index (toxic reactions, deaths reported); do not use in debilitated birds[25]
		1 g/gal drinking water × 1 day, repeat in 5-7 days[198]	Pheasants/*Syngamus trachea*
		0.52 g/gal (or 0.4 g/3 L) drinking water × 1 day; can repeat in 5-7 days[152]	Poultry/*Capillaria; Heterakis; Ascaridia*
		20-25 mg/kg SC[206]	Gamebirds
		20-50 mg/kg PO, SC once[25]	Waterfowl
		25-30 mg/kg[142]	Chicken/*Ascaridia dissimilis; H. gallinariu; Capillaria obsingnata*
		40 mg/kg PO once[66]	Chickens/PK; *Capillaria*

TABLE 6-3 Antiparasitic Agents Used in Backyard Poultry, Gamebirds, and Waterfowl. (cont'd)

Parasite	Agent	Dosage	Species/Comments
Helminths (cont'd)		265-525 mg/L drinking water × 1 day, repeat in 7-14 days[206]	Gamebirds, poultry
	Mebendazole (Telmin Suspension, Telmintic Powder, Schering-Plough)	—	Broad-spectrum ovicidal antihelmintic; primarily used for *Capillaria*[25]
		5-15 mg/kg PO q24h × 2 days[25,147]	Galliformes, waterfowl/nematodes
		1.2 mg/kg feed × 14 days[27]	Waterfowl/nematodes
	Milbemycin oxime (Interceptor, Novartis)	2 mg/kg PO, repeat in 28 days[96]	Galliformes/nematodes
	Praziquantel	5-10 mg/kg PO, SC q24h × 14 days[41]	Waterfowl/trematodes
		10 mg/kg PO[41]	Chickens
		10 mg/kg PO, SC for 14 days[25,41]	Waterfowl/trematodes
		10-20 mg/kg PO, SC repeat in 10 days[25,41]	Waterfowl/cestodes, trematodes
	Thiabendazole	—	Nematodes; acanthocephalans; generally less efficacious than fenbendazole; may be toxic to diving ducks[25]
		425 mg/kg feed × 14 days[206]	Pheasants
External parasites	Carbaryl 5% (Sevin Dust, Bayer)	—	No longer approved for use in poultry
	Cypermethrin (5%) (Max Con, Y-Tex)	60-120 mg/chicken topically over dorsal neck[8]	Chickens/effective against *Triatoma infestans*
	Ivermectin	—	See Helminths

[a]The FDA does not allow extralabel use of nitroimidazoles (all agents, including dimetridazole, ipronidazole, metronidazole, and others) and only labeled uses of approved sulfonamides are allowed in any food-producing animal species.[77,226]

[b]Anticoccidial drugs added to feed are not included in the table because they are used as preventive medication and not as a treatment. For current information on these medications in the United States, consult the regulations for food additives in 21 Code of Federal Regulation Part 558 for up-to-date information on approved products, at https://www.fda.gov/food/food-additives-petitions/food-additive-status-list. For current information in the European Union, consult the European Food Safety Authority at https://ec.europa.eu/food/safety/animal-feed/feed-additives/eu-register_en.

TABLE 6-4 Chemical Restraint/Anesthetic/Analgesic Agents Used in Backyard Poultry, Gamebirds, and Waterfowl.

Agent	Dosage	Species/Comments
Acetaminophen	10 mg/kg IM q24h × 7 days[106]	Chickens/mild pain; pyrexia; no adverse clinical signs; normal serum creatinine and uric acid; no gross or histopathologic changes in kidneys observed
	20–30 mg/kg per day via water × 7 days[187]	Chickens/PD; did not improve mobility or walking pace but did increase other behaviors such as preening and dust bathing in hens with keel bone fractures
Alfaxalone	10 mg/kg IM, IV[122]	Mallard ducks/PK, PD; dose did not provide appropriate anesthetic depth for invasive procedures; hyperexcitability during recorvery
	10-15 mg/kg IV[235]	Isa Brown chickens/achieved endotracheal intubation; induction quality poor
Alfaxalone (A)/ midazolam (Mi)	(A) 15 mg/kg IM + (Mi) 2.5 mg/kg IM[119]	Rhode Island Red hens/successful for radiographic positioning in 7 out of 12 birds; faster onset and longer duration that butorphanol + midazolam IM
Alphachloralose (Fisher Scientific)	30 mg/kg PO once[26]	Canada geese/immobilization of nuisance geese; prepare suspension in corn oil, inject into individual bread baits, and hand-toss to target individuals; onset approximately 60 min, duration up to 24 hr; low therapeutic index in chickens suggests only marginally safe in domestic species or for field applications where dosage difficult to control[132]
	250-430 mg/cup of bait[41,93]	Waterfowl (including Canada geese)/ immobilization
Atipamezole (Antisedan, Zoetis)	—	α_2 adrenergic antagonist; 1:1 volume reversal of dexmedetomidine and medetomidine is general rule; although the same effects would be expected as with medetomidine (no longer available but can be compounded), there are no data available on the efficacy of this volume of atipamezole reversal of dexmedetomidine in birds
	2.5-5 × medetomidine dose IM, IV[93,137]	Geese/righting reflex regained 2-10 min after administration; for reversal of dexmedetomidine and medetomidine (no longer commercially available, but can be compounded)
	0.18-0.28 mg/kg IV[136]	Mallard ducks
	0.25-0.38 mg/kg IM[137]	Mallard ducks
Atropine sulfate	0.1 mg/kg IM, IV q3-4h[25]	Waterfowl
Bupivacaine HCl	1.94 mg/kg IV[58]	Chickens/TD_{50}; dose with 50% probability of a clinically significant change in blood pressure in isoflurane-anesthetized chickens
	2 mg/kg infused SC[139]	Mallard ducks/PK; high plasma concentrations at 6 and 12 hr post administration, so delayed toxicity is possible

TABLE 6-4 Chemical Restraint/Anesthetic/Analgesic Agents Used in Backyard Poultry, Gamebirds, and Waterfowl. (cont'd)

Agent	Dosage	Species/Comments
Bupivacaine HCl (cont'd)	2-8 mg/kg perineurally[34]	Mallard ducks/variable effectiveness for brachial plexus nerve block
	2-10 mg/kg infused into incision site[161]	Eider ducks/high bupivacaine dose toxicity or cumulative toxicity of bupivacaine and ketoprofen may have occurred
	3 mg/0.3 mL saline injected intra-articular[100]	Chickens/arthritis
	5 mg/kg (with 10 µg/kg epinephrine) perineurally[74]	Chickens/unsuccessful brachial plexus nerve block
	50:50 mixture with dimethyl sulfoxide topically[81]	Chickens/topical anesthesia; applied to amputated beaks
Buprenorphine HCl	0.05-1 mg/kg intraarticular[79]	Chickens/PD; no significant antinociceptive effects
Butorphanol tartrate	0.5-2 mg/kg IM[160]	Harlequin ducks/no isoflurane-sparing effects detected when administered 15 min prior to induction;[160] 4 mg/kg IM caused severe adverse cardiopulmonary effects in guinea fowl[70]
	2 mg/kg IM q8-12h[1]	Chicken/as part of bimodal pain therapy with PO carprofen
	2 mg/kg IV q2h[202]	Broiler chickens/PK; plasma concentrations above the minimum effective concentration for analgesia in mammals for approximately 2 hr
	247 µg/kg/h via SC osmotic pump[46]	Common peafowl/PK; plasma butorphanol concentration was ≥60 µg/L for a mean of 85.6 hr
Butorphanol (B)/ midazolam (Mi)	(B) 1 mg/kg + (Mi) 1 mg/kg[74]	Chickens/adequate sedation for lateral recumbency
	(B) 3 mg/kg + (Mi) 2.5 mg/kg[119]	Rhode Island Red hens/not successful for radiographic positioning; slower onset and shorter duration compared to alfaxalone + midazolam IM
Detomidine (Dormosedan, Zoetis)	0.3 mg/kg IM[93,229]	Chickens, rock partridges/marked sedation; significant decrease in HR and RR; decrease in cloacal temperature; prolonged recoveries (260 ± 17.6 min) in partridges
Diazepam[a]	0.5-1 mg/kg IM, IV q8-12h[25]	Waterfowl/sedation; anticonvulsant; IM administration may cause severe muscle irritation and absorption may be delayed
	6 mg/kg IM[229]	Rock partridges/decrease in cloacal temperature; prolonged recoveries (149 ± 8.3 min)
Fentanyl citrate	0.5-1 mg/kg intraarticular[79]	Chickens/PD; no effect on pain behavior
	5 mg/kg transdermal (intrascapular skin)[234]	Guinea fowl/PK; plasma concentrations greater than those reported to be analgesic for dogs for at least 7 days; no longer available in the United States

Continued

TABLE 6-4 Chemical Restraint/Anesthetic/Analgesic Agents Used in Backyard Poultry, Gamebirds, and Waterfowl. (cont'd)

Agent	Dosage	Species/Comments
Fentanyl citrate (cont'd)	25 µg/h patch x 72 hr[56]	Chickens/PK; wide variability; placed over plucked skin on dorsum; reached human therapeutic levels by 2-4 hr post application[56]
Flumazenil	0.018-0.028 mg/kg IV[136]	Mallard ducks
	0.05 mg/kg IM[119]	Rhode Island Red hens
	0.05 mg/kg intranasally[93,137]	Mallard ducks
	0.1 mg/kg IM[54]	Quail/PD; reversed midazolam in 1.4-1.8 min
Isoflurane	1.1% ± 0.1%[69]	Chickens/minimum anesthetic concentration
	1.15%[145]	Chickens/minimum anesthetic concentration
	1.3%[134]	Ducks/minimum anesthetic concentration
Ketamine	15-25 mg/kg IM, IV[95]	Waterfowl/seldom used as sole agent because of poor muscle relaxation and prolonged (up to 3 hr), violent recovery; may produce excitation or convulsions in golden pheasants; may fail to produce general anesthesia in some species, including waterfowl
Ketamine (K)/ diazepam (D)[a]	(K) 10-40 mg/kg IV + (D) 1-1.5 mg/kg IM,[a] IV[127]	Waterfowl/induction or surgical anesthesia; rapid bolus may produce apnea, arrhythmia, and increased risk of death
	(K) 75 mg/kg IM + (D) 2.5 mg/kg IV[44,143]	Chickens[44]/diazepam given 10 min after ketamine; pain reflexes elicited at all times; recovery in 90-100 min
		Chickens (white leghorn cockerels)[143]/ diazepam administered 5 min before ketamine for typhlectomy; smooth induction/recovery; some limb contracture, hypothermia, hypoxia, hypercapnia
Ketamine (K)/ medetomidine (Me)	(K) 1.5-2 mg/kg + (Me) 60-85 µg/kg IM, IV[127]	Waterfowl/sedation; medetomidine no longer available in the United States but can be compounded; see dexmedetomidine
Ketamine (K)/ medetomidine (Me)/midazolam (Mi)	(K) 10 mg/kg + (Me) 50 µg/kg + (Mi) 2 mg/kg IV[136,137]	Mallard ducks/PD; medetomidine no longer available in the United States but can be compounded; anesthesia of 30-min duration; reverse with atipamezole, flumazenil intranasally; regimen considered unsafe due to acidosis, bradypnea, apnea, and in 1 out of 12 birds, death[137]
Ketamine (K)/ midazolam (Mi)	(K) 50 mg/kg IV + (Mi) 2 mg/kg IM[143]	Chickens (white leghorn cockerels)/midazolam administered 5 min before ketamine for typhlectomy; hypoxia, hypercapnia, torticollis, dyspnea, salivation noted; prolonged recovery (92-105 min)
Ketamine (K)/ xylazine (X)	(K) 10 mg/kg + (X) 2 mg/kg IV[143]	Chickens (white leghorn cockerels)/for typhlectomy; smooth induction/recovery; optimal to excellent surgical anesthesia
	(K) 20 mg/kg + (X) 1 mg/kg IV[135]	Pekin ducks/bradypnea, acidemia, hypoxemia, moderate hyperthermia

TABLE 6-4 Chemical Restraint/Anesthetic/Analgesic Agents Used in Backyard Poultry, Gamebirds, and Waterfowl. (cont'd)

Agent	Dosage	Species/Comments
Ketamine (K)/ xylazine (X) (cont'd)	(K) 25 mg/kg + (X) 1 mg/kg IM[212]	Guinea fowl/lateral recumbency 1-6 min; adequate anesthesia; arousal in 1.4 ± 0.7 min after yohimbine administration
Ketamine (K)/ xylazine (X)/ diazepam (D)[a]	(K) 25 mg/kg + (X) 3 mg/kg + (D) 4 mg/kg IM[a,159]	Roosters/use with caution; significant decreases in HR, RR, cloacal temperatures; prolonged recoveries (up to 4 hr)
Ketamine (K)/ xylazine (X)/ midazolam (Mi)	(K) 15 mg/kg + (X) 2.5 mg/kg + (Mi) 0.3 mg/kg IM[6]	Guinea fowl/midazolam improved anesthetic quality
Lidocaine	—	Chickens/administered lidocaine 6 mg/kg IV bolus over 2 min had no adverse effects[33]
	0.5-2 mg/kg intrathecal in the synsacrococcygeal space[112]	Chickens/regional anaesthesia of the pericloacal area
	2.5 mg/kg IV (give over 20 sec)[52]	Chickens/PK; under isoflurane anesthesia
	15 mg/kg (with 3.8 µg/kg epinephrine) perineurally[34]	Mallard ducks/variable effectiveness for brachial plexus nerve block
	20 mg/kg (with 10 µg/kg epinephrine) perineurally[74]	Chickens/unsuccessful brachial plexus nerve block
Methohexital sodium (Brevital, JHP Pharmaceuticals)	4-8 mg/kg IV[148]	Poultry
	5-10 mg/kg IV[148]	Ducks
Midazolam HCl	2 mg/kg IM[230]	Canada geese/sedation for 15-20 min
	2-6 mg/kg IM[54]	Quail/PD; mild to heavy sedation
	4-6 mg/kg IM[109]	Waterfowl
	5 mg/kg IV[49]	Turkeys, chickens, ring-necked pheasants, bobwhites/PK; rapid absorption; $t_{1/2}$ = 0.42, 1.45, 1.90, and 9.71 hr for turkeys, chickens, bobwhites, and pheasants, respectively
Morphine sulfate	1-3 mg/kg intra-articular[79]	Chickens/PD; no analgesic effect for arthritis noted; early work in chickens demonstrated confusing clinical dosage results
	2 mg/kg IV[201]	Chickens/PK; plasma concentrations greater than MEC for humans for 2 hr
	2.5-3 mg/kg SC, IM q4h[188]	Galliformes/analgesia
	10-20 mg/kg IM[72]	Japanese quail/PD; exhibited antinociceptive effects on foot withdrawal and pressure tests; no effect on locomotion, eating, or drinking at these doses
Propofol	5 mg/kg IV (induction); 0.5 mg/kg/min IV (maintenance)[197]	Wild turkeys/PD; anesthesia; intubation, ventilation, and supplemental oxygen strongly recommended[93,197]

Continued

TABLE 6-4 Chemical Restraint/Anesthetic/Analgesic Agents Used in Backyard Poultry, Gamebirds, and Waterfowl. (cont'd)

Agent	Dosage	Species/Comments
Propofol (cont'd)	6-14 mg/kg (induction); boluses prn[161]	Eider ducks/anesthesia with inhalant, bupivacaine, ketoprofen; significant mortality but high-dose bupivacaine toxicity or cumulative bupivacaine/ketoprofen toxicity may have occurred
	8 mg/kg IV (induction); 0.85 mg/kg/min IV (maintenance)[162]	Swans (mute)/PD
	8-10 mg/kg IV (induction); 1-4 mg/kg IV boluses prn (maintenance)[136-138]	Mallard ducks, canvasback ducks/PD; anesthesia
	9 mg/kg IV (induction); 1.2 mg/kg/min (maintenance)[192]	Hissex brown chickens/PD; admininstered for TIVA (total intravenous anesthesia) in combination with either methadone 6 mg/kg IM or nalbuphine 12.5 mg/kg IM[192]
	15 mg/kg IV (induction); 0.8 mg/kg/min IV (maintenance)[136]	Canvasback ducks/PD; some excitement during induction; two deaths; significant reduction in ventilation
Ropivacaine (Ropi 0.75%, Cristália Chemical & Pharmaceutical)	7.5 mg/kg perineurally[40]	Chickens/15 min to effect for brachial plexus nerve block; approximately 110 min anesthesia; no toxic effects noted at this dose
Sevoflurane	2.21 ± 0.32%[166]	Chickens/PD; minimum anesthetic concentration; dose-dependent hypotension noted
Tiletamine/ zolazepam (Telazol, Zoetis)	6.6 mg/kg IM[195]	Swans
	9-30 mg/kg IM[195]	Wood partridges/restraint
Tramadol HCl	7.5 mg/kg PO[29]	Peafowl/PK; only 2/6 birds reached human tramadol analgesic concentrations; 5/6 maintained O-desmethyl-tramadol (M1) concentrations above human analgesic concentrations for 10-12 hr and 3/6 for 24 hr; analgesia not evaluated
	30 mg/kg PO[24]	Muscovy ducks/PK, PD; maintained concentrations therapeutic for humans for at least 12-24 hr; effective at this dose for analgesia from induced arthritis based on ground reactive forces[24]
Xylazine	1 mg/kg IV[135]	Pekin ducks
	1-20 mg/kg IM, IV[41]	Waterfowl/sedation
	10 mg/kg IM[229]	Rock partridges/good sedation; significant decrease in respiratory rate; decrease in cloacal temperature; prolonged recoveries (205 ± 22.2 min)
Yohimbine HCl (Yobine, Lloyd)	—	α_2 adrenergic antagonist; excitement and mortality observed at doses >1 mg/kg[95]
	0.1-0.2 mg/kg IV[41]	Waterfowl

TABLE 6-4 Chemical Restraint/Anesthetic/Analgesic Agents Used in Backyard Poultry, Gamebirds, and Waterfowl. (cont'd)

Agent	Dosage	Species/Comments
Yohimbine HCl (Yobine, Lloyd) (cont'd)	1 mg/kg IV[212]	Guinea fowl/excitement and mortality observed in birds at doses >1 mg/kg[95]

[a]Diazepam is not soluble in aqueous solution; admixing with aqueous solutions or fluids can result in precipitation; administering SC or IM can be painful and irritating; for SC or IM administration, midazolam may be preferred.

TABLE 6-5 Nonsteroidal Antiinflammatory Agents Used in Backyard Poultry, Gamebirds, and Waterfowl.[a]

Agent	Dosage	Species/Comments
Aspirin (acetylsalicylic acid)	25 mg/kg IV[22,23]	Chickens, ducks, turkeys
	50 mg/kg PO[180]	Chickens, turkeys/PK; mean residue time 7 hr and 4.5 hr, respectively;[180] chickens/400 mg/kg PO × 14 days led to decreased weight gain and ventricular ulceration[180,181]
	50 mg/kg IV[180]	Chickens, turkeys/PK; mean residue time 6 hr and 3.3 hr, respectively
	100-200 mg/kg IM[101]	Chickens/partially reduced arthritic behaviors after 1 hr
Carprofen	1 mg/kg SC[149]	Chickens/improved locomotion for at least 90 min post injection
	15-25 mg/kg SC[39]	Chickens/PD; therapeutically effective treatment of induced articular pain at 6 hr
	30 mg/kg IM[101]	Chickens/PD; arthritis painful behaviors reduced 1 hr post treatment only with this high dose
	40 mg/kg body weight in feed[53]	Chickens/analgesia; dosage required to reach similar mammalian therapeutic plasma concentrations (8.3 µg/mL), but much lower plasma concentrations (0.28 µg/mL) provided some analgesia
Diclofenac	—	Chickens/toxic at dose of 2.5 mg/kg IM q24h × 7 days; severe clinical signs of renal toxicity and high mortality with increased serum creatinine and uric acid concentrations[106]
Flunixin meglumine	—	Potential nephrotoxicity; histologic glomerular changes were demonstrated in bobwhite quail given doses as low as 0.1 mg/kg (severity of lesions was directly correlated to dose);[114] IM administration caused muscle necrosis in mallard ducks[141]
	1.1 mg/kg IV[22]	Chickens, ducks, turkeys/long half-life
		Ostriches/short half-life; $t_{1/2}$ = 10 min
	3 mg/kg IM[101]	Chickens/PD; arthritis behaviors reduced 1 hr after treatment

Continued

TABLE 6-5 Nonsteroidal Antiinflammatory Agents Used in Backyard Poultry, Gamebirds, and Waterfowl.[a] (cont'd)

Agent	Dosage	Species/Comments
Flunixin meglumine (cont'd)	5 mg/kg IM[141]	Mallard ducks/PD; reduced thromboxane activity for 12 hr; muscle necrosis at injection site
	5 mg/kg IV[239]	Chickens/PK; $t_{1/2}$ = 3 hr
	1.3 mg/kg IV RLP once[186]	Chickens/pododermatitis; regional limb perfusion (RLP) into medial metatarsal vein with a tourniquet placed proximal to hock joint for 15 min[186]
Ketoprofen	1 mg/kg IM q24h × 1-10 days[22,23,25,93]	Waterfowl/arthritis
	2 mg/kg PO, SC, IM, IV[86]	Japanese quail/PK, PD; poor bioavailability and rapid clearance after PO or IM administration
	2-5 mg/kg PO, IM, IV q12-24h[161]	Eider ducks/high mortality in male ducks may be due to high bupivacaine dose or cumulative toxicity of bupivacaine and ketoprofen
	3 mg/kg IM q24h × 5 days[153]	Chickens/no adverse clinical signs; normal creatinine, uric acid, ALT, AST
	5 mg/kg IM q12h[140,141]	Mallard ducks/PD; inhibited thromboxane for approximately 12 hr
	5-10 mg/kg IM, IV[41]	Waterfowl
	12 mg/kg IM[101]	Chickens/reduced arthritic pain behaviors for 12 hr
Meloxicam	—	Administration of 5 mg/kg PO q12h resulted in acute renal tubular necrosis and gout in 7 of 11 treated hens[103]
	0.5 mg/kg IV[22,23]	Chickens, ducks, turkeys/PK; variable distribution
	0.5 mg/kg IV, PO[194]	Bilgorajska geese/PK; maintained plasma concentrations which provided analgesia in Hispaniolan Amazon parrots for 5 hr after PO administration
	1 mg/kg PO once[205]	Chickens/PK; $t_{1/2}$ = 2.8 hr; drug detected in egg white up to 4 days and egg yolk up to 8 days after dosing
	1 mg/kg PO q12h × 9 treatments[204]	Chickens/PK; 2-wk withdrawal time should be adequate to avoid drug residues in eggs meant for consumption
	1 mg/kg PO[24]	Muscovy ducks/PD; effective at this dose for analgesia from induced arthritis based on ground reactive forces
	2 mg/kg IM q12h × 14 days[200]	Japanese quail/PD; unremarkable histologic and minimal biochemical changes
	3-5 mg/kg SC[39]	Chickens/PD; therapeutically effective treatment of induced articular pain at 6 hr
Tepoxalin	30 mg/kg PO, IV[31]	Chickens/PK; rapidly metabolized; $t_{1/2}$ = 2.8 hr for PO and 1 hr for IV[31]

[a]Nonsteroidal antiinflammatory agents may potentially cause gastrointestinal upset and hemorrhage as well as adverse renal effects ranging from fluid retention to renal failure.

TABLE 6-6 Hormones and Steroids Used in Backyard Poultry, Gamebirds, and Waterfowl.

Agent	Dosage	Species/Comments
Deslorelin acetate (Suprelorin, Virbac)	—	Poultry/prohibited drug
	Two 4.7-mg or two 9.4-mg implants[155]	Turkey/reduces male aggression
	Two 4.7-mg or one 9.4-mg implants[176,177]	Quail/decreases egg production
Dexamethasone sodium phosphate	0.3 mg/kg IM, IV once[233]	Broiler chickens/PK; high clearance compared to mammals
Estradiol benzoate	1 mg/kg IM q24h × 12 days[98]	Mallard ducks/induces molt
Levonorgestrel depot form (Levonorgestrel, Sigma Chemical)	40 mg/kg SC[76,215]	Japanese quail, turkeys/halts egg laying but may cause ovostasis if already in oviduct; repeat in 60 days in turkeys
Levothyroxine	0.2 mg/kg PO q12-24h[25]	Treatment of hypothyroidism; induction of molt
Melatonin	10 mg implant[107]	Poultry/increases egg production
Prostaglandin E_2 (dinoprostone) (Prepidil Gel, Upjohn)	Applied topically to the uterovaginal sphincter[60]	Waterfowl/dystocia; relaxes uterovaginal sphincter
Tamoxifen citrate	40 mg/kg IM[98,207]	Galliformes, ducks/induces molt

TABLE 6-7 Nebulization Agents Used in Backyard Poultry, Gamebirds, and Waterfowl.[a]

Agent	Dosage	Species/Comments
Ceftriaxone	—	Poultry/prohibited drug
	40 mg/mL sterile water[111]	Poultry/PK
	40 mg/mL sterile water and DMSO[111]	Poultry/PK; 1 g ceftriaxone in 10 mL sterile water, plus 15 mL DMSO
	200 mg/mL sterile water and DMSO[111]	Poultry/PK; 4 g ceftriaxone in 10 mL sterile water, plus 10 mL DMSO
Lincomycin	250 mg aerosolized drug/m³ chamber × 15-30 min[42]	Chickens/PD; antibiotic; therapeutic concentrations in blood, lungs, and trachea for up to 24 hr
Oxytetracycline	1 g/m³ of air using a DeVilbiss ultrasonic nebulizer, or 0.075 g/m³ of air using a Fogmaster fogger[231]	Turkey poults
Tylosin	20 mg/mL in DMSO or distilled water × 1 hr[130,131]	Quail/PK

[a]Nebulization is an adjunct therapy indicated for rhinitis, sinusitis, tracheitis, pneumonia, airsacculitis, and syringeal aspergilloma, where there is air movement occurring in the patient's disease state; optimal particle size for deposition in the trachea is 2-10 μm; optimal particle size for peripheral airways is 0.5-5 μm; treatments of 30-45 min repeated q4-12h are recommended; caution: do not overhydrate airways.[32]

TABLE 6-8 Agents Used in the Treatment of Toxicologic Conditions of Backyard Poultry and Waterfowl.

Agent	Dosage	Species/Comments
Atropine sulfate	0.1 mg/kg IM, IV q3-4h[25]	Waterfowl/acetylcholinesterase toxicosis
Botulinum type C antitoxin (Botumink, United)	1 mL IP[146]	Waterfowl/not fully protective[189]
Calcium EDTA (edetate calcium disodium)	10-40 mg/kg IM, IV q12h × 5-10 days[25]	Waterfowl
	25-50 mg/kg IV q12h[83]	Geese
Deferiprone (Ferriprox, Apotex)	50 mg/kg PO q12h × 30 days[236]	Chickens/PK; iron chelation; may produce rust-colored urates; an orphan drug in the United States
Magnesium sulfate (Epsom salts)	500-1000 mg/kg PO q24h × 1-3 days[25]	Waterfowl/cathartic used in lead toxicosis to encourage passage of heavy metal particles[25]
Melatonin	10 mg/kg in feed[173]	Chickens/aflatoxin exposure; can also administer melatonin when aflatoxin is still in feed
D-penicillamine (Cuprimine, Merck; Depen, MedaPharmaceutical; Distamine, Eli Lilly)	55 mg/kg PO q12h × 7-14 days[25]	Waterfowl/heavy metal chelator (e.g., copper, lead, and zinc)
Pralidoxime mesylate (2-PAM) (Protopam, Wyeth-Ayerst)	100 mg/kg IM q24-48h or repeat once after 6 hr[25]	Waterfowl/reverses muscle weakness due to pesticide poisoning

TABLE 6-9 Nutritional/Mineral Support Used in Backyard Poultry, Gamebirds, and Waterfowl.[a]

Agent	Dosage	Species/Comments
Biotin	150 mg/ton[128]	Poultry/biotin deficiency
Calcium[b]	4-8 mg/kg feed (0.4%-0.8%)[168]	Growing Muscovy ducks
	8 mg/kg feed (0.8%)[168]	Growing Japanese quail
	8-10 mg/kg feed (0.8%-1%)[168]	Growing chickens
	18.8-32.5 mg/kg feed (1.88%-3.25%)[168]	Laying chickens/3.25% recommended for hens that lay eggs daily
	22.5 mg/kg feed (2.25%)[168]	Laying turkeys
Folic acid	50-100 µg IM[21]	Poultry chicks/treatment of deficiency; anemia improved in 4 days
	1 mg/kg feed[128]	Poultry/folic acid deficiency

TABLE 6-9 Nutritional/Mineral Support Used in Backyard Poultry, Gamebirds, and Waterfowl. (cont'd)

Agent	Dosage	Species/Comments
Iron dextran	10 mg/kg IM, repeat in 7-10 days prn[25,27]	Waterfowl/iron deficiency anemia
Niacin	55-70 mg/kg feed[128]	Chicken, turkeys, game fowl, waterfowl/niacin deficiency
Pantothenic acid	12 mg/kg feed[128]	Poultry/pantothenic acid deficiency
	2 mg (calcium pantothenate) + 0.5 mg riboflavin in 50 gal (190 L) water × 2-3 day[128]	Poultry/pantothenic acid deficiency
Riboflavin	10 mg/kg feed[128]	Poultry/riboflavin deficiency
Thiamine	4 mg/kg feed[128]	
Vitamin A or retinol (Animed, AHC Products)	8224 IU/L or 31,250 IU/gal water[171]	Poultry/for periods of reduced feed intake or stress, or vitamin A deficiency
Vitamin B_{12}	≤20 µg/g feed × 1-2 wk	Poultry/vitamin B_{12} deficiency
Vitamin C (ascorbic acid)	150 mg/kg PO q24h[91]	Willow ptarmigan chicks/PD; supplemental daily requirements over 265 mg/kg diet
	150 mg/kg feed[150]	Poultry
Vitamin D_3	11-30 min of direct sunlight/day[93]	Chickens/sufficient for endogenous synthesis of vitamin D
	2000 or 4000 IU/kg feed[20]	Chickens
Vitamin D_3 (Animed, AHC Products)	2056 IU/L or 7813 IU/gal water[171]	Poultry/for periods of reduced feed intake or stress, or vitamin D deficiency
Vitamin E 40% (Animed, AHC Products)	70 IU/L or 645 IU/gal water[171]	Poultry/for periods of reduced feed intake or stress, or vitamin E deficiency
Vitamin E/γ-linolenic acid (2%), linoleic acid (71%) (Derm Caps, DVM Pharmaceuticals)	4000 mg linolenic acid/kg feed[163]	Japanese quail/PD; reduces essential fatty acid deficient hepatic lipidosis
Vitamin K_1 (phytonadione)	0.1 mg/kg feed[108]	Turkeys/PD; as effective as 1-2 mg/kg in reducing plasma prothrombin time
Vitamin K_1 (menadione)	1-4 mg/ton feed[128]	Poultry/for vitamin K deficiency, double the dose

[a]Nutritional and mineral supplementation are uncommon in poultry fed commercially prepared diets that are formulated for their particular physiologic state. In general, in a primary nutritional deficiency at least 5% of the flock should display deficiency signs.

[b]Recommended dietary levels.

TABLE 6-10 Ophthalmologic Agents Used in Backyard Poultry and Waterfowl.[a]

Agent	Dosage	Species/Comments
Amphotericin B	125 µg/5 mL sterile water subconjunctiva[2]	Ducks (ornamental)/candidiasis of third eyelid
Amphotericin B ointment (4%) (formulated)	Topical q24h[2]	Ducks (ornamental)/candidiasis of third eyelid; administered in conjunction with systemic antifungal therapy
Ivermectin	0.005-0.05 mg topical q24h × 10 days[220]	Chicken/PD; conjunctival oxyspirurid (nematode) infection; no adverse effects were seen with topical use
Proparacaine (Ophthaine, Zoetis)	1-5 drops topically as needed[77]	Chickens/approved for all classes, including laying hens in the United States

[a]Variable amounts of skeletal muscle are present in the avian iris, giving birds voluntary control over pupil dilation. In many avian patients, the pupils are best dilated by restraining the animal in a dark room.

TABLE 6-11 Oncologic Agents Used in Backyard Poultry and Waterfowl.

Agent	Dosage	Species/Comments
Chlorambucil (Leukeran, GlaxoSmithKline)	1 mg/bird PO 2×/wk[169]	Pekin ducks/lymphocytic leukemia or lymphosarcoma; responded to treatment initially, but was euthanatized 1 mo after presentation because of respiratory distress and hemorrhages
Prednisone	1 mg/kg PO q12h[169]	Ducks/lymphoma; lymphocytic leukemia
Vincristine sulfate	0.5 mg/m^2 IV, then 0.75 mg/m^2 q7d × 3 treatments[169]	Ducks/lymphoma; lymphocytic leukemia

TABLE 6-12 Euthanasia Agents Used in Backyard Poultry, Gamebirds, and Waterfowl.[a]

Agent	Dosage	Comments
Argon	70% argon with 30% CO_2[11,184]	Conditionally acceptable method of euthanasia by American Veterinary Medical Association (AVMA) if used properly[11]
	90% argon with 2% residual oxygen[11,184]	Chickens/little to no aversion;[11,184] conditionally acceptable method of euthanasia by the AVMA if used properly[11]

TABLE 6-12 Euthanasia Agents Used in Backyard Poultry, Gamebirds, and Waterfowl. (cont'd)

Agent	Dosage	Comments
Carbon dioxide (CO_2)	>40%-70%[11]	Chickens/renders the bird unconscious prior to death; unconscious motor activity such as flapping of wings may damage tissues for necropsy and may be disconcerting to the observer; conditionally acceptable method of euthanasia by AVMA if used properly
Carbon monoxide (CO)	Minimum 6% concentration in a closed container[11]	Causes rapid unconsciousness; conditionally acceptable method of euthanasia by AVMA if used properly[11]
Inhalant anesthetics (e.g., isoflurane, sevoflurane)	Saturated cotton ball in closed container or face mask; high concentrations (5% or more) using vaporizer are preferred[11]	Rapid induction; wing flapping and vocalizing may occur; less tissue damage compared with other methods;[126,183] conditionally acceptable by AVMA as a sole method of euthanasia if high concentrations used and safety considerations to personnel followed;[11] can also be used to render birds unconscious prior to other methods of euthanasia[11,172]
Nitrogen	100% gas exposure[11]	Conditionally acceptable method of euthanasia by AVMA if used properly
	70% nitrogen with 30% CO_2[11,184]	Conditionally acceptable method of euthanasia by AVMA if used properly
Pentobarbital sodium	0.2-1 mL/kg IV[11]	Acceptable method by AVMA to give IV either conscious or unconscious (under anesthesia); conditionally acceptable method to give intraosseous or intracoelomically only if unconscious or under anesthesia; unacceptable to administer IM due to the low pH, which causes pain;[11,174] birds may react unpredictably with IV administration[11]
Potassium chloride	1-2 mmol/kg IV[11]	Unacceptable as a sole method of euthanasia; it is acceptable to administer this agent to a fully anesthetized bird or otherwise unconscious as a means to ensure death[11]

[a]The 2020 AVMA Guidelines for Euthanasia state that methods regarded as "Acceptable with Conditions" are equivalent to "Acceptable" methods of euthanasia when all criteria for application of a method can be met.[11] The AVMA acceptable method is administering a pentobarbital euthanasia solution IV in either an awake or unconscious bird. The AVMA conditionally acceptable methods include inhalant anesthetic overdose, argon, nitrogen, CO, CO_2, cervical dislocation, decapitation, gunshot, captive bolts (penetrating or nonpenetrating), and exsanguination as long as the conditions are met.

TABLE 6-13 Miscellaneous Agents Used in Backyard Poultry and Waterfowl.

Agent	Dosage	Species/Comments
Digoxin	0.0035 mg/kg IV q24h[7]	Turkeys
	0.0049 mg/kg IV q12h[7]	Poultry
	0.019 mg/kg IV q12[7]	Pekin ducks
Doxapram	10 mg/kg IV once[25]	Waterfowl
Methocarbamol	32.5 mg/kg PO q12h[188]	Swans/capture myopathy
	50 mg/kg IV (slow bolus)[188]	Swans/muscle relaxation; capture myopathy; may be given q12h for muscle relaxation
Metoclopramide	2 mg/kg IM, IV q8-12h[27]	Waterfowl/crop stasis; ileus; no PK or PD studies available
Nicarbazin (OvoControl, Innolytics)	125 mg/kg in feed or 8.4 mg/kg PO × 8 days[242] or formulated pellets provided at baiting stations[228]	Waterfowl/egg-hatch control; inhibits sperm receptor sites on the vitelline membrane to prevent fertilization of eggs; check federal and state permit requirements prior to use

TABLE 6-14 Hematologic and Serum Biochemical Values of Healthy Chickens and Turkeys.

Measurement	Standard Size Chicken (*Gallus gallus*) – White Leghorn[48,109]	Bantam Size Chicken (*Gallus gallus*) – Polish & Cochin[48]	Turkey (*Meleagris gallopavo*)[109]
Hematology			
PCV (%)	21-31	35-41	30-46
RBC (10^6/µL)	1.3-4.5	3-3.2	1.7-3.7
Hgb (g/dL)	10.8-14.1	12.3-14	8.8-13.4
MCV (fL)	100-139	116-127	112-168
MCH (pg)	25-48	—	32-49
MCHC (g/dL)	20-34	21-33	23-35
WBC (10^3/µL)	14.4-36.8	18-19.6	16-25.5
Heterophils (%)	11-23.5	26-29	29-52
Lymphocytes (%)	59-71	78-83	35-48
Monocytes (%)	3-13	2-3	3-10
Eosinophils (%)	0-16	1.2-2.7	0-5
Basophils (%)	0-6	1.2-2.5	1-9
H:L ratio	0-8	0.2-0.7	0.6-1.5
Chemistries			
ALT (U/L)	6-20	—	—
AST (U/L)	112-230	—	—

TABLE 6-14 Hematologic and Serum Biochemical Values of Healthy Chickens and Turkeys. (cont'd)

Measurement	Standard Size Chicken (*Gallus gallus*) – White Leghorn[48,109]	Bantam Size Chicken (*Gallus gallus*) – Polish & Cochin[48]	Turkey (*Meleagris gallopavo*)[109]
Calcium (mg/dL)	13.2-17.0	—	11.7-38.7
Cholesterol (mg/dL)	86-211	261-291	81-129
Creatinine (mg/dL)	0.9-1.8	—	0.8-0.9
GGT (U/L)	—	—	—
Glucose (mg/dL)	200-353	—	275-425
Phosphorus (mg/dL)	1.5-3.6	—	5.4-7.1
Potassium (mmol/L)	3.1-4.6	4.6-4.8	6-6.4
Protein, total (g/dL)	3.3-5.5	4.3-4.6	4.9-7.6
Albumin (g/dL)	1.3-2.8	1.7-3.07	3-5.9
Globulin (g/dL)	1.5-4.1	1.8-2.3	1.7-1.9
Sodium (mmol/L)	140-161	138-140	149-155
Chloride (mmol/L)	107-112	—	—
Uric acid (mg/dL)	2.5-8.1	—	3.4-5.2

TABLE 6-15 Hematologic and Serum Biochemical Values of Select Gamebirds (Galliformes).

Measurement	Quail (*Coturnix* spp.)[a,109,196]	Ring-necked Pheasant (*Phasianus colchicus*)[48,156]	Guinea Fowl (*Numida meleagris*)[48]
Hematology			
PCV (%)	30-45	—	
RBC ($10^6/\mu L$)	4-5.2	2.6-3.9	2.3-2.7
Hgb (g/dL)	10.7-14.3	8-18.9	12.4-14.7
MCV (fL)	60-100	94-131	151-162
MCH (pg)	23-35	—	
MCHC (g/dL)	28-39	43-50	32-35
WBC ($10^3/\mu L$)	12.5-24.6	21-63.5	3.1-39
Heterophils (%)	25-50	12-30	14-19
Lymphocytes (%)	50-70	63-83	75-83
Monocytes (%)	0.5-3.8	2-9	0.6-1.2
Eosinophils (%)	0-15	0	2.1-2.3
Basophils (%)	0-1.5	0-3	0.8-1.1
H:L ratio	0.4-1	0.1-2.1	—

Continued

TABLE 6-15 Hematologic and Serum Biochemical Values of Select Gamebirds (Galliformes). (cont'd)

Measurement	Quail (*Coturnix* spp.)[a,109,196]	Ring-necked Pheasant (*Phasianus colchicus*)[48,156]	Guinea Fowl (*Numida meleagris*)[48]
Chemistries			
ALT (U/L)	6.5-9.6	—	—
AST (U/L)	402-422	—	—
Calcium (mg/dL)	—	9.8-11	—
Cholesterol (mg/dL)	—	—	—
Creatinine (mg/dL)	0.01-0.08	—	—
GGT (U/L)	1.7-1.9	4.1-7.4	—
Glucose (mg/dL)	259-312	284-427	—
Phosphorus (mg/dL)	—	7.1-9.6	—
Potassium (mmol/L)	1.4	5.5-8.7	—
Protein, total (g/dL)	3.4-3.6	3.3-4.7	—
Albumin (g/dL)	1.3-1.5	1.5-2.3	—
Globulin (g/dL)	—	1.9-2.1	—
Sodium (mmol/L)	180	147-156	—
Uric acid (mg/dL)	5.4-5.5	5.6-6.1	—

[a]Except for phosphorus, protein (total), and sodium, biochemistry values are reported in 16-wk-old Japanese quail.

TABLE 6-16 Hematologic and Serum Biochemical Values of Select Anseriformes (Waterfowl).

Measurement	Canada Goose (*Branta canadensis*)[38,109]	Mallard Duck (*Anas platyrhynchos*)[61]	Wood Duck (*Aix sponsa*)[38]
Hematology			
PCV (%)	38-58	39-49	46 ± 3
RBC (10^6/μL)	1.6-2.7	2-3.8	2.8 ± 0.2
Hgb (g/dL)	12.7-19.1	7.4-15.6	15 ± 1
MCV (fL)	145-210	148-200	164 ± 14
MCH (pg)	53.7-70	—	—
MCHC (g/dL)	28-32	29-32	33 ± 4
WBC (10^3/μL)	13-21.8	23.4-24.8	25.6 ± 5.7
Heterophils (%)	39	26-38	—
Lymphocytes (%)	46	54-63	—
Monocytes (%)	6	1-4	—
Eosinophils (%)	2	0.2-0.4	—
Basophils (%)	7	0-4	—
H:L ratio	0.5-0.9	0.4-2	0.4-0.7

TABLE 6-16 Hematologic and Serum Biochemical Values of Select Anseriformes (Waterfowl). (cont'd)

Measurement	Canada Goose (*Branta canadensis*)[38,109]	Mallard Duck (*Anas platyrhynchos*)[61]	Wood Duck (*Aix sponsa*)[38]
Chemistries			
ALP (U/L)	72 ± 43	—	160-780
ALT (U/L)	43 ± 11	—	19-48
AST (U/L)	75 ± 17	—	45-123
Bile acids (μmol/L)			
RIA	—	—	22-60
Colorimetric	—	—	—
Calcium (mg/dL)	10.2 ± 0.7	—	7.6-10.4
Chloride (mmol/L)	105 ± 4	—	101-113
Cholesterol (mg/dL)	172 ± 28	—	—
CK (U/L)	—	—	110-480
Creatinine (mg/dL)	0.8 ± 0.3	—	0.3-0.4
GGT (U/L)	2 ± 3	—	0-2.9
Glucose (mg/dL)	210 ± 31	—	232-269
LDH (U/L)	301 ± 80	—	30-205
Phosphorus (mg/dL)	2.8 ± 0.9	—	1.8-4.1
Potassium (mmol/L)	3.4 ± 0.6	—	3.9-4.7
Protein, total (g/dL)	4.8 ± 0.7	—	2.1-3.3
Albumin (g/dL)	2.1 ± 0.2	—	1.5-2.1
Globulin (g/dL)	2.8 ± 0.6	—	0.6-1.2
A:G ratio	0.76 ± 0.13	—	1.5-3.6
Sodium (mmol/L)	142 ± 4	—	141-149
Uric acid (mg/dL)	8.3 ± 2.3	—	2.5-12.9

TABLE 6-17 Biologic and Physiologic Values of Select Galliformes.[164]

Species	Incubation Period (days)	Fledgling Age (days)	Sexual Maturity	Lifespan in Captivity (Maximum) (years)	Body Weight (kg)
Bobwhite quail	23	14	1 yr	6	0.14-0.17
Chickens	21	1	5-8 mo	15	2.6
Peafowl	28	7	3 yr (M) 1-3 yr (F)	25	4
Pheasant, ring-necked	23-28	7-12	1 yr	10-18	1.263
Turkeys (wild)	28	1	7.5-10 mo	13	6.8-11 (M) 3.6-5.4 (F)

TABLE 6-18 Biologic and Physiologic Values of Select Anseriformes (Waterfowl) Species.[27,164]

Species	Clutch Size	Incubation Period (days)	Fledgling (days)	Sexual Maturity (yr)	Longevity (yr)	Weight (kg)	Respiratory Rate (breaths/min)	Heart Rate (beats/min)
Bar-headed goose	3-8	28-30	55-60	3	20	2-3	13-40	80-150
Canada goose	2-10	28-30	40-48	2-3	—	3-10.9	—	—
Common eider	2-8	25-28	30-50	2-3	20	0.85-3.03	30-95	180-230
Common goldeneye	4-12	28-32	56-65	2-6	11-15	0.96-1.2 (M) 0.7-0.86 (F)	30-95	180-230
Eurasian wigeon	7-11	22-25	40-45	1-2	35	0.42-0.97	30-95	180-230
Hawaiian goose	1-5	29-31	90	2-3	17-28	1.8-2.3	13-40	80-150
Mallard	9-13	26-29	42-60	1	26	1.05-1.08	30-95	180-230
Mandarin duck	9-12	28-30	—	1	10-15	0.43-0.69	30-95	180-230
Muscovy	24-30	33-35	60-70	26-29	7-8	1.1-4.1[a]	30-95	180-230
Mute swan	5-12	36-38	60	3	19-30	9.2-14.3 (M) 7.6-10.6 (F)	13-40	80-150
Pink-footed goose	3-5	26-28	50-60	3	22	2.2-2.7	13-40	80-150
Tufted duck	9-10	25-29	49-56	1	—	0.75-1 (M) 0.6-0.9 (F)	30-95	180-230

[a]Average weight of wild Muscovy ducks; domesticated drakes may weigh as much as 6.8 kg.

TABLE 6-19 Select Nutritional Recommendations for Wild Waterfowl Rehabilitation.[191]

- Offer domestic waterfowl, mallard ducks, and Canada geese cracked corn, scratch grains, leafy greens, and nonmedicated waterfowl or poultry diet.
- Swans, particularly trumpeter swans, may refuse to eat for three or more days; place the swan in an isolated area with a slurry of food and fresh greens; do not disturb unless absolutely necessary.
- Offer water in a dish or bucket deep enough to allow the bird to submerge its entire neck before its bill touches the bottom of the container.
- Do not use galvanized metal containers because the zinc may leach into food and water.
- For ducklings, goslings, and cygnets, offer nonmedicated waterfowl or chick starter in shallow dishes and scattered on the floor of the enclosure.
- • Tiny pieces of bright fruit, like strawberries, or small, live mealworms may stimulate self-feeding in a hospital setting.

TABLE 6-20 Veterinary Feed Directive (VFD) Order Information.[227]

- A VFD is used for drugs given in feed of food animals. They are given exactly per label instructions in regard to dose, concentration, frequency, duration, and so forth, and is not for extralabel drug use. A VFD is valid up to 6 mo.

- According to the U.S. Food and Drug Administration (FDA), a valid VFD order is needed for any feed additive given to a food animal and must be associated with a Valid Client Patient Relationship (VCPR), and it must contain the following:
  - Veterinarian information (name, address, phone) with signature
  - Client information (name, address, phone)
  - Name of the drug, drug concentration, indications for use, and duration of use
  - Dose, withdrawal time
  - Where animals are located (premises) and type (species) and number of animals
  - Date issued, expiration date, indication for use
  - Specified verbiage: "Use of feed containing this VFD drug in a manner other than as directed on the labeling (extralabel use) is not permitted"

TABLE 6-21 List of Antimicrobials That Require a Veterinary Feed Directive (VFD) (as of November 2020).[a,225]

- Apramycin
- Avilamycin
- Chlortetracycline (CTC)
- Chlortetracycline/sulfamethazine
- Chlortetracycline/sulfamethazine/penicillin
- Erythromycin
- Florfenicol
- Hygromycin B
- Lincomycin
- Oxytetracycline/neomycin
- Sulfadimethoxine/ormetoprim
- Sulfamerazine
- Timicosin
- Tylosin
- Tylosin/sulfamethazine
- Tylovasin
- Virginiamycin

[a]List includes medically important antimicrobials approved for use in or on animal feed and require VFD and those that transitioned from over-the-counter (OTC) to VFD marketing status.

TABLE 6-22 Serologic Tests (Antibody Detection) for Poultry.[a,50]

Test	Test Type[b]	Comments
Avian encephalomyelitis	ELISA	Chickens
	AGID	All poultry species
Avian hemorrhagic enteritis	ELISA	Turkeys
Avian influenza	ELISA (screen test)	Chickens, turkeys, or multispecies (e.g., ducks & others)
	AGID	All avian species
Avian metapneumovirus	ELISA	Chickens, turkeys
	IFA	Chickens, turkeys
Avian reovirus	ELISA	Chickens
Bordetella avium	ELISA	Turkeys
Chlamydia psittaci	CF	All avian species
Infectious bronchitis virus	ELISA	Chickens
Infectious bursal disease virus	ELISA	Chickens
Mycoplasma gallisepticum	ELISA (screen test)	Chickens, turkeys
	SPAT (screen test)	All avian species
	HI	All avian species
Mycoplasma meleagridis	SPAT (screen test)	Turkeys
	HI	Turkeys
Mycoplasma synoviae	ELISA (screen test)	Chickens, turkeys
	SPAT (screen test)	All avian species
	HI	All avian species
Newcastle disease virus (paramyxovirus—type 1)	ELISA	Chicken, turkeys
	HI	All avian species
Ornithobacterium rhinotracheale	SPAT	
Paramyxovirus—type 2	HI	All avian species
Paramyxovirus—type 3	HI	All avian species
Paramyxovirus—type 7	HI	All avian species
Pasteurella multocida	ELISA	Chickens, turkeys
Salmonella pullorum/ S. gallinarum	SPAT, STAT (both screen tests)	All avian species
Salmonella pullorum/ S. gallinarum	MAT	All avian species

[a]Sample needed: 0.5 mL serum per test, in a glass or plastic tube with no anticoagulant additives (e.g., plain red top or serum separator), or fresh eggs

[b]AGID, Agar gel immunodiffusion; CF, complement fixation; ELISA, enzymelinked immunosorbent assay; IFA, immunofluorescent-antibody; HA, hemagglutination; HI, hemagglutinin inhibition; MAT, microagglutination test; SPAT, serum plate agglutination test; STAT, serum tube agglutination test.

TABLE 6-23 Rapid Tests for Detection of Regulatory Important Poultry and Waterfowl Diseases.[a]

Test	Test Type[b]	Sample Needed
Avian influenza	RT-PCR	Choanal, tracheal, cloacal swab; tissues
Avian paramyxovirus 1 (including exotic Newcastle disease)	RT-PCR	Tissues, nasal swab, cloacal swab
Avian pneumovirus	RT-PCR	Tissues, tracheal swab, cloacal swab
Chlamydia spp.	PCR	Affected tissues, swab, feces
Chlamydia psittaci	FA	Affected tissues (heart, liver, spleen)
Eastern equine encephalitis (EEE) virus	RT-PCR	Brain tissues, blood
Infectious laryngotracheitis virus	PCR	Oropharyngeal swab, trachea, lung
Mycoplasma spp.	PCR	Choanal swab
Mycoplasma gallisepticum	PCR	Tissues (swab)
Mycoplasma iowae	PCR	Tissues
Mycoplasma meleagridis	PCR	Tissues
Mycoplasma synoviae	PCR	Tissues
Salmonella pullorum or *Salmonella enteritidis*	PCR	Tissues
West Nile virus	PCR	Brain, blood

[a]Following a positive test from these, state and/or federal authorities are contacted, and additional testing may be performed by those agencies to further an epidemiologic investigation.
[b]FA, Fluorescent antibody; PCR, polymerase chain reaction; RT-PCR, reverse transcriptase polymerase chain reaction.

TABLE 6-24 Definitions of the Various Designations of Drugs in Food-Producing Animals According to the U.S. Food and Drug Administration (FDA) as They Pertain to Poultry.[10,226]

Designation	Definition	Example
Prohibited, group 1	Drugs with no allowable extralabel uses in any food-producing animal species[226]	Chloramphenicol, clenbuterol, diethylstilbestrol (DES), fluoroquinolone-class antibiotics, glycopeptides (all agents, including vancomycin), medicated feeds, nitroimidazoles (all agents, including dimetridazole, ipronidazole, metronidazole, and others), nitrofurans (all agents, including furazolidone, nitrofurazone, and others)
Prohibited, group 2	Drugs with restricted extralabel uses in food-producing animal species[226]	Adamantane and neuraminidase inhibitors (in all poultry, including ducks), cephalosporin-class of antibiotics except cephapirin (in all classes of chickens and turkeys), gentian violet (prohibited from use in food or feed of food-producing animals) and indexed drugs (some exceptions for minor use species); extralabel drug use (ELDU) restrictions apply to all production classes of major food animal species (no ELDU for purpose of disease prevention; no ELDU that involves unapproved dose, treatment duration, frequency, or administration route; agent must be approved for that species and production class); ELDU restrictions do not apply to minor-use food animal species

Continued

TABLE 6-24 Definitions of the Various Designations of Drugs in Food-Producing Animals According to the U.S. Food and Drug Administration (FDA) as They Pertain to Poultry. (cont'd)

Designation	Definition	Example
Extralabel drug use (ELDU)	—	Use in another species: trimethoprim sulfamethoxazole directly orally to a duck
	—	Use for a different indication: erythromycin administered as per label instructions but for pododermatitis rather than chronic respiratory disease
	—	Use at a different dose or frequency: administering spectinomycin for more than the first 3 days of life
	—	Use via a different route of administration: erythromycin directly orally, not in food or drinking water
	—	Contact www.farad.org for information regarding potential meat and egg withdrawal
Labeled drug	Used exactly as written on the label, including the species, duration, dose, concentration, frequency, route, and indication	Erythromycin (erythromycin thiocyanate [Gallimycin, Cross Vetpharm Group Ltd.]): 185 g/ton of feed to aid in the prevention and reduction of lesions and in lowering severity of chronic respiratory disease; feed for 5 to 8 days; do not use in birds producing eggs for food purposes; withdraw 48 hr before slaughter

TABLE 6-25 Water and Feed Consumption Rates for Backyard Poultry.[a]

Use (Age)	Water per 100 Birds (L)	Weight (kg)	Feed Expressed as %BW
Hens (nonlaying)	19	—	—
Hens (laying)	19-28	—	—
Chickens (4 wk)	7.6	—	—
Chickens (8 wk)	15.5	—	—
Chickens (12 wk)	21	—	—
—	—	0.23	14
—	—	0.45	11.4
—	—	0.68	9.7
—	—	1.59	6.7
—	—	2.5	5.0

[a]Estimated water consumption rates per 100 birds based on age and use. Estimated feed consumption rates for chickens based on weight of food eaten per day expressed as a percentage of body weight.[216]

TABLE 6-26 Sources of Information on Meat and Egg Withdrawal for Backyard Poultry and Waterfowl.[a]

Source	Comments
Food Animal Residue Avoidance and Depletion Program (www.farad.org)	Provides information on labeled drug meat and egg withdrawal times as well as an interactive section (VetGram) to ask about estimated meat and egg withdrawal times on extralabel drugs
Animal Drugs @ FDA (https://animaldrugsatfda.fda.gov/adafda/views/#/home/previewsearch)	Food and Drug Administration website listing all animal drug products approved for safety and effectiveness (a.k.a. the "Green Book"); updated monthly
Pharmacokinetics of Veterinary Drugs in Laying Hens and Residues in Eggs; a Review of the Literature[82]	Extensive review article on meat and egg withdrawal for many labeled and extralabeled drugs
Poultry Medications Formulary, US edition (www.elancodvm.com/professional-resources)	A continually updated resource on meat and egg withdrawal times for labeled drugs

[a]These sources of information are provided rather than quoting meat and egg withdrawal times because of frequently changing regulations. The status of any medication should be checked prior to administration.[77]

TABLE 6-27 Values Reported for Select Ophthalmic Diagnostic Tests in Select Galliformes.

Species	Intraocular Pressure (mmHg) by Rebound Tonometry	Phenol Red Thread Test (mm/15 sec ± SD)
Chicken, 3 wk old[182]	17.5 ± 0.1	—
Helmeted guinea fowl, 15-40 mo old[185]	9.1 ± 0.9	16.5 ± 1.3

TABLE 6-28 Select Vaccines Used in Backyard Poultry.[a]

Disease	Vaccine	Route[b]	Age Administered	Comments
Coccidiosis	Live attenuated	PO	1 day +	Chickens to use properly, must allow chick access to its own feces; do not treat concurrently with anticoccidial drugs[9,80,158]
Hemorrhagic enteritis	Live attenuated	PO (drinking water)	4-5 wk	Turkeys/reduces clinical signs of disease[9,158]
Infectious laryngotracheitis	Tissue Culture OriGen (TCO)	Eyedrop	6 wk	Chickens/do not develop permanent immunity until at least 6 wk of age; not typically given to backyard flocks unless there is a past history of the disease

Continued

TABLE 6-28 Select Vaccines Used in Backyard Poultry. (cont'd)

Disease	Vaccine	Route[b]	Age Administered	Comments
Marek's disease	HVT[c] serotype 3	SC, OV	1 day or in ovo	Chickens/typically given at hatchery; most common Marek's vaccine used in backyard flocks[158]
	Serotype 2	—	1 day	Chickens/naturally avirulent isolates[158]
	Rispens	—	1 day	Chickens/non-oncogenic strains of serotype[158]
Pox	Pigeon pox	WW	—	Chickens/mild vaccine; can be used at any age[158]

[a]Because of the adjuvants and carriers, many vaccines have a slaughter withdrawal time of 21 days; be sure to read and follow all label directions.
[b]DW, Drinking water; IN, intranasal; IO, intraocular; OV, in ovo; PO, per os; SC, subcutaneous; WW, wing web (chickens).
[c]HVT, Turkey herpesvirus vaccine.

REFERENCES

1. ______. Veterinary Information Network (VIN) message boards. Available at: https://www.vin.com/vin/. Accessed August 23, 2020.
2. Abrams GA, Paul-Murphy J, Murphy CJ. Conjunctivitis in birds. *Vet Clin North Am Exot Anim Pract*. 2002;5:287–309.
3. Abu-Basha EA, Idkaidek NM, AF Al-Shunnaq. Comparative pharmacokinetics of gentamicin after intravenous, intramuscular, subcutaneous and oral administration in broiler chickens. *Vet Res Commun*. 2007;31:765–773.
4. Abu-Basha EA, Idkaidek NM, Al-Shunnaq AF. Pharmacokinetics of tilmicosin (Provitil powder and Pulmotil liquid AC) oral formulations in chickens. *Vet Res Commun*. 2007;31:477–485.
5. Aguilar R, Redig P. Diagnosis and treatment of avian aspergillosis. In: Bonagura JD, Abbott JA, Abrams KL, eds. *Kirk's Current Veterinary Therapy XII: Small Animal Practice*. 12th ed. Philadelphia: WB Saunders; 1995.
6. Ajadi RA, Kasali OB, Makinde AF, et al. Effects of midazolam on ketamine-xylazine anesthesia in guinea fowl (*Numida meleagris galeata*). *J Avian Med Surg*. 2009;23:199–204.
7. Allen DG, Pringle JK, Smith DA. *Handbook of Veterinary Drugs*. 2nd ed. Philadelphia: Lippincott Williams & Wilkins; 1998.
8. Amelotti I, Catalá SS, Gorla DE. Response of Triatoma infestans to pour-on cypermethrin applied to chickens under laboratory conditions. *Memorias do Instituto Oswaldo Cruz*. 2009;104:481–485.
9. American Poultry Association. *Disease Guide*: The Poultry Site; 2020. https://thepoultrysite.com/disease-guide . Accessed July 2, 2020.
10. American Veterinary Medical Association. Extralabel drug use and AMDUCA: Faq. 2012; https://www.avma.org/extralabel-drug-use-and-amduca-faq . Accessed July 25, 2020.
11. American Veterinary Medical Association. *AVMA Guidelines for the Euthanasia of Animals: 2020 Edition*: Schaumburg, Illinois; 2020.
12. Anadón A, Bringas P, Martinez-Larraæaga MR, et al. Bioavailability, pharmacokinetics and residues of chloramphenicol in the chicken. *J Vet Pharmacol Therap*. 1994;17:52–58.
13. Anadón A, Martinez-Larrañaga MR, Diaz MJ. Pharmacokinetics of tetracycline in chickens after intravenous administration. *Poult Sci*. 1985;64:2273–2279.
14. Anadón A, Martínez-Larrañaga MR, Díaz MJ, et al. Pharmacokinetics of doxycycline in broiler chickens. *Avian Pathol*. 1994;23:79–90.

15. Anadón A, Martínez-Larrañaga MR, Díaz MJ, et al. Pharmacokinetics and residues of enrofloxacin in chickens. *Am J Vet Res.* 1995;56:501–506.
16. Anadón A, Martínez-Larrañaga MR, Díaz MJ, et al. Pharmacokinetic characteristics and tissue residues for marbofloxacin and its metabolite N-desmethyl-marbofloxacin in broiler chickens. *Am J Vet Res.* 2002;63:927–933.
17. Anadón A, Martínez-Larrañaga MR, Velez C, et al. Pharmacokinetics and residues of norfloxacin and its N-desethyl- and oxo-metabolites in broiler chickens. *Am J Vet Res.* 1992;53:2084–2089.
18. Animal and Plant Health Inspection Service. Live poultry. Animal Health; 2020. https://www.aphis.usda.gov/aphis/ourfocus/animalhealth/animal-and-animal-product-import-information/entry-requirements/sa_avian/importing-live-poultry/ct_live_poultry#:~:text=The%20U.S.%20Department%20of%20Agriculture,USDA%20to%20be%20pet%20birds . Accessed November 15, 2020.
19. Assis RCL, Luns FD, Beletti ME, et al. Histomorphometry and macroscopic intestinal lesions in broilers infected with *Eimeria acervulina. Vet Parasitol.* 2010;168:185–189.
20. Atencio A, Edwards Jr HM, Pesti G. Effects of vitamin D3 dietary supplementation of broiler breeder hens on the performance and bone abnormalities of the progeny. *Poult Sci.* 2005;84:1058–1068.
21. Austic RE, Scott M, Calnek BW, et al. Nutritional diseases. In: *Diseases of Poultry.* 10th ed. Ames, Iowa: Iowa State University Press; 1997:47–73.
22. Baert K, Backer PD. Disposition of sodium salicylate, flunixin and meloxicam after intravenous administration in broiler chickens. *J Vet Pharmacol Ther.* 2002;25:449–453.
23. Baert K, Backer PD. Comparative pharmacokinetics of three non-steroidal anti-inflammatory drugs in five bird species. *Comp Biochem Physiol Part C: Toxicol Pharmacol.* 2003;134:25–33.
24. Bailey RS, Sheldon JD, Allender MC, et al. Analgesic efficacy of tramadol compared with meloxicam in ducks (*Cairina moschata domestica*) evaluated by ground-reactive forces. *J Avian Med Surg.* 2019;33:133–140.
25. Bailey TA, Apo MM. Pharmaceutical products commonly used in avian medicine. In: Samour JH, ed. *Avian Medicine.* 3rd ed. St. Louis, MO: Elsevier; 2016:637–678.
26. Belant JL, Seamans TW. Comparison of three formulations of alpha-chloralose for immobilization of Canada geese. *J Wildl Dis.* 1997;33:606–610.
27. Beynon PH, Forbes NA, Harcourt-Brown N. *BSAVA Manual of Raptors, Pigeons and Waterfowl.* Ames, IA: Iowa State University Press; 1996.
28. Bishop Y. *The Veterinary Formulary.* 6th ed. London: Pharmaceutical Press; 2001.
29. Black PA, Cox SK, Macek M, et al. Pharmacokinetics of tramadol hydrochloride and its metabolite O-desmethyltramadol in peafowl (*Pavo cristatus*). *J Zoo Wildl Med.* 2010;41:671–676.
30. Black WD. A study of the pharmacodynamics of oxytetracycline in the chicken. *Poult Sci.* 1977;56:1430–1434.
31. Boever SD, Neirinckx E, Baert K, et al. Pharmacokinetics of tepoxalin and its active metabolite in broiler chickens. *J Vet Pharmacol Ther.* 2009;32:97–100.
32. Boothe DM. Drugs affecting the respiratory system. *Vet Clin North Am Exot Anim Pract.* 2000;3:371–394.
33. Brandão J, Da Cunha AF, Pypendop BH, et al. Cardiovascular tolerance of intravenous lidocaine in broiler chickens (*Gallus gallus domesticus*) anesthetized with isoflurane. *Vet Anaesth Analg.* 2015;42:442–448.
34. Brenner DJ, Larsen RS, Dickinson PJ, et al. Development of an avian brachial plexus nerve block technique for perioperative analgesia in mallard ducks (*Anas platyrhynchos*). *J Avian Med Surg.* 2010;24:24–34.
35. Burhenne J, Haefeli WE, Hess M, et al. Pharmacokinetics, tissue concentrations, and safety of the antifungal agent voriconazole in chickens. *J Avian Med Surg.* 2008;22:199–220.
36. Bush M, Locke D, Neal LA, et al. Pharmacokinetics of cephalothin and cephalexin in selected avian species. *Am J Vet Res.* 1981;42:1014–1017.

37. Byrne R, Davis C, Lister S. Prescribing for birds. In: Bishop Y, ed. *The Veterinary Formulary*. 6th ed. London: Pharmaceutical Press; 2001:43–56.
38. Campbell TW, Smith SA, Zimmerman KL. Hematology of waterfowl and raptors. In: Weiss DJ, Wardrop KJ, Schalm OW, eds. *Schalm's Veterinary Hematology*. 6th ed. Ames, IA: Blackwell Publishing; 2010:977–986.
39. Caplen G, Baker L, Hothersall B, et al. Thermal nociception as a measure of non-steroidal anti-inflammatory drug effectiveness in broiler chickens with articular pain. *Vet J*. 2013;198:616–619.
40. Cardozo LB, Almeida RM, Fiúza LC, et al. Brachial plexus blockade in chickens with 0.75% ropivacaine. *Vet Anaesth Analg*. 2009;36:396–400.
41. Carpenter NA. Anseriform and galliform therapeutics. *Vet Clin North Am Exot Anim Pract*. 2000;3:1–17.
42. Chaleva EI, Vasileva IV, Savova MD. Absorption of lincomycin through the respiratory pathways and its influence on alveolar macrophages after aerosol administration to chickens. *Res Vet Sci*. 1994;57:245–247.
43. Charlton BR. Poultry use guide. In: Charlton BR, ed. *Avian Disease Manual*. 6th ed. Athens, GA: American Association of Avian Pathologists; 2006:227–231.
44. Christensen J, Fosse RT, Halvorsen OJ, et al. Comparison of various anesthetic regimens in the domestic fowl. *Am J Vet Res*. 1987;48:1649–1657.
45. Chung HS, Jung WC, Kim DH, et al. Ceftiofur distribution in plasma and tissues following subcutaneously administration in ducks. *J Vet Med Sci*. 2007;69:1081–1085.
46. Clancy MM, KuKanich B, Sykes JM. Pharmacokinetics of butorphanol delivered with an osmotic pump during a seven-day period in common peafowl (*Pavo cristatus*). *Am J Vet Res*. 2015;76:1070–1076.
47. Clark CH, Thomas JE, Milton JL, et al. Plasma concentrations of chloramphenicol in birds. *Am J Vet Res*. 1982;43:1949–1953.
48. Cook JR, Heatley JJ. Galliformes. In: Heatley JJ, Russell KE, eds. *Exotic Animal Laboratory Diagnosis*. Hoboken, NJ: Wiley Blackwell; 2020:868–919.
49. Cortright KA, Wetzlich SE, Craigmill AL. Plasma pharmacokinetics of midazolam in chickens, turkeys, pheasants and bobwhite quail. *J Vet Pharmacol Therap*. 2007;30:429–436.
50. Crespo R, Shivaprasad HL. Interpretation of laboratory results and values. In: Greenacre CB, Morishita TY, eds. *Backyard Poultry Medicine and Surgery: A guide for Veterinary Practitioners*. Ames, IA: Wiley Blackwell; 2015:283–296.
51. Custer RS, Bush M, Carpenter JW. Pharmacokinetics of gentamicin in blood plasma of quail, pheasants, and cranes. *Am J Vet Res*. 1979;40:892–895.
52. Da Cunha AF, Messenger KM, Stout RW, et al. Pharmacokinetics of lidocaine and its active metabolite monoethylglycinexylidide after a single intravenous administration in chickens (*Gallus domesticus*) anesthetized with isoflurane. *J Vet Pharmacol Therap*. 2012;35:604–607.
53. Danbury TC, Weeks CA, Chambers JP, et al. Self-selection of the analgesic drug carprofen by lame broiler chickens. *Vet Rec*. 2000;146:307–311.
54. Day TK, Roge CK. Evaluation of sedation in quail induced by use of midazolam and reversed by use of flumazenil. *J Am Vet Med Assoc*. 1996;209:969–971.
55. Dein FJ, Monard DF, Kowalczyk DF. Pharmacokinetics of chloramphenicol in Chinese spot-billed ducks. *J Vet Pharmacol Therap*. 1980;3:161–168.
56. Delaski KM, Gehring R, Heffron BT, et al. Plasma concentrations of fentanyl achieved with transdermal application in chickens. *J Avian Med Surg*. 2017;31:6–15.
57. Devriese LA, Dutta GN. Effects of erythromycin-inactivating Lactobacillus crop flora on blood levels. *J Vet Pharmacol Therap*. 1984;7:49–53.
58. Digeronimo PM, Cunha AFD, Pypendop B, et al. Cardiovascular tolerance of intravenous bupivacaine in broiler chickens (*Gallus gallus domesticus*) anesthetized with isoflurane. *Vet Anaesth Analg*. 2017;44:287–294.

59. Dimitrova D, Moutafchieva R, Kanelov I, et al. Pharmacokinetics of tobramycin in ducks and sex-related differences. *Vet J*. 2009;179:462–464.
60. Doneley B. Disorders of the reproductive tract. In: Doneley B, ed. *Avian Medicine and Surgery in Practice: Companion and Aviary Birds*. 2nd ed. Boca Raton, CA: CRC Press; 2016:317–331.
61. Driver EA. Hematological and blood chemical values of mallard, *Anas platyrhynchos*, drakes before, during and after remige moult. *J Wildl Dis*. 1981;17:413–421.
62. Efstathopoulos N, Giamarellos-Bourboulis E, Kanellakopoulou K, et al. Treatment of experimental osteomyelitis by methicillin resistant *Staphylococcus aureus* with bone cement system releasing grepafloxacin. *Injury*. 2008;39:1384–1390.
63. El-Banna HA, El-Bahy MM, El-Zorba HY, et al. Anticoccidial efficacy of drinking water soluble diclazuril on experimental and field coccidiosis in broiler chickens. *J Vet Med A Physiol Pathol Clin Med*. 2005;52:287–291.
64. El-Gammal AA, Ravis WR, Krista LM, et al. Pharmacokinetics and intramuscular bioavailability of amikacin in chickens following single and multiple dosing. *J Vet Pharmacol Therap*. 1992;15:133–142.
65. El-Gendi AY, El-Banna HA, Abo Norag M, et al. Disposition kinetics of danofloxacin and ciprofloxacin in broiler chickens. *Dtsch Tierarztl Wochenschr*. 2001;108:429–434.
66. El-Kholy H, Kemppainen B, Ravis W, et al. Pharmacokinetics of levamisole in broiler breeder chickens. *J Vet Pharmacol Therap*. 2006;29:49–53.
67. Elanco. Flubenol 5%. In: Ltd EAP, ed. Elanco Australasia Pty Ltd; 2016.
68. Elviss NC, Williams LK, Jørgensen F, et al. Amoxicillin therapy of poultry flocks: effect upon the selection of amoxicillin-resistant commensal *Campylobacter* spp. *J Antimicrob Chemother*. 2009;64:702–711.
69. Escobar A, Rocha RWD, Pypendop BH, et al. Effects of methadone on the minimum anesthetic concentration of isoflurane, and its effects on heart rate, blood pressure and ventilation during isoflurane anesthesia in hens (*Gallus gallus domesticus*). *PLoS One*. 2016;28:1–12.
70. Escobar A, Valadão CaA, Brosnan RJ, et al. Cardiopulmonary effects of butorphanol in sevoflurane-anesthetized guinea fowl (*Numida meleagris*). *Vet Anaesth Analg*. 2014;41:284–289.
71. Espigol C, Artigas C, Palmada J, et al. Serum levels of doxycycline during water treatment in poultry. *J Vet Pharmacol Therap*. 1997;20:192–193.
72. Evrard HC, Balthazart J. The assessment of nociceptive and non-nociceptive skin sensitivity in the Japanese quail (*Coturnix japonica*). *J Neurosci Methods*. 2002;116:135–146.
73. Fernández-Varón E, Cárceles CM, Espuny A, et al. Pharmacokinetics of a combination preparation of ampicillin and sulbactam in turkeys. *Am J Vet Res*. 2004;65:1658–1663.
74. Figueiredo JP, Cruz ML, Mendes GM, et al. Assessment of brachial plexus blockade in chickens by an axillary approach. *Vet Anaesth Analg*. 2008;35:511–518.
75. Flinchum GB. Management of waterfowl. In: Harrison GJ, Lightfoot TL, eds. *Clinical Avian Medicine*. Palm Beach, FL: Spix Publishing; 2011:831–848.
76. Fontenot DK, Terrell SP, Neiffer DL, et al. Clinical trial of a depot form of levonorgestrel in domestic turkeys. *Proc Annu Conf Assoc Avian Vet*; 2002:43.
77. Food Animal Residue Avoidance & Depletion Program. Food animal residue avoidance databank (FARAD). Available at http://www.farad.org. Accessed July 25, 2020.
78. Gberindyer AF, Okpeh ER, Semaka AA. Pharmacokinetics of short- and long-acting formulations of oxytetracycline after intramuscular administration in chickens. *J Avian Med Surg*. 2015;29:298–302.
79. Gentle MJ, Hocking PM, Bernard R, et al. Evaluation of intraarticular opioid analgesia for the relief of articular pain in the domestic fowl. *Pharmacol Biochem Behav*. 1999;63:339–343.
80. Gerhold R. Parasitic diseases. In: Greenacre CB, Morishita TY, eds. *Backyard Poultry Medicine and Surgery: A Guide for Veterinary Practitioners*. Ames, IA: Wiley; 2015:297–320.
81. Glatz PC, Murphy LB, Preston AP. Analgesic therapy of beak-trimmed chickens. *Aust Vet J*. 1992;69:18.
82. Goetting V, Lee KA, Tell LA. Pharmacokinetics of veterinary drugs in laying hens and residues in eggs: a review of the literature. *J Vet Pharm Therap*. 2011;34:521–556.

83. Goto I, Jin K, Murase T, et al. Treatment of lead poisoning in wild geese. *J Am Vet Med Assoc.* 1992;200:1726–1729.
84. Goudah A, Abo El Sooud K, Abd El-Aty AM. Pharmacokinetics and tissue residue profiles of erythromycin in broiler chickens after different routes of administration. *Dtsch Tierarztl Wochenschr.* 2004;111:162–165.
85. Gracía-Ovando H, Chlostri L, Vania A, et al. HPLC residues of enrofloxacin and ciprofloxacin in eggs of laying hens. *J Vet Pharm Therap.* 1997;20:181–182.
86. Graham JE, Kollias-Baker C, Craigmill AL, et al. Pharmacokinetics of ketoprofen in adult Japanese quail (*Coturnix coturnix japonica*). *J Vet Pharm Therap.* 2005;28:399–402.
87. Griffith R, Yaeger M, Hostetter S, et al. Safety of fenbendazole in Chinese ring-necked pheasants (*Phasianus colchicus*). *Avian Dis.* 2014;58:8–15.
88. Hamamoto K, Koike R, Machida Y. Bioavailability of amprolium in fasting and nonfasting chickens after intravenous and oral administration. *J Vet Pharm Therap.* 2000;23:9–14.
89. Hamdy AH, Kratzer DD, Paxton LM, et al. Effect of a single injection of lincomycin, spectinomycin, and linco-spectin on early chick mortality caused by *E. coli* and *S. aureus*. *Avian Dis.* 1979;24:164–173.
90. Hamdy AH, Saif YM, Kasson CW. Efficacy of lincomycin-spectinomycin water medication on *Mycoplasma meleagridis* airsacculitis in commercially reared turkey poults. *Avian Dis.* 1982;26:227–233.
91. Hanssen I, Grav HJ, Steen JB, et al. Vitamin C deficiency in growing willow ptarmigan (*Lagopus lagopus lagopus*). *J Nutr.* 1979;109:2260–2276.
92. Haritova AM, Rusenova NV, Parvanov PR, et al. Integration of pharmacokinetic and pharmacodynamic indices of marbofloxacin in turkeys. *Antimicrob Agents Chemother.* 2006;50:3779–3785.
93. Hawkins MG, Guzman DS-M, Beaufrére H, et al. Birds. In: Carpenter JW, ed. *Exotic Animal Formulary*. 4th ed. St. Louis, MO: Elsevier; 2018:167–375.
94. Hawkins MG, Taylor IT, Byrne BA, et al. The pharmacokinetics and pharmacodynamics of orbifloxacin in Japanese quail (*Coturnix coturnix japonica*) following oral and intravenous administration. *J Vet Pharm Therap.* 2011;34:350–358.
95. Heard D. Anesthesia and analgesia. In: Altman R, Clubb S, Dorrestein G, eds. *Avian Medicine and Surgery*. Philadelphia, PA: WB Saunders; 1997:807–827.
96. Hedberg G, Bennett R. Preliminary studies on the use of milbemycin oxime in galliformes. *Proc Annu Conf Assoc Avian Vet*; 1994:261–264.
97. Heinen E, Dejong A, Scheer M. Antimicrobial activity of fluoroquinolones in serum and tissues in turkeys. *J Vet Pharm Therap.* 1997;20(Suppl 1):196–197.
98. Hines R, Kolattukuty PE, Sharkey P. Pharmacological induction of molt and gonadal involution in birds. *Proc Annu Conf Assoc Avian Vet*; 1993:127–134.
99. Hirsh DC, Knox SJ, Conzelman Jr GM, et al. Pharmacokinetics of penicillin-G in the turkey. *Am J Vet Res.* 1978;39:1219–1221.
100. Hocking PM, Gentle MJ, Bernard R, et al. Evaluation of a protocol for determining the effectiveness of pretreatment with local analgesics for reducing experimentally induced articular pain in domestic fowl. *Res Vet Sci.* 1997;63:263–267.
101. Hocking PM, Robertson GW, Gentle MJ. Effects of non-steroidal anti-inflammatory drugs on pain-related behaviour in a model of articular pain in the domestic fowl. *Res Vet Sci.* 2005;78:69–75.
102. Hope KL, Tell LA, Byrne BA, et al. Pharmacokinetics of a single intramuscular injection of ceftiofur crystalline-free acid in American black ducks (*Anas rubripes*). *Am J Vet Res.* 2012;73:620–627.
103. Houck E, Petritz O, Chen L, et al. Clinicopathologic, gross necropsy, and histopathologic effects of high-dose, repeated meloxicam administration in Rhode Island Red chickens (*Gallus gallus domesticus*). *J Avian Med Surg.* 2022. In press.
104. Hu J, Mcdougald LR. The efficacy of some drugs with known antiprotozoal activity against *Histomonas meleagridis* in chickens. *Vet Parasitol.* 2004;121:233–238.

105. Islam KM, Klein U, Burch DG. The activity and compatibility of the antibiotic tiamulin with other drugs in poultry medicine-a review. *Poult Sci*. 2009;88:2353–2359.
106. Jayakumar K, Mohan K, Narayana Swamy HD, et al. Study of nephrotoxic potential of acetaminophen in birds. *Toxicol Int*. 2010;17:86–89.
107. Jia Y, Yang M, Zhu K, et al. Melatonin implantation improved the egg-laying rate and quality in hens past their peak egg-laying age. *Sci Rep*. 2016;6:1–8.
108. Jin S, Sell JL. Dietary vitamin K1 requirements and comparison of biopotency of different vitamin K sources for young turkeys. *Poult Sci*. 2001;80:615–620.
109. Johnson-Delaney CA. *Exotic Companion Medicine Handbook for Veterinarians*. 2nd ed. Lake Worth, FL: Zoological Education Network; 2008.
110. Jordan FTW, Horrocks BK. The minimum inhibitory concentration of tilmicosin and tylosin for *Mycoplasma gallisepticum* and *Mycoplasma synoviae* and a comparison of their efficacy in the control of *Mycoplasma gallisepticum* infection in chickens. *Avian Dis*. 1997;41:802–807.
111. Junge RE, Naeger LL, Lebeau MA, et al. Pharmacokinetics of intramuscular and nebulized ceftriaxone in chickens. *J Zoo Wildl Med*. 1994;25:224–228.
112. Kazemi-Darabadi S, Akbari G, Shokrollahi S. Development and evaluation of a technique for spinal anaesthesia in broiler chickens. *N Z Vet J*. 2019;67:241–248.
113. Kempf I, Reeve-Johnson L, Gesbert F, et al. Efficacy of tilmicosin in the control of experimental Mycoplasma gallisepticum infection in chickens. *Avian Dis*. 1997;41:802–807.
114. Klein PN, Charmatz K, Langenberg J. The effect of flunixin meglumine (Banamine) on the renal function in northern bobwhite (*Colinus virginianus*): an avian model. *Proc Annu Conf Am Assoc Zoo Vet*; 1994:128–131.
115. Kline Y, Clemons KV, Woods L, et al. Pharmacokinetics of voriconazole in adult mallard ducks (*Anas platyrhynchos*). *Med Mycol*. 2011;49:500–512.
116. Knafo SE, Graham JE, Barton BA. Intravenous and intraosseous regional limb perfusion of ceftiofur sodium in an avian model. *Am J Vet Res*. 2019;80:539–546.
117. Knoll U, Glünder G, Kietzmann M. Pharmacokinetics of enrofloxacin and danofloxacin in broiler chickens. *J Vet Pharm Therap*. 1997;22:239–246.
118. Knoll U, Glünder G, Kietzmann M. Compare study of the plasma pharmacokinetics and tissue concentrations of danofloxacin and enrofloxacin in broiler chickens. *J Vet Pharm Therap*. 1999;22:239–246.
119. Knutson K, Petritz O, Thomson A, et al. Effects of intramuscular alfaxalone and midazolam compared with midazolam and butorphanol in Rhode Island Red hens (*Gallus gallus domesticus*). *Proc Annu Conf Assoc Avian Vet*; 2020.
120. Kollias GV, Zgola MM, Weinkle TK, et al. Amikacin sulfate pharmacokinetics in ring-necked pheasants (*Phasianus colchicus*): age and route dependent effects. *Proc Annu Conf Am Assoc Zoo Vet*; 1996:178–180.
121. Krautwald-Junghanns M-E, Schmidt V, Zebisch R. Relevance and treatment of coccidiosis in domestic pigeons (*Columba livia domestica*) with particular emphasis on toltrazuril. *J Avian Med Surg*. 2009;23:1–5.
122. Kruse TN, Messenger KM, Bowman AS, et al. Pharmacokinetics and pharmacodynamics of alfaxalone after a single intramuscular or intravascular injection in mallard ducks (*Anas platyrhynchos*). *J Vet Pharm Therap*. 2019;42:713–721.
123. Laczay P, Semjén G, Nagy G, et al. Comparative studies on the pharmacokinetics of norfloxacin in chickens, turkeys, and geese after a single oral administration. *J Vet Pharm Therap*. 1998;21:161–164.
124. Lashev L, Moutafchieva R, Kanelov I, et al. Pharmacokinetics of tobramycin in broiler chickens. *Trakia J Sci*. 2005;3:11–13.
125. Lashev LD, Mihailov R. Pharmacokinetics of apramycin in Japanese quail. *J Vet Pharmacol Therap*. 1994;17:394–395.
126. Latimer KS, Rakich PM. Necropsy examination. In: Ritchie BW, Harrison GJ, Harrison LR, eds. *Avian Medicine: Principles and Application*. Lake Worth, FL: Wingers Publishing; 1994:355–379.

127. Lawton M. Anesthesia. In: Beynon PH, Forbes NA, Harcourt-Brown N, eds. *BSAVA Manual of Raptors, Pigeons and Waterfowl*. Ames, IA: Iowa State University Press; 1996:79–88.
128. Leeson S. Vitamin deficiencies in poultry. *Merck Veterinary Manual*. Kenilworth, NJ: Merck & Co. Available at: https://www.merckvetmanual.com/poultry/nutrition-and-management-poultry/vitamin-deficiencies-in-poultry. Accessed July 26, 2020.
129. Lister S, Houghton-Wallace J. Backyard poultry 2. Veterinary care and disease control. *In Pract*. 2012;34:214–225.
130. Locke D, Bush M. Tylosin aerosol therapy in quail and pigeons. *J Zoo Anim Med*. 1984;15:67–72.
131. Locke D, Bush M, Carpenter JW. Pharmacokinetics and tissue concentrations of tylosin in selected avian species. *Am J Vet Res*. 1982;43:1807–1810.
132. Loibl MF, Clutton RE, Marx BD, et al. Alpha-chloralose as a capture and restraint agent of birds: therapeutic index determination in the chicken. *J Wildl Dis*. 1988;24:684–687.
133. Lublin A, Mechani S, Malkinson M, et al. Efficacy of norfloxacin nicotinate treatment of broiler breeders against *Haemophilus paragallinarum*. *Avian Dis*. 1993;37:673–679.
134. Ludders JW, Mitchell GS, Rode J. Minimal anesthetic concentration and cardiopulmonary dose response of isoflurane in ducks. *Vet Surg*. 1990;19:304–307.
135. Ludders JW, Rode J, Mitchell GS, et al. Effects of ketamine, xylazine, and a combination of ketamine and xylazine in Pekin ducks. *Am J Vet Res*. 1989;50(2):245–249.
136. Machin KL, Caulkett NA. Cardiopulmonary effects of propofol and a medetomidine-midazolam-ketamine combination in mallard ducks. *Am J Vet Res*. 1998;59:598–602.
137. Machin KL, Caulkett NA. Investigation of injectable anesthetic agents in mallard ducks (*Anas platyrhynchos*): a descriptive study. *J Avian Med Surg*. 1998;12:255–262.
138. Machin KL, Caulkett NA. Evaluation of isoflurane and propofol anesthesia for intraabdominal transmitter placement in nesting female canvasback ducks. *J Wildl Dis*. 2000;36(2):324–334.
139. Machin KL, Livingston A. Plasma bupivacaine levels in mallard ducks (*Anas platyrhynchos*) following a single subcutaneous dose. *Proc Annu Conf Am Assoc Zoo Vet/Am Assoc Wildl Vet/Assoc Rept Amph Vet/Nat Assoc Zoo Wildl Vet*; 2001:159–163.
140. Machin KL, Livingston A. Assessment of the analgesic effects of ketoprofen in ducks anesthetized with isoflurane. *Am J Vet Res*. 2002;63:821–826.
141. Machin KL, Tellier LA, Lair S, et al. Pharmacodynamics of flunixin and ketoprofen in mallard ducks (*Anas platyrhynchos*). *J Zoo Wildl Med*. 2001;32:222–229.
142. Macklin KS, Hauck R. Helminthiasis in poultry (nematode and cestode infections). *Merck Veterinary Manual*. Kenilworth, NJ: Merck & Co. Available at: https://www.merckvetmanual.com/poultry/helminthiasis/helminthiasis-in-poultry. Accessed July 28, 2020.
143. Maiti SK, Tiwary R, Vasan P, et al. Xylazine, diazepam and midazolam premedicated ketamine anaesthesia in white leghorn cockerels for typhlectomy. *J S Afr Vet Assoc*. 2006;77:12–18.
144. Marshall R. Avian anthelmintics and antiprotozoals. *Semin Avian Exot Pet Med*. 1993;2:33–41.
145. Martin-Jurado O, Vogt R, Kutter APN, et al. Effect of inhalation of isoflurane at end-tidal concentrations greater than, equal to, and less than the minimum anesthetic concentration on the bispectral index in chickens. *Am J Vet Res*. 2008;69:1254–1261.
146. Martinez R, Wobeser G. Immunization of ducks for type C botulism. *J Wildl Dis*. 1999;35:710–715.
147. Marx KL. Therapeutic agents. In: Harrison GJ, Lightfoot TL, eds. *Clinical Avian Medicine*. Palm Beach, FL: Spix Publishing; 2011:241–342.
148. Marx KL, Roston MA. *The Exotic Animal Drug Compendium: An International Formulary*. Trenton, NJ: Veterinary Learning Systems; 1996.
149. McGeown D, Danbury TC, Waterman-Pearson AE, et al. Effect of carprofen on lameness in broiler chickens. *Vet Rec*. 1999;144:668–671.
150. McKee JS, Harrison PC. Effects of supplemental ascorbic acid on the performance of broiler chickens exposed to multiple concurrent stressors. *Poult Sci*. 1995;74(11):1772–1785.

151. Migaki TT, Avakian AP, Barnes HJ, et al. Efficacy of danofloxacin and tylosin in the control of mycoplasmosis in chicks infected with tylosin-susceptible or tylosin-resistant field isolates of Mycoplasma gallisepticum. *Avian Dis*. 1993;37:508–514.
152. Mississippi State University Extension. Solutions and treatments. Available at: http://www.extension.msstate.edu/content/solutions-and-treatments. Accessed August 13, 2020.
153. Mohan K, Jayakumar K, Narayanaswamy HD, et al. An initial safety assessment of hepatotoxic and nephrotoxic potential of intramuscular ketoprofen at single repetitive dose level in broiler chickens. *Poult Sci*. 2012;91:1308–1314.
154. Mohiti-Asli M, Ghanaatparast-Rashti M. Dietary oregano essential oil alleviates experimentally induced coccidiosis in broilers. *Prev Vet Med*. 2015;120:195–202.
155. Molter CM, Fontenot DK, Terrell SP. Use of deslorelin acetate implants to mitigate aggression in two adult male domestic turkeys (*Meleagris gallopavo*) and correlating plasma testosterone concentrations. *J Avian Med Surg*. 2015;29:224–230.
156. Moreira dos Santos Schmidt E, Paulillo AC, Locatelli Dittrich R, et al. Serum biochemical parameters in the ring-necked pheasant (*Phasianus colchicus*) on breeding season. *Int J Poult Sci*. 2007;6(2):673–674.
157. Moreno L, Bistoletti M, Fernández H, et al. Albendazole treatment in laying hens: egg residues and its effects on fertility and hatchability. *J Vet Pharmacol Therap*. 2018;41:726–733.
158. Morishita TY, Porter RE. Gastrointestinal and hepatic diseases. In: Greenacre CB, Morishita TY, eds. *Backyard Poultry Medicine and Surgery: A Guide for Veterinary Practitioners*. Ames, IA: Wiley; 2015:297–320.
159. Mostachio GQ, De-Oliveira LD, Carciofi AC, et al. The effects of anesthesia with a combination of intramuscular xylazine–diazepam–ketamine on heart rate, respiratory rate and cloacal temperature in roosters. *Vet Anaesth Analg*. 2008;35:232–236.
160. Mulcahy DM, Stoskopf MK, Esler D. Lack of isoflurane-sparing effect of butorphanol in field anesthesia of harlequin ducks (*Histrionicus histrionicus*). *Proc Annu Conf Am Assoc Zoo Vet/Int Assoc Aquatic Anim Med*; 2000:532–533.
161. Mulcahy DM, Tuomi P, Larsen RS. Differential mortality of male spectacled eiders (*Somateria fischeri*) and king eiders (*Somateria spectabilis*) subsequent to anesthesia with propofol, bupivacaine, and ketoprofen. *J Avian Med Surg*. 2003;17:117–123.
162. Müller K, Holzapfel J, Brunnberg L. Total intravenous anaesthesia by boluses or by continuous rate infusion of propofol in mute swans (*Cygnus olor*). *Vet Anaesth Analg*. 2011;38:286–291.
163. Murai A, Furuse M, Okumura J. Involvement of (N-6) essential fatty acids and prostaglandins in liver lipid accumulation in Japanese quail. *Am J Vet Res*. 1996;57:342–345.
164. Museum of Zoology. Aves (on-line). Animal Diversity Web. Available at: https://animaldiversity.org/accounts/Aves/. Accessed November 6, 2020.
165. Naccari F, Salpietro DC, De Sarro A, et al. Tolerance and pharmacokinetics of ciprofloxacin in the chick: preliminary experience in subjects of pediatric age with urinary tract infections. *Res Commun Mol Pathol Pharmacol*. 1998;99:187–192.
166. Naganobu K, Fujisawa Y, Ohde H, et al. Determination of the minimum anesthetic concentration and cardiovascular dose response for sevoflurane in chickens during controlled ventilation. *Vet Surg*. 2000;29:102–105.
167. National Office for Animal Health (NOAH). Antibiotics for animals. Available at: http://www.noah.co.uk/medicine-topics/antibiotics-for-animals. Accessed August 13, 2020.
168. National Research Council U.S. *Subcommittee on Poultry Nutrition. Nutrient Requirements of Poultry*. 9th rev. ed. Washington, DC: National Academy Press; 1994.
169. Newell SM, McMillan MC, Moore FM. Diagnosis and treatment of lymphocytic leukemia and malignant lymphoma in a Pekin duck (*Anas platyrhyncos domesticus*). *J Assoc Avian Vet*. 1991;5:83–86.
170. Newman L, Sander J, et al. Poultry drug use guide. In: Boulianne M, Brash ML, Fitz-Coy SH et al., eds. *Avian Disease Manual*. 7th ed. Jacksonville, FL: American Association of Avian Pathologists; 2013:263–267.

171. North American Compendiums. Poultry medications formulary. Available at: https://bayer-all.cvpservice.com/prodindex/main?spcsId=4000. Accessed May 7, 2021.
172. Orosz S. Birds. *American Association of Zoo Veterinarians (AAZV). Guidelines for Euthanasia of Nondomestic Animals*. Yulee, FL: AAZV; 2006:46–49.
173. Ozen H, Karaman M, Ciğremiş Y, et al. Effectiveness of melatonin on aflatoxicosis in chicks. *Res Vet Sci*. 2009;86:485–489.
174. Paul-Murphy J, Koch VW, Briscoe JA, et al. Advancements in the management of the welfare of avian species. In: Speer B, ed. *Current Therapy in Avian Medicine and Surgery*. St. Louis, MO: Elsevier; 2016:669–718.
175. Pedersoli WM, Ravis WR, Askins DR, et al. Pharmacokinetics of single doses of gentamicin given intravenously and intramuscularly to turkeys. *J Vet Pharmacol Therap*. 1989;12: 124–132.
176. Petritz OA, Guzman DS-M, Hawkins MG, et al. Comparison of two 4.7-milligram to one 9.4-milligram deslorelin acetate implants on egg production and plasma progesterone concentrations in Japanese quail (*Coturnix coturnix japonica*). *J Zoo Wild Med*. 2015;46:789–797.
177. Petritz OA, Guzman DS-M, Paul-Murphy J, et al. Evaluation of the efficacy and safety of single administration of 4.7-mg deslorelin acetate implants on egg production and plasma sex hormones in Japanese quail (*Coturnix coturnix japonica*). *Am J Vet Res*. 2013;74:316–323.
178. Phalen D. Diagnosis and treatment of megabacteriosis in birds. *Vet Quart Rev*. 2001.
179. Phillips A, Fiorello CV, Baden RM, et al. Amphotericin B concentrations in healthy mallard ducks (*Anas platyrhynchos*) following a single intratracheal dose of liposomal amphotericin B using an atomizer. *Med Mycol*. 2017;56:322–331.
180. Poźniak B, Świtała M, Bobrek K, et al. Adverse effects associated with high-dose acetylsalicylic acid and sodium salicylate treatment in broilers. *Br Poult Sci*. 2012;53:777–783.
181. Poźniak B, Świtała M, Jaworski K, et al. Comparative pharmacokinetics of acetylsalicylic acid and sodium salicylate in chickens and turkeys. *Br Poult Sci*. 2013;54:538–544.
182. Prashar A, Guggenheim JA, Erichsen JT, et al. Measurement of intraocular pressure (IOP) in chickens using a rebound tonometer: quantitative evaluation of variance due to position inaccuracies. *Exp Eye Res*. 2007;85:563–571.
183. Rae MA. Diagnostic value of necropsy. In: Lightfoot TL, Harrison GJ, eds. *Clinical Avian Medicine*. Palm Beach, FL: Spix Publishing; 2006:661–678.
184. Raj ABM, Gregory NG, Wotton SB. Changes in the somatosensory evoked potentials and spontaneous electroencephalogram of hens during stunning in argon-induced anoxia. *Br Vet J*. 1991;147:322–330.
185. Rajaei SM, Mood MA. Measurement of tear production and intraocular pressure in healthy captive helmeted guinea fowl (*Numida meleagris*). *J Avian Med Surg*. 2016;30:324–328.
186. Ratliff CM, Zaffarano BA. Therapeutic use of regional limb perfusion in a chicken. *J Avian Med Surg*. 2017;31:29–32.
187. Rentsch AK, Rufener CB, Spadavecchia C, et al. Laying hen's mobility is impaired by keel bone fractures and does not improve with paracetamol treatment. *Appl Anim Behav Sci*. 2019;16:19–25.
188. Ritchie BW, Harrison GJ. Formulary. In: Ritchie BW, Harrison GJ, Harrison LR, eds. *Avian Medicine: Principles and Applications*. Lake Worth, FL: Wingers Publishing; 1994:457–478.
189. Rocke TE, Samuel MD, Swift PK, et al. Efficacy of a type C botulism vaccine in green-winged teal. *J Wild Dis*. 2000;36:489–493.
190. Rolinski Z, Kowalski C, Wlaz P. Distribution and elimination of norfloxacin from broiler chicken tissues and eggs. *J Vet Pharmacol Therap*. 1997;20:200–201.
191. Ruth I. *Wildlife Care Basics for Veterinary Hospitals: Before the Rehabilitator Arrives*. Humane Society of the United States (HSUS); 2012.
192. Santos EA, Monteiro ER, Herrera JR, et al. Total intravenous anesthesia in domestic chicken (*Gallus gallus domesticus*) with propofol alone or in combination with methadone, nalbuphine or fentanyl for ulna osteotomy. *Vet Anaesth Analg*. 2020;47:347–355.

193. Sarközy G, Semjén G, Laczay P, et al. Treatment of experimentally induced *Pasteurella multocida* in broilers and turkeys: comparative studies of different oral treatment regimens. *J Vet Med B Infect Dis Vet Public Health*. 2002;49:130–134.
194. Sartini I, Łebkowska-Wieruszewska B, Lisowski A, et al. Pharmacokinetic profiles of meloxicam after single IV and PO administration in Bilgorajska geese. *J Vet Pharmacol Therap*. 2020;43:26–32.
195. Schobert E. Telazol use in wild and exotic animals. *Vet Med*. 1987;82:1080–1088.
196. Scholtz N, Halle I, Flachowsky G, et al. Serum chemistry reference values in adult Japanese quail (*Coturnix coturnix japonica*) including sex-related differences. *Poult Sci*. 2009;88:1186–1190.
197. Schumacher J, Citino SB, Hernandez K, et al. Cardiopulmonary and anesthetic effects of propofol in wild turkeys. *Am J Vet Res*. 1997;58:1014–1017.
198. Schwartz LD. Internal parasites. In: Bengtson GD, ed. *Growers' Reference on Gamebird Health*. Okemis, MI: Avicon, Inc.; 1995:185–211.
199. Shannon L, Cox SK, Bailey J, et al. Pharmacokinetics and drug residue in eggs after multiple-day oral dosing of amoxicillin-clavulanic acid in domestic chickens. *J Avian Med Surg*. 2020;34:3–8.
200. Sinclair KM, Church ME, Farver TB, et al. Effects of meloxicam on hematologic and plasma biochemical analysis variables and results of histologic examination of tissue specimens of Japanese quail (*Coturnix japonica*). *Am J Vet Res*. 2012;73:1720–1727.
201. Singh PM, Johnson C, Gartrell B, et al. Pharmacokinetics of morphine after intravenous administration in broiler chickens. *J Vet Pharmacol Therap*. 2010;33:515–518.
202. Singh PM, Johnson C, Gartrell B, et al. Pharmacokinetics of butorphanol in broiler chickens. *Vet Rec*. 2011;168:588–591.
203. Soliman AM, Sedek M. Pharmacokinetics and tissue residues of tylosin in broiler chickens. *Pharmacol Pharm*. 2016;7:36–42.
204. Souza MJ, Bailey J, White M, et al. Pharmacokinetics and egg residues of meloxicam after multiple day oral dosing in domestic chickens. *J Avian Med Surg*. 2018;32:8–12.
205. Souza MJ, Bergman JB, White MS, et al. Pharmacokinetics and egg residues after oral administration of a single dose of meloxicam in domestic chickens (*Gallus domesticus*). *Am J Vet Res*. 2017;78:965–968.
206. Stadler CK, Carpenter JW. Parasites of backyard game birds. *Semin Avian Exot Pet Med*. 1996;5:85–96.
207. Stake PE. Tamoxifen induced forced-rest/molt in laying hens. *Poult Sci*. 1979;58:1111.
208. Stipkovits L, Burch DGS, Salyi G, et al. Study to test the compatibility of tetramutinfi given in feed at different levels with salinomycin (60 ppm) in chickens. *J Vet Pharmacol Therap*. 1997;20:191–192.
209. Tanner AC. Antimicrobial drug use in poultry. In: Prescott J, Baggot J, eds. *Antimicrobial Therapy in Veterinary Medicine*. 3rd ed. Ames, IA: Iowa State University Press; 2000:637–655.
210. Tanner AC, Avakian AP, Barnes HJ, et al. A comparison of danofloxacin and tylosin in the control of induced *Mycoplasma gallisepticum* infection in broiler chicks. *Avian Dis*. 1993;37:515–522.
211. Taylor S, Kenny J, Houston A, et al. Efficacy, pharmacokinetics and effect on egg-laying and hatchability of two dose rates of in-feed fenbendazole for the treatment of *Capillaria* species infections in chickens. *Vet Rec*. 1993;133:519–521.
212. Teare JA. Antagonism of xylazine hydrochloride-ketamine hydrochloride immobilization in guinea fowl (*Numidia meleagris*) by yohimbine hydrochloride. *J Wildl Dis*. 1987;23:301–305.
213. Teare JA, Schwark WS, Shin SJ, et al. Pharmacokinetics of a long-acting oxytetracycline preparation in ring-necked pheasants, great horned owls and Amazon parrots. *Am J Vet Res*. 1985;46:2639–2643.
214. Tekeli IO, Turk E, Corum DD, et al. Pharmacokinetics, bioavailability and tissue residues of doxycycline in Japanese quails (*Coturnix coturnix japonica*) after oral administration. *Food Addit Contam. Part A*. 2020:1–11.

215. Tell L, Shukla A, Munson L, et al. A comparison of the effects of slow release, injectable levonorgestrel and depot medroxyprogesterone acetate on egg production in Japanese quail (*Coturnix coturnix japonica*). *J Avian Med Surg.* 1999;13:23–31.
216. Tell LA. Regulatory considerations for medicine use in poultry. In: Greenacre CB, Morishita TY, eds. *Backyard Poultry Medicine and Surgery: A Guide for Veterinary Practitioners.* Ames, IA: Wiley; 2015:297–320.
217. Tell LA, Clemons KV, Kline Y, et al. Efficacy of voriconazole in Japanese quail (*Coturnix japonica*) experimentally infected with *Aspergillus fumigatus*. *Med Mycol.* 2010;48:234–244.
218. Tell LA, Craigmill AL, Clemons KV, et al. Studies on itraconazole delivery and pharmacokinetics in mallard ducks (*Anas platyrhynchos*). *J Vet Pharmacol Therap.* 2005;28:267–274.
219. Tell LA, Harrenstien L, Wetzlich S, et al. Pharmacokinetics of ceftiofur sodium in exotic and domestic avian species. *J Vet Pharmacol Therap.* 1998;21:85–91.
220. Thomas-Baker B, Dew RD, Patton S. Ivermectin treatment of ocular nematodiasis in birds. *J Am Vet Med Assoc.* 1986;189:1113.
221. Thuesen LR, Bertelsen MF, Brimer L, et al. Selected pharmacokinetic parameters for cefovecin in hens and green iguanas. *J Vet Pharmacol Therap.* 2009;32:613–617.
222. Turbahn A, De Jäckel SC, Greuel E, et al. Dose response study of enrofloxacin against *Riemerella anatipestifer* septicaemia in Muscovy and Pekin ducklings. *Avian Path.* 1997;26:791–802.
223. U.S. Food and Drug Administration. Animal drugs. Available at: https://animaldrugsatfda.fda.gov/adafda/views/#/home/previewsearch. Accessed August 14, 2020.
224. U.S. Food and Drug Administration. Cfr - code of Federal Regulations title 21. *U.S. Department of Health and Human Services,* ed. *21 CFR Part 530.41*; 2019.
225. U.S. Food and Drug Administration. Drugs with veterinary feed directive (VFD) marketing status. Available at: https://www.fda.gov/animal-veterinary/development-approval-process/drugs-veterinary-feed-directive-vfd-marketing-status. Accessed August 14, 2020.
226. U.S. Food and Drug Administration. Extralabel use and antimicrobials. Available at: https://www.fda.gov/animal-veterinary/antimicrobial-resistance/extralabel-use-and-antimicrobials. Accessed August 14, 2020.
227. U.S. Food and Drug Administration. Veterinary feed directive producer requirements. Available at: https://www.fda.gov/animal-veterinary/development-approval-process/veterinary-feed-directive-producer-requirements. Accessed November 6, 2020.
228. United States Department of Agriculture - Wildlife Services. Questions and answers: OvoControl. Wildlife damage. Available at: https://www.aphis.usda.gov/publications/wildlife_damage/content/printable_version/fs_ovocontrol.pdf. Accessed November 5, 2020.
229. Uzun M, Onder F, Atalan G, et al. Effects of xylazine, medetomidine, detomidine, and diazepam on sedation, heart and respiratory rates, and cloacal temperature in rock partridges (*Alectoris graeca*). *J Zoo Wildl Med.* 2006;37:135–140.
230. Valverde A, Honeyman VL, Dyson DH, et al. Determination of a sedative dose and influence of midazolam on cardiopulmonary function in Canada geese. *Am J Vet Res.* 1990;51:1071–1074.
231. Van Alstine WG, Dyer DC. Antibiotic aerosolization: tissue and plasma oxytetracycline concentrations in turkey poults. *Avian Dis.* 1985;29:430–436.
232. Villanúa D, Acevedo P, Höfle U, et al. Changes in parasite transmission stage excretion after pheasant release. *J Helminthol.* 2006;80:313–318.
233. Watteyn A, Wyns H, Plessers E, et al. Pharmacokinetics of dexamethasone after intravenous and intramuscular administration in broiler chickens. *Vet J.* 2013;195:216–220.
234. Waugh L, Knych HK, Cole G, et al. Pharmacokinetic evaluation of a long-acting fentanyl solution after transdermal administration in helmeted guinea fowl (*Numida meleagridis*). *J Zoo Wildl Med.* 2016;47:468–473.
235. White DM, Martinez-Taboada F. Induction of anesthesia with intravenous alfaxalone in two Isa brown chickens (*Gallus gallus domesticus*). *J Exot Pet Med.* 2019;29:119–122.
236. Whiteside DP, Barker IK, Conlon PD, et al. Pharmacokinetic disposition of the oral iron chelator deferiprone in the white leghorn chicken. *J Avian Med Surg.* 2007;21:110–120.

237. Wojick KB, Langan JN, Adkesson MJ, et al. Pharmacokinetics of long-acting ceftiofur crystalline-free acid in helmeted guineafowl (*Numida meleagris*) after a single intramuscular injection. *Am J Vet Res.* 2011;72:1514–1518.
238. Xie W, Zhang X, Wang T, et al. Pharmacokinetic analysis of cefquinome in healthy chickens. *Br Poult Sci.* 2013;54:81–86.
239. Yang F, Li GH, Meng XB, et al. Pharmacokinetic interactions of flunixin meglumine and doxycycline in broiler chickens. *J Vet Pharmacol Therap.* 2012;36:85–88.
240. Yang F, Si HB, Wang YQ, et al. Pharmacokinetics of doxycycline in laying hens after intravenous and oral administration. *Br Poult Sci.* 2016;57:576–580.
241. Yang F, Sun N, Zhao ZS, et al. Pharmacokinetics of doxycycline after a single intravenous, oral or intramuscular dose in Muscovy ducks (*Cairina moschata*). *Br Poult Sci.* 2015;56:137–142.
242. Yoder CA, Miller LA, Bynum KS. Comparison of nicarbazin absorption in chickens, mallards, and Canada geese. *Poult Sci.* 2005;84:1491–1494.
243. Yuan L, Sun J, Wang R, et al. Pharmacokinetics and bioavailability of cefquinome in healthy ducks. *Am J Vet Res.* 2011;72:122–126.
244. Zhao D-H, Wang X-F, Wang Q, et al. Pharmacokinetics, bioavailability and dose assessment of cefquinome against *Escherichia coli* in black swans (*Cygnus atratus*). *BMC Vet Res.* 2017;13:226.
245. Ziółkowsk H, Grabowski T, Jasiecka A, et al. Pharmacokinetics of oxytetracycline in broiler chickens following different routes of administration. *Vet J.* 2016;208:96–98.
246. Ziółkowski H, Jasiecka-Mikołajczyk A, Madej-Śmiechowska H, et al. Comparative pharmacokinetics of chlortetracycline, tetracycline, minocycline, and tigecycline in broiler chickens. *Poult Sci.* 2020;99:4750–4757.
247. Ziv G, Shem-Tov M, Glickman A, et al. Concentrations of amoxycillin and clavulanic acid in the serum of broilers during continuous and pulse-dosing of the drinking water. *J Vet Pharmacol Therap.* 1997;20(Suppl 1):183–184.
248. Ziv G, Shem-Tov M, Glickman A, et al. Serum oxytetracycline and chlortetracycline concentrations in broilers and turkeys treated with high doses of the drugs via the feed and water. *J Vet Pharmacol Therap.* 1997;20(Suppl 1):190–191.

Chapter 7 Sugar Gliders

Grayson A. Doss | Cathy A. Johnson-Delaney

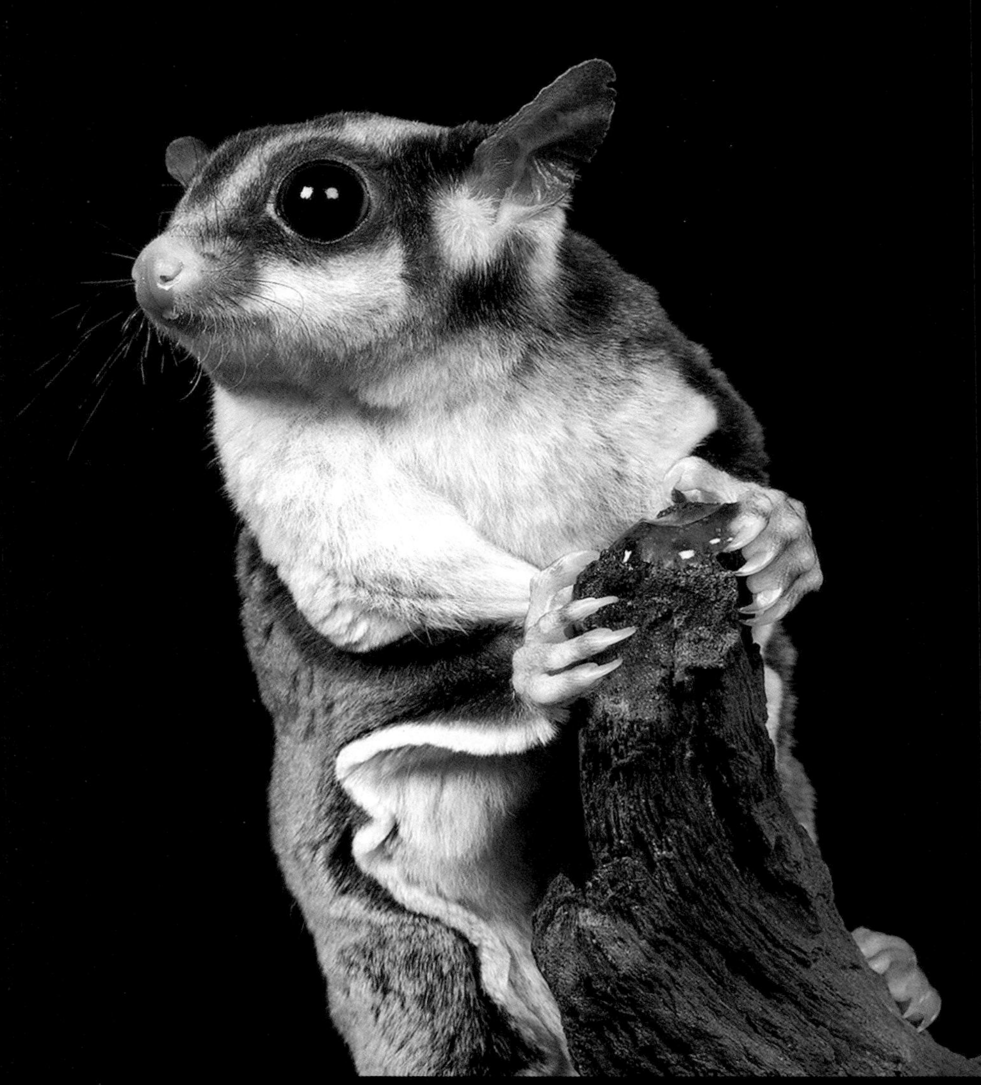

TABLE 7-1 Antimicrobial and Antifungal Agents Used in Sugar Gliders.

Agent	Dosage	Comments
Amikacin sulfate	3 mg/kg SC, IM q12h[30]	Severe gram-negative infections; administer SC fluids concurrently
	10 mg/kg SC, IM q12h × 5 days[3,32]	Gram-negative pneumonia
Amoxicillin	30 mg/kg PO, SC q12-24h[10,30,32]	
Amoxicillin/clavulanic acid	12.5 mg/kg PO, SC divided q12h[10,30,32]	
Cefovecin sodium (Convenia, Zoetis)	—	Not recommended due to high interspecies variability in PD
Cephalexin	30 mg/kg PO, SC divided q12-24h[30,32,34]	
Chloramphenicol	50 mg/kg PO q12h[10,30]	
Ciprofloxacin	10 mg/kg PO q12h[30]	
Clindamycin	5.5-10 mg/kg PO q12h[10] x 7-10 days[3]	Periodontal disease; sinusitis
Enrofloxacin	2.5-5 mg/kg PO, SC IM q12-24h[32]	Tissue necrosis can occur when administered parenterally; dilute for SC injection
	5 mg/kg PO, SC, IM q12h[7]	
	10 mg/kg PO q24h[3]	
Gentamicin	1.5-2.5 mg/kg SC, IM q12h[10,32]	Not recommend due to nephrotoxicity; amikacin preferred if an aminoglycoside is needed; if this is the only choice, then administer SC fluids concurrently
	2 mg/kg SC, IM divided q12-24h[7]	
Griseofulvin	20 mg/kg PO q24h × 30-60 days[32]	Dermatophytes; fungistatic; rarely used, as safer drug options available
Itraconazole	5-10 mg/kg PO q12h[32]	Dermatophytes
	5-10 mg/kg PO q24h[10,30]	
Lincomycin	30 mg/kg PO, SC, IM q24h[10,32]	Dose can be divided q12h
	30 mg/kg PO, IM q24h x 7 days[3]	Dermatitis
Marbofloxacin	2-5 mg/kg PO, SC, IM q24h[10]	
Metronidazole	25 mg/kg PO q12-24h × 7-10 days[32]	CNS toxicity possible at high doses or if underlying hepatic disorder; compound at 5 mg/mL in tutti-frutti flavor;[5] use the benzoate form
Nystatin	2000 U/kg PO q12h[5]	Candidiasis
	5000 U/kg PO q8h[32]	
	5000-10,000 U/kg PO q8h x 3-5 days[3,15]	Prevention of secondary yeast infection during antibiotic therapy[3]
	10,000 U/kg PO q8h x 7 days[3]	Oral candidiasis; higher doses of 50-100,000 U/kg PO used in some Australian wildlife hospitals[3]
Penicillin	22,000-25,000 U/kg SC, IM q12-24h[30,32]	

Continued

TABLE 7-1 Antimicrobial and Antifungal Agents Used in Sugar Gliders. (cont'd)

Agent	Dosage	Comments
Trimethoprim/ sulfamethoxazole	10-20 mg/kg PO q12-24h[32] 15 mg/kg PO q12h[3,30] 50 mg/kg PO q24h[7]	

TABLE 7-2 Antiparasitic Agents Used in Sugar Gliders.

Agent	Dosage	Comments
Albendazole (A) + levamisole (L)	(A) 23.75 mg/kg + (L) 37.5 mg/kg PO q7d x 2 treatments[3]	Nematodiasis
Carbaryl powder (5%)	Topical[30,32]	Ectoparasites; use sparingly; can be used in nest boxes
Fenbendazole	20-25 mg/kg PO q24h x 3 days[3]	Roundworms, hookworms, whipworms; cestodes
	20-50 mg/kg PO q24h × 3 days, repeat in 14 days[10,15,30,32]	Lower end of dosage range may be preferable
Imidacloprid	10 mg/kg topically q30d[1,15]	Fleas
Ivermectin	0.2 mg/kg SC, repeat in 7-14 days[30,32]	Roundworms, hookworms, whipworms; mites
	0.2 mg/kg SC q7d for up to 3 treatments[15]	Mites
	0.2-0.4 mg/kg PO, SC, repeat at 14 and 28 days[10]	Mites, nematodes
Levamisole	10 mg/kg PO[32]	
Metronidazole	25 mg/kg PO q12h[5,30]	Intestinal protozoa; compound at 5 mg/mL in tutti-frutti flavor[5]
	25 mg/kg PO q24h[11]	
Piperazine	50 mg/kg PO q24h[10]	GI nematodes; safe in pregnant animals
	100 mg/kg PO[11]	
Praziquantel	5-10 mg/kg PO, SC, repeat in 10-14 days[7]	Cestodes, trematodes
Pyrethrin powder	Topical[11]	Ectoparasites; use products safe for kittens
Selamectin (Revolution, Zoetis)	6-18 mg/kg topically, repeat in 30 days[5,30,34,37]	Ectoparasites other than *Demodex* spp.[37]
Toltrazuril	7 mg/kg PO q24h x 2 days[14]	Part of combination toxoplasmosis therapy; combined with clindamycin 12.5 mg/kg PO q12h at least 2 wk and trimethoprim/sulfamethoxazole 30 mg/kg PO q24h x 3 wk

TABLE 7-3 Chemical Restraint/Anesthetic Agents Used in Sugar Gliders.

Agent	Dosage	Comments
Acepromazine	—	See butorphanol, ketamine for combinations
Atropine	0.01-0.02 mg/kg SC, IM[10,30] 0.02-0.04 mg/kg SC, IM, IV[11]	
Bupivacaine	1-2 mg/kg (local infiltrate)[30]	Local anesthesia
Buprenorphine	—	Buprenorphine combination follows
Buprenorphine (Bu) + midazolam (Mi) + meloxicam (Mel)	(Bu) 0.01 mg/kg + (Mi) 0.1 mg/kg + (Mel) 0.2 mg/kg IM[7]	Give preemptively for the reduction of postsurgical self-mutilation
Butorphanol (Torbugesic, Fort Dodge)	0.4-1 mg/kg SC, IM[15] —	Sedation for minor procedures Butorphanol combinations follows
Butorphanol (B) + acepromazine (A)	(B) 1.7 mg/kg + (A) 1.7 mg/kg PO[16]	Postoperative sedation and analgesia to prevent self-trauma to incision site
Dexmedetomidine (Dexdomitor, Pfizer)	—	α-2 agonist that is the active optical enantiomer of racemic compound medetomidine; ½ the dose of medetomidine should be administered; limited data on safety or efficacy available
Diazepam	0.5-2 mg/kg PO, SC, IM[11,30]	Sedative, anticonvulsant; avoid parenteral injection if possible (use midazolam instead)
Flumazenil	0.05-0.1 mg/kg SC, IM[24]	Reversal of diazepam and midazolam
Glycopyrrolate	0.01-0.02 mg/kg SC, IM, IV[30]	Controls salivation during sedation
Isoflurane	5% induction; 1%-3% maintenance[7,25]	Anesthetic of choice
Ketamine	20 mg/kg IM[30] 30-50 mg/kg IM[32] —	Immobilization; combinations preferred for improved muscle relaxation Ketamine combinations follow
Ketamine (K) + acepromazine (A)	(K) 10 mg/kg + (A) 1 mg/kg SC[16] (K) 30 mg/kg + (A) 2 mg/kg SC, IM[32]	Postoperative sedation and analgesia to prevent self-trauma to incision site For immobilization
Ketamine (K) + medetomidine (Me)	(K) 2-3 mg/kg + (Me) 0.05-0.1 mg/kg SC, IM[32]	For immobilization (see medetomidine)
Ketamine (K) + midazolam (Mi)	(K) 10-20 mg/kg + (Mi) 0.35-0.5 mg/kg SC, IM[30,32]	
Ketamine (K) + xylazine (X)	(K) 10-25 mg/kg + (X) 5 mg/kg SC, IM[32]	
Lidocaine	<4 mg/kg local infiltration or topical[10]	Local anesthesia; dilute to avoid toxicity from accidental overdosing

Continued

TABLE 7-3 Chemical Restraint/Anesthetic Agents Used in Sugar Gliders. (cont'd)

Agent	Dosage	Comments
Medetomidine	—	No longer commercially available, but can be obtained through various compounding services; see dexmedetomidine; see ketamine for combination
Midazolam	—	Reversal with flumazenil; see buprenorphine, ketamine for combinations
	0.1-0.5 mg/kg SC, IM, intranasal[7,10,30,32,35]	Anxiolytic; anticonvulsant; preanesthetic; sedation
Sevoflurane	1%-5% to effect[32]	Anesthesia
Tiletamine/zolazepam (Telazol, Fort Dodge)	—	Do not use; neurological syndromes and death reported in squirrel gliders (*Petaurus norfolcensis*) at 10 mg/kg[12]
Xylazine	—	See ketamine for combination
Yohimbine	0.2 mg/kg SC, IM[32]	Reversal of xylazine

TABLE 7-4 Analgesic Agents Used in Sugar Gliders.

Agent	Dosage	Comments
Buprenorphine	0.005-0.01 mg/kg SC, IV q12h[3]	
	0.01-0.03 mg/kg PO, SC, IM q8-12h[30,32]	
	0.05 mg/kg IM[26]	
Butorphanol	0.1-0.5 mg/kg SC, IM q6-8h[30,32]	Higher dosages may cause sedation[15]
	0.4 mg/kg SC, IM[3]	
Carprofen	2 mg/kg PO q12h[27]	Nonsteroidal antiinflammatory
	4 mg/kg SC initial dose, then 2 mg/kg q24h x 2 doses[3]	
Flunixin	1 mg/kg SC, IM q12-24h up to 3 days[14]	
Gabapentin	3-5 mg/kg PO q8-24h[24]	Neurotropic pain; anxiolytic; may cause sedation at higher doses; start at lower dosage and titrate up to desired effect; useful in cases of self-mutilation
Ketoprofen	1 mg/kg SC[27]	
Meloxicam	0.1-0.2 mg/kg q24h PO, SC[11,32]	Nonsteroidal antiinflammatory
	0.2 mg/kg PO, SC q12h[30]	
	0.5 mg/kg PO q24h[26]	
Methadone	0.15-0.4 mg/kg SC q4-6h for 24-48 hr only[3]	Severe trauma cases
Tramadol	5-10 mg/kg PO, IM q12h[3]	

TABLE 7-5 Miscellaneous Agents Used in Sugar Gliders.

Agent	Dosage	Comments
Calcitonin	50-100 U/kg SC, IM[32]	Nutritional osteodystrophy; ensure serum calcium levels are normal prior to use; salmon origin
Calcium glubionate	150 mg/kg PO q24h[6,32]	Nutritional osteodystrophy; calcium deficiency; commercial product may no longer be available; can be compounded
Calcium gluconate	100 mg/kg SC q12h × 3-5 days; dilute in saline to 10 mg/mL[6,27]	Nutritional osteodystrophy; calcium deficiency
Cisapride	0.1-0.2 mg/kg PO q8h[3] 0.25 mg/kg PO, SC q8-24h[6,32]	Gastrointestinal prokinetic
Deslorelin	4.7 mg implant SC[3]	Contraceptive in female brushtailed possums; likely to be effective in gliders[3]
Dexamethasone	0.1-0.6 mg/kg SC, IM, IV[30] 0.2 mg/kg SC, IM, IV q12-24h[32]	Antiinflammatory allergies
Dextrose (20%)	2-5 mL/kg IV	Hypoglycemia, especially with diarrhea in pouch young[15]
Doxapram	2 mg/kg SC, IM, IV[30]	Respiratory stimulant; can also administer sublingually
Enalapril	0.5 mg/kg PO q24h[28,30]	ACE inhibitor used for heart disease
Epinephrine	0.003 mg/kg IV[28,30]	Stimulates heart; antagonizes effects of histamine; raises blood sugar
Fluoxetine (Prozac, Eli Lilly)	1 mg/kg PO q12h[27] 1-5 mg/kg PO q8h[24] 2-5 mg/kg PO q12h[21]	Self-mutilation; use liquid form
Furosemide	1-5 mg/kg PO, SC, IM q6-12h[6,10,11] 2-4 mg/kg PO, SC, IM[28]	Diuretic
Glucose (10% or 50%)	500-2000 mg glucose/kg IV[15]	Hypoglycemia, especially with diarrhea in pouch young[15]
Lactulose	150-750 mg/kg PO q8-12h[14]	Liver disease
L-carnitine	100 mg/kg PO q12h[32]	Cardiac disease[32]
Maropitant citrate (Cerenia, Zoetis)	0.2 mg/kg SC q24h[30]	Cooling of the injection may decrease SC injection site discomfort
Metoclopramide	0.05-0.1 mg/kg PO, SC, IM q6-12h prn[32] 0.5 mg/kg SC q12h prn[3,15]	Gastrointestinal prokinetic

Continued

TABLE 7-5 Miscellaneous Agents Used in Sugar Gliders. (cont'd)

Agent	Dosage	Comments
Pimobendan	0.3-0.5 mg/kg PO q12h[10]	Positive inotropic and vasodilatory effect; administration with food may reduce bioavailability
Prednisolone	0.1-0.2 mg/kg PO, SC, IM q24h[10,32] 0.2 mg/kg PO q12h[29,30]	Antiinflammatory
Vitamin A	500-5000 U/kg IM[32]	Skin disorders[32]
Vitamin B complex	0.01-0.2 mL/kg SC, IM[30,32]	Use small animal formulation; dilute; stings on injection so best to inject into a pocket of SC fluids
Vitamin E	10 U/kg SC[5] 25-100 U/animal/day[32]	Neurologic conditions
Vitamin K	2 mg/kg SC, PO q24-72h[30,32]	Adjunctive therapy for liver, cardiac, intestinal disease[11,32]
	2.5 mg/kg SC, then 5 mg/kg PO q24h for at least 14 days[3,15]	Anticoagulant rodenticide poisoning

TABLE 7-6 Hematologic and Plasma Biochemical Values of Sugar Gliders.[5]

Measurement	Reference Range[a–c]
Hematology	
Hematocrit, %	53 ± 6 (51–54)
RBC (10^6/µL)	8.6 ± 1.0 (8.3–8.8)
Hgb (g/dL)	16.3 ± 1.9 (15.8–16.9)
MCH (pg)	19.1 ± 1.1 (18.8–19.4)
MCHC (g/dL)	30.8 ± 0.7 (30.6–31.0)
MCV (fL)	64.1 ± 14.8 (60.2–68.1)
WBC (10^3/µL)	7.4 ± 7.7 (5.5–9.3)
Neutrophils (10^3/µL)	1.8 ± 1.5 (1.5–2.2)
Lymphocytes (10^3/µL)	5.4 ± 7.0 (3.7–7.2)
Monocytes (10^3/µL)	0.1 ± 0.1 (0.1–0.2)
Eosinophils (10^3/µL)	0.2 ± 0.2 (0.1–0.3)
Basophils (10^3/µL)	0.0 ± 0.0 (0.0–0.1)
Platelets (10^3/µL)	346 ± 201 (292–400)
Chemistries	
ALP (U/L)	102 ± 57 (89–137)
ALT (U/L)	117 ± 28 (97–137)

TABLE 7-6 Hematologic and Plasma Biochemical Values of Sugar Gliders. (cont'd)

Measurement	Reference Range[a–c]
Amylase (U/L)	2734 ± 890 (2117–3351)
AST (U/L)	77 ± 71 (54–100)
Bilirubin, total (mg/dL)	0.4 ± 1.3 (0.1–0.7)
Calcium (mg/dL)	8.7 ± 0.8 (8.5–8.9)
Chloride (mmol/L)	107 ± 7 (106–109)
Cholesterol (mg/dL)	118 ± 28 (112–124)
CPK (U/L)	1359 ± 972 (1081–1637)
Creatinine (mg/dL)	0.5 ± 0.3 (0.5–0.6)
Glucose (mg/dL)[c]	162 ± 45 (153–172)
Magnesium (mmol/L)	0.95 ± 0.25 (0.8–1.05)
Phosphorus (mg/dL)	5.2 ± 3.6 (4.4–6.1)
Potassium (mmol/L)	5.1 ± 2.3 (4.6–5.5)
Protein, total (g/dL)	6.9 ± 0.7 (6.7–7.0)
Albumin (g/dL)	3.9 ± 0.4 (3.1–4.6)
Globulin (g/dL)	3.0 ± 0.5 (2.9–3.1)
Sodium (mmol/L)	141 ± 11 (139–143)
Urea nitrogen (mg/dL)	17 ± 8 (15–18)

[a]All data in this table were obtained from healthy males; blood values later obtained from healthy females reportedly fell within those ranges (D. Brust, personal communication; 2019).
[b]Mean ± SD (ranges shown are the 95% confidence intervals after outliers were removed; statistically 90% of the population should have values within these limits).
[c]Glucose levels measured immediately after collection.

TABLE 7-7 Biologic and Physiologic Values of Sugar Gliders.[4,5,7,14,34,36]

Parameter	Normal Values
Average life span (wild)	
Male	4-5 years
Female	5-7 years
Maximum reported life span	
Captivity	15 years
Wild	9 years
Colony size (wild)	7 (avg) (1 dominant male, 2 subordinate males, 4 adult females)
Colony size (captivity)	Minimum 2 (more is better)
Adult weight	Male, 100-160 g Female, 80-135 g
Body length	16-21 cm (avg 17 cm)
Tail length	16.5-21 cm (avg 19 cm)
Heart rate	200-300 beats/min

Continued

TABLE 7-7 Biologic and Physiologic Values of Sugar Gliders. (cont'd)

Parameter	Normal Values
Respiratory rate	16-40 breaths/min
Cloacal temperature	36.2°C ± 0.4°C (97.2°F ± 0.7°F)
Torpor cloacal temperature	≤15°C (59°F)
Thermoneutral zone	27-31°C (81-88°F)
Basal metabolic rate (kcal $kg^{-0.75}$ d^{-1})	50 (weight in $kg)^{0.75}$
	Example: 128 g sugar glider
	BMR = 50 $(0.128)^{0.75}$ = 10.7 kcal daily
Estrus cycle	
Type	Seasonal polyestrus
Length	29 days
Gestation period	15-17 days
Litter size	1-4 (usually 2)
Birth weight	0.2 g
Pouch emergence	50-74 days (usually 60 days)
Weaning age	85-120 days (usually 100 days)
Dispersal from nest	7-10 months
Sexual maturity	Male: 12-14 months; female: 8-12 months
Adult dental formula	2 (I3/2: C1/0: P3/3: M4/4) = 40; diprotodont
GI retention time	29 hr (average)

TABLE 7-8 Urinalysis Values of Sugar Gliders.[5]

Measurement	Avg	Reference Interval[a,b]
Specific gravity	1.030	1.020-1.040 (103)
pH	6.2	6-6.3 (98)
Protein (mg/dL)	12	9.5-14.6 (82)

[a]Values shown are the 95% reference intervals after outliers were removed; analysis performed using IDEXX Vetlab UA.
[b]Sample size is presented in parentheses.

TABLE 7-9 Growth and Development of Sugar Gliders.[4,6,9]

Stage 1: In Pouch

Age (days)	Weight (g)	Head (mm)	Leg (mm)	Key Developmental Characteristics
1	0.2	—	—	Mouth and forelimbs most developed feature
20	0.8	11	6	Ears free from head; papillae of mystacial vibrissae (whiskers) visible

TABLE 7-9 Growth and Development of Sugar Gliders. (cont'd)

Stage 1: In Pouch (cont'd)

Age (days)	Weight (g)	Head (mm)	Leg (mm)	Key Developmental Characteristics
30	1.6	14	9	—
35	2	—	—	Mystacial vibrissae erupt; ears pigmented
40	3.2	17	12	Start to pigment on shoulders; eye slits present
50	6.2	20	16	Typical detachment from teat and emergence from pouch at 50-60 days

Stage 2: Out of Pouch (OOP)[a,b]

Age (weeks)	Weight (g)	Key Developmental Characteristics
1	8-18	Dorsal stripe developing; little to no fur; slick tail; closed eyes
2	12-22	Eyes open at approximately 17-21 days; fur lengthens
3	17-29	Very fine fur, except abdominal area; tail still slick; eyes still closed
4	18-35	Fur becoming more prominent; tail beginning to fluff; weaning begins
5	19-39	Complete fur coverage; light fur on abdominal area; tail continues to fill out
6	20-45	Tail fully fluffed out; abdominal area fully furred; mostly weaned
7	21-60	Very active at night; eating mainly solid foods
8	23-75	Fully self-sufficient and weaned

[a]On a practical level, estimating an exact out of pouch (OOP) date is often problematic because of the nocturnal nature of the animal and protectiveness of dam; pouch young often exhibit wide weight differentials at the same age; the most reliable method for estimating age is to visually assess key distinguishing characteristics of their physical development, especially the abdominal area and tail.[5]

[b]Once a pouch young is observed out of the pouch, age is typically measured in weeks.[2]

TABLE 7-10 Common Clinical Presentations of Sugar Gliders.

- Nutritional osteodystrophy
- Obesity
- Fractures
- Ocular injury
- Malnutrition
- Oral/dental disease
- Diarrhea
- Rectal/cloacal prolapse
- Respiratory disease
- Cystitis/urolithiasis
- Paracloacal gland impaction/infection
- Penile necrosis
- Pouch infection, mastitis
- Failure-to-thrive pouch young
- Self-mutilation
- Neoplasia
- Neurologic signs: tremors, seizures
- Renal disease

TABLE 7-11 Suggested Sugar Glider Diets.[8,17,18,23,25,38]

Feeding captive sugar gliders appropriately can be challenging for owners. There are a number of commercial sugar glider kibble diets currently on the market, although none are considered nutritionally complete without the addition of some produce items, nectars, or additional protein sources. The exact vitamin and mineral requirements for all life stages of captive sugar gliders have yet to be determined and many commercial diets have not been evaluated through extensive feeding trials. Variations in produce, carbohydrates, fiber, vitamins, and minerals in a diet may result in inconsistent or incomplete nutrition. Produce items should be finely chopped and mixed together so that the glider cannot pick out a favorite item. A large variety of items is recommended. Sugar gliders are hindgut fermenters of gums. They are omnivores, feeding on gum and sap, nectar and pollen from flowers, and insects. They can digest both simple sugars (nectar) and complex carbohydrates (gum) as sources of energy. Protein is obtained from pollen and insects. Their natural diet is relatively low in iron, so consumption of many human foods and even many commercial "sugar glider" diets or supplements may contribute to iron deposition and overload. The suggested dietary iron range is 40-85 mg/kg (dry matter basis). Commercial gum arabic (*Acacia*) is available as a dry powder and can be used along with captive diets. The complex carbohydrate in plant gums is likely beneficial for gut health. It can be offered in hollowed sticks that allow gliders to gouge out the gum.

Diet 1

Diet plan for a 100 g adult sugar glider, moderate activity levels. Food intake should be adjusted based on body weight and level of activity. Pregnant or lactating females will need the feed quantity increased by about 30%.

Component	Daily Quantity Per Glider	% of Diet
Fruit & vegetable mix[a]	20 g (2 heaping Tbs) diced fruits & vegetables with 2 g (1 level tsp) Wombaroo High Protein Supplement (Wombaroo Food Products, Glen Osmond, South Australia) mixed in	65%
Nectar mix (lory/lorikeet nectar; follow package instructions for mixing)	5 mL (1 tsp)	20%
Small carnivore food	2 g (1 level tsp) of prepared Wombaroo Small Carnivore Food made up as a moist crumble[b]	10%
Insects	1 g gut-loaded crickets, moths, or other invertebrates; mealworms should be used infrequently	5%

[a]Fruit & vegetable mix:

- 50%: vegetables (frozen-thawed peas, corn, carrots, beans; cucumbers, bell peppers, sweet potatoes)
- 25%: leafy greens (bok choy, organic dandelion greens)
- 25%: fruits (apple, pear, berries, stone fruit, cantaloupe, papaya, figs)
- Dice/chop together so the glider cannot just pick out its favorite bits.
- Note: a few days' worth at a time can be made and stored in a sealed container in the refrigerator.

[b]One author (CJ-D) has also used Insectivore Diet (Reliable Protein Products, Palm Desert, CA) or soaked Omnivore Diet (Mazuri Omnivore, St. Louis, MO) for this portion.

Diet 2[13]

Quantity is for 1 adult sugar glider. Quantity can be adjusted per the individual glider.

- 1 piece of Eukanuba Pet Food Dog Kibble
- 10 g mixed fruit and vegetables (apple, banana, corn, currants, figs, grapes, green beans, honeydew melon, mango, papaya, pear, peas, cantaloupe, stone fruit without pit, watermelon); cut into 10 mm cubes
- 3 mL nectar mix[a]
- 2 g fly pupae
- 2 g cooked corn kernels
- 2 mealworms

[a]Nectar mix: 320 mL hot water (not boiling), 60 g Wombaroo Honeyeater & Lorikeet Mix, and 60 g Wombaroo High Protein Supplement; mix well and freeze in suitable volumes for daily thawing/feeding (i.e., 3-5 mL/average adult glider).

TABLE 7-12 Feed Estimates for Hand-Rearing Sugar Gliders.[a-d,9]

Age (days)	Feed (mL/day)	Wombaroo Possum Milk Replacer
20	0.7	Formula “<0.8”
30	1.1	Formula “<0.8”
40	1.8	Formula “<0.8”
50	3	Formula “<0.8”
51-53	4 (3 mL [“<0.8”] + 1 mL [“>0.8”])	Transition from Formula “<0.8” to Formula “>0.8”
54-56	4 (2 mL [“<0.8”] + 2 mL [“>0.8”])	Transition from Formula “<0.8” to Formula “>0.8”
57-59	4 (1 mL [“<0.8”] + 3 mL [“>0.8”])	Transition from Formula “<0.8” to Formula “>0.8”
60	3	Formula “>0.8”
70	4	Formula “>0.8”
80	6	Formula “>0.8”
90	7	Formula “>0.8”
100	8	Formula “>0.8”

[a]Using Table 7-9, estimate the age of the sugar glider using developmental characteristics and weight measurements. Feed the volume listed according to the estimated age of the sugar glider. In emaciated pouch young, the head and leg measurement is a more accurate method to determine age than the animal's weight.
[b]Note that marsupial milk changes in composition and energy as the pouch young develops. Therefore, there are two formulas of Wombaroo Possum Milk Replacer (Wombaroo Food Products, Glen Osmond, South Australia) that are used for hand-rearing sugar gliders. Formula “<0.8” is for younger pouch young; Formula “>0.8” is for gliders out of the pouch. When a pouch young can climb out of the pouch and remain out for short periods, it then uses Formula “>0.8” entirely.
[c]Wombaroo Possum Milk Replacer “<0.8” and “>0.8” is available in the United States from Perfect Pets Inc., Redford, MI; (734) 461-1362; wombaroo.com or worldwide at wombaroo.com.au.
[d]For hand-rearing procedures, refer to Barnes[2] and Johnson-Delaney.[25]

TABLE 7-13 Drug Administration Sites in Sugar Gliders.

Route	Site	Recommended Maximum Volume (mL)
Intramuscular	Anterior thigh; triceps[22]	0.1; 0.05
Intranasal	Nostrils, tip head back	0.01-0.02
Intraosseous	Proximal tibia, give slowly	≥1
Intraperitoneal	This route usually reserved for pouch young;[15] mixed with warmed fluids, given slowly; risk of inadvertent organ puncture	Fluid volume based on 25 mL/kg
Intravenous	Lateral tail vein (as in rats) common site for catheterization; lateral saphenous vein can be used for single IV injection; administer slowly	IV catheter: ≥1 IV injection: up to 0.5
Subcutaneous	Dorsum; absorption may be delayed if administered in patagium	Permits large volumes

TABLE 7-14 Blood Collection Sites in Sugar Gliders.[24,25,33]

Collection volume: the rule of thumb is that total blood volume in mL is approximately 7-10% body weight in grams. *Example*: a 100 g sugar glider has 7-10 mL blood volume. In a healthy animal, up to 10% of circulating blood volume (0.7-1 mL) can be safely collected. In an ill animal, 1/4 to 1/3 of that volume (i.e., 0.17-0.25 mL) may be a safer collection volume. Clinicians should use their best judgement.

Venipuncture site[a]	Comments
Cranial vena cava	Place glider in dorsal recumbency; perform under chemical immobilization to inhibit movement; practice first on a cadaver to prevent inadvertent insertion into the atrium; insertion point is at the sternum and first rib, angled to the opposite hind leg
Jugular vein	Place glider in dorsal recumbency; perform under chemical immobilization to inhibit movement; occlude vein at the level of the thoracic inlet
Lateral saphenous vein	Place glider in sternal or lateral recumbency; vein located at lateral aspect of the tibia, just proximal to the tarsal joint
Lateral tail vein	Place glider in sternal or lateral recumbency; apply tourniquet at the tail base to help occlude and distend the vein
Ventral tail vein	Place glider in dorsal recumbency or in sternal recumbency with tail lifted off the table; vein is located on the ventral midline of the tail; insert the needle perpendicular to the skin close to the tail base until bone is encountered; withdraw slowly, applying negative pressure

[a]Venipuncture in sugar gliders usually requires chemical immobilization. A blind stick (relying on anatomic landmarks) is typically required.

TABLE 7-15 Cardiopulmonary Resuscitation in Sugar Gliders.[14,24]

1. Intubate (1.0-2.0 I.D. noncuffed endotracheal tubes will fit most adult gliders).
2. Ventilate at 20-30 breaths/min.
3. If cardiac arrest, initiate external cardiac massage at around 100 compressions/min.
4. Epinephrine can be administered at 0.2 mg/kg IV, IO, or intracardiac.
5. Initiate IV or IO fluid therapy.
6. If bradycardic, administer atropine at 0.05 mg/kg IV or IO.

TABLE 7-16 Fluid Therapy in Sugar Gliders.[14,24]

- Baseline requirement 60-100 mL/kg/day.
- Dehydration: add estimated percentage dehydrated in mL.
- If administering SC, can deliver 2% of body weight q6-12h; SC fluids may pool in the patagium.
- Hyaluronidase (150 IU/mL) at 0.5-1.0 mL/L of fluids can be added to improve absorption.
- Fluids should be delivered at body temperature.
- IV or IO routes are preferred to correct dehydration.

REFERENCES

1. Baker RT, Beveridge I. Imidacloprid treatment of marsupials for fleas (*Pygiopsylla hoplia*). *J Zoo Wildl Med.* 2001;32:391–392.
2. Barnes M. Sugar gliders. In: Gage LJ, ed. *Hand-Rearing Wild and Domestic Mammals.* Ames, IA: Iowa State Press; 2002:55–62.
3. Bodley K. Appendix 4. Drug Formulary. In: Vogelnest L, Portas T, eds. *Current Therapy in Medicine of Australian Mammals.* Clayton South, Vic: CSIRO Publishing; 2019:702–727.
4. Booth RJ. General husbandry and medical care of sugar gliders. In: Bonagura JD, ed. *Kirk's Current Veterinary Therapy XIII: Small Animal Practice.* Philadelphia, PA: WB: Saunders; 2000:1157–1163.
5. Brust DM. *Sugar Gliders: A Complete Veterinary Care Guide.* Sugarland, TX: Veterinary Interactive Publications; 2009.
6. Brust DM. What every veterinarian needs to know about sugar gliders. *Exotic DVM.* 2009;11:32–41.
7. Brust DM, Mans C. Sugar gliders. In: Carpenter JW, ed. *Exotic Animal Formulary.* 5th ed. St. Louis, MO: Elsevier; 2018:432–442.
8. Dierenfeld ES, Whitehouse-Tedd KM. Evaluation of three popular diets fed to pet sugar gliders (*Petaurus breviceps*): intake, digestion and nutrient balance. *J Anim Physiol Anim Nutr.* 2018;102:e193–e208.
9. Donneley B. Hand-rearing orphan marsupials. *Exot DVM.* 2002;4:79–82.
10. Hedley J. *BSAVA Small Animal Formulary. Part B: Exotic Pets.* 10th ed. Gloucester, UK: British Small Animal Veterinary Association; 2020.
11. Hess L. Sugar gliders. In: Aiello SE, ed. *Merck Veterinary Manual.* Kenilworth, NJ: Merck & Co.; 2016:2035–2043.
12. Holz P. Immobilization of marsupials with tiletamine and zolazepam. *J Zoo Wildl Med.* 1992;23(4):426–428.
13. Jackson S. *Personal communication*; 2020.
14. Jepson L. Sugar gliders. In: Jepson L, ed. *Exotic Animal Medicine: A Quick Reference Guide.* 2nd ed. St. Louis, MO: Elsevier; 2016:231–257.
15. Johnson R, Hemsley S. Gliders and possums. In: Vogelnest L, Woods R, eds. *Medicine of Australian Mammals.* Clayton South, Vic: CSIRO Publishing; 2008:395–437.
16. Johnson SD. Orchiectomy of the mature sugar glider (*Petaurus breviceps*). *Exot Pet Pract.* 1997;2:71.
17. Johnson-Delaney C. Feeding sugar gliders. *Exot DVM.* 1998;1:4.
18. Johnson-Delaney C. Marsupial nutrition and physiology. *Exot DVM.* 2002;4:75–77.
19. Johnson-Delaney CA. Marsupials. In: Johnson-Delaney CA, ed. *Exot Companion Medicine Handbook.* West Palm Beach, FL: Zoological Education Network; 2000.
20. Johnson-Delaney CA. Therapeutics of companion exotic marsupials. *Vet Clin North Am Exot Anim Pract.* 2000;3:173–181.
21. Johnson-Delaney CA. Practical marsupial medicine. *Annu Conf Assoc Exot Mam Vet*; 2006:51–60.
22. Johnson-Delaney CA. Marsupials. In: Meredith A, Johnson-Delaney CA, eds. *BSAVA Manual of Exotic Pets.* 5th ed. Gloucester, UK: British Small Animal Veterinary Association; 2010:103–126.
23. Johnson-Delaney CA. Captive marsupial nutrition. *Vet Clin North Am Exot Anim Pract.* 2014;17:415–447.
24. Johnson-Delaney CA. *Personal observation*; 2020.
25. Johnson-Delaney CA, et al. Sugar gliders. In: Quesenberry KE, Orcutt CJ, Mans C et al., eds. *Ferrets, Rabbits, and Rodents: Clinical Medicine and Surgery.* 4th ed. St. Louis, MO: Elsevier; 2021:385–400.
26. Keller KA, Nevarez JG, Rodriguez D, et al. Diagnosis and treatment of anaplastic mammary carcinoma in a sugar glider (*Petaurus breviceps*). *J Exot Pet Med.* 2014;23:277–282.

27. Kubiak M. Sugar gliders. In: Kubiak M, ed. *Handbook of Exotic Pet Medicine*. Oxford, UK: Wiley Blackwell; 2021:125–139.
28. Lennox AM. Emergency and critical care procedures in sugar gliders (*Petaurus breviceps*), African hedgehogs (*Atelerix albiventris*), and prairie dogs (*Cynomys* spp.). *Vet Clin North Am Exot Anim Pract*. 2007;10:533–555.
29. Lindemann DM, Carpenter JW, DeBey BM, et al. Concurrent adrenocortical carcinoma and hepatocellular carcinoma with hemosiderosis in a sugar glider (*Petaurus breviceps*). *J Exot Pet Med*. 2016;25:144–149.
30. Morrisey JK, Carpenter JW. Formulary. In: Quesenberry KE, Orcutt CJ, Mans C, et al., eds. *Ferrets, Rabbits, and Rodents: Clinical Medicine and Surgery*. 4th ed. St. Louis, MO: Elsevier; 2021:620–630.
31. Ness RD, Booth RJ. Sugar gliders. In: Quesenberry KE, Carpenter JW, eds. *Ferrets, Rabbits, and Rodents: Clinical Medicine and Surgery*. 2nd ed. St. Louis, MO: Saunders/Elsevier; 2004:330–338.
32. Ness RD, Johnson-Delaney C. Sugar gliders. In: Quesenberry KE, Carpenter JW, eds. *Ferrets, Rabbits, and Rodents: Clinical Medicine and Surgery*. 3rd ed. St. Louis, MO: Saunders/Elsevier; 2012:393–410.
33. Portas T. Appendix 2. Blood collection sites. In: Vogelnest L, Portas T, eds. *Current Therapy in Medicine of Australian Mammals*. Clayton South, Vic: CSIRO Publishing; 2019:691–695.
34. Pye GW, Carpenter JW. A guide to medicine and surgery in sugar gliders. *Vet Med*. 1999;94:891–905.
35. Rivas AE, Pye GW, Papendick R. Dermal hemangiosarcoma in a sugar glider (*Petaurus breviceps*). *J Exot Pet Med*. 2014;23:384–388.
36. Shaw M, Jarman A. Nutrition. In: Vogelnest L, Portas T, eds. *Current Therapy in Medicine of Australian Mammals*. Clayton South, Vic: CSIRO Publishing; 2019:225–248.
37. Vogelnest L. Dermatology. In: Vogelnest L, Portas T, eds. *Current Therapy in Medicine of Australian Mammals*. Clayton South, Vic: CSIRO Publishing; 2019:181–206.
38. Wombaroo Food Products, Glen Osmond, SA. Available at: www.wombaroo.com.au. Accessed Oct 5, 2020.

Chapter 8 Hedgehogs

Grayson A. Doss | James W. Carpenter

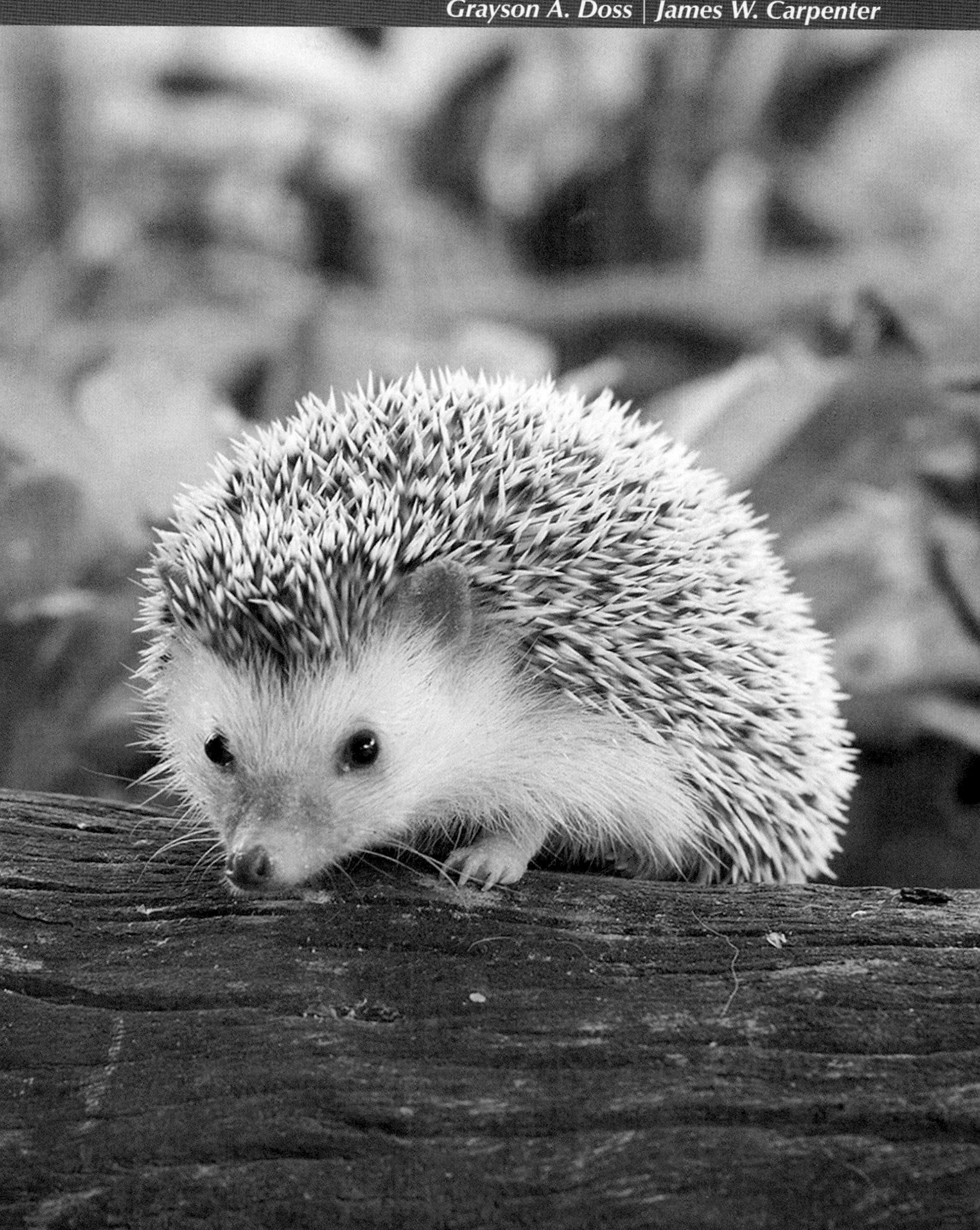

TABLE 8-1 Antimicrobial Agents Used in Hedgehogs.

Agent	Dosage	Comments
Amikacin	2.5-5 mg/kg IM q8-12h[45]	Maintain hydration due to the potential for nephrotoxicity with aminoglycosides
	5 mg/1 mL sterile saline × 15 min nebulization q12-24h[15]	Adjunct therapy for pneumonia[15]
	1 mg per 4 g powder[44]	Polymethylmethacrylate (PMMA) beads
Amoxicillin	15 mg/kg PO, SC, IM q12h[29,45,68]	Palatable to most hedgehogs[45]
Amoxicillin/clavulanic acid (Clavamox, Pfizer)	12.5 mg/kg PO q12h[25,34,52]	Palatable to most hedgehogs[45]
	12-25 mg/kg PO q8h[45]	
	25 mg/kg PO q8-12h[6]	
Ampicillin	10 mg/kg PO, IM q12-24h[29,34,68]	Not recommended as antimicrobial resistance common[32]
Cefovecin (Convenia, Zoetis)	8 mg/kg SC q5-6d[11a]	Third-generation cephalosporin; PK; no adverse effects were noted
Ceftiofur sodium	20 mg/kg SC q12-24h[34,45]	
	1 g per 20 mL powder[44]	Polymethylmethacrylate (PMMA) beads
Cephalexin	25 mg/kg PO q8h[45]	May make stools loose[32]
Chloramphenicol	30 mg/kg IM q12h[29,33]	Potentially toxic to humans; avoid human contact with medication[57]
	30-50 mg/kg PO, SC, IV q6-12h[25]	
	30-50 mg/kg PO q12h[34]	
	30-50 mg/kg SC, IM, IV, IO q12h[68]	
	50 mg/kg PO q12h[33,68]	
Chlorhexidine	Topical[68] q8-12h	Bacterial dermatitis; traumatic skin lesions; wound treatments; soaking (e.g., appendages); use properly diluted
Chlorhexidine shampoo	2%-3% shampoo[45]	Bacterial, mycotic dermatitis
Chlortetracycline	5-20 mg/kg PO q12h[51]	
Ciprofloxacin	5-20 mg/kg PO q12h[34,52]	
Clarithromycin	5.5 mg/kg PO q12h[52]	
Clindamycin	10 mg/kg PO q12h[45]	Anaerobes; dental disease; mix with food to improve palatability
Doxycycline	2.5-10 mg/kg PO, SC, IM q12h[52]	Concentration of active drug declines rapidly after 7 days in compounded formulations[56]
Enrofloxacin	2.5-10 mg/kg PO, SC, IM q12h[34,45,68]	Avoid administering more than a single dose IM; dilute if administering SC

TABLE 8-1 Antimicrobial Agents Used in Hedgehogs. (cont'd)

Agent	Dosage	Comments
Erythromycin	10 mg/kg PO, IM q12h[29,33]	Penicillin-resistant gram-positive cocci; *Mycoplasma*; *Pasteurella*; *Bordetella*; palatable to most hedgehogs
Gentamicin		Maintain hydration due to the potential for nephrotoxicity with aminoglycosides
	5 mg/1 mL sterile saline × 15 min nebulization q12-24h[15]	Adjunct therapy for pneumonia[15]
Gentamicin ophthalmic drops	Topical to cornea or conjunctiva[45] q4-8h[32,57]	Corneal abrasions or conjunctivitis; use as in dog or cat
Metronidazole	20 mg/kg PO q12h[25,29,34,45,52]	Anaerobes
Mupirocin (2%) (Muricin, Dechra)	Topical to cutaneous lesions q12-24h prn[45]	Bacterial dermatitis or traumatic skin lesions
Neomycin, polymyxin B, bacitracin ophthalmic ointment	Topical to cornea or conjunctiva[45] q6-12h[32,57]	Corneal abrasions or conjunctivitis; use as in dog or cat
Neomycin, thiabendazole, dexamethasone solution (Tresaderm, Merial)	Topical to cutaneous lesions or ear canal q12-24h prn[45]	Bacterial, mycotic dermatitis; otitis externa; antiinflammatory
Nystatin, neomycin, thiostrepton, triamcinolone cream (Panalog, Fort Dodge)	Topical to cutaneous lesions q12-24h prn[45]	Bacterial, mycotic dermatitis; antiinflammatory
Orbifloxacin (Orbax suspension, Intervet)	10-20 mg/kg PO q12-24h[27]	
Oxytetracycline	25-50 mg/kg PO q24h × 5-7 days[25,45] 50 mg/kg PO q12h[34]	*Bordetella*; may be administered in food
Oxytetracycline ophthalmic ointment (Terramycin, Pfizer)	Topical to cornea or conjunctiva[45] q6-12h[32,34,57]	Corneal abrasions or conjunctivitis; use as in dog or cat
Penicillin G procaine	40,000 IU/kg SC, IM q24h[29,52]	
Piperacillin	10 mg/kg SC q8-12h[25,34,45]	
Sulfadimethoxine	2-20 mg per day PO, SC, IM[29,33]	May have slight nephrotoxicity; treat for 2-5 days, off for 5 days, then repeat[29,33]
Trimethoprim/sulfa	30 mg/kg PO, SC, IM q12h[28,52,66]	Respiratory infections; trimethoprim/sulfamethoxazole is available in injectable form
Tylosin	10 mg/kg PO, SC q12h[33,52]	*Mycoplasma*; *Clostridium*; do not administer IM (causes muscle necrosis)[33]

TABLE 8-2 Antifungal Agents Used in Hedgehogs.

Agent	Dosage	Comments
Chlorhexidine	2%-3% shampoo q2-7d prn[25]	Dermatophytosis; not as effective as other topical therapies; not recommended as a sole agent for treating dermatophytosis[50]
Enilconazole	Topical q24h[52,71]	Dermatophytosis; dilute 1:50
	Dip in 1:50 solution q24h[52]	Dermatophytosis
Griseofulvin (microsize)	—	Dermatophytosis; rarely used as safer drug options available;[50,57] known teratogen in multiple species;[57] long-term therapy
	25-50 mg/kg PO q24h[25,30,34]	Dermatophytosis
	50 mg/kg PO q24h × 14-21 days[47]	
Itraconazole	5-10 mg/kg PO q12-24h[25,34,45]	Systemic mycoses; a safe, effective treatment option for dermatophytosis in small animals[50]
	10 mg/kg PO q12h[8]	European hedgehogs/dermatophytosis; administered in food; only 66% animals culture negative after 28 days, 85% after 42 days; safety not assessed
	10 mg/kg PO q24h × 20-30 days[20]	Cutaneous paecilomycosis
Ketoconazole	10 mg/kg PO q24h × 6-8 wk[47,68]	Dermatophytosis; *Candida*[34]
Lime sulfur	Topical[28]	Dermatophytosis
Nystatin	30,000 IU/kg PO q8-24h[45]	Yeast infections
Terbinafine	—	Considered a safe, effective treatment option for dermatophytosis in small animals[50]
	100 mg/kg PO q12h[8]	European hedgehogs/dermatophytosis; administered in food; 93% animals culture negative after 14 days, 99% after 28 days; safety not assessed

TABLE 8-3 Antiparasitic Agents Used in Hedgehogs.

Agent	Dosage	Comments
Amitraz	0.3% topical q7-14d × 2-3 treatments[43,45]	Mites (*Caparinia, Chorioptes*, etc.); may dilute; due to documented adverse effects in other species, use with caution[57]
Afoxolaner (A) + milbemycin oxime (MO) (NexGard Spectra, Merial)	(A) 2.5 mg/kg + (MO) 40 mg/kg PO once[53]	Demodicosis; safety not assessed
Fenbendazole	10-30 mg/kg PO q24h × 5 days[33,52]	Nematodes (i.e., *Crenosoma, Capillaria*)
	25 mg/kg PO q14d × 3 treatments[34]	Nematodes

TABLE 8-3 Antiparasitic Agents Used in Hedgehogs. (cont'd)

Agent	Dosage	Comments
Fipronil spray (Frontline, Merial)	Topical, repeat in 10-14 days for 1-3 treatments[34,42,52]	Mites; apply 1 light spray over spiny dorsum ('mantle')
Fluralaner (Bravecto, Merck)	15 mg/kg PO once[65]	*Caparinia;* safety not assessed
Imidacloprid	½ puppy/kitten dose topical q30d[25]	Fleas; apply to spined areas behind head
Imidacloprid 10% + moxidectin 1% (Advantage Multi for cats, Advocate for cats, Elanco)	0.1 mL/kg topical once[36]	*Caparinia*
Ivermectin	0.2-0.4 mg/kg PO, SC q7-14d × 3-5 treatments[17,25,52]	Ectoparasites, nematodes; resistant mite infestations not uncommon
	≤1 mg/kg[32] PO, SC	For resistant *Chorioptes*
Levamisole (1%)	10 mg/kg SC, repeat q48h; repeat prn q14d[6,34]	Nematodes, including lungworms; therapeutic margin of safety may be small[25]
	10-20 mg/kg SC, repeat q48h × 2-3 doses; repeat prn q14d[29]	Use 10 mg/kg if <300 g body weight, 20 mg/kg if >300 g body weight[29]
Lufenuron	½ puppy/kitten dose PO q30d[25]	Fleas
Mebendazole	15 mg/kg PO, repeat q14d[28]	Nematodes; do not use in animals with hepatic disease
	25 mg/animal <500 g q12h; 50 mg/animal >500 g q12h PO × 5 days, repeat q14-21d[29]	*Capillaria, Crenosoma, Brachylaernus, Hymenolepsis, Physaloptera*
Metronidazole	25 mg/kg PO q12h × 5 days[33,34,68]	Intestinal protozoa
Moxidectin (Cydectin, Bayer)	0.3 mg/kg SC q10d[55]	Notoedric mange
Permethrin (1%)	Topical[70]	Mites; apply once via fine mist; change bedding and clean cage
Praziquantel	7 mg/kg PO, SC, repeat q14d[28,68]	Cestodes; trematodes[29]
Sarolaner (Simparica, Zoetis)	2 mg/kg PO once[3]	*Caparinia*; safety not assessed
Selamectin (Revolution, Pfizer)	10-20 mg/kg topically[52]	Ectoparasites
	20-30 mg/kg topically q21-28d[17,17a]	External mites
Sulfadimethoxine	2-20 mg per day PO, SC, IM[29,33]	Coccidia; may have slight nephrotoxicity; treat for 2-5 days, off for 5 days, then repeat[29,33]
	10 mg/kg PO q24h × 5-7 days[45]	Coccidia
Toltrazuril	10 mg/kg PO q24h × 2 treatments then repeated q7d × 3 wk[30]	Coccidia (*Eimeria, Isospora*)

TABLE 8-4 Chemical Restraint/Anesthetic Agents Used in Hedgehogs.

Agent	Dosage	Comments
Acepromazine	0.1-1 mg/kg PO, SC, IM[25]	Sedative; hypotension may occur when used alone; atropine pretreatment may alleviate this effect
Alfaxalone	—	See midazolam for combination
Atipamezole (Antisedan, Zoetis)	0.3-0.5 mg/kg IM[52]	Reversal of medetomidine and dexmedetomidine
	1 mg/kg IM[4]	European hedgehogs; reversal of medetomidine
Atropine	0.01-0.05 mg/kg SC, IM[25,30,34]	Preanesthetic to decrease hypersalivation; potential adverse effects (e.g., increased salivary viscosity, decreased gastrointestinal motility) may outweigh benefits
Buprenorphine	—	See midazolam for combination
Butorphanol	—	See midazolam for combination
Dexmedetomidine (Dexdomitor, Zoetis)	0.02 mg/kg IM[40]	Avoid use in ill or debilitated animals as no reports of safety or efficacy available; reversible with atipamezole
Diazepam	—	Diazepam combination follows
Diazepam (D)/ketamine (K)	(D) 0.5-2 mg/kg + (K) 5-20 mg/kg IM[7]	Anesthesia; do not use in neck area where there is brown fat;[29] midazolam preferred for IM use
Fentanyl	—	See medetomidine for combination
Flumazenil	0.05 mg/kg SC, IM[22]	Reversal of midazolam and diazepam
Isoflurane	3%-5% induction[23,28a,68]	Anesthetic of choice; induction generally occurs in a chamber
	2%-3% maintenance[23,28a]	By mask, endotracheal tube, or small rabbit supraglottic airway device;[5,28a] lower maintenance levels may be sufficient for debilitated or premedicated animals
Ketamine	—	See midazolam, diazepam, and medetomidine for combinations; combinations follow
Ketamine (K)/ medetomidine (M)	(K) 5 mg/kg + (M) 0.1 mg/ kg IM[71]	Anesthesia; (M) reverse with atipamezole (0.3-0.5 mg/kg IM); see medetomidine
Ketamine (K)/ midazolam (Mi)	(K) 30 mg/kg + (Mi) 1 mg/ kg IM[22]	Partial reversal with flumazenil (0.05 mg/kg SC); can display hyperactivity during recovery; significant postsedation decrease in food intake; use caution in debilitated animals
Medetomidine	—	Medetomidine combination follows; not commercially available but can be obtained through select compounding pharmacies
	0.05-0.1 mg/kg IM[34,71]	Light sedation; reverse with atipamezole (0.3-0.5 mg/kg IM)
	0.2 mg/kg SC[6]	Heavy sedation; reverse with atipamezole (0.3-0.5 mg/kg IM)

TABLE 8-4 Chemical Restraint/Anesthetic Agents Used in Hedgehogs. (cont'd)

Agent	Dosage	Comments
Medetomidine (M)/ ketamine (K)/fentanyl (F)	(M) 0.2 mg/kg + (K) 2 mg/ kg + (F) 0.1 mg/kg SC[4]	European hedgehogs; anesthesia; good muscle relaxation; (M) reversed with atipamezole (1 mg/kg IM) and (F) reversed with naloxone (0.16 mg/kg IM); see medetomidine
Midazolam	—	Midazolam combinations follow; it is preferred over diazepam for SC, IM use
	0.5-1.0 mg/kg IM[40]	Sedation
Midazolam (Mi)/ alfaxalone (A)	(Mi) 1 mg/kg + (A) 3 mg/ kg SC[22]	Heavy sedation; administered deep SC (~1 cm) into the spiny dorsum ('mantle'); partial reversal with flumazenil (0.05 mg/kg SC)
	(Mi) 1 mg/kg + (A) 5 mg/ kg SC[15]	Heavy sedation to light anesthesia; administered deep SC (~1 cm) into the spiny dorsum ('mantle'); partial reversal with flumazenil (0.05 mg/kg SC)
Midazolam (Mi)/ buprenorphine (Bup)	(Mi) 0.25-0.5 mg/kg + (Bup) 0.03 mg/kg IM[39]	Preanesthetic for painful or stressful procedures
	(Mi) 0.5-1 mg/kg + (Bup) 0.03-0.05 mg/kg SC[15]	Preanesthetic for painful procedures
Midazolam (Mi)/ butorphanol (But)	(Mi) 0.5 mg/kg + (But) 0.5 mg/kg SC, IM[17]	Mild sedation; see butorphanol comments in Table 8-6
Midazolam (Mi)/ butorphanol (But)/ ketamine (K)	(Mi) 0.5-1 mg/kg + (But) 0.5 mg/kg + (K) 3-5 mg/kg SC, IM[17]	Mild to moderate sedation
Naloxone	0.04 mg/kg SC, IM[15]	Opioid reversal
	0.16 mg/kg SC, IM[4]	European hedgehogs; reversal of fentanyl
Propofol	6-8 mg/kg IV[24]	Anesthetic induction
Sevoflurane	To effect[25,34]	Anesthesia; may provide more rapid induction and plane changes than isoflurane
Tiletamine/zolazepam (Telazol, Zoetis)	1-5 mg/kg IM[25,34]	Sedation; anesthesia; recovery may be prolonged and/or rough
	10 mg/kg SC[21]	Heavy sedation to light anesthesia; deeper immobilization for 30 mg/kg dosage but significantly longer recovery times (>1h for 10 mg/kg, >3h for 30 mg/kg); flumazenil reversal did not have a significant effect on recovery time; no significant changes in post-sedation food intake
	30 mg/kg SC[21]	
Xylazine	0.5-1 mg/kg IM[34]	Anesthesia; may be given with ketamine; rarely indicated due to availability of safer, more efficacious injectable agents
Yohimbine	0.5-1 mg/kg IM[34]	Reversal of xylazine

TABLE 8-5 Chemical Immobilization Protocols for Hedgehogs.[a,b,5,15,17,21–23,28a]

- Isoflurane: light to surgical anesthesia; chamber induction (3-5%) followed by maintenance (2-3%) via face mask, endotracheal tube, or supraglottic airway device
- Alfaxalone-midazolam SC: heavy sedation to light anesthesia
- Ketamine-midazolam SC: heavy sedation to light anesthesia
- Tiletamine-zolazepam (Telazol) SC: heavy sedation to light anesthesia
- Midazolam-butorphanol-ketamine SC: mild to moderate sedation
- Midazolam-butorphanol SC: mild sedation

[a]Combinations containing midazolam can be partially reversed with flumazenil (0.05 mg/kg, SC).
[b]Dosages listed in Table 8-4.

TABLE 8-6 Analgesic/Antiinflammatory Agents Used in Hedgehogs.

Agent	Dosage	Comments
Buprenorphine hydrochloride	0.01 mg/kg SC q36h[18] 0.03-0.05 mg/kg SC q48h[18]	PD; administered deep SC (~1 cm) into the spiny dorsum ('mantle'); thermal analgesia model: severely painful conditions may warrant more frequent dosing; 0.05 mg/kg had more pronounced analgesic effect compared to 0.01 and 0.03 mg/kg dosages; administration of 0.05 mg/kg q24h × 3 doses had no effect on food intake
	0.01-0.05 mg/kg SC, IM q6-8h[34]	Analgesia
Butorphanol	0.05-0.4 mg/kg PO, SC, IM q6-12h prn[25]	Analgesia; when compared with other opiate analgesics, this drug is less useful for treating moderate to severe pain in small animals and has to be dosed more frequently
	0.2-0.5 mg/kg SC, IM q6-8h[34]	Analgesia
Carprofen	1 mg/kg PO, SC q12-24h[25]	Nonsteroidal; antiinflammatory
Dexamethasone	0.1-1.5 mg/kg IM[29]	Glucocorticoid; inflammation
Hydromorphone	0.1 mg/kg SC[63]	Preoperative analgesia
Meloxicam	0.2 mg/kg PO, SC q24h[1a,25,34,72]	Nonsteroidal; antiinflammatory; analgesic
	0.2 mg/kg SC q12h[1]	Recommendations are based on limited sample size and PK data
Methylprednisolone	1-2 mg/kg SC[45]	Glucocorticoid; antiinflammatory
Naloxone	0.04 mg/kg SC, IM[15]	Opioid reversal
	0.16 mg/kg SC, IM[4]	European hedgehogs; reversal of fentanyl
Prednisolone	0.5-2 mg/kg PO q12-24h[52]	Glucocorticoid; antiinflammatory
Tramadol	2-4 mg/kg PO q12h[27]	Synthetic μ-receptor opiatelike agonist
Triamcinolone	0.2 mg/kg SC, IM[25]	Glucocorticoid; antiinflammatory; no frequency given

TABLE 8-7 Miscellaneous Agents Used in Hedgehogs.

Agent	Dosage	Comments
Acyclovir	40-100 mg/kg PO q24h[30]	Herpes simplex infection
Aluminum hydroxide	100 mg/kg PO with each syringe feeding[58]	Renal failure; hyperphosphatemia
Atropine	0.05-0.2 mg/kg SC, IM[25]	Bradycardia
Bupivicaine	1.1 mg/kg diluted with saline 1:12[63]	Surgical site infiltration
Calcium gluconate (10%)	50 mg/kg IM[45]	Hypocalcemia, can cause tissue irritation
Calcium gluconate (23%)	100-150 mg/kg IV[39]	
L-carnitine	50 mg/kg PO q12h[12]	Cardiomyopathy
Carnivore Care (Oxbow)	2-3 mL PO[31]	Gavage feeding; slight sedation may facilitate
	Mix 1:1 with Critical Care Fine Grind (Oxbow)[1a]	Esophagostomy tube feedings
Cimetidine	10 mg/kg PO q8h[45]	Treatment of gastric ulcers
Doxapram	2-10 mg/kg IV, IP[25]	Respiratory stimulant; use with caution as can increase myocardial oxygen demand and decrease cerebral blood flow[57]
Emeraid Carnivore (Lafeber)	3 mL/100 g BW q6h	Mix 1:1 with Emeraid Omnivore per label
Enalapril	0.5-1 mg/kg PO q24h[12,45]	Vasodilator; heart failure
Epinephrine	0.003 mg/kg IV[39]	Cardiac arrest
Erythropoietin (Epogen, Amgen)	100 U/kg SC q48-72h[45]	Chronic anemia
Famotidine	1 mg/kg SC q24h[58]	Prevention or treatment of gastric ulcers
Furosemide	2.5-5 mg/kg PO, SC, IM q8h[52,71]	Edema; diuretic
	3-5 mg/kg SC, IM q6-8h[12,26]	Congestive heart failure
Glycopyrrolate	0.01-0.02 mg/kg SC[25]	Bradycardia
Hetastarch	5 mL/kg IV[39]	Give over 5-10 min; use cautiously in patients with renal dysfunction, congestive heart failure, or pulmonary edema[57]
Hyaluronidase	100-150 U/L[45]	Add to SC fluids; may facilitate fluid absorption
Iron dextran	25 mg/kg IM[71]	Anemia
Lactated Ringer's solution (LRS)	10-15 mL/kg IV[39]	Fluid replacement; dehydration; shock
	25 mL/kg SC q12h[72]	
	50-100 mL/kg q24h[31]	
Lactobacilli	½ tsp/kg q24h[29]	May aid in restoring gastrointestinal flora
Lactulose	0.3 mL/kg PO q8-12h[45]	Hepatic disease; constipation[32]
	150-750 mg/kg PO q8-12h[30]	Heaptic disease
Lysine	250-500 mg/kg PO q24h[30]	Herpes simplex infection

Continued

TABLE 8-7 Miscellaneous Agents Used in Hedgehogs. (cont'd)

Agent	Dosage	Comments
Metoclopramide	0.2-0.5 mg/kg PO, SC[45]	Regurgitation; antiemetic; GI motility enhancer[32]
	0.2-1.0 mg/kg SC q8h[30]	Antiemetic
Milk thistle (*Silybum marianum*)	4-15 mg/kg PO q8-12h[30]	Hepatoprotectant
Pimobendan	0.3 mg/kg PO q12h[12,26]	Congestive heart failure
Sucralfate	10 mg/kg PO q8-12h[52]	Gastrointestinal ulcers
Theophylline	10 mg/kg PO, IM q12h[45]	Bronchodilator
Thiamine	300 mg daily	Thiamine deficiency
Trilostane	2 mg/kg PO q24h[30]	Hyperadrenocorticism
Vitamin A	400 U/kg IM q24h × 10 days[29]	Skin disorders; excessive spine loss
Vitamin B complex	1 mL/kg SC, IM once[33,52]	CNS signs; paralysis of unknown origin; anorexia; use small animal formulation
	1-2 mg/kg thiamine content prn[30]	Thiamine deficiency
Vitamin C	50-200 mg/kg PO, SC q24h[29]	Deficiency; infections; gingivitis
	1 g ascorbic acid/L drinking water[29]	Change daily;[33] not recommended; alternative routes of supplementation preferred (oral pills or powder)[32]

TABLE 8-8 Hematologic and Serum Biochemical Values of Hedgehogs.

Measurement	Reference Range[69]	Reference Range[a,54]
Hematology		
PCV (%)	33 (21-47)	42.0 ± 0.9 (33.5-47.0)
RBC (10^6/μL)	4.8 (2.5-7.0)	5.0 ± 0.1 (4.3-6.0)
Hgb (g/dL)	10.9 (5.8-15.5)	13.1 ± 0.3 (10.7-14.9)
MCV (fL)	—	87.8 ± 1.8 (76.3-99.8)
MCH (pg)	—	27.1 ± 0.7 (22.5-31.4)
MCHC (g/dL)	—	30.9 ± 0.5 (27.7-35.2)
Platelets (10^3/μL)	226 (33-560)	—
WBC (10^3/μL)	9.7 (3.0-22.3)	15.0 ± 0.7 (11.5-21.7)
Neutrophils (10^3/μL)	4.4 (0.7-11.7)	9.5 ± 0.5 (6.1-14.6)
Lymphocytes (10^3/μL)	3.6 (0.9-8.9)	5.2 ± 0.4 (3.3-8.9)
Monocytes (10^3/μL)	0.4 (0-1.4)	0.2 ± 0.1 (0-0.8)
Eosinophils (10^3/μL)	1.0 (0-3.2)	0.2 ± 0 (0-0.3)
Basophils (10^3/μL)	0.3 (0-0.9)	0.1 ± 0 (0-0.2)

TABLE 8-8 Hematologic and Serum Biochemical Values of Hedgehogs. (cont'd)

Measurement	Reference Range	Reference Range
Chemistries		
ALP (U/L)	43 (6-94)	22.4 ± 1.0 (18.2-25.5)
ALT (U/L)	58 (21-160)	22.8 ± 1.4 (15.2-28.8)
Amylase (U/L)	477 (175-968)	—
AST (U/L)	37 (6-119)	33.5 ± 3.5 (19.0-65.6)
Bilirubin, total (mg/dL)	0.2 (0-0.8)	—
BUN (mg/dL)	29 (14-59)	47.1 ± 2.3 (34.3-57.3)
Calcium (mg/dL)	7.7 (5.3-9.7)	9.7 ± 0.3 (8.6-11.4)
Chloride (mmol/L)	113 (97-125)	—
Cholesterol (mg/dL)	147 (73-255)	132.5 ± 5.3 (100-150)
Creatine kinase (U/L)	800 (194-2093)	—
Creatinine (mg/dL)	0.4 (0.1-0.8)	0.7 ± 0.1 (0.5-1.0)
GGT (U/L)	4 (0-13)	—
Glucose (mg/dL)	81 (11-137)	86.1 ± 4.7 (60-125)
LDH (U/L)	353 (35-1313)	—
Phosphorus (mg/dL)	5.6 (3.1-9.3)	—
Potassium (mmol/L)	5.1 (3.6-7.2)	—
Protein, total (g/dL)	5.9 (4.2-7.5)	6.0 ± 0.2 (4.6-6.9)
Albumin (g/dL)	2.7	3.4 ± 0.2 (2.7-3.9)
Globulin (g/dL)	2.8 (1.3-4.2)	2.6 ± 0.2 (1.9-3.6)
Sodium (mmol/L)	143 (129-160)	—
Triglycerides (mg/dL)	36 (0-127)	37.8 ± 2.3 (30.8-46.2)

[a]Data collected from wild-caught animals.

TABLE 8-9 Endocrine Values of Hedgehogs.[69]

Measurement	Value
Total thyroxine (nmol/L)	24.5

TABLE 8-10 Urinalysis Values of Hedgehogs.[69]

Measurement	Reference Range
Specific gravity	1.036 (1.011-1.070)
pH	6.1 (5.0-7.5)

TABLE 8-11 Biological and Physiological Values of Hedgehogs.[1a,10,17,19,25,28,37,49,61,67,68,75]

Parameter	Biological and Physiological Values
Weight	Male, 400-600 g
	Female, 300-400 g
Life span	Avg 4-6 years, may live 8 years
Temperature, rectal	95.7-98.6°F (35.4-37°C)
Preferred environmental temperature	75-85°F (24-29°C)
	Temperatures < 60°F (16°C) may induce torpor state
Adult dental formula	2 (I3/2: C1/1: P3/2: M3/3) = 36; variations have been reported
Gastrointestinal system	Simple stomach; no cecum; transit time 12-16 hours
Heart rate	180-280 beats/min
Respiratory rate	25-50 breaths/min
Age at sexual maturity	61-68 days, both sexes
Reproductive life span	Male, throughout life
	Female, 2-3 years
Gestation	34-37 days
Milk composition	Protein, 16 g/100 g; carbohydrate, trace; fat, 25.5 g/100 g
Litter size	Avg 3-4 (range 1-7)
Birth weight	8-13 g
Eyes open	14-18 days
Deciduous teeth eruption	Begins on day 18; all deciduous teeth erupt by 9 weeks
Permanent teeth eruption	Begins at 7-9 weeks
Age at weaning	4-6 weeks (start eating solids at 3 weeks)
Endotracheal tube size	14 g over-the-needle IV catheter to 2.0 mm I.D.
Esophagostomy tube size	8 Fr

TABLE 8-12 Suggested Diets for Hedgehogs.[14,17,32,33,61,66]

The exact nutritional requirements of hedgehogs are unknown. Diets for captive animals have been developed taking into consideration their omnivorous nature, simple gastrointestinal tract, ability to digest chitin, poor digestibility of cellulose, propensity toward obesity, and lack of reports of specific nutritional problems (with the exception of lactose intolerance).

Hedgehogs in captivity will thrive on a base diet composed of approximately 30%-50% protein (dry matter basis) and 10%-20% fat. Because scientific studies regarding hedgehog nutritional needs are lacking, commercial diets appear to be the most balanced diet that a pet owner can offer. If a commercial hedgehog food is not used, a premium commercial feline (adults may use "lite" adult cat foods), ferret, or insectivore diet may be used. Dry foods may be advantageous to help with dental health as periodontal disease is fairly common in hedgehogs. It is inappropriate to use these commercial diets as a sole nutrition source. Supplement with small portions of cooked egg, pinky mice, vegetable and meat jarred human baby foods, gut-loaded crickets and mealworms,[a] chopped vegetables, and fruits. Dairy products, such as cottage cheese and milk, should be avoided, however, because of reports of lactose intolerance.

TABLE 8-12 Suggested Diets for Hedgehogs. (cont'd)

In general, pets should not be fed ad libitum as obesity is very common. Approximately 1-2 Tbs of food daily is a reasonable starting point for adults, with growing animals and reproductively active females being fed the usual diet ad libitum, and calcium-rich foods should be supplemented. Young or pregnant/lactating hedgehogs can also use kitten or ferret formulations. Hedgehogs are generally nocturnal eaters. Fresh water should be provided ad libitum in a shallow dish; animals can also learn to drink from sipper bottles.

In addition to the main diet, 1-2 tsp of varied moist foods (e.g., canned cat or dog food, cooked meat or egg, low-fat cottage cheese) and approximately ½ tsp of fruit (e.g., banana, grape, apple, pear, berries) or vegetables (e.g., beans, cooked carrots, squash, peas, tomatoes, leafy greens) should also be provided daily.[b] One key to balanced nutrition is to provide variety. Acceptable treats include mealworms, earthworms, waxworms, crickets, and cat treats; these may be hidden in the bedding to promote foraging behavior as environmental enrichment.

[a]Mealworms are high calorie, low calcium, and should be limited to 6-10 smaller mealworms, 2-3 times a week; 1-2 crickets (more if hedgehog is pregnant or lactating) can be fed a commercial, high-calcium, gut-loading cricket diet for a minimum of 12-24 hours after purchase before being fed to the hedgehog; other types of commercially available insects can also be fed. Insects can be dusted with a calcium supplement before feeding to hedgehogs.

[b]An alternative fruit/vegetable mix: chop together ½ tsp diced leafy dark greens (spinach, kale, leaf lettuce), ¼ tsp diced carrot, ¼ tsp diced apple, ¼ tsp diced banana, ¼ tsp diced grape or raisin, ¼ tsp vitamin/mineral powder (Vionate or crushed feline vitamin tab).

TABLE 8-13 Hand-Rearing Orphaned Hedgehogs.[17,67,68]

1. Leave neonates with the mother, if possible, for the first 24-72 hours for colostrum ingestion.
2. In cases of lactation failure or abandonment by the female, fostering the pups to another dam with similarly aged pups is generally successful.
3. Feed a canine milk replacer with added lactase (Lactaid, McNeil Nutritionals) using a 1-cc syringe with a catheter tip or an eye dropper.
4. Neonates should be fed as much as they will consume every 2-4 hours for about 3 weeks, then the time between feedings can be gradually lengthened; the newborns should gain 2-3 g/day during the first few weeks, about 4-5 g/day during the third and fourth weeks, and 7-9 g/day until they are 60 days old; at 4-6 weeks, parent- or hand-raised young should be weaned by offering canned dog or cat food, minced beef, or freshly molted mealworms.
5. The ambient temperature should be maintained at 90-95°F (32-35°C) for the first few weeks.
6. Manual stimulation is required for defecation and should be performed after each meal by massaging the ventrum and perineal area with a cloth or swab moistened in warm water.
7. Hand-rearing hedgehogs is often associated with high mortality.

TABLE 8-14 Common Injection and Venipuncture Sites in Hedgehogs.[17,17a,28,31,33,41,46]

Injection Sites	Comments
Subcutaneous	5-10 mL/site; common route for fluid therapy; flank at junction of furred skin and spined mantle or into mantle; large volumes possible (up to 100 mL/kg, split between multiple sites), although absorption may be prolonged with mantle administration
Intramuscular	0.5 mL/site; epaxials, anterior thigh, triceps; may require sedation; orbicularis up to 1 mL/site
Intravenous	Saphenous, jugular

Continued

TABLE 8-14 Common Injection and Venipuncture Sites in Hedgehogs. (cont'd)

Injection Sites	Comments
Intraperitoneal	Rarely used; 5-10 mL; requires immobilization for access; caudal right abdominal quadrant; can be used for fluid administration; risk of inadvertent organ puncture
Intraosseous	0.5-1 mL slow bolus; anterograde tibial (use tibial crest as landmark) or femoral (use trochanteric fossa as landmark) placement; requires chemical immobilization to place
Venipuncture Sites[a]	**Comments**
Saphenous	0.25-1 mL; the lateral saphenous crosses below the stifle; common site for catheterization with 24G-26G catheter
Jugular	Midcervical approach; 0.5-1 mL; more difficult in obese animals; proximal approach:[16] up to 1% of body weight; with needle positioned perpendicular to skin, insert the needle approximately 1 cm deep at notch formed by clavicle, manubrium, and neck
Cephalic	0.25-1 mL; on the dorsal forearm; common site for catheterization with 24G-26G catheter
Cranial vena cava	Up to 1% of body weight; risk of cardiac puncture; insert needle at notch formed between clavicle and manubrium

[a]Venipuncture in hedgehogs requires chemical immobilization. A blind stick (relying on anatomic landmarks) is typically required.

TABLE 8-15 Common Supportive Care Measures for Ill Hedgehogs.

- Thermal support: aim for ambient incubator temperatures of 80-85°F (27-30°C); forced-air heating devices and recirculating water blankets are useful for aggressive thermal support.
- Fluid therapy: SC fluids for mild to moderately dehydrated animals; place an indwelling IO (femoral, tibial) or IV (saphenous, jugular) catheter to provide fluid therapy for severely dehydrated or shocky animals.
- Nutritional support: presenting hedgehog kibble, wet cat/dog food, critical care formulas for carnivores, meat-flavored human baby food, and/or live insects may stimulate an anorectic hedgehog to eat; syringe feeding may be necessary—holding a hedgehog upright on its rump and using a 1-mL syringe with a plastic teat cannula to approach the mouth as the animal unrolls can increase success.
- Administering oral medications: PO administration of medications can be facilitated by using a small syringe with a plastic teat cannula and holding the hedgehog in an upright position; small amounts of medication can be administered by injecting it into waxworms (*Galleria mellonella*) or mixing it with a small amount of a preferred wet food item.
- Hospitalization: to avoid inducing torpor, provide a heat source in the enclosure and ensure the ambient temperature does not fall below 68°F (20°C); provide hiding areas in both the cooler and warmer areas of the enclosure and a water dish and water bottle; unless contraindicated, provide a close-walled running wheel; clean soiled areas daily.

TABLE 8-16 Preventive Medicine in Hedgehogs.[33]

- Have owners weigh hedgehogs weekly to prevent obesity and identify weight loss secondary to illness.
- Dental prophylaxis—routine brushing, scaling.
- Nails need periodic trimming.
- Annual to semiannual physical examination, including a complete oral exam.
- No routine vaccines recommended.
- Consider elective ovariohysterectomy due to high incidence of uterine pathology.
- Prevent chilling; provide heated environment with dry bedding.
- Microchip for personal identification.

TABLE 8-17 Common Differential Diagnoses Based on Physical Examination Findings.[2,11,13,17,25,30,32,35,38,48,59,60,74]

- Ataxia: severe weakness, brain neoplasia, intervertebral disk disease, wobbly hedgehog syndrome, herpes simplex infection.
- Cutaneous/subcutaneous masses: mammary neoplasia, lymphadenomegaly, cutaneous hemangiosarcoma, squamous cell carcinoma, papilloma, mast cell tumor, thyroid tumor.
- Dermatitis/spine loss: mange (*Caparinia*, *Chorioptes*, *Notoedres*), fungal dermatophytosis, bacterial pyoderma.
- Dyspnea: congestive heart failure, bacterial pneumonia, pulmonary metastases.
- Gastroenteritis: bacterial (*Salmonella*), lymphosarcoma, parasitic.
- Hematuria/hemorrhagic vulvar discharge: endometrial polyp, endometrial hyperplasia, endometrial neoplasia, bacterial cystitis.
- Limb or digit discoloration: fiber constriction injury, dermatitis.
- Oral cavity masses: squamous cell carcinoma, gingival hyperplasia, odontogenic fibroma.

TABLE 8-18 Confirmed Zoonotic Diseases Carried by Hedgehogs.[17,17a,62,64,73]

- Bacterial: *Salmonella* spp., *Yersinia pseudotuberculosis, Mycobacterium marinum*
- Mycotic: *Trichophyton erinacei, Trichophyton mentagrophytes, Microsporum* spp.

TABLE 8-19 Common Vocalizations in Hedgehogs.[25,61]

Snorting/huffing; hissing/grunting	Aggressive or warning sounds produced by sharp, vibrating exhalations through the nostrils; generally made when the animal is disturbed, when it encounters another animal, or when it is in the process of rolling up
Screaming	Severe distress call given when the animal is in distress or pain; can occur during scruffing or other forms of manual restraint[15]
Twittering/whistling	High-pitched sounds of neonates; whistling stimulates contact by the dam
Clucking	High-pitched contact call of the dam to neonates; also made by courting males
Snuffling	Made as hedgehogs search for food
Inaudible sounds	Hedgehogs can produce and hear sounds in the ultrasonic range, above the range of human hearing

TABLE 8-20 Cardiac Measurements in Hedgehogs.[a,9]

Radiographic Measurements[b]	Mean ± SD (Range)
AB/CD	1.38 ± 0.11 (1.24-1.59)
AB/H	0.88 ± 0.07 (0.74-1.01)
AB/R5-7	1.89 ± 0.29 (1.55-2.73)
CD/H	0.63 ± 0.04 (0.58-0.7)
VHS	8.16 ± 0.48 (7.25-8.75)
L/W	1.4 ± 0.11 (1.16-1.55)
L/C	1.64 ± 0.25 (1.38-2.13)
W/T	0.6 ± 0.03 (0.55-0.66)
W/C	1.17 ± 0.17 (1-1.45)

Continued

TABLE 8-20 Cardiac Measurements in Hedgehogs. (cont'd)

Echocardiographic Measurements[c]	Mean ± SD (Range)
IVSd (cm)	0.15 ± 0.01 (0.13-0.17)
IVSs (cm)	0.22 ± 0.02 (0.19-0.24)
LVIDd (cm)	0.74 ± 0.05 (0.67-0.84)
LVIDs (cm)	0.58 ± 0.03 (0.54-0.65)
LVFWd (cm)	0.16 ± 0.01 (0.14-0.18)
LVFWs (cm)	0.23 ± 0.02 (0.19-0.27)
FS (%)	21.45 ± 2.5 (17.4-26.8)
EPSS (cm)	0.11 ± 0.02 (0.09-0.14)
AO (cm)	0.36 ± 0.02 (0.31-0.4)
LA (cm)	0.56 ± 0.04 (0.51-0.62)
LA/AO ratio	1.55 ± 0.16 (1.37-1.92)
LVOT Vmax (m/sec)	0.489 ± 0.108 (0.296-0.662)
RVOT Vmax (m/sec)	0.335 ± 0.094 (0.236-0.512)
R-wave amplitude (mV)	0.22 ± 0.11 (0.08-0.5)
QRS duration (sec)	0.03 ± 0 (0.03-0.03)
Mean electrical axis	– 10 ± 13 (– 28 to 8)
Heart rate (beats/min)	200 ± 48 (100-260)

[a]n = 13; 5 male, 8 female; age range 6 mo-5 yr, 7 < 1 yr, 6 > 1 yr; measurements performed under isoflurane inhalant anesthesia.

[b]AB, Apicobasilar length of heart; CD, maximum width of heart perpendicular to AB; H, vertical depth of thorax from ventral border of spine to dorsal border of sternum at level of tracheal bifurcation; R5-7, distance from 5th rib cranial edge to 7th rib caudal edge; VHS, vertebral heart score; L, heart length; W, maximum width perpendicular to L; C, length of clavicle; T, thoracic width at level of 6th rib articulation with vertebral column.

[c]IVSd, interventricular septal thickness in diastole; IVSs, interventricular septal thickness in systole; LVIDd, left ventricular internal diameter in diastole; LVIDs, left ventricular internal diameter in systole; LVFWd, left ventricular free wall thickness in diastole; LVFWs, left ventricular free wall thickness in systole; FS, fractional shortening; EPSS, E-point-to-septal separation length; AO, aortic diameter in diastole; LA, left atrium internal dimension; LVOT, maximum velocity of left ventricular outflow; RVOT, maximum velocity of right ventricular outflow.

REFERENCES

1. Abad C, Cuerel J, Gilabert J, et al. Pharmokinetics of oral and subcutaneous meloxicam (Metcam™) in African pygymy hedgehogs (*Alelerix albiventris*). *Proc 3rd Internat Conf Avian, Herpetol Exot Mam Med. (ICARE)*; 2017:740.

1a. Adamovicz L, Bullen L, Saker K, et al. Use of an esophagostomy tube for management of traumatic subtotal glossectomy in an African pygmy hedgehog (*Atelerix albiventris*). *J Exot Pet Med.* 2016;25:231–236.

2. Allison N, Chang TC, Steele KE, et al. Fatal herpes simplex infection in a pygmy African hedgehog (*Atelerix albiventris*). *J Comp Pathol.* 2002;126:76–78.

3. Antelo J, Núñez C, Contreras L, et al. Use of sarolaner in African hedgehogs (*Atelerix albiventris*) infested with *Caparinia tripilis*. *J Exot Pet Med.* 2020;35:1–3.

4. Arnemo JM, Søli NE. Chemical immobilization of free-ranging European hedgehogs (*Erinaceus europaeus*). *J Zoo Wildl Med.* 1995;26:246–251.

5. Baldo CF, Boelke R. Rabbit supraglottic airway device (V-GEL) for successful airway control in a hedgehog (*Atelerix albiventris*). *Vet Anaesth Analg.* 2020;47:141–143.
6. Barbiers R. Insectivora (hedgehogs, tenrecs, shrews, moles) and Dermoptera (flying lemurs). In: Fowler M, Miller R, eds. *Zoo and Wild Animal Medicine.* 5th ed. Philadelphia, PA: WB Saunders; 2003:304–315.
7. Bennett R. Husbandry and medicine of hedgehogs. *Proc Exot Small Mam Med Mgt (Annu Conf Assoc Avian Vet)*; 2000:109–114.
8. Bexton S, Nelson H. Comparison of two systemic antifungal agents, itraconazole and terbinafine, for the treatment of dermatophytosis in European hedgehogs (*Erinaceus europaeus*). *Vet Dermatol.* 2016;27:500 -e133.
9. Black PA, Marshall C, Seyfried AW, et al. Cardiac assessment of African hedgehogs (*Atelerix albiventris*). *J Zoo Wildl Med.* 2011;42:49–53.
10. Brodie E, Brodie Jr E, Johnson J. Breeding the African hedgehog *Atelerix pruneri* in captivity. *Int Zoo Yearb.* 1982;22:195–197.
11. Chambers JK, Shiga T, Takimoto H, et al. Proliferative lesions of the endometrium of 50 four-toed hedgehogs (*Atelerix albiventris*). *Vet Pathol.* 2018;55:562–571.
11a. Cueral J, Abad C, Gilabert JA, et al. Pharmacokinetics of cefovecin (Convenia™) in African pygmy hedgehogs (*Atelerix albiventris*). *Proc 3rd Internat Conf Avian, Herpetol Exot Mam Med (ICARE)*; 2017:594.
12. Delk KW, Eshar D, Garcia E, et al. Diagnosis and treatment of congestive heart failure secondary to dilated cardiomyopathy in a hedgehog. *J Small Anim Pract.* 2014;55:174–177.
13. Demkowska-Kutrzepa M, Tomczuk K, Studzinska M, et al. *Caparinia tripilis* in African hedgehog (*Atelerix albiventris*). *Vet Dermatol.* 2015;26:73–75.
14. Dierenfeld ES. Feeding behavior and nutrition of the African pygmy hedgehog (*Atelerix albiventris*). *Vet Clin North Am Exot Anim Pract.* 2009;12:335–337.
15. Doss G. *Personal observation*; 2020.
16. Doss G. Proximal jugular venipuncture in African pygmy hedgehogs (*Atelerix albiventris*). *J Exot Pet Med.* 2020;35:94–96.
17. Doss G, Carpenter J, et al. African pygmy hedgehogs. In: Quesenberry K, Orcutt C, Mans C et al., eds. *Ferrets, Rabbits, and Rodents: Clinical Medicine and Surgery.* 4th ed. St. Louis, MO: Elsevier; 2021:401–415.
17a. Doss GA, Carpenter JW. Hedgehogs. *The MSD Veterinary Manual.* 12th ed. Rahway, NJ: Merck & Co. 2022. https://www.msdvetmanual.com/exotic-and-laboratory-animals/hedgehogs.
18. Doss G, Mans C. Antinociceptive efficacy and safety of subcutaneous buprenorphine hydrochloride in African pygmy hedgehogs (*Atelerix albiventris*). *J Am Vet Med Assoc.* 2020;257(6):618–623.
19. Hallam SL, Mzilikazi N. Heterothermy in the southern African hedgehog, *Atelerix frontalis*. *J Comp Physiol B.* 2011;181:437–445.
20. Han JI, Na KJ. Cutaneous paecilomycosis caused by *Paecilomyces variotii* in an African pygmy hedgehog (*Atelerix albiventris*). *J Exot Pet Med.* 2010;19:309–312.
21. Hausmann KE, Doss GA, Mans C. Subcutaneous tiletamine-zolazepam immobilization and effect of flumazenil reversal in African pygmy hedgehogs (*Atelerix albiventris*). *J Exot Pet Med.* 2021;36:42–46.
22. Hawkins S, Doss G, Mans C. Evaluation of subcutaneous alfaxalone-midazolam and ketamine-midazolam sedation protocols in African pygmy hedgehogs (*Atelerix albiventris*). *J Am Vet Med Assoc.* 2020;257:820–825.
23. Hawkins SJ, Doss GA, Mans C. Postanesthetic effects of two durations of isoflurane anesthesia in African pygmy hedgehogs (*Atelerix albiventris*). *J Exot Pet Med.* 2020;32:27–30.
24. Heard D. Insectivores (hedgehogs, moles, and tenrecs). In: West G, Heard D, Caulkett N, eds. *Zoo Animal and Wildlife Immobilization and Anesthesia.* 2nd ed. Ames, IA: John Wiley & Sons; 2014:529–531.
25. Heatley J. Hedgehogs. In: Mitchell MA, Tully TN Jr., eds. *Manual of Exotic Pet Practice.* St. Louis, MO: Saunders/Elsevier; 2009:433–455.

26. Hedley J, Benato L, Fraga G, et al. Congestive heart failure due to endocardiosis of the mitral valves in an African pygmy hedgehog. *J Exot Pet Med*. 2013;22:212–217.
27. Helmer PJ, Carpenter JW. Hedgehogs. In: Carpenter JW, ed. *Exotic Animal Formulary*. 5th ed. St. Louis, MO: Elsevier; 2018:443–458.
28. Hoefer HL. Hedgehogs. *Vet Clin North Am Small Anim Pract*. 1994;24:113–120.
28a. Huckins G, Doss GA, Ferreira TH. Evaluation of supraglottic airway device use during inhalation anesthesia in healthy African pygmy hedgehogs (*Atelerix albiventris*). *Vet Anaesth Analg*. 2021;48:517–523.
29. Isenbügel E, Baumgartner R. Diseases of the hedgehog. In: Fowler M, ed. *Zoo and Wild Animal Medicine: Current Therapy*. 3rd ed. Philadelphia, PA: WB Saunders; 1993:294–302.
30. Jepson L. Hedgehogs. In: Jepson L, ed. *Exotic Animal Medicine: A Quick Reference Guide*. 2nd ed. St. Louis, MO: Elsevier; 2016:198–230.
31. Johnson-Delaney C. Common procedures in hedgehogs, prairie dogs, exotic rodents, and companion marsupials. *Vet Clin North Am Exot Anim Pract*. 2006;9:415–435.
32. Johnson-Delaney C. What veterinarians need to know about hedgehogs. *Exot DVM*. 2007;9:38–44.
33. Johnson-Delaney C. *Exotic Companion Medicine Handbook for Veterinarians*. Lake Worth, FL: Zoological Education Network; 2008.
34. Johnson D. African pygmy hedgehogs. In: Meredith A, Johnson-Delaney C, eds. *BSAVA Manual of Exotic Pets*. 5th ed. Gloucester, UK: British Small Animal Veterinary Association; 2010:139–147.
35. Johnson D. Diagnosing and treating African pygmy hedgehogs. *Proc Atlantic Coast Vet Conf.*; 2004.
36. Kim KR, Ahn KS, Oh DS, et al. Efficacy of a combination of 10% imidacloprid and 1% moxidectin against *Caparinia tripilis* in African pygmy hedgehog (*Atelerix albiventris*). *Parasit Vectors*. 2012;5:158.
37. Landes E, Zentek J, Wolf P. Investigations on composition of milk and development of sucklings in hedgehogs. *Kleintierpraxis*. 1997;42:647–658.
38. LaRue MK, Flesner BK, Higbie CT, et al. Treatment of a thyroid tumor in an African pygmy hedgehog (*Atelerix albiventris*). *J Exot Pet Med*. 2016;25:226–230.
39. Lennox AM. Emergency and critical care procedures in sugar gliders (*Petaurus breviceps*), African hedgehogs (*Atelerix albiventris*), and prairie dogs (*Cynomys spp*). *Vet Clin North Am Exot Anim Pract*. 2007;10:533–555.
40. Lennox AM. Safe sedation and immobilization of unusual exotic species encountered in practice. *J Exot Pet Med*. 2014;23:363–368.
41. Lennox AM, Miwa Y. Anatomy and disorders of the oral cavity of miscellaneous exotic companion mammals. *Vet Clin North Am Exot Anim Pract*. 2016;19:929–945.
42. Leonatti S. *Ornithonyssus bacoti* mite infestation in an African pygmy hedgehog. *Exot DVM*. 2007;9:3–4.
43. Letcher JD. Amitraz as a treatment for acariasis in African hedgehogs (*Atelerix albiventris*). *J Zoo Anim Med*. 1988;19(1-2):24–29.
44. Levine BS. Review of antibiotic-impregnated polymethylmethacrylate beads in avian and exotic pets. *Exot DVM*. 2003;5(4):11–14.
45. Lightfoot T. Therapeutics of African pygmy hedgehogs and prairie dogs. *Vet Clin North Am Exot Anim Pract*. 2000;3:155–172.
46. Longley LA. Anaesthesia of other small mammals *Anaesthesia of Exotic Pets*. London, UK: Saunders; 2008:96–102.
47. Marshall KL. Fungal diseases in small mammals: therapeutic trends and zoonotic considerations. *Vet Clin North Am Exot Anim Pract*. 2003;6(2):415–427.
48. Mikaelian I, Reavill D. Spontaneous proliferative lesions and tumors of the uterus of captive African hedgehogs (*Atelerix albiventris*). *J Zoo Wildl Med*. 2004;35(2):216–220.
49. Morgan K, Berg B. Body temperature regulation and energy metabolism in pygmy hedgehogs. *Proc Annu Meet Soc Integr Comp Biol*;1998:150A.

50. Moriello KA, Coyner K, Paterson S, et al. Diagnosis and treatment of dermatophytosis in dogs and cats: clinical consensus guidelines of the world association for veterinary dermatology. *Vet Dermatol.* 2017;28:266 -e68.
51. Morrisey J, Carpenter J. Formulary. In: Quesenberry KE, Carpenter J, eds. *Ferrets, Rabbits, and Rodents: Clinical Medicine and Surgery.* 3rd ed. St. Louis, MO: Saunders/Elsevier; 2012:566–575.
52. Morrisey JK, Carpenter JW, et al. Formulary. In: Quesenberry Q, Orcutt C, Mans C et al., eds. *Ferrets, Rabbits and Rodents: Clinical Medicine and Surgery.* 4th ed. St. Louis, MO: Elsevier; 2021:620–630.
53. Núñez CR, Waisburd GS, Cordero AM, et al. First report of the use of afoxolaner/milbemycin oxime in an African pygmy hedgehog (*Atelerix albiventris*) with demodicosis caused by *Demodex canis* identified by molecular techniques. *J Exot Pet Med.* 2019;29:128–130.
54. Okorie-Kanu CO, Onoja RI, Achegbulu EE, et al. Normal haematological and serum biochemistry values of African hedgehog (*Atelerix albiventris*). *Comp Clin Path.* 2015;24:127–132.
55. Pantchev N, Hofmann T. Notoedric mange caused by *Notoedres cati* in a pet African pygmy hedgehog (*Atelerix albiventris*). *Vet Rec.* 2006;158:59–60.
56. Papich MG, Davidson GS, Fortier LA. Doxycycline concentration over time after storage in a compounded veterinary preparation. *J Am Vet Med Assoc.* 2013;242:1674–1678.
57. Plumb DC. *Plumb's Veterinary Drug Handbook.* 9th ed. Hoboken, NJ: Wiley-Blackwell; 2018.
58. Powers L. Subcutaneous implantable catheter for fluid administration in an African pygmy hedgehog. *Exot DVM.* 2002;4(5):16–17.
59. Raymond JT, Aguilar R, Dunker F, et al. Intervertebral disc disease in African hedgehogs (*Atelerix albiventris*): four cases. *J Exot Pet Med.* 2009;18:220–223.
60. Raymond JT, Clarke KA, Schafer KA. Intestinal lymphosarcoma in captive African hedgehogs. *J Wildl Dis.* 1998;34:801–806.
61. Reeve N. *Hedgehogs.* London, UK: T & AD Poyser; 1994.
62. Rhee DY, Kim MS, Chang SE, et al. A case of tinea manuum caused by *Trichophyton mentagrophytes* var. *erinacei*: the first isolation in Korea. *Mycoses.* 2009;52:287–290.
63. Rhody JL, Schiller CA. Spinal osteosarcoma in a hedgehog with pedal self-mutilation. *Vet Clin North Am Exot Anim Pract.* 2006;9:625–631.
64. Riley PY, Chomel BB. Hedgehog zoonoses. *Emerg Infect Dis.* 2005;11:1–5.
65. Romero C, Waisburd GS, Pineda J, et al. Fluralaner as a single dose oral treatment for *Caparinia tripilis* in a pygmy African hedgehog. *Vet Dermatol.* 2017;28(6):622 -e152.
66. Smith A. Husbandry and medicine of African hedgehogs (*Atelerix albiventris*). *J Small Exot Anim Med.* 1992;2:21–28.
67. Smith A. Neonatology of the hedgehog (*Atelerix albiventris*). *J Small Exot Anim Med.* 1995;3:15–18.
68. Smith A. General husbandry and medical care of hedgehogs. In: Bonagura JD, ed. *Kirk's Current Veterinary Therapy XIII: Small Animal Practice.* Philadelphia, PA: WB Saunders; 2000:1128–1133.
69. Species360 Zoological Information Management System. Retrieved from https://zims.Species360.org. Accessed October 15, 2020.
70. Staley EC, Staley EE, Behr MJ. Use of permethrin as a miticide in the African hedgehog (*Atelerix albiventris*). *Vet Hum Toxicol.* 1994;36:138.
71. Stocker L. *Medication for Use in the Treatment of Hedgehogs.* Ayelsbury, UK: Marshcliff; 1992.
72. Vuolo S, Whittington JK. Dystocia secondary to a perianal fetal hernia in an African hedgehog. *Exot DVM.* 2008;10:10–12.
73. Weishaupt J, Kolb-Mäurer A, Lempert S, et al. A different kind of hedgehog pathway: tinea manus due to *Trichophyton erinacei* transmitted by an African pygmy hedgehog (*Atelerix albiventris*). *Mycoses.* 2014;57:125–127.
74. Wozniak-Biel A, Janeczek M, Janus I, et al. Surgical resection of peripheral odontogenic fibromas in African pygmy hedgehog (*Atelerix albiventris*): a case study. *BMC Vet Res.* 2015;11:145.
75. Wrobel D, Brown SA. *The Hedgehog: An Owner's Guide to a Happy, Healthy Pet.* New York, NY: Howell Book House; 1997.

Chapter 9 Rodents

Jennifer Frohlich | Jörg Mayer

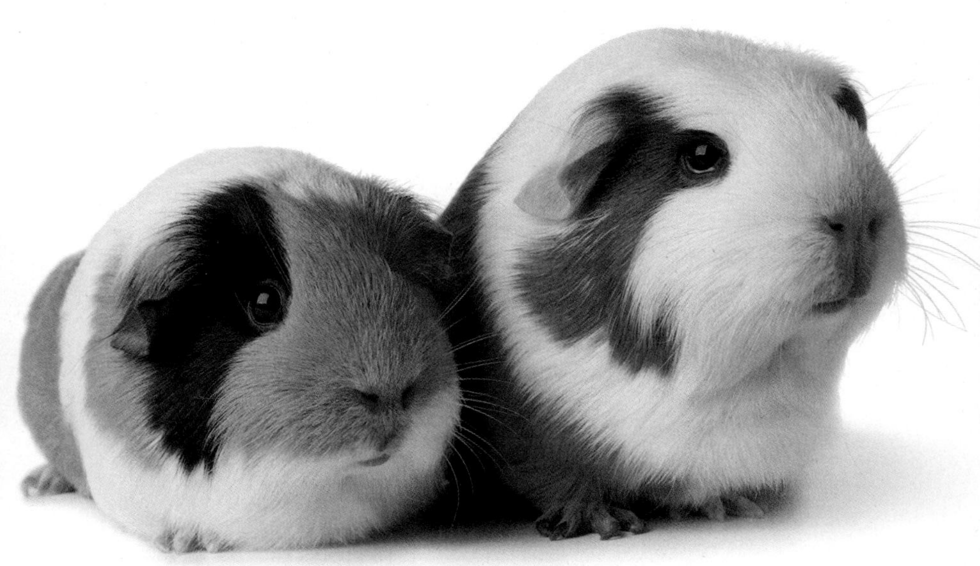

TABLE 9-1 Antimicrobial and Antifungal Agents Used in Rodents.[a]

Agent	Dosage	Comments
Amikacin	5-15 mg/kg SC, IM, IV q8-12h[122]	All species/also administer fluid therapy
	15 mg/kg IM q12h[118]	Guinea pigs/high peak dosing regimen as efficacious as divided regimen/PK
	16 mg/kg SC, IM, IV divided q8-24h[130]	All species/also administer fluid therapy
Amoxicillin	10-15 mg/kg PO q12h[168]	Rats
	25 mg/kg PO q12h[121]	Rats
	100-150 mg/kg IM, SC[122]	Rats, mice
	0.25 mg/mL drinking water × 7 days[112]	Mice/PK; only effective against highly susceptible bacteria, plasma levels reached <300 ng/mL[112]
Amoxicillin/ clavulanic acid	20 mg/kg PO q12h[130]	Mice, rats
Amphotericin B	0.11 mg/kg SC q24h [122,130]	Mice/use with caution; may cause renal toxicity
	0.43 mg/kg PO q24h [122,130]	Mice/candidiasis
	1.25-2.5 mg/kg SC q24h[122]	Guinea pigs/cryptococcosis
Ampicillin	—	Do not use orally in hamsters, guinea pigs, chinchillas; may cause enterocolitis[2]
	6-30 mg/kg PO q8h[122]	Gerbils
	20-100 mg/kg PO, SC, IM q8h[122]	Gerbils
	20-250 mg/kg PO q12h[168]	Rats
	25 mg/kg SC, IM q12h[122]	Rats, mice
	50-200 mg/kg PO q12h[122]	Rats, mice
Azithromycin	15-30 mg/kg PO q24h[48,130]	Most species, including guinea pigs, chinchillas, hamster
	50 mg/kg PO q12h × 14 days[122]	Rats, mice
	30 mg/kg PO q24h[11,28]	Chinchillas
Captan powder	1 tsp/2 cups dust[79] (10 mL/0.5 L)	Chinchillas/fungicide to prevent spread of dermatophytes between cagemates; add to dust box
Cephalexin	15 mg/kg SC, IM q12h[51]	Rats, mice
	15 mg/kg SC q12h[51]	Guinea pigs
	20mg/kg PO q8h[168]	Rats
	25 mg/kg SC q24h[130]	Hamsters, gerbils
	25 mg/kg IM q12-24h[122,168]	Guinea pigs
	60 mg/kg PO q12h[130]	Mice
Chloramphenicol	30-50 mg/kg PO q8-12h[48,130]	Most species
	200 mg/kg PO q12h[122]	Mice
	0.5 mg/mL drinking water[122]	Mice

Continued

TABLE 9-1 Antimicrobial and Antifungal Agents Used in Rodents. (cont'd)

Agent	Dosage	Comments
Chloramphenicol (cont'd)	0.83 mg/mL drinking water[122]	Gerbils
	1 mg/mL drinking water[122]	Guinea pigs
Ciprofloxacin	5-25 mg/kg PO q12-24h[122,130]	Chinchillas, guinea pigs/may cause arthropathies in young of any species
	10 mg/kg PO q12h[122]	Rats, mice
	10-20 mg/kg PO q12h[122]	Hamster
Clarithromycin	15 mg/kg PO q12h[8]	Chinchillas
Clindamycin	7.5 mg/kg SC q12h[130]	Most species/can cause diarrhea; do not give orally; avoid or use with caution in chinchillas and guinea pigs; good bone penetration
Doxycycline	2.5-5 mg/kg PO q12h[130]	All species/pneumonia; may give in combination with enrofloxacin; do not use in young and pregnant animals
	70-100 mg/kg SC, IM q7d[130]	Mice, rats/use long-acting formulation
	0.05 mg/mL drinking water × 7 days[112]	Mice/PK; failed to achieve effective plasma concentrations
Enilconazole	Dip in a 0.2% solution (1:50 dilution of 10% concentrate) q7d[2,130]	Dermatophytosis
	0.2% solution topical q3-4d[48]	All species/dermatophytosis
Enrofloxacin	—	Very high doses may cause arthropathies in young if given for a prolonged time; limit SC, IM injections; SC injections can be diluted in NaCl or lactated Ringer's solution
	5-20 mg/kg PO, SC, IM q12-24h[2,122,130]	Most species/may combine with doxycycline for chronic respiratory infections in rats
	10 mg/kg SC q12h[51]	Most species
	0.25 mg/mL drinking water × 7 days[112]	Mice/failed to achieve effective plasma concentrations; remains stable for 7 days
Enrofloxacin (E)/ doxycycline (D)	10 mg/kg (E) + 5 mg/kg (D) PO q12h[36]	Rats, chronic respiratory infection
Erythromycin	—	Do not use orally in chinchillas, guinea pigs. Use with caution in hamsters and gerbils.[78]
	10 mg/kg PO q24h[168]	Rats/chronic respiratory disease
	20 mg/kg PO q12h[122]	Mice, rats, hamsters
	0.13 mg/mL drinking water[122]	Hamsters/outbreaks of proliferative ileitis; use with caution: can cause enterotoxemia; equivalent to 500 mg/gal drinking water
Gentamicin	—	Use cautiously, nephrotoxic, ensure adequate hydration; consider use of amikacin instead
	2-5 mg/kg SC, IM q24h[122]	All species
	4-24 mg/kg SC, IM q12h[2]	All species
	20 mg/kg SC q24h[2]	Rats

TABLE 9-1 Antimicrobial and Antifungal Agents Used in Rodents. (cont'd)

Agent	Dosage	Comments
Itraconazole	2.5-10 mg/kg PO q24h[122,130]	Most species/in guinea pigs less effective than terbinafine for treatment of dermatophytosis[123]
	5 mg/kg PO q24h[48]	Guinea pigs/dermatophytosis; consider pulse therapy, 7 days on/off until culture negative[48]
	50-150 mg/kg PO q24h[122,130]	Mice/blastomycosis
Ketoconazole	10-40 mg/kg PO q24h × 14 days[130]	All species/systemic mycoses; candidiasis
Lime sulfur dip	Dip q7d × 4 treatments[130]	All species/dermatophytosis; dilute 1:40 with water
Marbofloxacin	2-5 mg/kg PO, SC, IM q24h[122]	All species/do not give during lactation, pregnancy or while growing; injectable can be given orally
	4 mg/kg PO, SC q24h[130]	
Metronidazole	—	Use with caution in chinchillas; objectionable taste may result in reduced food consumption
	10-20 mg/kg PO q12h[130]	Most species
	10-40 mg/kg PO q24h[130]	Mice, rats
	20-60 mg/kg PO q8-12h[2]	Prairie dogs
	40 mg/kg PO q24h[122]	Chinchillas, guinea pigs
	2.5 mg/mL drinking water × 5 day[21]	Mice
Neomycin	—	No absorption following oral administration, therefore not effective against systemic infections; extremely nephrotoxic following parenteral administration.
	15 mg/kg PO q12h[122]	Chinchillas, guinea pigs
	25 mg/kg PO q12h[122]	Mice, rats, hamsters
	0.5 mg/mL drinking water[122]	Hamsters
	2 mg/mL drinking water[51]	Mice, rats
	2.6 mg/mL drinking water[122]	Mice, rats, gerbils
Nystatin	60,000-90,000 U/kg PO q12h × 7-10 days[122]	Gastrointestinal mycoses (not absorbed from gastrointestinal tract)
Oxytetracycline	5 mg/kg IM q12h or 10-20 mg/kg PO q8h[122]	Guinea pigs
	10 mg/kg PO q8h[21]	Gerbils
	10-20 mg/kg PO q8h[122]	Mice, rats/Tyzzer's disease (mice); *Mycoplasma* pneumonia (rats)
	15 mg/kg IM q12h or 50 mg/kg PO q12h[122]	Chinchilla
	20-25 mg/kg IM q8-12h[122]	Hamsters, gerbils
	100 mg/kg SC q24h[153]	All species
	0.25-1 mg/mL drinking water[21]	Hamsters, mice, rats, gerbils
	200 mg/L drinking water × 30 days[168]	Rats/prophylactic treatment

Continued

TABLE 9-1 Antimicrobial and Antifungal Agents Used in Rodents. (cont'd)

Agent	Dosage	Comments
Oxytetracycline (cont'd)	400 mg/L drinking water × 10 days[168]	Rats/curative treatment
	3 g/L in drinking water[153]	Chinchillas, guinea pigs
Penicillin G (procaine)	22,000 U/kg SC, IM q24h[130]	Rats
Penicillin G (benzathine and procaine)	22,000 U/kg SC, IM q24h[122]	Most species
	50,000 U/kg SC q3-5 days[107,108]	Chinchillas, guinea pigs, degus
Sulfonamide + trimethoprim combinations	15-30 mg/kg PO, SC, IM q12-24h[122,130]	Most species
	25 mg/kg PO q12h[168]	Rats
	50-100 mg/kg PO, SC q24h[122]	Gerbils, rats, mice
	0.8 mg/mL drinking water[112]	Mice/failed to achieve effective plasma concentrations; remains stable for 7 days
Terbinafine	10-30 mg/kg PO q24h × 4-6 wk[130]	Most species/antifungal
	20 mg/kg PO q24h[123]	Guinea pigs/PD; dermatophytosis, more effective than itraconazole
Tetracycline	10 mg/kg PO q8-12h[130]	Guinea pigs, chinchillas/use with caution[130]
	10 mg/kg PO, SC q24h[48]	Guinea pig
	20 mg/kg PO q12h[2]	Most species
	30 mg/kg PO q6h[2]	Hamsters
	0.2-0.5 mg/mL drinking water × 7-10 days[168]	Rats
Trimethoprim/ sulfa	See sulfonamide + trimethoprim combinations	—
Tylosin	2-10 mg/kg PO, SC q12h[130]	Hamsters, gerbils/use with caution
	10 mg/kg PO q24h × 5 days[168]	Rats
	10 mg/kg PO, SC q12h[122,130,174]	Chinchillas, guinea pigs, mice, rats/toxicity reported in guinea pigs
	0.5 mg/mL (500 mg/L) drinking water[24]	Gerbils, hamsters, mice, rats/PD in rats;[24] toxicity in hamsters reported[9]
Vancomycin	20 mg/kg PO q24h[47]	Tyzzer's disease
Voriconazole	10 mg/kg PO q24h[29]	Guinea pigs/PD
	40 mg/kg PO 3 × /wk[162]	Mice/PD, PK

[a]Oral antibiotic treatment can result in enteritis and antibiotic-associated clostridial enterotoxemia, especially when antibiotics with a primary gram-positive spectrum are given. Chinchillas, guinea pigs, and hamsters are most susceptible. Also, direct toxicity due to streptomycin and dihydrostreptomycin occurs in gerbils, guinea pigs, hamsters, and mice. Procaine, included in some penicillin preparations, can be toxic to mice. Guinea pigs and chinchillas are highly susceptible to the ototoxic effects of chloramphenicol and aminoglycosides at dosages above those recommended clinically. Antibiotics implicated in antibiotic-associated clostridial enterotoxemia following oral administration include:[79,141]

- Chinchillas: penicillins (including ampicillin, amoxicillin), bacitracin, cephalosporins, clindamycin, erythromycin, lincomycin
- Guinea pigs: penicillins (including ampicillin, amoxicillin), cefazolin, clindamycin, erythromycin, lincomycin, dihydrostreptomycin, streptomycin, bacitracin, chlortetracycline, oxytetracycline, tetracycline, tylosin
- Hamsters: penicillins (including ampicillin, amoxicillin), bacitracin, cephalosporins, clindamycin, erythromycin, lincomycin, vancomycin, dihydrostreptomycin, streptomycin, tylosin

TABLE 9-2 Antiparasitic Agents Used in Rodents.

Agent	Dosage	Comments
Albendazole	5 mg/kg PO q12h[14]	Guinea pigs
Amitraz	1.4 mL/L (0.007%) topical q7-14d × 3 treatments[2,122,130]	Gerbils, hamsters/demodecosis; apply with cotton ball, brush; use with caution; not recommended in young
	1.4 mL/L local, repeat q14d[168]	Rats
	0.3% solution topically q7-14d × 3-6 treatments[122]	Guinea pigs, mites
Carbaryl powder (5%)	Topical q7d × 3 treatments[130]	Chinchillas, guinea pigs/ectoparasites
Dimetridazole	20-50 mg/kg PO q24h × 7 days[14]	Guinea pigs
	500 mg/L drinking water[14,152]	Degus, hamsters/*Trichomonas, Giardia*
	1 g/L drinking water × 40 days[14]	Chinchillas, degus, chipmunks, squirrels/*Giardia*
	1.2-10 mg/mL drinking water × 5 days[147]	Mice/trichomoniasis; not effective; use metronidazole or tinidazole instead[147]
	4 g/L drinking water × 7 days[14,168]	Rats, mice
Doramectin	0.2-0.5 mg/kg SC, q7-14d × 2-3 treatments[14]	Most species
Emodepside + praziquantel (Profender)	0.07-0.7 mL/kg topical[120]	Mice/PD; nematodes, cestodes; contains 21.4 mg/mL of emodepside + 85.9 mg/mL of praziquantel
Fenbendazole	20 mg/kg PO q24h × 5 days[14,168]	Rats, guinea pigs
	20-50 mg/kg PO q24h × 5 days[2,122,130]	All species/giardiasis; a lower dose is generally preferred, higher end for giardiasis only[122]
	25-150 ppm in feed × 5 days[168]	Mice/oxyurids
	50 ppm in feed × 5 days[168]	Mice/*Hymenolepis diminuta*
	300 ppm in feed × 5 days[168]	Mice/*Hymenolepis nana*
Fipronil	7.5 mg/kg topically q30-60d[122]	Most species/fleas, ticks, and lice
	1-2 spray pumps topical, repeat 1-2 q7-10d[48]	Guinea pigs
Fluralaner	10 mg/kg PO, SC, IP once or dipped in 100 ppm of a topical solution[72]	Guinea pigs/*Ornithodoros moubata* ticks and *Cimex lectularius* bed bugs Mice/*Ctenocephalides felis* fleas and *Myocoptes musculinus* mites
Imidacloprid	20 mg/kg topically q30d[122,130]	Most species/flea control
Imidacloprid 10%/ moxidectin 1% (Advocate, Bayer)	0.1 mL/animal topically[83,122,130]	Guinea pigs/ectoparasites (e.g., fleas, biting lice, mites)

Continued

TABLE 9-2 Antiparasitic Agents Used in Rodents. (cont'd)

Agent	Dosage	Comments
Imidacloprid 10%/ moxidectin 1% (Advocate, Bayer) (cont'd)	13 mg/kg (I) + 3 mg/kg (M) topically q7d × 8 wk[132]	Mice/*Demodex musculi*
	33 mg/kg topically × 2 days/wk q2wk[150]	Guinea pigs/cutaneous nematodes
Ivermectin	0.2-0.4 mg/kg PO, SC q7-14d[130]	Chinchillas, guinea pigs, hamsters, prairie dogs, mice, rats/ectoparasites; preferred dosage appears to be 0.4 mg/kg q7d (higher doses have also been reported); for *Demodex*, use q5-7d
	0.2-0.5 mg/kg SC, PO q7-14d[122]	Most species
	0.3 mg/kg PO q24h[163]	Hamsters/PD; demodicosis
	0.4 mg/kg SC q7d[15]	Hamsters/notoedric mites
	0.4 mg/kg SC, repeat q14d[42]	Guinea pigs/PD; effective against *Trixacarus caviae*
	Spray animals or topical drops[13]	Mice/clinical trial for mite control;[13] use 1% ivermectin diluted 1:100 with 1:1 propylene glycol:water (0.1 mg/mL); sprayed onto mice or topical behind ear
	8 mg/L drinking water × 4 days/wk × 5 wk[94]	Mice/pinworms
	25 mg/L drinking water × 4 days/wk × 5 wk[94]	Rats/pinworms
	48 mg/L drinking water × 3 days[52]	Rats/pinworms, *Giardia*, *Hymenolepis*
Levamisole	25 mg/kg SC[14]	Guinea pigs
Lime sulfur dip	Dip q7d × 6 wk[130]	All species/ectoparasites; dilute 1:40 with water
Mebendazole	20 mg/kg PO[14]	Guinea pigs
	40 mg/kg PO q7d × 21 days[2]	Mice, rats/pinworms
	50-60 mg/kg PO q12h × 5 days[14]	Chinchillas, degus, chipmunks
Metronidazole	10-20 mg/kg PO q12h or 40 mg/kg q24h[122]	Guinea pigs, chinchillas
	20-40 mg/kg PO q24h[122]	Rats, mice, gerbils, hamsters
	20-50 mg/kg PO q12-24h[130]	Gerbils, hamsters
	25 mg/kg PO q12h[14]	Guinea pigs, chinchillas
	50 mg/kg PO q12h × 5 days[122]	Chinchillas/giardiasis; may cause anorexia, use with caution
	50-60 mg/kg PO q12h × 5 days[168]	Rats
	2.5 mg/mL drinking water × 5 days[2,14,147]	Rats, mice/trichomoniasis
Moxidectin	—	See imidacloprid
	0.5 mg/kg topically[128]	Mice/fur mites; combine with cage/bedding change for best results

TABLE 9-2 Antiparasitic Agents Used in Rodents. (cont'd)

Agent	Dosage	Comments
Niclosamide	100 mg/kg PO q7d × 2 treatments[14]	Guinea pigs/*Hymenolepis* spp.
Nitenpyram (e.g., Capstar)	1 mg/kg PO once[122]	Most species/fleas, flystrike; safe in pregnant animals[122]
Permethrin	0.25% dust in cage[58]	All species/ectoparasites
	Cotton ball soaked in 5% solution[58]	Most species/place in cage 4-5 wk
Permethrin impregnated cotton ball, 7.4% solution (MiteArrest, Ecohealth Inc.)	2 cotton balls per cage q7d × 6 wk[170]	Mice/fur mites
	2-3 cotton balls per cage[109]	Voles/*Ornithonyssus bacoti*
Piperazine citrate	4-5 mg/mL drinking water × 7 days, off 7 days, on 7 days[122]	Rats, mice
	4-7 g/L drinking water[14]	Guinea pigs
	10 mg/mL drinking water × 7 days, off 7 days, on 7 days[122]	Guinea pigs, hamsters
Piperazine sulfate (Wazine, Fleming Laboratories)	100 mg/kg/day in drinking water × 7 days[33]	African pouched rats/nematodes
Ponazuril	30 mg/kg PO q48h × 2 treatments[60,111]	Prairie dogs/*Eimeria*
		Rats
Praziquantel	5-10 mg/kg PO, SC q10d × 2 treatments[48]	Guinea pigs
	6-10 mg/kg PO, SC repeat in 10 days[48,130]	All species/cestodes, trematodes
	30 mg/kg PO q14d × 3 treatments[122]	Gerbils, mice, rats
	30 mg/kg SC[33]	African pouched rats/cestodes
	140 ppm in feed × 7 days[2]	Mice
Pyrantel pamoate	15 mg/kg PO q14d × 2 treatments[33]	African pouched rats/nematodes
	50 mg/kg PO[130]	Most species/gastrointestinal nematodes
Pyrethrin powder	Topical 3 × /wk[130]	Gerbils, hamsters, mice, rats/ectoparasites
	Topical q7d × 3 treatments[130]	Chinchillas, guinea pigs/ectoparasites
Pyrethrin shampoo (0.05%)	Shampoo q7d × 4 treatments[130]	Hamsters, gerbils, mice, rats/fleas
Ronidazole	400 mg/L drinking water[14,168]	Rats, mice, gerbils
Selamectin	2.5 mg/animal topically[109]	Voles/*Ornithonyssus bacoti*
	10-12.4 mg/kg once[63]	Rats and mice/mites
	15 mg/kg topically once[42]	Guinea pigs/PD; effective against *Trixacarus caviae*
	15-30 mg/kg topically q21-28d × 2 treatments (q14d if Demodex)[47,48]	Most species/use 30 mg/kg with *Sarcoptes*
	20 mg/kg topically[34]	Patagonian cavy/*Otodectes cynotis*

Continued

TABLE 9-2 Antiparasitic Agents Used in Rodents. (cont'd)

Agent	Dosage	Comments
Sulfadimethoxine	15-100 mg/kg PO q24h × 3 days, off 5 days, on 3 days[14]	Guinea pigs
	25-50 mg/kg PO q24h × 10 days[130]	Most species
	50 mg/kg PO once, then 25 mg/kg q24h × 10-20 days	All species/coccidiosis
Sulfamerazine	1.5 mg/L drinking water × 10 days[14]	Chinchillas, degus, chipmunks, squirrels/coccidiosis
Sulfamethoxypyrazine	25 mg/kg PO q24h × 3-5 days[14]	Guinea pigs
Sulfamethazine	1-5 mg/mL drinking water[2]	All species/coccidosis
	1 mg/mL drinking water × 4 days, off 4 days × 3 treatments[14]	Chinchillas, degus, chipmunks, squirrels/coccidosis
Sulfaquinoxaline	1 mg/mL drinking water × 14-21 days[2,130]	All species/coccidiosis
Thiabendazole	100-200 mg/kg PO q24h × 5 days[14]	Guinea pigs
Tinidazole	50-100 mg/kg PO[107]	Prairie dogs/*Giardia*
	2.5 g/L drinking water[14,147]	Rats, mice, gerbil
Toltrazuril (Baycox, Bayer)	10 mg/kg PO q24h × 3 days, off 3-5 days, on 3 days[46,152,168]	Most species/drug of choice for coccidiosis; 2.5% solution has very low pH; needs to be diluted with equal parts water and propylene glycol (1:1:1);[155] 5% solution does not need to be diluted
	10-20 mg/kg PO q24h × 3 days, off 5 days, on 3 days[168]	Hamster/coccidiosis
	25 mg/L drinking water[14]	Most species

TABLE 9-3 Chemical Restraint/Anesthetic Agents Used in Rodents.

Agent	Dosage	Comments
Acepromazine	—	See ketamine for combinations
	0.5-1 mg/kg IM[130,172]	Most species
	0.5-2.5 mg/kg IM, SC, PO[122]	Rats
	0.5-5 mg/kg IM, SC, PO[122]	Guinea pigs, hamsters, mice/higher doses should only be given PO
Alfaxalone	—	Licensed for IV administration; can be administered IM, SC, IP; high doses needed, resulting in large volumes
	2-5 mg/kg IV[99]	Rats/anesthesia; mean duration <15 min
	5-10 mg/kg SC, IM administration[137]	Chinchillas/not effective
	10 mg/kg/h IV as CRI[73]	Rats/anesthesia maintenance after induction

TABLE 9-3 Chemical Restraint/Anesthetic Agents Used in Rodents. (cont'd)

Agent	Dosage	Comments
Alfaxalone (cont'd)	20 mg/kg IP[99]	Rats/anesthesia; 20-60 min; no induction in 30% of animals
	20 mg/kg IM or 120 mg/kg IP[122]	
	25-45 mg/kg IP[10]	Rats/light anesthesia; higher doses required in males
	40 mg/kg IM, IP[122]	Guinea pigs
	80 mg/kg IP[158]	Mice/surgical anesthesia for ~ 60 min
	100 mg/kg IP, SC[77]	Mice/anesthesia
Alfaxalone (A)/ butorphanol (B)	(A) 5 mg/kg + (B) 0.5 mg/kg IM[137]	Chinchilla/short term; inconsistent anesthesia (<20 min); significant post-anesthetic reduction in food intake and fecal output[137]
Alfaxalone (A)/ butorphanol (B)/ midazolam (M)	(A) 8 mg/kg + (B) 1 mg/kg + (M) 1 mg/kg IM[43]	Five-striped palm squirrel/anesthesia
Alfaxalone (A)/ dexmedetomidine (D)/ fentanyl (F)	(A) 20 mg/kg (females) or 60 mg/kg (males) + (D) 0.05 mg/kg + (F) 0.1 mg/kg IP[10]	Rats/anesthesia
Alfaxalone (A)/ ketamine (K)	(A) 6 mg/kg + (K) 40 mg/kg IM[43]	Five-striped palm squirrel/anesthesia
Alfaxalone (A)/ ketamine (K)/ dexmedetomidine (D)	(A) 6 mg/kg + (K) 20 mg/kg + (D) 0.1 mg/kg IM[43]	Five-striped palm squirrel/anesthesia
Alfaxalone (A)/ medetomidine (Me)/ butorphanol (B)	(A) 40-80 mg/kg + (Me) 0.3 mg/kg + (B) 5 mg/kg SC[77]	Mice/anesthesia; surgical anesthesia for 35-85 min dependent on alfaxalone dose; not effective after IP administration
Alfaxalone (A)/xylazine (X)	(A) 40-120 mg/kg + (X) 10 mg/kg SC, IP[41]	Mice/surgical anesthesia; results vary between sexes and strains; recommend SC for decreased mortality during laparotomy
	(A) 80 mg/kg + (X) 10 mg/kg IP[158]	Mice/surgical anesthesia for 80±18 min
Atipamezole (Antisedan, Pfizer)	5x the administered medetomidine dose, or 10x the administered dexmedetomidine dose, SC, IM[122]	Dexmedetomidine/medetomidine reversal
	0.15 mg/kg IM[43]	Five-striped palm squirrel/ dexmedetomidine reversal
	1 mg/kg SC[130]	All species
Atropine	0.04-0.4 mg/kg SC, IM[130]	Gerbils, hamsters, mice, rats/rats possess serum atropinesterase
	0.05-0.2 mg/kg SC, IM, IV[130]	Chinchillas, guinea pigs
	0.1-0.2 mg/kg SC, IM[122]	Chinchillas, guinea pigs

Continued

TABLE 9-3 Chemical Restraint/Anesthetic Agents Used in Rodents. (cont'd)

Agent	Dosage	Comments
Bupivacaine	0.5 mg/kg[3]	Guinea pigs/nerve blocks
	1-2 mg/kg local nerve block[122]	Guinea pig, rats/use with caution in mice, can cause neurotoxicity at a dose of 7 mg/kg[110]
	1 mg/kg + 0.1 mg/kg morphine (preservative free) epidural[122]	Limit volume to 0.33 mL/kg
	1.6 mg/kg epidural[122]	Anesthesia to level of L4
	2.3 mg/kg epidural[122]	Anesthesia to level of T11-13
Bupivacaine, extended release (Exparel, Pacira)	1 mg/kg SC[89]	Rats/1 dose lasts up to 4 days
Butorphanol	0.2 mg/kg SC[165]	Rats/sufentanil reversal
Dexmedetomidine (Dexdomitor, Orion)	—	α2 agonist similar to medetomidine; see ketamine for combination
Diazepam[a]	—	See ketamine for combinations
	0.5-5 mg/kg IM[122,a]	Guinea pigs
	2.5-5 mg/kg IM[122,a]	Chinchillas, hamsters, gerbils, rats, mice
Fentanyl/fluanisone (Hypnorm, Janssen)	—	Anesthesia
	0.2-0.6 mL/kg IM, IP[144]	Mice, rats
	0.5-1 mL/kg IM[122]	Guinea pigs
Fentanyl/fluanisone (F/f) + midazolam (Mi)	(F/f) 0.5 mL/kg + (Mi) 5 mg/kg SC[165]	Rats/anesthesia
Flumazenil	0.1 mg/kg SC[74]	Chinchillas/midazolam reversal
	0.1 mg/kg IM[43,80]	Five-striped palm squirrel, naked mole rat/midazolam reversal
Glycopyrrolate	0.01-0.02 mg/kg SC[81]	All species/excess oral or respiratory mucus
Isoflurane	2-5% induction then 0.25-4% maintenance[68,81,114,122,146]	All species/inhalant anesthetic
Ketamine	—	Avoid use alone due to high doses needed; ketamine combinations follow
	5-40 mg/kg IM[130]	Chinchillas, guinea pigs, hamsters/light sedation; heavy sedation at higher doses
	22-44 mg/kg IM[130]	Mice, rats/light sedation; heavy sedation at 44 mg/kg in mice and 25-40 mg/kg in rats
	40-100 mg/kg IM[130]	Gerbils/light sedation; heavy sedation at higher doses (marked individual variation)
Ketamine (K)/ acepromazine (A)	(K) 40 mg/kg + (A) 0.5 mg/kg IM[129]	Chinchillas/anesthesia; prolonged recovery
	(K) 50-150 mg/kg + (A) 2.5-5 mg/kg IM[127]	Mice, rats/lower end of doses preferred
Ketamine (K)/ acepromazine (A)/ xylazine (X)	(K) 60 mg/kg + (A) 1-2 mg/kg + (X) 5-7.5 mg/kg[5]	Rats/anesthesia; use lower end of dosing range for females

TABLE 9-3 Chemical Restraint/Anesthetic Agents Used in Rodents. (cont'd)

Agent	Dosage	Comments
Ketamine (K)/ dexmedetomidine (De)	(K) 2-4 mg/kg + (De) 0.025 mg/kg IM[122]	Most species/sedation
	(K) 3-5 mg/kg + (De) 0.05 mg/kg SC, IM[122]	Guinea pigs/short anesthesia
	(K) 4 mg/kg + (De) 0.015 mg/kg[38,56]	Chinchillas/anesthesia; provide supplemental oxygen; reverse with atipamezole[56]
	(K) 75 mg/kg + (De) 0.5 mg/kg IP[22]	Mice/less reliable than ketamine and medetomidine
	(K) 75 mg/kg + (De) 1 mg/kg IP[171]	Rats
Ketamine (K)/ dexmedetomidine (De)/ midazolam (Mi)	(K) 40 mg/kg + (De) 0.25 mg/kg + (Mi) 1.5 mg/kg IM[20]	Prairie dogs/anesthesia; short procedures
	(K) 20 mg/kg + (De) 0.06 mg/kg + (Mi) 1 mg/kg IM[80]	Naked mole rats/anesthesia; mean time 15 min
Ketamine (K)/ diazepam (D)[a]	(K) 20-40 mg/kg + (D) 1-2 mg/kg IM[79,a]	Chinchillas/anesthesia
Ketamine (K)/ medetomidine (Me)	(K) 2-4 mg/kg + (Me) 0.05 mg/kg IM[122]	Most species/sedation
	(K) 3-5 mg/kg + (Me) 0.1 mg/kg SC, IM[122]	Guinea pigs/short anesthesia
	(K) 4-5 mg/kg + (Me) 0.03 mg/kg[107]	Chinchillas/anesthesia; provide supplemental oxygen; reverse with atipamezole
	(K) 5 mg/kg + (Me) 0.06 mg/kg IM[74]	Chinchilla/anesthesia
	(K) 5-10 mg/kg + (Me) 0.02-0.04 mg/kg IM[82]	Degus/anesthesia; supplement with isoflurane if needed
	(K) 40 mg/kg + (Me) 0.5 mg/kg IM, IP[48,114,144]	Guinea pigs/20-30 min duration of anesthesia
	(K) 40-75 mg/kg + (Me) 1 mg/kg IP[32]	Mice/anesthesia; minor procedures; use the higher dose of ketamine in females; (Me) reversal is atipamezole
	(K) 75-90 mg/kg + (Me) 0.5 mg/kg IM, IP[114,144]	Rats, gerbils/surgical anesthesia; 20-30 min duration
	(K) 100 or 200 mg/kg + (Me) 0.25 mg/kg SC, IP[39,92]	Hamster (Syrian)/anesthesia
Ketamine (K)/ medetomidine (Me)/ buprenorphine (B)	(K) 20 mg/kg + (Me) 0.1 mg/kg + (B) 0.03 mg/kg IM[3]	Guinea pigs/premedication
Ketamine (K)/ midazolam (M)	(K) 5-10 mg/kg + (M) 0.5-1 mg/kg IM[130]	Chinchillas, guinea pigs/anesthesia
	(K) 40 mg/kg + (M) 1-2 mg/kg SC, IM, IP[48]	Rats/anesthesia

Continued

TABLE 9-3 Chemical Restraint/Anesthetic Agents Used in Rodents. (cont'd)

Agent	Dosage	Comments
Ketamine (K)/ midazolam (M)/ butorphanol (B)	(K) 5-10 mg/kg + (M) 0.2-0.4 mg/kg + (B) 0.3-0.5 mg/kg IM[82]	Degus/anesthesia; supplement with isoflurane if needed
Ketamine (K)/xylazine (X)	(K) 20-40 mg/kg + (X) 2 mg/kg IM[66]	Guinea pigs/light anesthesia
	(K) 40 mg/kg + (X) 2 mg/kg IM[74]	Chinchilla/anesthesia
	(K) 50 mg/kg + (X) 2 mg/kg IP[66]	Gerbils/anesthesia
	(K) 60 mg/kg + (X) 6 mg/kg IP[90]	Mice/anesthesia, <40 min
	(K) 80 mg/kg + (X) 5 mg/kg IM, IP[66]	Hamsters/anesthesia
	(K) 80 mg/kg + (X) 8 mg/kg IP[90]	Mice/anesthesia, <30 min
	(K) 100 mg/kg + (X) 5 mg/kg IM, IP[47]	Rats/anesthesia
	(K) 191 mg/kg + (X) 4.25 mg/kg SC[101]	Mice/anesthesia; surgical plane
Medetomidine	—	See ketamine for combinations
	0.1 mg/kg SC[87,106]	Hamsters/light to moderate sedation
	0.1-0.2 mg/kg SC[87,106]	Gerbils/light to moderate sedation
	0.15 mg/kg IM[16,48]	Rats, guinea pigs/sedation
	0.15-0.25 mg/kg IM[67]	Rats/sedation
	0.2-0.3 mg/kg SC[48]	Hamsters/sedation
Medetomidine (Me)/ butorphanol (B)	(Me) 0.1 mg/kg + (B) 2 mg/kg IM[16]	Rats/sedation
Medetomidine (Me)/ sufentanil (S)	(Me) 0.15 mg/kg + (S) 0.05 mg/kg SC[165]	Rats/anesthesia
Midazolam	—	See ketamine for combination
	0.4-2 mg/kg IM[172]	Guinea pigs, chinchillas
	1-2 mg/kg IM[130]	All species/preanesthetic
	2-3 mg/kg IM[172]	Rats, mice, gerbils
Midazolam (Mi)/ butorphanol (B)	(Mi) 0.2-0.8 mg/kg + (B) 0.3-0.5 mg/kg IM[82]	Degus/sedation
Midazolam (Mi) / medetomidine (Me)/ butorphanol (B)	(Mi) 1 mg/kg + (Me) 0.05 mg/kg + (B) 2 mg/kg IP[16]	Rats/sedation; completely reversible
	(Mi) 2 mg/kg + (Me) 0.15 mg/kg + (B) 2.5 mg/kg IP[93]	Rats/anesthesia; completely reversible
	(Mi) 4 mg/kg + (Me) 0.3 mg/kg + (B) 5 mg/kg IP[77,90]	Mice/anesthesia, <60 min; completely reversible
Midazolam (Mi)/ medetomidine (Me)/ fentanyl (F)	(Mi) 1 mg/kg + (Me) 0.05 mg/kg + (F) 0.02 mg/kg IM[74]	Chinchillas/anesthesia; completely reversible with flumazenil (0.1 mg/kg) + atipamezole (0.5mg/kg) + naloxone (0.05 mg/kg) SC[74]

TABLE 9-3 Chemical Restraint/Anesthetic Agents Used in Rodents. (cont'd)

Agent	Dosage	Comments
Midazolam (Mi)/ medetomidine (Me)/ fentanyl (F) (cont'd)	(Mi) 2 mg/kg + (Me) 0.15 mg/kg + (F) 0.005 mg/kg IM[4]	Rats/anesthesia; completely reversible with flumazenil (0.2 mg/kg) + atipamezole (0.75 mg/kg) + naloxone (0.12 mg/kg)
	(Mi) 2 mg/kg + (Me) 0.2 mg/kg + (F) 0.025-0.05 mg/kg IM[48]	Guinea pigs/anesthesia; completely reversible with flumazenil (0.1 mg/kg) + atipamezole (1 mg/kg) + naloxone (0.03 mg/kg)[48]
	(Mi) 3.3 mg/kg + (Me) 0.33 mg/kg + (F) 0.033 mg/kg SC[48]	Hamsters/anesthesia; completely reversible
Naloxone	0.01-0.1 mg/kg SC, IP[74,81,114,122]	All species/opioid reversal
	0.02 mg/kg/h IV[122]	Constant rate infusion (CRI)
Pentobarbital	—	Anesthesia; not recommended; marginal analgesia; autonomic depression; euthanasia dose is 150 mg/kg[122]
	30-45 mg/kg IP[66]	Guinea pigs, chinchillas, rats
	50 mg/kg IP[90]	Mice/anesthesia, <45 min; no surgical anesthesia achieved
	50-90 mg/kg IP[66]	Gerbils, hamsters, mice
Propofol	—	Anesthesia; induction
	3-5 mg/kg IV[130]	Guinea pigs, chinchillas, prairie dogs
	7.5-10 mg/kg IV[61,114,122]	Rats
	12-26 mg/kg IV[122]	
Sevoflurane	To effect[68]	Most species
Tiletamine/zolazepam (Telazol, Zoetis)	40-460 mg/kg IM[23]	Guinea pigs/anesthesia
	30 mg/kg IM IP[48]	Hamsters
	50-80 mg/kg IM[127]	Mice, rats
Tiletamine/zolazepam (T)/xylazine (X)	(T) 20 mg/kg + (X)10 mg/kg IP[81]	Gerbils/anesthesia
	(T) 30 mg/kg + (X) 10 mg/kg IM, IP[66]	Hamsters/anesthesia
Xylazine	—	See ketamine, tiletamine/zolazepam for combinations
	5-10 mg/kg SC, IM, IP[127]	Most species/may cause muscle necrosis when given IM
Yohimbine	0.5-1 mg/kg IV, IP[66]	All species/xylazine reversal

[a]Diazepam is not soluble in aqueous solution; admixing with aqueous solutions or fluids can result in precipitation; administering SC or IM can be painful and irritating; for SC or IM administration, midazolam may be preferred.

TABLE 9-4 Analgesic Agents Used in Rodents.

Agent	Dosage	Comments
Acetaminophen	50-100 mg/g SC[169]	Rats/effective for postoperative pain
	100 mg/kg PO[124]	Rats/PD
	200 mg/kg PO[51]	Mice, rats
	1-2 mg/mL drinking water[81]	All
Acetylsalicylic acid	50-150 mg/kg PO q4-8h[122]	All
	87 mg/kg PO[51]	Guinea pigs
	100 mg/kg PO[51,59]	Rats
	120 mg/kg PO q4h[51]	Mice
Buprenorphine	0.01-0.05 mg/kg SC, IM q6-12h[47,122]	Gerbils, hamsters
	0.01-0.05 mg/kg SC, IV q8-12h[51]	Rats
	0.03-0.05 mg/kg SC, IM, IV q8-12h[130]	Prairie dogs
	0.03-0.05 mg/kg SC or 0.5-0.6 mg/kg PO[50]	Rats
	0.05 mg/kg SC q8-12h[48,51]	Guinea pigs, chinchillas
	0.05 mg/kg q12h SC, IM[156]	Rats/PD, PK
	0.05-0.1 mg/kg SC q12h[51] or 0.1-0.2 mg/kg SC[50]	Mice
	0.1 mg/kg SC q12h[91]	Mice/PD; not sufficient analgesia following laparotomy
	0.1-0.25 mg/kg PO q8-12h[51]	Rats
	0.1-0.4 mg/kg PO[125,149]	Rats
	0.2 mg/kg IV q7h[149,151]	Guinea pigs/PK
	0.2 mg/kg q4h oral transmucosal[145]	Guinea pigs/PK
	0.2 mg/kg SC q4-6h[55]	Chinchillas/PD
	0.5 mg/kg SC q8h[48]	Hamsters
	1 mg/kg PO (mixed with 2 g/kg of Nutella)[76]	Rats/give 60 min prior to procedure
Buprenorphine, extended release (Animalgesics Labs)	0.48 mg/kg SC[135]	Guinea pigs/give 8-12 hr prior to procedure; 1 dose lasts up to 96 hr
	0.65 mg/kg SC q48h[85]	Rats/PD
Buprenorphine, sustained release (Buprenorphine SR, ZooPharm)	—	Injections site lesions have been reported; may not be absorbed if injected SC in immune-compromised animals[136]
	0.3-0.48 mg/kg SC[50]	Guinea pigs
	0.3-1.2 mg/kg SC q48-72h[30]	Rats/PD

TABLE 9-4 Analgesic Agents Used in Rodents. (cont'd)

Agent	Dosage	Comments
Buprenorphine, sustained release (Buprenorphine SR, ZooPharm) (cont'd)	0.6 mg/kg SC q48h[177]	Guinea pigs/reaches adequate plasma concentrations
	0.6 mg/kg SC q72h[91]	Mice/PD; sufficient postlaparotomy analgesia
	1.2 mg/kg SC q72-96h[85,156]	Rats/PD, PK
	1.5 mg/kg SC q48h[70]	Mice/PD
	2.2 mg/kg SC q24-48h[84]	Mice/PD, PK
Butorphanol	0.2-2 mg/kg q2-4h[7,130]	Most species
	1-2 mg/kg SC q4h[51]	Guinea pigs, rats, mice
	1-5 mg/kg SC q4h[47,122,130]	Gerbils, rats, mice, hamsters
Carprofen	—	Nonsteroidal antiinflammatory; high end of dosage reflects total daily dose; can be divided
	2-5 mg/kg PO, SC, IM, IV total daily dose in single or two divided doses[122]	All
	4 mg/kg SC q12-24h[125]	Guinea pigs, chinchillas
	5 mg/kg SC[47,51]	Rats, mice, gerbils
	5-10 mg/kg PO[103,172]	Rats, mice, gerbils
	5-15 mg/kg SC[148,149]	Rats/PD
	2 mg compounded flavored tablet (Bio-Serv)/1 tablet PO q 24h[178]	Rats
Celecoxib	10-20 mg/kg PO[124]	Rats/PD
Clonidine	0.25-0.5 mg/kg PO[59]	Mice
Codeine	40 mg/kg SC[119]	Rats/PD
Diclofenac	2.1 mg/kg PO[51]	Guinea pigs
	8 mg/kg PO[51]	Mice
	10 mg/kg PO[51]	Rats
Dipyrone	See metamizole	—
Duloxetine	30 mg/kg PO q24h[88]	Mice/PD
	10 mg/kg IP[88]	Mice/PD
Flunixin meglumine	—	Nonsteroidal anti-inflammatory; do not use in dehydrated animals
	2.5 mg/kg SC[125]	Most species
	2.5-5 mg/kg SC q12-24h[51]	Most species
Fentanyl	0.025-0.6 mg/kg SC[59]	Mice
	0.16 mg/kg SC[119]	Rats/PD
Firocoxib	10-20 mg/kg IP q24h[143]	Mice

Continued

TABLE 9-4 Analgesic Agents Used in Rodents. (cont'd)

Agent	Dosage	Comments
Gabapentin	10-30 mg/kg PO[88]	Mice/PD
	30 mg/kg PO q12h[126]	Prairie dogs/PK
	30 mg/kg PO q8h[122]	Rats
	50 mg/kg PO q24h[122]	Hamsters
	100 mg/kg IP q24h x 3 treatments[64]	Rats/effective pain relief without producing locomotor sedation
	90 mg compounded flavored tablet (Bio-Serv)/1 tablet PO q24h[178]	Rats
Hydrocodone	10-40 mg/kg SC[119]	Rats/PD
Hydromorphone	0.4 mg/kg SC < q2h[160]	Rats/PD
	2 mg/kg SC < q4h[45]	Chinchillas/PD
Ibuprofen	5-30 mg/kg SC[169]	Rats
	10 mg/kg PO q4h[51]	Guinea pigs
	15 mg/kg PO[51]	Rats
	30 mg/kg IP[131]	Rats/PD
	30 mg/kg PO[51]	Mice
	40 mg/kg PO[69]	Mice/PD
Indomethacin	2 mg/kg PO[51]	
	8 mg/kg PO[51]	Guinea pigs
Ketoprofen	—	Use with caution in rats; may induce gastrointestinal complications such as bleeding, ulcers, and erosions[157]
	1-2 mg/kg SC, IM q12-24h[122,130]	Chinchillas, guinea pigs
	2 mg/kg SC, IM q12h[130]	Prairie dogs
	5 mg/kg SC[51]	Rats, mice
	5-15 mg/kg SC[148]	Rats/ PD
	15-25 mg/kg SC[169]	Rats/effective for postoperative pain when given prophylactically
Meloxicam	≥ 0.5 mg/kg PO, SC q24h[130]	Chinchillas, guinea pigs, hamsters, gerbils
	1 mg/kg PO, SC[51,125]	Rats
	1-2 mg/kg PO q12-24h[7,122]	Rats
	1-5 mg/kg PO, SC q24h[130]	Mice
	5 mg/kg PO, SC[51]	Mice
Meloxicam, sustained release (Meloxicam SR, ZooPharm)	4 mg/kg SC q96h[156]	Rats/PD
Meperidine	10-20 mg/kg SC, IM q2-3h[51]	Guinea pigs, mice, rats
Methadone	0.5-3 mg/kg SC[40]	Rats/PD

TABLE 9-4 Analgesic Agents Used in Rodents. (cont'd)

Agent	Dosage	Comments
Methadone (cont'd)	1-2 mg/kg SC IM[7]	Mice
	1-4 mg/kg SC, IM[7]	Rats
	5-10 mg/kg IP[1]	Rats/PD
Metamizole	20-50 mg/kg PO, SC q6-12h[46,47]	Most species
	150 mg/kg PO[12]	Mice
Morphine	0.2 mg/kg intrathecal[166]	Rats
	1-3 mg/kg SC[87]	Mice/PD
	1-5 mg/kg SC[50]	Mice
	2-5 mg/kg SC, IM q4h[7,130]	Most species
	2-5 mg/kg SC, IM q4h[51]	Guinea pigs
	2.5 mg/kg SC q2-4h[51,122]	Rats, mice, hamsters
	5 mg/kg SC[50]	Guinea pigs
Nalbuphine	1-2 mg/kg IM q3h[51]	Guinea pigs, rats
	2-4 mg/kg IM q4h[51]	Mice
Oxycodone	10-40 mg/kg SC[119]	Rats/PD
Oxymorphone	0.2-0.5 mg/kg SC, IM q4h[51,125]	Guinea pigs, rats, mice
Palmitoylethanolamide and quercetine	10 mg/kg PO[19]	Rats/analgesia for osteoarthritis
Pentazocine	5-10 mg/kg SC q3-4h[51]	Rats, mice
	5-10 mg/kg q2-4h[122]	Gerbils, guinea pigs, hamsters, mice, rats
Pethidine	10-20 mg/kg SC, IM q2-3h[51,122]	Most species
Piroxicam	3.4-20 mg/kg PO[122]	Mice
Tolfenamic acid	2 mg/kg SC q24h[122]	Guinea pigs
	4 mg/kg PO, SC q24h x 3 doses max[46,47]	Most species
Tramadol	—	Oral route unlikely to be effective
	5 mg/kg SC IP[7,51]	Rats/mice
	5-40 mg/kg SC, IP[53]	Mice
	10-20 mg/kg PO, SC q8-12h[122]	Rats
	10-40 mg/kg SC q12h[122]	Mice
	10-40 mg/kg SC[45a]	Chinchillas/PD; no analgesic effects; side effects at >40 mg/kg
	20-40 mg/kg PO[50]	Rats
	20-80 SC mg/kg[173]	Mice/not effective analgesia if used a single agent in male mice
	40 mg/kg PO q24h[164]	Rats/has shown analgesic effects at that dose

TABLE 9-5 Cardiovascular Agents Used in Rodents.

Agent	Dosage	Comments
Atenolol (cont'd)	0.2-2 mg/kg PO q24h[83]	Most species/beta-blocker; hypertension and tachyarrhythmias
	2-10 mg/kg IV, IP q24h[122]	Mice
Atropine	0.05-0.5 mg/kg SC, IM[2,83]	All species/preanesthetic; cardiac problems
	0.1-0.2 mg/kg SC, IM[122]	Guinea pigs, chinchillas
Benazepril	0.05-0.1 mg/kg PO q24h[83,122]	Most species/ACE inhibitor; heart failure, hypertension, and chronic renal failure
	0.125-0.25 mg/kg PO q24h[46,47]	
Carvedilol	1-11 mg/kg PO q24h[122]	Hamsters/beta-blocker
	2-30 mg/kg PO q24h[122]	Rats/beta-blocker
Digoxin	0.005-0.01 mg/kg PO q12-24h[46-48]	Most species
	0.05-0.1 mg/kg PO q12-24h[114,122,130]	Hamsters/dilated cardiomyopathy
Diltiazem	0.5-1 mg/kg PO q12-24h[48,83]	Most species/calcium channel blocker; hypertension and hypertrophic cardiomyopathy
Dopamine	0.08 mg/kg IV prn[98]	Guinea pigs/hypotension, especially anesthetic related
Enalapril	0.5-1 mg/kg PO q24h[46,48]	ACE inhibitor; heart failure
Epinephrine (adrenaline)	0.003-0.1 mg/kg IV prn[48]	Guinea pigs/cardiac arrest
	0.01 mg/kg IV[122]	Most species
	0.1 mg/kg IV[130]	Most species
Etilefrine	0.5-1 mg/kg PO q6-8h[46]	Sympathomimetic
Furosemide	1-5 mg/kg PO, SC, IM q12-24h[46,47]	Most species/congestive heart failure
	1-4 mg/kg SC, IM q4-6h or 5-10 mg/kg SC, IM q12h[122]	Most species
Glyceryl trinitrate ointment (2%)	3 mm strip applied to inner pinna q6-12h[83,122]	Most species/congestive heart failure
Glycopyrrolate	0.01-0.02 mg/kg SC, IM, IV[122]	Most species/anticholinergic agent used for bradycardia; premedication
Imidapril hydrochloride	0.125-0.25 mg/kg PO q24h[46]	ACE inhibitor
Lidocaine	1-2 mg/kg IV or 2-4 mg/kg IT[83]	Most species/arrhythmias
Metildigoxin	0.005-0.01 mg/kg PO q24h[46]	Dilative cardiomyopathy; tachycardic arrhythmia
Pimobendan	0.2-0.4 mg/kg PO q12h[130]	Most species/inodilator for treating heart failure
	0.25 mg/kg PO q12h[46,47]	Most species
Propentofylline	0.125 mg/kg PO q24h[46]	ACE inhibitor
	10-25 mg/kg PO q12-24h[46,47]	Ischemia
Spironolactone	1 mg/kg PO q24h[142]	Chinchilla/case report
Taurine	100 mg/kg PO q12h × 8 wk[83]	Most species/cardiomyopathy
Verapamil	0.25-0.5 mg/kg SC q12h[122]	Hamsters/calcium channel blocker

TABLE 9-6 Emergency Drugs Used in Rodents.

Agent	Dosage	Comments
Atropine	0.05-0.1 mg/kg SC[46,47]	All species/bradycardia; some rats possess serum atropinesterase
	0.1-0.2 mg/kg SC, IM[122]	Chinchillas, guinea pigs
	Up to 10 mg/kg SC, IM, IV q20min[66,122]	All species/organophosphate toxicity
Calcium gluconate	100 mg/kg IM, IP once[48,114,138a]	Guinea pigs/dystocia; follow with 1 U oxytocin (see Table 9-7)
	100 mg/kg IM, IP once[122]	Chinchillas/hypocalcemic tetany; eclampsia
Charcoal (activated)	0.5-5 g/kg PO prn[122]	Acute poisoning with organophosphates and other pesticides
Dexamethasone	—	All species/antiinflammatory
	0.5-2 mg/kg SC, IM, IV[130]	
	0.6 mg/kg IM, IV[2,122]	Guinea pigs/pregnancy toxemia
	4-5 mg/kg SC, IM, IP, IV[114]	Shock
Diazepam	0.5-5 mg/kg IM, IV, IP[122]	All/treatment of seizures, sedation
Diphenhydramine	—	Antihistamine; anaphylaxis
	1-2 mg/kg PO, SC q12h[130]	All species
	1-5 mg/kg SC prn[122,130]	Guinea pigs
Dopamine	0.08 mg/kg IV[98]	Guinea pigs/hypotension
Doxapram	—	Respiratory stimulant
	2-5 mg/kg IV, IP, SC[48,122]	Guinea pigs
	5-10 mg/kg IV, IP[46,122]	Most species
Ephedrine	1 mg/kg IV[122]	Guinea pigs/antihistamine; stimulant
Epinephrine (adrenalin)	0.003-0.1 mg/kg IV prn[48]	Guinea pigs/cardiac arrest
	0.01 mg/kg IV[122]	Most species
	0.1 mg/kg IV[130]	Most species
Furosemide	—	Diuretic for edema, pulmonary congestion, ascites
	1-4 mg/kg SC, IM q4-6h[122]	Most species
	1-5 mg/kg PO, SC, IM q12-24h[46,47]	Most species/congestive heart failure
	5-10 mg/kg SC, IM q12h[122]	Most species
Glycopyrrolate	0.01-0.02 mg/kg SC, IM, IV[122]	Most species/anticholinergic agent used for bradycardia; premedication
Hetastarch	1-10 mL/kg IV[122]	Rats/hypotension; shock
	3 mL/kg IV, IO[102]	Shock; administer with hypertonic saline (3 mL/kg) over 10 min
Lactated Ringer's solution	10-25 mL/kg IV, IO[139]	Most species/give slowly over 5-10 min (if unsuccessful, administer IP)
Mannitol	0.3 g/kg/h IV[46]	Reduction of intracranial pressure, acute glaucoma, oliguric renal failure

Continued

TABLE 9-6 Emergency Drugs Used in Rodents. (cont'd)

Agent	Dosage	Comments
Prednisolone	10-20 mg/kg IM, IV, IP once[46]	Most species/shock
Saline, hypertonic (7.2-7.5%)	3 mL/kg IV, IO slow over 10 min[102]	Shock; administer with hetastarch (3 mL/kg) over 10 min

TABLE 9-7 Miscellaneous Agents Used in Rodents.

Agent	Dosage	Comments
Acetylcysteine	3 mg/kg PO, SC q12h[46,47]	Mucolytic
	2% solution nebulization over 30-60 min prn[122]	Injectable form can be used for nebulization, dilute in 0.9% NaCl
Aglepristone	10 mg/kg IM, SC on day 1, 2, and 8[122]	Guinea pigs/ progesterone antagonist for treatment of pyometra/metritis, pregnancy termination
	10-20 mg/kg SC q12h × 2 days, repeat after 8 days[48]	Hamster/pyometra
	10 mg/kg SC q24h × 2 treatments[47]	Rats, hamster, gerbils/pyometra
Aluminum hydroxide	20-40 mg/animal PO prn[122]	Guinea pigs/hyperphosphatemia caused by renal failure
Aminophylline	10 mg/kg PO q12-24hr[134]	Rats
	50 mg/kg PO, SC[122,130]	Guinea pigs
Amitriptyline	5-20 mg/kg PO q24h[122]	Rats/antidepressant; chronic antianxiety treatment
Asparaginase (L-Asparaginase)	400 IU/kg SC q7d[48]	Guinea pigs/lymphoma
	10,000 IU/m^2 SC, IM q21d[122]	Guinea pigs/lymphoma
Atropine (1%)/ phenylephrine (10%)	Topical to eyes[66]	All species/mydriasis for nonalbino eyes
Barium sulfate (1000 mg/mL)	5-10 mL/kg PO[46,47]	Most species/contrast studies; might need to be diluted with water (1:1)
Bromhexine	0.5 mg/kg PO q12-24h[46,47]	Bronchial secretolytic
	0.5-1 mg/kg PO q12-24h[48]	Guinea pigs
Cabergoline	10-50 µg/kg PO q12-24h[122]	Rats/pituitary adenoma
	0.6 mg/kg PO q72h[115]	
	12.5-15 µg/kg PO q24h × 4-6 days[46,47]	Most species/pseudopregnancy
Calcium EDTA	25-30 mg/kg SC q6-12h, 5 days on/5 day off cycle[122]	Lead or zinc intoxication; treat until blood levels within normal range at end of "off period"
	30 mg/kg SC q12h[79,130]	All species/lead chelation
Carbimazole	1-2 mg/kg PO q24h[46,117]	Guinea pigs/hyperthyroidism
Charcoal (activated)	1 g/kg PO[47]	Most species/use only in cases of toxicity (not with general diarrhea)

TABLE 9-7 Miscellaneous Agents Used in Rodents. (cont'd)

Agent	Dosage	Comments
Chlorpheniramine maleate	0.6 mg/kg PO q24h[2,122]	Guinea pigs/antihistamine
Cholestyramine	1 g/animal mixed with water PO q24h[122]	Guinea pig/gastrointestinal *Clostridium* overgrowth; decreases toxin absorption
Cimetidine	5-10 mg/kg PO, SC, IM, IV q6-12h[122]	All species/H_2-blocker; gastric and/or duodenal ulceration; esophagitis; gastroesophageal reflux
Cisapride	0.1-0.5 mg/kg PO q8-12h[48]	All species/may enhance gastrointestinal motility
	0.1-1 mg/kg PO q8-12h[122]	Chinchillas, guinea pigs
Clomipramine	16-32 mg/kg PO q12h[122]	Rats
Cyclophosphamide	300 mg/kg IP q24h[98]	Guinea pigs/antineoplastic
	300 mg/m² IP q24h[122]	
Cyclosporine	10 mg/kg PO q24h[122]	Rats
Cyproheptadine	0.5 mg/kg PO q12h[122]	Guinea pigs, chinchillas/appetite stimulation
Deslorelin acetate	4.7 mg implant/animal SC[96]	Guinea pigs/suppression of estrus
	4.7 mg implant/animal SC[154]	Guinea pigs/ovarian cysts; not effective against serous cysts
	4.7 mg implant/animal SC[6,27,65,159]	Rats/antigonadal effects for at least 12 mon[6,27]
Dexamethasone	—	Antiinflammatory
	0.5-2 mg/kg PO, SC, then decreasing dose q12h × 3-14 days[66]	All species
	0.6 mg/kg SC, IM, IV q24h[122]	Guinea pigs/pregnancy toxemia
Diazoxide	5-25 mg/kg PO q12h[75]	Guinea pigs/insulinoma
Diphenhydramine	—	Antihistamine; anaphylaxis
	1-2 mg/kg PO, SC q12h[130]	Chinchillas, hamsters, mice, rats
	1-5 mg/kg SC prn[122]	Guinea pigs
Diphenylhydantoin (Phenytoin)	25-50 mg/kg q12h[83]	Most species/seizures
Dorzolamide	1 drop of 1% solution q12h[122]	Rats/glaucoma
Ephedrine	1 mg/kg PO, IV prn[98,122]	Guinea pigs/antihistamine; anaphylaxis
Famotidine	0.4-0.5 mg/kg PO, SC, q24h[122]	Guinea pigs, chinchillas
Fluoxetine	5-10 mg/kg PO q24h[83]	Most species/for behavioral problems (i.e., fur chewing)
	1-1.5 mg/kg PO q24h[122]	Rats
Furosemide	1-5 mg/kg PO, SC, IM q12-24h[46,47]	Most species/congestive heart failure
	1-4 mg/kg SC, IM q4-6h or 5-10 mg/kg SC, IM q12h[122]	Most species
GnRH (e.g., gonadorelin)	20 µg/animal IM once[62]	Guinea pigs/ovarian cysts, short-acting formulations
	25 µg/animal q14d × 2 treatments[113]	Guinea pigs/ovarian cysts

Continued

TABLE 9-7 Miscellaneous Agents Used in Rodents. (cont'd)

Agent	Dosage	Comments
Heparin	5 mg/kg IV prn[98]	Guinea pigs/disseminated intravascular coagulation
Human chorionic gonadotropin (hCG)	100 U/kg SC q10-14 days × 3 treatments[46]	Guinea pigs/cystic ovaries
	100 U/kg SC q7d days × 3 treatments[122]	Guinea pigs/cystic ovaries
Insulin	1 U/kg SC q12h[122]	Chinchillas
	1-2 U/animal SC q12h[122]	Guinea pigs
	1-3 U/kg q12-24h SC; starting dose is 1 U/kg[46]	Guinea pigs, chinchillas, degus
	1-3 U/animal SC q12h[122]	Rats
	2 U/animal SC[122]	Hamsters, gerbils
Iodine, I-131 (radioactive)	1 mCi/animal SC once[117]	Guinea pigs/hyperthyroidism
Iodine (iohexol)	300 mg/kg IV[35]	Contrast IV radiographs (rat)
Kaolin pectin	0.2 mL PO q6-8h[2]	Guinea pigs/antidiarrheal
	1-2 mL/kg PO q2-6h[122]	
Lactulose	0.5 mL/kg PO q12h[122]	Most species/constipation; hepatic disorders
	2 mL/kg PO prn[46,47]	Most species/constipation
Leuprolide acetate depot (Lupron Depot, TAP Pharmaceuticals)	0.2-0.3 mg/kg IM q28d[133]	Guinea pigs/cystic ovaries
Levetiracetam	20 mg/kg PO q8h[122]	Prairie dogs/seizures
Levothyroxine	5 µg/kg PO q12h[122]	Most species/hypothyroidism
	10-20 µg/kg PO q24h[46]	Guinea pigs/hypothyroidism
Lomustine	10-15 mg/kg PO q21d[138a]	Guinea pigs
Loperamide	0.1 mg/kg PO q8h[66,122]	All species/diarrhea; limit use to avoid gastrointestinal stasis
Magnesium hydroxide	4 mg/kg PO[83]	Prevention of calcium oxalate uroliths
Maropitant	30 mg/kg PO[100]	Mice/no adverse reaction seen
	100 mg/kg PO[100]	Rats/no adverse reaction seen
Methimazole	0.5-2 mg/kg PO q24h[117]	Guinea pigs/hyperthyroidism
	1-3 mg/kg PO q8-24h[97]	Guinea pigs/hyperthyroidism
Metoclopramide	0.2-1 mg/kg PO, SC, IM q12h[130]	Most species
	0.5-1 mg/kg PO, SC q6-12h[122]	Guinea pigs/antiemetic and upper gastrointestinal prokinetic
	1-5 mg/kg q8-12h SC, PO[46,47]	
Metyrapone	8 mg/animal PO q24h × 4 wk[48,83]	Hamsters/hyperadrenocorticism
Milk thistle (*Silybum marianum*) (see Silymarin)	—	—

TABLE 9-7 Miscellaneous Agents Used in Rodents. (cont'd)

Agent	Dosage	Comments
Mitotane	5 mg/animal PO q24h × 4 wk[83]	Hamsters/hyperadrenocorticism
N-acetyl-L-cysteine (NAC)	200 mg/kg PO × 10 wk[31]	Mice/reduces inflammation associated with leishmaniasis
Octreotide	1.5 µg/kg PO q12h[35]	Rat/cardiomyopathy; reduces intestinal chyle production and chylous effusion
Oxytocin	0.2-3 U/kg SC, IM, IV[122]	All species/delayed parturition if unobstructed
	1 U/kg SC, IM[46,47]	All species
	1-2 U/animal IM[2]	Guinea pigs/uterine contraction; milk letdown
	6.25 U/kg SC[2]	Mice/milk letdown
Pentosan polysulphate	3 mg/kg SC q5-7d × 4 treatments[122]	Guinea pigs/osteoarthritis; idiopathic cystitis
Pentoxifylline	20 mg/kg IP injection q12h[104]	Guinea pig
Phenobarbital	5-20 mg/kg PO, IV, IP[130]	Guinea pigs/antiseizure medication; sedative
	5-25 mg/kg IV, IP q12-24h[122]	Guinea pigs, gerbils/seizures
Phenoxybenzamine	0.25 mg/kg PO q12h[107]	Guinea pigs/urolithiasis
Potassium citrate	10-30 mg/kg PO q12h[130]	Guinea pigs
Prednisone	0.5-2.2 mg/kg PO, SC, IM[130]	All species/antiinflammatory
Prednisolone	1-2 mg/kg PO, SC q12-24h[46,48]	Guinea pigs
Pseudoephedrine	1.2 mg/animal PO q12h[145]	Chinchillas/nasal and sinus decongestant
Ranitidine	5 mg/kg PO q12h[122]	Guinea pigs, chinchillas
S-adenosylmethionine (SAMe)	20-100 mg/kg PO q24h[122]	Most species
Sildenafil citrate	5 mg/kg PO q24h[95]	Rats
Silymarin (also known as milk thistle)	4-15 mg/kg PO q8-12h[83]	Most species/hepatic disorders
	50-200 mg/kg/day PO[25,161]	Rats
Sucralfate	25-50 mg/kg PO q6-8h[122]	All species/oral, esophageal, gastric, and duodenal ulcers
	25-100 mg/kg PO q8-12h[130]	
Terbutaline	5 mg/kg PO q12h[122,138]	Most species
Theophylline	2-3 mg/kg PO q8-12h[46,47]	Most species
	4-10 mg/kg PO q8-12h[48]	Guinea pigs
	10-20 mg/kg PO q8-12h[122]	Rats, prairie dogs
Thiamazol (and see methimazole)	1-2 mg/kg PO q24h[46]	
Thiamine	1 mg/kg feed[83]	Most species/thiamine deficiency
Toremifene	12 mg/kg PO q24h[83]	Rats/pituitary hyperplasia/adenoma

Continued

TABLE 9-7 Miscellaneous Agents Used in Rodents. (cont'd)

Agent	Dosage	Comments
Trilostane	2-4 mg/kg PO q12-24h[122,176]	Hyperadrenocorticism
TSH, human recombinant	100 μg IM[116]	Guinea pigs/thyroid function testing
Vitamin A	50-500 U/kg IM[122]	Guinea pigs, hamsters
	2000 U/animal[83]	Chinchillas/hypovitaminosis A
	2 μg vitamin A palmitate/g feed[122]	Hamsters
	10 mg β-carotene/kg of feed[122]	Guinea pigs
Vitamin B complex (small animal)	0.02-0.2 mL/kg SC, IM[122]	All species/B1 (100 mg/mL), B2 (2 mg/mL), B12 (0.1 mg/mL)
Vitamin C (ascorbic acid)	10-30 mg/kg PO, SC, IM[122]	Guinea pigs/maintenance
	50-100 mg/kg SC, PO[48]	Guinea pigs/treatment of deficiency
	100-200 mg/kg PO q24h[122]	Guinea pigs/hypovitaminosis C
	0.2-0.4 mg/mL drinking water[122]	Guinea pigs/prevents deficiency; change daily
Vitamin D	200-400 U/kg SC, IM[114]	All species
Vitamin E	50 mg/kg of feed[48]	Guinea pigs
Vitamin K1	1-5 mg/kg SC q12-24h[46,47]	Most species
	1-10 mg/kg IM q24h × 4-6 days[66]	All species/warfarin poisoning; menadiols not used in acute cases

TABLE 9-8 Common and Scientific Names of Rodents.[48]

Common Name	Other Common Names	Scientific Name
Chinchilla	Long-tailed chinchilla	*Chinchilla lanigera*
Chipmunk	Siberian chipmunk, Korean chipmunk	*Eutamias sibiricus*
Degu	Common degu	*Octodon degus*
Gerbil	Mongolian gerbil, Mongolian jird, clawed jird	*Meriones unguiculatus*
Guinea pig	Cavy, cuy	*Cavia porcellus*
Hamster, Chinese	Striped hamster	*Cricetulus griseus*
Hamster, dwarf	Russian dwarf hamster, Siberian dwarf hamster, Djungarian hamster	*Phodopus sungorus*
	Campbell dwarf hamster	*Phodopus campbelli*
	Roborowski dwarf hamster	*Phodopus roborovskii*
Hamster, golden	Syrian hamster	*Mesocricetus auratus*
Mouse	Common mouse	*Mus musculus*
Palm squirrel, five-striped	Northern palm squirrel	*Funambulus pennantii*
Prairie dog	Black-tailed prairie dog	*Cynomys ludovicianus*
Rat	Brown rat, Norway rat	*Rattus norvegicus*

TABLE 9-9 Hematologic and Serum Biochemical Values of Rodents.[43a,54,78,140]

Measurement	Mouse	Rat	Gerbil	Hamster	Guinea Pig	Chinchilla	Prairie Dog
PCV (%)	44 (42-44)	35-45	35-45	45-50	39-55	33-48	30-44
RBC (106/μL)	8.7-10.5	7-10	7-8	7-8	4-7	5.8-9.2	5.9-9.4
Hgb (g/dL)	13.4 (12.2-16.2)	12-18	14-16	16.6-18.6	11-17	10.5-15.2	6.44-14.8
WBC (103/μL)	8.4 (5.1-11.6)	5-23	7.5-10.9	7-10	2.9-14.4	2.1-17.6	3.3-10.5
Neutrophils (%)	18 (7-37)	10-50	22	18-40	12-63	4-58	43-87
x 10^3/μL	—	—	—	—	—	—	0.8-7.9
Lymphocytes (%)	69 (63-75)	50-70	75	56-80	30-80	31-95	8-54
x 10^3/μL	—	—	—	—	—	—	1.0-5.6
Monocytes (%)	1 (1-3)	0-10	0-4	2	0-9	0-14	0-12
x 10^3/μL	—	—	—	—	—	—	0-0.42
Eosinophils (%)	2 (1-4)	0-5	0-3	0-1	0-14	0-3	0-10
x 10^3/μL	—	—	—	—	—	—	0-0.5
Basophils (%)	0.5 (0-1.5)	0-1	0-1	0-1	0-1	0-1	0-2
ALT (U/L)	26-77	20-92	—	M: 45 ± 26 F: 53 ± 18.3	31-51	2-24	25 ± 16
ALP (U/L)	45-222	16-96	—	126 ± 6	68-71	22-247	74 ± 22 (45-128)
AST (U/L)	54-269	—	—	M: 61 ± 39 F: 53 ± 23	32-51	19-247	35 ± 11 (21-63)
Bile acids (μmol/L)	—	—	—	—	0-85	—	13 (2-24)
Bilirubin, total (mg/dL)	0.1-0.9	0.2-0.6	0.2-0.6	M: 0.3 ± 0.1 F: 0.3 ± 0.1	0.3-0.9	0-0.4	0.3 ± 0.1 (0.2-0.6)

Continued

TABLE 9-9 Hematologic and Serum Biochemical Values of Rodents. (cont'd)

Measurement	Mouse	Rat	Gerbil	Hamster	Guinea Pig	Chinchilla	Prairie Dog
BUN (mg/dL)	17-28	M: 19 ± 2 F: 21 ± 3	17-27	M: 23 ± 4 F: 28 ± 5	9-62	30-81	21-44
Calcium (mg/dL)	3.2-8	M: 12.0 ± 0.9 F: 12.1 ± 0.7	3.7-6.2	M: 12.6 ± 0.6 F: 13.2 ± 1.4	9.0-11.3	7.5-11.9	9.1 ± 0.4 (7.5-10.2)
Chloride (mmol/L)	82-114	M: 103 ± 2 F: 104 ± 2	—	M: 104 ± 3 F: 104 ± 4	94-111	105-126	98 ± 4 (85-108)
Cholesterol (mg/dL)	26-82	M: 119 ± 51 F: 119 ± 29	90-150	M: 143 ± 24 F: 158 ± 35	12-65	48-119	104 ± 26 (50-171)
Creatinine (mg/dL)	0.3-1	M: 0.7 ± 1 F: 0.7 ± 1	0.6-1.4	M: 0.4 ± 0.9 F: 0.5 ± 0.2	0.6-2.2	0.25-0.87	0.54 ± 0.1 (0.3-0.9)
Fructosamine (umol/L)	—	—	—	—	134-271	—	—
y-Glutamyl transferase (U/L)	—	—	—	—	0-13	—	—
Glucose (mg/dL)	62-175	M: 115 ± 17 F: 111 ± 17	50-135	M: 84 ± 19 F: 100 ± 17	89-287	53-249	318 ± 90 (138-510)
Phosphorus (mg/dL)	6-10.4	M: 7.3 ± 1.5 F: 5.8 ± 1.1	3.7-7	M: 5.4 ± 1.0 F: 5.5 ± 1.1	3.2-21.6	1.8-11.5	6.3 ± 0.9 (4.1-8.3)
Potassium (mmol/L)	5.1-10.4	M: 7.0 ± 0.7 F: 6.1 ± 0.7	3.3-6.3	M: 6.5 ± 0.8 F: 6.4 ± 0.7	4.5-8.8	3.3-6.1	5.1 ± 1.0 (3.6-8.0)
Protein, total (g/dL)	3.5-7.2	M: 7.0 ± 0.5 F: 7.5 ± 0.5	4.3-12.5	M: 6.3 ± 0.3 F: 5.9 ± 0.3	4.4-6.6	4.1-6.7	5.7 ± 0.8 (4.4-8.8)

TABLE 9-9 Hematologic and Serum Biochemical Values of Rodents. (cont'd)

Measurement	Mouse	Rat	Gerbil	Hamster	Guinea Pig	Chinchilla	Prairie Dog
Albumin (g/dL)	2.5-4.8	M: 3.4 ± 0.2 F: 4.0 ± 0.3	1.8-5.5	M: 4.3 ± 0.2 F: 4.1 ± 0.3	2.3-3.0	2.3-4.1	2.5 ± 1.1 (1.7-9)
Globulin (g/dL)	0.6	1.8-3	1.2-6	2.7-4.2	1.7-2.6	0.9-2.2	3.4-4.2
Sodium (mmol/L)	112-193	150 ± 3	141-172	148 ± 4	121-126	142-166	144-175
Triglycerides (mg/dL)	—	M: 266 ± 121 F: 249 ± 160	—	M: 209 ± 53 F: 212 ± 53	29-206	22-205	—
Other Parameters							
Partial thromboplastin time (PTT) (sec)	55-110	—	—	—	—	—	
Clotting time (min)	2-10	—	—	—	—	—	
Prothrombin time (sec)	7-19	—	—	—	—	8-10	
Activated partial thromboplastin time (sec)	—	—	—	—	—	19-26	
Fibrinogen (mg/dL)	—	—	—	—	—	224-626	

TABLE 9-10 Biologic and Physiologic Data of Rodents.[46,48,54,66,114]

Species	Life Span	Avg wt (g) (male/female)	Temperature°C (°F)	Heart Rate (beats/min)	Respiratory (breaths/min)
Chinchilla	10-20	450-600/550-800	36.1-37.8 (97-100)	200-240	40-80
Degu	5-7	170-350	37-39 (98.6-102.2)	240-390	80-150
Gerbil	3-4	65-130/70-100	37-39 (98.6-102.2)	260-450	70-130
Guinea pig	4-6	900-1500/700-1000	37.5-39.5 (99.5-103.1)	230-380	40-120
Hamster, Chinese	1.5-3	30-45/30-45	—	—	—
Hamster, golden	2-3	80-150/90-160	37-39 (98.6-102.2)	250-500	50-135
Hamster, Russian dwarf and Campbell	2-3	19-45/19-36	37-39 (98.6-102.2)	200-560	90-120
Hamster, Roborowski dwarf	1.5-2	20-28/18-23	37-39 (98.6-102.2)	200-560	90-120
Mouse	1.5-3	20-40/18-35	37-37.2 (98.8-99.3)	310-840 beats/min	70-220
Prairie dog	8-10	1000-2200/500-1500	35.4-39.1 (95.7-102.3)	150-320	30-60
Rat	1.5-3	350-500/250-350	37.5-39.5 (98.6-103.1)	300-500	70-120

TABLE 9-11 Blood Volumes of Rodents with Safe-Bleeding Volume Recommendations.[133]

Species	Blood Volume (Average)	Safe Venipuncture Volume
Gerbil	67 mL/kg	0.3 mL/animal
Guinea pig	75 mL/kg	7.7 mL/kg
Hamster	78 mL/kg	5.5 mL/kg
Mouse	79 mL/kg	7.7 mL/kg
Rat	64 mL/kg	5.5 mL/kg

TABLE 9-12 Urinalysis Reference Values of Rodents.[a,37,44,47,49,54,58,83]

Measurement	Chinchilla	Gerbil	Guinea Pig	Hamster	Mouse	Prairie Dog	Rat
Specific gravity	1.014->1.060	1.006-1.080	1.005-1.050	1.014-1.060	1.034-1.058	1.005-1.059	1.022-1.050
pH	8.5-9.5	6.2-8.2	8.4 ± 0.3	6.9-9	7.3-8.5	8-8.5	7.3-8.5
Protein[b] (mg/dL)	Present[b] (6-87)	Present[b]	Present[b]	Present[b]	Present[b]	Present[b] (6-124)	Present[b]
Crystals	Common, amorphous crystals predominant		Amorphous crystals predominant			Rare, amorphous	
Parasites	—	—	Cysts of *Klossiella cobaye* might be seen	—	—	—	*Trichosomoides crassicauda* (bladder threadworm), larvated ova in urine

[a]Values should be considered as guides; values are likely to vary between groups of animals according to such variables as strain, age, sex, fasting, and methodology.

[b]Proteinuria is a normal feature in most rodent species, and dipstick protein levels do not correlate with actual urinary protein levels in most species, in particular in the presence of alkaline urine.

TABLE 9-13 Reproductive Data for Rodents.[18,48,54,66,114,140]

Species	Estrus Cycle Length (days)	Gestation (days)	Litter Size	Birth Weight (g)	Age Eyes Open (days)	Weaning Age (days)	Breeding Life	Separate Adults Before Birth
Chinchilla	30-50	105-115	1-4	30-50	birth	36-48	—	—
Degu	18-21	87-93	1-10	10-20	2-3	35-42	—	—
Gerbil	4-6	24-26	1-12	2.5-3.5	16-20	21-28	15-20 months	No (mate for life)
Guinea pig	15-19	59-72	2-5	60-100	birth	21-28	3-4 years	No
Hamster	4-5	15-22	4-12	2-3	14-16	20-28	11-18 months	Yes
Mouse	4-5	19-21	10-12	0.5-1.5	10-14	21-28	12-18 months	No
Prairie dog	14-21	33-38	1-10	15	14	37-51	—	—
Rat	4-5	21-23	8-14	5-6	12-17	17-21	14 months	No

TABLE 9-14 Determining the Sex of Mature Rodents.[66,140]

Male	Female
• Anogenital distance is longer in the male • Manipulate prepuce to protrude penis • Palpate for testicles either in a scrotal sac (if present) or subcutaneous in inguinal region • Males have only two external openings in the inguinal area: – Anus – Urethral orifice at tip of penis • In very fat males, there may be a depression between the penis and anus; this depression can be obliterated by manipulating the skin in that area	• Anogenital distance is shorter in the female • Look for three external openings in the inguinal area: – Anus (most caudal opening) – Vaginal orifice (middle opening)-look carefully – Urethral orifice at tip of urethral papilla (most cranial opening) • The urethral papilla is located outside the vagina (unlike dogs and cats) • In very fat females or young females, the vaginal orifice may be either hidden by folds of skin (the former) or sealed (latter); gentle manipulation of the skin in this area will reveal the orifice

TABLE 9-15 Nutritional Data for Rodents.[9,48,114,140]

	Consumption (per 100 g BW/day)		Nutritional Recommendations			
Species	Food (g)	Water[166]	Minimum Fiber (%)	Carbo-hydrates (%)	Fat (%)	Protein (%)
Chinchilla	3-6	—	16-18	—	2-4	14-16
Gerbil	5-8	4-7	—	—	2-4	16-22
Guinea pig	6	10	16-18	16	—	18-30
Hamster	8-12	8-10	—	8	3-5	15-25
Mouse	12-18	15	—	45-55	5-25	16-20
Prairie dog	2-4	—	—	—	—	—
Rat	5-6	≥10-12	—	—	5-25	12-27

TABLE 9-16 Zoonotic Diseases in Rodents.[9,17,54,86]

Species	Potential Zoonotic Disease
Chinchilla	*Listeria monocytogenes*
	Lymphocytic choriomeningitis (LCM); rare
	Dermatophytes (*Trichophyton mentagrophytes, Microsporum canis, M. gypseum*)
	Baylisascaris procyonis
Gerbil	Salmonellosis; rare
	Hymenolepis nana; rare

Continued

TABLE 9-16 Zoonotic Diseases in Rodents. (cont'd)

Species	Potential Zoonotic Disease
Guinea pig	Allergies (cutaneous and respiratory) to dander and urinary proteins
	Bordetella, salmonellosis, *Yersinia pseudotuberculosis*, *Streptococcus*; rare
	Dermatophyte (*Trichophyton mentagrophytes*)
	Sarcoptic mites (*Trixacarus caviae*, *Sarcoptes scabei*)
Hamster	Salmonellosis, *Acinetobacter*
	Lymphocytic choriomeningitis (LCM); rare
	Dermatophytes (*Trichophyton mentagrophytes*, *Microsporum* spp.)
	Hymenolepis nana
Mouse	Allergies (cutaneous and respiratory) to dander and urinary proteins
	Salmonellosis; rare
	Lymphocytic choriomeningitis (LCM); rare
Prairie dog	*Clostridium piliforme*, *Pasteurella multocida*, salmonellosis, *Yersinia pseudotuberculosis*, *Y. pestis*, *Y. enterocolitica*
	Hantavirus (wild-caught), rabies virus (wild-caught)
	Dermatophytes (*Trichophyton mentagrophytes*, *Microsporum gypseum*)
	Various ectoparasites (mites, fleas, lice)
Rat	Allergies (cutaneous and respiratory) to dander and urinary proteins
	Leptospirosis, salmonellosis, cestodiasis, streptococcal infection
	Hemorrhagic fever, sylvatic plague (vector: rat fleas), St. Louis encephalitis (vector: *Liponyssus sylviarum*), rat bite fever (*Streptobacillus moniliformis*)

TABLE 9-17 Disease Testing in Rodents.[114]

Laboratory	Test
Animal Health Diagnostic Center College of Veterinary Medicine Cornell University 240 Farrier Rd. Ithaca, NY 14853, USA 607-253-3900 Email: diagcenter@cornell.edu www.diagcenter.vet.cornell.edu	Serum neutralization and direct fluorescence for canine distemper virus, *Giardia* and *Cryptosporidium* antigen ELISA, fungal serology
Charles River Research Animal Diagnostic Services 251 Ballardvale St. Wilmington, MA 01887, USA 800-338-9680 (US and Canada) 888-319-5343 (Europe) www.criver.com	Serology and PCR for rodents

TABLE 9-17 Disease Testing in Rodents. (cont'd)

Laboratory	Test
Comparative Pathology Laboratory University of California Davis 1000 Old Davis Rd, Bldg R-1 Davis, CA 95616, USA (530) 752-2832 Email: cpl@ucdavis.edu https://cpl.ucdavis.edu/	Anatomic and clinical pathology, serology, microbiology, parasitology, and molecular diagnostics
IDEXX BioAnalytics (was RADIL) 4011 Discovery Drive Columbia, MO 65201, USA 800-669-0825 Email: idexxbioanalytics@idexx.com https://www.idexxbioanalytics.com/animal-health-monitoring Europe: Email: idexxbioanalytics-europe@idexx.com http://www.idexxbioanalytics.eu	PCR, serology, microbiology, and pathology testing for rodents
University of Georgia 110 Riverbend Rd. Athens, GA 30602, USA 706-542-5812 https://vet.uga.edu/diagnostic-service-labs/infectious-diseases-lab/	PCR for *Salmonella* and *Pasteurella*, serology for *Pasteurella*, Aleutian disease virus ELISA
University of Miami–Comparative Pathology RMSB 1600 NW 10th Avenue Room 7101-A Miami, FL 33136, USA 800-596-7390 Email: compathlab@med.miami.edu http://cpl.med.miami.edu/	Serology for rodents, *Giardia* and *Cryptosporidium* antigen ELISA
Zoologix Inc 9811 Owensmouth Avenue, Suite 4 Chatsworth, CA 91311, USA 818-717-8880 Email: info@zoologix.com http://www.zoologix.com/	Extensive list of avian, primate, wildlife, and rodent PCR tests

TABLE 9-18 Endocrine Values in Rodents.[54,57,83]

Test	Guinea Pig	Syrian Hamster	Mouse	Rat
Free plasma cortisol (μg/dL)	0.6-5.8	0.5-1	—	—
Salivary cortisol[a] (ng/mL)	Baseline: 6.6 ± 3.4	—	—	—

Continued

TABLE 9-18 Endocrine Values in Rodents. (cont'd)

Test	Guinea Pig	Syrian Hamster	Mouse	Rat
Salivary cortiso[a] (ng/mL) (cont'd)	Post-ACTH stim: 157 ± 53	—	—	—
Total serum T4 (μg/dL)	2.26-5.82[57]	3.6	3.08-4.74	3.4-6.22
Free T4 (ng/dL)	1.26-2.03	3-7	—	2.212 ± 0.055
Total T3 (ng/dL)	39-44	45.45	84.42-110.39	M: 66 ± 35 F: 83 ± 3
Free T3 (ng/dL)	0.221-0.26	30-80	52-77.9	208.49 ± 8.55 (pg/dL)
Calcitonin (pg/mL)	—	—	—	200–1000
Parathyroid hormone (pg/mL)	—	—	—	M: 140-180 F: <50-400
1,25-Dihydroxy vitamin D (pg/mL)	—	—	—	M: 120 ± 24 F: 96 ± 17
Aldosterone (ng/dL)	—	—	—	M: 12-35 (late light period) 4-11 (middle light period) F: 25-35 (9-10 a.m.)
Progesterone (ng/mL)	—	1.0 (basal) 10-12 (proestrus) 6-8 (estrus, diestrus	5 (early proestrus) 35 (late proestrus, estrus)	1-5 (early proestrus) 40-50 (estrus) 20-30 (first diestrus day)
Estradiol (pg/mL)	—	5-10 (basal) 300–400 (proestrus)	1-5 (basal)	<10 (basal) 20-30 (2nd diestrus day) 40–50 (proestrus)
Testosterone (ng/mL)	—	1.5-2.0	1.5-2.0	3 (1330-1600 hr) <1 (2130 hr)

[a]For ACTH stimulation test, inject 20 U ACTH IM; repeat sample 4 hr postinjection.

TABLE 9-19 Echocardiographic Measurements in Rodents.[26,71,105,114,140,175]

Parameters	Chinchilla	Guinea Pig[a]	Hamster[a]	Mouse[a]	Rat[a]
Left ventricular internal diameter in diastole (mm)	Manual restraint: 5.9 ± 0.8 Isoflurane: 6.4 ± 0.5	6.49-7.21	3.7-4.5	3.48-3.66	5.93-6.43
Left ventricular internal diameter in systole (mm)	Manual restraint: 2.9 ± 0.6 Isoflurane: 3.8 ± 0.5	4.18-4.52	1.9-2.7	2.26-2.42	4.08-4.42

TABLE 9-19 Echocardiographic Measurements in Rodents. (cont'd)

Parameters	Chinchilla	Guinea Pig	Hamster	Mouse	Rat
Thickness of left ventricular free wall in diastole (mm)	1.8-3.1	1.44-2.06	0.9-1.1	0.41-0.43	1.12-1.7
Thickness of left ventricular free wall in systole (mm)	—	1.91-2.61	—	0.86-0.92	2.02-2.7
Thickness of interventricular septum in diastole (mm)	Manual restraint: 2.4 ± 0.4 Isoflurane: 2.6 ± 0.2	1.88-2.68	0.9-1.1	0.42-0.44	1.06-1.36
Thickness of interventricular septum in systole (mm)	—	2.22-3.38	—	0.89-0.93	1.4-1.9
Left atrial diameter (mm)	Manual restraint: 5.3 ± 0.6 Isoflurane: 4.9 ± 0.6 (cm)	4.61-5.29	—	—	—
Aortic diameter (mm)	Manual restraint: 4.1 ± 0.4 (cm) Isoflurane: 3.6 ± 0.5	4.4-4.9	—	—	—
FS, %	Manual restraint: 50 ± 8 Isoflurane: 40 ± 5	—	—	—	—
LA/Ao ratio[a]	Manual restraint: 1.28 ± 0.13 Isoflurane: 1.38 ± 0.2	—	—	—	—

[a]Measurements obtained in anesthetized animals.

TABLE 9-20 Electrocardiographic Measurements in Rodents.[71,167]

Parameters	Guinea Pig	Prairie Dog, Black Tailed
P wave duration (sec)	0.015-0.035	0.02-0.03
P wave amplitude	0.01	0.01-0.06
P-R interval (sec)	0.048-0.06	0.04-0.06
QRS duration (sec)	0.008-0.046	0.02
QRS wave amplitude	1.1-1.9	0.1-1.15
QT interval (sec)	0.106-0.144	0.1-0.14
T wave amplitude	0.062	—
Mean electrical axis (degrees)	120 to 180	–15 to +120

REFERENCES

1. Abreu M, Aguado D, Benito J, et al. Reduction of the sevoflurane minimum alveolar concentration induced by methadone, tramadol, butorphanol and morphine in rats. *Lab Anim.* 2012;46:200–206.
2. Adamcak A, Otten B. Rodent therapeutics. *Vet Clin North Am Exot Anim Pract.* 2000;3:221–237.
3. Aguiar J, Mogridge G, Hall J. Femoral fracture repair and sciatic and femoral nerve blocks in a guinea pig. *J Small Anim Pract.* 2014;55:635–639.
4. Albrecht M, Henke J, Tacke S, et al. Effects of isoflurane, ketamine-xylazine and a combination of medetomidine, midazolam and fentanyl on physiological variables continuously measured by telemetry in wistar rats. *BMC Vet Res.* 2014;10:198.
5. Alemán-Laporte J, Bandini LA, Garcia-Gomes MS, et al. Combination of ketamine and xylazine with opioids and acepromazine in rats: physiological changes and their analgesic effect analysed by ultrasonic vocalization. *Lab Anim.* 2020;54:171–182.
6. Alkis I, Cetin Y, Sendag S, et al. Long term suppression of oestrus and prevention of pregnancy by deslorelin implant in rats. *Bull Vet Inst Pulawy.* 2011;55:237–240.
7. Allweiler SI. How to improve anesthesia and analgesia in small mammals. *Vet Clin North Am Exot Anim Pract.* 2016;19:361–377.
8. Alper CM, Doyle WJ, Seroky JT, et al. Efficacy of clarithromycin treatment of acute otitis media caused by infection with penicillin-susceptible, -intermediate, and -resistant Streptococcus pneumoniae in the chinchilla. *Antimicrob Agents Chemother.* 1996;40:1889–1892.
9. Anderson NL. Pet rodents. In: Birchard SJ, Sherding RG, eds. *Saunders Manual of Small Animal Practice.* St. Louis, MO: Elsevier; 2006:1881–1909.
10. Arenillas M, Gomez De Segura IA. Anaesthetic effects of alfaxalone administered intraperitoneally alone or combined with dexmedetomidine and fentanyl in the rat. *Lab Anim.* 2018;52:588–598.
11. Babl FE, Pelton SI, Li Z. Experimental acute otitis media due to nontypeable *Haemophilus influenzae*: comparison of high and low azithromycin doses with placebo. *Antimicrob Agents Chemother.* 2002;46:2194–2199.
12. Bauer C, Schillinger U, Brandl J, et al. Comparison of pre-emptive butorphanol or metamizole with ketamine + medetomidine and s-ketamine + medetomidine anaesthesia in improving intraoperative analgesia in mice. *Lab Anim.* 2019;53:459–469.
13. Baumans V, Havenaar R, Van Herck H, et al. The effectiveness of Ivomec and Neguvon in the control of murine mites. *Lab Anim.* 1988;22:243–245.
14. Beck W, Pantchev N. *Praktische Parasitologie bei Heimtieren.* Hannover, Germany: Schluetersche Verlagsgesellschaft MBH & Co; 2006.
15. Beco L, Petite A, Olivry T. Comparison of subcutaneous ivermectin and oral moxidectin for the treatment of notoedric acariasis in hamsters. *Vet Rec.* 2001;149:324–327.
16. Bellini L, Banzato T, Contiero B, et al. Evaluation of three medetomidine-based protocols for chemical restraint and sedation for non-painful procedures in companion rats (*Rattus norvegicus*). *Vet J.* 2014;200:456–458.
17. Birchard SJ, Sherding RG. *Saunders Manual of Small Animal Practice.* 3rd ed. St. Louis, MO: Saunders Elsevier; 2006.
18. Bishop CR. Reproductive medicine of rabbits and rodents. *Vet Clin North Am Exot Anim Pract.* 2002;5:507–535.
19. Britti D, Crupi R, Impellizzeri D, et al. A novel composite formulation of palmitoylethanolamide and quercetin decreases inflammation and relieves pain in inflammatory and osteoarthritic pain models. *BMC Vet Res.* 2017;13:229.
20. Browning GR, Eshar D, Beaufrère H. Comparison of dexmedetomidine-ketamine-midazolam and isoflurane for anesthesia of black-tailed prairie dogs (*Cynomys ludovicianus*). *J Am Assoc Lab Anim Sci.* 2019;58:50–57.
21. Burgmann P, Percy DH. Antimicrobial drug use in rodents and rabbits. In: Prescott JF, Baggot JD, eds. *Antimicrobial Therapy in Veterinary Medicine.* 2nd ed. Ames, IA: Iowa State University Press; 1993:524–541.

22. Burnside WM, Flecknell PA, Cameron AI, et al. A comparison of medetomidine and its active enantiomer dexmedetomidine when administered with ketamine in mice. *BMC Vet Res*. 2013;9:48.
23. Cantwell SL. Ferret, rabbit, and rodent anesthesia. *Vet Clin North Am Exot Anim Pract*. 2001;4:169–190.
24. Carter KK, Hietala S, Brooks DL, et al. Tylosin concentrations in rat serum and lung tissue after administration in drinking water. *Lab Anim Sci*. 1987;37:468–470.
25. Cavaretta M. Therapeutic review: milk thistle. *J Exot Pet Med*. 2015;24:470–472.
26. Çetin N, Çetin E, Toker M. Echocardiographic variables in healthy guinea pigs anaesthetized with ketamine-xylazine. *Lab Anim*. 2005;39:100–106.
27. Cetin Y, Alkis I, Sendag S, et al. Long-term effect of deslorelin implant on ovarian pre-antral follicles and uterine histology in female rats. *Reprod Domest Anim*. 2013;48:195–199.
28. Chan KH, Swarts JD, Doyle WJ, et al. Efficacy of a new macrolide (azithromycin) for acute otitis media in the chinchilla model. *Arch Otolaryngol Head Neck Surg*. 1988;114:1266–1269.
29. Chandrasekar P, Cutright J, Manavathu E. Efficacy of voriconazole against invasive pulmonary aspergillosis in a guinea-pig model. *J Antimicrob Chemother*. 2000;45:673–676.
30. Chum HH, Jampachairsri K, Mckeon GP, et al. Antinociceptive effects of sustained-release buprenorphine in a model of incisional pain in rats (*Rattus norvegicus*). *J Am Assoc Lab Anim Sci*. 2014;53:193–197.
31. Crupi R, Gugliandolo E, Siracusa R, et al. N-acetyl-l-cysteine reduces leishmania amazonensis-induced inflammation in balb/c mice. *BMC Vet Res*. 2020;16:13.
32. Cruz JI, Loste JM, Burzaco OH. Observations on the use of medetomidine/ketamine and its reversal with atipamezole for chemical restraint in the mouse. *Lab Anim*. 1998;32:18–22.
33. Cullin CO, Sellers MS, Rogers ER, et al. Intestinal parasites and anthelmintic treatments in a laboratory colony of wild-caught African pouched rats. *Comp Med*. 2017;67:420–429.
34. Da Cruz CL, Alpino T, Kottwitz J. Recurrent ear mite (*Otodectes cynotis*) infestation in three related groups of patagonian cavies (*Dolichotis patagonum*). *J Zoo Wildl Med*. 2017;48:484–490.
35. Dias S, Anselmi C, Casanova M, et al. Clinical and pathological findings in 2 rats (*Rattus norvegicus*) with dilated cardiomyopathy. *J Exot Pet Med*. 2017;26:205–212.
36. Donnelly T. Mice and rats as pets *Merck Veterinary Manual*. 11th ed. Kenilworth, NJ: Merck & Co; 2016. https://www.merckvetmanual.com/en-ca/exotic-and-laboratory-animals/rodents/mice-and-rats-as-pets Accessed September 30, 2020.
37. Doss GA, Mans C, Houseright RA, et al. Urinalysis in chinchillas (*Chinchilla lanigera*). *J Am Vet Med Assoc*. 2016;248:901–907.
38. Doss GA, Mans C, Stepien RL. Echocardiographic effects of dexmedetomidine-ketamine in chinchillas (*Chinchilla lanigera*). *Lab Anim*. 2017;51:89–92.
39. Erhardt W, Wohlrab S, Kilic N, et al. Comparison of the anaesthesia combinations racemic-ketamine/medetomidine and s-ketamine/medetomidine in syrian golden hamsters (*Mesocricetus auratus*). *Vet Anaesth Analg*. 2001;28:212–213.
40. Erichsen HK, Hao J-X, Xu X-J, et al. Comparative actions of the opioid analgesics morphine, methadone and codeine in rat models of peripheral and central neuropathic pain. *Pain*. 2005;116:347–358.
41. Erickson RL, Blevins CE, Souza Dyer C, et al. Alfaxalone-xylazine anesthesia in laboratory mice. *J Am Assoc Lab Anim Sci*. 2019;58:30–39.
42. Eshar D, Bdolah-Abram T. Comparison of efficacy, safety, and convenience of selamectin versus ivermectin for treatment of Trixacarus caviae mange in pet guinea pigs (*Cavia porcellus*). *J Am Vet Med Assoc*. 2012;241:1056–1058.
43. Eshar D, Beaufrère H. Anesthetic effects of alfaxalone-ketamine, alfaxalone-ketamine-dexmedetomidine, and alfaxalone-butorphanol-midazolam administered intramuscularly in five-striped palm squirrels (*Funambulus pennantii*). *J Am Assoc Lab Anim Sci*. 2020;59:384–392.
43a. Eshar D, Gardhouse SM. Prairie dogs. In: Quesenberry KE, Orcutt CJ, Mans C et al., eds. *Ferrets, Rabbits and Rodents: Clinical Medicine and Surgery*. St. Louis, MO: Elsevier; 2021:334–344.

44. Eshar D, Pohlman LM, Harkin KR. Urine properties of captive black-tailed prairie dogs (*Cynomys ludovicianus*). *J Exot Pet Med.* 2016;25:213–219.
45. Evenson EA, Mans C. Analgesic efficacy and safety of hydromorphone in chinchillas (*Chinchilla lanigera*). *J Am Assoc Lab Anim Sci.* 2018;57:282–285.
45a. Evenson EA, Mans C. Antinociceptive efficacy and safety of subcutaneous tramadol in chinchillas (*Chinchilla langera*). *J Exot Pet Med.* 2019;28:98–104.
46. Ewringmann A, Gloeckner B. *Leitsymptome bei Meerschweinchen, Chinchilla und Degu.* Stuttgart, Germany: Enke; 2012.
47. Ewringmann A, Gloeckner B. *Leitsymptome bei Hamster, Ratte, Maus und Rennmaus.* Stuttgart, Germany: Enke; 2014.
48. Fehr M, Sassenburg L, Zwart P. *Krankheiten der Heimtiere.* 8th ed. Hannover, Germany: Schluetersche Verlagsgesellschaft; 2015.
49. Fisher PG. Exotic mammal renal disease: diagnosis and treatment. *Vet Clin North Am Exot Anim Pract.* 2006;9:69–96.
50. Flecknell P. Rodent analgesia: assessment and therapeutics. *Vet J.* 2018;232:70–77.
51. Flecknell PA. Analgesia and post-operative care. *Laboratory Animal Anaesthesia.* 2016:141–192.
52. Foletto VR, Vanz F, Gazarini L, et al. Efficacy and security of ivermectin given orally to rats naturally infected with *Syphacia* spp., *Giardia* spp. and *Hymenolepis nana. Lab Anim.* 2015;49:196–200.
53. Foley PL, Kendall LV, Turner PV. Clinical management of pain in rodents. *Comp Med.* 2019;69:468–489.
54. Fox JG, Anderson LC, Otto GM, et al. *Laboratory Animal Medicine.* 3rd ed. Amsterdam, Netherlands: Elsevier/Academic Press; 2015.
55. Fox L, Mans C. Analgesic efficacy and safety of buprenorphine in chinchillas (*Chinchilla lanigera*). *J Am Assoc Lab Anim Sci.* 2018;57:286–290.
56. Fox L, Snyder LB. Mans C. Comparison of dexmedetomidine-ketamine with isoflurane for anesthesia of chinchillas (*Chinchilla lanigera*). *J Am Assoc Lab Anim Sci.* 2016;55:312–316.
57. Fredholm DV, Cagle LA, Johnston MS. Evaluation of precision and establishment of reference ranges for plasma thyroxine using a point-of-care analyzer in healthy guinea pigs. *J Exot Pet Med.* 2012;21:87–93.
58. Frohlich J. Rats and mice. In: Quesenberry KE, Orcutt CJ, Mans C et al., eds. *Ferrets, Rabbits, and Rodents: Clinical Medicine and Surgery.* 4th ed. St. Louis, MO: Elsevier; 2021:345–367.
59. Gaertner DJ, Hallman TM, Hankenson FC, et al. Anesthesia and analgesia for laboratory rodents. In: Brown MJ, Danneman PJ, Karas AZ, eds. *Anesthesia and Analgesia in Laboratory Animals.* 2nd ed. San Diego, CA: Academic Press; 2008:239–297.
60. Gardhouse S, Eshar D. Diagnosis and successful treatment of Eimeria infection in a group of zoo-kept black-tailed prairie dogs (*Cynomys ludovicianus*). *J Zoo Wildl Med.* 2015;46:367–369.
61. Glen JB. Animal studies of the anaesthetic activity of ICI 35 868. *Br J Anaesth.* 1980;52:731–742.
62. Goebel T, Erwingmann A. *Heimtierkrankheiten: Kleinsaeuger, Amphibien, Reptilien.* Stuttgart, Germany: UTB Publishing; 2005.
63. Gönenç B, Sarimehmetoğlu HO, Iça A, et al. Efficacy of selamectin against mites (*Myobia musculi, Mycoptes musculinus and Radfordia ensifera*) and nematodes (*Aspiculuris tetraptera* and *Syphacia obvelata*) in mice. *Lab Anim.* 2006;40:210–213.
64. Griggs RB, Bardo MT, Taylor BK. Gabapentin alleviates affective pain after traumatic nerve injury. *Neuroreport.* 2015;26:522.
65. Grosset C, Peters S, Peron F, et al. Contraceptive effect and potential side-effects of deslorelin acetate implants in rats (*Rattus norvegicus*): preliminary observations. *Can J Vet Res.* 2012;76:209–214.
66. Harkness JE. *A Practitioner's Guide to Domestic Rodents.* Lakewood, CO: American Animal Hospital Association; 1993.
67. Hauptman K, Jekl V, Knotek Z. Use of medetomidine for sedation in the laboratory rat (*Rattus norvegicus*). *Act Vet Brno.* 2003;72:583–591.

68. Hawkins MG, Pascoe PJ. Anesthesia, analgesia and sedation of small mammals. In: Quesenberry KE, Orcutt CJ, Mans C et al., eds. *Ferrets, Rabbits and Rodents: Clinical Medicine and Surgery*. 4th ed. St. Louis, MO: Elsevier; 2021:536–558.
69. Hayes KE, Raucci Jr JA, Gades NM, et al. An evaluation of analgesic regimens for abdominal surgery in mice. *J Am Assoc Lab Anim Sci*. 2000;39:18–23.
70. Healy JR, Tonkin JL, Kamarec SR, et al. Evaluation of an improved sustained-release buprenorphine formulation for use in mice. *Am J Vet Res*. 2014;75:619–625.
71. Heatley JJ. Cardiovascular anatomy, physiology, and disease of rodents and small exotic mammals. *Vet Clin North Am Exot Anim Pract*. 2009;12:99–113.
72. Heckeroth AR, Lutz J, Mertens C, et al. Isoxazoline compositions and their use as antiparasitics. *Google Patents*. 2008. https://patents.google.com/patent/JP2017222692A/en Accessed May 2, 2021.
73. Heng K, Marx JO, Jampachairsi K, et al. Continuous rate infusion of alfaxalone during ketamine-xylazine anesthesia in rats. *J Am Assoc Lab Anim Sci*. 2020;59:170–175.
74. Henke J, Baumgartner C, Roltgen I, et al. Anaesthesia with midazolam/medetomidine/fentanyl in chinchillas (*Chinchilla lanigera*) compared to anaesthesia with xylazine/ketamine and medetomidine/ketamine. *J Vet Med A Physiol Pathol Clin Med*. 2004;51:259–264.
75. Hess LR, Ravich ML, Reavill DR. Diagnosis and treatment of an insulinoma in a guinea pig (*Cavia porcellus*). *J Am Vet Med Assoc*. 2013;242:522–526.
76. Hestehave S, Munro G, Pedersen TB, et al. Antinociceptive effects of voluntarily ingested buprenorphine in the hot-plate test in laboratory rats. *Lab Anim*. 2017;51:264–272.
77. Higuchi S, Yamada R, Hashimoto A, et al. Evaluation of a combination of alfaxalone with medetomidine and butorphanol for inducing surgical anesthesia in laboratory mice. *Jpn J Vet Res*. 2016;64:131–139.
78. Hillyer EV, Quesenberry KE, eds. *Ferrets, Rabbits, and Rodents: Clinical Medicine and Surgery*. Philadelphia, PA: W.B. Saunders; 1997.
79. Hoefer HL. Chinchillas. *Vet Clin North Am Small Anim Pract*. 1994;24:103–111.
80. Huckins GL, Eshar D, Shrader T, et al. Anesthetic effect of dexmedetomidine-ketamine-midazolam combination administered intramuscularly to zoo-housed naked mole-rats. *J Zoo Wildl Anim Med*. 2020;51:59–66.
81. Huerkamp M. Anesthesia and postoperative management of rabbits and pocket pets. In: Bonagura JD, ed. *Kirk's Current Veterinary Therapy XII Small Animal Practice*. Philadelphia, PA: W.B. Saunders; 1995:1322–1327.
82. Jekl V. Personal communication; 2016.
83. Jepson L. *Exotic Animal Medicine: A Quick Reference Guide*. New York, NY: WB Saunders; 2009.
84. Jirkof P, Tourvieille A, Cinelli P, et al. Buprenorphine for pain relief in mice: repeated injections vs sustained-release depot formulation. *Lab Anim*. 2015;49:177–187.
85. Johnson RA. Voluntary running-wheel activity, arterial blood gases, and thermal antinociception in rats after 3 buprenorphine formulations. *J Am Assoc Lab Anim Sci*. 2016;55:306–311.
86. Johnson-Delaney CA. Zoonotic parasites of selected exotic animals. *Sem Avian Exot Pet Med*. 1996;5:115–124.
87. Johnson-Delaney CA. Postoperative management of small mammals. *ExoticDVM*. 1999;1(5):19–21.
88. Jones CK, Peters SC, Shannon HE. Efficacy of duloxetine, a potent and balanced serotonergic and noradrenergic reuptake inhibitor, in inflammatory and acute pain models in rodents. *J Pharmacol Exp Ther*. 2005;312:726–732.
89. Kang SC, Jampachaisri K, Seymour TL, et al. Use of liposomal bupivacaine for postoperative analgesia in an incisional pain model in rats (*Rattus norvegicus*). *J Am Assoc Lab Anim Sci*. 2017;56:63–68.
90. Kawai S, Takagi Y, Kaneko S, et al. Effect of three types of mixed anesthetic agents alternate to ketamine in mice. *Exp Anim*. 2011;60:481–487.

91. Kendall LV, Wegenast DJ, Smith BJ, et al. Efficacy of sustained-release buprenorphine in an experimental laparotomy model in female mice. *J Am Assoc Lab Anim Sci.* 2016;55:66–73.
92. Kilic N, Henke J, Erhardt W. Ketamine/medetomidine-anaesthesia in the hamster: a clinical comparison between the subcutaneous and intraperitoneal way of application. *Tierärztliche Praxis Kleintiere.* 2004;32:384–388.
93. Kirihara Y, Takechi M, Kurosaki K, et al. Effects of an anesthetic mixture of medetomidine, midazolam, and butorphanol in rats-strain difference and antagonism by atipamezole. *Exp Anim.* 2016;65:27–36.
94. Klement P, Augustine JM, Delaney KH, et al. An oral ivermectin regimen that eradicates pinworms (*Syphacia* spp.) in laboratory rats and mice. *Lab Anim Sci.* 1996;46:286–290.
95. Knafo ES. Sildenafil citrate as a pulmonary protectant in chronic murine *Mycoplasma pulmonis* infection. *Proc Assoc Exot Mam Vet.* 2014;6.
96. Kohutova S, Jekl V, Knotek Z, et al. The effect of deslorelin acetate on the oestrous cycle of female guinea pigs. *Veterinarni Medicina.* 2015;60:155–160.
97. Kunzel F, Hierlmeier B, Christian M, et al. Hyperthyroidism in four guinea pigs: clinical manifestations, diagnosis, and treatment. *J Small Anim Pract.* 2013;54:667–671.
98. Laird KL, Swindle MM, Flecknell PA. *Handbook of Rodent and Rabbit Medicine.* New York, NY: Pergamon; 1996.
99. Lau C, Ranasinghe MG, Shiels I, et al. Plasma pharmacokinetics of alfaxalone after a single intraperitoneal or intravenous injection of Alfaxan® in rats. *J Vet Pharmacol Ther.* 2013;36: 516–520.
100. Le K. Maropitant. *J Exot Pet Med.* 2017;26:305–309.
101. Levin-Arama M, Abraham L, Waner T, et al. Subcutaneous compared with intraperitoneal ketamine-xylazine for anesthesia of mice. *J Am Assoc Lab Anim Sci.* 2016;55(6):794–800.
102. Lichtenberger M, Lennox AM. Critical care of the exotic companion mammal (with a focus on herbivorous species): the first twenty-four hours. *J Exot Pet Med.* 2012;21:284–292.
103. Liles JH, Flecknell PA. A comparison of the effects of buprenorphine, carprofen and flunixin following laparotomy in rats. *J Vet Pharmacol Ther.* 1994;17:284–290.
104. Lim AAT, Greinwald Jr JH, Lorenz F, et al. Poster 12: The effect of pentoxifylline on the healing of guinea pig tympanic membrane. *Otolaryngol–Head Neck Surg.* 1996;115(2):127.
105. Linde A, Summerfield NJ, Johnston MS, et al. Echocardiography in the chinchilla. *J Vet Intern Med.* 2004;18:772–774.
106. Longley L. Rodent anaesthesia. In: Longley L, ed. *Anaesthesia of Exotic Pets.* Philadelphia, PA: Saunders Elsevier; 2008:59–84.
107. Mans C. Personal communication; 2016.
108. Mans C, Jekl V. Anatomy and disorders of the oral cavity of chinchillas and degus. *Vet Clin North Am Exot Anim Pract.* 2016;19:843–869.
109. Mantovani S, Allan N, Pesapane R, et al. Eradication of a tropical rat mite (*Ornithonyssus bacoti*) infestation from a captive colony of endangered amargosa voles (*Microtus californicus scirpensis*). *J Zoo Wildl Med.* 2018;49:475–479.
110. Markova L, Umek N, Horvat S, et al. Neurotoxicity of bupivacaine and liposome bupivacaine after sciatic nerve block in healthy and streptozotocin-induced diabetic mice. *BMC Vet Res.* 2020;16:247.
111. Marroquin SC, Eshar D, Browning GR, et al. Diagnosis and successful treatment of Eimeria infection in a pair of pet domestic rats (*Rattus norvegicus*) with ponazuril. *J Exot Pet Med.* 2020;33:31–33.
112. Marx JO, Vudathala D, Murphy L, et al. Antibiotic administration in the drinking water of mice. *J Am Assoc Lab Anim Sci.* 2014;53:301–306.
113. Mayer J. The use of GnRH to treat cystic ovaries in a guinea pig. *Exotic DVM.* 2003;3:36.
114. Mayer J. Rodents. In: Carpenter JW, ed. *Exotic Animal Formulary.* 4th ed. St. Louis, MO: Saunders/Elsevier; 2013:476–516.
115. Mayer J, Sato A, Kiupel M, et al. Extralabel use of cabergoline in the treatment of a pituitary adenoma in a rat. *J Am Vet Med Assoc.* 2011;239:656–660.

116. Mayer J, Wagner R, Mitchell MA, et al. Use of recombinant human thyroid-stimulating hormone for evaluation of thyroid function in guinea pigs (*Cavia porcellus*). *J Am Vet Med Assoc.* 2013;242:346–349.
117. Mayer J, Wagner R, Taeymans O. Advanced diagnostic approaches and current management of thyroid pathologies in guinea pigs. *Vet Clin North Am Exot Anim Pract.* 2010;13:509–523.
118. Mcclure JT, Rosin E. Comparison of amikacin dosing regimens in neutropenic guinea pigs with *Escherichia coli* infection. *Am J Vet Res.* 1998;59:750–755.
119. Meert TF, Vermeirsch HA. A preclinical comparison between different opioids: antinociceptive versus adverse effects. *Pharmacol Biochem Behav.* 2005;80:309–326.
120. Mehlhorn H, Schmahl G, Frese M, et al. Effects of a combinations of emodepside and praziquantel on parasites of reptiles and rodents. *Parasitol Res.* 2005;97(Suppl 1):S65–S69.
121. Melo ME, Silva CA, De Souza Gomes WD, et al. Immediate tooth replantation in rats: effect of systemic antibiotic therapy with amoxicillin and tetracycline. *Clin Oral Invest.* 2016;20:523–532.
122. Meredith A. *BSAVA Small Animal Formulary: Part B: Exotic Pets.* Quedgeley, Gloucester, UK: British Small Animal Veterinary Association; 2015.
123. Mieth H, Leitner I, Meingassner JG. The efficacy of orally applied terbinafine, itraconazole and fluconazole in models of experimental trichophytoses. *J Med Vet Mycol.* 1994;32:181–188.
124. Millecamps M, Jourdan D, Leger S, et al. Circadian pattern of spontaneous behavior in monarthritic rats: a novel global approach to evaluation of chronic pain and treatment effectiveness. *Arthritis Rheum.* 2005;52:3470–3478.
125. Miller AL, Richardson CA. Rodent analgesia. *Vet Clin North Am Exot Anim Pract.* 2011;14:81–92.
126. Mills PO, Tansey CO, Genzer SC, et al. Pharmacokinetic profiles of gabapentin after oral and subcutaneous administration in black-tailed prairie dogs. *J Am Assoc Lab Anim Sci.* 2020;59:305–309.
127. Mitchell MA, Tully JrTN, eds. *Manual of Exotic Pet Practice.* St. Louis, MO: Saunders/Elsevier; 2009.
128. Mook DM, Benjamin KA. Use of selamectin and moxidectin in the treatment of mouse fur mites. *J Am Assoc Lab Anim Sci.* 2008;47:20–24.
129. Morgan RJ, Eddy LB, Solie TN, et al. Ketamine-acepromazine as an anaesthetic agent for chinchillas (*Chinchilla laniger*). *Lab Anim.* 1981;15:281–283.
130. Morrisey JK, Carpenter JW. Formulary. In: Quesenberry KE, Carpenter JW, eds. *Ferrets, Rabbits, and Rodents: Clinical Medicine and Surgery.* 4th ed. St. Louis, MO: Elsevier; 2021:620–630.
131. Munro G. Pharmacological assessment of the rat formalin test utilizing the clinically used analgesic drugs gabapentin, lamotrigine, morphine, duloxetine, tramadol and ibuprofen: Influence of low and high formalin concentrations. *Eur J Pharmacol.* 2009;605:95–102.
132. Nashat MA, Ricart Arbona RJ, Lepherd ML, et al. Ivermectin-compounded feed compared with topical moxidectin-imidacloprid for eradication of *Demodex musculi* in laboratory mice. *J Am Assoc Lab Anim Sci.* 2018;57:483–497.
133. Ness RD. Rodents. In: Carpenter JW, ed. *Exotic Animal Formulary.* 3rd ed. St. Louis, MO: Saunders/Elsevier; 2005:375–408.
134. Oglesbee BL. *Blackwell's Five Minute Veterinary Consult: Small Mammals.* 2nd ed. Chichester, West Sussex: Wiley-Blackwell; 2011.
135. Oliver VL, Athavale S, Simon KE, et al. Evaluation of pain assessment techniques and analgesia efficacy in a female guinea pig. *J Am Assoc Lab Anim Sci.* 2017;56:425–435.
136. Page CD, Sarabia-Estrada R, Hoffman RJ, et al. Lack of absorption of a sustained-release buprenorphine formulation administered subcutaneously to athymic nude rats. *J Am Assoc Lab Anim Sci.* 2019;58:597–600.
137. Parkinson L, Mans C. Anesthetic and postanesthetic effects of alfaxalone-butorphanol compared with dexmedetomidine–ketamine in chinchillas (*Chinchilla lanigera*). *J Am Assoc Lab Anim Sci.* 2017;56:290–295.
138. Petersen NT. Therapeutic review: Terbutaline. *J Exot Pet Med.* 2012;21:260–263.

138a. Pignon C, Mayer J. Guinea pigs. In: Quesenberry KE, Orcutt CJ, Mans C et al., eds. *Ferrets, Rabbits and Rodents: Clinical Medicine and Surgery*. 4th ed. St. Louis, MO: Elsevier; 2021:270–297.

139. Plunkett SJ. *Emergency Procedures for the Small Animal Veterinarian*. 3rd ed. London, UK: Elsevier; 2013.

140. Quesenberry K, Mans C, Orcutt C, et al. *Ferrets, Rabbits, and Rodents: Clinical Medicine and Surgery*. 4th ed. St. Louis, MO: Elsevier; 2021.

141. Quesenberry KE. Guinea pigs. *Vet Clin North Am Small Anim Pract*. 1994;24:67–87.

142. Ratliff C, Zaffarano B. Generalized edema and chylothorax in a 5-year-old female intact chinchilla (*Chinchilla lanigera*). *J Exot Pet Med*. 2017;26:219–223.

143. Reddyjarugu B, Pavek T, Southard T, et al. Analgesic efficacy of firocoxib, a selective inhibitor of cyclooxygenase 2, in a mouse model of incisional pain. *J Am Assoc Lab Anim Sci*. 2015;54:405–410.

144. Redrobe S. Imaging techniques in small mammals. *Sem Avian Exot Pet Med*. 2001;10:187–197.

145. Richardson VCG. *Diseases of Small Domestic Rodents*. Malden, MA: Blackwell Scientific; 1997.

146. Rivard AL, Simura KJ, Mohammed S, et al. Rat intubation and ventilation for surgical research. *J Invest Surg*. 2006;19:267–274.

147. Roach PD, Wallis PM, Olson ME. The use of metronidazole, tinidazole and dimetridazole in eliminating trichomonads from laboratory mice. *Lab Anim*. 1988;22:361–364.

148. Roughan JV, Flecknell PA. Behavioural effects of laparotomy and analgesic effects of ketoprofen and carprofen in rats. *Pain*. 2001;90:65–74.

149. Roughan JV, Flecknell PA. Behaviour-based assessment of the duration of laparotomy-induced abdominal pain and the analgesic effects of carprofen and buprenorphine in rats. *Behav Pharmacol*. 2004;15:461–472.

150. Röthig A, Hermosilla CR, Taubert A, et al. *Pelodera strongyloides* as a cause of severe erythematous dermatitis in 2 guinea pigs (*Cavia porcellus*). *J Exot Pet Med*. 2016;25:208–212.

151. Sadar MJ, Knych HK, Drazenovich TL, et al. Pharmacokinetics of buprenorphine after intravenous and oral transmucosal administration in guinea pigs (*Cavia porcellus*). *Am J Vet Res*. 2018;79:260–266.

152. Sassenburg L. Degu. In: Fehr M, Sassenburg L, Zwart P, eds. *Krankheiten der Heimtiere*. Hannover, Germany: Schluetersche Verlagsgesellschaft; 2015.

153. Schoeb TR. Respiratory diseases of rodents. *Vet Clin North Am Exot Anim Pract*. 2000;3:481–496.

154. Schuetzenhofer G, Goericke-Pesch S, Wehrend A. Effects of deslorelin implants on ovarian cysts in guinea pigs. *Schweizer Archiv für Tierheilkunde*. 2011;153:416–417.

155. Schweigart G. *Arzneimittelanwendung bei Nagetieren und Kanninchen*. 2nd ed. Berlin, Germany: Veterinärmedizinischer Fachverlag; 2009.

156. Seymour TL, Adams SC, Felt SA, et al. Postoperative analgesia due to sustained-release buprenorphine, sustained-release meloxicam, and carprofen gel in a model of incisional pain in rats (*Rattus norvegicus*). *J Am Asso Lab Ani Sci*. 2016;55:300–305.

157. Shientag LJ, Wheeler SM, Garlick DS, et al. A therapeutic dose of ketoprofen causes acute gastrointestinal bleeding, erosions, and ulcers in rats. *J Am Assoc Lab Anim Sci*. 2012;51:832–841.

158. Siriarchavatana P, Ayers JD, Kendall LV. Anesthetic activity of alfaxalone compared with ketamine in mice. *J Am Assoc Lab Anim Sci*. 2016;55:426–430.

159. Smith A, Asa C, Edwards B, et al. Predominant suppression of FSHβ-immunoreactivity after long-term treatment of intact and castrate adult male rats with the GnRH agonist deslorelin. *J Neuroendocrinol*. 2012;24:737–747.

160. Smith LJ, Valenzuela JR, Krugner-Higby LA, et al. A single dose of liposome-encapsulated hydromorphone provides extended analgesia in a rat model of neuropathic pain. *Comp Med*. 2006;56:487–492.

161. Soto C, Perez J, Garcia V, et al. Effect of silymarin on kidneys of rats suffering from alloxan-induced diabetes mellitus. *Phytomedicine*. 2010;17:1090–1094.
162. Sugar AM, Liu X-P. Efficacy of voriconazole in treatment of murine pulmonary blastomycosis. *Antimicrob Agents Chemother*. 2001;45:601–604.
163. Tani K, Iwanaga T, Sonoda K, et al. Ivermectin treatment of demodicosis in 56 hamsters. *J Vet Med Sci*. 2001;63:1245–1247.
164. Taylor BF, Ramirez HE, Battles AH, et al. Analgesic activity of tramadol and buprenorphine after voluntary ingestion by rats (*Rattus norvegicus*). *J Am Assoc Lab Anim Sci*. 2016;55:74–82.
165. Ter Horst EN, Krijnen PAJ, Flecknell P, et al. Sufentanil-medetomidine anaesthesia compared with fentanyl/fluanisone-midazolam is associated with fewer ventricular arrhythmias and death during experimental myocardial infarction in rats and limits infarct size following reperfusion. *Lab Anim*. 2018;52:271–279.
166. Thomas AA, Detilleux J, Sandersen CF, et al. Minimally invasive technique for intrathecal administration of morphine in rats: practicality and antinociceptive properties. *Lab Anim*. 2017;51:479–489.
167. Thomason JD, Eshar D, Zimmer Coyle C, et al. The static electrocardiogram in clinically healthy, anesthetized, zoo-kept black-tailed prairie dogs (*Cynomys ludovicianus*). *J Vet Cardiol*. 2015;17:293–297.
168. Visser C, Wijnbergen A, Bleich A. Maeuse und ratten. In: Fehr M, Sassenburg L, Zwart P, eds. *Krankheiten der Heimtiere*. Hannover, Germany: Schluetersche Verlagsgesellschaft; 2015.
169. Waite ME, Tomkovich A, Quinn TL, et al. Efficacy of common analgesics for postsurgical pain in rats. *J Am Assoc Lab Anim Sci*. 2015;54:420–425.
170. Weiss EE, Evans KD, Griffey SM. Comparison of a fur mite PCR assay and the tape test for initial and posttreatment diagnosis during a natural infection. *J Am Assoc Lab Anim Sci*. 2012;51:574–578.
171. Wellington D, Mikaelian I, Singer L. Comparison of ketamine-xylazine and ketamine-dexmedetomidine anesthesia and intraperitoneal tolerance in rats. *J Am Assoc Lab Anim Sci*. 2013;52:481–487.
172. Wenger S. Anesthesia and analgesia in rabbits and rodents. *J Exot Pet Med*. 2012;21:7–16.
173. Wolfe AM, Kennedy LH, Na JJ, et al. Efficacy of tramadol as a sole analgesic for postoperative pain in male and female mice. *J Am Assoc Lab Anim Sci*. 2015;54:411–419.
174. Wyre NR. Rats, chronic respiratory disease. In: Mayer J, Donnelly TM, eds. *Clinical Veterinary Advisor: Birds and Exotic Pets*. St. Louis, MO: W.B. Saunders; 2013:242–252.
175. Yang X-P, Liu Y-H, Rhaleb N-E, et al. Echocardiographic assessment of cardiac function in conscious and anesthetized mice. *Am J Physiol-Heart Circ Physiol*. 1999;277:H1967–H1974.
176. Zaheer OA, Beaufrère H. Treatment of hyperadrenocorticism in a guinea pig (*Cavia porcellus*). *J Exot Pet Med*. 2020;34:57–61.
177. Zanetti AS, Putta SK, Casebolt DB, et al. Pharmacokinetics and adverse effects of 3 sustained-release buprenorphine dosages in healthy guinea pigs (*Cavia porcellus*). *J Am Assoc Lab Ani Sci*. 2017;56:768–778.
178. Zude BP, Jampachaisri K, Pacharinsak C. Use of flavored tablets of gabapentin and carprofen to attenuate postoperative hypersensitivity in an incisional pain model in rats (*Rattus norvegicus*). *J Am Assoc Lab Anim Sci*. 2020;59:163–169.

Chapter 10 Rabbits

Peter Fisher | Jennifer E. Graham

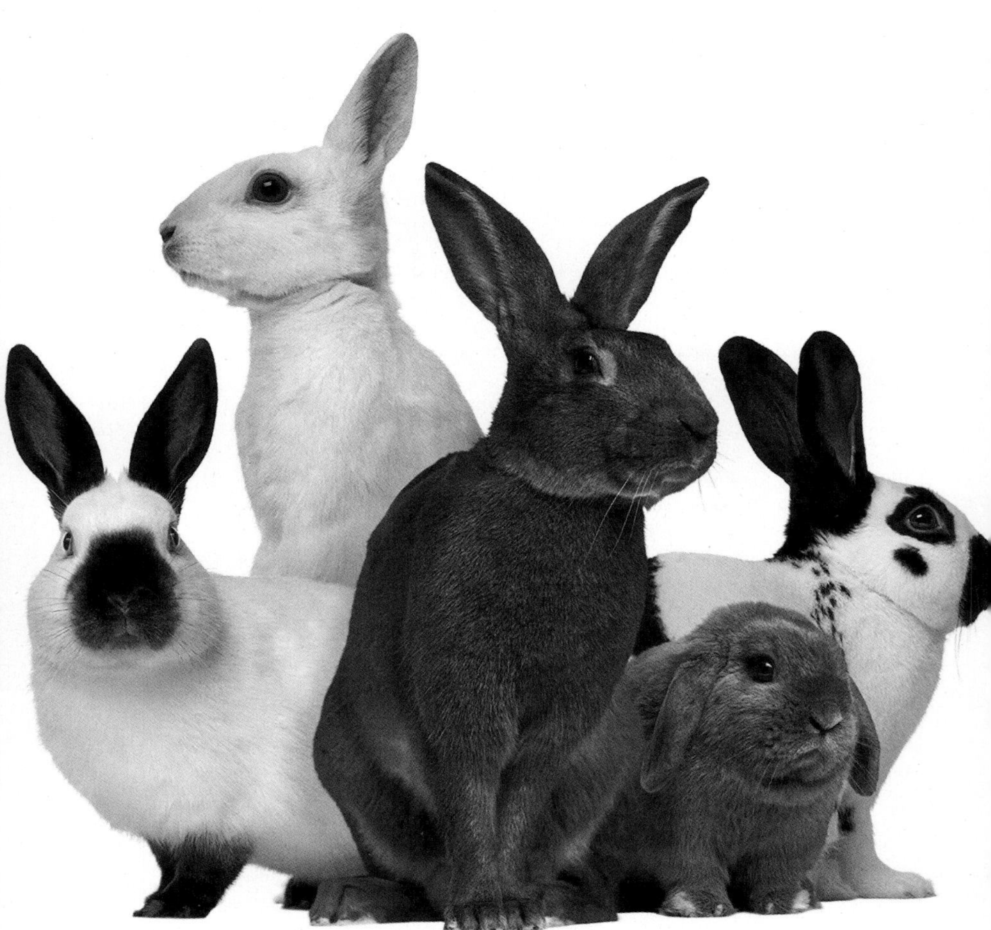

TABLE 10-1 Antimicrobial Agents Used in Rabbits.[a]

Judicious use of antimicrobials includes using an evidence-based approach in making decisions to use antimicrobial drugs, along with appropriate sample collection and culture techniques, and proper interpretation of culture and susceptibility data, dose selection, dosing interval, and length of treatment. For more information see the AVMA 2020 Committee on Antimicrobials report: Antibacterial resistant bacteria affecting animal health in the United States: https://www.avma.org/sites/default/files/2020-10/AntimicrobialResistanceFullReport.pdf.

Agent	Dosage	Comments
Amikacin	5-10 mg/kg SC, IM, IV divided q8-24h[194]	Increased efficacy and decreased toxicity when given once daily; for IV use, dilute in 4 mL/kg saline and give over 20 min
	1.25 g/20 g methylmethacrylate;[18] see www.kerrier.com for a calcium sulfate alternative to polymethylmethacrylate (PMMA)[b]	Place in bone after surgical debridement of jaw abscess
Azithromycin	4-5 mg/kg IM q48h × 7 days[34]	Effective against syphilis
	10 mg/kg IM, IV[62]	PK; fast and extensive tissue distribution followed by slow redistribution
	15-30 mg/kg PO q24h × 15 days[166]	Pulmonary infections
Cefazolin	20 mg/kg IV[71]	Perioperative use with gastrointestinal surgery
	2 g/20 g methylmethacrylate;[18] see www.kerrier.com for a calcium sulfate alternative to PMMA[b]	Place in bone after surgical debridement of jaw abscess
Cefotaxime	50 mg/kg IM q8h[192]	Pneumococcal endocarditis
Ceftazidime	50 mg/kg IM, IV q3h[1]	PK
	100 mg/kg IM q12h[256]	
Ceftiofur	2 g/20 g methylmethacrylate;[18] see www.kerrier.com for a calcium sulfate alternative to PMMA[b]	Place in bone after surgical debridement of jaw abscess
Ceftiofur crystalline free acid (100 mg/mL; Excede, Zoetis)	40 mg/kg SC q24-72h[81]	PK; minimal side effects with single injection[81]
Ceftriaxone	40 mg/kg IM q12h × 3 days[192]	Effective against *Treponema* (rabbit syphilis), pneumococcal endocarditis
	71 mg/kg IV q24h[46]	Pneumococcal pneumonia
Cephalexin	—	Oral cephalosporins are not recommended[166]
	15 mg/kg SC q12h[166]	Parenteral form not available in the United States; not generally recommended
	2 g/20 g methylmethacrylate;[18] see www.kerrier.com for a calcium sulfate alternative to PMMA[b]	Place in bone after surgical debridement of jaw abscess

Continued

TABLE 10-1 Antimicrobial Agents Used in Rabbits. (cont'd)

Agent	Dosage	Comments
Chloramphenicol	—	The use of chloramphenicol in food-producing animals is prohibited in the United States
	30-50 mg/kg PO, SC, IM, IV q8-24h[194]	
	55 mg/kg PO q12h × 4 wk[209]	Effective against *Treponema* (rabbit syphilis)
Chlortetracycline	50 mg/kg PO q24h[194]	
Ciprofloxacin[c]	—	May cause arthropathies in young animals[220]
	1 drop topical q8-12h[91]	Nasal pasteurellosis; maintains therapeutic levels in tear film for at least 6 hr after application (tears drain into nasal sinus)
	20 mg/kg q24h PO × 5 days[94]	PK; high tissue concentrations in kidneys, lung, spleen, liver, and muscle[94]
Difloxacin[c] (Dicural, Fort Dodge)	5 mg/kg IM, IV q24h[3]	PK; dose appropriate for *E. coli* infections
Doxycycline	2.5 mg/kg PO q12h[166]	
	4 mg/kg PO q24h[176]	
	2000 ppm in low-calcium diet[83]	PK; reaches target concentrations in major organs and mycobacteriosis lung lesions
Doxycycline hyclate	Suppository 10 mg/kg[42]	PK; similar half-life to intravenous administration (5 mg/kg)
Enrofloxacin[c]	—	May cause arthropathies in young dogs, but similar effects using standard dosages in rabbits have not been reported; SC and IM injections may cause muscle necrosis or sterile abscesses; dilute before giving parenterally
	5 mg/kg IM, IV q12-24h[61]	Angora rabbits/PK
	5 mg/kg PO, SC, IM, IV q12h[25,29]	PK;[25,29] clinical trial for pasteurellosis, × 14 days[25]
	5-20 mg/kg PO, IM q12h × 14-30 days[194]	Pasteurellosis
	15-20 mg/kg PO q12h[194]	Pasteurellosis; treat for a minimum of 14 days in mild infections and up to several months for chronic infections[194]
Florfenicol	—	In the United States, use of related drug chloramphenicol is prohibited in food-producing animals
	25 mg/kg IM, IV q6h[129]	PK
	30 mg/kg PO, IV q8h[2]	PK
Gentamicin	—	Seldom indicated; use with caution; see ophthalmic agents for intraocular use (Table 10-9)
	4 mg/kg SC, IM q24h[28]	

TABLE 10-1 Antimicrobial Agents Used in Rabbits. (cont'd)

Agent	Dosage	Comments
Gentamicin (cont'd)	5-8 mg/kg SC, IM, IV q8-24h[194]	Decreased toxicity when given once daily; for IV use, dilute in 4 mL/kg saline and give over 20 min
	1 g/20 g methylmethacrylate;[18] see www.kerrier.com for a calcium sulfate alternative to PMMA[b]	Place in bone after surgical debridement of jaw abscess
Marbofloxacin[c]	—	Lowest MIC of nine antibiotics tested against bacteria responsible for upper respiratory infections[207]
	2 mg/kg SC, IM, IV q24h[4,156]	PK; study performed during *Pasteurella* infection[4]
	5 mg/kg PO q24h × 10 days[38]	PK
Meropenem	Meropenem-impregnated PMMA beads;[56] see www.kerrier.com for a calcium sulfate alternative to PMMA[b]	Consider with methicillin-resistant *Staphylococcus aureus*;[56] retained in vitro antimicrobial activity and eluted drug for 2 weeks after vaporized hydrogen peroxide sterilization[56]
Metronidazole	5 mg/kg IV q12h[194]	Anaerobic infections; administer slowly
	20 mg/kg PO q12h × 3-5 days[194]	
	40 mg/kg PO q24h × 3 days[28,194]	
Minocycline	6 mg/kg IV q8h[170]	PK
Moxifloxacin[c]	5 mg/kg PO, IM q24h × 10 days[65]	PK; susceptible infections (some bacteria may require higher doses)
	40 mg/kg IV q12h × 2 doses, then q24h[180]	Bacterial meningitis
Netilmicin (Netromycin, Schering)	7 mg/kg IV q12h[212]	PK; induced renal tubular necrosis in 50% of animals
Ofloxacin (Ocuflox, Allergan)	20 mg/kg SC q8h[155]	Urogenital, skin, respiratory infections
Orbifloxacin[c]	20 mg/kg PO q24h × 7-21 days[247]	PK
Oxytetracycline	15 mg/kg IM q8h[159]	PK; anorexia and diarrhea at 30 mg/kg IM q8h; tissue irritation can occur
	25 mg/kg SC q24h[176]	
	50 mg/kg PO q12h[28,194]	
Penicillin	—	Do not give any form of penicillin orally to rabbits
Penicillin G	60,000 U/kg IM q12h[116]	PK
Penicillin G benzathine	42,000-60,000 U/kg IM q48h[84]	Benzathine penicillin achieves lower serum levels than other forms and is effective against only highly susceptible organisms
	42,000-84,000 U/kg SC q7d × 3 wk[196]	
Penicillin G procaine	42,000-84,000 U/kg SC, IM q24h[196]	
	60,000 U/kg IM q8h[248]	PK

Continued

TABLE 10-1 Antimicrobial Agents Used in Rabbits. (cont'd)

Agent	Dosage	Comments
Rifampin (R)/ azithromycin (A)	(R) 40 mg/kg PO q12h + (A) 50 mg/kg PO q24h[222]	*Staphylococcus* osteomyelitis
Rifampin (R)/ clarithromycin (C)	(R) 40 mg/kg + (C) 80 mg/kg PO q12h[222]	*Staphylococcus* osteomyelitis
Silver sulfadiazine cream (Silvadene, Marion)	Topical q12-24h	Does not cause diarrhea if ingested
Sulfadimethoxine	10-15 mg/kg PO q12h[194]	
Sulfamethazine	1 mg/mL drinking water[28]	
	5-10 g/kg feed[28]	
Sulfaquinoxaline	1 mg/mL drinking water[28]	
	0.6 g/kg feed[28]	
Tetracycline	50-100 mg/kg PO q8-12h[194]	
	250-1000 mg/L drinking water[84]	Therapeutic levels not achieved even at 800-1600 mg/L;[187] 250 mg/L not effective in clinical trial for pasteurellosis[176]
Tilmicosin (Micotil, Elanco)	12.5 mg/kg PO q24h × 7 days[80]	PK; macrolide antibiotic; use with caution
	25 mg/kg SC once[194]	Pasteurellosis; use cautiously (at least one rabbit death and several human deaths have been reported; has been associated with anemia and leukopenia)
Tobramycin	1 g/20 g methylmethacrylate;[18] see www.kerrier.com for a calcium sulfate alternative to PMMA[b]	Place in bone after surgical debridement of jaw abscess
	10% in calcium sulfate pellets[169]	Biodegradable implants for treatment of osteomyelitis
Trimethoprim/sulfa	15 mg/kg PO q12h[28]	
	30 mg/kg PO, SC, IM q12h[166]	
	15-30 mg/kg PO q12-24h[194]	Rabbits treated with 40 mg/kg PO q12h demonstrated a ~50% drop in tear production at end of 2 wk study period[15]
	30-48 mg/kg SC q12h[194]	
Tylosin	10 mg/kg, SC, IM q12-24h[194]	
Vancomycin	50 mg/kg IV q8h[170]	PK
	10 mg vancomycin and 50 mg DL-lactide-co-glycolide copolymer[238]	Antibiotic beads; osteomyelitis; effective locally for 56 days

[a]There is a potential for antibiotic-induced enterotoxemia following administration of some antimicrobial agents (see Table 10-23). Appetite and fecal character must be monitored closely during and following therapy.
[b]www.kerrier.com is an alternate to PMMA. This is medical grade calcium sulfate that does not act as a foreign body.
[c]The use of fluoroquinolones in food-producing animals is strictly prohibited in the United States. Do not use these drugs in rabbits that may be consumed by humans.

TABLE 10-2 Antifungal Agents Used in Rabbits.[a]

Agent	Dosage	Comments
Albaconazole	5 mg/kg PO q24h[163]	Cryptococcal meningitis
	50 mg/kg PO q24h[33]	Disseminated *Scedosporium prolificans*
Amphotericin B	—	Severe fungal infections; use in combination with fluconazole;[210] potentially nephrotoxic and hepatotoxic
• Desoxycholate form	1 mg/kg IV q24h[194,210]	Invasive aspergillosis
• Liposomal form	5 mg/kg IV q24h[190]	
Clotrimazole (Lotrimin, Bayer)	Topical q24h × 14-28 days[194]	Localized dermatophytosis
Fluconazole	5 mg/kg PO q24h[163]	Cryptococcal meningitis
	25-43 mg/kg IV (slow) q12h[150,194]	Systemic fungal disease
	38 mg/kg PO q12h[11]	*Aspergillus* keratitis
	80 mg/kg PO q24h × 21 days[224]	Coccidioidal meningitis; controlled but did not cure
	80 mg/kg PO q24h × 7 days[109]	Serum and extravascular levels superior to ketoconazole
Griseofulvin	12.5-25 mg/kg PO q12-24h × 30-45 days[196]	Advanced cases of dermatophytosis; decrease dose by 50% if using ultra-microsize form (Gris-PEG, Allergan Herbert), which has better absorption
	15-25 mg/kg PO q24h, or divided q12h × 30 days[105]	At high doses may cause bone marrow suppression and panleukopenia
Itraconazole	5-10 mg/kg PO q24h × 30 days[194]	Dermatophytosis
	10 mg/kg slow IV infusion[137]	PK; eliminated slowly
	20-40 mg/kg PO q24h[244]	*Aspergillus* pneumonia
	40 mg/kg PO q24h[185]	Invasive aspergillosis
Ketoconazole	10-40 mg/kg PO q24h × 14 days[64]	Dermatophytosis
	35 mg/kg PO q12h × 7 days[109]	Ineffective in systemic candidiasis rabbit model
Lime sulfur (2%-3%)	Topical q5-7d × 4 wk[194]	Dermatophytosis; use with caution
	Topical 1:32 dilution with water 2 ×/wk[105]	
Micafungin	0.25-2 mg/kg IV q24h[190]	Systemic candidiasis
Nystatin	20 mg/kg PO q12h × 10 days[118]	*Cyniclomyces guttulatus* gastrointestinal yeast overgrowth
Posaconazole	6 mg/kg PO q24h[189]	*Aspergillus* pneumonia
	20 mg/kg PO q24h[244]	*Aspergillus* pneumonia
Terbinafine	—	Best used as part of combination therapy; little activity when used as a single agent[127,224]

Continued

TABLE 10-2 Antifungal Agents Used in Rabbits. (cont'd)

Agent	Dosage	Comments
Terbinafine (cont'd)	10 mg/kg PO q24h[105]	Dermatophytosis
	10-30 mg/kg PO q24h[166]	Dermatophytosis
	100 mg/kg PO q12h × 21 days[224]	Less effective than fluconazole for coccidioidal meningitis
Terbinafine (T)/ amphotericin B (A)	(T) 100 mg/kg PO q24h + (A) 0.4 mg/kg IV q24h[127]	Invasive aspergillosis
Voriconazole	—	The short terminal elimination half-life of less than 1 hr in the rabbit indicates that the efficacy of voriconazole is less than optimal in this species;[203] however, voriconazole is effective as a topical antifungal ophthalmic preparation in the rabbit (see Table 10-9)

[a]Antifungal protocols using amphotericin B administered intravenously or itraconazole, fluconazole, or ketoconazole administered orally alone or in combination for deep mycotic infections have been based on those used successfully in the dog and may be adequate treatment options in the rabbit; however, this hypothesis requires confirmation and validation.[24a] Certain antifungal protocols have not caused death in rabbit models, even when given for extended periods.[33,185,189,190,210]

TABLE 10-3 Antiparasitic Agents Used in Rabbits.[a]

Agent	Dosage	Comments
Albendazole	7.5-20 mg/kg PO q24h × 3-14 days[194]	Potential treatment for encephalitozoonosis; use cautiously, deaths have been reported[90]
	20 mg/kg PO q24h × 10 days[194]	
	30 mg/kg PO q24h × 30 days, then 15 mg/kg q24h × 30 days[194]	*Encephalitozoon cuniculi*-induced phacoclastic uveitis
	150 mg/kg PO once	PK; q24h dosing appropriate; quickly and mainly oxidized in the liver to albendazole sulphoxide, an active metabolite which undergoes a second and slower irreversible metabolism to form sulfur dioxide, an inactive metabolite[30]
Amprolium (9.6%)	0.5 mL/pint drinking water × 10 days[194]	Coccidiosis
Carbaryl powder 5%	Topically q7d[166]	Ectoparasites; use sparingly
Cyromazine 6% (Rearguard, Novartis)	Topically q6-10wk[118]	Preventive for myiasis
Decoquinate (Deccox, Rhone-Poulenc)	62.5 ppm in feed[96]	Coccidiosis
Diclazuril	4 mg/kg SC[184]	
	1 ppm in feed[239]	PD; intestinal and hepatic coccidiosis

TABLE 10-3 Antiparasitic Agents Used in Rabbits. (cont'd)

Agent	Dosage	Comments
Doramectin	0.2 mg/kg IM once[121,194]	*Psoroptes* mites
	0.3 mg/kg SC[88]	PD
	0.4 mg/kg SC[60]	Topical spot-on ivermectin more effective[60]
Emodepside 2.1%/ praziquantel 8.6% (Profender, Bayer)	0.14 mL/kg topically once[194]	*Trichostrongylus colubriformis*; studies performed in laboratory animals (e.g., rats, rabbits) suggest that emodepside may interfere with fetal development in those species[194]
Eprinomectin	0.2-0.3 mg/kg SC once[183]	*Psoroptes* mites
	2 mg/kg topically once[249]	*Psoroptes* mites
Febantel/ pyrantel pamoate/ praziquantel (Drontal Plus, Bayer)	½ tablet/5 kg PO once[162]	Use tablet for puppies and small dogs (2-25 lb); effective against nematodes and cestodes
Fenbendazole	—	On rare occasions, anemia and arteritis have been reported[90]
	5-20 mg/kg PO q24h × 5 days; repeat in 14 days[162,166]	Nematodes; use 20 mg/kg for *Passalurus ambiguous*
	20 mg/kg PO q24h × 7 days before and 2 days after mixing rabbits[229]	Preventive against encephalitozoonosis
	20 mg/kg PO q24h × 28 days[194,229]	Treatment for encephalitozoonosis
Fipronil (Frontline, Merial)	Contraindicated[165,166]	Can cause neurologic disease and death; blocks GABA receptors in CNS by preventing chloride ion uptake[191]
Fluralaner (Bravecto, Merck)	25 mg/kg PO once[221]	*Psoroptes cuniculi* treatment
Imidacloprid (Advantage, Bayer)	10-16 mg/kg or 1 cat dose topically q30d[110,166]	Flea adulticide; use single 0.4 mL dose, 10% solution
Imidacloprid (I) 10%/ moxidectin (M) 1% (Advantage Multi for Cats, Bayer)	(I) 10 mg/kg + (M) 1 mg/kg topically q4wk × 3 treatments[118]	*Psoroptes* mites
Imidacloprid 8.8%/ permethrin 44% (Advantix, Bayer)	11-16.6 mg/kg topically once[19]	*Leporacarus gibbus* (rabbit fur mite)
Ivermectin	—	Ectoparasites
	0.1-0.2 mg/kg SC, repeat in 14 days[22]	Ear mites; clinical trial
	0.2-0.44 mg/kg PO, SC repeat in 8-18 days[194]	*Psoroptes* (ear mites)
	0.3-0.4 mg/kg SC, repeat in 14 days[194]	*Sarcoptes scabiei* (sarcoptic mange); *Notoedres cati*
	0.4 mg/kg SC q80h × 3 doses[122]	Sarcoptic mange
Lime sulfur (2%-3%)	1-2 dips/wk × 28 days[196]	Ectoparasites; young animals
	Dip q7d × 4-6 wk[166]	

Continued

TABLE 10-3 Antiparasitic Agents Used in Rabbits. (cont'd)

Agent	Dosage	Comments
Lufenuron (Program, Novartis)	30 mg/kg PO q30d[194]	Flea larvicide
Metronidazole	20 mg/kg PO q12h[166]	Antiprotozoal agent
Monensin (CoBan 60, Elanco)	0.002%-0.004% in feed[96]	Coccidiosis; coccidiostat
Moxidectin	0.2 mg/kg PO, repeat in 10 days[194,243]	Psoroptic mange
	0.3 mg/kg SC[88]	PK
Oxibendazole	30 mg/kg PO q24h × 7-14 days, then 15 mg/kg PO q24h for 30-60 days[194]	Encephalitozoonosis; no highly effective treatment has been identified; bone marrow suppression has been reported with the use of benzimidazoles, so an intratreatment CBC is recommended[90]
Piperazine	100 mg/kg PO q24h × 2 days[194]	Use with citrate formulation
	200-500 mg/kg PO × 2 days[194]	Adults; use with adipate formulation
	750 mg/kg PO × 2 days[194]	Juveniles; wash perianal area
Praziquantel	5-10 mg/kg PO once; may repeat in 10 days[194]	Cestodes, trematodes
Pyrantel pamoate	5-10 mg/kg PO, SC, IM, repeat in 14 days[166]	
	5-10 mg/kg PO, repeat in 14-21 days[194]	
Pyrethrins	Topically as directed for puppies/ kittens q7d[166]	Flea control
Selamectin (Revolution, Zoetis)	12 mg/kg topically at base of neck once[125]	Cheyletiellosis
	20 mg/kg topically q7d[37]	PK/flea infestation; further studies are needed to assess long-term safety in rabbits at this dose following repeated application[37]
	30 mg (8-14 mg/kg) topically q30 days × 2 doses[63,133]	Sarcoptic mange
	30 mg (6-18 mg/kg) topically once[133,161]	*Psoroptes*
Sulfadimethoxine	50 mg/kg PO once, then 25 mg/kg q24h × 10-20 days[166]	Coccidiosis
Sulfadimidene	100-233 mg/L drinking water[95]	Coccidiosis
Sulfamerazine	100 mg/kg PO[84]	Coccidiosis
	0.05%-0.15% in drinking water[84]	
Sulfamethazine	100 mg/kg PO q24h[84]	Coccidiosis
	0.77 g/L drinking water[84]	
	0.5%-1% in feed[84]	
Sulfamethoxine	50 mg/kg PO once, then 25 mg/kg PO q24h × 10-20 days[26]	Coccidiosis

TABLE 10-3 Antiparasitic Agents Used in Rabbits. (cont'd)

Agent	Dosage	Comments
Sulfaquinoxaline	0.1%-0.15% in drinking water[84]	Coccidiosis; treatment
	1 mg/mL in drinking water[166]	
	125-250 ppm in feed[96]	
Thiabendazole	25-50 mg/kg PO[84]	
Toltrazuril	2.5-5 mg/kg PO[194,199]	Intestinal coccidiosis; a single oral dose of toltrazuril 2.5 mg/kg or 5 mg/kg PO reduced oocyte counts by 98.1% and 99.6%, respectively[194]
	10 mg/kg PO[108]	PK;[126] coccidiosis due to *Eimeria tenella*[108]
	25 ppm in drinking water (or 25 mg/kg PO) q24h × 2 days, repeat after 5 days[95]	Coccidiosis
	50 ppm in drinking water[31]	Hepatic coccidiosis due to *Eimeria stiedae*

[a]Genetic evidence of a mitochondrial-type chaperone combined with phylogenetic analysis of multiple gene sequences support a relationship between the microsporida (e.g., *Encephalitozoon cuniculi*) and atypical fungi with extreme host dependency.[20a]

TABLE 10-4 Chemical Restraint/Sedative/Anesthetic/Analgesic Agents Used in Rabbits.[a,b]

Agent	Dosage	Comments
Acepromazine	—	See butorphanol, ketamine, ketamine/xylazine for combinations
	0.1-0.5 mg/kg SC[194]	15 min before anesthetic induction; may cause hypotension/hypothermia;[194] no analgesia
	0.25-1 mg/kg IM[166]	Preanesthetic; sedative; tranquilizer
	0.25-2 mg/kg SC, IM, IV[194]	
	1 mg/kg IM[194]	Tranquilization; effect should begin 10 min after administration and last for 1 to 2 hours[194]
	1-5 mg/kg SC, IM[84]	Preanesthetic; lower end of dose range is preferred
Acetaminophen (Tylenol, McNeil)	—	Short-term use only; use with caution as associated with liver failure[151]
	200-500 mg/kg PO[84]	Analgesia
	1-2 mg/mL drinking water[68]	
Acetaminophen/codeine (120 mg/12 mg per 5 mL)	1 mL elixir/100 mL drinking water[251]	Analgesia

Continued

TABLE 10-4 Chemical Restraint/Sedative/Anesthetic/Analgesic Agents Used in Rabbits. (cont'd)

Agent	Dosage	Comments
Acetylsalicylic acid (aspirin)	5-20 mg/kg PO q24h[194]	Antiinflammatory; for low grade analgesia
	10-100 mg/kg PO q8-12h[166]	
	100 mg/kg PO q8-24h[41]	
Alfaxalone[c] (Alfaxan, Alfaxan Multidose, Alfaxan IDX, Jurox)	—	Neurosteroid anesthetic; IV dose-dependent respiratory depression; no analgesic properties; oxygenation prior to administration recommended
	0.5-1 mg/kg IM[147]	For additional sedation when combined with midazolam, an opioid, and ketamine[147]
	1 mg/kg IV slowly to effect[147]	Anesthetic induction when used in conjunction with preanesthetic sedatives (i.e., midazolam 0.5 mg/kg, hydromorphone 0.1 mg/kg, ketamine 7 mg/kg, and dexmedetomidine 0.005 mg/kg combined in single syringe and given IM)[147]
	2-3 mg/kg IV[93]	Anesthetic induction; give slow to effect
	4 mg/kg IV[193]	Dilute with 5% dextrose and give over 1 min for smooth induction that allows intubation[193]
	4-6 mg/kg IM[112]	Deep sedation; longer duration of action with higher dose
	5 mg/kg IM, IV[157]	PK
	6 mg/kg IM[23]	
Alfaxalone (A)/ butorphanol (B)	(A) 6 mg/kg IM + (B) 0.3 mg/kg IM[23]	Consistent sedation and short-term anesthesia
Alfaxalone (A)/ butorphanol (B)/ dexmedetomidine (De)	(A) 6 mg/kg + (B) 0.3 mg/kg + (De) 0.2 mg/kg IM[23]	Consistent sedation and short-term anesthesia; longer effects with dexmedetomidine[23]
Alfaxalone (A)/ dexmedetomidine (De)	(A) 5 mg/kg IM + (De) 100 µg/kg IM[157]	PK; moderate sedation with (A) alone; deep sedation with (A) + (De)
	(A) 6 mg/kg + (De) 0.2 mg/kg IM[23]	Consistent sedation and short-term anesthesia; longer effects with dexmedetomidine[23]
Alfaxalone (A)/ midazolam (Mi)	(A) 6 mg/kg + (Mi) 1 mg/kg IM[23]	Consistent sedation and short-term anesthesia
Alfaxalone (A)/ hydromorphone (H)/ dexmedetomidine (De)	(A) 5 mg/kg + (H) 0.1 mg/kg + (De) 0.005 mg/kg IM[198a]	Allowed successful intubation in 3/5 rabbits; good short term anesthesia; did not cause a decrease in respiratory rate or apnea[198a]
	(A) 7 mg/kg + (H) 0.1 mg/kg + (De) 0.005 mg/kg IM[198a]	Allowed successful intubation in 4/5 rabbits; good short term anesthesia; did not cause a decrease in respiratory rate or apnea[198a]
Atipamezole (Antisedan, Orion)	Give same volume SC, IV, IP as medetomidine or dexmedetomidine (5 × medetomidine or 10 × dexmedetomidine dose in mg)[166]	Dexmedetomidine and medetomidine[e] reversal
	0.25 mg/kg IV[194]	
	0.5 mg/kg SC, IM[194]	
	1 mg/kg SC, IM, IV[166]	

TABLE 10-4 Chemical Restraint/Sedative/Anesthetic/Analgesic Agents Used in Rabbits. (cont'd)

Agent	Dosage	Comments
Atropine	—	Many rabbits possess serum atropinase, hence very high doses are often administered; glycopyrrolate often preferred
	0.1-0.5 mg/kg SC, IM[166]	
	0.1-3 mg/kg SC[96]	
	10 mg/kg SC q20min[194]	To treat organophosphate toxicity
Bupivicaine 0.125%, 0.5%	—	Local and regional anesthetic techniques; concentrations of 0.125% or less produce a good sensory block with least motor effect; epidural anesthesia; dilute with preservative-free saline only; total volume should not exceed 0.33 mL/kg[98]
	1 mg/kg[98]	Injectable epidural; use 0.125% preparation;[98] loco-regional anesthesia; maximum recommended dose[213] (see Table 10-6)
	2 mg/kg[146]	
Bupivicaine liposome injectable suspension (Exparel, Pacira Pharm)	9, 18, 30 mg/kg[202a] once injected around brachial plexus	PK; single-dose toxicology study; well tolerated; minimal inflammation in adipose; no nerve damage
Buprenorphine	—	Partial agonist that exerts significant actions at the mu opioid receptor; duration of analgesia may be dose dependent; only suitable for mild to moderate pain;[217] may cause respiratory depression,[13] suppressed food consumption, and fecal output;[8,44] metabolites of buprenorphine should be considered when determining analgesic doses;[8] see midazolam for combination
	0.01-0.05 mg/kg SC, IM, IV q6-12h[41,166]	Analgesia
	0.012 mg/kg[98]	Epidural anesthesia; dilute with preservative-free saline only; total volume should not exceed 0.33 mL/kg[98]
	0.02-0.1 mg/kg SC, IM, IV[145]	Preanesthetic
	0.03 mg/kg IM q12h[44]	Decreased food consumption and fecal output
	0.05 mg/kg SC[8] once	PK; analgesia
	0.06 mg/kg IV q8h[217]	Only suitable for mild to moderate pain
Buprenorphine SR-LAB (1 mg/mL, ZooPharm)	0.12 mg/kg SC[51]	Compounded formulation of sustained-release buprenorphine
Buprenorphine SR (Zoo Pharm)	0.15 mg/kg SC[8] once	PK; analgesia

Continued

TABLE 10-4 Chemical Restraint/Sedative/Anesthetic/Analgesic Agents Used in Rabbits. (cont'd)

Agent	Dosage	Comments
Buprenorphine High Concentration (HC) (Simbadol, Zoetis)	0.24 mg/kg SC q8h[231]	A high concentration buprenorphine that binds to opiate receptors with high affinity and high receptor avidity resulting in slow disassociation from the opiate receptor; substantial variability based on PK study; rapid absorption; no notable side effects
	0.24 mg/kg IM once[8]	PK; may not be an appropriate analgesic; adverse neurologic signs in 2 rabbits
Butorphanol	—	See ketamine/xylazine and midazolam for combinations; mixed agonist/antagonist with low intrinsic activity at the mu receptor and strong agonist activity at kappa and sigma receptors; duration of analgesia may be dose dependent; use lower doses IV
	0.1-0.5 mg/kg SC, IM, IV q2-4h[41,194]	Analgesia
	0.1-1 mg/kg SC, IM, IV q2-6h [166]	Doses up to 2 mg/kg may be given[166]
	0.3-0.5 mg/kg SC, IM, IV q2-4h[215]	
Butorphanol (B)/ acepromazine (A)	(A) 0.5 mg/kg + (B) 0.5 mg/kg SC, IM[73]	
Carprofen	—	Nonsteroidal anti-inflammatory; chronic osteoarthritis or degenerative joint disease
	1-2.2 mg/kg PO q12h[41]	
	1-5 mg/kg PO q12-24h[95,166]	
	2-4 mg/kg PO q12-24h[13]	
	2-4 mg/kg SC q24h[41]	
	4 mg/kg SC, IM q24h[13]	
Dexmedetomidine (Dexdomitor, Orion)	—	See ketamine/fentanyl and midazolam/ hydromorphone/ketamine for combinations; α_2 agonist similar to medetomidine;[e] reverse with atipamezole
	0.005 mg/kg IM[141]	Preanesthetic when combined with ketamine
	0.035-0.05 mg/kg IM[141]	Induction/maintenance when combined with ketamine
Dexmedetomidine (De)/midazolam (Mi)/butorphanol (B)	(De) 0.1 mg/kg + (Mi) 2 mg/ kg + (B) 0.4 mg/kg IN[211]	Deep sedation; administered via catheter inserted intranasally (IN) to level of medial aspect of eye[211]
Diazepam[d]	—	Benzodiazepine sedative; IV route preferred;[d] see ketamine for combination
	0.5-2 mg/kg IM, IV[166,194]	For sedation
	1 mg/kg intracavernous[55]	Seizures; alternative to IV route
	1-3 mg/kg IM[96]	Preanesthetic; tranquilizer
	1-5 mg/kg IM, IV[41]	Preanesthetic; tranquilizer

TABLE 10-4 Chemical Restraint/Sedative/Anesthetic/Analgesic Agents Used in Rabbits. (cont'd)

Agent	Dosage	Comments
Etomidate	1-2 mg/kg[141,145]	Give slow to effect for anesthetic induction; short-acting induction agent; good choice with cardiac patients
Fentanyl	—	Mu opioid agonist; analgesia; see ketamine/dexmedetomidine and medetomidine[e]/midazolam for combinations
	Six target plasma concentrations (2, 4, 8, 16, 32, 64 ng/mL) IV[232]	In isoflurane-anesthetized rabbits, reduced MAC and improved mean arterial pressure and cardiac output[232]
	0.0074 mg/kg IV[41]	
Fentanyl patch	12.5 µg/h patch/3 kg rabbit × 3 days[41]	Do not cut patches; may cause drowsiness when initially applied
	25 µg/h patch/3 kg rabbit × 3 days[75]	Rapid hair coat regrowth after clipping; decreased plasma concentrations of fentanyl; use of a depilatory agent leads to early and rapid absorption of fentanyl, causing undue sedation in some rabbits and lack of sustained plasma concentrations for the desired 3-day period[75]
Fentanyl/fluanisone (Hypnorm, Janssen)	0.2-0.3 mL/kg SC, IM[95,196]	Premedication; analgesia; sedation
Flumazenil	0.01-0.1 mg/kg IM, IV[32]	Reversal for benzodiazepines
	0.05 mg/kg IV[208]	Antagonizes sedative effects of midazolam (1.2 mg/kg IV); repeat in 20 min if resedation occurs[208]
Flunixin meglumine	—	Analgesia; nonsteroidal antiinflammatory
	0.3-2 mg/kg PO, IM, IV q12-24h[186]	Use for no more than 3 days
	1.1 mg/kg SC, IM, IV q12-24h[194]	
	1-2 mg/kg SC q12-24h[100]	
Gabapentin	—	Neuropathic pain analgesic; indicated for adjunctive treatment of chronic or neurogenic pain in dogs and cats at 3 mg/kg PO q24h and for ancillary therapy of refractory seizures in dogs at 10-30 mg/kg PO q8h[194]
	3-5 mg/kg PO q12-24h[166]	
	25 mg/kg SC[131]	Dose used to approximate plasma concentrations in humans
Glycopyrrolate	—	Anticholinergic; premedication to prevent salivation and bradycardia
	0.01-0.02 mg/kg SC[166]	
	0.01-0.1 mg/kg SC, IM[194]	
	0.02 mg/kg IV, IO, intratracheally[104]	

Continued

TABLE 10-4 Chemical Restraint/Sedative/Anesthetic/Analgesic Agents Used in Rabbits. (cont'd)

Agent	Dosage	Comments
Hydromorphone	—	Opioid analgesic; mainly a mu agonist with less affinity for delta receptors
	0.05-0.2 mg/kg SC, IM q6-8h[36]	
	0.1-0.2 mg/kg SC, IM, IV q6-8h[120]	
Ibuprofen	—	Analgesia; nonsteroidal anti-inflammatory; may have gastrointestinal side effects
	2-7.5 mg/kg PO q4h[166]	
Isoflurane	3%-5% induction, 1.5%-1.75% maintenance[84]	MAC = 2.05%; prior use of a sedative or injectable induction agent(s) is recommended, as use of preanesthetic agent or combinations will lower the MAC of inhalants
	3%-5% induction, 2%-3% maintenance[96]	
Ketamine	—	NMDA receptor antagonist; should be administered in combination with other agents; combinations to follow
	1-10 mg/kg IM[142]	
	7-10 mg/kg IM[141,143]	Preanesthetic; add to midazolam/opioid combination if additional sedation required[143]
	15-20 mg/kg IV[84]	
	20 mg/kg IM[141]	Anesthetic induction, maintenance
	20-50 mg/kg IM[84]	60 min of sedation
Ketamine (K)/ acepromazine (A)	(K) 25-40 mg/kg + (A) 0.25-1 mg/kg IM, IV[100]	Anesthesia
Ketamine (K)/ dexmedetomidine (De)/fentanyl (F)	(De) 0.02 mg/kg + (K) 5 mg/kg + (F) 0.01 mg/kg IM[206]	May result in mild respiratory depression, respiratory acidosis, and hypoxemia; supplemental oxygen recommended
Ketamine (K)/ diazepam (D)[d]	(K) 20-35 mg/kg IM, IV + (D) 0.5-2 mg/kg IM, IV[194]	Anesthesia; if used, drugs should be administered in separate syringes
	(K) 20-40 mg/kg IM, IV + (D) 1-5 mg/kg IM, IV[100]	Anesthesia; follow with inhalant as needed
	(K) 30-40 mg/kg IM + (D) 2-5 mg/kg IM[73]	Surgical anesthesia; lower end of dose range for (D) is preferred; less preferable than aforementioned (K)/(D) combinations
Ketamine (K)/ medetomidine (Me)[e]	(K) 5 mg/kg IV+ (Me) 0.35 mg/kg IM[102]	Surgical anesthesia
	(K) 15 mg/kg + (Me) 0.25 mg/kg SC,[179] IM[73,92]	Anesthetic induction; laryngospasm common
Ketamine (K)/ midazolam (Mi)	(K) 15 mg/kg IM + (Mi) 3 mg/kg IM[92]	Anesthetic induction

TABLE 10-4 Chemical Restraint/Sedative/Anesthetic/Analgesic Agents Used in Rabbits. (cont'd)

Agent	Dosage	Comments
Ketamine (K)/ midazolam (Mi)/ hydromorphone (H)/ dexmedetomidine (De)	(K) 7 mg/kg + (Mi) 0.5 mg/kg + (H) 0.1 mg/kg + (De) 0.005 mg/kg IM[141]	Preanesthetic
Ketoprofen	—	Nonsteroidal antiinflammatory
	1 mg/kg IM q12-24h[186]	Musculoskeletal pain; nonsteroidal antiinflammatory
	3 mg/kg SC, IM q24h[32]	Estimated duration of action 12-24 hr[74]
Ketoprofen 2.5% topical gel (Menarini, France)	Apply topically q6-12h[10]	PK; musculoskeletal pain
Lidocaine	—	Amide local anesthetic; local, regional, topical, and epidural anesthesia; see Table 10-5
• 1.5% injectable	0.4 mL/kg epidural[204]	Epidural anesthesia
• 2% injectable	1 mg/kg[140]	
	2 mg/kg[213]	Maximum recommended dose for local anesthesia; see Table 10-6
	2-3 mg/kg[145]	
• 10% injectable	Topical to glottis	Facilitates intubation
Lidocaine 2.5%/ prilocaine 2.5% (Emla cream)	Topical to skin	Facilitates IV catheter placement
Maropitant citrate (Cerenia, Zoetis)	1 mg/kg SC, IV[181]	PK; plasma concentrations similar to levels considered therapeutic in dogs
	2 mg/kg SC q24h × 3-5 days[40]	Neurokinin (NK1) receptor antagonist; gastrointestinal (visceral) and arthritic pain; can be administered long term q48h or 3 × weekly as needed[40]
Medetomidine[e]	—	Medetomidine is no longer commercially available in the United States
	0.1-0.5 mg/kg IM[242]	Sedation
Medetomidine (Me)[e]/fentanyl (F)/ midazolam (Mi)	(Me) 0.2 mg/kg + (F) 0.02 mg/kg + (Mi) 1 mg/kg IM[103]	Anesthesia; endotracheal intubation and supplemental oxygen are required
Medetomidine (Me)[e]/propofol (P)	(Me) 0.35 mg/kg IM + (P) 3 mg/kg IV[102]	Surgical anesthesia; note high medetomidine dose
Meloxicam	—	Nonsteroidal antiinflammatory; analgesia; antipyretic; used for osteoarthritis and postoperative pain; palatable PO form
	1 mg/kg PO q24h[77]	PK; dose required to achieve plasma levels associated with analgesia in other species; clinical efficacy was not evaluated

Continued

TABLE 10-4 Chemical Restraint/Sedative/Anesthetic/Analgesic Agents Used in Rabbits. (cont'd)

Agent	Dosage	Comments
Meloxicam (cont'd)	1 mg/kg PO q24h × 29 days[48]	PK; safety studies indicated may be safe for long-term use in rabbits
Midazolam	—	Benzodiazepine sedative; may reverse with flumazenil; more potent, shorter action than diazepam; water soluble; rapidly absorbed and less painful than diazepam when given IM; combinations to follow
	0.25-0.5 mg/kg IM[104]	When combined with an opioid
	0.25-1 mg/kg SC, IM, IV[59]	Minor procedures
	0.25-2 mg/kg SC, IM, IV[166]	Sedation; preanesthetic
Midazolam (Mi)/ buprenorphine (Bpr)	(Mi) 0.5 mg/kg + (Bpr) 0.01-0.05 mg/kg SC, IM[104]	Add ketamine (1-10 mg/kg) for additional sedation
Midazolam (Mi)/ butorphanol (B)	(Mi) 0.5 mg/kg + (B) 0.2-0.4 mg/kg SC, IM[104]	Add ketamine (1-10 mg/kg) for additional sedation and analgesia
	(Mi) 0.5-1 mg/kg + (B) 0.25-0.5 mg/kg IM[154]	Add ketamine 5-10 mg/kg IM for additional sedation and analgesia
Midazolam (Mi)/ butorphanol (B)/ alfaxalone (A)	(Mi) 1 mg/kg + (B) 1 mg/kg + (A) 2 mg/kg IM[128a]	Sufficient sedation for radiographic acquisition
Midazolam (Mi)/ butorphanol (B)/ ketamine (K)	(Mi) 1 mg/kg + (B) 1 mg/kg + (K) 5 mg/kg IM[128a]	Sufficient sedation for radiographic acquisition; faster recovery times and higher sedation scores than (Mi) + (B) + (A) (alfaxalone)
	(Mi) 1-2 mg/kg + (B) 1-1.5 mg/kg +/- (K) 3-7 mg/kg IM[80a]	Excellent sedation protocol for non-painful procedures; (Mi) can be reversed, if needed
Midazolam (Mi)/ dexmedetomidine (De)	(Mi) 0.2 mg/kg + (De) 25 µg/kg IM[16]	Deep sedation
Midazolam (Mi)/ hydromorphone (H)/ketamine (K)	(Mi) 1-2 mg/kg + (H) 0.3 mg/kg +/- (K) 3-7 mg/kg IM[80a]	Excellent drug combination for painful procedures or as a preanesthetic; (Mi) and (H) can be reversed, if needed
Midazolam (Mi)/ ketamine (K)	(Mi) 0.2 mg/kg + (K) 30 mg/kg IM[16]	Sedation
Midazolam (Mi)/ oxymorphone (O)	(Mi) 0.5 mg/kg + (O) 0.05-0.2 mg/kg SC, IM[104]	Add ketamine (1-10 mg/kg) for additional sedation
Morphine	—	Analgesic; mu receptor agonist; decreases gastrointestinal transit time[47]
	0.1 mg/kg[36,98,194]	Epidural anesthesia; dilute with preservative-free saline only; total volume should not exceed 0.33 mL/kg[98]
	0.5-2 mg/kg SC, IM q2-4h[36,166]	Analgesia
	2-5 mg/kg SC, IM q2-4h[32,194]	
	10 mg/kg IM[47]	Decreased gastrointestinal transit time and affected stomach and cecum motility[47]

TABLE 10-4 Chemical Restraint/Sedative/Anesthetic/Analgesic Agents Used in Rabbits. (cont'd)

Agent	Dosage	Comments
Naloxone	0.01-0.1 mg/kg IM, IV[32]	Mu opioid antagonist; narcotic reversal; note that analgesic effects are also reversed; avoid use following painful procedure as sudden awareness of pain may predispose to breath holding, increased catecholamine release, and fatal arrhythmias[32]
	0.01-0.02 mg/kg SC, IM, IV, IP[194]	Repeat as necessary
Naproxen	2.4 mg/mL in drinking water × 21 days[194]	Septic arthritis pain; inflammation in rabbits (extralabel)[194]
Oxymorphone	0.05-0.2 mg/kg SC, IM q6-12h[100,166]	Analgesia
	0.1-0.3 mg/kg SC, IM, IV q3-4h[13,194]	
Piroxicam	0.1 – 0.2 mg/kg PO q8h × 21 days[194]	Analgesia; nonsteroidal anti-inflammatory
Propofol	—	Intravenous nonbarbituate anesthetic; slow IV; lower dose after premedicated, higher dose when used alone; see medetomidine[e] for combination
	5-14 mg/kg slow IV to effect or 20 mg/kg/min CRI[194]	Not recommended as sole agent for anesthesia maintenance
	6-8 mg/kg IV induction, followed by 0.8-1 mg/kg/min CRI[205]	Anesthetic induction and maintenance; premedicated with dexmedetomidine (20 µg/kg IM), ketamine (5 mg/kg IM), fentanyl (10 µg/kg IM)[205]
	7.5-15 mg/kg IV[43]	Slow IV to effect
	12.5 mg/kg IV, IO followed by 1 mg/kg/min CRI[158]	Anesthetic induction and maintenance
	16 ± 5 mg/kg IV[6]	Anesthetic induction
Sevoflurane	To effect[6]	Anesthesia; MAC = 3.7%[214]
	6%-8% induction, 1%-3% maintenance	Prior use of a sedative or injectable induction agent is recommended, as use of preanesthetic combinations will lower the MAC of inhalants
Tiletamine/zolazepam (Telazol, Zoetis)	3 mg/kg IM[96]	Sedation prior to gas anesthetic; tiletamine causes severe renal tubular necrosis at 32 mg/kg and mild nephrosis at 7.5 mg/kg;[52] not generally recommended for use in rabbits
Tramadol	—	Pharmacokinetic data reported to be variable, data on clinical efficacy lacking[13]
	4.4 mg/kg IV[57]	Did not result in isoflurane-sparing effects[57]
	5 mg/kg q2h PO[219]	Improved pain management when used in conjunction with meloxicam[219]
	5 mg/kg SC, IV q8h[41]	
	5-15 mg/kg PO q8-12h[41]	

Continued

TABLE 10-4 Chemical Restraint/Sedative/Anesthetic/Analgesic Agents Used in Rabbits. (cont'd)

Agent	Dosage	Comments
Tramadol (cont'd)	10 mg/kg PO q12-24h[13]	Recommendation based on personal experience and anecdotal reports
	11 mg/kg PO[225]	PK; did not achieve adequate plasma concentrations for analgesia based on human levels
Yohimbine	0.2-1 mg/kg IM, IV[84]	$Alpha_2$-adrenergic antagonist; xylazine reversal

[a]See Table 10-5 for Constant Rate Infusion (CRI) protocols.

[b]Drugs and doses chosen depend on individual patient requirements and health status, procedure planned, and level of sedation desired. Combination of drugs are mixed in one syringe unless otherwise indicated. Atipamezole may be used to reverse dexmedetomidine or medetomidine, flumazenil may be used to reverse midazolam, and naloxone may be used to reverse opioids.

[c]The rabbit is considered a food animal in the USA and as such Alfaxan Multidose and Alfaxan Multidose IDX are not registered or indexed for use in the rabbit, respectively, and therefore use in the rabbit is considered off label in the USA. Both Alfaxan and Alfaxan Multidose are approved for use in pet rabbits in the United Kingdom. Alfaxan Multidose is also approved for use in pet rabbits in the in the following countries: Austria, Belgium, Finland, France, Hungary, Ireland, Italy, Netherlands, Norway, Portugal, Slovak Republic, Sweden, and Switzerland.

[d]Diazepam is not soluble in aqueous solution; admixing with aqueous solutions or fluids can result in precipitation; administering SC or IM can be painful and irritating; for SC or IM administration, midazolam may be preferred.

[e]Medetomidine is no longer commercially available in the United States, although it may be obtained from select compounding services.

TABLE 10-5 Constant Rate Infusion (CRI) Protocols Used in Rabbits.[a]

Agent(s)	Loading Dose IV	CRI Rate IV Per Hour Unless Noted
Butorphanol	0.2-0.4 mg/kg[98]	0.1-0.2 mg/kg[194]
		0.2-0.4 mg/kg[98]
Fentanyl	5-10 µg/kg[98]	10-30 µg/kg[98]
		30-100 µg/kg/min[32]
Ketamine	2-5 mg/kg[98]	0.3-1.2 mg/kg[98]
Ketamine (K)/ butorphanol (B)	(K) 0.4-0.5 mg/kg + (B) 0.02-0.06 mg/kg[143]	(K) 0.6 mg/kg + (B) 0.1-0.2 mg/kg[143]
	(K) 0.4-0.5 mg/kg + (B) 0.02-0.06 mg/kg[144]	(K) 0.4-1 mg/kg + (B) 0.1-0.2 mg/kg[144]
Ketamine (K)/fentanyl (F)	(K) 0.4-0.5 mg/kg + (F) 0.005 mg/kg[143]	(K) 0.6 mg/kg (0.4-1) + (F) 0.005-0.02 mg/kg[143]
Ketamine (K)/ hydromorphone (H)	(K) 0.4-0.5 mg/kg + (H) 0.05 mg/kg[143]	(K) 0.6 mg/kg (0.4-1) + (H) 0.025-0.05 mg/kg[143]
	(K) 0.4-0.5 mg/kg + (H) 0.05 mg/kg[144]	(K) 0.4-1 mg/kg + (H) 0.025-0.05 mg/kg[144]
Lidocaine	2 mg/kg[216]	50 or 100 µg/kg/min[216]; both CRI doses decreased the isoflurane MAC[216]; 100 µg/kg/hr × 48 hr: long-term analgesia with minimal risk of anorexia or gastrointestinal stasis[217]

[a]Surgical fluid rate is 10 mL/kg/h IV.[143]

TABLE 10-6 Locoregional Anesthesia Sites Used in Rabbits.

Loco-regional anesthesia (LRA) has been shown to provide a superior quality of analgesia compared to opioid-based protocols, decreases perioperative opioid consumption, and allows earlier recovery of bowel function. Some nerves can be blocked blindly, whereas deeper structures need guidance with peripheral nerve stimulation (PNS) or ultrasound (US).[213] Maximum recommended doses are 2 mg/kg lidocaine and 1 mg/kg bupivacaine.[213]

Block name	Area of Analgesia	Anatomical Landmarks
Infiltration/line block	Surgical site analgesia	Along incision site; pre- or intraoperatively
Epidural	Hindlimb, tail, perineum	For lumbosacral epidural; sternal recumbency, wings of ilium, lumbosacral space
Rostral infraorbital nerve block	Dental procedures; upper incisor teeth, upper lip, and surrounding tissue	Entrance of infraorbital canal
Mental nerve block	Dental procedures; cranial mandible and lower lip	Entrance of the mental foramen just in front of first premolar
Inferior alveolar nerve block	Dental procedures; mandibular cheek teeth and adjacent soft tissues	Extraoral approach with peripheral nervous system (PNS) guidance; needle inserted at level of the temporomandibular joint and advanced in a rostromedial direction until contraction of masticatory muscles is seen
Maxillary nerve block	Dental procedures	Lateral recumbency; needle inserted in a dorsomedial direction just caudal to facial tuberosity and ventral to zygomatic arch
Ear LRA	External ear canal and pinna	PNS guidance; needle inserted caudodorsal border of coronoid process of mandible and external acoustic meatus; block auriculotemporal (branch of trigeminal nerve) and caudal auricular (branch of facial nerve); blindly; greater auricular (branch of second cervical nerve): needle inserted in a caudocranial direction, cranially to the atlas wings, parallel to them, between the wings and the maxillary vein
Ear LRA	For total ear canal ablation with or without bulla osteotomy	PNS guidance; block mandibular nerve at level of temporomandibular joint and auriculopalpebral nerves
Eye LRA	Retrobulbar block; enucleation	Needle (bent at 20°angle) inserted at lateral canthus; follow wall of orbit until access orbital fascia; ultrasound-guided (US) technique for periconal ocular blockade
Brachial plexus block	Forelimb analgesia; surgeries of elbow, antebrachium, and carpus	Brachial plexus originates from roots of C6-T1 and emerges in the ventral border of scalenus muscle; PNS guidance alone or combined with US; axillary approach: lateral recumbency, affected leg up; needle inserted medial to acromion in a cranial-caudal direction in a parallel line to jugular vein
Sciatic nerve block	Surgery of hindlimb	PNS or US-guided; proximal lateral approach: lateral recumbency, affected leg up; landmarks are greater trochanter and ischiatic tuberosity

Continued

TABLE 10-6 Locoregional Anesthesia Sites Used in Rabbits (cont'd)

Block name	Area of Analgesia	Anatomical Landmarks
Femoral nerve block	Surgery of hindlimb	PNS or US-guided; inguinal approach: lateral recumbency with affected leg abducted; nerve cranial to femoral artery
Transversus abdominis plane block	Abdominal wall and parietal perineum; celiotomy procedures in humans include appendectomy, hysterectomy, and large bowel resection; literature lacking for rabbit	US-guided; cranial subcostal and caudal approaches depending on surgery; goal is to place LA between and internal oblique and transversus abdominis muscles
Erector spinae block	Acute or chronic pain; used in human medicine following abdominal, thoracic, and spinal surgery	US-guided; anesthetize the medial and lateral branches of dorsal branches of spinal nerves; goal is to place LA in interfascial plane between erector spinae muscles and transverse process of thoracic or lumbar vertebrae

TABLE 10-7 Chemotherapeutic Agents Used in Rabbits.[a,b]

Agent	Dosage	Comments
Carboplatin	150-180 mg/m² IV q21-28d[53,78,101,240]	Platinum product; neutropenia, gastrointestinal toxicity; decrease dose if renal failure
Chlorambucil (Leukeran, GlaxoSmithKline)	2 mg/kg PO q48h[153]	Alkylating agent; used in combination with prednisolone to treat chronic lymphocytic leukemia in a rabbit
Cyclophosphamide	50-60 mg/m² PO q24h × 2-3d/wk[101,240] 100-200 mg/m² IV q1-3wk[101,240] (often combined with doxorubicin)	Alkylating agent; neutropenia, hemorrhagic cystitis, gastrointestinal toxicity; repeat cyclophosphamide injections have been associated with renal failure in rabbits[7]
Doxorubicin	1 mg/kg IV q14-21d[53,240]	Antitumor antibiotic; renal failure, cardiac toxicity, neutropenia, tissue necrosis at extravasation sites; doxorubicin administered IV to male rabbits at doses of 3 mg/kg (50 mg/m²) q7d × 10 wk without causing cardiac injury but resulted in aplastic anemia, significant body weight loss, nephrotoxicity, and high premature mortality[128]
L-asparaginase	400 U/kg SC, IM[53,101,240]	Single IV dose at 10,000 IU/kg induced hyperinsulinemia insulin-resistant diabetic syndrome in rabbits; consider avoiding IV route[135]
Lomustine (CCNU)	50 mg/m² PO q3-6wk[101,167,240]	Alkylating agent; adverse effects neutropenia, hepatotoxicity, nephrotoxicity; used to treat mediastinal lymphoma in a rabbit;[177] rabbit died of renal failure 21 days after 2nd treatment;[167] used to treat cutaneous lymphoma in a rabbit[167]

TABLE 10-7 Chemotherapeutic Agents Used in Rabbits. (cont'd)

Agent	Dosage	Comments
Melphalan	0.1 mg/kg PO q24h × 10 days, then 0.05 mg/kg PO q24h[134]	Alkylating agent; used to treat multiple myeloma in a rabbit[134]
Mitoxantrone	5-6 mg/m² IV q21d[53,101,240]	Antitumor antibiotic; neutropenia, gastrointestinal toxicity, renal failure
Prednisone	0.5-2 mg/kg PO q12-24h[7,53,101,188]	Use with caution; may cause immunosuppression and predispose to pasteurellosis or encephalitozoonosis; concurrent gastroprotectant advised; may cause PU/PD, polyphagia, dermatologic effects; used as adjunct therapy in rabbits with thymoma undergoing radiation therapy, but benefit not noted;[7,53] prednisolone used as sole treatment for 6 rabbits with mediastinal neoplasia with survival from diagnosis 2.5-30.8 mo;[188] survival times of 18 rabbits with thymoma which were administered prednisolone alone were significantly longer compared to those rabbits receiving no treatment[182a]
Toceranib phosphate (Palladia, Zoetis)	3 mg/kg PO 3 × weekly[201]	M/W/F toceranib used with prednisolone for 83 days to manage metastatic carcinoma
Vincristine	0.5-0.7 mg/m² IV q7-14d[53]	Vinca alkaloid; tissue damage with extravasation, gastrointestinal toxicity, neutropenia, peripheral neuropathy; neurotoxic effects of vincristine well studied in rabbits[69,168,174]

[a]Because of the lack of data on efficacy of chemotherapeutics in rabbits, potential risks must be considered before treatment. Recommend routine hematologic examination and *E. cuniculi* testing prior to treatment. Lethal *E. cuniculi* infection reported in rabbits secondary to immunosuppressive effects of chemotherapy.[107]
[b]Body surface area = $(K * W^{2/3})/10^4$, where K = 9.9 and W = weight in grams.[255]

TABLE 10-8 Cardiovascular Agents Used in Rabbits.

Agent	Dosage	Comments
Atenolol	0.3 mg/kg PO q24h[181b] 0.5-2 mg/kg PO q24h[241] 1.5 mg/kg PO q12h[181b] 8.5 mg/kg PO q24h[50]	Negative inotrope; beta-blocker; to reduce heart rate and treat supraventricular and ventricular arrhythmias;[241] used in conjunction with methimazole for maximum effect on thyroid hormones
Atropine	0.05-3 mg/kg IM[72] 0.1-0.5 mg/kg SC, IM[166]	Parasympatholytic; repeat injections may be needed due to atropine esterase activity q10-20min[241]
Benazepril	0.25-0.5 mg/kg PO q24h[241]	Vasodilator; potentially less toxic than enalapril
Chlorothiazide	20-40 mg/kg PO[241]	Diuretic
Digoxin	0.0005-0.07 mg/kg PO q24-48h[241] 0.005-0.01 mg/kg PO q12-24h[166] 0.02 mg/kg PO[72] 0.03 mg/kg PO q12h[181b] 0.07 mg/kg PO[72]	Positive inotrope; congestive heart failure; atrial fibrillation

Continued

TABLE 10-8 Cardiovascular Agents Used in Rabbits. (cont'd)

Agent	Dosage	Comments
Diltiazem	0.5-1 mg/kg PO q12-24h[166,241] 4 mg/kg PO q8h[181b] 24 mg/kg PO q12h[181b]	Negative inotrope; calcium channel blocker for hypertrophic cardiomyopathy; to reduce heart rate and treat supraventricular and ventricular arrhythmias[241]
Dobutamine	5-15 µg/kg/min[241]	Positive inotrope; constant rate infusion
Dopamine	5-15 µg/kg/min[241]	Positive inotrope; constant rate infusion
Enalapril	0.1-0.5 mg/kg q24-48h[118,241] 0.18-0.5 mg/kg PO q12-24h[181b]	Vasodilator; monitor for hypotensive side effects
Epinephrine	0.2-0.4 mg/kg IM, IV, intratracheally[194]	Cardiac arrest
Furosemide	—	Loop diuretic
	0.3-2 mg/kg SC, IM, IV[95] prn	
	1-4 mg/kg PO, SC q8, 12, or 24h[181b]	
	1-4 mg/kg SC, IM, IV q4-6h[194,241] prn	Pulmonary edema
	2-5 mg/kg PO, SC, IM, IV q12h[241]	Congestive heart failure
Glycopyrrolate	0.01-0.02 mg/kg SC, IM[72] 0.01-0.1 mg/kg SC, IM, IV[72,241]	Parasympatholytic
Hydrochlorothiazide	1 mg/kg PO q12h[181b]	Diuretic
	1-4 mg/kg PO q12h[241]	Diuretic
Lidocaine	1-2 mg/kg IV (bolus)[72,198,241]	Cardiac arrhythmia
	2-4 mg/kg intratracheally[198]	Cardiac arrhythmia
Norepinephrine	0.5-1 µg/kg/min[236]	Effective in treating isoflurane-related hypotension
Pimobendan	0.1-0.3 mg/kg PO q12-24h[72,166,241]	Phosphodiesterase inhibitor; increases cardiac contractility with dilated cardiomyopathy or valvular disease
	0.2-1 mg/kg PO q8, 12, or 24h[181b] 2 mg/kg PO[181a]	
Sotalol	1.7 mg/kg PO q12h[181b]	Cardiac arrythmia (both atrial and ventricular)
Spironolactone	1-2 mg/kg PO q12h[241]	Diuretic; has been associated with leukopenia in humans[181b]
Verapamil	8-16 mg/kg PO + 0.5-2 mg/kg SC q24h[194]	Slow-channel calcium blocking agent

TABLE 10-9 Ophthalmologic Agents Used in Rabbits.

Agent	Dosage	Comments
Amphotericin B (liposomal form) (A)/moxifloxacin (Mo)	(A) 10 µg in 0.05 mL + (Mo) 100 µg in 0.05 mL intravitreally[49]	(Mo) strongly augments efficacy of (A)
Atropine 1%	Topical to eyes q12h prn[123,194]	Mydriasis; systemic effects are possible; may be ineffective in rabbits with pigmented irises or those that produce atropinase[250]

TABLE 10-9 Ophthalmologic Agents Used in Rabbits. (cont'd)

Agent	Dosage	Comments
Azithromycin 1% (Azasite, Akorn)	Topical to eyes q12h × 2 days, then q24h × 5 days[5]	Bacterial conjunctivitis
Besifloxacin 0.6% (Besivance, Bausch & Lomb)	Topical to eyes q12h[195]	Fluoroquinolone; bacterial conjunctivitis/endophthalmitis;[172] minimal systemic absorption
Betaxolol 0.5% (Betoptic, Alcon)	Topical to eyes q12h[124]	Glaucoma; effectively decreases intraocular pressure in rabbits
Ciprofloxacin 0.3% (Ciloxan, Alcon)	Topical to eyes q8-12h[123,194] 2 drops topical q1h for 7-14 hr[182]	Susceptible infections Ocular penetration injuries; good penetration into aqueous and vitreous humor
Cyclosporine A 0.05% (Restasis, Allergan)	Topical to eyes q12h[233]	Dry eye due to autoimmune dacryoadenitis
Cyclosprine A 0.2% (Optimmune, Merck)	Topical to eyes q12h[234]	Shown to increase tear production in rabbits; may inhibit recurrence of precorneal membranous occlusion postoperatively[82]
Dexamethasone 0.1% (Santen)	1 drop q12h x 2 days, then 1 drop on day 3[9]	PK; corneal distribution superior to oral prednisolone[9]
Diclofenac sodium 0.1%	Topical to eyes[246] Topical to eyes q12h[152]	Nonsteroidal antiinflammatory Blepharitis[250]
Dorzolamide 2% (Trusopt, Merck)	Topical to eyes q8-12h[123,152]	Glaucoma
Doxycycline monohydrate	2.5 mg/kg PO q12h[152]	*Encephalitozoon cuniculi*-induced glaucoma
Fluconazole	37.5 mg/kg PO q12h[11]	*Aspergillus* keratitis
Flurbiprofen sodium 0.03%	Topical to eyes[130]	Nonsteroidal antiinflammatory; blepharitis[250]
Flurbiprofen 7.66 mg/mL	0.1 mL injected intravitreally[20]	PK; short half-life; uveal inflammation
Fusidic acid (Fucithalmic, Leo)	Topical to eyes q12-24h[95]	Bacterial conjunctivitis
Gatifloxacin 0.3% (Zymar, Allergan)	Topical to eyes q8h[195]	Bacterial conjunctivitis; no longer available in the United States
Gentamicin (Tiacil, Virbac)	Topical to eyes q8h[95]	Bacterial conjunctivitis
Gentamicin injectable solution (100 mg/mL)	8 mg per eye intravitreally[254]	Decreases IOP in nonresponsive glaucoma; alternative to enucleation; retinotoxic; not used in visual eye[254]
Ketorolac tromethamine 0.1%	Topical to eyes[246]	Nonsteroidal antiinflammatory; blepharitis[250]
Levofloxacin 0.5%, 1.5%	Single dose	In vitro PK model 1.5% greater antibiotic efficacy than 0.5% against *Staphylococcus epidermidis*[230]

Continued

TABLE 10-9 Ophthalmologic Agents Used in Rabbits. (cont'd)

Agent	Dosage	Comments
Marbofloxacin (Marbocyl FD, Vetoquinol)	4 mg/kg IV[200]	Penetration of marbofloxacin into the aqueous and vitreous humor after IV administration was significantly enhanced by intraocular inflammation
Methylsulfonylmethane (MSM) ophthalmic 15% (Alcon)	Topical to eyes q12h[152]	*Encephalitozoon cuniculi*-induced glaucoma
Moxifloxacin 0.5% (Vigamox, Alcon)	Topical to eyes q6h[160,172]	Bacterial conjunctivitis; good aqueous concentration with both oral and ophthalmic administration; oral better for vitreous concentration[79]
Micafungin 0.1%	0.5 mL subconjunctivally q24h × 3 wk[106]	*Candida* keratitis
Neomycin/bacitracin/ polymyxin B	Topical to eyes q6h[123]	Susceptible infections; corneal ulceration
Neomycin/polymyxin B/ dexamethasone	Topical to eyes q6h	Eosinophilic keratitis
Penicillin G	40,000 U/kg SC q7d × 3 treatments[82]	*Treponema cuniculi*-induced blepharitis
Phenylephrine 10%	Topical to eyes[115]	Mydriasis
Prednisolone acetate 1%	Topical to eyes q6-12h[123]	Inflammation of eyes; rabbits are a corticosteroid-sensitive species
	Topical to eyes q12h[152]	*Encephalitozoon cuniculi*-induced glaucoma
Prednisolone	0.25 mg/kg q24h PO × 3 days[9]	PK; similar conjunctival concentration of corticosteroid with topical dexamethasone
Prednisolone liposomes	4 mg/mL; 0.1 mL injected subconjunctivally[252]	Capable of inducing sustained anti-inflammatory action; better than eyedrops[252]
Ripasudil 1%	50 µ/L once in each eye[114]	PK; a selective Rho-associated coiled-coil containing protein kinase (ROCK) inhibitor; glaucoma and ocular hypertension; penetrated most ocular tissues; maximum levels in 15 min[114]
Terbinafine 0.2%	2 drops, repeated in 5 min[228]	PK; corneal and aqueous humor levels at concentrations adequate for fungal inhibition[228]
Terbinafine 1% ointment	Topical q6h × 8 wk[21]	Keratomycosis; compounded
Timolol 0.5% (Timoptic, Merck)	Topical to eyes q12h[124]	Glaucoma
Tobramycin 0.3%	Topical to eyes q6h[21]	Bacterial ulcerative keratitis

TABLE 10-9 Ophthalmologic Agents Used in Rabbits. (cont'd)

Agent	Dosage	Comments
Triamcinolone liposomes	4 mg/mL; 0.1 mL injected subconjunctivally[252]	Capable of inducing sustained anti-inflammatory action; better than eyedrops[252]
Tropicamide 1%	Topical to eyes[96]	Mydriasis; 1 drop in affected eye(s) q8-12h to achieve dilation (not rabbit specific)[194]
Trovafloxacin 0.5%	Topical to eyes[12]	Broad spectrum; safe for intravitreal injection up to 25 µg
Vancomycin 0.3%, 1%	Topical to eyes q2h for 10 hr each day × 5 days[58]	Commercially available product not available in the United States; compounded from injectable form of vancomycin; used to treat methicillin-resistant *Staphylococcus aureus*
Voriconazole	Topical to eyes q12h;[226] topical to eyes q2-3h initially[194]	Fungal keratitis; compounded to a 1% voriconazole solution[194]

TABLE 10-10 Miscellaneous Agents Used in Rabbits.

Agent	Dosage	Comments
Activated charcoal (1 g/5 mL water)	1 g/kg PO q4-6h[113,173]	May reduce intestinal absorption of toxins
Aluminum hydroxide	30-60 mg/kg PO q8-12h[27]	Phosphorus binder; hyperphosphatemia due to renal failure
Barium	10-14 mL/kg PO[196]	Gastrointestinal contrast studies qs 50:50 with water
Bethanechol	5 mg/kg q8h[139]	Aids bladder contractility; reduces detrusor atony
Bio-Sponge (Platinum Performance)	Equine paste PO to effect	Rabbit dysbiosis; di-tri-octahedral smectite (a clay mineral) decreased *Clostridium perfringens* exotoxins in vitro[136]
Blood transfusion (whole blood)	10-20 mL/kg given no faster than 22 mL/kg/h	Cross-matching advised, especially for repeated transfusions
Calcium EDTA (edetate calcium disodium) (Calcium Disodium Versenate, 3M)	25 mg/kg PO, SC q8h x 14 days[245] 27 mg/kg SC, IV q6-12h[166]	Chelation therapy; diluted to <10 mg/mL with 0.45% NaCl/2.5% dextrose
Calcium gluconate	5-10 mL/rabbit PO, IM[87]	Dystocia; when uterine inertia suspected
Chlorpheniramine maleate	0.2-0.4 mg/kg PO q12h[95]	Antihistamine
Cholestyramine (Questran Light, Squibb)	2 g/rabbit PO q24h × 18-21 days[166,194]	Ion exchange resin for toxin absorption following inappropriate antibiotic administration; use for treating enterotoxemia; gavage with 20 mL water; may result in constipation
Chondroitin sulfate (Cosequin, Nutramax)	Used empirically at feline dose[237]	Arthritis; nutraceutical

Continued

TABLE 10-10 Miscellaneous Agents Used in Rabbits. (cont'd)

Agent	Dosage	Comments
Cimetidine	5-10 mg/kg PO, SC, IM, IV q6-12h[194]	Gastric and duodenal ulcers
	5-10 mg/kg PO q8-12h[194]	
Cisapride	0.5 mg/kg PO q6-12h[194]	Enhances gastrointestinal motility; must be compounded in United States; may be synergistic if used with ranitidine (0.5 mg/kg q24h IV)[194]
Cosyntropin	5 µg/kg IV[43a]	Synthetic form of ACTH; leads to substantial increase in serum cortisol up to 60 min postadministration; total dose of 125 µg subjectively leads to significant lethargy up to 8 hr after administration
Cyclizine	8 mg/rabbit PO q12h[95]	Vertigo associated with torticollis
Cyproheptadine	1-4 mg/rabbit PO q12-24h[89]	Possible appetite stimulant
Deslorelin (Suprelorin F 4.7 mg, Virbac)	4.7 mg gonadotrophin-releasing hormone agonist slow-release implant (GNRH A-SRI) SC[218]	Contraception: male unreliable; female >9 mo may develop endometritis and/or endometrial hyperplasia[218]
Dexamethasone	—	Corticosteroids are seldom indicated in rabbits; rabbits are a corticosteroid-sensitive species; use with extreme caution and consider concurrent administration of a gastroprotective agent
	0.2-0.6 mg/kg SC, IM, IV[166]	Antiinflammatory; use with caution
	0.5 mg/kg IM q24h x 5 days[157a]	Well tolerated; 5-day dosing suppressed leukocytes, in particular the T cells ($P \leq 0.003$); rabbits did not show any adverse clinical signs throughout the study[157a]
Dexamethasone sodium phosphate (SP) 4 mg/mL	1 mg/kg IM[66]	Used in emergency tracheal stent placement
Diphenhydramine	1-2 mg/kg PO q12h[194]	
	2 mg/kg PO, SC q8-12h[166]	Antihistamine; torticollis
	2 mg/kg IV[194]	Prior to blood transfusion
Epoetin alpha, recombinant (Epogen, Amgen)	50-150 U/kg SC q2-3d[194]	Biosynthetic form of erythropoietin; adjunctive treatment of anemia; use until PCV is normal, then q7d for at least 4 wk
Famotidine	0.5-1 mg/kg PO, SC, IV q12-24h[67,194]	H_2-receptor antagonist used to reduce gastrointestinal acid production
	1 mg/kg IV q24h[194]	Stress-induced ulcer prevention
Fecal transfaunation	Mix fresh cecotrophs with warm saline, strain through gauze, and administer by gavage	Dysbiosis; placement of E-collar on donor facilitates collection of sample
Ferrous sulfate	4-6 mg/kg PO q24h[68]	Iron deficiency anemia
Furosemide	—	Loop diuretic
	0.3-2 mg/kg SC, IM, IV[194] prn	
	1-4 mg/kg IM, IV q4-6h[194]	Pulmonary edema

TABLE 10-10 Miscellaneous Agents Used in Rabbits. (cont'd)

Agent	Dosage	Comments
Furosemide (cont'd)	2-5 mg/kg PO, SC, IM, IV q12h[194] prn	Congestive heart failure
Hetastarch (Hespan, DuPont)	5 mL/kg IV given over 5-10 min; repeat if necessary[149] 20 mL/kg IV[171]	Volume expansion in hypoproteinemic patients; may be of benefit in endotoxemia; see Table 10-22 for more details
Hydroxyzine	2 mg/kg PO q8-12h[166]	Antihistamine; antipruritic
Iron dextran	4-6 mg/kg IM once[166]	Iron deficiency anemia (treatment or prevention)
Lactated Ringer's solution or other appropriate fluid of choice	3-4 mL/kg/h + [% dehydration × kg × 1000 mL][86] 100-150 mL/kg/day CRI or divided SC q6-12h[149]	Maintenance + dehydration fluid requirements (mL); treatment for shock; see Table 10-22 for more details Maintenance fluid support
Levetiracetam (Keppra, UCB)	20 mg/kg PO q8h[17]	Anticonvulsant; dosage not established in rabbits but PK are similar to those in dogs
Loperamide	0.1 mg/kg PO q8h × 3 days, then q24h × 2 days[194]	Reduce gut motility; enteropathies (nonspecific diarrhea); give in 1 mL water
Manuka honey	Topical wound dressing	Effects on osmolarity, pH, hydrogen peroxide production, and nutrient content promotes healing
Maropitant citrate (Cerenia, Zoetis)	1 mg/kg SC, IV[181] 2 mg/kg SC q24h × 3-5 days, then q48h or 3 × weekly if needed[40]	PK; plasma concentrations similar to levels considered therapeutic in dogs May be helpful in arthritis or inflammatory conditions; reduces visceral pain
Meclizine	2-12 mg/kg PO q24h[194] 12.5-25 mg/kg PO q8-12h[117]	Reduces disorientation and rolling with torticollis
Methimazole	1.25 mg total dose q12h PO[50] 1.4 mg/kg q24h PO[50]	Treatment of hyperthyroidism Most significant effect on thyroid hormone levels when used in conjunction with atenolol 8.5 mg/kg q24h PO[50]
Metoclopramide	0.2-0.5 mg/kg PO, SC q6-8h[166] 0.2-1 mg/kg PO, SC, IM q8-24h[194] 0.5 mg/kg PO, SC q6-8h[166]	Stimulates gastrointestinal motility
Mirtazapine	0.3-0.5 mg/kg PO q24h[197]	Appetite stimulant; dosage not established in rabbits; cat dose given here
Nandrolone (Deca-Durabolin, Organon)	2 mg/kg SC, IM[95]	Anabolic steroid; appetite stimulant; adjunct to treatment for anemia, especially in chronic renal failure
Norepinephrine	0.5-1 µg/kg/min[236]	Effective in treating isoflurane-related hypotension
Omeprazole	20 mg/kg SC q12h[138]	Proton pump inhibitor used as a gastroprotective agent; note: standard small animal and equine dose is 0.5-1 mg/kg

Continued

TABLE 10-10 Miscellaneous Agents Used in Rabbits. (cont'd)

Agent	Dosage	Comments
Oxytocin	0.1-3 U/kg SC, IM[166]	Use in delayed, but unobstructed parturition; agalactia
	0.57-4.6 U/kg IM in 1-2 U increments[87]	Dystocia; when uterine inertia suspected
Polysulfated glycosaminoglycan (Adequan, Luitpold)	2.2 mg/kg SC, IM q3d × 21-28 days, then q14d[194]	Noninfectious, traumatic, or degenerative joint disease
Potassium citrate	33 mg/kg q8h[166]	Urinary calculi; may decrease calcium-based stone formation
Prazosin	0.5 mg/rabbit PO q12h[139]	Urethral sphincter relaxation
Prednisolone	—	See dexamethasone; rarely indicated; steroid-sensitive species (may have secondary immunosuppressive effects)[191]
	0.25-0.5 mg/kg PO q12h × 3 days, then q24h × 3 days, then q48h[196]	Treatment of nonresponsive torticollis, when negative for pasteurellosis; give antibiotics concurrently
	0.5-2 mg/kg PO q12h[194]	Antiinflammatory
	1 mg/kg q24h PO[188]	Cranial mediastinal neoplasia; alternative to euthanasia
Prednisone	—	See dexamethasone; rarely indicated
	0.5-2 mg/kg PO[194]	Antiinflammatory
Prochlorperazine	0.2-0.5 mg/kg PO q8h[95]	Torticollis; doses as high as 30 mg/kg q8h are used to treat labyrinthine disorders in humans
Ranitidine	0.5 mg/kg IV q24h with cisapride (0.5 mg/kg PO q8h)[194]	Prokinetic
	2-5 mg/kg PO, SC, IV q12h[175,194]	Gastric ulceration (often in inappetant rabbits)
Sevelamer	Dosage not established in animals	Cat dosage is 200-400 mg per dose PO q8h with meals;[194] phosphorus binder for hyperphosphatemia associated with chronic renal failure; consider monitoring coagulation parameters, as vitamin K absorption may be affected; drug is not absorbed systemically so toxicity is unlikely
Silymarin (milk thistle)	4-15 mg/kg PO q8-12h[119]	Nutraceutical used as an adjunctive treatment for liver disease; hepatoprotectant; dosage not established for rabbits; suggested dose for small animals
Stanozolol	0.5-2 mg PO once[194]	Stimulates appetite following surgery or illness; may be available from compounding pharmacy
Succimer (DMSA)	1050 mg/m^2 PO × 1 wk, then 700 mg/m^2 × 2 wk[253]	Lead toxicity
Sucralfate	25 mg/kg PO q8-12h[166]	Gastrointestinal ulcers; may interfere with other orally administered drugs

TABLE 10-10 Miscellaneous Agents Used in Rabbits. (cont'd)

Agent	Dosage	Comments
Terbutaline	0.01 mg/kg SC q12h[66]	Bronchodilator; treats breathing problems caused by asthma and bronchitis
Verapamil	2.5-25 μg/kg/h IP[227]	Postoperative administration decreases adhesion formation; see Table 10-8 for cardiac use
	8-16 mg/kg PO plus 0.5-2 mg/kg SC q24h[194]	Slow-channel calcium blocking agent
Vitamin A	500-1000 U/kg IM[166]	
Vitamin B complex	0.02-0.4 mL/rabbit SC, IM q24h[89]	Possible appetite stimulant; vitamin B deficiency
Vitamin C (ascorbic acid)	100 mg/kg PO q12h[194]	Soften stools (may reduce cecal absorption of clostridial endotoxins);[194] nutritional supplement
Vitamin K	1-10 mg/kg PO, SC q24h prn[166]	Select bleeding disorders and toxicities; vitamin K is fat soluble; give PO formulations in oil

TABLE 10-11 Hematologic and Serum Biochemical Values of Rabbits.[24]

Biochemical Parameter	Reference Interval[d]	Mean ± SD[d]	Range (Min-Max)[f]
Hematocrit, %	31.3–43.3	32.1 ± 2.7	20.6–39.6
Erythrocytes, × 10^6/μL	4.5–6.9	5.7 ± 0.5	3.9–7.0
Hemoglobin, g/dL	11.0–14.4	12.3 ± 1.0	7.8–15.4
Mean corpuscular hemoglobin, pg/cell	19.4–23.8	21 ± 1	18–23
Mean corpuscular hemoglobin concentration, g/dL	32.3–34.5	33.6 ± 0.6[a]	31.1–37.0[a]
Mean corpuscular volume, $μm^3$	59.0–70.1	63.7 ± 3.1[a]	59.0–70.1[a]
Platelets, × 10^3/μL	134–567[c]	400 ± 89	192–662
White blood cells, × 10^3/μL	4.1–10.8[c]	7.2 ± 2.5	2.4–12.8
Neutrophils, × 10^3/μL	—	4.5 ± 2.3	1.1–7.4
Neutrophils, %		52 ± 12	21–73
Lymphocytes, × 10^3/μL	—	2.1 ± 1.4	0.5–6.5
Lymphocytes, %		29 ± 14	9–64
Monocytes, × 10^3/μL	—	1.1 ± 0.6	0–3.7
Monocytes, %		15 ± 5	1–32
Eosinophils, × 10^3/μL	—	0.01 ± 0.01	0–0.03
Eosinophils, %		0 ± 0.1	0–0.7
Basophils, × 10^3/μL	—	0.1 ± 0.1	0–0.4
Basophils, %	—	2 ± 1	0–7

Continued

TABLE 10-11 Hematologic and Serum Biochemical Values of Rabbits. (cont'd)

Biochemical Parameter	Reference Interval[d]	Mean ± SD[d]	Range (Min-Max)[f]
Alkaline phosphatase, U/L	6–14	10 ± 2	—
Alanine transferase, U/L	52–80	66 ± 7	—
Amylase, IU/L	82–343[g]	—	—
Aspartate aminotransferase, U/L	48–96	72 ± 12	—
Bile acids, µmol/L	26–34[g]	—	—
Bilirubin (total), mg/dL	0.1–0.5	0.3 ± 0.04	—
Calcium, mg/dL	7.6–12.2	10.0 ± 1.2	
Chloride, mmol/L	—	102 ± 3[f]	96–109[f]
Cholesterol, mg/dL	6–65[g]	—	—
Creatine kinase, U/L	23–247	135 ± 56	—
Creatinine, mg/dL	1.0–2.2	1.6 ± 0.3	—
Gamma-glutamyltransferase, U/L	0–7	3 ± 2	—
Glucose, mg/dL	109–161	135 ± 13	—
Lactate dehydrogenase, U/L	59–205[e]	107 ± 44[e]	—
Lipase, IU/L	38–210[g]	—	—
Magnesium, mg/dL	1.9–3.2[g]	—	—
Phosphorous, mg/dL	3.0-6.2[e]	4.7 ± 0.8[e]	—
Potassium, mmol/L	—	4.2 ± 0.3[f]	3.4-5.1[f]
Total protein, g/dL	6.1-7.7	6.9 ± 0.4	—
Albumin, g/dL	2.8–4.0	3.4 ± 0.3	—
Globulin, g/dL	2.1–3.7[g]	—	—
Sodium, mmol/L	—	143 ± 3[f]	138-148[f]
Triglycerides, mg/dL	22-188[g]	—	—
Urea nitrogen, mg/dL	9-29	19 ± 5	—

[a]n = 110 young male New Zealand white rabbits, 2.5-97.5 percentile values.
[b]n = 58 nulliparous does.
[c]90% confidence intervals; n = 54 mixed sex pet rabbits, age range 5 months-10 years.
[d]n =120 adult males.
[e]Plasma samples; 2.5 and 97.5 percentile values; n = 110 young adult males.
[f]Plasma samples; min-max values given if n < 100; n = 60 young adult males.
[g]90% confidence interval; plasma samples; n = 60 mixed-sex pet rabbits, age range 5 months-10 years.
SD, Standard deviation.

TABLE 10-12 Reference Intervals for Venous Blood Samples Analyzed with the i-STAT EC8+[a] in Rabbits.[24,b]

Analyte	95% Reference Interval
pH	7.25–7.53
pCO_2, mmHg	28.9–52.9
HCO_3^-,mmol/L	17.0–32.5
tCO_2, mmol/L	18–34
BE_{ecf}, mmol/L	−10 to 8
Na, mmol/L	136–147
K, mmol/L	3.4–5.7
Cl, mmol/L	93–113
AnGap, mmol/L	11–26
Hematocrit, %	29–46
Hemoglobin, g/dL	9.8–15.5
Blood urea nitrogen, mg/dL	9–33
Glucose, mg/dL	93–245

[a]Abbot Point of Care, Princeton, NJ.
[b]Data from Ardiaca M, Bonvehi C, Montesinos A. Point-of-care blood gas and electrolyte analysis in rabbits. *Vet Clin North Am Exot Anim Pract.* 2013;16:175-195.

TABLE 10-13 Rabbit Blood Glucose and Sodium Levels as Prognostic Indicators.[119]

Physiologic State	Blood Glucose (mg/dL)	Sodium (mmol/L)	Osmolarity[a] (mOsm/L)	Tonicity[a] (mOsm/L)
Normal	76-148	136-147	284-312	278-302
Stress (e.g., handling)	144-180	—	—	—
Severe disease (e.g., enterotoxemia, mucoid enteropathy, GI obstruction)	360-540	<129 carries a 2.3 times mortality risk	—	—
Diabetes mellitus	540-601	—	—	—

[a]Osmolarity and tonicity may be used to differentiate true hyponatremia from pseudohyponatremia (may occur with hyperlipidemia, severe liver disease, or congestive heart failure).
Calculated tonicity:
Ton (mOsm/L) = 2 × Na (mmol/L) + glucose (mg/dL)/18
Calculated osmolarity:
P_{osm} (mOsm/L) = 2 × Na (mmol/L) + glucose (mg/dL)/18 + BUN (mg/dL)/2.8

TABLE 10-14 Biologic and Physiologic Data of Rabbits.[96]

Parameter	Normal Values
Adult body weight, male (buck)	1.5-5 kg
Adult body weight, female (doe)	1.5-6 kg
Birth weight	30-80 g
Respiratory rate	30-60 breaths/min

Continued

TABLE 10-14 Biologic and Physiologic Data of Rabbits. (cont'd)

Parameter	Normal Values
Tidal volume	4-6 mL/kg
Heart rate	130-325 beats/min
Rectal temperature	38.5-40°C (101.3-104°F)
Life span	5-6 yr (up to 15 yr)
Food consumption	50 g/kg/day
Water consumption	100 mL/kg/day
Gastrointestinal transit time	4-5 hr
Breeding onset, male	6-10 mo
Breeding onset, female	4-9 mo
Breeding life of female	4 mo to 3.75 yr
Reproductive cycle	Induced ovulation
Gestation period	29-35 days
Litter size	4-10
Weaning age	4-6 wk
Dental formula	I2/1 C0/0 P3/2 M3/3

TABLE 10-15 Urinalysis Values in Rabbits.[24,196,202]

Measurement	Normal Values
Urine volume	
Large breeds	20-350 mL/kg/day
Medium breeds	130 mL/kg/day
Specific gravity	1.003-1.036
pH	8-9
Crystals	Ammonium magnesium phosphate, calcium carbonate monohydrate, anhydrous calcium carbonate, calcium oxalate
Casts, epithelial cells, or bacteria	Absent to rare
Erythrocytes	0
Leukocytes	0-25
Albumin	Occasional in young rabbits
Protein:creatinine ratio	0.11-0.47
Protein (mg/dL)	0-30
Protein (Multistix dipsticks)	Negative to +++
Bilirubin, mg/dL	0
Glucose	0
Ketones, mg/dL	0-15
Urobilinogen, mg/dL	0-1

TABLE 10-16 Electrocardiographic (ECG) Values in Rabbits.[178]

Parameter	New Zealand White Rabbits (awake)[a] (N = 100: 44 M; 56 F)		Client-Owned Fancy, Fur, and Crossbreeds (awake)[b] (N = 46: 24 M [8 intact]; 22 F [8 intact])	
	Mean ± SD	Range	Mean ± SD	Range
Age, mo	—	6 (all)	—	2–84
Body weight, kg	2.62 ± 0.20	2.1–3.0	—	1.1–7.9
Heart rate, beats/min	243 ± 34	154– 330	264 ± 34	198–330
P wave amplitude, mV	0.05 ± 0.02	0.01–0.13	0.08 ± 0.02	0.04–0.12
P wave duration, s	0.032 ± 0.004	0.021–0.045	0.03 ± 0.01	0.01–0.05
P-R interval, s	0.050 ± 0.006	0.036–0.072	0.06 ± 0.01	0.04–0.08
R wave amplitude, mV	0.18 ± 0.09	0.04–0.42	0.21 ± 0.09	0.03–0.39
QRS duration, s	0.056 ± 0.004	0.043–0.066	0.04 ± 0.01	0.02–0.06
Q-T interval, s	0.143 ± 0.012	0.115–0.173	0.12 ± 0.02	0.08–0.16
T wave amplitude, mV	0.16 ± 0.07	0.01–0.51	0.11 ± 0.03	0.05–0.17
Mean electrical axis	—	−60° to 180°[c]	19° ± 31°	−43° to 80°

[a]*J Exot Pet Med.* 2015;24(2):223-234.
[b]*Vet Rec.* 2010;167:961-965.
[c]In 85% of rabbits, the mean electrical axis was -30° to 90°.

TABLE 10-17 Echocardiographic Measurements (M-mode and 2-dimensional) in Clinically Normal New Zealand White Rabbits.[a,b,178]

Parameter	Awake (N = 100)[d]	Sedated[c] (N = 26)[e]
Body weight, kg	2.6 ± 0.2	2.3 ± 0.4
Age, mo	6 (all)	4 - 5
Sex	44 M; 56 F	26 M; 0 F
Heart rate, beats/min	227 ± 36	263 ± 37 (Doppler)
IVSd, mm	2.74 ± 0.51	2.65 ± 0.31
IVSs, mm	4.01 ± 0.70	3.63 ± 0.34
LVIDd, mm	13.28 ± 1.91	13.51 ± 1.05
LVIDs, mm	8.32 ± 1.47	8.64 ± 0.82
LVFWd, mm	2.78 ± 0.54	2.25 ± 0.29
LVFWs, mm	3.56 ± 0.52	3.15 ± 0.38
FS, %	37.17 ± 4.99	36.01 ± 4.31
EF, %	71.12 ± 6.32	69.58 ± 5.33
LA, mm	8.62 ± 1.02 (2D)	7.49 ± 1.14
Ao, mm	7.90 ± 0.77 (2D)	6.57 ± 0.46

Continued

TABLE 10-17 Echocardiographic Measurements (M-mode and 2-dimensional) in Clinically Normal New Zealand White Rabbits. (cont'd)

Parameter	Awake (N = 100)	Sedated[c] (N = 26)
LA/Ao	1.09 ± 0.10 (2D)	1.15 ± 0.19
EPSS, mm	—	1.41 ± 0.25

[a]Values are mean ± standard deviation except for age and sex.
[b]All values are M-mode derived unless indicated otherwise (2D).
[c]Sedated with ketamine (20 mg/kg SC) and midazolam (2 mg/kg SC).
[d]*J Exot Pet Med.* 2015;24(2):223-234.
[e]*Vet J.* 2009;181:326-331.
Ao, Aorta diameter; EF, ejection fraction; EPSS, E-point to septal separation; FS, fractional shortening; IM, intramuscularly; IVSd, interventricular septum in diastole; IVSs, interventricular septum in systole; LA, left atrial diameter; LVIDd, left ventricular internal diameter in diastole; LVIDs, left ventricular internal diameter in systole; LVFWd, left ventricular free wall in diastole; LVFWs, left ventricular free wall in systole; SC, subcutaneously.

TABLE 10-18 Treatments Used in the Management of Rabbit Gastrointestinal Syndrome (RGIS).[a]

Agent	Dosage	Comments
Buprenorphine	0.01-0.05 mg/kg SC, IM, IV q6-12h[166]	Analgesia
Buprenorphine SR	0.12 mg/kg SC q72h[51]	Analgesia
Butorphanol	0.1 – 1 mg/kg SC, IM, IV q2-6h[166]	Analgesia; doses up to 2 mg/kg may be given
Cisapride	0.5 mg/kg PO q8-12h[194]	Enhances gastrointestinal motility; compounded in United States
Cyproheptadine HCl	1-4 mg/rabbit PO q12-24h[89]	Possible appetite stimulant
Enrofloxacin	5-10 mg/kg PO, SC, IM, IV q12h[25,29,175]	Suspected primary bacterial enteritis (rare in rabbits); dilute when administering parenterally
Famotidine	0.5-1 mg/kg PO, SC, IV q12-24h[67,194]	H_2-receptor antagonist used to reduce gastrointestinal acid production
Fluid therapy	Weight (kg) × % dehydration × 1000 mL = fluid deficit divided into SC boluses or divided IV per hr over 12-24 hr[89]	Add deficit to maintenance requirement of 3-4 mL/kg/h; see Tables 10-21 and 10-22 for more information
	60-90 mL/kg × 1 hr	Shock therapy
	100-150 mL/kg/day constant rate infusion or divided SC q6-12h	Maintenance fluid support
Herbivore critical care diet (Oxbow Animal Health)	Follow manufacturer's instructions for reconstitution; feed 45 mL/kg/day PO divided q8h	Syringe feeding; use fine grind (Oxbow Animal Health) for nasogastric tubes
Hydromorphone	0.05-0.2 mg/kg SC, IM, IV q6-8h[36]	Analgesia
Lidocaine	2 mg/kg IV loading dose given over 5 min followed by 60-100 µg/kg/min[216]	CRI for severe, refractory cases of RGIS
	100 mg/kg/min × 2 days[217]	Better surgical and postoperative outcome than buprenorphine

TABLE 10-18 Treatments Used in the Management of Rabbit Gastrointestinal Syndrome (RGIS). (cont'd)

Agent	Dosage	Comments
Maropitant citrate (Cerenia, Zoetis)	1 mg/kg SC, IV[181]	PK
	2 mg/kg SC q24h × 3-5 days; then q48h or 3 × weekly if needed[40]	May be helpful in inflammatory conditions; reduces visceral pain
	10 mg/kg SC[209a]	PK (n = 3); achieved plasma concentrations similar or higher to those found in dogs at 1 and 2 mg/kg SC[209a]
Meloxicam	1 mg/kg PO q24h[39,235]	NSAID; use only if well hydrated with normal renal parameters
Metoclopramide	0.01-0.09 mg/kg/h IV[194]	CRI
	0.2-1 mg/kg PO, SC q6-8h[166]	Stimulates gastrointestinal motility
Metronidazole	5 mg/kg slow IV q12h[194]	
	20 mg/kg PO q12h for 3-5 days[194]	For suspected clostridial overgrowth and enterotoxemia
Midazolam	0.25-0.5 mg/kg IM, IV[104]	Antianxiety; may also stimulate appetite
Ranitidine	2-5 mg/kg PO, SC, IV q12h[175,194]	Gastric ulceration (often in inappetent rabbits)
Simethicone	65-130 mg/animal PO q1h × 2-3 treatments[132]	May reduce abdominal discomfort associated with excess gas
Thermal support	Provide thermal support if body temperature <99°F[89]	Avoid overheating
Trimebutine	1.5 mg/kg PO, IV[148]	Enhance gastrointestinal motility; not available in the United States; oral available in Canada
Vitamin B Complex	0.02-0.4 mL/rabbit SC, IM q24h[89]	Possible appetite stimulant

[a]Concurrent to treatment, it is important to correct the cause (e.g., boredom, stress, excessive shedding, inadequate dietary roughage, nutritional deficiency or imbalance, disease, toxin, obesity). Surgical intervention is no longer considered the primary treatment option and is rarely indicated except in cases of complete obstruction.

TABLE 10-19 Rabbit Feeding Recommendations.[35,223]

>70% high-fiber hay offered ad libitum	Mixed grass hays; orchard, meadow, timothy, etc., or high-quality grass clippings
	Provide alfalfa (high protein and calcium) during growth stages/ lactation, then discontinue
<25% high-fiber uniform pellets	¼ cup pellets per 2.3 kg (5 lb) BW divided into 2 meals/day for 5 days/ wk; preferred pellet for adult rabbit maintenance is timothy-based or timothy blend with ≥ protein, 0.5-1% calcium, and 20-29% fiber
5% fresh greens	Chopped, dark, fibrous, leafy greens and vegetables (kale, mustard greens, carrot tops, parsley, dandelion greens, romaine lettuce, cilantro, collard greens, Swiss chard, bib or red-tipped lettuce)
<5% treats	Small amount of fresh or dried fruit or hay-based treats several times/wk
Fresh clean water	Ad libitum
Feeding for life stages	Growing rabbits and females in late gestation may consume 2x food of adult rabbit at maintenance; does in pregnancy may decrease food intake briefly; lactating does may consume 3x maintenance

TABLE 10-20 Rabbit Vascular Access.[164]

Collection Site	Advantages	Disadvantages
Lateral saphenous vein	• Easily visualized • Easily accessible	• Vein is mobile, requires stabilization • Vein may collapse during aspiration • Sedation may facilitate venipuncture
Cephalic vein	• Good for collecting small to moderate volumes of blood	• May not be easily visualized • Vein is mobile, requires stabilization • Sedation desirable to prevent injury to limb and visual stress to rabbit • Skin may be contaminated with exudates from upper respiratory tract (URT) infection—foreleg used in grooming • Shorter length in smaller breeds, hard to access
Jugular vein	• Good for collecting larger volumes of blood	• Not easily visualized in obese rabbits or females with large dewlaps • Sedation/anesthesia recommended • Short-nosed/dwarf breeds and rabbits with URT infections may become dyspneic when the neck is extended back during restraint
Central auricular artery	• Easily visualized • Easily accessible • Vessel is not mobile • Does not require sedation/anesthesia • Rapid collection of large volume of blood	• May require topical application of local anesthetic to prevent arteriospasm • If damage is done to the artery, blood supply to the pinna will be compromised • Hematoma formation and bruising can occur
Marginal ear vein	• Easily visualized • Easily accessible • Vessel is not mobile • Does not require sedation/anesthesia • Good for collecting small volumes of blood	• The vein is small and easily collapsed with rapid aspiration • May be too small in smaller breeds or young rabbits • Cannot collect a large volume of blood • May result in thrombosis and sloughing of skin over site • Hematoma formation and bruising can occur

TABLE 10-21 Correction of Dehydration Deficits.[86]

- Estimate percent dehydration:
  - 4%-5% Dry MM
  - 5%-7% Mild skin tenting, dry MM
  - 7%-9% Moderate skin tenting, dry MM
  - >10% Sunken eyes, altered mentation, significant skin tenting, dry MM
- Calculating deficits: % dehydration × kg × 1000 mL = fluid requirements (mL)
- Add maintenance requirements: 3-4 mL/kg/hr plus on-going losses (diarrhea, etc.)
- Replacing losses based on CV status:
  - Acute loss of <24 hr, unstable CV status: replace deficit over 4-6 hr
  - Chronic loss >24 hr, stable CV status: replace over 12-24 hr
  - Assess response to rehydration with serial body weight and urine output

CV, Cardiovascular; MM, mucous membranes.

TABLE 10-22 Cardiopulmonary Resuscitation and Shock Therapy Agents Used in Rabbits.[a]

Agent	Dosage	Comments
Atipamezole	1 mg/kg SC,IM,IV[166]	α_2 adrenergic antagonist; reversal of dexmedetomidine or medetomidine anesthesia
Atropine	0.1-0.5 mg/kg IV[166]	Parasympatholytic; repeat injections may be needed due to atropine esterase activity q10-20min[241]
Dextrose	50% 1 mL/kg diluted 1:4 1V, IO[86] (5% dextrose can be added as needed to additional fluids based on serial blood glucose measurements[86])	Used in patients with hypoglycemia and/or hyperkalemia; reserve for patients highly suspected of or diagnosed with hypoglycemia
Dobutamine	5-15 μg/kg/min[241]	Positive inotrope; constant rate infusion
Dopamine	5-15 μg/kg/min[241]	Positive inotrope; constant rate infusion
Doxapram	5-10 mg/kg IV, IM q15min[166]	Respiratory stimulant; side effects can be significant (e.g., cardiac arrhythmias, muscle fasciculation, seizures), therefore its use should be limited to patients that cannot be intubated or otherwise allow control of ventilation
Epinephrine	0.2-0.4 mg/kg IM, IV, intratracheally[194]	Cardiac arrest
Fluid therapy	Crystalloids, isotonic: 10-15 mL/kg boluses IV, IO[86] Crystalloids, hypertonic: 3-4 mL/kg slow bolus × 10 min IV, IO[86]	Colloids, crystalloids, blood, etc.; can be used alone or in combination to treat hypovolemia and shock; crystalloids (isotonic, saline): primarily used to restore blood volume and promote perfusion; crystalloids (hypertonic): treatment and/or prevention of cerebral edema
	Colloids: 3-5 mL/kg bolus over 5-10 min IV, IO[86]	Colloids (e.g., hetastarch, dextran 70): promote rapid expansion of intravascular volume (smaller volumes needed compared to crystalloids); blood or blood products: primarily used to treat (severe) anemia
Flumazenil	0.01-0.1 mg/kg IV/IO[32]	Benzodiazepine antagonist; used to reverse the effects of benzodiazepines such as midazolam and diazepam
	0.05 mg/kg IV[208]	0.05 mg/kg IV flumazenil antagonized sedative effects of midazolam (1.2 mg/kg IV); repeat in 20 min if resedation occurs[208]
Furosemide	—	Loop diuretic
	1-4 mg/kg SC, IM, IV q4-6h[194,241]	Pulmonary edema
	2-5 mg/kg PO, SC, IM, IV q12h prn[194]	Congestive heart failure
Glycopyrrolate	0.01-0.02 mg/kg SC, IM[166,241] 0.01-0.1 mg/kg SC, IM, IV, IO[86,241]	Parasympatholytic
Lidocaine	1-2 mg/kg IV, IO (bolus)[166,241] 2-4 mg/kg intratracheally[198]	Cardiac arrhythmia

Continued

TABLE 10-22 Cardiopulmonary Resuscitation and Shock Therapy Agents Used in Rabbits. (cont'd)

Agent	Dosage	Comments
Naloxone	0.04 mg/kg IM, IV, IO[86]	Narcotic reversal; mu opioid agonist
Sodium bicarbonate	0.5-1 mEq/kg IV/IO q10 min; calculation of exact amount: mEq = BW (kg) × 0.3 × deficit; provide ½ deficit initially and reevaluate[111] 2 mEq/kg IV, IP[97]	Ketoacidosis; can be considered in patients with severe preexisting metabolic acidosis, extreme hyperkalemia, calcium channel blocker overdose, prolonged cardiopulmonary cerebral resuscitation (CPCR) (>10 min) and/or in case of significant bicarbonate loss (e.g., via kidney or gastrointestinal tract)
Vasopressin	0.5-4.0 mU/kg/min IV CRI[86] 0.8 U/kg IV, IO[86]	Nonadrenergic vasopressor; use in case of ventricular fibrillation, asystole, or pulseless electrical activity (PEA); can follow with epinephrine

[a]Drugs and doses are selected depending on individual patient requirements and health status, procedure planned, and level of sedation desired. Combination of drugs are mixed in one syringe unless otherwise indicated. Atipamezole may be used to reverse dexmedetomidine or medetomidine, flumazenil may be used to reverse midazolam, and naloxone may be used to reverse opioids.

TABLE 10-23 Drugs Reported to Be Toxic in Rabbits.[a]

Drug	Comments
Amoxicillin[175]	Enteritis; enterotoxemia
Amoxicillin/clavulanic acid[175]	Enteritis; enterotoxemia
Ampicillin[175]	Enteritis; enterotoxemia, high risk especially if given orally
Baytril otic (Bayer)[14]	Hearing impairment/ototoxic in middle ear with perforated tympanum
Benzimidazoles (fenbendazole, oxibendazole, albendazole)[90]	Bone marrow suppression reported; recommend intratreatment CBC to r/o anemia, leukopenia, thrombocytopenia
Cephalosporins[175]	Enteritis; enterotoxemia if given orally
Clindamycin[175]	Enteritis; enterotoxemia, high risk
Erythromycin[175]	Enteritis; enterotoxemia
Fipronil[166]	Blocks GABA receptors in CNS; can cause neurologic disease and death
Lincomycin[175]	Enteritis; enterotoxemia, high risk
Penicillin[175]	Enteritis; enterotoxemia if given orally
Procaine[175]	May be fatal at doses of 0.4 mg/kg
Tiletamine[52,85]	Nephrotoxic

[a]There have also been some reports of antibiotic-related colitis in rabbits given penicillin/streptomycin, trimethoprim/sulfamethoxazole, tetracycline, and gentamicin.

TABLE 10-24 Clinical Signs and Behavioral Changes Used in the Assessment of Pain in Rabbits.[a]

Clinical Signs	Behavioral Changes
Change of body posture; tensing of abdominal muscles, pressing abdomen onto ground	Decreased grooming activity; piloerection; unkempt and ruffled fur coat
Change of body posture; tucking of abdomen, hunched body; abdominal splinting on palpation	Decreased interest in food or cessation of food intake
Eyelids squinted; lack of focus; orbit may be retracted or bulging	Decreased frequency and duration of exploring/searching
Muzzle and nares contracture; increased intensity associated with level of pain	Decreased frequency and duration of movement or response to stimuli
Increased teeth grinding (bruxism)	Decreased conspecific interaction
Ears pinned back, held close to head	Irritable or aggressive temperament
Increased heart rate; increased frequency and depth of respirations	Stiff gait, lameness, staggering; difficulty finding comfortable resting position
Decreased body weight over time	Decreased fecal output or decreased size of fecal pellets

[a]Modified from Fisher (2010).[70]

TABLE 10-25 Sensitivity and Specificity Calculators for IgM and IgG Titers and CRP Levels Relative to the Diagnosis of Suspected *Encephalitozoon cuniculi* Infections in Pet Rabbits.[a,45]

IgM ≥ 1:64	IgG ≥ 1:512	CRP > 38 mg/L	Sensitivity (%)	Specificity (%)	Positive Predictive Value (%)	Negative Predictive Value (%)
+	ND	ND	69	75	88	48
ND	+	ND	62	78	88	44
ND	ND	+	40	89	90	38
+	+	ND	58	89	92	41
+	ND	+	27	100	100	34
ND	+	+	22	97	95	32
+	+	+	20	100	100	32

[a]CRP, C-reactive protein; ND, results of analyte not included in analysis.

REFERENCES

1. Abd El-Aty AM, Goudah A. Abo El-Sooud K. Pharmacokinetics, intramuscular bioavailability and tissue residue profiles of ceftazidime in a rabbit model. *Dtsch Tierarztl Wochenschr.* 2001;108:168–171.
2. Abd El-Aty AM, Goudah A, Abo El-Sooud K, et al. Pharmacokinetics and bioavailability of florfenicol following intravenous, intramuscular, and oral administration in rabbits. *Vet Res Commun.* 2004;28:515–524.

3. Abd El-Aty AM, Goudah A, Ismail M, et al. Disposition kinetics of difloxacin in rabbits after intravenous and intramuscular injection of Dicural. *Vet Res Commun*. 2005;29:297–304.
4. Abo-El-Sooud K, Goudah A. Influence of *Pasteurella multocida* infection on the pharmacokinetic behavior of marbofloxacin after intravenous and intramuscular administrations in rabbits. *J Vet Pharmacol Ther*. 2009;33:63–68.
5. Akpek EK, Vittitow J, Verhoeven RS, et al. Ocular surface distribution and pharmacokinetics of a novel ophthalmic 1% azithromycin formulation. *J Ocul Pharmacol Ther*. 2009;25:433–440.
6. Allweiler S, Leach MC, Flecknell PA. The use of propofol and sevoflurane for surgical anaesthesia in New Zealand white rabbits. *Lab Anim*. 2010;44:113–117.
7. Andres K, Kent M, Seidlecki C, et al. The use of megavoltage radiation therapy in the treatment of thymoma in rabbits: 19 cases. *Vet Comp Oncol*. 2012;10:82–94.
8. Andrews DD, Fajt VR, Baker KC, et al. A comparison of buprenorphine, sustained-release buprenorphine, and high-concentration buprenorphine in male New Zealand white rabbits. *J Am Assoc for Lab Anim Sci*. 2020;59(5):546–556.
9. Araki-Sasaki K, Katsuta O, Mano H, et al. The effects of oral and topical corticosteroid on rabbit corneas. *BMC Ophthalmol*. 2016;16 article #160.
10. Audeval-Gerard C, Nivet C, el Amrani A, et al. Pharmacokinetics of ketoprofen in rabbits after single topical application. *Eur J Drug Metab Pharmacokinet*. 2000;25:227–230.
11. Avunduk AM, Beuerman RW, Warnel ED, et al. Comparison of efficacy of topical and oral fluconazole treatment in experimental *Aspergillus* keratitis. *Curr Eye Res*. 2003;26:113–117.
12. Barequet IS, Denton P, Osterhout GJ, et al. Treatment of experimental bacterial keratitis with topical trovafloxacin. *Arch Ophthalmol*. 2004;122:65–69.
13. Barter LS. Rabbit analgesia. *Vet Clin North Am Exot Anim Pract*. 2011;14:93–104.
14. Bateman FL, Kirejczk SGM, Stewart GV, et al. Effects of an enrofloxacin-silver sulfadiazine emulsion in the ears of rabbits with perforated tympanic membranes. *Am J Vet Res*. 2019;80(4):325–334.
15. Bedard KM. Ocular surface disease in rabbits. In: Czerwinski SL, ed.; 2019. *Vet Clin North Am Exot Anim Pract: Medical and Surgical Management of Ocular Surface Disease in Exotic Animals*. 22:1–14.
16. Bellini L, Banzato T, Contiero B, et al. Evaluation of sedation and clinical effects of midazolam with ketamine or dexmedetomidine in pet rabbits. *Vet Rec*. 2014;175:372.
17. Benedetti M, Coupez R, Whomsley R, et al. Comparative pharmacokinetics and metabolism of levetiracetam, a new anti-epileptic agent, in mouse, rat, rabbit, and dog. *Xenobiotic*. 2004;34:281–300.
18. Bennett RA. Treatment of abscesses in the head of rabbits. *Proc North Am Vet Conf*; 1999:821–823.
19. Birke L, Molina P, Baker D, et al. Comparison of selamectin and imidacloprid plus permethrin in eliminating *Leporacarus gibbus* infestation in laboratory rabbits. *J Am Assoc Lab Anim Sci*. 2009;48:757–762.
20. Blazaki S, Tsika C, Tzatzrarakis M, et al. Pharmacokinetics and efficacy of intraocular flurbiprofen. *Graefes Arch Clin Exp Ophthalmol*. 2017;255(12):2375–2380.
21. Bourguet A, Guyonnet A, Donzel E, et al. Keratomycosis in a pet rabbit (*Oryctolagus cuniculus*) treated with topical 1% terbinafine ointment. *Vet Ophthalmol*. 2015;6:1–6.
22. Bowman DD, Fogelson ML, Carbone LG. Effect of ivermectin on the control of ear mites (*Psoroptes cuniculi*) in naturally infested rabbits. *Am J Vet Res*. 1992;53:105–109.
23. Bradley MP, Doerning CM, Nowland MH, et al. Intramuscular administration of alfaxalone alone or in combination for sedation and anesthesia in rabbits (*Oryctolagus cuniculus*). *J Assoc Lab Anim Sci*. 2019;58(2):216–222.
24. Brandao J, Graham J, Quesenberry K, et al. Basic approach to veterinary care of rabbits. In: Quesenberry KE, Orcutt CJ, Mans C, et al., eds. *Ferrets, Rabbits and Rodents: Clinical Medicine and Surgery*. 4th ed. St. Louis, MO: Elsevier; 2021:150–161.
25. Broome RL, Brooks DL, Babish JG, et al. Pharmacokinetic properties of enrofloxacin in rabbits. *Am J Vet Res*. 1991;52:1835–1841.

26. Brown SA. Intermittent soft stools in rabbits. *Proc North Am Vet Conf*; 1996:849–850.
27. Brown SA. Rabbit urinary tract disease. *Proc North Am Vet Conf*; 1997:785–787.
28. Burgmann P, Percy DH. Antimicrobial drug use in rodents and rabbits. In: Prescott JF, Baggot JD, eds. *Antimicrobial Therapy in Veterinary Medicine*. Ames, IA: Iowa State University Press; 1993:524–541.
29. Cabanes A, Arboix M, Anton JMG, et al. Pharmacokinetics of enrofloxacin after intravenous and intramuscular injection in rabbits. *Am J Vet Res*. 1992;53:2090–2093.
30. Cai Z-T, Galletis P, Lu Y, et al. Pharmacokinetics of albendazole in New Zealand white rabbits: oral versus intraperitoneal administration. *Anticancer Res*. 2007;27:417–422.
31. Cam Y, Atasever A, Eraslan G, et al. Experimental infection in rabbits and the effect of treatment with toltrazuril and ivermectin. *Exp Parasitol*. 2008;119:164–172.
32. Cantwell S. Ferret, rabbit, and rodent anesthesia. In: Heard D, ed. 2001. *Vet Clin North Am Exot Anim Pract*. 4:169–191.
33. Capilla J, Yustes C, Mayayo E, et al. Efficacy of albaconazole (UR-9825) in treatment of disseminated *Scedosporium prolificans* infection in rabbits. *Antimicrob Agents Chemother*. 2003;47:1948–1951.
34. Carceles CM, Fernandez-Varon E, Marin P, et al. Tissue disposition of azithromycin after intravenous and intramuscular administration to rabbits. *Vet J*. 2007;174:154–159.
35. Carpenter JW. Personal communication; 2020.
36. Carpenter JW, Hawkins MG. Personal communication; 2020.
37. Carpenter JW, Dryden M, KuKanich B. Pharmacokinetics, efficacy, and adverse effects of selamectin following topical administration in flea-infested rabbits. *Am J Vet Res*. 2012;73:562–566.
38. Carpenter JW, Pollock CG, Koch DE, et al. Single- and multiple-dose pharmacokinetics of marbofloxacin after oral administration to rabbits. *Am J Vet Res*. 2009;70:522–526.
39. Carpenter JW, Pollock CG, Koch DE, et al. Single- and multiple-dose pharmacokinetics of meloxicam after oral administration to the rabbit (*Oryctolagus cuniculus*). *J Zoo Wildl Med*. 2009;40:601–606.
40. Chen S. Personal communication; 2016.
41. Chitty J. Formulary. In: Harcourt-Brown F, Chitty J, eds. *BSAVA Manual of Rabbit Surgery, Dentistry and Imaging*. Gloucestershire, UK: BSAVA Press; 2013:430–431.
42. Christ AP, Biscaino PT, Lourenco RL, et al. Development of doxycycline hyclate suppositories and pharmacokinetic study in rabbits. *Eur J Pharm Sci*. 2020;142:105141.
43. Cockshott ID, Douglas EJ, Plummer GF, et al. The pharmacokinetics of propofol in laboratory animals. *Xenobiotica*. 1992;22:369–375.
43a. Conner C, Di Girolamo N, Kanda I, et al. Intravenous cosyntropin optimal dose determination in rabbits. *Proc ExoticsCon*; 2021;191.
44. Cooper CS, Metcalf-Pate KA, Barat CE, et al. Comparison of side effects between buprenorphine and meloxicam used postoperatively in Dutch belted rabbits (*Oryctolagus cuniculus*). *J Am Assoc Lab Anim Sci*. 2009;48:279–285.
45. Cray C, McKenny S, Perritt E, et al. Utility of IgM titers with IgG and C-reactive protein quantitation in the diagnosis of suspected *Encephalitozoon cuniculi* infection in rabbits. *J Exot Pet Med*. 2015;24:356–360.
46. Croisier-Bertin D, Piroth L, Charles PE, et al. Ceftaroline versus ceftriaxone in a highly penicillin-resistant pneumococcal pneumonia rabbit model using simulated human dosing. *Antimicrob Agents Chemother*. 2011;55:3557–3563.
47. Deflers H, Bolen G, Gandar F, et al. Influence of morphine on the rabbit gastrointestinal tract. *Proc Assoc Exot Mam Vet Conf*; 2014.
48. Delk KW, Carpenter JW, KuKanich B, et al. Pharmacokinetics of meloxicam administered orally to rabbits (*Oryctolagus cuniculis*) for 29 days. *Am J Vet Res*. 2014;75:195–199.
49. Deren YT, Ozdek S, Kalkanci A, et al. Comparison of antifungal efficacies of moxifloxacin, liposomal amphotericin B, and combination treatment in experimental *Candida albicans* endophthalmitis in rabbits. *Can J Microbiol*. 2010;56:1–7.

50. DiGeronimo PM, Brandao J. Update on thyroid disease in rabbits and guinea pigs. In: Wyre NR, Chen S, eds. *Vet Clin North Am Exot Anim Pract: New and Emerging Diseases: an Update.* 2020;23:373–381.
51. DiVencenti L, Meirelles LAD, Westcott RA. Safety and clinical effectiveness of a compounded sustained-release formulation of buprenorphine for postoperative analgesia in New Zealand white rabbits. *J Am Vet Med Assoc.* 2016;248:795–801.
52. Doerning BJ, Brammer DW, Chrisp CE, et al. Nephrotoxicity of tiletamine in New Zealand white rabbits. *Lab Anim Sci.* 1992;42:267–269.
53. Donnelly TM. Rabbit with cutaneous lymphoma: chemotherapy options and drug doses. *VIN Vet-to-Vet Message Boards*; 2014. www.vin.com. http://www.vin.com/Members/Boards/DiscussionViewer.aspx?documentid=6413492&ViewFirst=1. Accessed November 9, 2020.
54. Donnelly TM, Vella D. Basic anatomy, physiology, and husbandry of rabbits. In: Quesenberry KE, Orcutt CJ, Mans C, et al., eds. *Ferrets, Rabbits and Rodents: Clinical Medicine and Surgery.* 4th ed. St. Louis, MO: Elsevier; 2021:131–149.
55. Dundaroz R, DeGim T, Sizlan A, et al. Intracavernous application of diazepam: an alternative route of the seizure treatment—an experimental study in rabbits. *Pediatr Int.* 2002;44:163–167.
56. Durham ME, Elfenbein JR. Evaluation of vaporized hydrogen peroxide sterilization on the in vitro efficacy of meropenem-impregnated polymethyl methacrylate beads. *Am J Vet Res.* 2019;80(1):45–50.
57. Egger CM, Souza MJ, Greenacre CB, et al. Effect of intravenous administration of tramadol hydrochloride on the minimum alveolar concentration of isoflurane in rabbits. *Am J Vet Res.* 2009;70:945–949.
58. Eguchi H, Shiota H, Oguro S, et al. The inhibitory effect of vancomycin ointment on the manifestation of MRSA keratitis in rabbits. *J Infect Chemother.* 2009;15:279–283.
59. Eid R. Therapeutic review: midazolam. *J Exot Pet Med.* 2018;27(1):46–51.
60. Elhawary NM, ShSGH Sorour, El-Abasy MA, et al. A trial of doramectin injection and ivermectin spot-on for treatment of rabbits artificially infested with the ear mite "*Psoroptes cuniculi*". *Pol J Vet Sci.* 2017;20(3):521–525.
61. Elmas M, Uney K, Yazar E, et al. Pharmacokinetics of enrofloxacin following intravenous and intramuscular administration in Angora rabbits. *Res Vet Sci.* 2007;82:242–245.
62. Escudero E, Fernandez-Varon E, Marin P, et al. Pharmacokinetics and tissue tolerance of azithromycin after intramuscular administration to rabbits. *Res Vet Sci.* 2006;81(3):366–372.
63. Farmaki R, Koutinas AF, Papazahariadou MG, et al. Effectiveness of a selamectin spot-on formulation in rabbits with sarcoptic mange. *Vet Rec.* 2009;164:431–432.
64. Fehr M. Zoonotic potential of dermatophytosis in small mammals. *J Exot Pet Med.* 2015;24:308–316.
65. Fernandez-Varon E, Bovaira MJ, Espuny A, et al. Pharmacokinetic-pharmacodynamic integration of moxifloxacin in rabbits after intravenous, intramuscular and oral administration. *J Vet Pharmacol Ther.* 2005;28:343–348.
66. Ferris RL, Quesenberry KE, Weisse CW. Outcome of intraluminal tracheal stent placement for tracheal stenosis in a rabbit (*Oryctolagus cuniculus*). *J Exot Pet Med.* 2019;31C:23–27.
67. Fiorello CV. Personal communication; 2011.
68. Fiorello CV, Divers SJ. Rabbits. In: Carpenter JW, ed. *Exotic Animal Formulary.* 4th ed. St. Louis, MO: Elsevier; 2013:518–559.
69. Fiori MG, Schiavinato A, Lini E, et al. Peripheral neuropathy induced by intravenous administration of vincristine sulfate in the rabbit. An ultrastructural study. *Toxicol Pathol.* 1995;23:248–255.
70. Fisher P. Standards of care in the 21st century: the rabbit. *J Exot Pet Med.* 2010;19:22–35.
71. Fisher PG. Personal communication; 2020.
72. Fitzgerald BC, Dias S, Martorell J. Cardiovascular drugs in avian, small animal and reptile medicine. *Vet Clin North Am Exot Anim Pract: Therapeutics.* 2018;21:399–442.
73. Flecknell P. Anaesthesia and perioperative care. In: Meridith A, Flecknell P, eds. *BSAVA Manual of Rabbit Medicine and Surgery.* 2nd ed. Gloucestershire, UK: BSAVA Press; 2006:154–165.

74. Flecknell P. Analgesia and perioperative care. *Proc World Vet Conf. 2008*; accessed via Veterinary Information Network.
75. Foley P, Henderson A, Bissonette E, et al. Evaluation of fentanyl transdermal patches in rabbits: blood concentrations and physiologic response. *Comp Med.* 2001;51:239–244.
76. Fowler A. Hand-rearing small mammals: facts and fallacies. *Proc Conf Annu Assoc Exot Mam Vet*; 2019:459–468.
77. Fredholm DV, Carpenter JW, KuKanich B, et al. Pharmacokinetics of meloxicam in rabbits after oral administration of single and multiple doses. *Am J Vet Res.* 2013;74:636–641.
78. Froehlich F, Forbes N, Stidworthy M, et al. Malignant mixed Müllerian tumor of the uterus in a domestic rabbit (*Oryctolagus cuniculus*) and subsequent intravenous chemotherapy with carboplatin. *Proc Conf Annu Assoc Exot Mam Vet*; 2016:503–504.
79. Fukuda M, Shibata N, Osada H, et al. Vitreous and aqueous penetration of orally and topically administered moxifloxacin. *Ophthalmic Res.* 2011;46:113–117.
80. Gallina G, Lucatello L, Drigo I, et al. Kinetics and intrapulmonary disposition of tilmicosin after single and repeated oral bolus administrations to rabbits. *Vet Res Commun.* 2010;34:S69–S72.
80a. Gardhouse S. Unpublished data. 2022.
81. Gardhouse S, Sanchez-Migallon Guzman D, Cox S, et al. Pharmacokinetics of ceftiofur crystalline free acid in New Zealand white rabbits (*Oryctolagus cuniculus*). *Am J Vet Res.* 2017;78(7):796–803.
82. Gelatt KN. Exotic animal ophthalmology. In: Gelatt KN, ed. *Essentials of Veterinary Ophthalmology*. Oxford, UK: Blackwell; 2005:413–438.
83. Gengenbacher M, Zimmerman MD, Sarathy JP, et al. Tissue distribution of doxycycline in animal models of tuberculosis. *Antimicrob Agents Chemother.* 2020;64(5):e02479-19.
84. Gillett CS. Selected drug dosages and clinical reference data. In: Manning PJ, Ringler DH, Newcomer CE, eds. *The Biology of the Laboratory Rabbit*. 2nd ed. San Diego, CA: Academic Press; 1994:467–472.
85. Girolamo ND, Selleri P. Disorders of the urinary and reproductive systems. In: Quesenberry KE, Orcutt CJ, Mans C, et al., eds. *Ferrets, Rabbits and Rodents: Clinical Medicine and Surgery*. 4th ed. St. Louis, MO: Elsevier; 2021:201–219.
86. Gladden JN, Lennox AM. Emergency and critical care of small mammals. In: Quesenberry KE, Orcutt CJ, Mans C, et al., eds. *Ferrets, Rabbit, and Rodents: Clinical Medicine and Surgery*. 4th ed. St. Louis, MO: Elsevier; 2021:595–608.
87. Gleeson MD, Sanchez-Migallon Guzman D, Paul-Murphy JR. Clinical and pathological findings for rabbits with dystocia: 10 cases (1996-2016). *J Am Vet Med Assoc.* 2019;254(8):953–959.
88. Gokbulut C, Biligili A, Kart A, et al. Plasma dispositions of ivermectin, doramectin and moxidectin following subcutaneous administration in rabbits. *Lab Anim.* 2010;44:138–142.
89. Graham JE. Personal observation; 2020.
90. Graham JE, Garner MM, Reavill DR. Benzimidazole toxicosis in rabbits: 13 cases (2003-2011). *J Exot Pet Med.* 2014;23:188–195.
91. Green LC, Callegan MC, Engel LS, et al. Pharmacokinetics of topically applied ciprofloxacin in rabbit tears. *Jpn J Ophthalmol.* 1996;40:123–126.
92. Grint NJ, Murison PJ. A comparison of ketamine-midazolam and ketamine-medetomidine combinations for induction of anaesthesia in rabbits. *Vet Anaesth Analg.* 2008;35:113–121.
93. Grint NJ, Smith HE, Senior JM. Clinical evaluation of alfaxalone in cyclodextrin for the induction of anaesthesia in rabbits. *Vet Rec.* 2008;163:395–396.
94. Hanan MS, Riad EM, el-Khouly NA. Antibacterial efficacy and pharmacokinetic studies of ciprofloxacin on *Pasteurella multocida* infected rabbits. *Dtsch Tierarztl Wochenschr.* 2000;107(4):151–155.
95. Harcourt-Brown F. *Textbook of Rabbit Medicine*. Oxford, UK: Butterworth-Heinemann; 2002.

96. Harkness JE, Wagner JE. *The Biology and Medicine of Rabbits and Rodents*. 4th ed. Philadelphia, PA: Williams & Wilkins; 1995.
97. Harrenstien L. Critical care of ferrets, rabbits, and rodents. *Semin Avian Exotic Pet Med*. 1994;3:217–228.
98. Hawkins MG. Advances in exotic mammal clinical therapeutics. *J Exot Pet Med*. 2014;23:39–49.
99. Hawkins MG, Vernau W, Drazenovich TL, et al. Results of cytologic and microbiologic analysis of bronchoalveolar lavage fluid in New Zealand white rabbits. *Am J Vet Res*. 2008;69(5):572–578.
100. Heard DJ. Anesthesia, analgesia, and sedation of small mammals. In: Quesenberry KE, Carpenter JW, eds. *Ferrets, Rabbits, and Rodents: Clinical Medicine and Surgery*. 2nd ed. St. Louis, MO: WB Saunders; 2004:356–369.
101. Heatley JJ, Smith AN. Spontaneous neoplasms of lagomorphs. *Vet Clin North Am Exot Anim Pract*. 2004;7:561–577.
102. Hellebrekers LJ, de Boer EJW, van Zuylen MA, et al. A comparison between medetomidine-ketamine and medetomidine-propofol anaesthesia in rabbits. *Lab Anim*. 1997;31:58–69.
103. Henke J, Astner S, Brill T, et al. Comparative study of three intramuscular anaesthetic combinations (medetomidine-ketamine, medetomidine-fentanyl-midazolam and xylazine-ketamine) in rabbits. *Vet Anaesth Analg*. 2005;32:261–270.
104. Hernandez-Divers SJ, Lennox AM. Sedation and anesthesia in exotic companion mammals. *Proc Annu Conf Assoc of Avian Vet*; 2009:287–298.
105. Hess L, Tater K. Rabbits: dermatologic diseases. In: Quesenberry KE, Carpenter JW, eds. *Ferrets, Rabbits and Rodents: Clinical Medicine and Surgery*. 3rd ed. St. Louis, MO: Elsevier; 2012:232–244.
106. Hiraoka T, Kaji Y, Wakabayashi T, et al. Comparison of micafungin and fluconazole for experimental *Candida* keratitis in rabbits. *Cornea*. 2007;26:336–342.
107. Horvath M, Leng L, Stefkovic M, et al. Lethal encephalitozoonosis in cyclophosphamide-treated rabbits. *Acta Vet Hung*. 1999;47:85–93.
108. Hu L, Liu C, Shang C, et al. Pharmacokinetics and improved bioavailability of toltrazuril after oral administration to rabbits. *J Vet Pharmacol Ther*. 2010;33:503–506.
109. Hughes CR, Bennet RL, Tuna IC, et al. Activities of fluconazole (UK 49,858) and ketoconazole against ketoconazole-susceptible and -resistant *Candida albicans*. *Antimicrob Agents Chemother*. 1988;32:209–212.
110. Hutchinson MJ, Jacobs DE, Bell GD, et al. Evaluation of imidacloprid for the treatment and prevention of cat flea (*Ctenocephalides felis felis*) infestations on rabbits. *Vet Rec*. 2001;148:695–696.
111. Huynh M, Boyeaux A, Pignon C. Assessment and care of the critically ill rabbit. In: Fordham M, Roberts BK, eds. *Vet Clin North Am Exot Anim Pract: Emergency and Critical Care*. 2019; 19(2):379–409.
112. Huynh M, Poumeyrol S, Pignon C, et al. Intramuscular administration of alfaxalone for sedation in rabbits. *Vet Rec*. 2015;176:255–260.
113. Idid S, Lee C. Effects of fuller's earth and activated charcoal on oral absorption of paraquat in rabbits. *Clin Exp Pharmacol Physiol*. 1996;23:679–681.
114. Isobe T, Kasai T, Kawai H. Ocular penetration and pharmacokinetics of ripasudil following topical administration to rabbits. *J Ocular Pharm Ther*. 2016;32(7):405–414.
115. Ivey E. Personal communication; 2002.
116. Jekl V, Hauptman A, Minarikova A, et al. Pharmacokinetic study of benzylpenicillin potassium after intramuscular administration in rabbits. *Vet Rec*. 2016;179:18.
117. Jenkins J. *Rabbit Drug Doses*. Lakewood, CO: American Animal Hospital Association; 1995.
118. Jepson L. *Exotic Animal Medicine: A Quick Reference Guide*. Philadelphia, PA: Saunders/Elsevier; 2009.
119. Jepson L. Rabbits. In: Jepson L, ed. *Exotic Animal Medicine: A Quick Reference Guide*. 2nd ed. St. Louis, MO: Elsevier; 2016:42–87.

120. Johnston MS. Clinical approaches to analgesia in ferrets and rabbits. *J Exot Pet Med.* 2005;14:229–235.
121. Kanbur M, Atalay O, Ica A, et al. The curative and antioxidative efficiency of doramectin and doramectin+vitamin AD_3E treatment on *Psoroptes cuniculi* infestation in rabbits. *Res Vet Sci.* 2008;85:291–293.
122. Kaya D, Inceboz T, Kolatan E, et al. Comparison of efficacy of ivermectin and doramectin against mange mite (*Sarcoptes scabiei*) in naturally infested rabbits in Turkey. *Vet Ital.* 2010;46:51–56.
123. Kern TJ. Rabbit and rodent ophthalmology. *Semin Avian Exot Pet Med.* 1997;6:138–145.
124. Kiel JW, Patel P. Effects of timolol and betaxolol on choroidal blood flow in the rabbit. *Exp Eye Res.* 1998;67:501–507.
125. Kim SH, Lee JY, Jun HK, et al. Efficacy of selamectin in the treatment of cheyletiellosis in pet rabbits. *Vet Dermatol.* 2008;19:26–27.
126. Kim MS, Lim JH, Hwang YH, et al. Plasma disposition of toltrazuril and its metabolites, toltrazuril sulfoxide and toltrazuril sulfone, in rabbits after oral administration. *Vet Parasitol.* 2010;169:51–56.
127. Kirkpatrick WR, Vallor AC, McAtee RK, et al. Combination therapy with terbinafine and amphotericin B in a rabbit model of experimental invasive aspergillosis. *Antimicrob Agents Chemother.* 2005;49:4751–4753.
128. Klimtova I, Simunek T, Mazurova Y, et al. Comparative study of chronic toxic effects of danorubicin and doxorubicin in rabbits. *Hum Exp Toxicol.* 2002;21:649–657.
128a. Knutson K, Balko J, Thomson A, et al. Effects of intramuscular alfaxalone-butorphanol-midazolam compared with ketamine-butorphanol-midazolam in New Zealand white rabbits (*Oryctolagus cuniculus*). *Proc ExoticsCon;* 2021:341.
129. Koc F, Ozturk M, Kadioglu Y, et al. Pharmacokinetics of florfenicol after intravenous and intramuscular administration in New Zealand white rabbits. *Res Vet Sci.* 2009;87:102–105.
130. Kosravi E, Elena P, Hariton C. Allergic conjunctivitis and uveitis models: reappraisal with some marketed drugs. *Inflamm Res.* 1995;44:47–54.
131. Kozer E, Levicheck Z, Hoshino N, et al. The effect of amitriptyline, gabapentin, and carbamazepine on morphine-induced hypercarbia in rabbits. *Anaesth Analg.* 2008;107:1216–1222.
132. Krempels D, Cotter M, Stanzione G. Ileus in domestic rabbits. *Exot DVM.* 2000;2:19–21.
133. Kurtdede A, Karaer Z, Acar A, et al. Use of selamectin for the treatment of psoroptic and sarcoptic mite infestation in rabbits. *Vet Dermatol.* 2007;18:18–22.
134. Laniesse D, Beaufrére H, James F, et al. Multiple myeloma in a 6-year-old rabbit. *Proc Conf Annu Assoc Exot Mam Vet*; 2016:505.
135. Lavine RI, Dicintio DM. l-Asparaginase-induced diabetes mellitus in rabbits. *Diabetes.* 1980;29:528–531.
136. Lawler JB, Hassel DM, Magnuson RJ, et al. Adsorptive effects of di-tri-octahedral smectite on *Clostridium perfringens* alpha, beta and beta-2 exotoxins and equine colostral antibodies. *Am J Vet Res.* 2008;69(2):233–239.
137. Lee JH, Shin JH, Lee MG. Pharmacokinetics, blood partition, and tissue distribution of itraconazole. *Res Commun Mol Pathol Pharmacol.* 2004;115-116:203–215.
138. Lee M, Kallal S, Feldman M. Omeprazole prevents indomethacin-induced gastric ulcers in rabbits. *Aliment Pharmacol Ther.* 1996;10:571–576.
139. Lempert M. Urinary obstruction due to prostatic abscess in a young neutered rabbit. *J Exot Pet Med.* 2019;29C:15–21.
140. Lennox AM. Clinical technique: small exotic companion mammal dentistry- anesthetic considerations. *J Exot Pet Med.* 2008;17:102–106.
141. Lennox AM. Protocols and tips for anesthesia and analgesia for rabbit and rodent dentistry and orofacial surgery. *Proc Assoc Exot Mam Vet Conf*; 2012:77–78.
142. Lennox AM. Sedation and local anesthesia as an alternative to general anaesthesia in exotic companion mammals. *Proc Brit Small Anim Vet Cong*; 2013.

143. Lennox AM. Sedation, anesthesia and analgesia in the critical exotic surgery patient. *Proc Internat Vet Emer Crit Care Symp*; 2013.
144. Lennox AM. The use of constant rate infusion analgesia in exotic companion mammals. *Proc Assoc Exot Mam Vet Conf*; 2013.
145. Lennox AM. Anesthesia and analgesia for dentistry of rabbits and rodents. *Proc Am Board Vet Pract Conf*; 2014.
146. Lennox AM. Anesthesia and analgesia for critical exotic companion mammals. *Proc Internat Vet Emer Crit Care Symp*; 2015.
147. Lennox AM. Introducing alfaxalone into exotic companion mammal practice. *Proc Assoc Exot Med Vet Conf*; 2015:321–323.
148. Lennox AM.Personal communication; 2016.
149. Longley L. *Anaesthesia of Exotic Pets*. Philadelphia, PA: Saunders/Elsevier; 2008.
150. Louie A, Liu QF, Drusano GL, et al. Pharmacokinetic studies of fluconazole in rabbits characterizing doses which achieve peak levels in serum and area under the concentration-time curve values which mimic those of high-dose fluconazole in humans. *Antimicrob Agents Chemother*. 1998;42:1512–1514.
151. Maciejewska-Paszek I, Pawlowska-Góral K, Kostrzewski M, et al. The influence of small doses of paracetamol on rabbit liver. *Exp Toxicol Pathol*. 2007;59:139–141.
152. Maguire R, Gallinato MJ. Novel treatment of *Encephalitozoon cuniculi*-induced glaucoma in a rabbit. *Proc Assoc Exot Mam Vet Conf*; 2011:125.
153. Malka S, Britton B. Diagnosis and treatment of chronic lymphocytic leukemia in a pet rabbit (*Oryctolagus cuniculus*). *Proc Conf Annu Assoc Exot Mam Vet*; 2018:585.
154. Mans C. Personal communication; 2016.
155. Marangos MN, Zhu Z, Nicolau DP, et al. Disposition of ofloxacin in female New Zealand white rabbits. *J Vet Pharmacol Ther*. 1997;20:17–20.
156. Marín P, Álamo LF, Escudero E, et al. Pharmacokinetics of marbofloxacin in rabbit after intravenous, intramuscular, and subcutaneous administration. *Res Vet Sci*. 2013;94:698–700.
157. Marin P, Belda E, Laredo FG, et al. Pharmacokinetics and sedative effects of alfaxalone with and without dexmedetomidine in rabbits. *Res Vet Sci*. 2020;129:6–12.
157a. Mayer J, Aguilar LAB, Walth GB, et al. Clinical tolerance of dexamethasone in New Zealand white rabbits. *Proc ExoticsCon;* 2021:197–198.
158. Mazaheri-Khameneh R, Sarrafzadeh-Rezaei F, Asri-Rezaei S, et al. Comparison of time to loss of consciousness and maintenance of anesthesia following intraosseous and intravenous administration of propofol in rabbits. *J Am Vet Med Assoc*. 2012;241:73–80.
159. McElroy DE, Ravis WR, Clark CH. Pharmacokinetics of oxytetracycline hydrochloride in rabbits. *Am J Vet Res*. 1987;48:1261–1263.
160. McGee DH, Holt WF, Kastner PR, et al. Safety of moxifloxacin as shown in animal and in vitro studies. *Surv Ophthalmol*. 2005;50:S46–S54.
161. McTier TL, Hair JA, Walstrom DJ, et al. Efficacy and safety of topical administration of selamectin for treatment of ear mite infestation in rabbits. *J Am Vet Med Assoc*. 2003;223:322–324.
162. Mencke N, Bach T. Managing gastrointestinal helminths in small mammals. *Comp Cont Educ Pract*. 2007;29:13–16.
163. Miller JL, Schell WA, Wills EA, et al. In vitro and in vivo efficacies of the new triazole albaconazole against *Cryptococcus neoformans*. *Antimicrob Agents Chemother*. 2004;48:384–387.
164. Moore DM, Zimmerman K. Hematological assessment in pet rabbits. *Vet Clin North Am Exot Anim Pract*. 2015;18:9–19.
165. Morrisey JK, Carpenter JW. Formulary. In: Quesenberry KE, Carpenter JW, eds. *Ferrets, Rabbits, and Rodents: Clinical Medicine and Surgery*. 3rd ed. St. Louis, MO: Elsevier; 2012:566–575.
166. Morissey JM, Carpenter JW. Appendix: Formulary. In: Quesenberry KE, Orcutt CJ, Mans C, et al., eds. *Ferrets, Rabbits and Rodents: Clinical Medicine and Surgery*. 4th ed. St. Louis, MO: Elsevier; 2021:620–630.

167. Morrison J, Craft Q. Treatment of cutaneous lymphoma in a lop rabbit (*Oryctolagus cuniculus*). *Proc Conf Annu Assoc Exot Mam Vet*; 2019:538.
168. Muzylak M, Maslinska D. Neurotoxic effect of vincristine on the ultrastructure of hypothalamus in rabbits. *Folia Histochem Cytobiol.* 1992;30:113–117.
169. Nelson CL, McLaren SG, Skinner RA, et al. The treatment of experimental osteomyelitis by surgical debridement and the implantation of calcium sulfate tobramycin pellets. *J Orthop Res.* 2002;20:643–647.
170. Nicolau DP, Freeman CD, Nightingale CH, et al. Pharmacokinetics of minocycline and vancomycin in rabbits. *Lab Anim Sci.* 1993;43:222–225.
171. Nielson VG, Tan S, Brix AE, et al. Hextend (hetastarch solution) decreases multiple organ injury and xanthine oxidase release after hepatoenteric ischemia-reperfusion in rabbits. *Crit Care Med.* 1997;25(9):1565–1574.
172. Norcross EW, Sanders ME, Moore Q, et al. Comparative efficacy of besifloxacin and other fluoroquinolones in a prophylaxis model of penicillin-resistant *Streptococcus pneumoniae* rabbit endophthalmitis. *J Ocul Pharmacol Ther.* 2010;26:237–243.
173. Ofoefule SI, Onuoha LC, Okonta MJ, et al. Effect of activated charcoal on isoniazid absorption in rabbits. *Boll Chim Farm.* 2001;140(3):183–186.
174. Ogawa T, Mimura Y, Kato H, et al. The usefulness of rabbits as an animal model for the neuropathological assessment of neurotoxicity following the administration of vincristine. *Neurotoxicology.* 2000;21:501–511.
175. Oglesbee B, Lord B. Gastrointestinal diseases of rabbits. In: Quesenberry KE, Orcutt CJ, Mans C, et al., eds. *Ferrets, Rabbits and Rodents: Clinical Medicine and Surgery.* 4th ed. St. Louis, MO: Elsevier; 2021:174–187.
176. Okerman L, Devriese LA, Gevaert D, et al. In vivo activity of orally administered antibiotics and chemotherapeutics against acute septicaemic pasteurellosis in rabbits. *Lab Anim.* 1990;24:341–344.
177. Onuma M, Kondo H, Ishikama M, et al. Treatment with lomustine for mediastinal lymphoma in a rabbit. *J Jpn Vet Med Assoc.* 2009;62:69–71.
178. Orcutt C, Malakoff R. Cardiovascular disease. In: Quesenberry KE, Orcutt CJ, Mans C, et al., eds. *Ferrets, Rabbits and Rodents: Clinical Medicine and Surgery.* 4th ed. St. Louis, MO: Elsevier; 2021:174–187.
179. Orr HE, Roughan JV, Flecknell PA. Assessment of ketamine and medetomidine anaesthesia in the domestic rabbit. *Vet Anaesth Analg.* 2005;32:271–279.
180. Ostergaard C, Sorensen TK, Knudsen JD, et al. Evaluation of moxifloxacin, a new 8-methoxyquinolone, for treatment of meningitis caused by a penicillin-resistant pneumococcus in rabbits. *Antimicrob Agents Chemother.* 1998;42:1706–1712.
181. Ozawa SM, Hawkins MG, Drazenovich TL, et al. Pharmacokinetics of maropitant citrate in New Zealand white rabbits (*Oryctolagus cuniculus*). *Am J Vet Res.* 2019;80(10):963–968.
181a. Ozawa S, Sanchez-Migallon Guzman D, Hawkins M, et al. Pharmacokinetics of pimobendan in New Zealand white rabbits (*Oryctolagus cuniculus*). *Proc ExoticsCon;* 2021:200.
181b. Ozawa S, Sanchez-Migallon Guzman D, Keel K, et al. Clinical and pathological findings in rabbits with cardiovascular disease: 59 cases (2001-2018). *J Am Vet Med Assoc.* 2021;259(7):764–776.
182. Ozturk F, Kurt E, Inan UU, et al. The effects of prolonged acute use and inflammation on the ocular penetration of topical ciprofloxacin. *Int J Pharm.* 2000;204:97–100.
182a. Palmer A, Wu CC, Miwa Y, et al. Outcomes and survival times of client-owned rabbits diagnosed with thymoma and treated with either prednisolone or radiotherapy, or left untreated. *J Exot Pet Med.* 2021;38:35–43.
183. Pan B, Wang M, Xu F, et al. Efficacy of an injectable formulation of eprinomectin against *Psoroptes cuniculi*, the ear mange mite in rabbits. *Vet Parasitol.* 2006;137:386–390.
184. Pan BL, Zhang YF, Suo X, et al. Effect of subcutaneously administered diclazuril on the output of *Eimeria* species oocysts by experimentally infected rabbits. *Vet Rec.* 2008;162:153–155.

185. Patterson TF, Fothergill AW, Rinaldi MG. Efficacy of itraconazole solution in a rabbit model of invasive aspergillosis. *Antimicrob Agents Chemother.* 1993;37:2307–2310.
186. Paul-Murphy J, Ramer JC. Urgent care of the pet rabbit. *Vet Clin North Am Exotic Anim Pract.* 1998;1:127–152.
187. Percy DH, Black WD. Pharmacokinetics of tetracycline in the domestic rabbit following intravenous or oral administration. *Can J Vet Res.* 1988;52:5–11.
188. Perez K, Chen S, Antinoff N. Use of prednisolone in six rabbits (*Oryctolagus cuniculus*) with cranial mediastinal disease. *Proc Conf Annu Assoc Exot Mam Vet*; 2017:252–253.
189. Petraitiene R, Petraitis V, Groll AH, et al. Antifungal activity and pharmacokinetics of posaconazole (SCH 56592) in treatment and prevention of experimental invasive pulmonary aspergillosis: correlation with galactomannan antigenemia. *Antimicrob Agents Chemother.* 2001;45:857–869.
190. Petraitis V, Petraitiene R, Groll AH, et al. Comparative antifungal activities and plasma pharmacokinetics of micafungin (FK463) against disseminated candidiasis and invasive pulmonary aspergillosis in persistently neutropenic rabbits. *Antimicrob Agents Chemother.* 2002;46:1857–1869.
191. Petritz OA. Therapeutic contraindications in exotic pets. In: van Zeeland YRA, ed. *Vet Clin North Am Exot Anim Pract: Therapeutics.* 2018;21:327–340.
192. Pichardo C, Docobo-Pérez F, Pachón-Ibáñez ME, et al. Efficacy of beta-lactam against experimental pneumococcal endocarditis caused by strains with different susceptibilities to penicillin. *J Antimicrob Chemother.* 2005;56:732–737.
193. Pignon C. Personal communication; 2016.
194. Plumb DC. *Plumb's Veterinary Drug Handbook.* 9th ed. Ames, IA: Wiley Blackwell; 2018.
195. Proksch JW, Ward KW. Ocular pharmacokinetics/pharmacodynamics of besifloxacin, moxifloxacin, and gatifloxacin following topical administration to pigmented rabbits. *J Ocul Pharmacol Ther.* 2010;26:449–458.
196. Quesenberry KE. Rabbits. In: Birchard SJ, Sherding RG, eds. *Saunders Manual of Small Animal Practice.* Philadelphia, PA: WB Saunders; 1994:1345–1362.
197. Quimby JM, Gustafson DL, Samber BJ, et al. Studies on the pharmacokinetics and pharmacodynamics of mirtazapine in healthy young cats. *J Vet Pharmacol Ther.* 2011;34:388–396.
198. Ramer JC, Paul-Murphy J, Benson KG. Evaluating and stabilizing critically ill rabbits – Part II. *Comp Cont Educ Pract.* 1999;21:36–40.
198a. Reabel SN, Queiroz-Williams P, Creamer J, et al. Assessment of intramuscular administration of alfaxalone combined with hydromorphone and dexmedetomidine for endoscopic-guided orotracheal intubation in domestic rabbits (*Oryctolagus cuniculus*). *J Am Vet Med Assoc.* 2021;259:1148–1153.
199. Redrobe S, Gakos G, Elliot SC, et al. Comparison of toltrazuril and sulphadimethoxine in the treatment of intestinal coccidiosis in pet rabbits. *Vet Rec.* 2010;167:287–290.
200. Regnier A, Schneider M, Concordet D, et al. Intraocular pharmacokinetics of intravenously administered marbofloxacin in rabbits with experimentally induced acute endophthalmitis. *Am J Vet Res.* 2008;69:410–415.
201. Renna C, Malka S. Management of metastatic abdominal carcinoma in a rabbit (*Oryctolagus cuniculus*) with toceranib (palladia) and prednisolone. *Proc Conf Annu Assoc Exot Mam Vet*; 2017:254–255.
202. Reusch B, Murray J, Papsouliotis K, et al. Urinary protein:creatinine ratio in rabbits in relation to their serological status to *Encephalitozoon cuniculi*. *Vet Rec.* 2009;164:293–295.
202a. Richard BM, Newton P, Ott LR, et al. The safety of Exparel® (Bupivacaine Liposome Injectable Suspension) administered by peripheral nerve block in rabbits and dogs. *J Drug Deliv.* 2012. doi:10.1155/2012/962101 published on line.
203. Roffey SJ, Cole S, Comby P, et al. The disposition of voriconazole in mouse, rat, rabbit, guinea pig, dog, and human. *Drug Metab Dispos.* 2003;31:731–741.
204. Rosenthal K. Epidural anesthesia. *Proc North Am Vet Conf*; 1996:876

205. Rota S, Briganti A, Portela DA, et al. Anesthesia and recovery time in rabbits (*Oryctolagus cuniculus*) premedicated with dexmedetomidine, ketamine and fentanyl and maintained with an infusion of propofol. *Proc Assoc Exot Mam Vet Conf*; 2012:3.
206. Rota S, Briganti I, Tayari A, et al. Effect of dexmedetomidine-fentanyl-ketamine anesthesia on arterial gas analysis in rabbits (*Oryctolagus cuniculus*). *Proc Assoc Exot Mam Vet*; 2013.
207. Rougier S, Galland D, Boucher S, et al. Epidemiology and susceptibility of pathogenic bacteria responsible for upper respiratory tract infections in pet rabbits. *Vet Microbiol.* 2006;115:192–198.
208. Rousseau-Blass F, Cribb AE, Pang DSJ, et al. A pharmacokinetic-pharmacodynamic study of intravenous midazolam and flumazenil in adult New Zealand white-Californian rabbits (*Oryctolagus cuniculus*). *J Assoc Am Lab Anim Sci.* 2021. doi:10.30802/AALAS-20-000084.
209. Saito K, Hasegawa A. Chloramphenicol treatment for rabbit syphilis. *J Vet Med Sci.* 2004;66:1301–1304.
209a. Sadar MJ, McGee WK, Au GG, et al. Pilot pharmacokinetics of a higher dose of subcutaneous maropitant administration in healthy domestic rabbits (*Oryctolagus cuniculus*). *J Exot Pet Med.* 2022;41:1–2.
210. Sanati H, Ramos C, Bayer A, et al. Combination therapy with amphotericin B and fluconazole against invasive candidiasis in neutropenic-mouse and infective-endocarditis rabbit models. *Antimicrob Agents Chemother.* 1997;41:1345–1348.
211. Santangelo B, Micieli F, Mozzillo T, et al. Transnasal administration of a combination of dexmedetomidine, midazolam, and butorphanol produces deep sedation in New Zealand white rabbits. *Vet Anaesth Analg.* 2016;43(2):209–214.
212. Santos M, Arevalo M, Colino CI, et al. Study on pharmacokinetics and nephrotoxicity of netilmicin in rabbits using a new dosage regimen. *Methods Find Exp Clin Pharmacol.* 1997;19:53–59.
213. Scarabelli S. Loco-regional anesthesia in rabbits. *Proc Conf Annu Assoc Exot Mam Vet*; 2019:444–452.
214. Scheller MS, Daidman LJ, Partridge BL. MAC of sevoflurane in humans and the New Zealand white rabbit. *Can J Anesth.* 1988;35:153–156.
215. Schnellbacher R. Butorphanol. *J Exot Pet Med.* 2010;19:192–195.
216. Schnellbacher RW, Carpenter JW, Mason DE, et al. Effects of lidocaine administration via continuous rate infusion on the minimum alveolar concentration of isoflurane in New Zealand white rabbits (*Oryctolagus cuniculus*). *Am J Vet Res.* 2013;74:1377–1384.
217. Schnellbacher RW, Divers SJ, Comolli JR, et al. Effects of intravenous administration of lidocaine and buprenorphine on gastrointestinal tract motility and signs of pain in New Zealand white rabbits after ovariohysterectomy. *Am J Vet Res.* 2017;78(12):1359–1371.
218. Schoemaker NJ. Gonadotrophin-releasing hormone agonists and other contraceptive medications in exotic companion animals. In: van Zeeland YRA, ed. *Vet Clin North Am Exot Anim Pract: Therapeutics.* 2018;21:443–464.
219. Schott R. Assessing pain-suppressed behaviors in injured eastern cottontail rabbits (*Sylvilagus floridanus*) using meloxicam with and without tramadol. *Proc Conf Annu Assoc Exot Mam Vet*; 2016:493.
220. Sharpnack DD, Mastin JP, Childress CP, et al. Quinolone arthropathy in juvenile New Zealand white rabbits. *Lab Anim Sci.* 1994;44:436–442.
221. Sheinberg G, Romero C, Heredia R, et al. Use of oral fluralaner for treatment of *Psoroptes cuniculi* in 15 naturally infected rabbits. *Vet Derm.* 2017;28(4):393–e91.
222. Shirtliff M, Mader J, Calhoun J. Oral rifampin plus azithromycin or clarithromycin to treat osteomyelitis in rabbits. *Clin Orthop.* 1999;359:229–236.
223. Smith S. Gastrointestinal physiology and nutrition of rabbits. In: Quesenberry KE, Orcutt CJ, Mans C, et al., eds. *Ferrets, Rabbits and Rodents: Clinical Medicine and Surgery.* 4th ed. St. Louis, MO: Elsevier; 2021:162–173.

224. Sorensen KN, Sobel RA, Clemons KV, et al. Comparative efficacies of terbinafine and fluconazole in treatment of experimental coccidioidal meningitis in a rabbit model. *Antimicrob Agents Chemother*. 2000;44:3087–3091.
225. Souza MJ, Greenacre CB, Cox SK. Pharmacokinetics of orally administered tramadol in domestic rabbits (*Oryctolagus cuniculus*). *Am J Vet Res*. 2008;69:979–982.
226. Sponsel W, Chen N, Dang D, et al. Topical voriconazole as a novel treatment for fungal keratitis. *Antimicrob Agents Chemother*. 2006;50:262–268.
227. Steinleitner A, Lambert H, Kazensky C, et al. Reduction of primary postoperative adhesion formation under calcium channel blockade in the rabbit. *J Surg Res*. 1990;48:42–45.
228. Sun XG, Wang ZX, Wan ZQ, et al. Pharmacokinetics of terbinafine in the rabbit ocular tissues after topical administration. *Ophthal Res*. 2007;39:81–83.
229. Suter C, Muller-Doblies UU, Hatt JM, et al. Prevention and treatment of *Encephalitozoon cuniculi* infection in rabbits with fenbendazole. *Vet Rec*. 2001;148:478–480.
230. Suzuki T, Yamamoto T, Ohashi Y. The antibacterial activity of levofloxacin eye drops against staphylococci using in vitro pharmacokinetic model in the bulbar conjunctiva. *J Infect Chemother*. 2016;22(6):360–365.
231. Sypniewski LA, Maxwell LK, Moody D, et al. Pharmacokinetic evaluation of sustained-release buprenorphine in the domestic rabbit. *Proc Conf Annu Assoc Exot Mam Vet*; 2017:256.
232. Tearney CC, Barter LS, Pypendop BH. Cardiovascular effects of equipotent doses of isoflurane alone and isoflurane plus fentanyl in New Zealand white rabbits (*Oryctolagus cuniculus*). *Am J Vet Res*. 2015;76(7):591–598.
233. Thomas P, Samant D, Zhu Z, et al. Long-term topical cyclosporine treatment improves tear production and reduces keratoconjunctivitis in rabbits with induced autoimmune dacryoadenitis. *J Ocul Pharmacol Ther*. 2009;25:285–291.
234. Toshida H, Nakayasu K, Kanai A. Effect of cyclosporine A eyedrops on tear secretion in the rabbit. *Jpn J Ophthalmol*. 1998;42:168–173.
235. Turner P, Chen H, Taylor W. Pharmacokinetics of meloxicam in rabbits after single and repeat oral dosing. *Comp Med*. 2006;56:63–67.
236. Uccello O, Sanchez A, Valverde A, et al. Cardiovascular effects of increasing doses of norepinephrine on isoflurane-induced hypotension in healthy rabbits. *Proc Conf Annu Assoc Exot Mam Vet*; 2019:531.
237. Uebelhart D, Thonar EJ, Zhang JW, et al. Protective effect of exogenous chondroitin 4,6-sulfate in the acute degradation of articular cartilage in the rabbit. *Osteoarthr Cartilage*. 1998;6:6–13.
238. Ueng SW, Yuan LJ, Lee N, et al. In vivo study of hot compressing molded 50:50 poly (DL-lactide-co-glycolide) antibiotic beads in rabbits. *J Orthop Res*. 2002;20:654–661.
239. Vanparijs O, Hermans L, van der Flaes L, et al. Efficacy of diclazuril in the prevention and cure of intestinal and hepatic coccidiosis in rabbits. *Vet Parasitol*. 1989;32:109–117.
240. van Zeeland Y. Rabbit oncology: diseases, diagnostics and therapeutics. *Vet Clin North Am Exot Anim Pract: Exotic Animal Oncology*. 2017;20(1):135–182.
241. van Zeeland YRA, Schoemaker NJ. Diagnosis and treatment of cardiovascular disease in small mammals. *Proc Conf Annu Assoc Exot Mam Vet*; 2018:607–616.
242. Varga M. Anaesthesia and analgesia. In: *Textbook of Rabbit Medicine*. 2nd ed. Oxford, UK: Butterworth Heinemann Elsevier; 2014:178–202.
243. Wagner R, Wendlberger U. Field efficacy of moxidectin in dogs and rabbits naturally infested with *Sarcoptes* spp., *Demodex* spp., and *Psoroptes* spp. mites. *Vet Parasitol*. 2000;93:149–158.
244. Walsh TJ, Petraitis V, Petraitiene R, et al. Experimental pulmonary aspergillosis due to *Aspergillus terreus*: pathogenesis and treatment of an emerging fungal pathogen resistant to amphotericin B. *J Infect Dis*. 2003;188:305–319.
245. Walter KM, Bischoff K, de Matos R. Severe lead toxicosis in a lionhead rabbit. *J Med Toxicol*. 2017;13:91–94.

246. Waterbury L, Flach A. Comparison of ketorolac tromethamine, diclofenac sodium, and loteprednol etabonate in an animal model of ocular inflammation. *J Ocul Pharmacol Ther.* 2006;22:155–159.
247. Watson MK, Wittenburg LA, Bui CT, et al. Pharmacokinetics and bioavailability of orbifloxacin oral suspension in New Zealand white rabbits (*Oryctolagus cuniculus*). *Am J Vet Res.* 2015;76:946–951.
248. Welch WD, Lu YS, Bawdon RE. Pharmacokinetics of penicillin-G in serum and nasal washings of *Pasteurella multocida*-free and -infected rabbits. *Lab Anim Sci.* 1987;37:65–68.
249. Wen H, Pan B, Wang F, et al. The effect of self-licking behavior on pharmacokinetics of eprinomectin and clinical efficacy against *Psoroptes cuniculi* in topically administered rabbits. *Parasitol Res.* 2010;106:607–613.
250. Williams DL. Common features of exotic animal ophthalmology. In: Williams DL, ed. *Ophthalmology in Exotic Pets.* Oxford, UK: Wiley-Blackwell; 2012:9–14.
251. Wixson SK. Anesthesia and analgesia. In: Manning PJ, Ringler DH, Newcomer CE, eds. *The Biology of the Laboratory Rabbit.* 2nd ed. San Diego, CA: Academic Press; 1994.
252. Wong CW, Czarny B, Metselaar JM, et al. Evaluation of subconjunctival liposomal steroids for treatment of experimental uveitis. *Sci Report.* 2018;8:6604. doi:10.1038/s41598-018-24545-2.
253. Yu GY, Yan CH, Yu XG, et al. Effects of chelation therapy with succimer in young rabbits of moderate lead poisoning. *Zhonghua Yu Fang Yi Xue Za Zhi.* 2009;43:8–13.
254. Yuschenkoff D, Graham J, Pumphrey SA. Diagnosis and treatment of glaucoma in client-owned rabbits (*Oryctolagus cuniculus*): 16 eyes from 11 rabbits (2008-2019). *J Exot Pet Med.* 2020;34:67–71.
255. Zehnder AM, Hawkins MG, Trestrail EA, et al. Calculation of body surface area via computed tomography-guided modeling in domestic rabbits (*Oryctolagus cuniculus*). *Am J Vet Res.* 2012;73(12):1859–1863.
256. Zhou JY, Xu PF, Chen H, et al. Therapeutic effect of ceftazidime in a rabbit model of peritonitis caused by *Escherichia coli* producing CTX-M-14 extended-spectrum beta-lactamase. *Zhonghua Jie He He Hu Xi Za Zhi.* 2005;28:689–693.

Chapter 11 Ferrets

Jeffrey R. Applegate, Jr. | Craig A. Harms

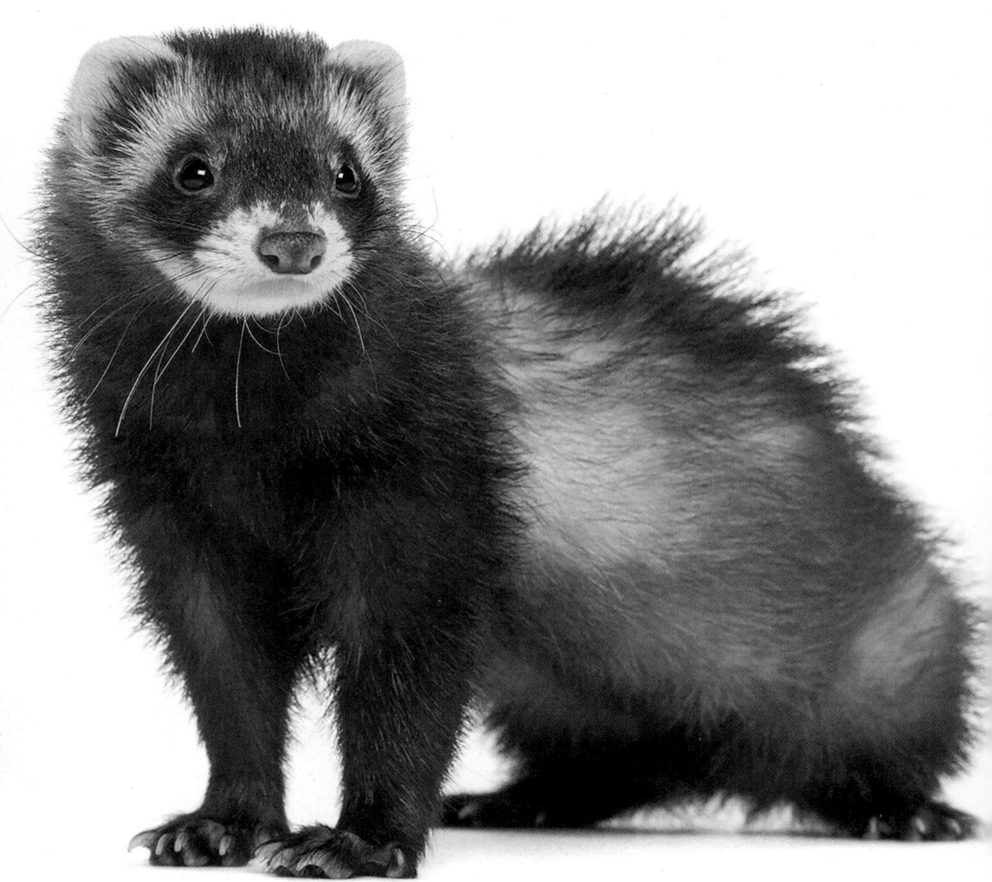

TABLE 11-1 Antimicrobial Agents Used in Ferrets.

Agent	Dosage	Comments
Amikacin	8-16 mg/kg SC, IM, IV divided q8-24h[88]	Potentially ototoxic and nephrotoxic
Amoxicillin	20 mg/kg PO, SC q12h[51]	
	30 mg/kg PO q8h × 21 days[35]	*Helicobacter*, can use with metronidazole and bismuth subsalicylate
Amoxicillin/ clavulanic acid (Clavamox, Zoetis)	13-25 mg/kg PO q8-12h[51]	
	18.75 mg per jill PO q12h[34]	*E. coli*-induced mastitis
Ampicillin	5-30 mg/kg SC, IM, IV q8-12h[11,85]	
Azithromycin	5 mg/kg PO q24h[100]	
Cefadroxil	15-20 mg/kg PO q12h[12]	
Cefovecin (Convenia, Zoetis)	8 mg/kg SC q2-3d[46]	Second-generation parenteral cephalosporin; long-acting antibiotic
Cephalexin	15-30 mg/kg PO q8-12h[88]	
Cephaloridine	10-25 mg/kg SC, IM q24h × 5-7 days[88]	Dermatitis
Chloramphenicol	25-50 mg/kg PO, SC, IM, IV q12h[88]	14-day minimum for proliferative bowel disease
	50 mg/kg SC, IM q12h[34]	For treatment of mastitis
Ciprofloxacin	10-30 mg/kg PO q24h[88]	Mix 500 mg tablet in 10 mL water (50 mg/mL); flavor for improved acceptance
Clarithromycin	12.5 mg/kg PO q8-12h × 14 days[76]	*Helicobacter*, use with ranitidine bismuth citrate
	50 mg/kg PO q24h or divided q12h × 14 days[85]	*Helicobacter*, use with omeprazole (or ranitidine) and metronidazole
Clindamycin	5.5-10 mg/kg PO q12h[88]	Anaerobic infections; bone and dental disease
	12.5 mg/kg PO q12h[88]	Toxoplasmosis
Cloxacillin	10 mg/kg PO, IM, IV q6h[10]	
Doxycycline	10 mg/kg PO q12h[88]	May help with ferret systemic coronavirus infection
Enrofloxacin (Baytril, Bayer)	—	SC and IM injections may cause muscle necrosis or sterile abscesses; dilute before giving parenterally.
	5 mg/kg PO, IM q12h[34]	For treatment of mastitis
	5-10 mg/kg PO, SC, IM q12h[88]	IM for short term (generally one injection); injectable form can be given PO in palatable liquid; liquid for PO can also be compounded
	10-20 mg/kg PO, SC, IM q12-24h[123]	
Erythromycin	10 mg/kg PO q6h[10]	
	220 g/ton feed[88]	Controlling *Campylobacter* diarrhea in large groups

Continued

TABLE 11-1 Antimicrobial Agents Used in Ferrets. (cont'd)

Agent	Dosage	Comments
Gentamicin	2 mg/kg PO q12h × 10-14 days[44]	Parenteral form can be given PO; proliferative colitis that is nonresponsive to chloramphenicol[21,44]
	2-5 mg/kg SC, IM, IV q12-24h[12,22]	If given IV, dilute with saline and administer over 20 min
Lincomycin	11 mg/kg PO q8h[88]	
Metronidazole	15-20 mg/kg PO q12h[11]	Anaerobic infections; can use with amoxicillin and bismuth subsalicylate for *Helicobacter*
	20 mg/kg PO, IV q12h[93]	Used in combination with amoxicillin and bismuth subsalicylate for *Helicobacter* gestritis
Neomycin	10-20 mg/kg PO q6h[10,22]	Potential nephrotoxicity and neuromuscular blockage
Netilmicin (Netromycin, Schering)	6-8 mg/kg SC, IM, IV q24h[88]	Severe staphylococcal infections
Nitazoxanide (Alinia, Romark Laboratories)	5 mg/kg PO q12h[55]	Cryptosporidiosis
Oxytetracycline	20 mg/kg PO q8h[10,12,22]	
Penicillin G (sodium or potassium)	20,000 U/kg IM q12h[71]	
	40,000 U/kg SC, IM q24h[10,12,11,88]	
Pentamidine isethionate	3-4 mg/kg SC q48h[55]	*Pneumocystis* pneumonia
Pyremethamine	0.5 mg/kg PO q12h[55]	Combine with trimethoprim sulfa (30 mg/kg PO q12h) and folic acid (3-5 mg/kg PO q24h) for treatment of toxoplasmosis
Sulfadimethoxine	25 mg/kg PO, SC, IM q24h[88]	
	30-50 mg/kg PO q12-24h[12]	
Sulfamethazine	1-5 mg/mL drinking water[58]	
Sulfasoxazole	50 mg/kg PO q8h[88]	
Sulfathalidine	Mix in food at dose of 1 g/day/kg body weight[21]	Opioid useful for management of *Salmonella* and to reduce shedding in colonies
Tetracycline	20-25 mg/kg PO q8-12h[10,22]	
Trimethoprim/sulfa	5 mg/kg PO q24h[34]	Pyelonephritis
	15 mg/kg IV q12h[6]	
	15-30 mg/kg PO, SC q12h[51]	Dosage amount of combined drugs
Tylosin (Tylan, Elanco)	5-10 mg/kg PO, SC, IM, IV q12h[12,22,85]	

TABLE 11-2 Antifungal Agents Used in Ferrets.

Agent	Dosage	Comments
Amphotericin B	0.15 mg/kg IV 3 × /wk × 2-4 mo[55]	Cryptococcosis
	0.25-1 mg/kg IV q24h or q48h until total dose of 7-25 mg has been given[55]	
	0.4-0.8 mg/kg IV q7d[10]	Blastomycosis; monitor for azotemia; total dose 7-25 mg
Fluconazole	50 mg/kg PO q12h[88]	
Griseofulvin	25 mg/kg PO q12-24h[88]	Refractory dermatomycosis; use with lime sulfur dips q7d
Itraconazole	1.5 mg/kg PO q24h[73]	Invasive nasal cryptococcosis
	10 mg/kg PO q12h[42]	Histoplasmosis
	10-20 mg/kg PO q24h[118]	Cryptococcosis
	25-33 mg/kg PO q24h[55,125]	
Ketoconazole	10-50 mg/kg PO q12-24h[71]	
Lime sulfur	Dip q7d[51]	Dermatomycosis; see griseofulvin

TABLE 11-3 Antiviral Agents Used in Ferrets.

Agent	Dosage	Comments
Amantadine (Symmetrel, Endo Labs)	6 mg/kg as aerosol q12h[5,55]	Influenza; experimental antiviral
Hyperimmune serum	1 mL/animal IV once[97]	Canine distemper virus infection; use serum from a healthy, appropriately vaccinated ferret
Oseltamivir phosphate (Tamiflu, Genentech)	5-10 mg/kg PO q12h × 10 days[63]	Influenza
Zanamivir (Relenza, GlaxoSmithKline)	0.3-1 mg/kg via inhalation q12h[63]	Influenza
	12.5 mg/kg intranasal only[5]	Influenza; greater effect if used with amantadine

TABLE 11-4 Antiparasitic Agents Used in Ferrets.

Agent	Dosage	Comments
Amitraz (Mitaban, Upjohn)	0.0125% topical solution q7d × 3 treatments, then 0.0375% q7d × 3 treatments[92]	Demodecosis secondary to other illness
	0.03% topical solution to affected area q7d × 3-6 treatments[88]	Demodecosis; use full concentration

Continued

TABLE 11-4 Antiparasitic Agents Used in Ferrets. (cont'd)

Agent	Dosage	Comments
Amprolium	19 mg/kg PO q24h[12]	Coccidiosis
	100 mg/kg PO in food or water for 7 days[55]	*Isospora* spp.
Carbaryl powder (5%)	Topical q7d × 3-6 treatments[12]	Ectoparasites
Decoquinate	0.5 mg/kg PO for ≥ 2 wk[100]	Coccidiosis; larger groups of ferrets
Fenbendazole	20 mg/kg PO q24h × 5 days[85]	
	50 mg/kg PO q24h × 30 days[1]	*Mesocestoides* infection
Fipronil (Frontline, Boehringer Ingelheim)	1 pump of spray or $^1/_5$ -½ of cat pipette topical q60d[84]	Flea adulticide
	0.2-0.4 mL/animal topically q30d[123]	
Fipronil/S-methoprene (Frontline Combo/ Frontline Plus, Boehringer Ingelheim)	0.5 mL/animal (50 mg fipronil/60 mg S-methoprene) topically to back of neck[46]	Flea adulticide and larval development inhibitor
Imidacloprid (Advantage, Bayer)	10 mg/kg topically[69]	Fleas; PD
	0.1-0.4 mL topically q30d[71]	Flea adulticide; use small cat/kitten vial
Imidacloprid/ moxidectin (Advantage Multi, Bayer)	1.9-3.3 µg/kg topically q30d[100]	Heartworm prevention
Ivermectin	0.02 mg/kg PO, SC q30d[119]	Heartworm prevention
	0.05 mg/kg PO q30d until negative testing[119]	Recommended treatment for heartworms; give prednisolone (1 mg/kg q24h) concurrently
	0.05-0.3 mg/kg PO q24h × 1 mo after negative skin scraping[6]	Demodecosis
	0.2-0.5 mg/kg SC q14d × 3 treatments[51]	Sarcoptic mange
	0.4 mg/kg PO, SC, repeat in 14-28 days[51,106]	Ear mites, ticks
	0.5-1 mg/kg in ears, repeat in 14 days12[51]	Ear mites; half dose in each ear; treat cats and dogs in house concurrently
Lime sulfur	Dip 1:40 dilution q7d × 6 wk[44]	Demodectic mange
Lufenuron (Program, Novartis)	10 mg/kg SC[55]	Flea larvicide
	30 mg/kg PO in food[55]	
	30-45 mg/kg PO q30d[62]	
Mebendazole	50 mg/kg PO q12h × 2 days[55]	Nematodes

TABLE 11-4 Antiparasitic Agents Used in Ferrets. (cont'd)

Agent	Dosage	Comments
Melarsomine dihydrochloride (Immiticide, Merial)	2.5 mg/kg IM once, repeat in 30 days with 2 treatments 24 hr apart[12]	Heartworm adulticide; less commonly used; use prednisone (1 mg/kg q24h × 4 mo) following treatment
Metronidazole	15-20 mg/kg PO q12h × 14 days[10]	Gastrointestinal protozoa
Milbemycin oxime (Interceptor, Novartis)	1.15-2.33 mg/kg PO q30d[114]	Heartworm preventive
Moxidectin	0.17 mg SC once[100]	Heartworm adulticide
Paromomycin	165 mg/kg PO q12h × 5 days[100]	Cryptosporidiosis; possible treatment; use with caution, severe renal disease possible
Piperazine citrate	50-100 mg/kg PO q14d[88]	Intestinal nematodes
Praziquantel (Droncit, Bayer)	5-10 mg/kg PO, SC, repeat in 10[88]-14d[10]	Cestodes
	25 mg/kg PO × 3 days[100]	Trematodes
Pyrantel pamoate	4.4 mg/kg PO, repeat in 14 days[12]	
Pyrethrins	Topical q7d prn[84]	Fleas; use products safe for puppies and kittens
Pyrimethamine	0.5 mg/kg PO q12h[55]	Toxoplasmosis; antiprotozoal
Selamectin (Revolution, Zoetis)	6-18 mg/kg topically[85,86,88,100]	Ectoparasites (fleas, lice, most mites except *Demodex*)
	15 mg topically q30d[29]	Ear mites, fleas; PD
	45 mg/ferret topically[82]	Ear mites; although this dose has been reported in a PD study, it appears that lower doses (see previous) are also effective
Sulfadimethoxine	20-50 mg/kg PO q24h[7]	Coccidia
	50 mg/kg PO, then 25 mg/kg q24h × 9 days[10]	
	0.5 mL/kg of a 12.5% solution mixed into drinking water[95]	For treatment of enteric coccidiosis in a large group of ferrets
Thiabendazole/ dexamethasone/ neomycin (Tresaderm, Merial)	2 drops in each ear q24h × 7 days, off 7 days, on 7 days[94]	Ear mites

TABLE 11-5 Chemical Restraint/Anesthetic Agents Used in Ferrets.

Agent	Dosage	Comments
Acepromazine	—	See ketamine for combination
	0.1-0.25 mg/kg SC, IM[10,32]	Preanesthetic; light sedation
	0.1-0.5 mg/kg SC, IM[66]	Rapid onset of sedation if given IM; doses above 0.2 mg/kg are associated with prolonged recovery times and hypothermia
	0.2-0.5 mg/kg SC, IM[32]	Tranquilization
Alfaxalone (Alfaxan, Jurox)	5 mg/kg IV[39]	Anesthetic induction; PD
	5-15 mg/kg IM[58]	Sedative
Alfaxalone (A)/ butorphanol (B)	(A) 2.5 mg/kg + (B) 0.2 mg/kg[82a]	Moderate sedation
	(A) 5 mg/kg + (B) 0.2 mg/kg[82a]	Marked sedation, more clinically useful than lower dose alfaxalone, mild transient hypotension and hypoxemia
Atipamezole (Antisedan, Zoetis)	0.4 mg/kg IM[88] 1 mg/kg SC, IV, IP[31]	Dexmedetomidine and medetomidine reversal; give same volume SC, IV, IP as medetomidine or dexmedetomidine (5 × medetomidine or 10 × dexmedetomidine dose in mg)
Atropine	0.04-0.05 mg/kg SC, IM, IV[30,45,51]	Preanesthetic; bradycardia; hypersalivation
Bupivacaine	1 mg/kg epidurally[87]	Epidural anesthesia; analgesia
	1-1.5 mg/kg SC infiltrate[57]	Local anesthesia; lasts several hr
Butorphanol	Loading dose 0.05-0.2 mg/kg; maintenance 0.1-0.4 mg/kg/hr[44]	Constant-rate infusion (CRI) for perioperative analgesia; see ketamine, midazolam, and tiletamine/zolazepam for combinations
Dexmedetomidine (Dexdomitor, Zoetis)	0.04-0.1 mg/kg IM[46]	α_2 agonist; not commonly used because of bradycardia and other side effects
Diazepam[a]	—	See ketamine for combinations; drug is slowly and incompletely absorbed following IM administration
	0.5 mg/kg PO, IM, IV q6-8h[99]	Smooth muscle relaxation in urethral obstruction cases
	0.5-1.5 mg/kg/h constant-rate infusion[54]	Seizure control
	1 mg/animal IV[51]	Seizure control; 1-2 boluses
	2 mg/kg SC, IM[55]	Tranquilization; seizure control
Detomidine (Dormosedan Gel; Zoetis)	2-4 mg/m^2 transmucosal (0.16-0.48 mg/kg)[97a]	Sedation; administer on maxillary gingiva with micropipette; causes hyperglycemia; may reverse with atipamezole at 0.4 mg/kg IM
Enflurane	2% maintenance[28]	Anesthesia
Etomidate	1 mg/kg IV[57]	Induction and intubation of critically ill animal
Fentanyl citrate/ fluanisone (Hypnorm, Janssen)	0.3 mg/kg IM[28]	Anesthesia; not available in the United States
Fentanyl/droperidol (Innovar-Vet, Schering Plough)	0.15 mL/kg IM[32]	Minor surgical procedures; deep sedation

TABLE 11-5 Chemical Restraint/Anesthetic Agents Used in Ferrets. (cont'd)

Agent	Dosage	Comments
Glycopyrrolate	0.01 mg/kg IM[45]	Preanesthetic; bradycardia; hypersalivation
Isoflurane	To effect[65]	Inhalant anesthesia
Ketamine	—	Ketamine combinations follow
	10-20 mg/kg IM[32]	Tranquilization; induction
	30-60 mg/kg IM[32]	Anesthesia; when used alone, high doses cause poor muscle relaxation, rough recoveries, and convulsions; not recommended as a sole agent
Ketamine (K)/ acepromazine (A)	(K) 20-35 mg/kg + (A) 0.2-0.35 mg/kg SC, IM[51]	Anesthesia
Ketamine (K)/ dexmedetomidine (De)	(K) 5 mg/kg IM + (De) 0.03 mg/kg IM[109]	Medetomidine no longer commercially available; dexmedetomidine at half the dose of medetomidine may be effective
Ketamine (K)/ diazepam (D)[a]	(K) 10-20 mg/kg + (D) 1-2 mg/kg IM[51]	Anesthesia; poor analgesia[61]
	0.1 mL/kg IV[28]	Induction; allows intubation with premedication; use equal volumes of (K) at 100 mg/mL and (D) at 5 mg/mL[a]
Ketamine (K)/ medetomidine (Me) or dexmedetomidine (De)/butorphanol (B)	(K) 5 mg/kg + (Me) 0.08 mg/kg or (De) 0.04 mg/kg + (B) 0.2 mg/kg IM[65]	Medetomidine no longer commercially available; induction or total injectable anesthesia; allows for intubation; 60-80 min of surgical plane of anesthesia
Ketamine (K)/ midazolam (M)	(K) 5-10 mg/kg + (M) 0.25-0.5 mg/kg IV[86]	
	0.1 mL/kg IV[28]	Induction; use equal volumes of (K) at 100 mg/mL and (M) at 5 mg/mL
Ketamine (K)/ xylazine (X)	(K) 10-25 mg/kg + (X) 1-2 mg/kg IM[51,83]	Anesthesia; avoid in sick animals; may result in cardiac arrhythmias
Lidocaine	1-2 mg/kg total SC[57]	Local anesthesia; use 1%-2% solution; lasts 15-30 min
Midazolam (Versed, Roche)	—	See ketamine for combination; can be reversed with flumazenil at same volume
	0.25-0.3 mg/kg SC, IM[55]	Mild sedation; premedication
	0.25-0.5 mg/kg SC, IM, IV[88]	
Midazolam (M)/ butorphanol (B)	(M) 0.2 mg/kg + (B) 0.2 mg/kg IM[17,98]	Good sedation; premedication for minor procedures (i.e., ultrasonography, endoscopy, etc.); if needed, can follow with gas anesthesia or IV propofol; can reverse midazolam with flumazenil
Naloxone (Narcan, Dupont)	0.01-0.03 mg/kg IM, IV[16]	Reversal of opioids; up to 1 mg/kg may be used
	0.04 mg/kg SC, IM, IV[12]	
Propofol	1-3 mg/kg IV[65]	Induction when premedicants are used; bradypnea or apnea and hypoxia common; intubation and oxygen insufflation are recommended
	2-10 mg/kg IV[55]	Induction
Sevoflurane	To effect[86]	Inhalant anesthesia

Continued

TABLE 11-5 Chemical Restraint/Anesthetic Agents Used in Ferrets. (cont'd)

Agent	Dosage	Comments
Tiletamine/zolazepam (Telazol, Fort Dodge)	—	Tiletamine/zolazepam combinations follow
	12-22 mg/kg IM[96]	Minor surgical procedures at 22 mg/kg; recovery may be prolonged at higher doses; poor muscle relaxation; rarely indicated
Tiletamine/zolazepam (T)/xylazine (X)	(T) 3 mg/kg + (X) 3 mg/kg IM[67]	Small injection volume; rapid and smooth induction; allows for endotracheal intubation
Tiletamine/zolazepam (T)/xylazine (X)/ butorphanol (B)	(T) 1.5 mg/kg + (X) 1.5 mg/kg + (B) 0.2 mg/kg IM[67]	Small injection volume; rapid and smooth induction; allows for endotracheal intubation; analgesia; profound cardiorespiratory depression necessitates oxygen insufflation
Tiletamine/zolazepam (T)/dexmedetomidine (De)/butorphanol (B)	0.03 mL/kg IM of prepared solution (see comment)[65]	Telazol powder is reconstituted with 2.5 mL of dexmedetomidine (0.5 mg/mL) and 2.5 mL of butorphanol (10 mg/mL) to form final volume of 5 mL
Xylazine	—	See ketamine and tiletamine/zolazepam for combinations
	0.1-0.5 mg/kg SC, IM[88]	Tranquilization; may cause hypotension, bradycardia, and arrhythmias; use with care in sick animals
	2 mg/kg IM[66]	Rapid immobilization within 3-5 min; associated with arrhythmias, hypotension, bradycardia
Yohimbine (Yobine, Lloyd)	0.2-0.5 mg/kg IV[16]	Xylazine reversal
	0.5-1 mg/kg IM[16,88,116]	

[a]Diazepam is not soluble in aqueous solution; admixing with aqueous solutions or fluids can result in precipitation; administering SC or IM can be painful and irritating; for SC or IM administration, midazolam may be preferred.

TABLE 11-6 Analgesic Agents Used in Ferrets.

Agent	Dosage	Comments
Acetylsalicylic acid (aspirin)	0.5-22 mg/kg PO q8-24h[51]	Analgesia; antiinflammatory; antipyretic; cannot be compounded as molecule is unstable in aqueous solution
Amantadine	3-5 mg/kg PO[46]	May potentiate other analgesics via NMDA antagonist action
Bupivacaine	1-2 mg/kg SC[65]	
Buprenorphine	12 μg/kg epidurally[44]	Epidural analgesia/anesthesia
	0.01-0.05 mg/kg oral transmucosal, SC, IM, IV q6-12h[45,65]	Analgesia
	0.04 mg/kg IM q4-6h[60]	PK
Butorphanol	—	See ketamine, midazolam, and tiletamine/zolazepam (see Table 11-5) for anesthetic combinations
	0.05-0.5 mg/kg SC, IM q8-12h[12,65]	Analgesia; lower end of dose may be too low for clinical effect; higher end of dose range may cause profound sedation
	0.3 mg/kg SC q2-4h[60]	PK

TABLE 11-6 Analgesic Agents Used in Ferrets. (cont'd)

Agent	Dosage	Comments
Carprofen (Rimadyl, Zoetis)	1-5 mg/kg PO q12-24h[12,44] 4 mg/kg SC[65]	Nonsteroidal antiinflammatory; use caution in animals with gastritis or enteritis
Fentanyl citrate	1.25-5 μg/kg/h IV via constant-rate infusion[44,46]	Postoperative analgesia
	10-30 μg/kg/h IV via constant-rate infusion[44,46]	Perioperative analgesia; administer after loading dose of 5-10 μg/kg IV
Flunixin meglumine (Banamine, Schering)	0.3-2 mg/kg PO, SC, IV q12-24h[13,45,88,]	Nonsteroidal antiinflammatory; use caution in animals with gastritis or enteritis; use caution in using drug more than 5 days continuously; mix injectable form with palatable syrup for PO
Gabapentin	3-5 mg/kg PO q8-24h[87]	Neurotropic pain; may cause sedation at higher doses
Hydromorphone	0.1 mg/kg SC q1-2h[60] 0.1-0.2 mg/kg SC, IM, IV[71]	Opioid; PK
Ibuprofen	1 mg/kg PO q12-24h[86]	Nonsteroidal antiinflammatory
Ketamine	0.1-0.4 mg/kg/h IV via constant-rate infusion[44]	Postoperative analgesia
	0.3-1.2 mg/kg/h IV via constant-rate infusion[44]	Perioperative analgesia; administer after 2-5 mg/kg IV loading dose
Ketoprofen (Ketofen, Fort Dodge)	1-3 mg/kg PO, SC, IM q24h[88]	Nonsteroidal antiinflammatory; use caution with gastritis or enteritis or if using >5 days
Meloxicam	0.1-0.3 mg/kg PO, SC, IM q24h[53,55,57]	Nonsteroidal antiinflammatory; monitor liver and kidney values
	0.2 mg/kg SC[19a]	PK; achieved plasma concentrations considered effective in other species; maximum plasma concentration higher and elimination slower for males
Meperidine (Demerol, Winthrop-Breon)	5-10 mg/kg SC, IM, IV q2-4h[55]	Analgesia
Morphine	0.1 mg/kg epidurally[44]	Analgesia
	0.2-5 mg/kg SC, IM q2-6h[16,45]	SC administration of 1 mg/kg associated with emesis, excitability, and ptyalism[71]
Nalbuphine (Nubain, Endo Labs)	0.5-1.5 mg/kg IM, IV q2-3h[55]	Analgesia
Oxymorphone	0.05-0.2 mg/kg SC, IM, IV q8-12h[45,57]	Analgesia
Pentazocine (Talwin, Sanofi Winthrop)	5-10 mg/kg IM q4h[45]	Analgesia
Tramadol	5-10 mg/kg PO q12-24h[55]	Analgesia; synergistic with nonsteroidal antiinflammatories

TABLE 11-7 Cardiopulmonary Agents Used in Ferrets.

Agent	Dosage	Comments
Aminophylline	4 mg/kg PO, IM, IV q12h[88]	Bronchodilator
Amlodipine (Norvasc, Pfizer)	0.2-0.4 mg/kg PO q12h[58]	Vasodilator
Atenolol (Tenormin, ICI)	3.125-6.25 mg/kg PO q24h[89]	β-adrenergic blocker for hypertrophic cardiomyopathy
Atropine	0.02-0.04 mg/kg SC, IM, IV[46]	Bradycardia
	0.04-0.05 mg/kg SC, IM, IV q12h[88]	
	0.1 mg/kg intratracheal[58]	
Benazepril	0.25-0.5 mg/kg PO q24h[89]	Vasodilator; less nephrotoxic than enalapril
Captopril (Capoten, Squibb)	1/8 of 12.5 mg tablet/animal PO q48h[58]	Vasodilator; starting dose, gradually increase to q12-24h; can cause lethargy
Digoxin (Cardoxin, Evsco)	0.005-0.01 mg/kg PO q12-24h[89]	Positive inotrope; dilated cardiomyopathy, atrial fibrillation, supraventricular tachycardia; monitor serum levels
Diltiazem (Cardizem, Marion Merrill Dow)	1.5-7.5 mg/kg PO q12h[89]	Calcium channel blocker: hypertrophic cardiomyopathy, atrial fibrillation
Dobutamine	0.01 mL/animal IV prn[58]	Hypotension; 12. 5 mg/mL solution
Doxapram	2-5 mg/kg IM, IV[88]	Respiratory stimulant
Enalapril (Enacard, Merck)	0.25-0.5 mg/kg PO q24-48h[89]	Vasodilator for dilated cardiomyopathy; do not use with concurrent renal disease
Epinephrine	0.02 mg/kg SC, IM, IV, intratracheal[88]	Cardiac arrest; anaphylactic reactions (including vaccine reactions)
	0.2 mg/kg IV, intracardiac, IO[55]	
	0.2-0.4 mg/kg diluted in 0.9% NaCl[55] intratracheal	Administer during cardiopulmonary arrest
Furosemide	1-4 mg/kg PO, SC, IM, IV q8-12h[89]	Diuretic; use high dose in fulminant heart failure
	2-3 mg/kg IM, IV q8-12h followed by 1-2 mg/kg PO q12h for long-term management[119]	Emergency management of fulminant heart failure
Isoproterenol	20-25 µg/animal SC, IM q4-6h[119]	Positive chronotrope to increase ventricular rate in third-degree AV block
	40-50 µg/animal PO q4-6h[119]	
Metaproterenol	0.25-1 mg/kg PO q12h[119]	Positive chronotrope to increase ventricular rate in third-degree AV block
Nitroglycerin (2% Ointment; Nitrol, Savage)	1/16-1/8 inch (1.6-3.2 mm)/animal q12-24h[119]	Vasodilator for cardiomyopathy; apply to shaved inner thigh or pinna

TABLE 11-7 Cardiopulmonary Agents Used in Ferrets. (cont'd)

Agent	Dosage	Comments
Pimobendan	0.25-1.25 mg/kg PO q12h[55] 0.5-1.25 mg/kg PO q12h[119] 0.625-1.25 mg/kg q12h[71]	Phosphodiesterase inhibitor; increases cardiac contractility with dilated cardiomyopathy or mitral valve disease
Propranolol (Inderal, Wyeth-Ayerst)	0.2-1 mg/kg PO q8-12h[58]	β-blocker for hypertrophic cardiomyopathy; may cause lethargy, loss of appetite
Pseudophedrine	5 mg/kg PO q8h[119]	Positive chronotrope to increase ventricular rate in third-degree AV block
Terbutaline	2.5-5 mg/kg PO q12-24h[58]	Bronchodilator

TABLE 11-8 Endocrine and Reproductive Disease Agents Used in Ferrets.

Agent	Dosage	Comments
Anastrazole (Arimidex, AstraZeneca Pharmaceuticals)	0.1 mg/kg PO q24h[108,122]	Estrogen inhibitor; precursor hormones blocked by inhibition of aromatase enzyme; use until signs resolve, then 7 days on, 7 days off, etc.; pregnant owners should avoid handling agent
Bicalutamide (Casodex, AstraZeneca Pharmaceuticals)	5 mg/kg PO q24h[108,122]	Testosterone inhibitor; competitively inhibits androgen by binding to receptors in target tissues; use until clinical signs resolve, then 7 days on, 7 days off, etc.; pregnant owners should avoid handling agent
Buserelin	1.5 µg/animal IM q24h × 2 days[46]	GnRH analog; suppresses signs of estrus
Cabergoline	5 µg/kg PO q24h × 5 days[57]	Pseudopregnancy
Deoxycorticosterone pivalate (DOCP)	2 mg/kg IM q21d[40]	Treatment of adrenal insufficiency following bilateral adrenalectomy
Deslorelin (Suprelorin, Virbac Animal Health)	—	Long-acting GnRH analog that may suppress LH and FSH; used to control signs of adrenal disease; given as a subcutaneous implant approximately once yearly; only the 4.7 mg is available in the United States
	2.7 mg implant SC[70]	Alternative to spay/neuter; the 2.7 mg implant is not available in the United States
	3 mg or 4.7 mg SC[70,121]	The 3 mg implant is not available in the United States
	4.7 mg implant SC[55]	Treatment of adrenal disease; lasts 10-18 mo
	9.4 mg implant SC[55]	Treatment of adrenal disease; lasts 16-48 mo; not available in the United States
Dexamethasone	0.5 mg/kg SC, IM, IV[13]	
	1 mg/kg IM[51]	Post adrenalectomy; follow with prednisone
Diazoxide (Proglycem, Medical Market Specialties)	5-30 mg/kg PO q12h[77,107] 10 mg/kg PO q24h or divided q8-12h[49,51]	Insulinoma; insulin blocker; can cause hypertension, lethargy, depression, nausea

Continued

TABLE 11-8 Endocrine and Reproductive Disease Agents Used in Ferrets. (cont'd)

Agent	Dosage	Comments
Finasteride (Proscar, Merck)	5 mg/kg PO q24h[107]	Inhibits conversion of testosterone to active form of dihydrotestosterone; also used in treatment of prostatic enlargement
Fludrocortisone	0.05-0.1 mg/kg PO q24h or divided q12h[112]	Mineralocorticoid replacement after adrenal gland removal
Flutamide (Eulexin, Schering)	5-10 mg/kg PO q12-24h[13,19,112]	Androgen inhibitor; reduces enlarged periurethral prostate tissue; lifetime treatment; associated with mammary tumors
Glucagon	15 ng/kg/min IV constant-rate infusion[8]	Emergency management of hypoglycemia secondary to insulinoma
Gonadotropin-releasing hormone (GnRH) (Cystorelin, Sanofi)	20 μg/animal IM[34]	Termination of estrus after day 10 of estrus; repeat in 2 wk prn
Human chorionic gonadotropin (hCG) (Pregnyl, Organon)	—	Use 10 or more days after onset of estrus to induce ovulation and prevent hyperestrogenemia; repeat in 1-2 wk prn
	50-100 U/animal IM[34]	
	200-1000 U/animal IM[10,107]	
Insulin, glargine	0.5 U/animal SC q12h[48]	
Insulin, NPH	0.1 U/animal SC q12h[68]	
	0.5-1 U/kg (or to effect) SC[46]	Diabetes mellitus; diabetic ketoacidosis; monitor blood glucose
Insulin, ultralente	0.1 U/animal SC q24h[107]	Diabetes mellitus; monitor blood glucose
Leuprolide acetate (Lupron, AbbVie)	—	Long-acting GnRH analog that may cause an initial stimulation, then suppression of LH and FSH; palliative treatment of adrenal disease (will not resolve tumor); administer q28d until clinical signs regress, then treatment interval can be up to 6-8 wk; lifetime treatment; higher dosage may shrink prostate within 12-48 hr, which may improve urine flow in cases of urethral obstruction; must be prepared in aliquots and frozen (although the effects of freezing on drug efficacy are questionable) until used; expensive
	1 mg IM q60-75d;[19] 3 mo depot	Adrenal disease
Leuprolide acetate (Lupron), Depot 30 day (TAP)	100-150 μg/kg IM q4-8wk[2,120]	
	250 μg/kg IM q4-8wk[56]	
Leuprolide acetate (Lupron), Depot 4 month (TAP)	250 μg/kg IM[99]	
	2 mg/kg SC, IM q16wk[122]	
Levothyroxine	50-100 μg/animal q12h[125]	Hypothyroidism (uncommon in ferrets)

TABLE 11-8 Endocrine and Reproductive Disease Agents Used in Ferrets. (cont'd)

Agent	Dosage	Comments
Melatonin	0.5-1 mg/animal PO q24h[104] prn	Symptomatic treatment of hyperadrenocorticism; may not affect tumor growth
	5.4 mg implant SC[90]	Should last 6-12 mo
Mitotane (o,p′-DDD) (Lysodren, Bristol-Myers)	—	Hyperadrenocorticism in other species; results in ferrets have been unsatisfactory and therefore, use is not recommended
Octreotide (Sandostatin, Novartis)	1-2 μg/kg SC q8-12h[46]	Somatostatin analogue; potential treatment for insulinomas
Oxytocin	0.2-3 U/kg SC, IM[11]	Expels retained fetuses; stimulates lactation
Prednisone	0.25 mg/kg PO q12h × 5 days, then 0.1 mg/kg q12h × 10 days[51]	Postoperative adrenalectomy; after initial dose of dexamethasone
	0.25-1 mg/kg PO divided q12h[49,51]	Insulinoma; gradually increase to 4 mg/kg/day prn; up to 2 mg/kg/day when given with diazoxide
	0.5 mg/kg PO q12h × 7-10 days, then q24h × 7-10 days, then q48h × 7-10 days[91]	Postoperative adrenalectomy
Proligestone	50 mg SC[99]	Induce ovulation when jill has been in estrus for 10 days; not available in the United States
Prostaglandin F_2-α (Lutalyse, Upjohn)	0.1-0.5 mg/animal IM prn[7]	Metritis; expels necrotic debris
	0.5 mg/animal IM[7]	Can induce delivery on day 41 if only one kit; follow with 6 U oxytocin 1-4 hr later
Thyroid-stimulating hormone (TSH)	1 U/animal IV[61]	Blood for T_4 measurement taken 120 min later
Trilostane (Vetoryl, Dechra)	2 mg/kg PO q12h[55]	May be useful for treating pituitary-dependent hyperadrenocorticism or adrenal-dependent hyperadrenocorticism; reduces synthesis of adrenal androgens
Yeast, brewer's	$^1/_8$-$^1/_4$ tsp (0.6-1.2 mL)/animal PO q12h[51]	Source of chromium to stabilize glucose and insulin for animals with insulinomas

TABLE 11-9 Chemotherapy Agents Used in Ferrets.[a]

Agent	Dosage	Comments
Bleomycin (Blenoxane, BristolMyersSquibb)	10-20 U/m² SC[43,58]	Treatment of squamous cell carcinoma
Chlorambucil (Leukeran, Glaxo)	1 mg/kg PO q7d[124] 20 mg/m² PO[124]	Antineoplastic; in chemotherapy protocols for lymphoma[a]

Continued

TABLE 11-9 Chemotherapy Agents Used in Ferrets. (cont'd)

Agent	Dosage	Comments
Cyclophosphamide	10 mg/kg PO, SC[124]	Antineoplastic; use at higher dose for salvage treatment of lymphoma[a]
	200 mg/m² PO, SC × 4 consecutive days weekly[124]	
	250 mg/m² PO q4-5wk[79]	Part of a noninvasive protocol for treatment of lymphoma[a]
Cytarabine (Cytosar-U, Zoetis)	300 mg/m² q8wk[79]	Part of a noninvasive protocol for treatment of lymphoma[a]
	1 mg/animal PO, SC q24h × 2 days[2]	
Doxorubicin	1 mg/kg IV q21d × 4 treatments[4,124]	Antineoplastic agent; lymphoma;[a] salvage treatment
Isotretinoin	2 mg/kg PO q24h[4,124]	Cutaneous epitheliotropic lymphoma
L-asparaginase	400 U/kg SC, IM[124]	Antineoplastic,[a] hypersensitivity reactions possible, pretreat with diphenhydramine (1 mg/kg IM) or dexamethasone (0.5 mg/k SC, IM, IV)
	10,000 U/m² SC q7d × 3 treatments[79]	Part of a noninvasive chemotherapy protocol[a]
Methotrexate	0.5 mg/kg IV[124]	Antineoplastic[a]
	0.8 mg/kg IM[79]	Part of noninvasive protocol for treatment of lymphoma[a]
Procarbazine	50 mg/m² PO q24h × 14 days[79]	Part of a noninvasive protocol for treatment of lymphoma[a]
Vincristine	0.12-0.2 mg/kg IV[124]	Lymphoma[a]

[a]See Table 11-19 Chemotherapy Protocols for Lymphoma in Ferrets.

TABLE 11-10 Miscellaneous Agents Used in Ferrets.[a]

Agent	Dosage	Comments
Acetylcysteine	20 mg/mL solution diluted with saline and nebulized 30-60 min prn[46]	Mucolytic
Activated charcoal	1-3 g/kg PO[88]	Orally administered adsorbent for gastrointestinal tract toxins/drug overdoses
Apomorphine	0.04 mg/kg SC[25]	Emetic
	0.1-.0.2 mg/kg SC[64]	
Atropine	5-10 mg/kg SC, IM[58]	Organophosphate toxicity
Azathioprine (Imuran, GlaxoSmithKline)	0.9 mg/kg PO q24-72h[14]	Immunosuppressive agent; may use in chronic hepatitis; with prednisone and sucralfate for chronic inflammatory bowel disease[52]
Barium (30%)	8-13 mL/kg PO[111]	Gastrointestinal contrast study

TABLE 11-10 Miscellaneous Agents Used in Ferrets. (cont'd)

Agent	Dosage	Comments
Barium (60%)	17 mL/kg PO[113]	Followed 30 min later by 42 mL/kg of air for a double-contrast gastrointestinal study
Bismuth subcitrate, colloidal	6 mg/kg PO q12h[58]	In combination with enrofloxacin at 4.25 mg/kg q12h for *Helicobacter*
Bismuth subsalicylate (Pepto-Bismol, Procter & Gamble)	17.5 mg/kg PO q8-12h[58]	Gastrointestinal ulcers; may help prevent *Helicobacter* colonization
Budesonide (Entocort, AstraZeneca)	0.5 mg/kg or up to 1 mg/ferret PO q24h[46,58]	Steroid may have use as single-agent treatment for inflammatory bowel disease
Calcium EDTA	20-30 mg/kg SC q12h[88]	Treatment of heavy metal toxicosis
Chitosan	0.5 mg/kg on food q12h[46]	Intestinal phosphorus and uremic toxin absorbent; cellulose-like biopolymer from exoskeletons of marine invertebrates
Chlorpheniramine (Chlor-Trimeton, Squibb)	1-2 mg/kg PO q8-12h[58]	Antihistamine; controls sneezing and coughing when they interfere with eating or sleeping
Cimetidine (Tagamet, SmithKline)	5-10 mg/kg PO, SC, IM, IV q6-8h[13,50,51,72]	H_2 blocker; inhibits acid secretion; gastrointestinal ulcers; unpalatable; give IV (slow)
Cisapride (Propulsid, Janssen)	0.5 mg/kg PO q8-12h[88]	Antiemetic; motility enhancer; not currently available in the United States; must be compounded
Cobalamin	25 µg/kg SC q7d × 6 wk, then q14d × 6 wk, then q30d[53]	Chronic diarrhea; with cobalamin malabsorption
Cyclosporine	4-6 mg/kg PO q12h[74]	Pure red cell aplasia
Cyproheptadine (Periactin, Merck)	0.5 mg/kg PO q12h[46]	Appetite stimulation
Dexamethasone sodium phosphate	2 mg/kg IM, IV[41]	Anaphylactic reaction to vaccine
	4-8 mg/kg IM, IV[20]	Shock therapy
Dextrose 50%	0.25-2 mL IV[20]	Bolus for hypoglycemia; give to effect
	1.25%-5% IV[20]	Infusion for hypoglycemic or inappetant animal
Diatrizoate meglumine/ Diatrizoate sodium (RenoCal-76)	2.3 mL/kg IV[113]	Excretory urography
Diphenhydramine	0.5-2 mg/kg PO, IM, IV q8-12h[20,75]	Antihistamine; controls sneezing and coughing when they interfere with eating or sleeping; give at high dose IM prevaccination when previous reaction occurred or for treatment of vaccine reaction
Doxapram	2-5 mg/kg IV, IM[88]	Respiratory stimulant
Epinephrine	0.02 mg/kg SC, IM, IV, IT[88]	Severe vaccine reaction; cardiac arrest

Continued

TABLE 11-10 Miscellaneous Agents Used in Ferrets. (cont'd)

Agent	Dosage	Comments
Epoetin alfa (Epogen, Amgen)	50-150 U/kg IM, SC q48-72h[46,88]	Stimulates erythropoiesis; after desired PCV is reached, administer q7d × ≥4 wk for maintenance
Famotidine (Pepcid, Merck)	0.25-0.5 mg/kg PO, SC, IV q24h[88]	Inhibits acid secretion; gastrointestinal ulcers
	2.5 mg PO, SC, IV q24h[55]	
Flunixin meglumine (Banamine, Schering)	2.5 mg/animal SC, IM q12h prn[34]	Reduce inflammation in mastitis
Fluoxetine	3 mg/kg PO q24h[24]	Hyperactivity, aggression (treatment with behavioral modification)
Flurbiprofen sodium	1-2 drops q12-24h[55]	Ophthalmic inflammation
Glutamine	—	Amino acid; L form available OTC as a nutritional supplement
	0.5 g/kg PO divided daily[46]	Enterocyte supplementation with starvation
Hairball laxative, feline	1-2 mL/animal PO q48h[58]	Trichobezoar prophylaxis
Hydrocortisone sodium succinate	25-40 mg/kg IV[46]	Shock
Hydrogen peroxide (3%)	2.2 mL/kg PO[58]	Emetic
Hydroxyzine (Atarax, Roerig)	2 mg/kg PO q8h[88]	Antihistamine; pruritus; may cause drowsiness
Interferon-α	10^7 units IV or intranasal q24h × several days[63]	Adjunctive therapy for influenza
Iohexol	0.25-0.5 mL/kg[58] injected epidurally at the L5-L6 intervertebral disc space	Myelography (CT or MRI preferred if available)
	10 mL/kg PO[58]	Gastrointestinal contrast study; can dilute 1:1 with water
Ipecac (7%)	2.2-6.6 mL/animal PO[58]	Emetic
Iron dextran	10 mg/animal IM once[46]	Iron deficiency anemia; hemorrhage
Kaolin/pectin	1-2 mL/kg PO q2-6h prn[58]	Gastrointestinal protectant
Lactulose syrup (10 g/15 mL)	0.15-0.75 mL/kg PO q12h[46]	Absorption of blood ammonia in hepatic disease; may cause soft stools at higher dose
Loperamide	0.2 mg/kg PO q12h[58]	Antidiarrheal
Mannitol	0.5-1 g/kg IV[20]	Give over 20 min
Maropitant citrate (Cerenia, Zoetis)	1 mg/kg PO q24h[52]	Antiemetic
Metoclopramide	0.2-1 mg/kg PO, SC, IM q6-8h[88]	Antiemetic; motility enhancer
Milk thistle (*Silybum marianum*)	4-15 mg/kg PO q8-12h[55]	Herbal; empiric; hepatoprotective

TABLE 11-10 Miscellaneous Agents Used in Ferrets. (cont'd)

Agent	Dosage	Comments
Misoprostol (Cytotech, Searle)	1-5 µg/kg PO q8h[46]	Gastric ulcers
Nandrolone decanoate	1-5 mg/kg IM q7d[46]	Anabolic steroid
Nutri-Cal (EVSCO)	1-3 mL/animal PO q6-8h[58]	Nutritional supplement
Omeprazole (Prilosec, Astra Merck)	0.7 mg/kg PO q24h[36]	*Helicobacter*; proton pump inhibitor; decreases gastric secretion of HCl
	1 mg/kg PO q12h[52]	*Helicobacter* adjunct therapy, gastric acid suppressant
	4 mg/kg PO q24h[55]	*Helicobacter*; use with clarithromycin and metronidazole
Ondansetron	1 mg/kg PO q12-24h[46]	Antiemetic
Penicillamine	10 mg/kg PO q24h[55]	Copper toxicity
Pentoxifylline (Pentoxil, Upsher-Smith)	20 mg/kg PO q12h[52]	Supportive treatment for ferret systemic coronavirus
Pet-Tinic (Zoetis)	0.2 mL/kg PO q24h[51]	Nutritional/iron supplement for anemia; extrapolated from label dose for dogs and cats
Phenobarbital	1-2 mg/kg PO q8-12h[71,88]	Seizure control
	3 mg/kg slow IV up to 18-24 mg/kg first 24 hr, then 3 mg/kg q12h[54]	Seizure control
Phenoxybenzamine (Dibenzyline, SmithKline Beecham)	0.5-1 mg/kg PO q12h[46]	α-adrenergic antagonist; smooth muscle relaxation for urethral obstruction; potential gastrointestinal or cardiovascular side effects
Potassium bromide	—	Seizure control
	22-30 mg/kg q24h PO[54]	Dose if used with phenobarbital
	70-80 mg/kg q24h PO[54]	Dose if used alone
Prazosin (Minipress, Zoetis)	0.05-0.1 mg/kg PO q8h[46]	α-adrenergic antagonist; smooth muscle relaxation for urethral obstruction; potential for gastrointestinal and cardiovascular side effects
Prednisone	0.5 mg/kg PO q12-24h[89]	Use during and following heartworm adulticide treatment; thromboembolism
	0.5 mg/kg PO q12h; 1 mg/kg PO q24h; 40 mg/m² PO q24h; or 2 mg/kg PO q24h × 1 wk then q48h[124]	Palliative therapy for lymphosarcoma[a] or chronic inflammatory bowel disease; taper dose as appropriate
	1.25-2.5 mg/kg PO q24h[52]	Eosinophilic gastroenteritis; treat until clinical signs abate; gradually decrease to q48h
	1.5 mg/kg PO q24h × 7 days, then taper to 0.8 mg/kg PO q24h[78]	Management of eosinophilic gastroenteritis
	1 mg/kg PO q12h[52]	Chronic inflammatory bowel disease; use with azathioprine and sucralfate

Continued

TABLE 11-10 Miscellaneous Agents Used in Ferrets. (cont'd)

Agent	Dosage	Comments
Pyridostigmine (Mestinon, Bausch)	1 mg/kg PO q8h[23]	Oral cholinesterase inhibitor for potential treatment of myasthenia gravis
	1 mg/kg PO q8-12h[3]	Myasthenia gravis; overdose possible with long-term use
Ranitidine bismuth citrate (Pylorid, Glaxo Wellcome)	24 mg/kg PO q8h[76]	*Helicobacter*; use in combination with clarithromycin; not available in the United States
Ranitidine HCl (Zantac, Glaxo Wellcome)	2.5-3.5 mg/kg PO q12h[55,58]	Inhibits acid secretion; gastrointestinal ulcers
Ropinirol (Clevor, Orion)	3.75 mg/m^2 instilled in eye[115]	Emetic approved for use in dogs, not validated in ferrets; dosing would require micropipette or dilution; dopamine receptor agonist; reverse if necessary with metoclopramide 0.5 mg/kg SC
S-adenosylmethionine (SAMe) (Vetri-SAMe, VetriScience Labs)	20-100 mg/kg PO q24h[46]	Adjunctive treatment for liver disease; hepatoprotectant; improves synthesis of glutathione and other compounds important for liver function
Stanozolol (Winstrol, Upjohn)	0.5 mg/kg PO, SC q12h[58]	Anemia; anabolic steroid; use with caution in hepatic disease
Sucralfate (Carafate, Hoechst Marion Roussel)	25-125 mg/kg PO q8-12h[88]	Gastrointestinal ulcers; give before meals; requires acidic pH
	100 mg/kg PO q6h[52]	With prednisone and azathioprine for chronic inflammatory bowel disease
Sulfasalazine	62.5-125 mg PO q8-24h[46]	Management of colitis
Theophylline elixir	4.25-10 mg/kg PO q8-12h[46]	Bronchodilator
Trientine (Syprine, Valeant)	10 mg/kg PO q12h[55]	Chelating agent used for copper toxicosis
Ursodiol (Actigall, Ciba)	15 mg/kg PO q12h[14]	Treatment of chronic hepatopathies
Vitamin A (retinol palmitate)	50,000 U/animal IM q24h × 2 treatments[105]	Reduced mortality secondary to canine distemper virus infection
Vitamin B complex	1-2 mg/kg IM prn[88]	Dose based on thiamine content
Vitamin C	50-100 mg/kg PO q12h[55]	Adjunct therapy for lymphoma
Vitamin K	2.5 mg/kg SC, then 1-2.5 mg/kg PO divided q8-12h × 5-7 days[46]	First-generation rodenticide toxicity (e.g., warfarin class)
	2.5-5 mg/kg SC, then 2.5 mg/kg PO divided q8-12h × 3-4 wk[46]	Inandione or unknown anticoagulant toxicity
	5 mg/kg SC, then 2.5 mg/kg PO divided q8-12h × 3 wk[46]	Second-generation rodenticide toxicity (e.g., brodifacoum class)

[a]See Table 11-19 Chemotherapy Protocols for Lymphoma in Ferrets.

TABLE 11-11 Hematologic and Biochemical Values of Ferrets.[a,33,47]

Measurements	Normal Values
Hematology	
PCV (%)	40-70
RBC (10^6/μL)	7.4-13.0
Hgb (g/dL)	13.9-21.9
MCV (fL)	50-61
MCH (pg)	16.1-19.3
MCHC (g/dL)	28.7-33.7
WBC (10^3/μL)	3.0-16.7
Neutrophils (10^3/μL [%])	0.9-7.4 [17-82]
Band cells (10^3/μL [%])	0.0-0.1 [0-1.2]
Lymphocytes (10^3/μL [%])	0.6-10.5 [13-81]
Monocytes (10^3/μL [%])	0-0.5 [0.0-6.5]
Eosinophils (10^3/μL [%])	0.0-0.7 [0.0-5.7]
Basophils (10^3/μL [%])	0.0-0.2 [0.0-1.4]
Platelets (10^3/μL)	171-1280
Biochemistries	
ALP (U/L)	13-142
ALT (U/L)	49-243
Amylase (U/L)	19-62
AST (U/L)	40-143
Bile acids (μmol/L)	0-29
Bilirubin, total (mg/dL)	0.0-0.2
BUN (mg/dL)	13-47
Calcium (mg/dL)	8.0-10.4
Chloride (mmol/L)	108-120
Cholesterol (mg/dL)	93-274
CK (U/L)	94-731
Creatinine (mg/dL)	0.3-0.9
GGT (U/L)	0.2-14.0
Glucose (mg/dL)	54-153
Iron (μg/dL)	65-314
LDH (U/L)	154-1781
Lipase (U/L)	73-351
Magnesium (mg/dL)	2.2-3.4
Phosphorus (mg/dL)	3.1-9.6
Potassium (mmol/L)	3.9-5.9

Continued

TABLE 11-11 Miscellaneous Agents Used in Ferrets. (cont'd)

Measurements	Normal Values
Protein, total (g/dL)	5.5-7.8
Albumin (g/dL)	2.8-4.4
Sodium (mmol/L)	140-170
Triglycerides (mg/dL)	44-248

[a]Conscious pet ferrets (n = 94-106 of various ages and hair coat types, age 11 wk–9 yr, intact and neutered males and females) sampled from the lateral saphenous vein. Additional clinical pathology reference intervals are available subdivided by sex, hair coat, and age categories.[33] Anesthesia can alter some values, including PCV, RBC, hemoglobin, plasma protein and glucose.

TABLE 11-12 Biologic and Physiologic Data of Ferrets.[27,33,37,38,65,101,110]

Parameter	Normal Values
Adult body weight, male	1-2 kg
Adult body weight, female	0.65-0.95 kg
Birth weight	6-12 g
Weight at 10 days	30 g average
Weight at 21 days	10x birth weight
Sexual maturity	6-12 mo (usually first spring after birth)
Reproductive cycle	Induced ovulator
Gestation period	39-42 days
Litter size	1-18 (average 8)
Weaning age	6-8 wk
Eyes and ears open	28-34 days
Life span	6-8 (up to 12) yr
Food consumption	50-75 g/day (or 140-190 g/day semimoist; dry preferred for dental health)
Water consumption	75-100 mL/day
Gastrointestinal transit time	2.5-4 hr
Maintenance caloric needs	200-300 kcal/kg/day
Dental formula	2(I 3/3 C 1/1 P 3/3 M 1/2) = 34
Deciduous teeth erupt	20-28 days
Permanent teeth erupt	50-74 days
Stomach capacity (distended)	50 mL/kg
Heart rate	200-400 beats/min
Systolic blood pressure	95-155 mmHg
Diastolic blood pressure	51-87 mmHg
Mean blood pressure	69-109 mmHg
Blood volume	60-80 mL (5%-7% body weight)

TABLE 11-12 Biologic and Physiologic Data of Ferrets. (cont'd)

Parameter	Normal Values
Respiratory rate	33-36 breaths/min
Tidal volume	10-11 mL/kg
Endotracheal tube size	2-3 mm ID
Rectal temperature	37.8-40°C (100-104°F)
Intraocular pressure	22.8 ± 5.5 mmHg

TABLE 11-13 Protein Electrophoresis Values of Ferrets.[81]

Measurements	Normal Values
Total protein (g/dL)	5.6-7.2
Albumin (g/dL)	3.3-4.1
$Alpha_1$ globulins (g/dL)	0.33-0.56
$Alpha_2$ globulins (g/dL)	0.36-0.60
Beta globulins (g/dL)	0.83-1.2
Gamma globulins (g/dL)	0.3-0.8
A:G	1.3-2.1

TABLE 11-14 Coagulation Values of Ferrets.[9,102]

Measurements	Normal Values
Prothrombin time (PT) (sec)	10.6-12.7
Partial thromboplastin time (PTT) (sec)	16.5-22.3
Fibrinogen (mg/dL)	90-164
Antithrombin activity (%)	69-115
Clotting time (glass tubes) (min)	2.0+/-0.5

TABLE 11-15 Blood Gases, pH, Lactate, and Ionized Mineral Values of Ferrets.[126]

Measurement	Normal Values[a]
pH	7.341 (7.274-7.415)
pCO_2 (mmHg)	46.8 (35.2-59.1)
pO_2 (mmHg)	51.0 (30.0-69.2)
SO_2 (%)	74.5 (55.3-93.3)
TCO_2 (mmol/L)	26.9 (22.6-31.6)
HCO_3^- (mmol/L)	25.3 (21.3-30.0)
Lactate (mmol/L)	0.9 (0.3-1.5)
iCa (mmol/L)	1.24 (1.14-1.35)
iMg (mmol/L)	0.56 (0.44-0.66)

[a]Medians and reference intervals.

TABLE 11-16 Hormone Values of Ferrets.[15,47,80,112]

Measurements	Normal Values
Adrenal	
Androstenedione - neutered M&F (nmol/L)	<0.1-15
Androstenedione - intact F (nmol/L)	20-96
Estradiol - neutered M&F (pmol/L)	30-108
Estradiol - intact F (pmol/L)	122-210
17-hydroxyprogesterone - neutered M&F (nmol/L)	<0.1-0.8
17-hydroxyprogesterone - intact F (nmol/L)	2.3-13.1
Cortisol[a] (µg/dL) [nmol/L]	0.0-3.7 [0.0-101.5]
Thyroid	
Thyroxine (T_4) resting (µg/dL) [nmol/L]	1.24-3.26 [15.9-42.0]
Thyroxine (T_4) 4 hr after rhTSH 100 µg/kg IM (µg/dL) [nmol/L]	2.32+/-0.64 [29.9+/-8.2]
Triiodothyronine (T_3) (ng/dL) [nmol/L]	29-78 [0.45-1.2]
Parathyroid	
Intact parathyroid hormone (PTH) (pmol/L)	2.2-24.4
Ionized calcium (mmol/L)	1.09-1.25
25-hydroxyvitamin D (nmol/L)	61-138
Pancreatic Islets	
Insulin (µU/mL) [pmol/L]	4.5-42.8 [32-300]

[a]Cosyntropin at 1 µg/kg caused a 3-to-4-fold increase in plasma cortisol concentration.

TABLE 11-17 Urinalysis Values of Ferrets.[26,33,102,103,117]

Measurements	Male	Female
Volume (mL/24 hr)	26 (8-48)	28 (8-140)
Sodium (mmol/24 hr)	1.9 (0.4-6.7)	1.5 (0.2-5.6)
Potassium (mmol/24 hr)	2.9 (1-9.6)	2.1 (0.9-5.4)
Chloride (mmol/24 hr)	2.4 (0.7-8.5)	1.9 (0.3-7.8)
pH	5.0-6.5[a]	5.0-7.5[a]
Protein (mg/dL, by strip)	30-100 (1+ to 2+)	Trace-30 (trace to 1+)
Exogenous creatinine clearance (mL/min/kg)	—	3.32 ± 2.16
Inulin clearance (mL/min/kg)	—	3.02 ± 1.78
Specific gravity	1.034-1.070	1.026-1.060

[a]Urine pH can vary according to diet; normal urine pH in ferrets on a high-quality, meat-based diet is approximately 6.

TABLE 11-18 **Proposed Schedule of Vaccinations and Routine Prophylactic Care for Ferrets.**[11,18,75,87,102,103,a]

Age	Recommendations
4-6 wk	CDV[b] vaccination if dam is unvaccinated
6-8 wk	CDV[b,c] vaccination if dam was vaccinated; physical examination; fecal examination
10-11 wk	CDV[b-d] vaccination; physical examination; fecal examination
12-14 wk	CDV[b-d] vaccination; rabies vaccination;[e] physical examination; fecal examination (optional)
4-8 mo	Spay/castrate; fecal examination; remove musk glands (optional); start heartworm and flea prevention (endemic areas)
1 yr	CDV[b,f] booster; rabies booster;[e] physical examination; dental prophylaxis and fecal examination if indicated; CBC; heartworm and flea prevention
2 yr	CDV[b,f,g] booster; rabies booster;[e] physical examination; dental prophylaxis and fecal examination if indicated; CBC; heartworm and flea prevention
3 yr and older (every 6 mo)	CDV[b,f,g] booster (annual); rabies booster[e], (annual); physical examination; dental prophylaxis and fecal examination if indicated; CBC; serum chemistries, including fasting blood glucose; heartworm and flea prevention

[a]Vaccine reactions may occur; see Table 11-10 (dexamethasone, diphenyhydramine, epinephrine) for prevention and treatment of vaccine reactions.
[b]CDV, canine distemper vaccine; Purevax (Merial) and NeoVac FD are the only CDV vaccines approved for use in ferrets; if these are unavailable, other vaccines which have been used include Novibac DPv (Merck) and Recombitek (Merial).
[c]Purevax is recommended to be administered at 8 wk, then every 3 wk for 3 doses.
[d]Vaccinations are generally administered at 2-3 wk intervals until the ferret is 12-14 wk of age.
[e]Only a killed virus vaccine (Imrab 3, Rhône Merieux) should be used. Vaccines should be separated by several days to reduce vaccine reactions.
[f]In previously unvaccinated adults, an initial series of two vaccinations given 14-28 days apart should be given.
[g]Rabies and distemper titers are under evaluation and may alter the revaccination schedule of older animals.

TABLE 11-19 **Chemotherapy Protocols for Lymphoma in Ferrets.**[a]

Protocol I[79]			
Week	**Day**	**Agent**	**Dosage**
1	1	Prednisone	1-2 mg/kg PO q12h and continued throughout therapy
	1	Vincristine	0.025 mg/kg IV
	3	Cyclophosphamide	10 mg/kg PO, SC
2	8	Vincristine	0.025 mg/kg IV
3	15	Vincristine	0.025 mg/kg IV
4	22	Vincristine	0.025 mg/kg IV
	24	Cyclophosphamide	10 mg/kg PO, SC
7	46	Cyclophosphamide	10 mg/kg PO, SC
9	63	Prednisone	Gradually decrease dose to 0 over the next 4 wk

Continued

TABLE 11-19 Chemotherapy Protocols for Lymphoma in Ferrets. (cont'd)

Protocol II[b]		
Week	**Agent**	**Dosage**
1	Vincristine	0.025 mg/kg IV
	L-asparaginase	400 U/kg IP
	Prednisone	1 mg/kg PO q24h and continued throughout therapy
2	Cyclophosphamide	10 mg/kg SC
3	Doxorubicin	1 mg/kg IV
4-6	As weeks 1-3 above, but discontinue L-asparaginase	—
8	Vincristine	0.025 mg/kg IV
10	Cyclophosphamide	10 mg/kg SC
12	Vincristine	0.025 mg/kg IV
14	Methotrexate	0.5 mg/kg IV
Protocol III[79]		
Week	**Agent**	**Dosage**
1	L-asparaginase	10,000 U/m^2 SC
	Cytoxin	250 mg/m^2 PO, SC (in 50 mL/kg of NaCl SC)
	Prednisone	2 mg/kg PO daily for 7 days, then q48h throughout therapy
2	L-asparaginase	10,000 U/m^2 SC
	Perform CBC[c]	
3	L-asparaginase	10,000 U/m^2 SC
	Cytosar	300 mg/m^2 SC × 2 days (dilute 100 mg with 1 mL H_2O)
4	Perform CBC[c]	
5	Cytoxin	250 mg/m^2 PO, SC (in 50 mL/kg of NaCl SC)
7	Methotrexate	0.8 mg/kg IM
8	Perform CBC[c]	
9	Cytoxin	250 mg/m^2 PO, SC (in 50 mL/kg of NaCl SC)
11	Cytosar	300 mg/m^2 SC × 2 days (dilute 100 mg with 1 mL H_2O)
	Leukeran	1 tablet/animal PO or ½ tablet/animal PO × 2 days
12	Perform CBC[c]	
13	Cytoxin	250 mg/m^2 PO, SC (in 50 mL/kg of NaCl SC)
15	Procarbazine	50 mg/m^2 PO q24h × 14 days
16	Perform CBC[c]	
17	Perform CBC[c]	
18	Cytoxin	250 mg/m^2 PO, SC (in 50 mL/kg of NaCl SC)
20	Cytosar	300 mg/m^2 SC × 2 days (dilute 100 mg with 1 mL H_2O)
	Leukeran	1 tablet/animal PO or ½ tablet/animal PO × 2 days
23	Cytoxin	250 mg/m^2 PO, SC (in 50 mL/kg of NaCl SC)
26	Procarbazine	50 mg/m^2 PO q24h × 14 days
27	Perform CBC[c] and chemistry panel	If not in remission, continue weeks 20-26 for 3 cycles

TABLE 11-19 Chemotherapy Protocols for Lymphoma in Ferrets. (cont'd)

Protocol IV[4]		
Week	**Agent**	**Dosage**
3 days	L-asparaginase	400 U/kg SC (premedicate with diphenhydramine)
1	Vincristine	0.12 mg/kg IV
	Prednisone	1 mg/kg PO q24h continue throughout therapy
	Cyclophosphamide	10 mg/kg PO
2	Vincristine	0.12 mg/kg IV
3	Vincristine	0.12 mg/kg IV
4	Vincristine	0.12 mg/kg IV
	Cyclophosphamide	10 mg/kg PO
7, 10, 13, etc.	Vincristine	0.12 mg/kg IV
	Cyclophosphamide	10 mg/kg PO
		Continue therapy every 3 wk for 1 yr, then decrease to every 4-6 wk
Rescue treatment (after failure of standard treatments)	Doxorubicin	1-2 mg/kg IV (over 20 min)

[a]CBC should be checked weekly during therapy; after therapy is discontinued, continue to monitor CBC and do physical examination at 3-mo intervals.

[b]Protocol is continued in sequence biweekly after week 14, making the therapy protocol less intensive.

[c]If CBC shows severe myelosuppression, reduce dosage by 25% for all subsequent treatments of the previously used myelosuppressive drug.

TABLE 11-20 Conversion of Body Weight (kg) to Body Surface Area (BSA) (m^2).[59,79]

Body Weight (kg)	Body Surface Area (m^2)
0.5	0.063
0.6	0.071
0.7	0.078
0.8	0.086
0.9	0.093
1.0	0.099
1.1	0.106
1.2	0.112
1.3	0.118
1.4	0.124
1.5	0.130
1.6	0.136

Continued

TABLE 11-20 Conversion of Body Weight (kg) to Body Surface Area (BSA) (m^2). (cont'd)

Body Weight (kg)	Body Surface Area (m^2)
1.7	0.141
1.8	0.147
1.9	0.152
2.0	0.158
2.1	0.163
2.2	0.168
2.3	0.173
2.4	0.178
2.5	0.183

BSA (m^2) = 0.94 x (body weight in g)$^{2/3}$ x 10^{-4}; formula validated for weight range of 620-1850 g.[59]

REFERENCES

1. Ahlgrim KA. Personal communication; 2003.
2. Antinoff N. Neoplasia in ferrets. In: Bonagura JD, ed. *Kirk's Current Veterinary Therapy XIII: Small Animal Practice*. Philadelphia, PA: WB Saunders; 2000:1149–1152.
3. Antinoff N. Diagnosis and successful treatment of myasthenia gravis in a ferret. *Proc ExoticsCon*. 2015:367.
4. Antinoff N, Hahn K. Ferret oncology: diseases, diagnostics, and therapeutics. *Vet Clin North Am Exot Anim Pract*. 2004;7:579–626.
5. Barron HW, Rosenthal KL. Respiratory diseases. In: Quesenberry KE, Carpenter JW, eds. *Ferrets, Rabbits, and Rodents: Clinical Medicine and Surgery*. 3rd ed. St. Louis, MO: Saunders/Elsevier; 2012:78–85.
6. Beaufrère H, Neta M, Smith DA. Demodectic mange associated with lymphoma in a ferret. *J Exot Pet Med*. 2009;18:57–61.
7. Bell JA. Periparturient and neonatal diseases. In: Quesenberry KE, Carpenter JW, eds. *Ferrets, Rabbits, and Rodents: Clinical Medicine and Surgery*. 2nd ed. St. Louis, MO: WB Saunders; 2004:50–57.
8. Bennett KR, Gaunt MC, Parker DL. Constant rate infusion of glucagon as an emergency treatment for hypoglycemia in a domestic ferret (*Mustela putorius furo*). *J Am Vet Med Assoc*. 2015;246:451–454.
9. Benson KG, Paul-Murphy J, Hart AP, et al. Coagulation values in normal ferrets (*Mustela putorius furo*) using selected methods and reagents. *Vet Clin Pathol*. 2008;37:286–288.
10. Besch-Williford CL. Biology and medicine of the ferret. *Vet Clin North Am Small Anim Pract*. 1987;17:1155–1183.
11. Brown SA. Ferrets. In: Jenkins JR, Brown SA, eds. *A Practitioner's Guide to Rabbits and Ferrets*. Lakewood, CO: American Animal Hospital Association; 1993:43–111.
12. Brown SA. Clinical techniques in the ferret. *Semin Avian Exot Pet Med*. 1997;6:75–85.
13. Brown SA, Antinoff N, Bauck L, Boyer TH, et al. Ferret drug dosages. *Exotic Formulary*. 2nd ed. Lakewood, CO: American Animal Hospital Association; 1999:43–61.
14. Burgess M, Garner M. Clinical aspects of inflammatory bowel disease in ferrets. *Exot DVM*. 2002;4(2):29–34.

15. Cannizo SA, Rick M, Harrison TM, et al. Parathyroid hormone, ionized calcium, and 25-hydroxyvitamin D concentrations in the domestic ferret (*Mustela putorius furo*). *J Exot Pet Med.* 2017;26:294–299.
16. Cantwell SL. Ferret, rabbit, and rodent anesthesia. *Vet Clin North Am Exotic Anim Pract.* 2001;4:169–191.
17. Carpenter JW. Personal observation; 2017.
18. Carpenter JW, Harms CA, Harrenstien L. Biology and medicine of the domestic ferret: an overview. *J Small Exot Anim Med.* 1994;2:151–162.
19. Chen S, Michels D, Culpepper E. Nonsurgical management of hyperadrenocorticism in ferrets. *Vet Clin North Am Exot Anim Pract.* 2014;17:35–49.
19a. Chinnadurai SK, Messenger KM, Papich MG, et al. Meloxicam pharmacokinetics using nonlinear mixe-effects modeling in ferrets after single subcutaneous administration. *J Vet Pharmacol Ther.* 2014;37:382–387.
20. Chitty JR, Johnson-Delaney CA. Emergency care. In: Johnson-Delaney CA, ed. *Ferret Medicine and Surgery*. Boca Raton, FL: CRC Press; 2017:113–125.
21. Coburn DR, Morris JA. The treatment of *Salmonella typhimurium* infection in ferrets. *Cornell Vet.* 1949;39:198–201.
22. Collins BR. Antimicrobial drug use in rabbits, rodents, and other small mammals *Antimicrobial Therapy in Caged Birds and Exotic Pets.* Trenton, NJ: Veterinary Learning Systems; 1995:3–10.
23. Couturier J, Huynh M, Boussarie D, et al. Autoimmune myasthenia gravis in a ferret. *J Am Vet Med Assoc.* 2009;235:1462–1466.
24. Desmarchelier MR. Clinical psychopharmacology for the exotic animal practitioner. *Vet Clin Exot Anim.* 2021;24:17–35.
25. Dunayer E. Toxicology of ferrets. *Vet Clin North Am Exot Anim Pract.* 2008;11:301–314.
26. Eshar D, Wyre NR, Brown DC. Urine specific gravity values in clinically healthy young pet ferrets (*Mustela furo*). *J Small Anim Pract.* 2012;53:115–119.
27. Evans H, An NQ. Anatomy of the ferret. In: Fox JG, Marini RP, eds. *Biology and Diseases of the Ferret.* 3rd ed. Ames, IA: Wiley Blackwell; 2014:23–67.
28. Evans AT, Springsteen KK. Anesthesia of ferrets. *Semin Avian Exot Pet Med.* 1998;7:48–52.
29. Fisher M, Beck W, Hutchinson MJ. Efficacy and safety of selamectin (Stronghold®/Revolution®) used off-label in exotic pets. *Int J Appl Res Vet Med.* 2007;5:87–96.
30. Flecknell PA. *Laboratory Animal Anesthesia.* San Diego, CA: Academic Press; 1987.
31. Flecknell PA. Medetomidine and atipamezole: potential uses in laboratory animals. *Lab Anim.* 1997;26:21–25.
32. Fox JG. Anesthesia and surgery. In: Fox JG, ed. *Biology and Diseases of the Ferret.* Philadelphia, PA: Lea and Febiger; 1988:289–302.
33. Fox JG. Normal clinical and biological parameters. In: Fox JG, Marini RP, eds. *Biology and Diseases of the Ferret.* 3rd ed. Ames, IA: Wiley Blackwell; 2014:157–185.
34. Fox JG, Bell JA. Diseases of the genitourinary system. In: Fox JG, Marini RP, eds. *Biology and Diseases of the Ferret.* 3rd ed. Ames, IA: Wiley Blackwell; 2014:335–361.
35. Fox JG, Lee A. The role of *Helicobacter* species in newly recognized gastrointestinal diseases of animals. *Lab Anim Sci.* 1997;47:222–227.
36. Fox JG, Marini RP. *Helicobacter mustelae* infection in ferrets: pathogenesis, epizootiology, diagnosis, and treatment. *Semin Avian Exot Pet Med.* 2001;10:36–44.
37. Fox JG, Bell JA, Broome R. Growth and reproduction. In: Fox JG, Marini RP, eds. *Biology and Diseases of the Ferret.* 3rd ed. Ames, IA: Wiley Blackwell; 2014:187–209.
38. Fox JG, Schultz CS, Boler BMV. Nutrition of the ferret. In: Fox JG, Marini RP, eds. *Biology and Diseases of the Ferret.* 3rd ed. Ames, IA: Wiley Blackwell; 2014:123–143.
39. Giral M, Garcia-Olma DC, Gomez-Juarez M, et al. Anaesthetic effect in the ferret of alfaxalone alone and in combination with medetomidine or tramadol: a pilot study. *Lab Anim.* 2014;48:313–320.

40. Goett SD, Degner DA. Suspected adrenocortical insufficiency subsequent to bilateral adrenalectomy in a ferret. *Exot DVM*. 2003;5(1):15–18.
41. Greenacre CB. Incidence of adverse events in ferrets vaccinated with distemper or rabies vaccine: 143 cases (1995-2001). *J Am Vet Med Assoc*. 2003;223:663–665.
42. Greenacre CB, Dowling M, Nobrega-Lee M. Histoplasmosis in a group of domestic ferrets (*Mustela putorius furo*). *Proc ExoticsCon*. 2015:363.
43. Hamilton TA, Morrison WB. Bleomycin chemotherapy for metastatic squamous cell carcinoma in a ferret. *J Am Vet Med Assoc*. 1991;198:107–108.
44. Hawkins MG. Advances in exotic mammal clinical therapeutics. *Vet Clin North Am Exot Anim Pract*. 2015;18:323–327.
45. Heard DJ. Principles and techniques of anesthesia and analgesia for exotic practice. *Vet Clin North Am Small Anim Pract*. 1993;23:1301–1327.
46. Hedley J. *Small Animal Formulary-Part B: Exotic Pets*. 10th ed. Gloucester, UK: British Small Animal Veterinary Association; 2020.
47. Hein J, Spreyer F, Sauter-Louis C, et al. Reference ranges for laboratory parameters in ferrets. *Vet Rec*. 2012;171:218.
48. Hess L. Insulin glargine treatment of a ferret with diabetes mellitus. *J Am Vet Med Assoc*. 2012;241:1490–1494.
49. Hillyer EV. Ferret endocrinology. In: Kirk RW, Bonagura JD, eds. *Kirk's Current Veterinary Therapy XI: Small Animal Practice*. Philadelphia, PA: WB Saunders; 1992:1185–1188.
50. Hillyer EV. Gastrointestinal diseases of ferrets (*Mustela putorius furo*). *J Small Exot Anim Med*. 1992;2:44–45.
51. Hillyer EV, Brown SA. Ferrets. In: Birchard SJ, Sherding RG, eds. *Saunders Manual of Small Animal Practice*. Philadelphia, PA: WB Saunders; 1994:1317–1344.
52. Hoefer HL. Gastrointestinal diseases of ferrets. In: Quesenberry KE, Orcutt CJ, Mans C et al., eds. *Ferrets, Rabbits, and Rodents: Clinical Medicine and Surgery*. 4th ed. St. Louis, MO: Elsevier; 2021:27–38.
53. Hoppes SM. The senior ferret. *Vet Clin North Am Exot Anim Pract*. 2010;13:107–121.
54. Huynh M, Piazza S. Musculoskeletal and neurologic diseases. In: Quesenberry KE, Orcutt CJ, Mans C et al., eds. *Ferrets, Rabbits, and Rodents: Clinical Medicine and Surgery*. 4th ed. St. Louis, MO: Elsevier; 2021:117–130.
55. Jepson L. Ferrets. In: Jepson L, ed. *Exotic Animal Medicine: A Quick Reference Guide*. 2nd ed. St. Louis, MO: Elsevier; 2016:1–42.
56. Johnson D. Current therapies for ferret adrenal disease. *Proc Atlantic Coast Vet Conf*. 2006:1–7.
57. Johnson-Delaney C. Ferrets: anaesthesia and analgesia. In: Keeble E, Meredith A, eds. *BSAVA Manual of Rodents and Ferrets*. Gloucester, UK: British Small Animal Veterinary Association; 2009:245–253.
58. Johnson-Delaney CA. Formulary. *Ferret Medicine and Surgery*. Boca Raton, FL: CRC Press; 2017:457–467.
59. Jones KL, Granger LA, Kearney MT, et al. Evaluation of a ferret-specific formula for determining body surface area to improve chemotherapeutic dosing. *Am J Vet Res*. 2015;76:142–148.
60. Katzenbach JE, Wittenburg LA, Allweiler SI, et al. Pharmacokinetics of single-dose buprenorphine, butorphanol, and hydromorphone in the domestic ferret (*Mustela putorius furo*). *J Exot Pet Med*. 2018;27:95–102.
61. Keeble E. Endocrine diseases in small mammals. *In Pract*. 2001;23(10):570–585.
62. Kelleher SA. Skin disease of ferrets. *Semin Avian Exot Pet Med*. 2002;11:136–140.
63. Kiupel M, Perpinan D. Viral diseases of ferrets. In: Fox JG, Marini RP, eds. *Biology and Diseases of the Ferret*. 3rd ed. Ames, IA: Wiley Blackwell; 2014:439–517.
64. Knox AP, Strominger NL, Battles AH, et al. Behavioral studies of emetic sensitivity in the ferret. *Brain Res Bull*. 1993;31:477–484.
65. Ko JC, Marini RP. Anesthesia. In: Fox JG, Marini RP, eds. *Biology and Diseases of the Ferret*. 3rd ed. Ames, IA: Wiley Blackwell; 2014:259–283.

66. Ko JC, Heaton-Jones TG, Nicklin CF, et al. Comparison of sedative and cardiorespiratory effects of diazepam, acepromazine, and xylazine in ferrets. *J Am Anim Hosp Assoc.* 1998;34:234–241.
67. Ko JC, Nicklin CF, Montgomery T, et al. Comparison of anesthetic and cardiorespiratory effects of tiletamine-zolazepam-xylazine and tiletamine-zolazepam-xylazine-butorphanol in ferrets. *J Am Anim Hosp Assoc.* 1998;34:164–174.
68. Kolmstetter CM, Carpenter JW, Morrisey JK. Diagnosis and treatment of ferret endocrine diseases. *Vet Med.* 1995:1104–1110 Dec:.
69. Larsen KS, Siggurdsson H, Mencke N. Efficacy of imidacloprid, imidacloprid/permethrin and phoxim for flea control in the Mustelidae (ferrets, mink). *Parasitol Res.* 2005;97:S107–S112.
70. Lennox A. Alternative surgical options for elective altering in exotic companion mammals. *ExoticsCon.* 2015:435–444.
71. Lewington JH. Appendix. In: Lewington JH, ed. *Ferret Husbandry, Medicine and Surgery.* Oxford, UK: Butterworth Heinemann; 2000:273–282.
72. Lightfoot TL. Common ferret syndromes. *Proc North Am Vet Conf.* 1999:839–842.
73. Malik R, Martin P, McGill J, et al. Successful treatment of invasive nasal cryptococcosis in a ferret. *Aust Vet J.* 2000;78:158–159.
74. Malka S, Hawkins MG, Zabolotzky SM, et al. Immune-mediated pure red cell aplasia in a domestic ferret. *J Am Vet Med Assoc.* 2010;237:695–700.
75. Marini RP. Physical examination, preventive medicine, and diagnosis in the ferret. In: Fox JG, Marini RP, eds. *Biology and Diseases of the Ferret.* 3rd ed. Ames, IA: Wiley Blackwell; 2014:235–258.
76. Marini RP, Fox JG, Taylor NS, et al. Ranitidine bismuth citrate and clarithromycin, alone or in combination, for eradication of *Helicobacter mustelae* infection in ferrets. *Am J Vet Res.* 1999;60:1280–1286.
77. Marini RP, Ryden EB, Rosenblad WD, et al. Functional islet cell tumor in six ferrets. *J Am Vet Med Assoc.* 1993;202:430–433.
78. Maurer KJ, Fox JG. Diseases of the gastrointestinal system. In: Fox JG, Marini RP, eds. *Biology and Diseases of the Ferret.* 3rd ed. Ames, IA: Wiley Blackwell; 2014:363–375.
79. Mayer J, Erdman SE, Fox JG. Diseases of the hematopoietic system. In: Fox JG, Marini RP, eds. *Biology and Diseases of the Ferret.* 3rd ed. Ames, IA: Wiley Blackwell; 2014:311–334.
80. Mayer J, Wagner R, Mitchell MA, et al. Use of recombinant human thyroid-stimulating hormone for thyrotropin stimulation testing in euthyaroid ferrets. *J Am Vet Med Assoc.* 2013;243:1432–1435.
81. Melillo A. Applications of serum protein electrophoresis in exotic mammals. *Vet Clin North Am Exot Anim Pract.* 2013;16:211–225.
82. Miller DS, Eagle RP, Zabel S, et al. Efficacy and safety of selamectin in the treatment of *Otodectes cynotis* infestation in domestic ferrets. *Vet Rec.* 2006;159:748.
82a. Milloway MC, Posner LP, Balko JA. Sedative and cardiorespiratory effects of intramuscular alfaxalone and butorphanol at two dosages in ferrets (*Mustela putorius furo*). *J Zoo Wildl Med.* 2021;51:841–847.
83. Moreland AF, Glaser C. Evaluation of ketamine, ketamine-xylazine and ketamine-diazepam anesthesia in the ferret. *Lab Anim Sci.* 1985;35:287–290.
84. Morrisey JK. Parasites of ferrets, rabbits, and rodents. *Semin Avian Exotic Pet Med.* 1996;5:106–114.
85. Morrisey JK. Ectoparasites of ferrets and rabbits. *Proc North Am Vet Conf*; 1998:844–845.
86. Morrisey JK. Ferrets: therapeutics. In: Keeble E, Meredith A, eds. *BSAVA Manual of Rodents and Ferrets.* Gloucester, UK: British Small Animal Veterinary Association; 2009:237–244.
87. Morrisey JK. Personal observation; 2011.
88. Morrisey JK, Carpenter JW. Formulary. In: Quesenberry KE, Orcutt CJ, Mans C et al., eds. *Ferrets, Rabbits, and Rodents: Clinical Medicine and Surgery.* 4th ed. St. Louis, MO: Elsevier; 2021:620–630.

89. Morrisey JK, Malakoff RL, Quesenberry KE, et al. Cardiovascular and other diseases. *Ferrets, Rabbits, and Rodents: Clinical Medicine and Surgery*. 4th ed. St. Louis, MO: Elsevier; 2021:55–70.
90. Murray J. Melatonin implants: an option for use in the treatment of adrenal disease in ferrets. *J Exot Mammal Med Surg*. 2005;3(1):1–6.
91. Neuwirth L, Isaza R, Bellah J, et al. Adrenal neoplasia in seven ferrets. *Vet Radiol Ultrasound*. 1993;34:340–346.
92. Noli C, VanderHorst HH, Willemse T. Demodicosis in ferrets. *Vet Quart*. 1996;18:28–31.
93. Oglesbee BL, Lord B. Gastrointestinal diseases. In: Quesenberry KE, Carpenter JW, eds. *Ferrets, Rabbits, and Rodents: Clinical Medicine and Surgery*. 4th ed. St Louis, MO: WB Saunders; 2004:174–187.
94. Patterson MM, Kirchain SM. Comparison of three treatments for control of ear mites in ferrets. *Lab Anim Sci*. 1999;49:655–657.
95. Patterson MM, Fox JC, Eberhard ML. Parasitic diseases. In: Fox JG, Marini RP, eds. *Biology and Diseases of the Ferret*. 3rd ed. Ames, IA: Wiley Blackwell; 2014:553–572.
96. Payton AJ, Pick JR. Evaluation of a combination of tiletamine and zolazepam as an anesthetic for ferrets. *Lab Anim Sci*. 1989;39:243–246.
97. Perpinan D, Ramis A, Tomas A, et al. Outbreak of canine distemper in domestic ferrets (*Mustela putorius furo*). *Vet Rec*. 2008;163:246–250.
97a. Phillips BE, Harms CA, Messenger KM. Oral transmucosal detomidine gel for the sedation of the domestic ferret (*Mustela putorius furo*). *J Exot Pet Med*. 2015;24:446–454.
98. Pinon C, Huynh M. Flexible gastrointestinal endoscopy in ferrets. *Proc ExoticsCon*. 2015:459–463.
99. Pollock CG. Disorders of the urinary and reproductive systems. In: Quesenberry KE, Carpenter JW, eds. *Ferrets, Rabbits, and Rodents: Clinical Medicine and Surgery*. 3rd ed. St. Louis, MO: Saunders/Elsevier; 2012:46–61.
100. Powers LV. Bacterial and parasitic diseases of ferrets. *Vet Clin North Am Exot Anim Pract*. 2009;12:531–561.
101. Powers LV, Perpinan D. Basic anatomy, physiology, and husbandry of ferrets. In: Quesenberry KE, Orcutt CJ, Mans C et al., eds. *Ferrets, Rabbits, and Rodents: Clinical Medicine and Surgery*. 4th ed. St. Louis, MO: Elsevier; 2021:1–12.
102. Quesenberry KE. Basic approach to veterinary care. In: Hillyer EV, Quesenberry KE, eds. *Ferrets, Rabbits, and Rodents: Clinical Medicine and Surgery*. Philadelphia, PA: WB Saunders; 1997:14–25.
103. Quesenberry KE, de Matos R. Basic approach to veterinary care of ferrets. In: Quesenberry KE, Orcutt CJ, Mans C et al., eds. *Ferrets, Rabbits, and Rodents: Clinical Medicine and Surgery*. 4th ed. St. Louis, MO: Elsevier; 2021:13–26.
104. Ramer JC, Benson KG, Morrisey JK, et al. Effects of melatonin administration on the clinical course of adrenocortical disease in domestic ferrets. *J Am Vet Med Assoc*. 2006;229:1743–1748.
105. Rodeheffer C, von Messling V, Milot S, et al. Disease manifestations of canine distemper virus infection in ferrets are modulated by vitamin A status. *J Nutr*. 2007;137:1916–1922.
106. Rosenthal K. Ferrets. *Vet Clin North Am Small Anim Pract*. 1994;24:1–23.
107. Rosenthal K. Endocrine disorders of ferrets: insulinoma and adrenal gland disease. *Annu Waltham/OSU Symp Treat Small Anim Dis: Exotics Proc 21st*; 1997:35–38.
108. Rosenthal K. Adrenal gland disease in ferrets. *Proc North Am Vet Conf*. 2000:1015–1016.
109. Rosenthal KL. Personal communication; 2011.
110. Sapienza JS, Porcher D, Collins BR, et al. Tonometry in clinically normal ferrets (*Mustela putorius furo*). *Prog Vet Comp Ophthalmol*. 1991;1:291–294.
111. Schwarz LA, Solano M, Manning A, et al. The normal upper gastrointestinal examination in the ferret. *Vet Radiol Ultrasound*. 2003;44:165–172.
112. Shoemaker NJ, van Zeeland YRA, Quesenberry KE, et al. Endocrine diseases of ferrets. *Ferrets, Rabbits, and Rodents: Clinical Medicine and Surgery*. 4th ed. St. Louis, MO: Elsevier; 2021:77–91.

113. Silverman S, Tell LA. *Radiology of Rodents, Rabbits, and Ferrets: an Atlas of Normal Anatomy and Positioning*. St. Louis, MO: Elsevier Saunders; 2005.
114. Stahl SJ. Personal communication; 2003.
115. Suokko M, Saloranta L, Lamminen T, et al. Ropinirole eye drops induce vomiting effectively in dogs: a randomized, double-blind, placebo-controlled clinical study. *Vet Rec*. 2019. doi:10.1136/vetrec-2018-104953.
116. Sylvina TJ, Berman NG, Fox JG. Effects of yohimbine on bradycardia and duration of recumbency in ketamine/xylazine anesthetized ferrets. *Lab Anim Sci*. 1990;40:178–182.
117. Thornton PC, Wright PA, Sacra PJ, et al. The ferret, *Mustela putorius furo*, as a new species in toxicology. *Lab Anim*. 1979;13:119–124.
118. Vella D. Cryptococcosis. In: Mayer J, Donnelly TM, eds. *Clinical Veterinary Advisor: Birds and Exotic Pets*. St. Louis, MO: Elsevier Saunders; 2013:439.
119. Wagner RA. Diseases of the cardiovascular system. In: Fox JG, Marini RP, eds. *Biology and Diseases of the Ferret*. 3rd ed. Ames, IA: Wiley Blackwell; 2014:401–419.
120. Wagner RA, Bailey EM, Schneider JF, et al. Leuprolide acetate treatment of adrenocortical disease in ferrets. *J Am Vet Med Assoc*. 2001;218:1272–1274.
121. Wagner RA, Piche CA, Jöchle W, et al. Clinical and endocrine responses to treatment with deslorelin acetate implants in ferrets with adrenocortical disease. *Am J Vet Res*. 2005;66:910–914.
122. Weiss C. Medical management of ferret adrenal tumors and hyperplasia. *Exot DVM*. 1999;1.5:38–39.
123. Williams BH. Therapeutics in ferrets. *Vet Clin North Am Exot Anim Pract*. 2000;3:131–153.
124. Williams BH, Wyre NR. Neoplasia in ferrets. In: Quesenberry KE, Orcutt CJ, Mans C et al., eds. *Ferrets, Rabbits, and Rodents: Clinical Medicine and Surgery*. 4th ed. St. Louis, MO: Elsevier; 2021:92–108.
125. Wyre NR, Michels D, Chen S. Selected emerging diseases in ferrets. *Vet Clin North Am Exot Anim Pract*. 2013;16:469–493.
126. Yuschenkoff D, Graham J, Sharkey L, et al. Reference interval determination of venous blood gas, hematologic, and biochemical parameters in healthy sedated, neutered ferrets (*Mustela putorius furo*). *J Exot Pet Med*. 2021;36:25–27.

Chapter 12 Miniature Pigs

Kristie Mozzachio | Louisa Asseo

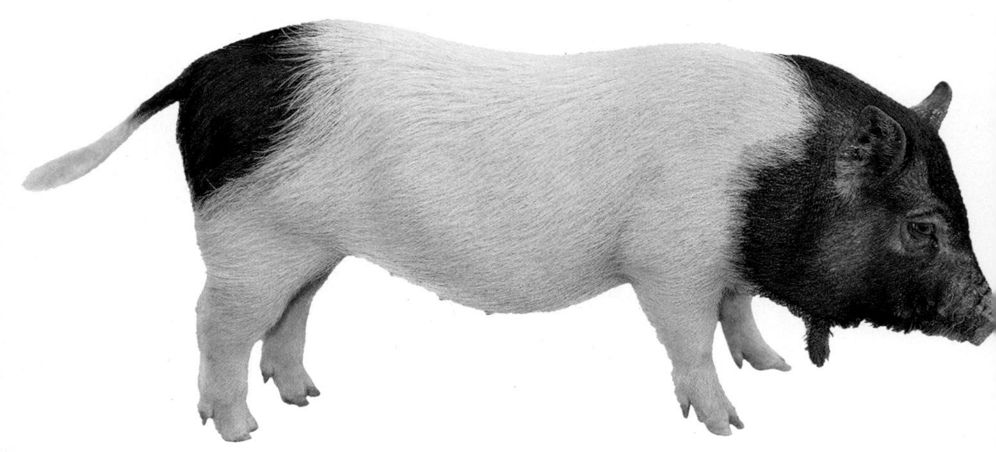

TABLE 12-1 Antimicrobial Agents Used in Miniature Pigs.[a,b]

Agent	Dosage	Comments
Amoxicillin	10-22 mg/kg PO q12-24h[19] 11-13 mg/kg PO q24h[5]	
Amoxicillin/clavulanate (Clavamox, Pfizer)	11-13 mg/kg PO q24h[13] 12.5-25 mg/kg PO q12h[31,c]	
Ampicillin	10-20 mg/kg SC, IM, IV q6-8h[19,31,c] 20 mg/kg SC, IM q8h[5] 20-40 mg/kg PO q8h[31,c]	
Apramycin (Apralan, Elanco)	10-20 mg/kg PO q12-24h[13]	
Ceftiofur	3-10 mg/kg IM q24h[13]	No more than 2 mL/injection site[d]
• Hydrochloride (Excenel, Zoetis)	3-5 mg/kg IM q24h × 3 days[19,31]	
• Sodium (Naxcel, Zoetis)	3-5 mg/kg IM q24h × 3 days[19,31]	
• Long acting (Excede, Zoetis)	5 mg/kg IM[31,d]	
Cephalexin	10-30 mg/kg PO q6-12h[31,c]	Extralabel administration of cephalosporins to food-producing animals in the US is a violation of FDA regulations; use approved cephalosporins (i.e., ceftiofur) or other beta-lactam antibiotic instead
Clindamycin	11-33 mg/kg PO q12h[31,c]	Tusk abscesses
Doxycycline	10-20 mg/kg PO q12h[31]	Tick-associated illness
	20 mg/kg PO q24h × 3 wk[31]	For *Lawsonia intracellularis*
Enrofloxacin (Baytril-S, Bayer)	7.5 mg/kg SC, IM[d]	Use per label instructions as extralabel use prohibited in food-producing animals
Florfenicol (Nuflor, Intervet)	15 mg/kg IM q24-48h[13,31]	
• Nuflor 2.3% concentrate solution	400 mg/gal drinking water × 5 days[31]	
Gentamicin	—	Aminoglycosides should not be administered to food-producing animals, with the exception of specifically licensed products[31]
	5 mg/kg PO q24h[13] 10-15 mg/kg SC, IM q24h[31]	
	1.1-2.2 mg/kg × 3 days in drinking water[31]	Colibacillosis and swine dysentery
Lincomycin	11 mg/kg IM q12-24h[19,31]	*Mycoplasma*
	8.4 mg/kg q24h in drinking water × 5-10 days[19,31]	Swine dysentery

Continued

TABLE 12-1 Antimicrobial Agents Used in Miniature. (cont'd)

Agent	Dosage	Comments
Metronidazole	—	Prohibited in food-producing animals
	12-15 mg/kg PO q12h × 8 days[31,c]	*Giardia*
	15 mg/kg PO q12h[31,c]	Anaerobes
Neomycin	10 mg/kg PO q6h[13]	
	11 mg/kg PO q24h[5]	
Oxytetracycline	6.6-11 mg/kg, up to 10-20 mg/kg IM q24h[5,31]	
	20 mg/kg IM q48h[31]	
	44-55 mg/kg PO q24h[5]	
• Long acting (Liquamycin LA-200, Zoetis)	1.4-2.3 mg/kg q24h IM × maximum 4 days[d]	
	19.8 mg/kg IM once[d]	When retreatment is impractical[d]
Penicillin G, procaine	15,000-25,000 U/kg IM q24h[31]	
	20,000-45,000 U/kg IM q24h[13]	
Spectinomycin (Spectogard Scour-Chek, Bimeda)	6.6-22 mg/kg IM q12-24h[31]	
	11 mg/kg PO q12h × 3-5 days[32]	Bacterial enteritis
Tetracycline	10-20 mg/kg IM q24h[13]	Enteritis and pneumonia
	11 mg/kg q12h or 22 mg/kg q24h in water or as a bolus[31]	
Trimethoprim/sulfadiazine	15 mg/kg PO q12h[31,c]	
	30 mg/kg PO q24h[19]	
Trimethoprim/sulfamethoxazole	15 mg/kg PO q12h[31,c]	
	30 mg/kg PO q12-24h[31,c]	
Tulathromycin (Draxxin, Zoetis)	2.5 mg/kg IM as a single injection[31]	Draxxin 25 formulation available for small pigs
Tylosin (Tylan, Elanco)	8.8 mg/kg IM q12h[31]	Arthritis, erysipelas, swine dysentery
	9 mg/kg IM q12-24h[13]	

[a]Established withdrawal times are not specifically listed here but can be found in the source references, if available; the range for antimicrobials is a 3- to 42-day withdrawal period.

[b]Products labeled for administration to swine should be considered before extralabel use of alternative drugs. The American Medicinal Drug Use Clarification Act (AMDUCA) list of prohibited and restricted drugs in food animals can be found at www.farad.org.

[c]Authors' note: in the past, in the absence of published dosages specific to swine, the authors have often found it necessary to rely upon canine dosages published by Papich (2016) when treating pet pigs. This has generally been found to be safe and effective.

[d]From product insert.

TABLE 12-2 Antiparasitic Agents (External Parasites) Used in Miniature Pigs.[a,b]

Agent	Dosage	Comments
Coumaphos (Co-Ral spray, Bayer)	Mix according to label instructions and apply topically to the point of runoff; do not make applications less than 10 days apart[c]	Lice; repeat treatment necessary as there is no ovicidal activity – repeat when adults emerge in 12-20 days; mini pigs may prefer powder over liquid forms[28]
• Co-Ral 1% Livestock Dust, Bayer	Apply not more than 1 oz. (3 level Tbs) per pig as a uniform coat to the head, shoulders, and back by use of a shaker can; do not make applications less than 10 days apart[c]	
Doramectin (Dectomax, Zoetis)	0.3 mg/kg IM[17,31,c]	Mites, lice, larval flies; use same as ivermectin; may cause less discomfort than ivermectin when injected[28]
Fipronil (Frontline Spray, Merial)	Apply spray to affected areas (usually axilla, inguinal area, behind the ears, and perineum); reapply when/if needed, but no sooner than 30 days[4,28]	Ticks; extralabel in swine
Ivermectin	0.3 mg/kg PO, SC, IM[6,7,17,31]	Mites, lice; repeat in 10-14 days for a total of 2-3 doses for sarcoptic mange; PO dosing ineffective for treating sarcoptic mange; may cause pain on injection[4,28]
Permethrin (Swine-Guard, Y-Tex)	Apply topically per label directions (2.5 cc per 85-169 lbs; 5 cc per 170-254 lbs) across back of head and ears, down midline of neck, over shoulders[c]	Mites, lice, flies, mosquitoes; various products available, some concentrates require mixing, others are ready to use; follow label directions; mini pigs may prefer powder over liquid forms[28]
• Permectrin Fly and Louse Dust 2 lb Shaker Can, Bayer	Topically apply 1 oz per pig[c]	
Phosmet (Prolate/Lintox, Wellmark International)	Mix according to label directions and apply topically once; may be repeated in 14 days[c]	Mites, lice

[a]Established withdrawal times are not specifically listed here but can be found in the source references, if available; the range for antiparasitic agents is a zero- to 24-day withdrawal period.
[b]Products labeled for administration to swine should be considered before extralabel use of alternative drugs. The American Medicinal Drug Use Clarification Act (AMDUCA) list of prohibited and restricted drugs in food animals can be found at www.farad.org.
[c]From product insert.

TABLE 12-3 Antiparasitic Agents (Internal Parasites) Used in Miniature Pigs.[a,b]

Agent	Dosage	Comments
Doramectin (Dectomax, Zoetis)	0.3 mg/kg IM[17,31,d]	Use same as ivermectin; may cause less discomfort than ivermectin when injected[28]
Fenbendazole (Safe-Guard, Intervet)	3 mg/kg PO q24h × 3 days[20]	One of the few antiparastic agents effective against whipworms
	9 mg/kg PO in divided doses over 3-12 days[16,17,d]	
Ivermectin	0.3 mg/kg PO, SC, IM[6,17,31]	
• Ivomec Premix (Boehringer Ingelheim – Canada)	0.1 mg/kg PO in feed × 7 days[16,17,d]	
Levamisole	8 mg/kg PO in drinking water[17,31]	Unpalatable in feed so typically administered in water[16]
Piperazine	275-440 mg/kg PO in feed or drinking water once[16,17]	
	110 mg/kg PO in drinking water[31]	
Pyrantel	6.6 mg/kg PO, repeat prn[6,7]	
	22 mg/kg PO in feed, once[31]	Administer for 3 consecutive days to remove adult roundworms; administer continuously to address larval forms;[16] can give ½ of this dose initially if suspect high parasite burden; in 7-10 days, repeat with full dose[28]
Sulfadimethoxine (Albon, Zoetis)	55 mg/kg PO as loading dose followed by 27.5 mg/kg PO q12h[31,c]	Coccidia

[a]Established withdrawal times are not specifically listed here but can be found in the source references, if available; the range for antiparasitic agents is a zero- to 24-day withdrawal period.
[b]Products labeled for administration to swine should be considered before extra-label use of alternative drugs. The American Medicinal Drug Use Clarification Act (AMDUCA) list of prohibited and restricted drugs in food animals can be found at www.farad.org.
[c]Authors' note: in the past, in the absence of published dosages specific to swine, the authors have often found it necessary to rely upon canine dosages published by Papich (2016) when treating pet pigs. This has generally been found to be safe and effective.
[d]From product insert.

TABLE 12-4 Chemical Restraint/Anesthetic Agents Used in Miniature Pigs.[a-c]

Agent	Dosage	Comments
Acepromazine	—	See Tiletamine/zolazepam for combinations
	0.03-0.1 mg/kg IM[26]	
	0.1-0.45 mg/kg IM[5]	Tranquilization; slow onset of action; inconsistent results
	0.2-0.5 mg/kg IM[24]	Onset 20-30 min

TABLE 12-4 Chemical Restraint/Anesthetic Agents Used in Miniature Pigs. (cont'd)

Agent	Dosage	Comments
Acepromazine (A)/ ketamine (K)	(A) 0.5 mg/kg + (K) 15 mg/kg SC, IM[10]	Give acepromazine 10 min prior to ketamine
	(A) 0.5-1.1 mg/kg IM, followed in 15 min by (K) 15-33 mg/kg IM[7]	
	(A) 1.0 mg/kg + (K) 22-27 mg/kg SC, IM[24]	
	(A) 1.1 mg/kg + (K) 33 mg/kg SC, IM[37]	
Alfaxalone	5-6 mg/kg IM[26]	
	6 mg/kg IV[26]	
Alfaxalone(Al)/ dexmedetomidine (Dex)	(Al) 5 mg/kg + (Dex) 10 μg/kg IM[34]	Onset of action 3-4 min; sedation smooth
Atipamezole	For IM dose, see comments	Reverses detomidine and dexmedetomidine, and potentially other α_2-adrenergic agonists; actual volume is same as volume used for detomidine (1 mg/mL) or dexmedetomidine (0.5 mg/mL)
	IM or IV: 0.32 mg/kg for small animals (4 kg); 0.23 mg/kg for medium-sized animals (11 kg); up to 0.14 mg/kg for large-sized animals (45 kg)[31]	
Atropine	0.02-0.05 mg/kg SC, IM, IV[37]	Anesthesia adjunct; increases heart rate, decreases GI and respiratory secretions
Azaperone (Stresnil, Schering-Plough)	—	See etomidate and ketamine for combinations
	0.25-2 mg/kg IM[7,24,30]	Light sedation; no ataxia up to 0.5 mg/kg dose
	1-2 mg/kg IM[3]	Onset 5-15 min; duration of action 60-120 min
	2-8 mg/kg SC, IM[12,30,37]	
Azaperone (Az)/ketamine (K)/midazolam (Mi)	(Az) 2 mg/kg + (K) 15 mg/kg + (Mi) 0.3 mg/kg IM[26]	
Azaperone (Az)/midazolam (Mi)/± atropine (At)	(Az) 4 mg/kg + (Mi) 0.5 mg/kg ± (At) 0.04 mg/kg IM[5]	Moderate to deep sedation; no analgesia
Azaperone (Az)/midazolam (Mi)	(Az) 4 mg/kg + (Mi) 1 mg/kg IM[26]	
Azaperone (Az)/xylazine (X)	(Az) 2 mg + (X) 2 mg/kg IM[26]	
Butorphanol	—	See detomidine, dexmedetomidine, ketamine, medetomidine, tiletamine/ zolazepam, and xylazine for combinations; see Table 12-5 for analgesic doses

Continued

TABLE 12-4 Chemical Restraint/Anesthetic Agents Used in Miniature Pigs. (cont'd)

Agent	Dosage	Comments
Detomidine (Dormosedan, Zoetis) (De)/butorphanol (B)/midazolam (Mi)	(De) 0.06-0.125 mg/kg + (B) 0.3-0.4 mg/kg + (Mi) 0.3-0.4 IM[30]	Rapid, smooth induction with excellent relaxation
Dexmedetomidine (Dexdomitor, Zoetis) (Dex)	—	See ketamine for combinations
Dexmedetomidine (Dexdomitor, Zoetis) (Dex)/midazolam (Mi)/butorphanol (B)	(Dex) 0.01-0.04 mg/kg + (Mi) 0.1-0.3 mg/kg + (B) 0.2-0.4 mg/kg IM[4,27,28]	Can substitute xylazine (1 mg/kg) for dexmedetomidine
Diazepam	—	See ketamine for combinations
	0.1-0.5 mg/kg PO[24,30]	Calming for car trip or veterinary examination
	0.44-2.0 mg/kg/hr IV CRI[24]	CRI
	0.5-1.5 mg/kg IV[38]	Sedation; rarely used in conscious pigs since venous access is extremely difficult
	0.5-2 mg/kg IM[5]	Effective muscle relaxation
Etomidate (E)/azaperone (Az)	(E) 2-4 mg/kg + (Az) 2-4 mg/kg IM[26]	
Etomidate (E)/xylazine (X)	(E) 2-4 mg/kg + (X) 1-2 mg/kg IM, IV[26]	
Fentanyl	—	See propofol for combinations
	0.02-0.04 mg/kg SC, IM, IV q2h[31]	
Fluids–crystalloid	3-10 mL/kg/hr IV[42]	
	10-15 mL/kg/hr IV[2]	
Flumazenil	0.02 mg/kg IV[31]	Benzodiazepine (midazolam, diazepam) reversal; use with caution if ketamine is only other agent being used
	1 mg/10-15 mg midazolam IM[9]	
Glycopyrrolate	0.004-0.01 mg/kg SC, IM, IV[37]	Anesthesia adjunct; increases heart rate, decreases GI and respiratory secretions; use with caution as heart may be overtaxed; atropine preferred
Ketamine	Used alone, results in poor muscle relaxation, poor visceral analgesia, and rough recovery (hyperkinesia, severe and prolonged ataxia, distress vocalizations), especially IM; use with other agents	See acepromazine, medetomidine, tiletamine/zolazepam, and xylazine for combinations
	4-6 mg/kg IV[26]	
Ketamine (K)/azaperone (Az)	(K) 15 mg/kg + (Az) 2 mg/kg SC, IM[12,37]	

TABLE 12-4 Chemical Restraint/Anesthetic Agents Used in Miniature Pigs. (cont'd)

Agent	Dosage	Comments
Ketamine (K)/ dexmedetomidine (Dex)	(K) 10 mg/kg + (Dex) 10 μg/kg IM[34]	Onset of action 3-4 min
Ketamine (K)/diazepam (D)	(K) 10-15 mg/kg +(D) 0.5-2 mg/ kg IM[10]	Good muscle relaxation
	(K) 10-15 mg/kg + (D) 1-2 mg/ kg IM[3]	Onset 10 min; duration of action 20-40 min
	(D) 1-2 mg/kg IM, followed by (K) 12-20 mg/kg IM[6]	Short-term anesthesia; prolong with (K) 2-4 mg/kg IV prn; minimal analgesia; smoother recovery than ketamine alone
	(K) 15-20 mg/kg + (D) 2 mg/kg IM, SC[12,37]	
Ketamine (K)/ medetomidine (Me)	(K) 10 mg/kg + (Me) 0.08-0.1 mg/ kg IM[26]	
Ketamine (K)/ medetomidine (Me)/ butorphanol (B)	(K) 2-10 mg/kg + (Me) 80 μg/ kg + (B) 0.2 mg/kg IM[3]	Onset 1-5 min; duration of action 60-120 min
Ketamine (K)/midazolam (Mi)	(K) 10-15 mg/kg + (Mi) 0.1-0.5 mg/kg IM[3]	Onset 5-10 min; duration of action 20-40 min
Ketamine (K)/xylazine (X)	(K) 10 mg/kg + (X) 1 mg/kg IM[27]	
	(X) 2.2 mg/kg IM, followed by (K) 12-20 mg/kg IM[6]	Short-term anesthesia; prolong with (K) 2-4 mg/kg IV prn
	(K) 15-20 mg/kg + (X) 2 mg/kg SC, IM[5,12,37]	Anesthesia; rough recovery
Ketamine (K)/xylazine (X)/ butorphanol (B)	(K) 5 mg/kg + (X) 2 mg/kg + (B) 0.22 mg/kg IM[5]	Anesthesia; butorphanol enhances analgesia
Ketamine (K)/xylazine (X)/ midazolam (Mi)	(K) 5-10 mg/kg + (X) 1 mg/ kg + (Mi) 0.2 mg/kg IM[27]	Can substitute xylazine with dexmedetomidine (Dex) at 10-40 μg/kg
	(K) 20 mg/kg + (X) 2 mg/kg + (Mi) 0.25 mg/kg IM[3]	Onset 5-10 min; duration of action 70-100 min
Ketamine (K)/xylazine (X)/ oxymorphone (O)	(K) 2 mg/kg + (X) 2 mg/kg + (O) 0.075 mg/kg IV[37]	
Medetomidine	—	See ketamine, propofol, and tiletamine/zolazepam for combinations
	0.01 mg/kg IM[3]	
	0.02-0.04 mg/kg IV[24]	
	0.04-0.08 mg/kg IM[24]	
Midazolam	—	See azaperone, detomidine, dexmedetomidine, ketamine, and xylazine for combinations
	0.1-0.5 mg/kg IM, IV[12,37]	Sedation

Continued

TABLE 12-4 Chemical Restraint/Anesthetic Agents Used in Miniature Pigs. (cont'd)

Agent	Dosage	Comments
Midazolam (cont'd)	0.2 mg/kg IV[44]	
	0.2-0.4 mg/kg intranasal[24]	
	0.2-0.5 mg/kg IM[24]	
Naloxone	0.5-2 mg/kg IV[37]	Narcotic reversal; given to effect prn
Pentobarbital	20-40 mg/kg IV[12,37]	Anesthesia with some analgesia
Propofol	2-5 mg/kg IV[10,26]	Induction
	4-8 mg/kg/hr IV CRI[10]	CRI maintenance
Propofol (P)/fentanyl (F)	(P) 2 mg/kg + (F) 0.005 mg/kg IV[26]	
	(P) 11 mg/kg/hr CRI + (F) 2.5 mg/kg q30min IV[3]	Immediate onset of action
Propofol (P)/medetomidine (Me)	(P) 2-4 mg/kg + (Me) 0.02-0.04 mg/kg IV[26]	
Thiamylal	6-18 mg/kg IV[26]	
	6.6-30 mg/kg IV[12,37]	Induction
Thiopental	10-20 mg/kg IV[3]	
Tiletamine/zolazepam (Telazol, Fort Dodge)	Poor muscle relaxation; may cause rough recovery; avoid using as sole agent	Tiletamine/zolazepam combinations follow
Tiletamine/zolazepam (T)/ketamine (K)/acepromazine (A)	(T) 4.4 mg/kg + (K) 2.2 mg/kg + (A) 0.03 mg/kg IM[3]	Onset 2-4 min; duration of action 40-50 min
Tiletamine/zolazepam (T)/ketamine (K)/xylazine (X)	—	Reconstitute (T) (500 mg) with (K) 2.5 mL (100 mg/mL) and (X) 2.5 mL (100 mg/mL) instead of sterile water; mixture has 50 mg/mL each of tiletamine, zolazepam, ketamine, xylazine; rough recovery
	0.03 mL/kg IM[28]	Heavy sedation; useful prior to euthanasia
	(T) 4.4 mg/kg + (K) 2.2mg/kg + (X) 2.2 mg/kg IM[10]	Duration of action 45-90 min; apnea can occur; intubation possible
Tiletamine/zolazepam (T)/medetomidine (Me)	(T) 5 mg/kg + (Me) 0.05 mg/kg IV[26]	
Tiletamine/zolazepam (T)/xylazine (X)	(T) 3-6 mg/kg + (X) 0.5-2.2 mg/kg IM[10]	Apnea may occur; intubation possible; good analgesia
	(T) 4.4 mg/kg + (X) 4.4 mg/kg SC, IM[37]	
	(T) 4.4-6 mg/kg + (X) 1.1-4.4 mg/kg IM[9]	Anesthesia; rapid induction; poor muscle relaxation; may have rough recovery

TABLE 12-4 Chemical Restraint/Anesthetic Agents Used in Miniature Pigs. (cont'd)

Agent	Dosage	Comments
Tiletamine/zolazepam (T)/ xylazine (X)/butorphanol (B)	(T) 0.6 mg/kg + (X) 2-3 mg/kg + (B) 0.3-0.4 mg/kg IM[30]	
	(T) 4.4 mg/kg + (X) 2.2 mg/kg + (B) 0.22 mg/kg SC, IM[37]	
Xylazine	—	See also azaperone, etomidate, ketamine, and tiletamine/zolazepam for combinations
	0.5-3 mg/kg IM[6]	Sedation; tranquilization; some analgesia; deep sedation seldom encountered
Xylazine (X)/butorphanol (B)/midazolam (Mi)	(X) 2-3 mg/kg + (B) 0.3-0.4 mg/kg + (Mi) 0.3-0.4 mg/kg IM[30]	Antagonize xylazine with atipamezole or yohimbine and butorphanol with naltrexone; xylazine or midazolam can be administered as a premedicant or concurrently
Xylazine (X)/ketamine (K)	(X) 1-2 mg/kg + (K) 5-10 mg/kg IM[10]	
	(X) 1-2 mg/kg + (K) 10-12 mg/kg IM[26]	
	(X) 2 mg/kg + (K) 20 mg/kg IM[3]	Onset 7-10 min; duration of action 20-40 min
Yohimbine	0.11 mg/kg IV[31]	
	0.25-0.5 mg/kg SC, IM[31]	α_2-antagonist (xylazine, dexmedetomidine, detomidine reversal)

[a]Established withdrawal times are not specifically listed here but can be found in the source references, if available.
[b]Products labeled for administration to swine should be considered before extralabel use of alternative drugs. The American Medicinal Drug Use Clarification Act (AMDUCA) list of prohibited and restricted drugs in food animals can be found at www.farad.org.
[c]Authors' note: in the past, in the absence of published dosages specific to swine, the authors have often found it necessary to rely upon canine dosages published by Papich (2016) when treating pet pigs. This has generally been found to be safe and effective.

TABLE 12-5 Analgesic/Antiinflammatory Agents Used in Miniature Pigs.[a,b]

Agent	Dosage	Comments
Acetaminophen	15 mg/kg PO q8h[31,c]	
	325-500 mg/adult pig q8-12h[29]	
Acetylsalicylic acid (aspirin)	10 mg/kg PO[22]	
	10-20 mg/kg PO q6-8h[29,31,37]	Also antiinflammatory and antipyretic; use enteric coated tablets
Bupivicaine (multi-vesicular liposomal)	Infiltrate surgical site with 100-200 mg/site[31,c]	Local anesthetic
Buprenorphine	0.01-0.05 mg/kg SC, IM q8-12h[37]	
	0.01-0.1 mg/kg IM, IV q12h[22]	
	0.02-0.03 mg/kg SC q8-10h[22]	
	0.05-0.1 mg/kg IM q8-12h[12]	
	0.12 mg/kg IM q7-24h[22]	
Butorphanol	0.1-0.3 mg/kg SC, IM q4-6h[5,12,22]	
	0.1-0.3 mg/kg SC, IM q8-12h[37]	
	0.1-0.4 mg/kg IM, IV[22]	
	0.2-0.4 mg/kg SC, IM, IV q2-6h[29]	
Carprofen[d]	1-4 mg/kg SC q24h[5]	
	2 mg/kg SC q24h[37]	
	2.2 mg/kg SC q12h[29]	
	2-3 mg/kg PO, SC, IM q12h[12,22,37]	
	4 mg/kg PO q24h[22]	
	4.4 mg/kg SC q24h[29]	
Etodolac[d]	10-15 mg/kg PO q24h[29]	
Fentanyl	0.005-0.01 mg/kg SC, IM, IV q2h[31,c]	
	0.02-0.05 mg/kg IM q2h[12]	
	0.02-0.05 mg/kg IM, IV prn[29]	
	0.02-0.1 mg/kg/h IV CRI[29]	CRI
	0.05 mg/kg IM, IV q4h[22]	
	0.05 mg/kg IV loading dose for CRI 0.03-0.1 mg/kg/h[22]	CRI
Fentanyl, transdermal patch	12.5 or 25 µg/h/27-82 kg[29]	Intense or prolonged pain or when oral or injectable analgesics are not an option; apply 12 hr before surgery;[29] may last up to 72 hr
	50-100 µg/h q48-72h[22]	Higher doses may cause paradoxical excitement[4,28]

TABLE 12-5 Analgesic/Antiinflammatory Agents Used in Miniature Pigs. (cont'd)

Agent	Dosage	Comments
Flunixin meglumine (Banamine-S, Merck)[d]	1-2 mg/kg SC q24h[5]	
	1-4 mg/kg SC, IM, IV q12h[22]	
	1.1 mg/kg SC, IM, IV q12-24h[29]	
	2.2 mg/kg IM once[31]	
Gabapentin	5-15 mg/kg PO q12h, then increase gradually to as high as 40 mg/kg PO q8-12h prn[28,31,c]	
Hydromorphone	0.05 mg/kg IV[22]	
	0.1-0.2 mg/kg IV q2h[29]	
	0.2 mg/kg SC, IM q4-6h[29]	
Ibuprofen[d]	10 mg/kg PO q6-8h[29]	
Ketoprofen[d]	1 mg/kg PO q24h up to 5 days[29,31,c]	
	1-3 mg/kg PO, SC, IM q24h[37]	
	3 mg/kg PO, SC, IM, IV q24h[5,11,29,31]	
Meloxicam[d]	0.1-0.2 mg/kg PO q24h[22]	
	0.1-0.4 mg/kg PO q24h[29]	
	0.4 mg/kg PO, SC, IM q24h[11,29,37]	
Meperidine (Demerol, Pfizer)	0.4-1 mg/kg IV[22]	
	2 mg/kg IM, IV q2-4h[22]	
	2-10 mg/kg IM q4h[12]	
	10 mg/kg SC q8h[37]	
Methadone	0.1-0.2 mg/kg IV[22]	
Morphine	0.05-0.1 mg/kg IV q4-6h[22]	
	0.2-0.5 mg/kg IM q4h[27]	
	0.2 mg/kg SC, IM q4h[29]	
Oxymorphone	0.1-0.2 mg/kg SC, IM, IV, re-dose at 0.05-0.1 mg/kg q1-2h[29]	
	0.15 mg/kg IM q4h[12,22]	
	0.15 mg/kg SC, IM q8-12h[37]	
Phenylbutazone	4 mg/kg IV q24h[29,31]	Also antiinflammatory and antipyretic
	4-8 mg/kg PO q12h[29]	
	5-20 mg/kg PO q12h[37]	
	10-20 mg/kg PO q12h[12]	
Prednisone	0.5-1 mg/kg PO q12-24h initially, then taper to q48h[29]	Antiinflammatory

Continued

TABLE 12-5 Analgesic/Antiinflammatory Agents Used in Miniature Pigs. (cont'd)

Agent	Dosage	Comments
Sufentanil	0.005-0.01 IM, IV q4h[22]	
	0.007 mg/kg IV loading dose for CRI, then 0.015-0.03 mg/kg/h[22]	CRI
Tramadol	1-4 mg/kg PO q8h[22]	
	1.6 mg/kg IM q2-3h[22]	
	2-4 mg/kg PO q6-24h[29]	
	5 mg/kg IM[22]	

[a]Established withdrawal times are not specifically listed here but can be found in the source references, if available.
[b]Products labeled for administration to swine should be considered before extralabel use of alternative drugs. The American Medicinal Drug Use Clarification Act (AMDUCA) list of prohibited and restricted drugs in food animals can be found at www.farad.org.
[c]Authors' note: in the past, in the absence of published dosages specific to swine, the authors have often found it necessary to rely upon canine dosages published by Papich (2016) when treating pet pigs. This has generally been found to be safe and effective.
[d]Potential exists for gastrointestinal upset and gastric ulcers, although these are uncommon in the pet pig; should be given with food and gastrointestinal protectants.

TABLE 12-6 Emergency Agents Used in Miniature Pigs.[a-c]

Agent	Dosage	Comments
Activated charcoal	1 g/kg PO[14]	Absorbent for toxins
Atropine	0.02-0.05 mg/kg SC, IM, IV[26,37]	
	0.05 mg/kg IV[2]	Bradycardia
	0.4 mg/kg IM[3]	Bradycardia; anticholinergic
	2 mg in 5-10 mL saline intratracheal[26]	Bradycardia; 9-30 min to onset of action
Azumolene	2 mg/kg IV[26]	Malignant hyperthermia
Dantrolene	1-5 mg/kg IV[3]	Malignant hyperthermia
Dexamethasone	0.5-1.0 mg/kg IV[3]	Shock
	0.6 mg/kg IV[35]	Airway inflammation
• Sodium phosphate	0.3 mg/kg IM, IV[7,43]	
Diphenhydramine	0.5-1.0 mg/kg IM as single dose[31]	
Dopamine	2-20 µg/kg/min IV CRI[2]	Hypotension
	15 µg/kg/min IV CRI[26]	Hypotension
Doxapram	5-10 mg/kg IV[2]	Hypoventilation
Epinephrine	0.02 mg/kg IV[2]	
Fluids		
• Crystalloid fluids	90 mL/kg IV[42]	
• Dextrose	10 mL/kg of 10% solution IP[7]	
	20 mL/kg of 5% solution IP[7]	

TABLE 12-6 Emergency Agents Used in Miniature Pigs. (cont'd)

Agent	Dosage	Comments
Fluids (cont'd)		
• Dextrose in lactated Ringer's	0.4% IV CRI[18]	Prevention of hypoglycemia in juvenile pigs
• Hetastarch	1-2 mL/kg IV[26]	Hypovolemia; hypoproteinemia
• Hypertonic saline (7.2%)	4 mL/kg IV over 3-10 min[42]	
• Mannitol	0.25-1.0 g/kg (20% solution) IV over 1 hr[31]	Hyperosmotic diuretic; cerebral edema
• Saline (7.5%) in 6% dextran	1-2 mL/kg IV[26]	Hemorrhagic hypovolemia
Flumazenil	0.01 mg/kg IV[24]	Benzodiazepine (midazolam, diazepam) reversal; use with caution if ketamine is only other agent being used
	0.02 mg/kg IV[31]	
	1 mg/10-15 mg midazolam IM[9]	
Furosemide	2.5-5.0 mg/kg SC, IM, IV q8h[14]	Diuretic
Glycopyrrolate	0.004-0.01 mg/kg SC, IM, IV[26,37]	Bradycardia; anticholinergic
	0.02 mg/kg IM[3]	
Hydrogen peroxide	1 mL/5 kg PO[38]	Induces vomiting; some animals may require larger dose; often ineffective[28]
Ipecac (syrup)	7-15 mL/animal PO[38]	Induces vomiting; often ineffective[28]
Lidocaine	50 µg/kg/min IV CRI[2]	
	0.5-2.0 mg/kg IV[23]	Postresuscitative arrhythmias
	2-4 mg/kg IV[2]	
Naloxone	0.5-2 mg/kg IM, IV[24,37]	Opioid reversal
	4 mg IV total[24]	
Propanolol	0.04-0.06 mg/kg IV[2]	Tachycardia

[a]Established withdrawal times are not specifically listed here but can be found in the source references, if available.
[b]Products labeled for administration to swine should be considered before extralabel use of alternative drugs. The American Medicinal Drug Use Clarification Act (AMDUCA) list of prohibited and restricted drugs in food animals can be found at www.farad.org.
[c]Authors' note: in the past, in the absence of published dosages specific to swine, the authors have often found it necessary to rely upon canine dosages published by Papich (2016) when treating pet pigs. This has generally been found to be safe and effective.

TABLE 12-7 Miscellaneous Agents Used in Miniature Pigs.[a-c]

Agent	Dosage	Comments
Dinoprost (Lutalyse, Zoetis)	5 mg/animal IM[7]	Induces parturition in 24-30 hr when given within 3 days of expected parturition; causes abortion after 12 days of gestation
	8 mg dose initially followed by 5 mg dose 12 hr later (in a 25 kg pig)[20]	For inducing estrus; estrus should occur 3-7 days later
Famotidine	0.1-0.2 mg/kg PO, SC, IM, IV q12h[31,d]	Reduce gastric acid secretion

Continued

TABLE 12-7 Miscellaneous Agents Used in Miniature Pigs. (cont'd)

Agent	Dosage	Comments
Glucosamine (G)/ chondroitin sulfate (C)	(G) 4 mg/kg + (C) 1.3 mg/kg PO q12h[29]	Maintenance dose
	(G) 12 mg/kg + (C) 3.8 mg/kg PO q12h × 4 wk[29]	Loading dose
	(G) 44 mg/kg/day PO[31,d]	For animals that do not respond; can also load with higher dose of glucosamine
Iron dextran	25 mg/animal IM in first few days of life; may repeat in 2-3 wk[33]	Iron deficiency in baby pigs; uncommon in miniature pigs so rarely used as a part of routine management practices but may be useful for treatment of anemia
Kaolin/pectin	1-2 mL/kg PO q2-6h[31,d]	Antidiarrheal
Maropitant citrate (Cerenia, Zoetis)	1 mg/kg SC, or 2 mg/kg PO q24h[31,d]	Antiemetic
	8 mg/kg PO q24h[28,31,d]	To prevent motion sickness[31]; often effective at lower, antiemetic dose[28]
Methocarbamol	44 mg/kg PO q8h on day one, then 22-44 mg/kg PO q8h[31,d]	Muscle relaxant for treatment of pain associated with spasm or myopathy (i.e., intervertebral disc disease)
Metoclopramide	0.2-0.5 mg/kg q6-8h PO, IM, IV[28,31,d]	Prevent postoperative ileus; start with the lower end of the dose to prevent cramping
Omeprazole	20 mg/animal PO q24h or 1-2 mg/kg PO q24h[31,d]	Treat and prevent GI ulcers in sick, stressed, or hospitalized pigs
Oxytocin	5-10 U/animal IM[20,31]	Dystocia if not obstructed
	10-20 U/animal IM[7]	
Pantoprazole	0.5-0.6 mg/kg PO q24h[31,d]	Treat and prevent GI ulcers in sick, stressed, or hospitalized pigs
Pentobarbital	100-150 mg/kg IV[5]	Euthanasia
	>150 mg/kg IV[12,37]	
	1 mL/4.5 kg (1 mL/10 lb) IV[28,31,d]	
Polysulfated glycosaminoglycan (Adequan, Novartis)	4.4 mg/kg IM q7d × 4 treatments, then q14d × 8 treatments, then q30d prn[4]	Antiarthritic agent; may not see results until after 3-4 treatments
	4.4 mg/kg IM, twice weekly, for up to 4 wk[31,d]	
Sucralfate	0.5-1 g PO q8-12h[31,d]	Prevents/treats ulcers; crush tablets and mix as suspension
Terbinafine	30-40 mg/kg q24h PO (with food) for 2-3 wk[31,d]	Treatment of dermatophyte infection

[a]Also see Table 12-6 (Emergency Agents Used in Miniature Pigs).
[b]Established withdrawal times are not specifically listed here but can be found in the source references, if available.
[c]Products labeled for administration to swine should be considered before extralabel use of alternative drugs. The American Medicinal Drug Use Clarification Act (AMDUCA) list of prohibited and restricted drugs in food animals can be found at www.farad.org.
[d]Authors' note: in the past, in the absence of published dosages specific to swine, the authors have often found it necessary to rely upon canine dosages published by Papich (2016) when treating pet pigs. This has generally been found to be safe and effective.

TABLE 12-8 Hematologic and Serum Biochemical Values of Miniature Pigs.

Measurement	Mean (Reference Range)[8,a]	Mean (Reference Range)[5,b]	Mean (Reference Range)[15,c]
Hematology			
PCV (%)	36 (22-50)	—	—
Hematocrit (%)	—	32-61	35-56
RBC (10^6/μL)	5.7 (3.6-7.8)	5.30-9.25	5.6-9.3
Hgb (g/dL)	12 (7.8-16.2)	9-17	10.9-17.0
MCV (fL)	63 (55-71)	40-73	46.0-72.5
MCH (pg)	21 (18-24)	15.2-26.4	13.7-24.3
MCHC (g/dL)	33.5 (31-36)	29.4-37.9	29.6-34.5
Platelets (10^3/μL)	310 (204-518)	148-898	152-845
WBC (10^3/μL)	11.5 (5.2-17.9)	4.4-26.4	6.9-32.4
Neutrophils (10^3/μL)	5.7 (0-11.4)	—	1.8-6.4
Band cells (10^3/μL)	0.03 (0-0.19)	—	0.0-24.6
Lymphocytes (10^3/μL)	5.3 (0.8-9.8)	—	2.1-17.3
Monocytes (10^3/μL)	0.2 (0-0.67)	—	0.2-1.3
Eosinophils (10^3/μL)	0.14 (0-0.73)	—	0-1.5
Basophils (10^3/μL)	0.15 (0-0.61)	—	0-0.5
Fibrinogen (g/L)	2 (1-4)	—	—
Chemistries			
ALP (U/L)	65 (27-160)	—	166-576
ALT (U/L)	53 (11-95)	20-106	—
AST (U/L)	32 (16-64)	13-53	15-90
Bilirubin, total (mg/dL)	0.25 (0.2-0.45)	0.0-0.3	0.1-0.41
BUN (mg/dL)	9.7 (4.2-15.1)	—	5.7-29
Calcium (mg/dL)	—	8.6-12.6	9.3-11.7
Chloride (mmol/L)	110 (106-113)	94-140	95-114
Creatine kinase (U/L)	701 (213-2852)	37-6000	—
Creatinine (mg/dL)	1.7 (1-2.3)	0.5-2.0	0.5-1.1
GGT (U/L)	35 (15-56)	25-86	20.4-96.4
Glucose (mg/dL)	105 (60-175)	43-153	56-123
Phosphorus (mg/dL)	—	4.9-9.8	5.0-10.7
Potassium (mmol/L)	4.3 (3.7-5)	3.5-7.4	3.9-7.7
Protein, total (g/dL)	7.7 (6.6-8.9)	6.0-9.4	4.9-9.4
Albumin (g/dL)	4.3 (3.6-5)	2.9-5.6	2.9-5.6
Globulin (g/dL)	—	1.4-5.2	1.4-3.7
Sodium (mmol/L)	144 (139-149)	132-153	139-153
TCO_2 (mEq/L)	24 (8-31)	—	20-29

[a]n = 100, 2- to 10-year-old healthy Vietnamese potbellied pigs.
[b]Combined ranges for adult Yucatan micro pigs, Gottingen, Sinclair, Yucatan, and Hanford mini pigs weighing 35-70 kg and 70-90 kg.
[c]Combined ranges for male and female Hanford, Yucatan micro pigs, and male and female Gottingen mini pigs.

TABLE 12-9 Urinalysis Reference Values for Miniature Pigs.[1,20,28,41]

Parameter	Reference Value
Specific gravity	1.010-1.050
pH	6.9 (range 5-8)
Color	Yellow-dark amber; may be slightly cloudy
Protein	Negative to trace
Red blood cells (per HPF)	0-5
White blood cells (per HPF)	0-5
Crystals	Common, occasionally pathologic;[28] calcium oxalate or triple phosphate crystals
Bacteria	Numerous in voided samples; only significant if numerous WBCs also present

TABLE 12-10 Biologic and Physiologic Data of Miniature Pigs.[5,6,15,20,25,29]

Parameter	Value
Life expectancy	14-21 yr (avg 15-18)
Respiratory rate (breaths/min)	
Newborn	50-60
Weaned pigs	25-40
10-15 wk	30-40
15-26 wk	25-35
Adult	12-18
Heart rate (beats/min)	
Newborn	200-250
Weaned pigs	90-100
10-15 wk	80-90
15-26 wk	75-85
Adult	70-80
Rectal temperature	37.6-39°C (99.7-102.2°F); diurnal variation in body temperature exists; temperature decreases as age increases
Weight	
Birth	250-450 g
Adult	34-91 kg (avg 55)
Reproduction	
Puberty	
• Boars	3 mo of age
• Gilts	3.5-4 mo of age
Estrous cycle	17-25 days (avg 21)
Standing heat duration	1-3 days
Ovulation	
• Gilts	24-36 hr after onset of estrus
• Sows	30-44 hr after onset of estrus
Gestation length	112-116 days (avg 114)
Litter size	2-15 piglets (avg 6-8)

TABLE 12-11 Preventive Medicine Recommendations for Miniature Pigs.[6,15,20,28,40]

Recommended Vaccinations	
All pigs	
• Erysipelas	8-12 wk of age; repeat in 3-4 wk; revaccinate pets semiannually or annually and 3 wk before breeding
• Leptospirosis	8-12 wk of age; repeat in 3-4 wk; revaccinate pets semiannually or annually and 3 wk before breeding; substantial risk of high fever after use[20]
• Rabies	Off-label use but recommended if at risk of exposure; 14-16 wk of age; revaccinate annually
Vaccines listed below are options to consider if and when environment, likelihood of exposure, herd management practices, and diseases historically identified dictate. However, miniature pigs infrequently suffer from most of the diseases important in commercial swine.	
Breeder pigs	
• Parvovirus	5-6 mo of age; repeat in 3-4 wk; revaccinate 3-8 wk before breeding; boars should be revaccinated semiannually
At-risk pigs	
• Colibacillosis (baby pig scours) (*E. coli*)	Sows: 5 and 2 wk before first farrowing, and 2 wk before each subsequent farrowing
• Other enteritides (rotavirus, TGE virus, *Clostridium, Salmonella*)	Sows: 5 and 2 wk before farrowing
• Atrophic rhinitis (*Bordetella bronchiseptica, Pasteurella multocida* [types A and D])	Sows: 7 and 3 wk before first farrowing, and 3 wk before each subsequent farrowing
	Piglets: 1 wk of age; repeat in 3 wk
	Boars: semiannually or annually
• Pneumonia (*Actinobacillus pleuropneumoniae*)	Sows: 5 and 2 wk before farrowing
	Piglets: 3-8 wk of age; repeat in 3 wk
• Pneumonia (*Mycoplasma hyopneumoniae*)	Sows: 5 and 2 wk before first farrowing, and 2 wk before each subsequent farrowing
	Piglets: 1 wk of age; repeat in 2-3 wk
	Boars: semiannually or annually
• Tetanus toxoid	Vaccinate after surgery or trauma or annually when exposure is likely; pigs are a relatively tetanus-resistant species and disease is rare
Other Procedures	
Tetanus antitoxin	Administer 500-1500 U (depending on body weight) after surgery, dental procedure, or trauma; if not current on tetanus vaccine and where exposure is likely
Castration	2-3 mo of age and older
Ovariohysterectomy or ovariectomy	3-4 mo of age and older, but may be performed as early as 6 wk of age

Continued

TABLE 12-11 Preventive Medicine Recommendations for Miniature Pigs. (cont'd)

Other Procedures (cont'd)	
Tusk (canine) removal	Not recommended
Tusk (canine) trimming	As needed
Hoof trimming	Every 3-6 mo
Fecal examination	Yearly for pets; twice yearly minimum for breeding herd or sanctuary

TABLE 12-12 Blood Collection Sites in Miniature Pigs.[28,30,36,38,41]

Venipuncture Site	Comments
Cranial vena cava/right brachiocephalic vein	Anesthesia required for safety
Right external jugular vein	Short, fat neck of most pet pigs makes this challenging; best if pig is anesthetized; advance a ≥1.5-inch needle cranially in the jugular furrow, angled slightly medially while applying slight negative pressure
Cephalic vein	Thick skin makes this difficult; cutdown may be required; reasonable choice for catheterization for fluid or medication administration if pig is sedated or moribund
Radial vein	Can be easily sampled in a properly restrained, awake patient; vein runs along medial aspect of front leg and landmarks are readily palpable
Lateral auricular vein	Easiest in debilitated or very cooperative pigs; good for obtaining very small blood samples; recommended for most routine catheterization
Subcutaneous abdominal vein	Easy to visualize and access in most large, cooperative pigs
Coccygeal (tail) vein	Performed as in the bovine

TABLE 12-13 Recommendations for Feeding Miniature Pigs.[4,28,39]

- Miniature pet pigs should be offered feeds made specifically for the miniature pig (i.e., Mazuri Mini Pig Feed) but also do well on livestock or equine feeds; commercial swine feed should be avoided as it can lead to excessive weight gain.
- A rate of 1%-2% of the pig's body weight daily, depending upon life stage, is usually appropriate, *or*
  - Piglet: ½ cup per 15-20 lb per day;
  - Adult: 1 cup per 50-80 lb per day.
- The pig's current body condition should be the most important consideration when determining how much to feed.
- Divide daily ration into 2-3 meals daily when possible; ideally, broadcast food on a grassy area, or place in food-dispensing toys or in rooting boxes.

REFERENCES

1. Almond GW, Stevens JB. Urinalysis techniques for swine practitioners. *Compend Contin Educ Vet.* 1995;17:121-129.
2. Alstrup AKO. Anaesthesia and analgesia. In: *Ellegaard aard Göttingen Minipigs.* Arhus, Denmark: PET Centre, Aarhus University Hospital; 2010:42-43.
3. Anderson DE, Mulon PY. Anesthesia and surgical procedures in swine. In: Zimmerman JJ, Karriker LA et al., eds. *Diseases of Swine.* 11th ed. Hoboken, NJ: Wiley Blackwell; 2019:171-196.
4. Asseo L. *Personal observation*; 2021.
5. Bollen PJA, Hansen AK, Alstrup AKO. *The Laboratory Swine.* 2nd ed. Boca Raton, FL: CRC Press; 2010:11-13, 45-71.
6. Braun WF, Jr. Potbellied pigs: general medical care. In: Bonagura JD, ed. *Kirk's Current Veterinary Therapy XII—Small Animal Practice.* Philadelphia, PA: WB Saunders; 1995:1388-1392.
7. Braun Jr WF, Casteel SW. Potbellied pigs – miniature porcine pets. *Vet Clin N Am: Small Anim Pract.* 1993;23:1149-1177.
8. Brockus CW, Mahaffey EA, Bush S, et al. Hematologic and serum biochemical reference intervals for Vietnamese potbellied pigs (*Sus scrofa*). *Comp Clin Path.* 2005;13:162-165.
9. Calle PP, Morris PJ. Anesthesia for nondomestic suids. In: Fowler ME, Miller RE, eds. *Zoo and Wild Animal Medicine: Current Therapy 4.* Philadelphia, PA: WB Saunders; 1999:639-646.
10. Carr J, Chen S-P, Connor JF, et al. Clinical examination. In: *Pig Health.* Boca Raton, FL: CRC Press; 2018:1-52.
11. Carr J, Chen S-P, Conner JF, et al. Pig health maintenance. In: *Pig Health.* Boca Raton, FL: CRC Press; 2018:383-468.
12. Flecknell P, Lofgren JLS, Dyson MC, et al. Preanesthesia, anesthesia, analgesia, and euthanasia. In: Fox JG, Anderson LC, Otto G, et al., eds. *Laboratory Animal Medicine.* 3rd ed. St. Louis, MO: Elsevier; 2015:1162-1168.
13. Friendship RM. Antimicrobial drug use in swine. In: Giguère S, Prescott JF, Baggot JD, et al., eds. *Antimicrobial Therapy in Veterinary Medicine.* 4th ed. Ames, IA: Blackwell Publishing; 2006:535-543.
14. George L. *Veterinary Management of Miniature Pigs.* Davis, CA: School of Veterinary Medicine University of California, Davis; 1993:44-46.
15. Helke KL, Ezell PC, Duran-Struuck R, et al. Biology and diseases of swine. In: Fox JG, Anderson LC, Otto G, et al., eds. *Laboratory Animal Medicine.* 3rd ed. St. Louis, MO: Elsevier; 2015:695-769.
16. Jacela JY, DeRouchey JM, Tokach MD, et al. Feed additives for swine: fact sheets – carcass modifiers, carbohydrate-degrading enzymes and proteases, and anthelmintics. *J Swine Health Prod.* 2009;17(6):325-332.
17. Karriker LA, Coetzee JF, Friendship RM, et al. Drug pharmacology, therapy, and prophylaxis. In: Zimmerman JJ, Karriker LA, Ramirez A, et al., eds. *Diseases of Swine.* 11th ed. Hoboken, NJ: John Wiley and Sons; 2019:168.
18. Keibl C, Kerbl M, Schlimp CJ. Comparison of Ringer's solution with 0.4% glucose or without in intraoperative infusion regimens for the prevention of hypoglycemia in juvenile pigs. *Lab Anim.* 2014;48(2):170-176.
19. Langston VC. Antimicrobial use in food animals (Table 5). In: Howard JL, Smith RA, eds. *Current Veterinary Therapy 4—Food Animal Practice.* Philadelphia, PA: WB Saunders; 1999:26.
20. Lawhorn B. Potbellied pigs. In: Aiello SE, ed. *The Merck Veterinary Manual.* 11th ed. Kenilworth, NJ: Merck and Co; 2016:1929-1937.
21. Lawhorn B. *Personal communication*; 2010.
22. Lin HC. Pain management for farm animals. In: Lin HC, Walz P, eds. *Farm Animal Anesthesia.* Ames, IA: Wiley Blackwell; 2014:174-214.
23. Lin HC. Perioperative monitoring and management of complications. In: Lin HC, Walz P, eds. *Farm Animal Anesthesia.* Ames, IA: Wiley Blackwell; 2014:110-135.

24. Lin HC. Standing sedation and chemical restraint. In: Lin HC, Walz P, eds. *Farm Animal Anesthesia*. Ames, IA: Wiley Blackwell; 2014:39-59.
25. Lord LK, Wittum TE, Anderson DE, et al. Resting rectal temperature of Vietnamese potbellied pigs. *J Am Vet Med Assoc*. 1999;215:342-344.
26. Malavasi LM. Swine. In: Grimm KA, Lamont LA, Tranquilli WJ, et al., eds. *Veterinary Anesthesia and Analgesia: The Fifth Edition of Lumb and Jones*. Ames, IA: Wiley Blackwell; 2015:928-940.
27. Messenger K. *Personal communication*; 2015.
28. Mozzachio K. *Personal observation*; 2021.
29. Mozzachio K, Tynes VV. Recognition and treatment of pain in pet pigs. In: Eggers CM, Love L, Doherty T, eds. *Pain Management in Veterinary Practice*. Ames, IA: Wiley Blackwell; 2014:383-389.
30. Padilla LR, Ko JC. Nondomestic suids. In: West G, Heard D, Caulkett N, eds. *Zoo Animal and Wildlife Immobilization and Anesthesia*. 2nd ed. Ames, IA: Wiley Blackwell; 2014:773-785.
31. Papich MG. *Saunders Handbook of Veterinary Drugs*. 4th ed. St. Louis, MO: Elsevier; 2016.
32. Plumb DC. *Plumb's Veterinary Drug Handbook*. 9th ed. Stockholm, WI: PharmaVet, Inc.; 2018.
33. Reeves DE. Neonatal care of miniature pet pigs. In: Reeves DE, ed. *Care and Management of Miniature Pet Pigs*. Santa Barbara, CA: Veterinary Practice Publishing Co; 1993:41-45.
34. Santos M, Bertran de Lis BT, Tendillo FJ. Effects of intramuscular dexmedetomidine in combination with ketamine or alfaxalone in swine. *Vet Anaesth Analg*. 2016;43(1):81-85.
35. Shao JI, Lin CH, Yang YH, et al. Effects of intravenous phosphodiesterase inhibitors and corticosteroids on severe meconium aspiration syndrome. *J Chin Med Assoc*. 2019;82(7):568-575.
36. Snook CS. Use of the subcutaneous abdominal vein for blood sampling and intravenous catheterization in potbellied pigs. *J Am Vet Med Assoc*. 2001;219:809-810.
37. Swindle MM, Sistino JJ. Anesthesia, analgesia, and perioperative care. In: Swindle MM, Smith AC, eds. *Swine in the Laboratory*. 3rd ed. Boca Raton, FL: CRC Press; 2016:39-87.
38. Tynes VV. Emergency care for potbellied pigs. *Vet Clin North Am Exot Anim Pract*. 1998;1:177-189.
39. Tynes VV. Potbellied pig husbandry and nutrition. *Vet Clin North Am Exot Anim Pract*. 1999;2:193-207.
40. Tynes VV. Vaccinating the pet potbellied pig. *Exot DVM*. 2000;2.1:11-13.
41. Van Metre DC, Angelos SM. Miniature pigs. *Vet Clin North Am Exot Anim Pract*. 1999;2:519-537.
42. Walz P. Fluid therapy. In: Lin HC, Walz P, eds. *Farm Animal Anesthesia*. Ames, IA: Wiley Blackwell; 2014:215-227.
43. Wyns H, Meyer E, Watteyn A et al. Pharmacokinetics of dexamethasone after intravenous and intramuscular administration in pigs. *Vet J*. 2013;198(1):286-288.
44. Zacharioudaki A, Lelovas P, Sergentanis TN, et al. Induction of anaesthesia with remifentanil after bolus midazolam administration in Landrace/large white swine. *Vet Anaesth Analg*. 2017;44(6):1353-1362.

Chapter 13 Primates

Terri Parrott | James W. Carpenter

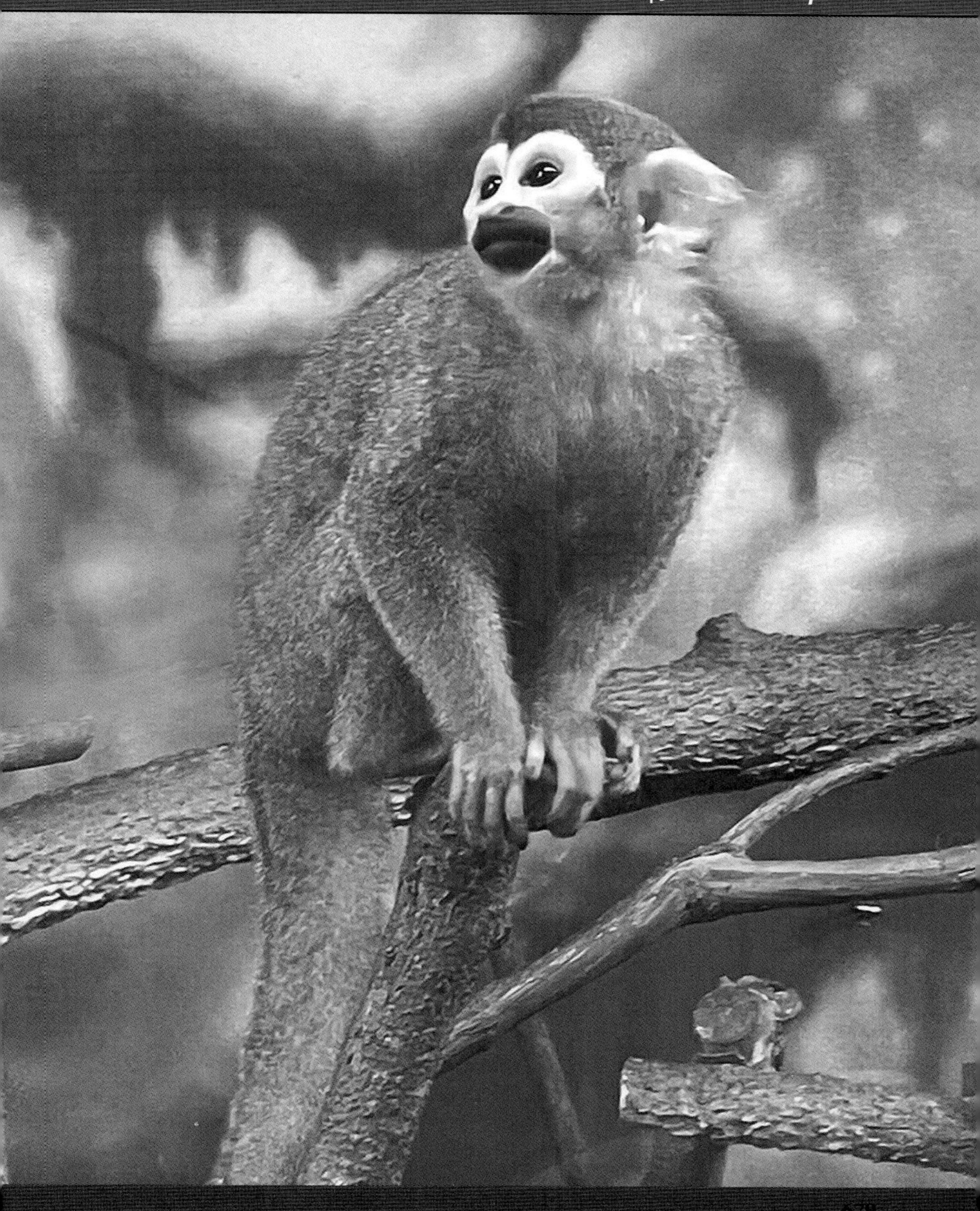

TABLE 13-1 Antimicrobial Agents Used in Primates.

Agent	Dosage	Species/Comments
Amikacin	—	Amikacin use as first-line therapy is limited due to poor oral absorption and short half-life and serious renal and vestibular toxicities
	2.3 mg/kg IM q24h[6]	Chimpanzees
	5 mg/kg IM q8h[6]	Monkeys
	15 mg/kg inhalation q24h × 7 days[69,110]	Monkeys/mycobacteriosis, gram-negative pneumonia (extrapolation human studies)
Amoxicillin	6.7-13.3 mg/kg PO, IM q8h[6]	Monkeys
	10 mg/kg PO q12h[130]	Macaques/combination treatment for *Helicobacter pylori* with clarithromycin
	10-15 mg/kg PO q12h[11]	Brown lemurs
	10-20 mg/kg PO q12h[143]	Prosimians
	11 mg/kg PO, IM q12h[109]	Monkeys, lemurs
	62.5 mg/animal PO q12h[109]	Lemurs
	500 mg/animal PO, IM, IV q8h[6]	Chimpanzees
Amoxicillin trihydrate/clavulanic potassium	6.7-13.3 mg/kg PO q8h[6]	Monkeys
	13.75 mg/kg PO q12h[6]	Chimpanzees
	15 mg/kg PO q12h[56]	
Ampicillin	10-30 mg/kg SC, IM, IV q6-8h[11,143]	Prosimians, brown lemurs
	20 mg/kg PO, IM, IV q8h[6]	Chimpanzees
	25-50 mg/kg/day IM, IV divided q6-8h[6]	Monkeys
	150-200 mg/kg/day IM, IV divided q3-4h[6]	Monkeys/meningitis, septicemia
Ampicillin/sulbactam	50 mg/kg IV (over 30 min) q12h[85,110]	Macaques/susceptible gram-negative infections such as *Klebsiella* and some MRSA infections
Azithromycin	—	In humans, associated with increased cardiac arrhythmogenicity;[117] use with caution in older great apes
	5-10 mg/kg PO q24h[6,11,143]	Chimpanzees, prosimians
	25 mg/kg PO q24h × 7 days, or 40 mg/kg PO q24h × 7 days, or 70 mg/kg PO q24h × 4 days[116]	Macaques/antimalarial
	30-50 mg/kg IM q12h × 7-14 days[65]	Drug of choice for *Campylobacter*-associated diarrhea
	40 mg/kg PO q24h once then 20 mg/kg × 5 days[109]	Monkeys

TABLE 13-1 Antimicrobial Agents Used in Primates. (cont'd)

Agent	Dosage	Species/Comments
Cefazolin sodium	8-16 mg/kg IM q8h[11]	Brown lemurs
	10-30 mg/kg IM, IV q8h[143]	Prosimians
	20 mg/kg IM, IV q8h[6]	Monkeys
	25 mg/kg IM, IV q12h[6,109] × 7-10 days	Chimpanzees, rhesus macaques, monkeys
Cefotaxime	50 mg/kg IM, IV q8h[56]	Third-generation cephalosporin
Cefovecin (Convenia, Pfizer)	—	Half-life of this drug in squirrel monkeys, cynomologus macaques, and rhesus macaques is much shorter than in dogs and cats and is not suitable for use as a long-acting antibiotic[13,107]
	10 mg/kg IM q≥5d[18]	Ring-tailed lemur
Ceftazidime	50 mg/kg IM, IV q8h[6]	Monkeys
	1 g IM, IV q6-12h[6]	Chimpanzees
Ceftiofur sodium (Naxcel, Zoetis)	1.1-2.2 mg/kg IM q24h[11,143]	Prosimians, brown lemurs
	2 mg/kg IM q24h[6]	Chimpanzees
Ceftiofur CFA (Excede, Zoetis)	5 mg/kg SC once[125]	Rhesus macaques/PK; with plasma concentrations >0.2 µg/mL × ≥2 days
	6 mg/kg SC once[53]	Ring-tailed lemur (n=1)/postsurgical
	20 mg/kg SC once[81,125]	Lion-tailed macaques[81]/*Streptococcus* toxic shock
		Rhesus macaques[125]/PK; with plasma concentrations >0.2 µg/mL × ≥7 days
Ceftriaxone	25-100 mg/kg IM, IV q12h[109,110]	Monkeys, siamangs
	50-100 mg/kg IM q12-24h[6]	Chimpanzees
Cephalexin	20 mg/kg PO q12h[11]	Brown lemurs
	30 mg/kg PO q12h[6]	Monkeys
	1-4 g q8-12h PO[6]	Chimpanzees
Chloramphenicol palmitate	—	Classified as a hazardous drug by the National Institute for Occupational Safety & Health (NIOSH); PPE should be used accordingly
	25 mg/kg PO q8h[6]	Monkeys (infants)/use with extreme caution
Chloramphenicol sodium succinate	20 mg/kg IM q12h[6]	Chimpanzees
	33.3 mg/kg IM q8h[6]	Monkeys
	50 mg/kg SC q8h[6]	Chimpanzees
Ciprofloxacin	10 mg/kg PO q12h[6]	Monkeys
	10-20 mg/kg PO q12h[56]	Marmosets
	16-20 mg/kg PO q12h[6]	Chimpanzees

Continued

TABLE 13-1 Antimicrobial Agents Used in Primates. (cont'd)

Agent	Dosage	Species/Comments
Clarithromycin	10 mg/kg PO q12h × 10 days[130]	Macaques/combined treatment of *Helicobacter pylori;* see amoxicillin
	20 mg/kg PO q24h[12]	Macaques/PK
	250-500 mg/animal PO q12h × 7-14 days[6]	Chimpanzees
Clindamycin	10 mg/kg PO q24h[56]	Lincosamide antibiotic
	12.5 mg/kg IM q8h[6]	Monkeys
	150-300 mg/animal PO q6h[6]	Chimpanzees
	300-600 mg/animal IM q8-12h[6]	Chimpanzees
Doxycycline	2-5 mg/kg PO q12h[6]	Chimpanzees
	2.5 mg/kg PO q12h × 1 day, then 2.5 mg/kg PO q24h[6]	Monkeys
	3-4 mg/kg PO q12h[56]	
	5-10 mg/kg PO q12h[143]	Prosimians
Enrofloxacin	5 mg/kg IM q24h[109]	Monkeys; SC and IM injections may cause muscle necrosis or sterile abscesses; dilute before giving parenterally; PO is generally preferred
	5 mg/kg PO, SC q12h × 10 days[56,109]	
	5 mg/kg PO, IM q12-24h[6]	Chimpanzees, monkeys; see comments above
Erythromycin	15-20 mg/kg/day IM q12h[6]	Monkeys
	30-50 mg/kg IM q12h[109]	Monkeys
	35 mg/kg PO q8h[6]	Monkeys
Ethambutol	15 mg/kg, then 25 mg/kg PO q24h[6]	Chimpanzees/antituberculosis drug
Florfenicol	50 mg/kg IM q48h[34]	Macaques
Flurofamide	25 mg/animal PO q12h × 3 doses[65]	Common marmosets/*Ureaplasma*; bacterial urease inhibitor
Furazolidone	10 mg/kg PO q12h[3]	Monkeys
	100 mg/animal PO q6h[6]	Chimpanzees
Gentamicin	2-4 mg/kg IM, IV q12h[6]	Monkeys, chimpanzees
	3 mg/kg IM q6-8h[141]	Baboons/PK
	3-5 mg/kg SC, IM q24h[109]	Monkeys
Isoniazid	5 mg/kg PO q24h[6]	Monkeys
	30-50 mg/kg PO q24h × 9 mo[6]	Chimpanzees/active tuberculosis
	300 mg PO q24h[6]	Chimpanzee/prophylaxis; treat concurrently with rifampin
Levofloxacin	—	In humans, associated with increased cardiac arrhythmogenicity;[117] use with caution in older great apes
	500 mg PO q24h[6]	Chimpanzees

TABLE 13-1 Antimicrobial Agents Used in Primates. (cont'd)

Agent	Dosage	Species/Comments
Lincomycin	5-10 mg/kg IM q12h[56]	Monkeys
Marbofloxacin	2-5 mg/kg PO q24h[59]	Marmosets
Metronidazole	—	Treatment of anaerobic infections
	15 mg/kg IV loading dose, then 7.5 mg/kg q8h (do not exceed 4 g/day)[110,112]	Monkeys, tamarins/anaerobic infections (e.g., skin, CNS, bone and joint, endocarditis, bacteremia)
	25 mg/kg PO q24h[143]	Prosimians
	25 mg/kg PO q12h[6]	Chimpanzees
	50 mg/kg PO q12h[6]	Monkeys
Minocycline	4 mg/kg PO[6]	Monkeys
	200 mg, then 100 mg, IV (slow)[6]	Chimpanzees
	200 mg PO q12h[6]	Chimpanzees
Neomycin	50 mg/kg PO q12h[6]	Monkeys
Ofloxacin	200-400 mg/animal PO, IV constant rate infusion[6]	Chimpanzees
Oxacillin	16.7 mg/kg IM q8h[6]	Monkeys
Oxytetracycline	10 mg/kg SC, IM q24h[6]	Monkeys
	25-50 mg/kg PO[6]	Monkeys
	250-300 mg/day PO, IM divided q8-24h[6]	Chimpanzees
Penicillin G, benzathine	20,000-60,000 U/kg IM q12-24h[6]	Monkeys
Penicillin G, procaine	20,000-40,000 U/kg SC, IM q12h[6]	Monkeys
	22,000 U/kg IM q24h[6]	Chimpanzees
Penicillin VK (penicillin V potassium)	11 mg/kg PO q6h[6]	Chimpanzees
Rifampin	22.5 mg/kg PO q24h × 6 wk, then 15 mg/kg PO q24h × 1 yr[56]	Wide spectrum of antimicrobial activity, including *Mycobacterium tuberculosis*
	600 mg PO, IV q24h[6]	Chimpanzees/tuberculosis; treat concurrently with or without isoniazid
Streptomycin	1-2 g/day PO divided q6-24h[6]	Chimpanzees
	2.5-5 mg/kg IM q12h[6]	Monkeys
Sulfadimethoxine	50 mg/kg first day, then 25 mg/kg IM q24h[6]	Monkeys
Tetracycline	20 mg/kg PO q8h[6]	Monkeys
	20-25 mg/kg PO q8-12h[6]	Chimpanzees

Continued

TABLE 13-1 Antimicrobial Agents Used in Primates. (cont'd)

Agent	Dosage	Species/Comments
Ticarcillin/ clavulanate	65-100 mg/kg IV q8h[6]	Monkeys
	200-300 mg/kg/day IM, IV, divided q4-6h[6]	Chimpanzees
Trimethoprim/sulfa	30 mg/kg PO, IM q24h[11]	Prosimians
Trimethoprim/ sulfadiazine	15 mg/kg PO q12h[92]	Marmosets, capuchins, lemurs
	30 mg/kg SC, IM q24h[53]	Marmosets, capuchins, lemurs
Trimethoprim/ sulfamethoxazole	4 mg/kg PO, SC q8h[6]	Monkeys
	15 mg/kg PO q12h[59]	Marmosets
	24 mg/kg PO q12h[53]	Monkeys/shigellosis
	25 mg/kg PO, IM q12h[143]	Prosimians
	800 mg/animal PO q12h[6]	Chimpanzees
Tylosin	2 mg/kg IM q24h[6]	Monkeys
	20 mg/kg IM q24h × 10 days[19]	Rhesus macaques/chronic diarrhea
Vancomycin	20 mg/kg IM, IV q12h[6]	Monkeys
	500 mg/animal PO q6h × 7-10 days; can give IV slow[6]	Chimpanzees

TABLE 13-2 Antifungal Agents Used in Primates.

Agent	Dosage	Species/Comments
Amphotericin B	150 µg/kg IV 3 ×/wk × 2-4 mo[65]	Common marmosets
Fluconazole	7 mg/kg PO q24h[104]	Guenon (n=1)/*Cryptococcus*
	25 mg/kg/day PO[109,151]	Mandrills, tamarins, marmosets/*Candida*
Flucytosine	12.5-37.5 mg/kg PO q6h[6]	Chimpanzees
Griseofulvin	20 mg/kg PO q24h[6]	Monkeys
	25 mg/kg PO q24h × 30-60 days[109]	Common marmosets/dermatophytosis
	200 mg/kg PO q24h[6]	Monkeys
	500 mg/day PO divided q6-24h[6]	Chimpanzees
Itraconazole	5-10 mg/kg PO q12h[65]	Common marmosets/dermatophytosis
	10 mg/kg PO q24h[53]	Marmosets, capuchins, lemurs/fungal (yeast) gastroenteritis

TABLE 13-2 Antifungal Agents Used in Primates. (cont'd)

Agent	Dosage	Species/Comments
Ketoconazole	5-10 mg/kg PO q12h[6] × 30 days[109]	Monkeys
	10-30 mg/kg PO q24h × 60 days[65]	Common marmosets
	200-400 mg/day PO[6]	Chimpanzees
Nystatin	100,000 U/animal PO q8h[6]	Monkeys
	100,000-200,000 U/kg PO q24h × 10 days[65,109]	Monkeys, common marmosets/*Candida*
	500,000-1,000,000 U/animal PO q8h[6]	Chimpanzees
Pentamidine isethionate	4 mg/kg IM, IV q24h × 14 days[1]	Great apes/*Pneumocystis;* slow IV infusion; associated with profound hypotension, cardiac arrhythmias
Terbinafine	8.25 mg/kg PO q24h × 30 days[70]	Monkeys (*Cercopithicus* sp.)
Voriconizole	5 mg/kg PO q12h × 21-30 days[109]	Monkeys/aspergillosis

TABLE 13-3 Antiparasitic Agents Used in Primates.

Agent	Dosage	Species/Comments
Albendazole	10 mg/kg PO[11]	Brown lemurs
	10 mg/kg PO q24h × 6 wk[65]	Common marmosets/*Encephalitozoon cuniculi*
	20 mg/kg PO q12h × 5 days[77]	Geoffroy's tamarins (n=3)/*Angiostrongylus;* treat concurrently with prednisolone
	25 mg/kg PO q12h × 5 days[26,53]	New World primates, Old World primates/*Filaroides*, *Giardia*, gastrointestinal nematodes
	28.5 mg/animal PO q12h × 10 days × 3 treatments q10d[149]	Red-ruffed lemur (n=1)/cysticercosis; administer with praziquantel (SC)
	50 mg/kg PO q12h × 16 days[50,65]	Common marmosets, cotton-topped tamarins/*Acanthocephalus* sp.
	100 mg/kg PO q12h × 3 days, then repeat 2 × weekly × 4 treatments[50,65]	Common marmosets, cotton-topped tamarins/*Acanthocephalus* sp.
Amitraz	250 ppm dip × 2-5 min duration q14d × 4 treatments or until resolution of skin lesions[26,64]	Red-handed tamarins (n=2)/demodectic mange; no hair clipping or bathing; not rinsed after treatment; dried by hot air; ataxia (transient)
Benznidazole (Exeltis USA)	25 mg PO q12h × 60 days[93]	*Trypanosoma cruzi*; n=1; no obvious negative effects

Continued

TABLE 13-3 Antiparasitic Agents Used in Primates. (cont'd)

Agent	Dosage	Species/Comments
Bunamidine	25-100 mg/kg PO once[26]	New World primates, Old World primates/ cestodes
Chloroquine	2.5-5 mg/kg IM q24h × 4-7 days[26]	New World primates, Old World primates/*Plasmodium;* follow with primaquine; give drugs separately to prevent toxicity
	5 mg/kg PO, IM q24h × 14 days[26]	New World primates, Old World primates/*Entamoeba histolytica*
	10 mg/kg PO, IM once, then 5 mg/kg 6 hr later; repeat q24h × 2 days; then primaquine or mefloquine[53]	New World primates, Old World primates/ give chloroquine and primaquine separately to prevent toxicity (see primaquine, mefloquine)
	10 mg/kg via nasogastric tube day 1 AM; 5 mg/kg via nasogastric tube day 1 PM, days 2 and 3 q24h[6]	Monkeys
Clindamycin	12.5 mg/kg PO, IM q12h × 28 days[26]	New World primates, Old World primates/ toxoplasmosis
	12.5-25 mg/kg PO q12h × 28 days[53]	New World primates, Old World primates/ toxoplasmosis
Diethylcarbamazine (not commercially available in USA)	6-50 mg/kg PO q24h × 6-21 days[53]	Owl monkeys, squirrel monkeys/filariasis
Diiodohydroxyquinoline (iodoquinol)	12 mg/kg PO q8h × 10-20 days[6]	Monkeys
	12-16 mg/kg PO q8h × 10-21 days[53]	Great apes (infants, juveniles)/*Balantidium coli*
	20 mg/kg PO q12h × 21 days[53]	Adult great apes/*Balantidium*; use with metronidazole 30-50 mg/kg PO q12h × 5-10 days
	630 mg PO q8h × 20 days[6]	Chimpanzees
Dithiazanine sodium	10-20 mg/kg PO q24h × 3-10 days[53]	New World primates, Old World primates/*Strongyloides;* low margin of safety
Doxycycline	5 mg/kg PO q12h × 1 day, then 2.5 mg/kg PO q24h[53]	New World primates, Old World primates/*Balantidium*
Fenbendazole	10-20 mg/kg PO q24h × 30 days[65]	Common marmosets/*Encephalitozoon cuniculi*
	10-25 mg/kg PO q24h × 3-10 days[26]	New World primates, Old World primates/*Anatrichosoma cynomolgi*
	20 mg/kg PO q24h × 7 days[26]	New World primates, Old World primates/*Prosthenorchis*
	20 mg/kg PO q24h × 14 days[26]	New World primates, Old World primates/*Strongyloides, Filaroides,* gastrointestinal nematodes
	25 mg/kg PO once, repeat in 7 days[26]	New World primates, Old World primates/*Ancylostoma*

TABLE 13-3 Antiparasitic Agents Used in Primates. (cont'd)

Agent	Dosage	Species/Comments
Fenbendazole (cont'd)	50 mg/kg PO q24h × 3 days,[36,119] repeat in 2 wk[109]	Baboons/gastrointestinal nematodes; *Trichuris trichiura*
		New World primates/*Capillaria hepatica*
	50 mg/kg PO q24h × 3-14 days[26]	New World primates, Old World primates
	50 mg/kg PO q24h × 5 days[65]	Common marmosets/*Baylisascaris*
	50 mg/kg PO q24h × 14 days[26,65]	Common marmosets/*Filaroides* sp., *Trichospiura leptostoma*
	50 mg/kg PO q24h × 3 days, repeat in 3 wk[6]	Chimpanzees, monkeys/for monkeys, repeat in 3 mo
	50 mg/kg PO q2wk until infection resolved[65]	Common marmosets/*Capillaria hepatica*
Fipronil (9.8% solution)	0.2 mL/kg topically q6wk[26]	Prosimians/*Cuterebra* sp., ticks
Fluralaner (Bravecto, Merck)	30-35 mg/kg PO once[31]	Tamarins/acaricide; demodicosis; tablets should be crushed and placed in desired food items (e.g., grapes)
Ivermectin	0.2 mg/kg PO,[6,11] SC,[6,17,67] IM[11,109]	Chimpanzees, monkeys, brown lemurs
	0.2 mg/kg PO, SC, IM, repeat in 10-14 days[26,53]	Monkeys/*Strongyloides* sp., *Gonglyonema* sp., *Pneumonyssus* sp., Anoplura lice
	0.2 mg/kg SC or topically, repeat after 4 wk[65]	Common marmosets/*Anatrichosoma, Sarcoptes, Demodex, Dipetalonema,* pentastomids
	0.2-0.4 mg/kg PO, SC, IM q7d[53]	Prosimians
	0.3 mg/kg PO q7d × 4 treatments[67]	Callitrichids/*Gongylonema* sp.
Levamisole	2.5 mg/kg PO q24h × 14 days[53]	Prosimians/*Physaloptera*
	5 mg/kg PO, repeat in 21 days[53]	New World primates, Old World monkeys/*Strongyloides, Trichuris, Spiruroides*
	7.5 mg/kg SC, repeat in 14 days[53]	New World primates, Old World primates/*Trichuris, Ancylostoma*
Mebendazole	3 mg/kg PO q24h × 10 days[26]	New World primates, Old World primates/*Ancylostoma*
	10-20 mg/kg PO[10] q12h × 3 days	Brown lemurs, prosimians/gastrointestinal nematodes
	15 mg/kg PO q24h × 3 days[26,53]	New World primates, Old World monkeys/*Strongyloides, Necator, Pterygodermatites, Trichuris*
	22 mg/kg PO q24h × 3 days, repeat in 14 days[26,53] or repeat in 3 wk[53]	New World primates, Old World monkeys/*Strongyloides*
		Common marmosets/*Giardia*

Continued

TABLE 13-3 Antiparasitic Agents Used in Primates. (cont'd)

Agent	Dosage	Species/Comments
Mebendazole (cont'd)	40 mg/kg PO q24h × 3 days, repeat 3-4 × /year for prevention[53]	New World primates, Old World primates/ *Pterygodermatites* sp., *Trichuris*, *Strongyloides*, acanthocephalans
	50 mg/kg PO q12h × 3 days[6]	Monkeys
	70 mg/kg PO q24h × 3 days[26]	New World primates/oral spiruridiasis
	100 mg/animal PO q12h × 3 days[6]	Chimpanzees, monkeys
	100 mg/kg PO q12h × 3 days, repeat in 3 wk[6]	Monkeys/*Trichurus*
Mefloquine	25 mg/kg PO once via nasogastric tube[6]	Monkeys
	Active infection: 1250 mg PO once; preventive: 250 mg PO q7d[26]	Chimpanzees
Metronidazole	10-16.7 mg/kg PO q8h × 5-10 days[26]	New World primates, Old World primates/*Giardia*
	17.5-25 mg/kg PO q12h × 10 days[26]	Enteric flagellates and amoebas
	20 mg/kg PO q12h[65]	Common marmosets/*Entamoeba*
	25 mg/kg PO q12h × 5 days[26]	New World primates, Old World primates/*Giardia*
	25 mg/kg PO q12h × 10 days[53,98]	New World primates, Old World monkeys, great apes/*Giardia*, *Entamoeba*, *Balantidium*, *Tritrichomonas*
	25 mg/kg PO q24h[143]	Prosimians
	30-50 mg/kg PO q24h × 5-10 days[65]	Common marmosets/*Giardia*
	30-50 mg/kg PO q12h × 5-10 days[53]	Great apes/*Balantidium coli;* use with diiodohydroxyquin 20 mg/kg PO q12h × 21 days
	35 mg/kg PO q24h × 3 days[111]	Macaques/*Trichomonas vaginalis*
Milbemycin oxime	1 mg/kg PO q24h q30d × 3 mo[119]	Baboons/*Trichuris trichiura*
Moxidectin	0.5 mg/kg PO, IM once[26]	New World primates, Old World primates/*Strongyloides*
Niclosamide	37.5 mg PO q24h × 5 days[6]	Monkeys
	100 mg/kg PO once[26]	New World primates, Old World primates/ intestinal cestodiasis
Nifurtimox	15-20 mg/kg PO q8h × 90 days[65]	Common marmosets/*Trypanosoma cruzi*
Nitazoxanide	5 mg/kg PO q24h[65]	Common marmosets/*Cryptosporidium*
	25 mg/kg PO q24h × 5-7 days[143]	Prosimians/protozoa

TABLE 13-3 Antiparasitic Agents Used in Primates. (cont'd)

Agent	Dosage	Species/Comments
Oxytetracycline (LA-200)	10 mg/kg SC, IM q24h[53]	New World monkeys (i.e., marmosets), lemurs
	20-33 mg/kg IM q24h[53]	Black and white lemurs, ring-tailed lemurs, thick-tailed bush babies/n=captive collection of primates with outbreak of tularemia and remaining asymptomatic animals treated with IM dose if orals not taken (see tetracycline)
Paromomycin	10-20 mg/kg PO q12h × 5-10 days[26]	New World primates, Old World primates/*Balantidium coli*
	12.5-15 mg/kg PO q12h × 5-10 days[26]	New World primates/amoebae; minimal enteric absorption
	15 mg/kg PO q12h × 28 days[54,65]	Common marmosets (n=2)/*Cryptosporidium*
	100 mg/kg PO q24h × 10 days[26]	Cercopithecids
Piperazine	65 mg/kg PO q24h × 10 days[56]	Antiascaridial anthelmintic
Praziquantel	5 mg/kg IM[109]	Cestodes
	5 mg/kg PO, SC, IM once[6,109]	Monkeys
	20 mg/kg PO, IM once[53]	New World primates (i.e., marmosets), Old World monkeys, lemurs/cestodes
	20 mg/kg PO q8h × 1 day[6]	Chimpanzees
	23 mg/animal PO q10d × 3 treatments[149]	Red ruffed lemur (n=1)/subcutaneous cysticercosis; treat concurrently with albendazole
	40 mg/kg PO, IM[109]	New World primates, Old World monkeys/trematodes
Primaquine	0.3 mg/kg PO q24h × 14 days[6,53]	New World primates, Old World monkeys/*Plasmodium;* treat in conjunction with chloroquine; treat separately to prevent toxicity
Pyrantel pamoate	5-10 mg/kg PO,[11] repeat in 2 wk[143]	Brown lemurs, prosimians/nematodes
	10 mg/kg PO, repeat in 3 wk[6]	Chimpanzees
	11 mg/kg PO once, repeat in 10 days[53]	New World primates, Old World monkeys/pinworms (oxyurids; i.e., *Trichuris*)
Pyrimethamine	0.5 mg/kg PO q12h[65]	Common marmosets/*Encephalitozoon cuniculi;* treat concurrently with trimethoprim/sulfamethoxazole and folic acid for encephalitozoonosis or toxoplasmosis
	2 mg/kg PO q24h × 3 days, then 1 mg/kg PO q24h × 28 days[53]	Great apes/toxoplasmosis; treat concurrently with sulfadiazine
	10 mg/kg PO q24h[26]	*Plasmodium*; folic acid antagonist so monitor for deficiency

Continued

TABLE 13-3 Antiparasitic Agents Used in Primates. (cont'd)

Agent	Dosage	Species/Comments
Pyrvinium	5 mg/kg PO once, repeat q6mo[26]	New World primates, Old World primates/ pinworms
Quinacrine	2 mg/kg PO q8h × 7 days (max 300 mg/day)[53]	Great apes/*Giardia*
	2-10 mg/kg PO q8h × 5-7 days[26,53]	New World primates, Old World primates/*Giardia*; lower dose may cause gastrointestinal upset in squirrel monkeys; at higher doses, reported to be 70-95% effective
Ronnel	55 mg/kg PO or topically q72h × 4 treatments, then q7d × 3 mo[26,53]	New World primates, Old World monkeys/lung mites, ectoparasites
Sulfadiazine	50 mg/kg PO q6h[53]	Great apes/toxoplasmosis; maximum dose of 6 g/animal/day; treat in conjunction with pyrimethamine but separately to avoid toxicity
	100 mg/kg PO q24h[26,53]	New World primates, Old World monkeys/ toxoplasmosis; treat in conjunction with pyrimethamine but separately to avoid toxicity
Sulfadimethoxine	50 mg/kg PO once, then 25 mg/kg q24h[26,53]	New World primates, Old World monkeys/ coccidiosis
Tetracycline	16.5-20 mg/kg PO q12h[53]	Black and white lemurs, ring-tailed lemurs, thick-tailed bush babies/n=captive collection of primates with outbreak of tularemia and remaining asymptomatic animals treated with IM dose if orals not taken (see oxytetracycline)
Thiabendazole	50 mg/kg PO[10] q24h × 2 days[6,26]	Brown lemurs, infant monkeys/*Necator*
	50 mg/kg PO × 3-5 days[143]	Prosimians/nematodes
	75-100 mg/kg PO q24h once, repeat in 21 days[26]	New World primates, Old World primates
	100 mg/kg PO q24h[6]	Monkeys (adult)
	100 mg/kg PO once, repeat in 3 wk[109]	*Strongyloides*
	750-1500 mg/animal PO q24h × 2 days or 7 days[6,26]	Chimpanzees/visceral larval migrans
Tinidazole	40-45 mg/kg PO q24h × 6 days[11,43]	Prosimians/protozoa
	150 mg/kg PO once, then 77 mg/kg PO on day 4[65,79]	Marmosets/*Giardia*
Toltrazuril	7 mg/kg PO q24h × 2 days[65]	Common marmosets/toxoplasmosis; treat concurrently with trimethoprim/sulfamethoxazole
Trimethoprim/ sulfadiazine	15 mg/kg PO q12h[53]	New World primates, Old World monkeys/ toxoplasmosis
Trimethoprim/ sulfamethoxazole	30 mg/kg PO q12h ≥3 wk[65]	Common marmosets/*Encephalitozoon cuniculi;* treat concurrently with folic acid and pyrimethamine for encephalitozoonosis or toxoplasmosis

TABLE 13-4 Chemical Restraint/Anesthetic/Analgesic[a] Agents Used in Primates.

Agent	Dosage	Species/Comments
Acepromazine	—	See ketamine for combination
	0.1-0.5 mg/kg IM, IV[6]	Monkeys
	0.5-1 mg/kg PO,[53] SC, IM[6]	Marmosets, lemurs, capuchins/tranquilization; no reversal
Acetaminophen	5-10 mg/kg PO q6h[65,115]	New World primates, common marmosets, juvenile macaques/pyrexia, mild pain
	6 mg/kg PO q8h[6]	Monkeys
	10 mg/kg PO[53]	Sumatran orangutan (n=1)/before blood transfusion
	10-15 mg/kg PO q8-12h[53,144]	Prosimians
	15-20 mg/kg rectal[115]	
	360 mg PO prn for pain[53]	Chimpanzee (n=1)/postoperative pain; fractures
	500-1000 mg/animal PO q8h[6]	Chimpanzees
Acetaminophen/ codeine suspension (120 mg/12 mg per 5 mL)	10-15 mL PO q6h[6]	Chimpanzees
Alfaxalone	—	Macaques/see alphaxalone/alphadolone and midazolam/medetomidine combinations
	12 mg/kg IM[56]	Small primates (e.g., marmosets)
Alphaxalone/ alphadolone	5-8 mg/kg IM[89]	Light sedation
	12-18 mg/kg IM[146]	Small primates/heavy sedation; additional dose (6-9 mg/kg IV) produces surgical anesthesia; peak effect in 5 min and lasts 45 min; volume is too large to be useful for larger primates
Atipamezole (Antisedan, Zoetis)	IM use only per label	Specific α_2-adrenergic antagonist; more specific for medetomidine and dexmedetomidine than for xylazine; as a general rule, atipamezole is dosed at the same volume of medetomidine or dexmedetomidine; atipamezole dose is 5 × dose of medetomidine or 10 × dose of dexmedetomidine on mg basis
	0.15-0.3 mg/kg IM, IV[6,115]	Chimpanzees; use lower dose in monkeys and baboons
	0.2 mg/kg IV[115]	Squirrel monkeys
	0.25 mg/kg IM, IV[115]	Macaques
Bupivacaine (0.5%)	2 mg/kg (max); 1.3 mg/kg mixed with 1:200,000 epinephrine[57]	Rhesus macaques/regional anesthesia for dentistry and orofacial surgery
	2 mg/kg maximum perineurally[39,57]	Macaques/local anesthetic

Continued

TABLE 13-4 Chemical Restraint/Anesthetic/Analgesica Agents Used in Primates. (cont'd)

Agent	Dosage	Species/Comments
Buprenorphine	—	Opioid agonist-antagonist; analgesia
	0.005-0.01 mg/kg SC,[62] IM, IV q6-12h[45,57,109]	Rhesus macaques, marmosets, great apes
	0.005-0.03 mg/kg IM, IV q6-12h[65]	Common marmosets
	0.01 mg/kg IM, IV q6-8h[105,115]	Macaques/PK; not to exceed 0.3 mg/animal IM q8h in chimpanzees
	0.01-0.02 mg/kg SC, IM, IV q8-12h[144]	Prosimians
	0.03 mg/kg IM q12h[71,105] or IV bolus[71]	Macaques/PK
	Sustained-release: 0.2 mg/kg SC once[105]	Macaques/single injection; plasma concentrations 0.1 ng/mL
Butorphanol	—	In primates, butorphanol behaves more as an agonist with intermediate efficacy; may cause profound respiratory depression; reverse with naloxone if needed; see dexmedetomidine and ketamine for combinations
	0.01-0.02 mg/kg SC, IM, IV q6-12h[65]	Common marmosets
	0.013 mg/kg IM q8h[22]	Rhesus macaques
	0.02 mg/kg SC, IM, IV q8h[6,53]	New World primates, marmosets, lemurs/ may cause profound respiratory depression; antagonize with naloxone if needed
	0.02 mg/kg SC q6h[109]	New World primates
	0.05 mg/kg IM q8h[6]	Monkeys
	0.1-0.4 mg/kg IM[11]	Brown lemurs
	0.1-0.4 mg/kg SC, IM, IV q3-4h[144]	Prosimians
Butorphanol (B)/ dexmedetomidine (De)/ketamine (K)	(B) 0.3-0.4 mg/kg + (De) 0.02 mg/kg + (K) 3-5 mg/kg IM[143,144]	Prosimians/can exchange ketamine with 0.2-0.3 mg/kg IM midazolam
Clonazepam	—	Benzodiazepine; anxiolytic, sedative, skeletal muscle relaxant, anticonvulsant; taming effect in aggressive primates; as a preanesthetic, administer 1 hr prior to induction; availability of orally dissolving tablets (ODT) makes dosing in primates easier than with other dosage forms; often placed in grapes
	0.25-3 mg/kg PO[28]	Chimpanzees, colobus monkeys, gibbons, macaques, and presumably many other species; some species have responded to 0.2 mg/kg PO; place ODT in food items (e.g., grapes)

TABLE 13-4 Chemical Restraint/Anesthetic/Analgesica Agents Used in Primates. (cont'd)

Agent	Dosage	Species/Comments
Dexmedetomidine	0.01 mg/kg IM[8,129]	Tamarins, macaques/dose should be 1/2 that of medetomidine; frequently used in combination with alfaxalone and ketamine for sedation; reverse with atipamezole; see butorphanol, ketamine, and midazolam for combinations
Dexmedetomidine (De)/midazolam (M)/ butorphanol (B)	(De) 10 µg/kg + (M) 0.5 mg/ kg + (B) 0.3 mg/kg IM[42]	Brown howler monkeys/anesthesia, analgesia, deep sedation; fast recovery
Diazepam[b]	—	Often used with ketamine; see ketamine combination[b]
	0.25-0.5 mg/kg PO, IV[11,143]	Prosimians, lemurs
	0.25-0.5 mg/kg IM, IV[6]	Chimpanzees
	0.5-1 mg/kg PO[6]	Chimpanzees
	0.5-2.5 mg/kg IV[144]	Prosimians
	1 mg/kg IM, IV, PO[45,53]	Marmosets, New World monkeys
	5 mg/animal PO[29,53]	Gorillas (juvenile)
	5-30 mg q12-24h PO[53]	Rapid effect and well tolerated for animals that display inappropriate fear, anxiety, or mild forms of self-injury during introductions
	10-40 mg PO total in juice 1-2 hr prior to anesthesia[53]	Adult chimpanzees/decrease anxiety
Droperidol	2.5-10 mg/animal IM[6]	Chimpanzees/given 30-60 min prior to procedure
Etomidate	0.1 mg/kg/min IV constant rate infusion[41]	Rhesus macaques/injectable nonbarbiturate anesthetic maintenance
	1 mg/kg IV[41]	Rhesus macaques/induction
Fentanyl	—	Produced respiratory depression and analgesia at dosages as low as 2 µg/kg IV;[138] apnea was seen consistently at 60 µg/kg
	0.05-0.15 µg/kg IM prn[6]	Monkeys
	1-2 µg/kg as an adjunct to general anesthesia; 50-150 µg/kg as sole anesthetic[25]	Great apes
	1-30 µg/kg/h IV constant rate infusion[143,144]	Prosimians
	4-8 µg/kg/h transdermal patch[89]	Monitor for respiratory depression
	5-10 µg/kg IV bolus[115] or IV constant rate infusion[6,39]	Rhesus macaques, baboons, chimpanzees
	10-25 µg/kg/h IV constant rate infusion[115]	

Continued

TABLE 13-4 Chemical Restraint/Anesthetic/Analgesica Agents Used in Primates. (cont'd)

Agent	Dosage	Species/Comments
Fentanyl (cont'd)	10-15 µg/kg PO as lollipops[29]	Orangutans, gorillas/adequate sedation in 30-45 min; chimpanzees suboptimal effects
	25 µg/kg/h (5-10 kg); 50 µg/kg/h (10 kg) q48-72h[6]	Monkeys/transdermal patch
Fentanyl/droperidol (Innovar-Vet, Janssen)	0.05 mL/kg IM[6]	New World primates
	0.1-0.3 mL/kg IM[6]	Chimpanzees, monkeys
Flumazenil	0.02 mg/kg IV[53,115,144]	Patas monkeys, prosimians/benzodiazepine antagonist
	0.02-0.1mg/kg IV[53]	Great apes
	0.025 mg/kg IV[29]	Chimpanzees, gorillas/did not significantly enhance speed or quality of recovery
Gabapentin	12.8-13.5 mg/kg PO q8h[24,110,122]	Monkeys, chimpanzees
Hydrocodone bitartrate	5 mg/animal PO q4-6h prn[6]	Chimpanzees
Hydromorphone	0.2 mg/kg IM q4h, IV bolus q4h[72]	Rhesus macaques/PK; may cause whole-body pruritus; short-acting pain relief with sedation
Isoflurane	1-2% maintenance[109]	Maintenance of surgical plane of anesthesia
	1%-3% maintenance[115]	Marmosets, chimpanzees
	3-5% induction[56]	Higher concentration required for unpremedicated patients
Ketamine	—	Tranquilization; anesthesia; mg/kg dose increases as size of animal decreases; causes seizures in lemurs when used as sole agent so not recommended for use alone in prosimians; not recommended as sole agent; not reversible; see butorphanol, dexmedetomidine, medetomidine, midazolam, and tiletamine/zolazepam for combinations
	Loading dose of 0.5 mg/kg IV then 0.001 mg/kg/min CRI (24 hr)[110,129]	Monkeys, siamangs, tamarins/good for postsurgical pain control; can combine with opioids at reduced doses; often used with dexmedetomidine
	5 mg/kg IV[6]	Monkeys
	5-12 mg/kg IM[106]	Monkeys
	5-15 mg/kg IM, IV[53,144]	Prosimians
	5-15 mg/kg PO, IM, IV or rectally[25]	Great apes/in general, 6-10 mg/kg should allow safe initial immobilization
	5-20 mg/kg IM[53]	Chimpanzees/rapid induction; minimal cardiovascular and respiratory changes; not reversible; short duration of action

TABLE 13-4 Chemical Restraint/Anesthetic/Analgesica Agents Used in Primates. (cont'd)

Agent	Dosage	Species/Comments
Ketamine (cont'd)	5-40 mg/kg IM[6]	Chimpanzees
	10 mg/kg IM[6]	Monkeys
	10-15 mg/kg IM[6]	New World primates
Ketamine (K)/ acepromazine (A)	(K) 4 mg/kg + (A) 0.2 mg/kg IM[53]	Western baboons/be aware of possible aggression among males during recovery
Ketamine (K)/ detomidine (Det)	(K) 9.6 mg/kg + (Det) 0.32 mg/kg PO[96]	Gorillas
	(K) 10 mg/kg + (Det) 0.5 mg/kg PO[96]	Gorillas (n=6), mandrill baboons (n=7)/reduced the reaction to darting
Ketamine (K)/ dexmedetomidine (De)	(K) 2-4 mg/kg + (De) 0.02-0.03 mg/kg IM[26]	Medium to large primates
Ketamine (K)/ diazepam[b] (D)	(K) 10 mg/kg + (D) 0.2-0.4 mg/kg IM[106]	Baboons/best to administer diazepam[b] PO 1 hr prior to ketamine IM
	(K) 15 mg/kg + (D) 1 mg/kg IM[89]	See comments above
Ketamine (K)/ medetomidine[c] (Me)	—	Medetomidine is no longer commercially available; can be compounded;[c] replaced with dexmedetomidine; recoveries can be quite sudden even without reversal
	(K) 2 mg/kg + (Me) 0.03-0.04 mg/kg IM[25]	Chimpanzees
	(K) 2-4 mg/kg + (Me) 0.04-0.06 mg/kg IM[26]	Medium to large primates
	(K) 2-5 mg/kg + (Me) 0.02-0.05 mg/kg IM[53]	Chimpanzees/antagonize with atipamezole 0.1-0.25 mg/kg IM
	(K) 2-6 mg/kg + (Me) 0.03-0.06 mg/kg IM[6]	Chimpanzees
	(K) 3 mg/kg + (Me) 0.02-0.03 mg/kg IM[29]	Orangutans
	(K) 3-4 mg/kg + (Me) 0.15 mg/kg IM[87,106,115,137]	Macaques, capuchins
	(K) 5 mg/kg + (Me) 0.01 mg/kg IM[65]	Common marmosets
	(K) 5 mg/kg + (Me) 0.05 mg/kg IM[106]	Japanese macaques
	(K) 5-7.5 mg/kg IM + (Me) 0.05-0.1 mg/kg IM, IV[53,106]	Use higher dosages for smaller primates
	(K) 10-15 mg/kg + (Me) 0.1 mg/kg[89]	Light anesthesia; add isoflurane or half dose of ketamine if needed; lower dose in large primates

Continued

TABLE 13-4 Chemical Restraint/Anesthetic/Analgesica Agents Used in Primates. (cont'd)

Agent	Dosage	Species/Comments
Ketamine (K)/ medetomidine[c] (Me)/ butorphanol (B)	—	Medetomidine is no longer commercially available; can be compounded;[c] replaced with dexmedetomidine (1/2 the mg dosage)
	(K) 2-3 mg/kg + (Me) 0.02-0.03 mg/kg + (B) 0.2-0.4 mg/kg IM[39]	Great apes
	(K) 3 mg/kg + (Me) 0.04 mg/kg + (B) 0.4 mg/kg IM[145,150]	Patas monkeys, ring-tailed lemurs/anesthesia; long duration of action
Ketamine (K)/ midazolam (Mi)	(K) 1-2 mg/kg + (Mi) 0.03 mg/kg IM[29]	Orangutans
	(K) 2.5 mg/kg + (Mi) 0.25 mg/kg IM[29]	Chimpanzees
	(K) 4-20 mg/kg IM + (Mi) 0.05-0.2 mg SC, IM[62]	
	(K) 5 mg/kg + (Mi) 0.1 mg/kg IM[115]	Baboons
	(K) 8 mg/kg + (Mi) 0.2 mg/kg IM[10,115]	Macaques/up to 1 mg/kg IM of midazolam
	(K) 9 mg/kg + (Mi) 0.05 mg/kg IM[29]	Gorillas
	(K) 10 mg/kg + (Mi) 1 mg/kg IM[48,106]	Marmosets
	(K) 15 mg/kg + (Mi) 0.05-0.09 mg (lower body weight)[57] or 0.05-0.15 mg (higher body weight) IV[115]	
Ketamine (K)/ tiletamine-zolazepam (T)	(K) 1-3 mg/kg + (T) 2-4 mg/kg IM[25]	Great apes/combination reduces amount of ketamine needed for induction
Ketamine (K)/ xylazine (X)	(K) 5 mg/kg + (X) 0.5-1 mg/kg IM[106]	Monkeys
	(K) 5-7 mg/kg + (X) 1-1.4 mg/kg IM[29]	Orangutans
	(K) 5-10 mg/kg + (X) 0.25-0.3 mg/kg SC, IM[62]	
	(K) 7 mg/kg + (X) 0.6 mg/kg IM[6,115]	Monkeys, macaques
	(K) 10 mg/kg + (X) 0.25 mg/kg IM for 45 min sedation, or (X) 2 mg/kg IM for138 min sedation[115]	Macaques
	(K) 10-20 mg/kg IM + (X) 3 mg/kg IM[6]	New World primates
	(K) 15-20 mg/kg IM + (X) 1 mg/kg IM[29,115]	Chimpanzees

TABLE 13-4 Chemical Restraint/Anesthetic/Analgesica Agents Used in Primates. (cont'd)

Agent	Dosage	Species/Comments
Lidocaine	0.025 mg/kg/min CRI[110]	New World primates, siamangs/postsurgical pain control; do not use with epinephrine
	2-4 mg/kg local block[25]	Great apes/preferred to bupivacaine for dental procedures
	6 mg/kg maximum perineurally[39]	Macaques/local anesthetic
Medetomidine[c]	—	Medetomidine is a more selective, potent and specific α_2-agonist than xylazine; can be compounded; replaced with dexmedetomidine; see ketamine, midazolam, and tiletamine/zolazepam for combinations
	0.01-0.035 mg/kg IM[6]	Monkeys
	0.1 mg/kg PO[29]	Great apes
	0.1 mg/kg SC, IM[115]	Squirrel monkeys, baboons
	0.15 mg/kg IM[115]	Macaques
Medetomidine[c] (Me)/ midazolam (Mi)	(Me) 0.03-0.06 mg/kg + (Mi) 0.3 mg/kg IM[58,106]	Macaques/can use dexmedetomidine (1/2 dosage); can use in combination with alfaxalone (2 mg/kg IM)[58]
Meperidine	2 mg/kg IM[115]	Macaques
	2-4 mg/kg IM,[115] IV q30-60 min[6] or q2-4h[56]	Baboons, monkeys/analgesia
	50-150 mg/animal PO[115] q3-4h prn[6]	Chimpanzees
Midazolam	—	See butorphanol, ketamine, and medetomidine for combinations
	0.05-0.1 mg/kg IM, slow IV[6]	Monkeys
	0.1-0.3 mg/kg IM,[11,144] IV[144]	Brown lemurs, prosimians
	0.1-0.5 mg/kg IM[109]	With ketamine, helps prevent seizures in lemurs
	0.7-1.2 mg/kg PO[29]	Gorillas, chimpanzees, orangutans
	1-2.5 mg/animal IV, or 5 mg/ animal IV[6]	Chimpanzees
	3 mg/kg PO[8]	Macaques
Morphine	0.01-0.1 mg/kg IV[6,115]	Chimpanzees
	0.1-2 mg/kg SC, IM q3-6h[59]	Marmosets
	0.15 mg/kg epidurally[115]	Baboons
	1 mg/kg PO, SC, IM, IV q4h[53]	New World monkeys, marmosets, lemurs/ may cause profound respiratory depression; antagonize with naloxone as needed
	1-2 mg/kg SC,[115] IM, IV q4h[6,115]	Monkeys, squirrel monkeys, macaques, baboons
	1-2 mg/kg SC, IM q6h[65]	Common marmosets

Continued

TABLE 13-4 Chemical Restraint/Anesthetic/Analgesica Agents Used in Primates. (cont'd)

Agent	Dosage	Species/Comments
Nalbuphine	2.5-5 mg/kg IM q3-4h[6]	Monkeys/agonist-antagonist opioid
	10 mg SC, IM, IV q3-6h prn[6]	Chimpanzees
Naloxone	—	Opioid antagonist/reversal; short acting; a second dose may be necessary to avoid the return of respiratory depression
	0.01-0.05 mg/kg IM, IV[53,65,110]	New World monkeys, common marmosets, lemurs
	0.015 mg/kg SC, IM, IV[6,115]	Chimpanzees
	0.02 mg/kg IM[144]	Prosimians
	0.1 mg/kg SC, IM, IV prn[6]	Monkeys
	0.1-0.2 mg SC, IM prn[115]	Macaques, baboons, squirrel monkeys, common marmosets
Naloxone intranasal spray (2 mg/0.1 mL)	0.04-1 mg/kg IN[114]	New World primates/opioid overdoses; repeat every 3 min to effect
Nitrous oxide (N_2O)	Up to 60% with O_2[62]	Not acceptable as sole agent
Oxymorphone	—	Opioid analgesia
	0.025 mg/kg SC, IM, IV q4-6h[6]	New World primates
	0.075 mg/kg IV bolus[74]	New World primates, titi monkeys (n=4), rhesus macaques (n=4)/PK
	0.075 mg/kg IM, IV q4-6h[115]	Squirrel monkeys, marmosets
	0.15 mg/kg SC, IM, IV q4-6h[6,74,109,115]	Old World primates, macaques, baboons, monkeys
	1-1.5 mg/animal SC, IM q4-6h[6,115]	Chimpanzees
Pentobarbital (pentobarbitone sodium)	—	The product has considerable variation between species; severe respiratory depression; inability to modulate depth of anesthesia; should be used for euthanasia only, not for sedation
Propofol	—	Dose to maintain anesthesia in great apes 5-10 × less than human dose; use sterile technique due to vehicle
	0.3-0.5 mg/kg/min constant rate infusion[114]	Baboons, macaques
	1-2 mg/kg IV bolus followed by constant-rate infusion to effect[6,115]	Chimpanzees
	2 mg/kg IV bolus[91]	Neonatal rhesus macaques (n=4)/induction
	2-4 mg/kg/min IV constant rate infusion[115]	Baboons

TABLE 13-4 Chemical Restraint/Anesthetic/Analgesica Agents Used in Primates. (cont'd)

Agent	Dosage	Species/Comments
Propofol (cont'd)	2 mg/kg/min IV[49]	Capuchins/induction
	2-5 mg/kg IV bolus;[65] maintenance with 0.3-0.4 mg/kg/min IV constant rate infusion[115]	Common marmosets, macaques
	2.5-5 mg/kg IV bolus; maintenance with 0.3-0.4 mg/kg/min constant rate infusion[6]	Monkeys
	2.5-5 mg/kg IV bolus[109]	Baboons, macaques/induction
	3-6 mg/kg IV[144]	Prosimians
	5 mg/kg IV bolus at 0.6 mg/kg/min[97]	Japanese macaques (n=5)/stepdown started at 0.6 mg/kg/min, then 0.3 mg/kg/min × 10 min, then 0.2 mg/kg/min × 100 min
	5-10 mg/kg IV, then 0.3-0.6 mg/kg IV constant rate infusion[45]	Marmosets
Sevoflurane	8% induction; 2.5% maintenance[89]	1 MAC = 2% inhalation[115]
Thiamylal sodium	15-25 mg/kg IV to effect[6]	Monkeys/barbiturate anesthesia
Thiopental	—	Barbiturate anesthesia
	5-7 mg/kg IV if combined with ketamine[115]	Macaques
	15-17 mg/kg/h IV constant rate infusion[115]	Baboons
	25 mg/kg IV to effect[6]	Monkeys
Tiletamine-zolazepam	—	Can concentrate in vial; see ketamine and medetomidine for combinations
	1-2.5 mg/kg IM[6]	New World primates
	2-5 mg/kg IM[26]	New World primates, Old World primates
	2-6 mg/kg IM[29,115]	Chimpanzees, gorillas, orangutans (up to 6.9 mg/kg)
	3-5 mg/kg IM[6,53,109,115,144]	Great apes, prosimians/restraint only; antagonize zolazepam with flumazenil 0.02 mg/kg IV
	4-6 mg/kg IM[115]	Macaques, baboons
	5-8 mg/kg IM[6]	Chimpanzees, monkeys
	10 mg/kg[106,115,121]	Squirrel monkeys, chimpanzees
	16 mg/kg PO once[53]	Chimpanzee/given PO in a cola drink; recumbent within 7 min; response to external stimuli within 40 min

Continued

TABLE 13-4 Chemical Restraint/Anesthetic/Analgesica Agents Used in Primates. (cont'd)

Agent	Dosage	Species/Comments
Tiletamine-zolazepam (T)/ medetomidine[c] (Me)	(T) 0.8-2.3 mg/kg + (Me) 0.02-0.06 mg/kg IM[29,106]	Orangutans, monkeys, gibbons, macaques
	(T) 1-3 mg/kg + (Me) 0.02-0.06 mg/kg[106]	Monkeys, macaques, gibbons
	(T) 1.25 mg/kg + (Me) 0.03 mg/kg IM[115]	Chimpanzees
	(T) 2 mg/kg + (Me) 0.03 mg/kg IM[121]	Chimpanzees
	(T) 3 mg/kg + (Me) 0.05 mg/kg IM[100]	Chimpanzees
	(T) 3 mg/kg IM + (Me) 0.1 mg/kg PO[100]	Chimpanzees
Tramadol	—	Management of mild to moderate acute pain and as an adjunctive analgesic in the management of chronic osteoarthritis
	1-4 mg/kg PO q12h[144]	Prosimians
	1.5 mg/kg IV q24h[73]	Rhesus macaques/PK; sedation, pruritus
	3 mg/kg PO[73]	Rhesus macaques/PK; PO bioavailability poor; oral dosages of 4-20 × this dose may be required for analgesia
Xylazine	—	See ketamine for combination
	0.5-6 mg/kg IM[6]	Monkeys
	1.1 mg/kg IV[6]	Chimpanzees
	2.2 mg/kg IM[6]	Chimpanzees
Yohimbine[d]	0.1 mg/kg IM, IV[6]	Monkeys, chimpanzees (0.11 mg/kg)
	0.125-0.25 mg/kg IM[29]	Chimpanzees
	0.5 mg/kg IV or 1 mg/kg IM[115]	Macaques/xylazine reversal

[a]For other analgesic agents (nonsteroidal antiinflammatory agents), see Table 13-5.
[b]Diazepam is not soluble in aqueous solution; admixing with aqueous solutions or fluids can result in precipitation; administering SC or IM can be painful and irritating; for SC or IM administration, midazolam may be preferred.
[c]Medetomidine is no longer commercially available, although it can be obtained from select compounding services (e.g., Wildlife Pharmaceuticals, www.zoopharm.net); limited data on the efficacy and safety of dexmedetomidine in primates; the effects of the v/v use of the two drugs may not be equivalent, so the dose of dexmedetomidine may need to be adjusted based on clinical response.
[d]Limited availability; may need to be compounded.

TABLE 13-5 Nonsteroidal Antiinflammatory Agents (NSAIDs) Used in Primates.

Agent	Dosage	Species/Comments
Acetylsalicylic acid (aspirin)	—	Analgesic; antipyretic; avoid aspirin-based products during viral infections due to concerns of Reyes syndrome[102]
	5-10 mg/kg PO q4-6h[6,53,65]	Monkeys, common marmosets, chimpanzees (use q6h; antipyretic)
	10-20 mg/kg PO q8-12h[144]	Prosimians
	20 mg/kg PO q8-12h[6]	Monkeys
	20 mg/kg PO q12h[5]	Rhesus macaques/platelet aggregation was significantly decreased
Carprofen	2 mg/kg PO q12h[6]	Chimpanzees, monkeys
	2-4 mg/kg PO, SC q12-24h[53,62,65,115]	New World monkeys, marmosets, lemurs/ analgesia, antipyretic; half-life varies with species; COX-1 selectivity
	3-4 mg/kg IV, SC once[44]	Macaques/preoperatively
Celecoxib	200 mg/animal PO q12-24h[6]	Chimpanzees/COX-2 NSAID
Deracoxib (Deramaxx, Eli Lilly)	2 mg/kg PO q24h[6]	Chimpanzees/COX-2 NSAID; chronic use
	4 mg/kg PO q24h[6]	Chimpanzees
Flunixin meglumine	0.25-0.5 mg/kg SC, IM, IV q24h[144]	Prosimians
	0.3-1 mg/kg SC, IV q24h[53]	New World monkeys, marmosets, lemurs/anti-inflammatory, antipyretic
	0.5-2 mg/kg SC, IM, IV q12h[109]	New World monkeys/analgesic
	1 mg/kg IM q12h[39]	Rhesus macaques
	2 mg/kg IM q12h[6]	Monkeys
Ibuprofen	7 mg/kg PO q12h[6,115]	Old World primates, New World primates/mild analgesia
	10 mg/kg PO q8-12h[144]	Prosimians
	10-20 mg/kg PO q12h[109]	New World monkeys (e.g., marmosets), Old World monkeys/can be used in conjunction with acetaminophen
	20 mg/kg PO q24h[53,65]	Common marmosets
	200-400 mg/animal PO q8h[6]	Chimpanzees
	200-800 mg/animal PO 8-12h[53]	Western lowland gorillas, chimpanzees
Ketoprofen	1 mg/kg IM q24h[53]	Squirrel monkeys
	2 mg/kg IM q24h[29]	Gorilla (n=1)
	2 mg/kg IM, IV q24h[6,109]	Chimpanzees, monkeys
	2 mg/kg PO, SC, IM, IV[144]	Prosimians/reduce to 1 mg/kg q24h after first dose
	5 mg/kg IM q24h[39]	Monkeys

Continued

TABLE 13-5 Nonsteroidal Antiinflammatory Agents (NSAIDs) Used in Primates. (cont'd)

Agent	Dosage	Species/Comments
Ketorolac	0.5-1 mg/kg[106] SC, IM q8-12h × 4 days[62]	Monkeys, gibbons
	15-30 mg/animal IM[115]	Baboons
	30 mg/animal PO q6h[6,115]	Chimpanzees
	60 mg/animal PO once[6]	Chimpanzees
Meloxicam	0.1 mg/kg PO q24h[15]	Cynomolgus macaques/PK; sustained-release formation (0.6 mg/kg SC) achieved adequate steady-state plasma concentration for 2-3 days; PO formulation limited use
	0.1-0.2 mg/kg SC q24h[45] up to 3 days[115]	Marmosets, rhesus macaques
	0.2 mg/kg IM q24h[15]	Cynomolgus macaques/PK; see above dose for cynomolgus macaques; IM provided adequate plasma concentrations for 12-24 hr
	0.2-0.3 mg/kg PO, SC, IM q24h × 4 days[62]	Use lower dose in common marmosets, macaques
	0.3 mg/kg PO, SC q24h[5]	Rhesus macaques/platelet aggregation was not affected
Naproxen	5 mg/kg PO q24h[6]	Chimpanzees

TABLE 13-6 Antipsychotic, Antianxiety, Antiaggressive, and Antiseizure Agents Used in Primates.

Agent	Dosage	Species/Comments
Carbamazepine	50 mg/animal PO q8-12h[51]	Gorilla (infants)/epilepsy
Deslorelin (Suprelorin, Virbac)	1-2 (6 mg) implants SC[53]	Lion-tailed macaques/reduce aggression (6 mg)
Diazepam	0.5-1 mg/kg IM, IV[6]	Monkeys/seizures; not soluble in aqueous solution; admixing with aqueous solutions or fluids can result in precipitation; administering IM can be painful and irritating; for IM administration, midazolam may be preferred
	5-30 mg q12-24h PO[53]	Reduce anxiety short term; rapid effect and well tolerated for animals that display inappropriate fear, anxiety, or mild forms of self-injury during introductions; appears to work better than lorazepam (0.5-3 mg PO q24h)
	10-40 mg PO total in juice 1-2 hr prior to anesthesia[53]	Adult chimpanzees/decrease anxiety
Diphenylhydantoin	2.5 mg/kg PO q24h[56]	Epilepsy; adverse effects may include ataxia, vomiting, etc.

TABLE 13-6 Antipsychotic, Antianxiety, Antiaggressive, and Antiseizure Agents Used in Primates. (cont'd)

Agent	Dosage	Species/Comments
Fluoxetine	0.5-1 mg/kg PO q24h[6]	Chimpanzees
	0.5-8 mg/kg PO q24h[109]	Smaller species may require higher dosage
	2 mg/kg PO q24h[84] × 1-4 wk[46]	Rhesus macaques (n=6)/reduction of self-biting behavior, but not self-directed stereotypes; venlafaxine ineffective
	3 mg/kg PO q24h[131]	Juvenile rhesus macaques
	10 mg/kg PO q24h[127]	Rhesus macaques
Gabapentin	12.8-13.5 mg/kg PO q8h[24,110,122]	Monkeys, chimpanzees/anticonvulsant, anxiolytic, sedative
Guanfacine	—	Self-injurious behavior; decreased agitation without profound sedation
	0.3 mg/kg PO, IM q12h × 5-10 days followed by gradual reduction to 0.15 mg/kg q24h over 30 days[90]	Baboon (n=1)/recurrence controlled by returning to 0.3 mg/kg q12h
	0.5 mg/kg PO, IM q12h × 5-10 days followed by gradual reduction to 0.25 mg/kg q24h over 30 days[90]	Macaques (n=2)/recurrence controlled by returning to 0.5 mg/kg q12h
Haloperidol	0.03-0.05 mg/kg IM q12h[6]	Monkeys
	0.5-5 mg PO q8-12h[6]	Chimpanzees
	60 mg/animal PO q24h[118]	Gorilla (n=1)/antipsychotic; treat concurrently with sulpiride; extrapyramidal symptoms; neuroleptic malignant syndrome is a rare but potential side effect
Levetiracetam	6 mg/kg PO q12h (extrapolated)[51]	Great apes (bonobo); used 250 mg PO q12h in a bonobo/seizures
	150 mg/kg IV[30]	Rhesus macaques/seizures
Midazolam	0.1-0.5 mg/kg IM[109]	With ketamine helps prevent seizures in lemurs
Mirtazapine	15 mg/animal PO q24h[21]	Mandrill (n=1)/anti-anxiety
Paroxetine	1-7.5 mg/kg PO q24h[113]	Rhesus monkeys
Phenobarbital	1-6 mg/kg PO[6]	Monkeys/seizures
	2 mg/kg IV[6]	
Phenytoin	2.5 mg/kg PO q12h, increase prn[6]	Monkeys/anticonvulsant
	125 mg PO q8h, increase prn[6]	Chimpanzees
Sulpiride	400-800 mg/animal PO q24h[118]	Gorilla (n=1)/antipsychotic; treat concurrently with haloperidol; extrapyramidal symptoms; neuroleptic malignant syndrome is a rare but potential side effect

Continued

TABLE 13-6 Antipsychotic, Antianxiety, Antiaggressive, and Antiseizure Agents Used in Primates. (cont'd)

Agent	Dosage	Species/Comments
Tryptophan	100 mg/kg PO q12h[142]	Macaques/self-injurious behavior; add to flavored commercial primate treat
Zonisamide	40 mg/kg SC q24h[147]	Not for first-line epilepsy treatment; experimental in marmosets for refractory seizures (abortifacient in cynomologus monkeys on days 21-45 days gestation at 10 mg/kg PO)
Zuclopenthixol (Clopixol, Lundbeck)	0.1-0.36 mg/kg PO q12h[29]	Gorillas/antipsychotic drug; not approved for use in the United States
	10-25 mg/animal PO q8h[118]	Gorilla (n=1)/aggression; tapered with a decrease of 5 mg/wk; antipsychotic; extrapyramidal symptoms; neuroleptic malignant syndrome is a rare but potential side effect

TABLE 13-7 Miscellaneous Agents Used in Primates.

Agent	Dosage	Species/Comments
Acetylcysteine	20 mg/mL solution (dilute with saline); nebulize 30-60 min prn (e.g., q6-12h)[56]	Mucolytic; decreases the viscosity of bronchial secretions
Albuterol sulfate inhalation aerosol 0.083%	Nebulize q12-24h[110]	Monkeys, marmosets/1 mL/2 mL saline dilution
Allopurinol	200-600 mg/animal PO q24h[6]	Chimpanzees
Aminophylline	10 mg/kg IV[6,43]	Chimpanzees, lemurs
	25-100 mg/animal PO q24h[6]	Monkeys
Amlodipine	0.1 mg/kg PO q24h[6]	Chimpanzees/antihypertensive agent
Atropine sulfate	0.01 mg/kg IM[29]	Orangutan (n=1)
	0.02-0.04 mg/kg SC, IM, IV[6,115]	Chimpanzees, monkeys, marmosets/for marmosets, use higher dose
	0.02-0.05 mg/kg SC, IM, IV[6,65,68]	Chimpanzees, macaques, baboons, common marmosets
	0.04 mg/kg IM[29]	Gorillas
	2-5 mg/animal IM[29]	Chimpanzees (juvenile)
Azathioprine	1-2 mg/kg PO q24h[6]	Monkeys/immunosuppressive agent; purine antagonist
	1-2.5 mg/kg PO q24h[6]	Chimpanzees
Benazepril	0.25-0.5 mg/kg PO q24h[65]	Common marmosets/less nephrotoxicity than enalapril
Bisacodyl	10-15 mg PO prn[6]	Chimpanzees

TABLE 13-7 Miscellaneous Agents Used in Primates. (cont'd)

Agent	Dosage	Species/Comments
Bismuth subsalicylate	30 mL PO prn[6]	Chimpanzees
	40 mg/kg PO q8-12h[6]	Monkeys
Budesonide	0.5 mg/animal PO q24h × 8 wk, then 0.75 mg PO q24h × 8 wk[65]	Common marmosets/marmoset wasting syndrome
Calcitonin	10 U/kg q48h × 3 wk[65]	Common marmosets/must be normocalcemic
Calcitriol	0.03 mg/kg PO q24h[6]	Chimpanzees
Calcium glubionate	23 mg/kg PO q12h[65]	Common marmosets/metabolic bone disease
Calcium gluconate	200 mg/kg SC, IM, IV[6]	Chimpanzees/hypocalcemia; hyperkalemia; prophylaxis and therapy of nutritional secondary hyperparathyroidism
Carvedilol	3.125 mg PO q12h × 2 wk, then 6.25 mg PO q12h, increase prn[6]	Chimpanzees
Chlorphenamine	0.5 mg/kg PO q24h[56]	Allergic disease; prevention and early treatment of anaphylaxis
Cimetidine	5-10 mg/kg PO[65]	Common marmosets/*Helicobacter*
	10 mg/kg PO, IM q8h[6]	Monkeys/gastrointestinal ulceration
	300 mg/animal PO, IM, slow IV q6-8h[6]	Chimpanzees
Cisapride	0.15 mg/kg PO q12h[40]	Orangutan (n=1)/not commercially available; must be compounded
Dapsone	50 mg/animal PO q24h; 100 mg/animal PO q24h[6]	Chimpanzees/use higher dose with *Mycobacterium leprae* (leprosy)
Deslorelin (Suprelorin, Virbac)	1-2 (6 mg) implants SC[53]	Lion-tailed macaques/reduce aggression (6 mg); only the 4.7 mg implant is commercially available in the United States
	4.7 mg SC implant effective for 6 mo; 9.4 mg SC implant effective for 12 mo[65,124]	GnRH antagonist implant; need secondary contraception of megesterol acetate (not medroxyprogesterone acetate) for 7 days prior to and postimplantation; only the 4.7 mg implant is commercially available in the United States
Dexamethasone	0.25-1 mg/kg PO, IM q24h[6]	Monkeys
	0.5-2 mg/kg SC, IM, IV once[56]	Cerebral edema
Digoxin	0.002-0.012 mg/kg PO, IM, IV divided q12-24h[6,56]	Monkeys/maintenance dose
	0.005-0.01 mg/kg PO q12h or IV prn[6]	Chimpanzees
	0.01 mg/kg PO q24h[65]	Common marmosets/congestive heart failure
Diphenhydramine	5 mg/kg/day PO, IM,[43] IV, daily total may be divided q6-8h[6]	Monkeys, lemurs
	25-50 mg/animal PO, IM, IV q6-8h[6]	Chimpanzees

Continued

TABLE 13-7 Miscellaneous Agents Used in Primates. (cont'd)

Agent	Dosage	Species/Comments
Dobutamine	2.5-10 µg/kg/min IV constant rate infusion[6]	Chimpanzees, monkeys/adrenergic β_1 agonist; increases cardiac output
Docusate sodium (DSS)	10-40 mg/animal PO[6]	Monkeys
	50-200 mg/animal PO[6]	Chimpanzees
Dopamine	2-5 µg/kg/min IV constant rate infusion[6]	Chimpanzees, monkeys/low to moderate doses; positive inotropic effects and renal vasodilation
	2-10 µg/kg/min IV constant rate infusion[25]	Great apes/stimulates dopaminergic, α and β adrenergic receptors; positive inotrope that significantly can improve blood pressures intraoperatively
	5-15 µg/kg/min IV constant rate infusion[6]	Monkeys
Doxapram	2 mg/kg IV[6]	Chimpanzees/respiratory stimulant
Duloxetine	30-60 mg/kg PO q12h[82]	Drill (n=1)/serotonin-norepinephrine reuptake inhibitor
Enalapril	0.015-0.125 mg/kg PO q12-24h[95]	Gorilla (n=1)/antihypertensive
	0.3 mg/kg PO, IV q24h[6,56]	Chimpanzees/ACE inhibitor; balanced vasodilator
	0.5 mg/kg PO q48h[65]	Common marmosets
Enoxaparin sodium	20 mg/animal SC q24h × 10 days, repeat in 2 mo[140]	Rhesus macaque (n=1)/deep vein thrombosis; low-molecular-weight heparin
Ephedrine	0.1-0.5 mg/animal SC, IM, IV, IC[6]	Monkeys
	1.25-2.5 mg/kg IV[115]	Macaques, baboons/vasopressor; safest during maternal hypotension
	2.5 mg/kg IV bolus[115]	Use when hypotension is accompanied by bradycardia
Epinephrine	0.1-0.5 mg/animal SC, IM, IV, IC[6]	Monkeys
	0.2-0.4 mg/kg diluted in 5 mL sterile water,[65] IT if ≥3 kg or 1:10,000 dilution[47]	Common marmosets/cardiac arrest
	0.2-1 mg/animal SC, IM; 0.5-10 mg IV, IC[6]	Chimpanzees
Erythropoietin	50-100 U/kg SC, IV 3 ×/wk[56]	Stimulates division and differentiation of red blood cells; once desired PCV is reached, administer q7d × ≥4 wk for maintenance
Exenatide (Bydureon, AstroZeneca)	0.13 mg/kg SC q30d[66]	Tamarins/n=1; glucagon-like peptide-1 mimetic; extended release; treatment of diabetes mellitus in NHP that do not respond to oral antihyperglycemics and in which daily SC insulin is not feasible

TABLE 13-7 Miscellaneous Agents Used in Primates. (cont'd)

Agent	Dosage	Species/Comments
Famotidine	0.5-0.8 mg/kg PO q24h[56]	Management of gastric and duodenal ulcers and esophagitis; more potent than cimetidine, but has poorer PO bioavailability (37%)
Fluids	Initial fluids IV, 4 mL/kg/h up to 10 kg (add 2 mL/kg/h for additional mass); renal and gastrointestinal loss, calculate for insensible losses (300-400 mL/m²/day) plus measured losses in 4-hr increments[114]	Appropriate choices of fluids to start are D5W 0.45% saline or lactated Ringer's to start and adjust with chemistries and electrolyte/blood gas parameters
	Severe volume depletion (acute blood loss), IV isotonic fluid bolus at 20-60 mL/kg; hypoglycemia should be corrected at 0.25 g/kg (2.5 mL/kg of 10% dextrose or 1 mL/kg of 25% dextrose) with reassessment after administration[78,110]	Off-label extrapolation and usage from pediatric medicine
Folic acid	15 µg/kg PO q24h[6]	Monkeys
	500 µg/kg PO[6]	Chimpanzees
Furosemide	1-2 mg/kg PO, IM, IV[6]	Chimpanzees/diuresis; congestive heart failure; pulmonary edema
	1-4 mg/kg PO, SC q12h[65]	Common marmosets/congestive heart failure
	1-4 mg/kg IV[6]	Monkeys
	2-4 mg/kg IM q8h[6]	Monkeys
Glipizide	0.38-2 mg/kg PO q12h[53]	Ring-tailed lemurs, Bengal slow loris/may combine with other oral hypoglycemics
Glycopyrrolate	—	Decreases oral and bronchial secretions; helps manage bradycardia caused by potent opioids
	0.004 mg/kg IM, IV[6]	Chimpanzees
	0.004-0.008 mg/kg IM[6]	Monkeys
	0.005-0.01 mg/kg IM[29,115]	Macaques, baboons, chimpanzees
	0.01 mg/kg IM[22,29]	Rhesus macaques, orangutans
	1 mg/animal PO q8h[6]	Chimpanzees
GnRH immunocontraceptive vaccine (GonaCon, USDA Wildlife Services)	500 µg dose IM[38]	Vervet monkeys/1 of 3 monkeys (adjuvant 1) cycled at 33 wk; 3 of 3 monkeys (adjuvant 2) cycled 25 wk; both had localized swelling at injection site
Guaifenesin	10-20 mL PO q4-6h[6]	Chimpanzees
Heparin	5000-10,000 units IV q6h[6]	Chimpanzees
	10,000-20,000 units SC q12h[6]	

Continued

TABLE 13-7 Miscellaneous Agents Used in Primates. (cont'd)

Agent	Dosage	Species/Comments
Human chorionic gonadotropin (hCG)	250 U/animal IM once[56]	Induces follicular maturation, ovulation, and development of the corpus luteum in females; stimulates testosterone production in males[56]
	5000-10,000 U IM[6]	Chimpanzees
Hydrochlorothiazide	1 mg/kg PO q24h[6]	Chimpanzees
Hydrocortisone sodium succinate	5 mg/kg IM, IV q12h[6]	Chimpanzees
Insulin, NPH	0.1 U/animal SC q12h[65]	Common marmosets/glucose monitoring
	0.25-0.5 U/kg SC q24h[6]	Chimpanzees/starting dose; diabetes mellitus; diabetic ketoacidosis
	0.5 U/kg SC q24h[109]	New World monkeys (*Cebus*)/advisable to start with this dose and reevaluate with blood glucose
Iohexol (nonionic iodinated contrast)	3 mL/kg IV[133]	Rhesus monkey/CT scan
Iron dextran	10 mg/kg IM q7d[6]	Monkeys
	11-22 mg/kg IM[6]	Chimpanzees
Isoproterenol	0.05-2 μg/kg/min IV constant rate infusion[6]	Monkeys/nonselective β-adrenergic agonist
	0.1-1 μg/kg/min IV constant rate infusion or 0.02-0.06 mg IV bolus[6]	Chimpanzees
Lactulose	0.25-1.1 mL/kg PO q8-12h[65]	Common marmosets
Leuprolide acetate (Lupron, Abbott)	Effective contraception for 1-6 mo[124]	New World primates/GnRH antagonist implant; need secondary contraception of megesterol acetate (not medroxyprogesterone) for 7 days prior to and post implant placement
	0.3 mg/kg IM q4wk[6]	
	3.75 mg/animal suspension q30d × 6 mo[63]	Allen's swamp monkey (n=1)/uterine fibroids and ovarian cysts
Levothyroxine	0.05 mg/animal PO q24h; incremental changes of 0.025 mg q24h at 30-day intervals up to 0.1 mg q24h[83]	Gorilla (n=1)/hypothyroidism; monitor TSH and T_4 q6-8wk
Lidocaine	0.7-1.4 mg/kg IV prn[6]	Monkeys
	1-1.5 mg/kg IV[6] prn	Chimpanzees/maximum of 3 mg/kg
	1-2 mg/kg IV bolus[65,115]	Common marmosets
	20-50 μg/kg/min IV constant rate infusion[115]	Ventricular arrhythmia
Liraglutide	0.015 mg SC q24h[117a]	Macaques/diabetes; longer-acting GLP-1R agonists available
Lisinopril	0.25-0.5 mg/kg PO q24h[6]	Chimpanzees
Loperamide	0.04 mg/kg PO q8h[6]	Monkeys
	4 mg/animal PO prn[6]	Chimpanzees

TABLE 13-7 Miscellaneous Agents Used in Primates. (cont'd)

Agent	Dosage	Species/Comments
Mannitol (25%)	0.25-0.5 g/kg IV over 5-10 min[6]	Monkeys/diuretic
	0.5-1 g/kg IV constant rate infusion[6]	Chimpanzees
	1.65-2.2 g/kg IV over 20 min[6]	Monkeys/cerebral edema
Maropitant	1 mg/kg SC,[136] IV[110]	Macaques, siamangs/reduction of emesis
Medroxyprogesterone acetate (Depo-Provera, Pfizer)	2.5-5 mg/kg IM[124]	Old World primates/contraception for 45-90 days; higher doses for smaller species
	5 mg/kg IM q40-60d[53]	Lemurs/seasonal contraceptive; may last longer in other species
	5 mg/kg IM[11,124]	Prosimians/contraception for 30-45 days, during breeding season (Nov-Mar)
	5-10 mg/animal PO q24h × 5-10 days[6]	Monkeys/contraceptive
	20 mg/kg IM[124]	New World primates/contraception for 30 days
	150 mg/animal IM q3mo[6] or q30d[37]	Chimpanzees, monkeys/contraceptive; rhesus macaques/endometriosis
Megestrol acetate	800 mg/animal PO q24h[6]	Chimpanzees
Melengestrol acetate implant (MGA, WildPharm)	—	Implant must not be autoclaved; can be ethylene oxide sterilized, then degassed for 2 wk before surgical placement; available only in United States
	0.06 g/kg[124]	Great apes, gibbons
	0.1 g/kg[124]	Old World primates, except Colobinae (0.15 g/kg)
	0.25 g/kg[124]	Lemurs
	0.4 g/kg[124]	Howler monkeys
	0.5 g/kg[124]	Spider monkeys, saki monkeys, cebids
	0.7 g/kg[124]	New World primates other than howler, spider, saki, capuchin, squirrel monkeys/not recommended in *Callimico*
	1 g/kg[124]	Squirrel monkeys
Metformin	5-10 mg/kg PO q12h[65,109]	New World monkeys (i.e., common marmosets)/oral hypoglycemic
Metoclopramide	0.2-0.5 mg/kg PO, IM q8-24h[6,56]	Monkeys/antiemetic; stimulates motility of upper gastrointestinal tract
	0.4 mg/kg PO,[25] IM, slow IV q8-24h[6]	Chimpanzees
Milk thistle (silymarin)	4-15 mg/kg PO q8-12h[65]	Common marmosets

Continued

TABLE 13-7 Miscellaneous Agents Used in Primates. (cont'd)

Agent	Dosage	Species/Comments
Mirtazapine	0.5 mg/kg transdermal (topically) to aura pinnae q24h × 14 days[94]	Macaques/hyporexia; appetite stimulant
Misoprostol	5 µg/kg PO q6h; 1-3 µg/kg intravaginal[6]	Chimpanzees
Mupirocin (2% ointment; Bactroban, Hanall Biopharma)	Apply ointment to nares q24h[76]	Cynomolgus macaques/useful in treating methicillin-resistant *Staphylococcus aureus*; use sterile dry swabs
Nitroglycerin (2% ointment)	3 mm topically q12-24h[65]	Common marmosets/congestive heart failure
	7.5 mg topically q8h[6]	Chimpanzees
Nitroprusside	0.3-10 µg/kg/min IV constant rate infusion[6]	Chimpanzees
Norepinephrine	0.05-0.1 µg/kg/min IV constant rate infusion[115]	Hypotension
	0.2-0.4 µg/kg/min IV constant rate infusion[6]	Chimpanzees
Omeprazole	0.4 mg/kg PO q12h × 10 days[130]	Macaques/management of gastric and duodenal ulcers and esophagitis; quadruple treatment of *Helicobacter pylori;* see amoxicillin (TABLE 13-1)
Ondansetron	0.1 mg/kg slow IV q24h[110]	Monkeys/nausea, antiemetic; sedation common side effect
	1 mg/kg SC q24h[110]	
	4 mg/animal PO prophylaxis 30 min[52]	Macaques/antiemetic
Oxytocin	0.5-1 U/min IV constant rate infusion[6]	Chimpanzees
	1-2 U/animal IM, IV q20min × 4 doses[56,65]	Common marmosets
	2 U/animal prn[6]	Monkeys
	5-30 U/animal SC, IV prn[6]	Chimpanzees
PGF_2 alpha	1 mg/kg IM q24h[6]	Monkeys
Phentolamine mesylate	5-10 mg SC, IV[6]	Chimpanzees/antihypertensive
Phenylephrine	1-2 µg/kg IV bolus, followed by 0.5-1 µg/kg/min IV constant rate infusion[115]	Drug of choice to treat isoflurane-induced hypotension
Pimobendan	0.2 mg/kg PO q24h[65]	Common marmosets/congestive heart failure
Polysulfated glycosaminoglycan (Adequan, Luitpold Pharmaceuticals)	2 mg/kg IM q3-5d × 2-3 mo[6]	Monkeys/chondroprotective agent in the adjunctive management of arthritis
	2-3 mg/kg IM q4d × 2 mo[6]	Chimpanzees

TABLE 13-7 Miscellaneous Agents Used in Primates. (cont'd)

Agent	Dosage	Species/Comments
Potassium chloride	0.5-1 mmol (mEq)/kg/h IV[6]	Chimpanzees, monkeys
	20-100 mmol (mEq) PO q24h[6]	Chimpanzees, monkeys
Prednisolone sodium succinate	1 mg/kg PO q24h[65]	Common marmosets/myelofibrosis
	10 mg/kg IM, IV[6,103]	Chimpanzees, monkeys, lemurs
Prednisone	0.5 mg/kg PO, SC, IM q24h[56]	Antiinflammatory
	≤2 mg/kg PO, SC, IM q24h[56]	Allerg, autoimmune disease
Probencid	1 g/animal PO q12h × 7 days[6]	Chimpanzees
Procainamide	12.5 mg/kg PO q6h[6]	Chimpanzees
Prochlorperazine	0.12 mg/kg IM, IV[6]	Monkeys/antiemetic
	5-10 mg PO, IM, IV q8-24h[6]	Chimpanzees
Propanolol	0.25-1 mg/kg PO q8-12h[6]	Chimpanzees
Quinidine	100-200 mg/animal PO q8-12h[6]	Chimpanzees
Ranitidine	0.5 mg/kg PO q12h[6]	Monkeys/management of gastric and duodenal ulcers and esophagitis
	150 mg/animal PO q8-12h[6]	Chimpanzees
Ribavirin	150 mg/kg IM q24h × 6 days[50]	Callitrichid hepatitis virus
S-adenosylme-thionine (SAM-e) (Denosyl, Nutramax)	18 mg/kg PO q24h[6]	Chimpanzees
Spironolactone	20-300 mg/day divided q8-24h[6]	Chimpanzees
Stanozolol	—	Anabolic steroid; no longer marketed in the United States; improves appetite and promotes weight gain; rarely indicated; little evidence for efficacy increasing appetite
	2 mg/animal PO q6-8h[6]	Chimpanzees
	5-10 mg/kg IM q4-7d[6]	Monkeys
Sucralfate	0.5 g/animal PO; maintenance, q12h; active ulcer, q6h × 4-6 wk[6]	Monkeys/prevent or treat esophageal, gastric, and duodenal ulcers
	1 g/animal PO q12h[6]	Chimpanzees
Telmisartan	1 mg/kg PO[65]	Common marmosets/protein-losing nephropathy
Terbutaline	0.05 mg/kg IM, IV[25]	Great apes/bronchodilator
	5 mg/animal PO q24h[6]	Chimpanzees
Theophylline	5 mg/kg, then 2-4 mg/kg PO q6-8h[6]	Chimpanzees

Continued

TABLE 13-7 Miscellaneous Agents Used in Primates. (cont'd)

Agent	Dosage	Species/Comments
Triamcinolone	0.2-2 mg/kg IM prn[6]	Monkeys
Vitamin B_{12}	0.7 µg q24h x 3 mo[59]	Marmosets/marmoset wasting syndrome
	3-5 mL PO, IM, IV[6]	Chimpanzees
Vitamin C (ascorbic acid)	—	Vitamin C is an essential nutrient for nonhuman primates; useful in times of increased oxidative stress, in cachexic patients, and in those requiring nutritional support
	1-4 mg/kg PO q24h[65,101]	Scurvy should be treated with 25-50 mg/kg daily until clinical signs resolve and dietary consumption of adequate vitamin C is restored
	3-6 mg/kg PO q24h to prevent scurvy[109]	
	4-25 mg/kg PO q24h[6]	Chimpanzees
	25 mg/kg PO q12h[56]	
	30 mg/kg IM q24h[6]	Monkeys
	30-100 mg/kg PO, SC q24h[56]	
Vitamin D_3	—	Vitamin D is an essential nutrient for nonhuman primates;[14] elevated concentration that is not D_2 is required for New World primates; useful in management of hypocalcemia
	20 U/kg PO q24h[6]	Chimpanzees
	125 U/100g diet[101]	New World primates, callitrichids/UVB light
	2000 U/kg PO[65]	Common marmosets
	5000 U ergocalciferol depot (sesame oil) IM once at age 4 mo and ergocalciferol 400 U PO q24h from age 4 mo until weaning[68]	Infant chimpanzees/prevention of rickets
Vitamin E	3.75 U/kg IM q3d w/Se (1.15 mg/kg) IM q24h × 30 days[56]	Myopathy
	3.75 U/kg PO q24h[6]	Chimpanzees
Vitamin K_1	—	Used in treating toxicity due to coumarin and its derivatives; vitamin K_1 deficiencies; prolonged anorexia
	1 mg/kg PO, IM q8h[6]	Chimpanzees
	1-5 mg/animal IM q24h[6]	Monkeys
Zinc	2.5 mg/animal PO q24h × 3 days[6]	Monkeys
	75 mg PO q12h prn[6]	Chimpanzees

TABLE 13-8 Hematologic and Serum Biochemical Values of Primates.[26,49,61,65,80,86,98,128,132,134,143,148]

Measurement	Baboon (*Papio* sp.)	Capuchin Monkey (*Cebus* sp.)	Chimpanzee (*Pan troglodytes*)	Common Marmoset (*Callithrix jacchus*)[b]	Guenon (*Cercopithecus* sp.)	Pygmy Marmoset (*Cebuella pygmaea*)
Hematology[a]						
PCV (%)	45	45-53	38-51	M=43; F=41	40 (30-53)	42 (26-56)
RBC (10^6/μL)	4.5-4.8	6	4.7-6.4	M=5.7; F=5.7	5.2 (4.1-6.9)	6.4 (3.9-8.6)
Hgb (g/dL)	13	14-17	7.6-10.7	M=16.1; F=15.0	13.1 (10.0-17.3)	13.3 (7.9-17.7)
WBC (10^3/μL)	14.1	5-24	7.3-15.7	M=8.1; F=7.4	5.9 (2.1-13.9)	7.7 (2.8-16.7)
Neutrophils (%)	60.5	55	3.0-10.7[a]	M=43; F=54	38 (5-81)	58.5 (23.8-83.7)
Lymphocytes (%)	36	41	2.0-7.3[a]	M=51; F=40	52 (16-82)	37.5 (8.8-77.3)
Monocytes (%)	1.5	1.8	65-572[a]	M=3.3; F=3.6	5 (1-13)	3.1 (0.0-9.6)
Eosinophils (%)	1.5	1.6	69-630[a]	M=0.4; F=0.5	4 (0-17)	2.2 (0.0-9.5)
Basophils (%)	0.4	<1	0-24[a]	M=0.8; F=1.5	1 (0-3)	0.9 (0.0-6.8)
Platelets (10^3/μL)	406	108-187	130-379	M=281; F=281	343 (59-653)	488 (137-894)
Chemistries						
ALP (U/L)	248 ± 152	M=35-891; F=31-835	95 (39-443)	80 (44-115)	173 (31-625)	172 (13-484)
ALT (U/L)	12-20	13-43	20.5-62.1	8.9 (3.8-14.0)	58 (20-150)	15 (2-50)
Amylase (U/L)	243 ± 78	M=37-918; F=38-771	33 (9-93)	231 (175-288)	253 (101-447)	417
AST (U/L)	22-28	21-57	12.1-56.6	125 (88-161)	46 (14-109)	44 (5-134)
Bilirubin (mg/dL)	0.3-0.4	0-4	0.2-0.6	0.2 (0.1-0.2)	0.3 (0.1-0.9)	0.2 (0.0-0.7)
BUN (mg/dL)	8-14	24-44	8.3-17.8	19.9 (14.2-25.6)	16 (6-32)	17 (5-38)
Calcium (mg/dL)	8-10	10	7.8-10.5	9.0 (7.6-10.5)	9 (8-10)	9.2 (6.0-12.8)

Continued

TABLE 13-8 Hematologic and Serum Biochemical Values of Primates. (cont'd)

Measurement	Baboon (*Papio* sp.)	Capuchin Monkey (*Cebus* sp.)	Chimpanzee (*Pan troglodytes*)	Common Marmoset (*Callithrix jacchus*)[b]	Guenon (*Cercopithecus* sp.)	Pygmy Marmoset (*Cebuella pygmaea*)
Chloride (mmol/L)	99 ± 4	108 ± 2	103(94-11)	108 (102-113)	110 (100-119)	107 (80-124)
Cholesterol (mg/dL)	60-134	170-254	167-296	148 (88-197)	128 (73-228)	164 (52-323)
CK (U/L)	39 ± 175	M=115-1009; F=131-964	179 (56-689)	281 (77-1802)	453 (45-1536)	600 (62-2056)
Creatinine (mg/dL)	1 ± 0.3	M=35-130; F=32-116	1 (0.5-1.5)	0.2 (0.1-0.4)	0.8 (0.4-1.3)	0.5 (0.1-1.1)
GGT (U/L)	39 ± 11	M=23-94; F=33-132	26 (10-58)	6.0 (0.7-11.3)	151 (56-313)	10 (0.0-36)
Glucose (mg/dL)	80-95	44-94	66-118	113 (70-156)	119 (43-249)	148 (18-318)
Lipase (U/L)	5 ± 4	M=52-124; F=51-164	30 (1-70)	33 (18-48)	128 (16-249)	—
Phosphorus (mg/dL)	5.5-8.5	7	1.5-4.9	3.6 (2.7-4.5)	5.0 (5.8-9.6)	5.9 (1.7-15.5)
Potassium (mmol/L)	3.9 ± 0.6	M=2.3-6.6; F=2.9-5.7	3.9 (2.8-5.3)	3.1 (2.7-3.5)	3.8 (2.7-5.6)	3.8 (1.9-7.1)
Protein, total (g/dL)	6-7	7.5-8.7	6.7-8.4	5.8 (5.2-6.4)	6.3 (4.9-7.4)	6.5 (4.1-9.3)
Globulin (g/dL)	3.6 ± 0.6	—	3.6 (2.3-5.1)	3.3 (3.3-4.2)	2.1 (0.1-3.5)	2.4 (0.7-4.2)
Sodium (mmol/L)	149 ± 3	M=130-163; F=140-158	141 (133-151)	149 (147-153)	151 (141-163)	150 (123-163)
Triglyceride (mg/dL)	66 ± 16	M=13-214; F=19-197	90 (33-221)	42 (22-102)	100 (18-436)	137

Measurement	Rhesus Macaque (*Macaca mulatta*)	Ring-tailed Lemur (*Lemur catta*)	Spider Monkey (*Ateles* spp.)	Squirrel Monkey (*Saimiri sciureus*)	Tamarin (*Saguinus* spp.)
Hematology					
PCV (%)	39-43	44-57	35-40	43-56	45
RBC (10^6/μL)	4.5-6	6.7-8.6	5.5	7.1-10.9	6.6

TABLE 13-8 Hematologic and Serum Biochemical Values of Primates. (cont'd)

Measurement	Rhesus Macaque (*Macaca mulatta*)	Ring-tailed Lemur (*Lemur catta*)	Spider Monkey (*Ateles* spp.)	Squirrel Monkey (*Saimiri sciureus*)	Tamarin (*Saguinus* spp.)
Hgb (g/dL)	12.7	13.8-17.2	16	12.9-17	15.5
WBC (10^3/µL)	11.5-12.4	4.8-12.5	10-12	5.1-10.9	12.6-14.4
Neutrophils (%)	20-56	1.2-7.5[a]	52	36-66	43-64
Lymphocytes (%)	40-76	1.7-5.7[a]	40	27-55	34-49
Monocytes (%)	0-2	0-0.8[a]	3	0-6	2-5
Eosinophils (%)	1-3	0-0.7[a]	5	0-11	1-1.2
Basophils (%)	0-1	0-0.1[a]	0-1	<1	0.1
Platelets (10^3/µL)	130-144	161-379	239-343	112	331-650
Chemistries					
ALP (U/L)	956 ± 460	114 ± 42	45-449	358 ± 175	25-448
ALT (U/L)	145-171	36-154	8-78	59-99	7-14
Amylase (U/L)	—	1034 ± 183	87-1270	516 ± 189	0-2146
AST (U/L)	20-34	12-80	42-210	56-118	49-59
Bilirubin (mg/dL)	0.1-0.7	0.2-1	0.1-1.0	0.1-0.5	0.1-0.3
BUN (mg/dL)	14-20	13-29	26	23-39	6-12
Calcium (mg/dL)	8-11	8.8-10.4	13	8-10	10
Chloride (mmol/L)	107 ± 4	104 ± 4	95-113	—	97-118
Cholesterol (mg/dL)	94-162	1.6-3.0	76-278	127-207	69
CK (U/L)	—	4508 ± 2960	0-939	562 ± 1380	—
Creatinine (mg/dL)	0.7 ± 0.2	M=72 ± 14; F=80 ± 18	0.4-1.5	0.9 ± 0.2	0.2-1.2
GGT (U/L)	73 ± 20	13.4 ± 3.7	0-20	56 ± 150	0-14
Glucose (mg/dL)	53-87	66-222	82	52-108	125-189
LDH (U/L)	201-665	—	0-1578	271-490	0-1578
Lipase (U/L)	—	45 ± 31	42 (3-82)	—	—
Phosphorus (mg/dL)	4-6	3.3-6.7	2.1-8.5	3.3-7.7	3-6
Potassium (mmol/L)	3.6 ± 0.4	M=3.3 ± 0.6; F=3.7 ± 0.6	2.9(2.6-3.2)	5.7 ± 1.0	2.2-6.4
Protein, total (g/dL)	6.1-7.1	6.5-8.1	10.2	6.9-8.1	6.2-8.6
Globulin (g/dL)	—	15 ± 4	0.9-4.3	—	1.4-5.8
Sodium (mmol/L)	145 ± 4	145 ± 6.7 143 ± 3	134(86-182)	150 ± 7	132-163
Triglyceride (mg/dL)	67 ± 47	43 ± 10	34-204	75 ± 33	—

[a]These values are reported as absolute differential as 10^3/µL for more accuracy when they were available.
[b]Data from reference 3 includes ranges from ±2 standard deviations of the mean (in parenthesis); n=41.[80]

TABLE 13-9 Biologic and Physiologic Data of Primates.[7,26,29,47,98,123,143]

Measurement	Baboon (*Papio* sp.)	Capuchin Monkey (*Cebus* sp.)	Chimpanzee (*Pan troglodytes*)	Common Marmoset (*Callithrix jacchus*)	Rhesus Macaque (*Macaca mulatta*)	Ring-tailed Lemur (*Lemur catta*)	Spider Monkey (*Ateles* sp.)	Squirrel Monkey (*Saimiri sciureus*)	Tamarin (*Saguinus* sp.)
Temperature°C (°F)	37-39 (98.6-103.1)	37-38.5 (98.6-101.3)	34.6-38.7 (94.3-101.7)	38.4-39.1 (101.1-102.4)	37-39 (98.6-103.1)	37.9-38.1 (100.2-100.6)	—	37-38.5 (98.6-101.3)	—
Respiratory (breaths/min)	22-35	30-50	20-60	36-44	35-50	30-60	—	20-50	—
Heart rate (beats/min)	85-90	165-225	60-200	204-399	98-122	168-210	—	200-350	—
Avg adult wt (kg) M/F	14-41; males 50% larger	3.5-3.9/2.5-3	45-90/40-80	0.34-0.35	6-11/4-9	2-3	6-10/6-8	0.75-1.1	0.225-0.9
Estrus length (days)	32-36	18-23	28-53	16-30	24-40	39	26	7-16	15
Gestation (days)	154-193	180	215-239	141-145	144-210	130-136	225-232	140-180	140
Weaning age (days)	180-450	270	1440	40-120	210-420	90-120	365	180	60-90
Median life expectancy (yr)	30-45	50	31.7-37.4	8-12	18-23.8	16.5	24.4	14.6	11.5

TABLE 13-10 Identifying Characteristics of Small Nonhuman Primates by their Taxonomic Classification.[26,47,123,143]

Characteristic	Prosimians	New World Monkeys (Platyrrhini)	Old World Monkeys (Catarrhini)
Tapetum	Yes	—	—
Moist rhinarium	Yes	—	—
Specialized scent glands	Yes	—	—
Uterus	Bicornuate	Simplex	Simplex
Placenta	Epitheliochorial	Hemochorial	Hemochorial
Closed orbits	—	Yes	Yes
Incisor comb	Yes	—	—
Dental formula	2.1.3.3./2.1.3.3. (36)	2.1.3.3./2.1.3.3. (36)	2.1.2.3./2.1.2.3. (32)
Grooming claw	Yes	—	—
Prehensile tail	—	Yes	—
Nostrils	At end of rhinarium	Round, directed laterally	Narrowed, directed ventrally
Claws or nails	Claws	Claws	Nails
Ischial callosities	—	—	Yes

TABLE 13-11 Venous Access Sites and Average Volumes Drawn (Healthy Animals).[33,109,132]

Common Marmoset (*Callithrix jacchus*)	Ring-tailed Lemur (*Lemur catta*)	Squirrel Monkey (*Saimiri sciureus*)	Tufted Capuchin (*Cebus apella*)
Femoral, jugular veins; 0.5-1% total body weight; maximum one-time sample; ex: 1-3 mL (adults)	Femoral, saphenous, jugular veins; maximum sample size 0.5-1% total body weight (one sample); ex: 5-10 mL (adult male)	Femoral, saphenous veins; maximum sample size not to exceed 0.5-1% total body weight (one sample); ex: 2-4 mL (adults)	Femoral, saphenous, cephalic, jugular veins; maximum sample size not to exceed 0.5-1% total body weight (one sample); ex: 2.7-6 mL (adults)

TABLE 13-12 Urinalysis Values of Primates.[a,16,27,80,86,88,108–110,132]

Measurement	Chimpanzee (*Pan troglodytes verus*)	Common Marmoset (*Callithrix jacchus*)	Cynomolgus Monkey (*Macaca fascicularis*)	Goeldi's Monkey (*Callimico goeldii*)	Rhesus Macaque (*Macaca mulatta*)	Squirrel Monkey (*Saimiri peruviensis*)	White-handed Gibbon (*Hylobates lar*)
Specific gravity	—	1.026	1.010-1.030	1.011-1.025	1.013	—	—
Glucose (mg/dL)	Negative	Negative-trace	1.6-3.6	Negative	Negative	0-1+	50
Ketones (mg/dL)	Negative	Negative	Negative	Negative	Negative	0-2+	Negative
Bilirubin (mg/dL)	Negative	Negative	Negative	Negative	Negative	Negative	Negative
Blood (RBC/uL)	Negative-80 (increased with menstruation)	Negative-+++	Negative	Negative	Negative	0-4+	Negative-trace
Urobilinogen (mg/dL)	Negative-0.2	Normal	Normal	Normal	0.2	Negative	Normal
pH	5-9	5-8.5	5-9	6-8.5	7.9	6-8.5	5-9 (mean 7.5)
Urine protein:creatinine (UPC)	—	12.3	0.003-0.160	0.1	—	0.13-2.36	—
Protein (mg/dL)	Negative-3	0-1.3	0.16-7.88	1+	Negative	9-53	Negative
Leukocytes/µL	Negative-500 (higher in F in estrus)	0-2	Negative	0-2	Negative	0-1+	Negative-positive

[a]Free-catch (dipstick) ± quantitative (RBC, leukocytes, UPC).

TABLE 13-13 Blood Gas Values and Lactate of Primates.[32,49,99,132,139]

Blood Gas Measurement (arterial, unless indicates venous)	Baboon (*Papio hamadryas, Papio cynocephalus*)	Capuchin (*Sapajus apella*) (propofol vs tiletamine/ zolazepam)	Cynomolgus Monkey (*Macaca fascicularis*)	Ring-tailed Lemur (*Lemur catta*) (venous)	Siamang (*Symphalangus syndactylus*)	Spider Monkey (*Ateles* sp.)	Squirrel Monkey (*Saimiri sciureus*)
pH	7.2	7.24 ± 0.06 7.19 ± -0.02	7.4 ± 0.05	—	7.33	7.29	7.20 ± 0.02
pCO_2 (mmHg)	66.4	47.7 ± 9.7 48.0 ± 3.5	36.2 ± 4.2	—	42.2	43.6	23.5 ± 1.6
pO_2 (mmHg)	85.6	476 ± 64 598 ± 47	90.5 ± 9.2	—	153	88.4	114.0 ± 2.9
HCO_3 (mmol/L)	22.1	19.4 ± 3.3 17.7 ± 1.1	22.8 ± 3.3	—	21.3	20.7	8.9 ± 0.4
Base excess (BE) (mmol/L)	-0.7	-6.9 ± 3.2 -9.1 ± 1.0	-2.2 ± 4.1	—	—	—	-17.2 ± 0.5
TCO_2 (mmol/L)	24.2	—	23.2 ± 4.0	25.7 ± 3.3	22.6	22.1	9.6 ± 0.4
AnGap (mmol/L)	—	—	16.2 ± 3.6	22.6 ± 1.3	—	—	—
O_2SAT (%)	96.1	99.9 ± 0.1 99.8 ± 0.1	96.8 ± 0.9	—	—	—	95.8 ± 0.7
Na^+ (mmol/L)	137	147 ± 6 151 ± 3	148 ± 3	144 ± 3	—	135-150	150 ± 7
Cl^- (mmol/L)	—	—	108 ± 2	100 ± 5	—	95-113	—
K^+ (mmol/L)	3.2	4.6 ± 1.2 5.2 ± 0.6	3.7 ± 0.4	3.6 ± 0.5	—	2.2-6.4	5.7 ± 1.0
Ca^{++} (mg/dL), total serum	—	8.4 ± 0.4 8.4 ± 0.4	4.1 ± 0.3	7.6 ± 0.4	—	7.9-10.9	9.6 ± 0.1
Lactate (mmol/L)	—	0.6 ± 0.01 0.77 ± 0.28	—	—	—	—	—

TABLE 13-14 Clotting Parameters of Primates.[2,120,132]

Clotting Parameters	African Green Monkey (*Chlorocebus aethiops*)	Baboon (*Papio* sp.)	Common Marmoset (*Callithrix jacchus*)	Cynomolgus Monkey (*Macaca fasicularis*)	Ring-tailed Lemur (*Lemur catta*)	Squirrel Monkey (*Saimiri sciureus*)	Tamarin (*Sanguinus labiatus*)
Antithrombin III (sec)	—	—	—	11.7	—	—	—
Clotting times (glass) (min)	3	3.1	—	—	—	2	—
Fibrinogen (mg/dL)	—	—	215-399 (mean=307)	245	—	—	230-560 (mean=390)
Partial thromboplastin time (PTT) (sec)	24.2	36.5	M=35.7; F=36.3	28.2	29	25.4	M=31.7; F=32.7
Platelets × $10^3/mm^2$	308 ± 82	297 ± 117	298-682 (mean=490)	354 ± 76	240	516 ± 67	296-564 (mean=430)
Prothrombin (PT) (sec)	13.5	16.2	M=5.7; F=5.6	11.7	12	8.3	M=7.1; F=7.1

TABLE 13-15 ECG Intervals and Durations.[9,65,126]

Species	P Wave Duration (sec)	PR Interval (sec)	QT Interval (sec)	QRS Duration (sec)
Baboon (*Papio* sp.)	0.02-0.06	0.05-0.09	0.13-0.19	0.01-0.05
Capuchin monkey (*Cebus* sp.)	0.02-0.04	0.07-0.09	0.14-0.16	0.01-0.03
Chimpanzee (*Pan troglodytes*)	<0.12	0.104-0.242	0.327-0.445	0.059-0.103
Common marmoset (*Callithrix jacchus*)	0.021-0.029	0.052-0.062	0.088-0.156	—
Rhesus macaque (*Macaca mulatta*)	0.03-0.05	0.08-0.1	0.18-0.22	0.02-0.04
Squirrel monkey (*Saimiri sciureus*)	0.02-0.04	0.05-0.07	0.14-0.16	0.01-0.03

TABLE 13-16 Preventive Medicine Recommendations for Primates.[1,26,57,60,65,98]

Procedure	Schedule	Comments
Routine examination	Annually for small or medium nonhuman primates; q2-3yr for great apes	Routine: physical examination, hemogram, serum biochemical analysis, serum banking, rectal culture, mycobacterial screening, radiographs, ultrasound By institution history: viral serology, vaccination
	Tuberculin skin testing (Intradermal Mammalian Old Tuberculin, Synbiotics)	Typically, the test is placed intrapalpebrally so test site can be examined without restraint; an alternative site, or used for subsequent screening, is the areolar area; following test placement, test is evaluated visually at 24, 48, and 72 hr; a positive reaction is erythema, edema, induration, or combination of these signs persisting for >48 hr; false-positives (especially in orangutans) and false-negatives (anergic animals) can occur; comparative testing with evaluation of hemogram, comparative antigens (e.g., avian purified protein derivative), thoracic radiographs, mycobacterial culture of tracheal or gastric lavage assists interpretation; imported primates to the United States have testing dictated by Centers for Disease Control and Prevention with three negative intradermal tests required over a 30-day interval; for all caretakers, tuberculin screening for in-contact staff is recommended annually; comparative testing could include serologic testing for gamma interferon, but often this methodology is not available reliably as a commercial test for nonhuman primates; although it is available for humans, these products were not validated for nonhuman primates
	0.05 mL ID via 27 ga needle; test annually[61]	Commonly used dose reduction for callitrichids and similar-sized New World primates; see previous comments
Fecal parasite examination	q3-12mo based on collection history or when abnormal fecal quality is present	Direct wet mount of fresh feces for protozoa; flotation and/or sedimentation procedures for parasite ova; trichrome stains can be used to identify protozoal cysts; direct staining of fecal smears for cell populations
Fecal culture	At collection entry; at routine examination schedule; based on collection history or when abnormal fecal quality is present	Culture for *Salmonella*, *Shigella*, *Campylobacter*, *Yersinia;* may take multiple samples to identify asymptomatic carriers of *Salmonella* or *Shigella*

TABLE 13-17 Immunization Recommendations for Primates.[a]

Species	Immunization	Dose/Schedule	Comments
Prosimians	—	—	There are no specific recommendations for prosimians[144]
	Rabies	—	Killed vaccine only; consider with elevated exposure risk situations[144]
	Tetanus	Tetanus toxoid	Used in some institutions;[144] of note, current preparations are combined with *Diphtheria* prophylaxis
New World primates	Measles	—	Measles in New World primates is a severe disease that may be associated with epizootics of high morbidity and mortality; in callitrichids, the virus targets the intestinal tract;[80] in the United States, only an attenuated measles/mumps/rubella vaccine is available; however, it is rarely recommended due to declined human incidence of this disease and extensive vaccination of humans[26,80]
	Rabies	Volume of vaccine adjusted by body size:[26] callitrichids, 0.05-0.1 mL; medium-sized primates, 0.25 mL;[109] larger primates, 0.5 mL	Used by some institutions in rabies-endemic areas; use only killed virus preparation[109]
		1 mL dose of killed vaccine IM (quadriceps muscle) days 2,7,12,19,33 post exposure and single dose of human rabies immunoglobulin IM 5 days post exposure[75]	Capuchin monkeys/post exposure prophylaxis in monkeys that had direct contact with rabid bats; animals developed and maintained levels of rabies virus neutralizing antibody >0.05 U/mL by 67 days post exposure[75]
	Tetanus	Volume of tetanus toxoid adjusted by body size:[26] callitrichids, 0.05-0.1 mL; medium-sized primates, 0.25 mL; larger primates, 0.5 mL	New World monkeys are susceptible to *Clostridium tetani*;[26] of note, current preparations are combined with *Diphtheria* prophylaxis
Old World primates	Measles	—	In the United States, only an attenuated measles/mumps/rubella vaccine is available; however, it is rarely recommended due to declined human incidence of this disease and extensive vaccination of humans[26]
	Rabies	Volume of vaccine adjusted by body size:[26] medium-sized primates, 0.25 mL; larger primates, 0.5 mL	Used by some institutions in rabies-endemic areas; use only killed virus preparation

Continued

TABLE 13-17 Immunization Recommendations for Primates. (cont'd)

Species	Immunization	Dose/Schedule	Comments
	Tetanus	Volume of tetanus toxoid adjusted by body size:[26] medium-sized primates, 0.25 mL; larger primates, 0.5 mL	Old World monkeys are susceptible to tetanus;[26,135] of note, current preparations are combined with *Diphtheria* prophylaxis
Great apes	Measles	MMR II (live-attenuated product; Merck): 12-15 mo; 4-6 yr of age[98]	Optional;[98] risk of shedding live virus and susceptibility of pregnant females and fetus is unquantified, but rubella component has fetal concerns labeled in pregnant humans; from Attenuvax (Merck) product vaccine, seroconversion occurred in Western lowland gorillas and persisted for at least 11 yr following 1, 2, or 3 vaccinations on individuals at 12 mo, 15 mo, and 10 yr of age or 2 doses separated by 2-4 wk for unvaccinated, seronegative adults[20]
	Polio	Inactivated poliovirus: 2, 4, 6-18 mo; 4-6 yr[98]	Although human adult vaccination in the United States is no longer considered necessary, catchup protocols exist for pediatric patients
	Rabies	—	Used by some institutions in rabies-endemic areas; use only killed virus preparation[98]
	Tetanus	*Diphtheria*, tetanus, pertussis (DTaP): 2, 4, 6, 15-18 mo; 11-12 yr; q10yr[98]	Based on human schedule; of note, current products are combined with *Diphtheria* prophylaxis

[a]Vaccination protocols are highly individualized to institutional risk with considerations of potential exposure, age of animals, outdoor housing, access to humans, and community health profiles of the in-access human population.[98] As of this writing, the SARS-CoV-2 pandemic has affected captive collections of nonhuman primates. Successful vaccine trials using rhesus macaques have been documented. Recent treatment of a captive gorilla population has also been successful with vaccination studies in progress.[4,35] Additionally, killed vaccine products are strongly encouraged whenever possible with caution of live or attenuated products for monitoring for vaccine-induced disease. It also should be noted that immunoprophylaxis products vary with availability to the medical community and human health issues and, therefore, absolute recommendations are not possible. Sources to consider for planning a program-specific approach include: www.cdc.gov, American Academy of Pediatrics publications,[3] *Conn's Current Therapy* (published annually),[23] *AAZV's Infectious Diseases of Concern to Captive and Free-Ranging Animals in North America,*[50] and species care guidelines available on www.aza.org.

TABLE 13-18 Nonhuman Primate Laboratories.

Antech Diagnostics
17672-B Cowan Avenue, Irvine, CA 92614, USA
ANTECH West: 1-800-745-4725; ANTECH East: 1-800-872-1001; ANTECH Test Express: 1-888-397-8378
http://www.antechdiagnostics.com/Main/TestGuide.aspx

Arbovirus Diagnostic Laboratory
3156 Rampart Road, Fort Collins, CO 80521, USA
970-221-6400
http://www.cdc.gov/ncezid/dvbd/specimensub/arboviral-shipping.html

B Virus Research and Resource Laboratory
Dr. Julia Hilliard
Georgia State University, Viral Immunology Center, 161 Jesse Hill Jr Dr., Atlanta, GA 30303, USA
For emergency: 404-358-8168
http://biotech.gsu.edu/virology/Diagnostics/diagnostics.html

BioReliance, Serology/PCR Laboratories
14920 Broschart Rd., Rockville, MD 20850, USA
1-877-615-7275
http://www.bioreliance.com/us/services

Centers for Disease Control and Prevention
1600 Clifton Rd. Atlanta, GA 30329, USA
800-232-4636
http://www.cdc.gov/

Clinical Parasitology Diagnostic Service Laboratory
University of Tennessee College of Veterinary Medicine, 2407 River Drive, Knoxville, TN 37996, USA
865-974-8387
https://vetmed.tennessee.edu/vmc/dls/Pages/default.aspx

Colorado State University Veterinary Diagnostic Laboratory
2450 Gillette Drive, Ft. Collins, CO 80526, USA
970-297-1281
http://csu-cvmbs.colostate.edu/vdl/Pages/default.aspx

Comparative Pathology Laboratory
University of Miami, Clinical Research Building, 1120 NW 14th Street, 14th Floor, Suite 1409 Miami, FL 33136, USA
305-243-7284
http://www.pathology.med.miami.edu/clinical-pathology

Diagnostic Center for Population and Animal Health (DCPAH)
Clinical Pathology Laboratory, A215 Veterinary Medical Center, Michigan State University, East Lansing, MI 48824, USA
517-353-1683
https://cvm.msu.edu/vdl/laboratory-sections/clinical-pathology

IDEXX Laboratories, Inc.
One IDEXX Drive, Westbrook, ME 04092, USA
1-207-556-0300
1-800-548-6733
https://www.idexx.com/en/about-idexx/idexx-products-and-services/

Continued

TABLE 13-18 Nonhuman Primate Laboratories. (cont'd)

Infectious Diseases Laboratory
University of Georgia College of Veterinary Medicine
110 Riverbend Rd., Riverbend North, Room 150, University of Georgia, Athens, GA 30602, USA
Lab: 706-542-5812
https://vet.uga.edu/diagnostic-service-labs/infectious-diseases-lab/

Infectious Disease Pathology Activity
CDC (MS-G32), 1600 Clifton Rd, NE, Atlanta, GA 30333, USA
1-800-232-4636

Kansas State University Diagnostic Laboratory
Kansas State University, 1800 Denison Avenue, Manhattan, KS 66506, USA
785-532-5650
http://www.ksvdl.org/

Louisiana Animal Disease Diagnostic Laboratory
School of Veterinary Medicine, 1909 Skip Bertman Drive, Room 1519, Baton Rouge, LA 70803, USA
225-578-9778
http://www.lsu.edu/vetmed/laddl/index.php

MiraVista Diagnostics
4705 Decatur Blvd., Indianapolis, IN 46241, USA
317-856-2681
1-888-841-8387
https://miravistavets.com/veterinaray-fungal-infections/

New York State Veterinary Diagnostic Laboratory
Cornell University, 240 Farrier Rd, Ithaca, NY 14852, USA
607-253-3900
https://www.vet.cornell.edu/animal-health-diagnostic-center

North Carolina State University College of Veterinary Medicine Vector Borne Disease Diagnostic Laboratory
1060 William Moore Drive, Room 462A Raleigh, NC 27607, USA
919-513-6461
https://cvm.ncsu.edu/research/labs/diagnostic-testing-labs/

Northwest ZooPath
207 North Harkness St., Everson, WA 98247, USA
360-794-0630
http://www.zoopath.com/

Pathogen Detection Laboratory
California National Primate Research Center, University of California, One Shields Avenue, Davis, CA 95616 USA
530-752-0447
https://cnprc.ucdavis.edu/

Primate Diagnostic Services Laboratory (PDSL)
Washington National Primate Research Center
University of Washington, 3018 Western Ave, Seattle, WA 98121, USA
206-543-0440
https://www.wanprc.org/

Texas A&M Veterinary Medical Diagnostic Laboratory
483 Agronomy Rd., College Station, TX 77840, USA
979-845-3414
888-646-5623
https://tvmdl.tamu.edu/

TABLE 13-18 Nonhuman Primate Laboratories. (cont'd)

The Fungus Testing Laboratory Department of Pathology 7703 Floyd Curl Dr. Room 330E, San Antonio, TX 78229, USA 210-567-4131 https://lsom.uthscsa.edu/pathology/reference-labs/fungus-testing-laboratory/
UC Davis Coccidioidomycosis Serology Laboratory, 3416 One Shields Avenue, Tupper Hall, Davis, CA 95616, USA 530-752-1757 https://health.ucdavis.edu/valley-fever/serology-lab/index.html
USDA-APHIS-VS-NVSL 1920 Dayton Ave. (packages), Ames, IA 50010, USA 515-337-7568 https://www.aphis.usda.gov/aphis/ourfocus/animalhealth/lab-info-services/
Veterinary Molecular Diagnostics, Inc. 5989 Meijer Dr., Suite 5, Milford, OH 45150, USA 513-576-1808 http://www.vmdlabs.com/
Virus Reference Laboratories, Inc. (VRL) P.O. Box 40100, 7540 Louis Pasteur Road, San Antonio, TX 78229, USA 877-615-7275 http://vrlsat.com/vrl-test-list/
Zoological Pathology Program 3300 Golf Road, Brookfield, IL 60513, USA 312-585-9050 http://vetmed.illinois.edu/vet-resources/veterinary-diagnostic-laboratory/zoological-pathology-program/
Zoologix Inc. 9811 Owensmouth Avenue, Suite 4, Chatsworth, CA 91311, USA 818-717-8880 http://www.zoologix.com/primate/index.htm

REFERENCES

1. Abee CR, Mansfield K, Tardiff S, eds. *Nonhuman Primates in Biomedical Research Diseases.* 2nd ed. San Diego, CA: Elsevier; 2012:147–148.
2. Abilogaard CF, Harrison J, Johnson CA. Comparative study of blood coagulation in nonhuman primates. *J Appl Physiol.* 1971;30(3):400–405.
3. American Academy of Pediatrics. https://www.aap.org/. Accessed November 2020.
4. American Association of Zoo Veterinarians (member communication). Accessed February 2021.
5. Anderson KE, Austin J, Escobar EP, et al. Platelet aggregation in rhesus macaques (*Macaca mulatta*) in response to short-term meloxicam administration. *J Am Assoc Lab Anim Sci.* 2013;52:590–594.
6. Association of Primate Veterinarians. *Nonhuman Primate Formulary.* https://www.primatevets.org/education. Accessed November 15, 2020.
7. Association of Zoos and Aquariums. *Species Survival Statistics.* https://www.aza.org/assets/2332/survival_statistics_library_-_expires_1_dec_ 2016.pdf. Accessed November 18, 2020.
8. Astrid CS, Pulley JA, Roberts NW, et al. Four preanesthetic oral sedation protocols for rhesus macaques (*Macaca mulatta*). *J Zoo Wildl Med.* 2004;35(4):497–502.

9. Atencia R, Revuelta L, Somauroo JD, et al. Electrocardiogram reference intervals for clinically normal wild-born chimpanzees (*Pan troglodytes*). *Am J Vet Res*. 2015;76:688–693.
10. Authier S, Chaurand F, Legaspi M, et al. Comparison of three anesthetic protocols for intraduodenal drug administration using endoscopy in rhesus monkeys (*Macaca mulatta*). *J Am Assoc Lab Anim Sci*. 2006;45:73–79.
11. AZA Prosimian Taxon Advisory Group. *Eulemur Care Manual*. Silver Spring, MD: Association of Zoos and Aquariums; 2013.
12. Badyal DK, Garg SK. Effect of clarithromycin on the pharmacokinetics of carbamazepine in rhesus monkeys. *Methods Find Exp Clin Pharmacol*. 2000;22:581–584.
13. Bakker J, Thuesen LR, Braskamp G, et al. Single subcutaneous dosing of cefovecin in rhesus monkeys (*Macaca mulatta*): a pharmacokinetic study. *J Vet Pharmacol Ther*. 2011;34:464–468.
14. Bartlett SL, Chen TC, Murphy H, et al. Assessment of serum 25-hydroxy vitamin D concentrations in two collections of captive gorillas (*Gorilla gorilla gorilla*). *J Zoo Wildl Med*. 2017;48:144–151.
15. Bauer C, Frost P, Kirschner S. Pharmacokinetics of 3 formulations of meloxicam in cynomolgus macaques (*Macaca fascicularis*). *J Am Assoc Lab Anim Sci*. 2014;53:502–511.
16. Beaman BA, Hesemeyer WJ, Dominy NJ, et al. Sterile pyuria in a population of wild white-handed gibbons (*Hylobates lar*). *Am J Primatol*. 2009;71:880–883.
17. Bentzel DE, Bacon DJ. Comparison of various anthelmintic therapies for the treatment of *Trypanoxyuris microon* infection in owl monkeys (*Aotus nancymae*). *J Comp Med*. 2007;57:206–209.
18. Bertelsen MF, Thuesen LR, Bakker J, et al. Limitations and usages of cefovecin in zoological practices. *Proc Int Conf Dis Zoo Wild Anim*. 2010:140–141.
19. Blackwood RS, Tarara RP, Christe KL, et al. Effects of the macrolide drug tylosin on chronic diarrhea in rhesus macaques (*Macaca mulatta*). *J Comp Med*. 2008;58:81–87.
20. Blasier MW, Travis DA, Barbiers R. Retrospective evaluation of measles antibody titers in vaccinated captive gorillas (*Gorilla gorilla gorilla*). *J Zoo Wildl Med*. 2005;36:198–203.
21. Bodley K, Ley J. Management of behavioral disorders in zoo primates: two cases at Melbourne Zoo. *Proc Annu Conf Am Assoc Zoo Vet*. 2014:73.
22. Bohm RP, Rockar RA, Ratterree MS, et al. A method of video-assisted thorascopic surgery for collection of thymic biopsies in rhesus monkeys (*Macaca mulatta*). *Contemp Topics Lab Anim Sci*. 2000;39:24–26.
23. Bope ET, Kellerman RD, eds. *Conn's Current Therapy 2016*. Philadelphia, PA: Elsevier; 2016.
24. Bourgeois SR, Vazquez M, Brasky K, et al. Combination therapy reduces self-injurious behavior in a chimpanzee (*Pan troglodytes*): a case report. *J Appl Anim Welfare Sci*. 2007;10(2):123–140.
25. Brainard B, Darrow EJ. Sedation and anesthesia in the great apes - an overview. *Proc Annu Conf Am Assoc Zoo Vet*. 2013:26–35.
26. Calle PP, Joslin JO. New World and Old World monkeys. In: Miller RE, Fowler RE, eds. *Zoo and Wild Animal Medicine*. St. Louis, MO: Elsevier; 2015;8:301–335.
27. Cannizzo SA, Langan JN, Warneke M, et al. Evaluation of in-house urine dipstick, reference laboratory urinalysis, and urine protein: creatinine ratio from a colony of callimicos (*Callimico goeldii*). *J Zoo Wildl Med*. 2016;47(4):977–983.
28. Carpenter JW. Unpublished data. 2021.
29. Cerveny S, Sleeman J. Great apes. In: West G, Heard D, Caulkett N, eds. *Zoo Animal and Wildlife Immobilization and Anesthesia*. 2nd ed. Ames, IA: John Wiley & Sons; 2014:573–584.
30. Cheng L, Lei S, Chen SH, et al. Pretreatment with intravenous levetiracetam in the rhesus monkey *Coriaria* lactone-induced status epilepticus model. *J Neuro Sci*. 2015;348(1-2):111–120.
31. Churgin SM, Lee FK, Groenvold K, et al. Successful treatment of generalized demodicosis in red-handed tamarins (*Saguinus midas*) using a single administration of oral fluralaner. *J Zoo Wildl Med*. 2018;49(2):470–474.
32. Cissik JH, Hankins GD, Hauth JC, et al. Blood gas, cardiopulmonary, and urine electrolyte reference values in the pregnant yellow baboon (*Papio cynocephalus*). *Am J Primatol*. 1986;11:277–284.

33. Colby LA, Nowland MH, Kennedy LH. *Clinical Laboratory Medicine: An Introduction*. 5th ed. Hoboken, NJ: Wiley Blackwell; 2020:371–415.
34. Cook AL, St Claire M, Sams R. Use of florfenicol in non-human primates. *J Med Primatol*. 2004;33:127–133.
35. Corbett KS, Flynn B, Foulds JR. Evaluation of the mRNA-1273 vaccine against SARS-CoV-2 in nonhuman primates. *New Engl J Med*. 2020;383:1544–1555.
36. Correia J, Noiva R, Pissarra H, et al. Four cases of *Calodium hepaticum* infection in non-human primates from the Lisbon Zoological Garden, Portugal. *Proc Int Conf Dis Zoo Wild Anim*. 2011:13–22.
37. Cruzen CL, Baum ST, Colman RJ. Glucoregulatory function in adult rhesus macaques (*Macaca mulatta*) undergoing treatment with medroxyprogesterone acetate for endometriosis. *J Am Assoc Lab Anim Sci*. 2011;50:921–925.
38. Dascanio JJ, Hegler A, Hall E, et al. Efficacy of gonadotropin-releasing hormone (GnRH) vaccine (GonaCon™) on reproduction function in female vervet monkeys (*Chlorocebus aethiops*). *Proc Annu Conf Am Assoc Zoo Vet*. 2014:180.
39. DiVincenti L. Analgesic use in nonhuman primates undergoing neurosurgical procedures. *J Am Assoc Lab Anim Sci*. 2013;52:10–16.
40. Emerson JA, Walden HS, Peters RK, et al. Eosinophilic meningoencephalomyelitis in an orangutan (*Pongo pygmaeus*) caused by *Angiostrongylus cantonensis*. *Vet Qtly*. 2013;33(4):191–194.
41. Fanton JW, Zar SR, Ewert DL, et al. Cardiovascular responses to propofol and etomidate in long-term instrumented rhesus monkeys (*Macaca mulatta*). *J Comp Med*. 2000;5:303–308.
42. Fagundes N, Castro ML, Silva RA, et al. Comparison of midazolam and butorphanol combined with ketamine or dexmedetomidine for chemical restraint in howler monkeys (*Alouatta guariba clamitans*) for vasectomy. *J Med Primatol*. 2020;49(4):179–187.
43. Feeser P, White F. Medical management of *Lemur catta*, *Varecia variegata*, and *Propithecus verreauxi* in natural habitat enclosures. *Proc Annu Conf Am Assoc Zoo Vet/Am Assoc Wildl Vet*. 1992:320–323.
44. Flecknell PA. Clinical experience with NSAIDs in macaques. *Lab Primate Newsl*. 2004;44:4.
45. Flecknell PA. *Laboratory Animal Anaesthesia*. 4th ed. Netherlands: Elsevier Science; 2015.
46. Fontenot MB, Musso MW, McFatter RM, et al. Dose-finding study of fluoxetine and venlafaxine for the treatment of self-injurious and stereotypic behavior in rhesus macaques (*Macaca mulatta*). *J Am Assoc Lab Anim Sci*. 2009;48:176–184.
47. Fortman JD, Hewett TA, Bennett BT. *The Laboratory Nonhuman Primate*. Boca Raton, FL: CRC Press; 2002.
48. Furtado MM, Nunes AL, Intelizano TR, et al. Comparison of racemic ketamine versus (S+) ketamine when combined with midazolam for anesthesia of *Callithrix jacchus* and *Callithrix penicillata*. *J Zoo Wildl Med*. 2010;41:389–394.
49. Galante R, Carvalho ER, Muniz J, et al. Comparison between total intravenous anesthesia with propofol and intermittent bolus of tiletamine-zolazepam in a capuchin monkey (*Sapajus apella*). *Braz J Vet Res*. 2019;39(4):271–277.
50. Gamble KC, Clancy MM, eds. *Infectious Diseases of Concern to Captive and Free-Ranging Animals in North America*. 2nd ed. Yulee, FL: Infectious Disease Committee, American Association of Zoo Veterinarians; 2013.
51. Gerlach T, Clyde VL, Morris GL, et al. Alternative therapeutic options for medical management of epilepsy in apes. *J Zoo Wildl Med*. 2011;42(2):291–294.
52. Graham M, Mutch L, Kittredge JA, et al. Management of adverse side-effects after chemotherapy in macaques as exemplified be streptozotocin: case studies and recommendations. *J Lab Anim*. 2012;46:178–192.
53. Hahn A. *Zoo and Wild Animal Formulary*. Hoboken, NJ: Wiley Blackwell; 2019:81–118.
54. Hahn NE, Capuano SV. Successful treatment of cryptosporidiosis in 2 common marmosets (*Callithrix jacchus*) by using paromomycin. *J Am Assoc Lab Anim Sci*. 2010;49:873–875.
55. Harwood JH, Listrani P, Wagner JD. Nonhuman primates and other animal models in diabetes research. *J Diab Sci Tech*. 2012;6(3):503–514.

56. Hedley J, ed. *BSAVA Small Animal Formulary-Part B: Exotic Pets*. 10th ed. Quedgeley, UK: British Small Animal Veterinary Association; 2020.
57. Hellebrekers LJ, Hedenqvist P. Laboratory animal analgesia, anesthesia, and euthanasia. In: Hau J, Schapiro SJ, eds. *Handbook of Laboratory Animal Science*. Vol 1. 3rd ed. Boca Raton, FL: CRC Press; 2011;1:485–534.
58. Henri GM, Bertrand J, Sandersen C, et al. A combination of alfaxalone, medetomidine and midazolam for chemical immobilization of rhesus macaque (*Macaca mulatta*). *J Med Primatol*. 2017;46(6):332–336.
59. Hopper J. Common marmosets. In: Kubiak M, ed. *Handbook of Exotic Pet Medicine*. Hoboken, NJ: Wiley Blackwell; 2021:27–42.
60. Hrapkiewicz K, Medina L. *Nonhuman Primates Clinical Laboratory Animal Medicine*. 3rd ed. Ames, IA: Blackwell Publishing; 2007:280–329.
61. Ihrig M, Tassinary LG, Bernacky B, et al. Hematologic and serum biochemical reference intervals for the chimpanzee (*Pan troglodytes*) categorized by age and sex. *J Comp Med*. 2001;51:30–37.
62. Institutional Animal Care and Use Committee of the University of California San Francisco. *Nonhuman Primate Formulary. Anesthesia and Analgesia in Laboratory Animals at UCSF*. http://www.iacuc.ucsf.edu/Proc/awNHPFrm.asp. Accessed December 18, 2016.
63. Jafarey Y, Hanley C, Berlinski R, et al. Management of uterine fibroids and ovarian cysts with leuprolide acetate in an Allen's swamp monkey (*Allenopithecus nigroviridus*). *Proc Annu Conf Am Assoc Zoo Vet*. 2012:236.
64. James SB, Raphael BL. Demodicosis in red-handed tamarins (*Saguinus midas*). *J Zoo Wildl Med*. 2000;31:251–254.
65. Jepson L. *Exotic Animal Medicine: A Quick Reference Guide*. 2nd ed. St. Louis, MO: Elsevier; 2016.
66. Johnson JG, Langan JN, Gilor C. Treatment of diabetes mellitus in a golden lion tamarin (*Leontopithecus rosalia*) with the glucagon-like peptide-1 mimetic exenatide. *J Zoo Wildl Med*. 2016;47(3):903–906.
67. Johnson-Delaney CJ. Parasites of captive nonhuman primates. *Vet Clin North Am Exot Anim Pract*. 2009;12:563–581.
68. Junge RE, Gannon FH, Porton I, et al. Management and prevention of vitamin D deficiency rickets in captive-born juvenile chimpanzees (*Pan troglodytes*). *J Zoo Wildl Med*. 2000;31:361–369.
69. Kazuma Y, Makoto I, Namkoong H, et al. The efficacy, safety, and feasibility of inhaled amikacin for the treatment of difficult-to-treat non-tuberculous mycobacterial lung diseases. *BMC Infect Dis*. 2017;17:558:1–9.
70. Keeble EJ, Neuber A, Hume CL, et al. Medical management of *Trichophyton* dermatophytosis using a novel treatment regime in L'Hoest's monkeys (*Cercopithecus lhoesti*). *Vet Rec*. 2010;167(22):862–864.
71. Kelly KR, Pypendop BH, Christe KL. Pharmacokinetics of buprenorphine following intravenous and intramuscular administration in male rhesus macaques (*Macaca mulatta*). *J Vet Pharmacol Ther*. 2014;37:480–485.
72. Kelly KR, Pypendop BH, Christe KL. Pharmacokinetics of hydromorphone after intravenous and intramuscular administration in male rhesus macaques (*Macaca mulatta*). *J Am Assoc Lab Anim Sci*. 2014;53:512–516.
73. Kelly KR, Pypendop BH, Christe KL. Pharmacokinetics of tramadol following intravenous and oral administration in male rhesus macaques (*Macaca mulatta*). *J Vet Pharmacol Ther*. 2015;38:375–382.
74. Kelly KR, Pypendop BH, Grayson JK, et al. Pharmacokinetics of oxymorphone in titi monkeys (*Callicebus* spp.) and rhesus macaques (*Macaca mulatta*). *J Am Assoc Lab Anim Sci*. 2011;50:212–220.
75. Kenny DE, Knightly F, Baier J, et al. Exposure of hooded capuchin monkeys (*Cebus apella cay*) to rabid bat at a zoological park. *J Zoo Wildl Med*. 2001;32(1):123–126.

76. Kim TM, Park H, Lee KW, et al. A simple way to eradicate methicillin-resistant *Staphylococcus aureus* in cynomolgus macaques (*Macaca fascicularis*). *Comp Med.* 2017;67(4):356–359.
77. Kottwitz JJ, Perry KK, Rose HH, et al. *Angiostrongylus cantonensis* infection in captive Geoffroy's tamarins (*Saguinus geoffroyi*). *J Am Vet Med Assoc.* 2014;245:821–827.
78. Koyfman A, Waseem M. *Pediatric Dehydration.* 2018; https://emedicine.medscape.com/article/801012. Accessed July 15, 2020.
79. Kramer JA, Hachey AM, Wachtman LM, et al. Treatment of giardiasis in common marmosets (*Callithrix jacchus*) with tinidazole. *J Comp Med.* 2009;59:174–179.
80. Kramer R, Burns M. Normal clinical and biological parameters of the common marmoset (*Callithrix jacchus*). In: Marini R, Wachtman LM, Tardif SD, et al., eds. *The Common Marmoset in Captivity and Biomedical Research.* San Diego, CA: Elsevier; 2019:93–104.
81. Kummrow MS, Mätz-Rensing K. High mortality due to streptococcal toxic shock syndrome in a captive colony of lion-tailed macaques (*Macaca silenus*). *Proc Joint Conf Am Assoc Zoo Vet/Euro Assoc Zoo Wildl Vet/Int Zoo Wildl.* 2016:159–160.
82. Kummrow MS, Schwittlick U, Wohlsein P, et al. Treatment of suspected diabetes type I induced polyneuropathy in a drill (*Mandrillus leucophaeus*). *Proc Int Conf Dis Zoo Wildl Anim.* 2011:23.
83. Lair S, Crawshaw GJ, Mehren KG, et al. Diagnosis of hypothyroidism in a western lowland gorilla (*Gorilla gorilla gorilla*) using human thyroid-stimulating hormone assay. *J Zoo Wildl Med.* 1999;30(4):537–540.
84. Laudenslager ML, Clarke AS. Antidepressant treatment during social challenge prior to 1 year of age affects immune and endocrine responses in adult macaques. *Psychiatry Res.* 2000;95:25–34.
85. Lee JI, Kim S, Kim A, et al. Acute necrotic stomatitis associated with methicillin-resistant *Staphylococcus aureus* infection in newly acquired rhesus macaque (*Macaca mulatta*). *J Med Primatol.* 2011;40(3):188–193.
86. Lee JI, Shin JS, Lee JE, et al. Reference values of hematology, chemistry, electrolytes, blood gas, coagulation time and urinalysis in the Chinese rhesus macaques (*Macaca mulatta*). *J Xenotransplantation.* 2012;19(4):1–15.
87. Lee VK, Flynt KS, Haag LM, et al. Comparison of the effects of ketamine, ketamine-medetomidine, and ketamine-midazolam on physiologic parameters and anesthesia-induced stress in rhesus (*Macaca mulatta*) and cynomolgus (*Macaca fascicularis*) macaques. *J Am Assoc Lab Anim Sci.* 2010;49:57–63.
88. Leendertz SAJ, Metzger S, Skjerve E, et al. A longitudinal study of urinary dipstick parameters in wild chimpanzees (*Pan troglodytes verus*) in Cote d' lvoire. *Am J Primatol.* 2010;72(8):689–698.
89. Longley L. Non-human primate anesthesia In: *Anesthesia of Exotic Pets.* Philadelphia, PA: Saunders Elsevier; 2008:103–111.
90. Macy JD, Beattie TA, Morgenstern SE, et al. Use of guanfacine to control self-injurious behavior in two rhesus macaques (*Macaca mulatta*) and one baboon (*Papio anubis*). *J Comp Med.* 2000;50:419–425.
91. Martin LD, Dissen GA, McPike MJ, et al. Effects of anesthesia with isoflurane, ketamine, or propofol on physiologic parameters in neonatal rhesus macaques (*Macaca mulatta*). *J Am Assoc Lab Anim Sci.* 2014;53:290–300.
92. Masters N. Primates. In; Meredith A, Johnson-Delaney C, eds. *BSAVA Manual of Exotic Pets.* 5th ed. Quedgeley, UK: British Small Animal Veterinary Association; 2010:148-166.
93. McCain S, Sim RR, Weidner B, et al. Diagnosis and treatment of Chagas disease (*Trypanosoma cruzi*) in a naturally infected De Brazza's monkey (*Cercopithecus neglectus*) in Alabama. *Proc Annu Conf Am Assoc Zoo Vet.* 2019:35–36.
94. Mendoza KA, Stockinger DE, Cukrov MJ, et al. Effects of transdermal mirtazapine on hyporexic rhesus and cynomolgus macaques (*Macaca mulatta* and *Macaca fascicularis*). *J Med Primatol.* 2021;50(2):128–133.
95. Miller CL, Schwartz AM, Barnhart MD, et al. Chronic hypertension with subsequent congestive heart failure in a western lowland gorilla (*Gorilla gorilla gorilla*). *J Zoo Wildl Med.* 1999;30(2):262–267.

96. Miller M, Weber M, Mangold B, et al. Use of oral detomidine and ketamine for anesthetic induction in nonhuman primates. *Proc Annu Conf Am Assoc Zoo Vet*. 2000:179–180.
97. Miyabe-Nishiwaki T, Masui K, Kaneko A, et al. Evaluation of the predictive performance of a pharmokinetic model for propofol in Japanese macaques (*Macaca fuscata fuscata*). *J Vet Pharmacol Ther*. 2013;36:169–173.
98. Murphy HW. Great apes. In: Miller RE, Fowler ME, eds. *Zoo and Wild Animal Medicine*. 8th ed. St. Louis, MO: Elsevier; 2015:336–354.
99. Nakayama S, Koie H, Kanayama K, et al. Establishment of reference values for complete blood count and blood gases in cynomolgus monkeys (*Macaca fasicularis*). *J Vet Med Sci*. 2017;79(5):881–888.
100. Naples LM, Langan JN, Kearns KS. Comparison of the anesthetic effects of oral transmucosal versus injectable medetomidine in combination with tiletamine-zolazepam for immobilization of chimpanzees (*Pan troglodytes*). *J Zoo Wildl Med*. 2010;41:50–62.
101. National Research Council of the Academies. Vitamins. In: *Nutrient Requirements of Nonhuman Primates*. 2nd ed. Washington, DC: The National Academic Press; 2003:113–149.
102. National Reye's Syndrome Foundation. Aspirin Lists. http://reyessyndrome.org/aspirinlists.html. Accessed December 18, 2016.
103. Nevitt BN, Langan JN, Adkesson MJ, et al. Multifocal *Cryptococcus neoformans* var. *neoforms*: infection, treatment, and monitoring by serial computed tomography in a Schmidt's red-tailed guenon (*Cercopithecus ascanius schmidti*). *J Zoo Wildl Med*. 2013;44(3):728–736.
104. Niederwerder MC, Stalis IH, Campbell GA, et al. Gastric pneumatosis with associated eosinophilic gastritis in four black and white ruffed lemurs (*Varecia variegata variegata*). *J Zoo Wildl Med*. 2013;44(1):79–86.
105. Nunamaker EA, Halliday LC, Moody DE, et al. Pharmacokinetics of 2 formulations of buprenorphine in macaques (*Macaca mulatta* and *Macaca fascicularis*). *J Am Assoc Lab Anim Sci*. 2013;52:48–56.
106. Ølberg RA, Sinclair M. Monkeys and gibbons. In: West G, Heard D, Caulkett N, eds. *Zoo Animal and Wildlife Immobilization and Anesthesia*. Ames, IA: John Wiley & Sons; 2014:561–571.
107. Papp R, Popovic A, Kelly N, et al. Pharmacokinetics of cefovecin in squirrel monkey (*Saimiri sciureus*), rhesus macaques (*Macaca mulatta*), and cynomolgus macaques (*Macaca fascicularis*). *J Am Assoc Lab Anim*. 2010;49(6):805–808.
108. Park HK, Cho JW, Lee BS, et al. Reference values of clinical pathology parameters in cynomolgus monkeys (*Macaca fascicularis*) used in preclinical studies. *J Lab Anim Res*. 2016;32(2):79–86.
109. Parrott T. Nonhuman primates. *The Merck Veterinary Manual*. 11th ed. Whitehouse Station, NJ: Merck and Co; 2016. www.merckvetmanual.com/ (revised January 2020).
110. Parrott T. Personal observation. 2020.
111. Patton DL, Cosgrove YT, Agnew KJ, et al. Development of a nonhuman primate model *Trichomonas vaginalis* infection. *Sex Transm Dis*. 2006;33:743–746.
112. PDR.NET. Metronidazole for treatment of serious anaerobic infections (e.g., skin and skin structure infections, CNS infection including meningitis, and brain abscess, bone and joint infections). Accessed October 15, 2020.
113. Peterson EN, Bechgaard E, Sortwell RJ, et al. Potent depletion 5HT from monkey whole blood by a new 5HT uptake inhibitor, paroxetine (FG 7051). *Eur J Pharmacol*. 1978;52(1):115–119.
114. Poliquin PG, Biondi M, Ranadheera C, et al. Delivering prolonged intensive care to a nonhuman primate: A high fidelity animal model of critical illness. *Sci Rep*. 2017;7(1):1204.
115. Popilskis SJ, Lee DR, Elmore DB. Anesthesia and analgesia in nonhuman primates. In: Fish RE, Brown MJ, Danneman PJ, et al., eds. Anesthesia and analgesia in nonhuman primates. *Anesthesia and Analgesia in Laboratory Animals*. 2008:336–363.
116. Puri SK, Singh N. Azithromycin: antimalarial profile against blood- and sporozoite-induced infections in mice and monkeys. *J Exp Parasitol*. 2000;94:8–14.
117. Rao GA, Mann JR, Shoaibi A, et al. Azithromycin and levofloxacin use and increased risk of cardiac arrhythmia and death. *Ann Fam Med*. 2014;12:121–127.

117a. Raubertas R, Beech J, Watson W, et al. Decreased complexity of glucose dynamics in diabetes in rhesus monkeys. *Sci Rep.* 2019;9(1):1438.
118. Redrobe SP. Neuroleptics in great apes, with specific reference to modification of aggressive behavior in a male gorilla. In: Fowler ME, Miller RE, eds. *Zoo and Wild Animal Medicine.* 6th ed. St. Louis, MO: Saunders Elsevier; 2008:243–250.
119. Reichard MV, Wolf RF, Carey DW, et al. Efficacy of fenbendazole and milbemycin oxime for treating baboons (*Papio cynocephalus anubis*) infected with *Trichuris trichiura. J Am Assoc Lab Anim Sci.* 2007;46(2):42–45.
120. Rhu J, Lee KW, Kim KS, et al. Coagulation biomarkers in healthy male cynomolgus macaque monkeys (*Macaca fascicularis*). *J Xenotransplantation.* 2019;26:1–8.
121. Rodriguez del Rio Lopez P, Sanchez C, Stembridge M, et al. Comparison of indirect blood pressure values in chimpanzees (*Pan troglodytes*) anesthetized with two anesthetic protocols: tiletamine-zolazepam and tiletamine-zolazepam-medetomidine. *Proc Annu Conf Am Assoc Zoo Vet.* 2014:31.
122. Romero E, Hasselschwert D. The use of gabapentin in a juvenile chimpanzee following arm amputation. *J Am Assoc Lab Anim Sci.* 2014;53(1):100–101.
123. Rowe N. *The Pictorial Guide to the Living Primates.* New York, NY: Pogonias Press; 1996.
124. Saint Louis Zoo. *Contraception Methods.* Rodriguez del Rio Lopez P, Sanchez C, et al. https://www.stlzoo.org/animals/scienceresearch/reproductivemanagementcenter/contraception-recommendatio/contraceptionmethods. Accessed December 18, 2016.
125. Salyards GW, Knych HK, Hill AE, et al. Pharmacokinetics of ceftiofur crystalline free acid in male rhesus macaques (*Macaca mulatta*) after subcutaneous administration. *J Am Assoc Lab Anim Sci.* 2015;54:557–563.
126. Sasseville VG, Hotchkiss CE, Levesque PC, et al. Hematopoietic, cardiovascular, lymphoid and mononuclear phagocyte systems of nonhuman primates. In: Abee C, Mansfield K, Tardif SD, et al., eds. *Nonhuman Primates in Biomedical Research: Diseases.* 2nd ed. London, UK: Elsevier; 2012:357–384.
127. Sawyer EK, Howell LL. Pharmacokinetics of fluoxetine in rhesus macaques following multiple routes of administration. *J Pharm.* 2011;88:44–49.
128. Schuurman HJ, Smith HT, Cozzi E. Reference values for clinical chemistry and clinical hematology parameters in baboons. *Xenotransplantation.* 2004;11:511–516.
129. Selmi AL, Mendes GM, Figueiredo JP, et al. Comparison of medetomidine-ketamine and dexmedetomadine-ketamine anesthesia in golden-headed lion tamarins (*Leontopithecus chrysomelas*). *Can Vet J.* 2004;45(6):481–485.
130. Semrau A, Gerold S, Frick JS, et al. Non-invasive detection and successful treatment of a *Helicobacter pylori* infection in a captive rhesus macaque. *J Lab Anim.* 2017;51(2):208–211.
131. Shrestha BA, Nelson EE, Liow JS, et al. Fluoxetine administration to juvenile monkeys: effects on the serotonin transporter and behavior. *Am J Psych.* 2014;171(3):323–331.
132. Smith M, Heatley JJ. Callitrichids (Chap.13); Clark SD. Lemurs (Chap. 14); Albertelli MA. Other small New World monkeys (Chap. 15). In: Heatley JJ, Russell KE, eds. *Exotic Animal Laboratory Diagnosis.* Hoboken, NJ: Wiley Blackwell; 2020:211–254.
133. Soroori S, Molazem M, Mokhtari R, et al. Ratio of the bronchial lumen to pulmonary artery diameter in rhesus macaques (*Macaca mulatta*) without clinical pulmonary disease. *J Am Assoc Lab Anim Sci.* 2019;58(1):83–86.
134. Species360 Zoological Information Management System. https://zims.Species360.org. Accessed October 15, 2020.
135. Springer DA, Phillippi-Falkenstein K, Smith G. Retrospective analysis of wound characteristics and tetanus development in captive macaques. *J Zoo Wildl Med.* 2009;40:95–102.
136. Steinbach JR, MacGuire J, Chang S, et al. Assessment of pre-operative maropitant citrate use in macaque (*Macaca fasicularis* and *Macaca mulatta*) for neurosurgical procedures. *J Med Prim.* 2018;47(3):178–184.

137. Sun FJ, Wright DE, Pinson DM. Comparison of ketamine versus combination of ketamine and medetomidine in injectable anesthetic protocols: chemical immobilization in macaques and tissue reaction in rats. *Contemp Topics Lab Anim Sci.* 2003;42:32–37.
138. Valverde CR, Mama KR, Kollias-Baker C, et al. Pharmacokinetics and cardiopulmonary effects of fentanyl in isoflurane-anesthetized rhesus monkeys (*Macaca mulatta*). *Am J Vet Res.* 2000;61:931–934.
139. Wallach J, Boever W. *Diseases of Exotic Animals: Medical and Surgical Management.* Philadelphia, PA: WB Saunders; 1983:3–133.
140. Wathen AB, Myers DD, Zajkowski P, et al. Enoxaparin treatment of spontaneous deep vein thrombosis in a chronically catheterized rhesus macaque (*Macaca mulatta*). *J Am Assoc Lab Anim Sci.* 2009;48:521–526.
141. Watson JR, Stoskopf MK, Rozmiarek H, et al. Kinetic study of serum gentamicin concentrations in baboons after single dose administration. *Am J Vet Res.* 1991;52:1285–1287.
142. Weld KP, Mench JA, Woodward RA, et al. Effect of tryptophan treatment on self-biting and central nervous system serotonin metabolism in rhesus monkeys (*Macaca mulatta*). *Neuropsychopharmacology.* 1998;19(4):314–321.
143. Williams CV. Prosimians. In: Miller RE, Fowler ME, eds. *Zoo and Wild Animal Medicine.* 8th ed. St. Louis, MO: Elsevier; 2015:291–301.
144. Williams CV, Junge RE. Prosimians. In: West G, Heard D, Caulkett N, eds. *Zoo Animal and Wildlife Immobilization and Anesthesia.* 2nd ed. Ames, IA: John Wiley & Sons; 2014:551–559.
145. Williams CV, Glenn KM, Levine JF, et al. Comparison of the efficacy and cardiorespiratory effects of medetomidine-based anesthetic protocols in ring-tailed lemurs (*Lemur catta*). *J Zoo Wildl Med.* 2003;34:163–170.
146. Wolfensohn S, Honess P. Physical well-being. In: *Handbook of Primate Husbandry and Welfare.* Ames, IA: Blackwell; 2005:59–98.
147. Yabe H, Choudhury ME, Kuba M, et al. Zonisamide increases dopamine turnover in the striatum of mice and common marmosets treated with MPTP. *J Pharm Sci.* 2010;114:298–303.
148. Yamada N, Sato J, Kanno T, et al. Morphological study of progressive glomerulonephropathy in common marmosets (*Callithrix jacchus*). *Toxicol Pathol.* 2013;41:1106–1115.
149. Young LA, Morris PJ, Keener L, et al. Subcutaneous *Taenia crassiceps* cysticercosis in a red-ruffed lemur (*Varecia variegata rubra*). *Proc Annu Conf Am Assoc Zoo Vet.* 2000:251–252.
150. Zikusoka GK, Horne WA, Levine J, et al. Comparison of cardiorespiratory effects of medetomidine-butorphanol-ketamine and medetomidine-butorphanol-midazolam in patas monkeys (*Erythrocebus patas*). *J Zoo Wildl Med.* 2003;34(1):47–52.
151. Zoller M. Mucocutaneous candidiasis in a mandrill (*Mandrillus sphinx*). *J Comp Path.* 2012;147:381–385.

Chapter 14 Native Wildlife

Erica A. Miller | Nicki Rosenhagen

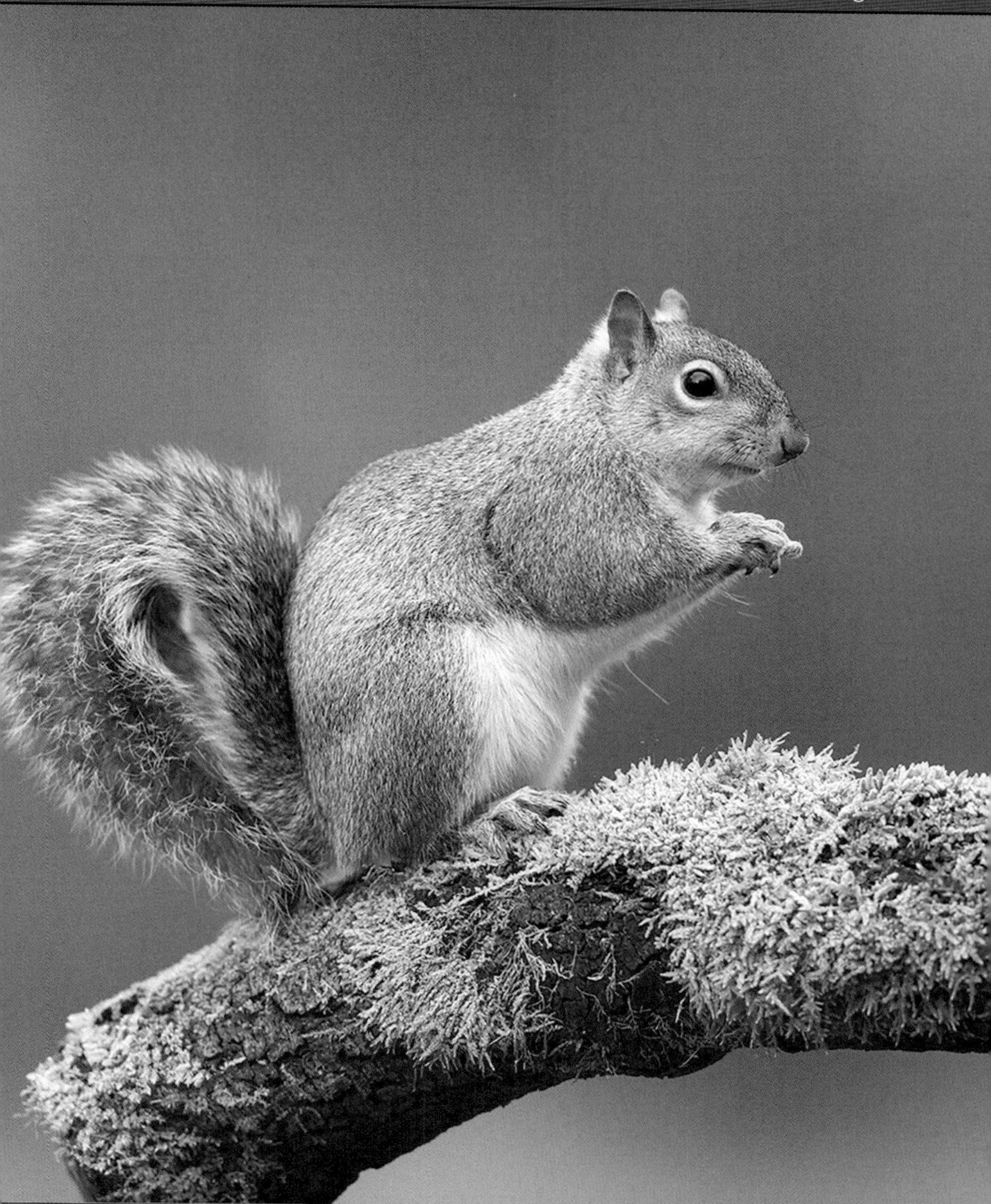

TABLE 14-1 Checklist for the Care of Sick, Injured, or Orphaned Wildlife.[a,b,15,31,34,35,41,60]

The information contained within this section is designed to help a veterinarian triage and provide basic stabilizing care to injured or orphaned wildlife. The veterinarian is strongly encouraged to transfer these animals to, or consult with, experienced wildlife veterinarians or permitted wildlife rehabilitators as soon as possible. In addition, any individual working with wildlife should check with state or provincial and federal officials on permit requirements. In the event of bites inflicted by rabies vector species (RVS) or other wild mammals showing neurologic signs to persons or domestic pets, the local health department should be contacted regarding appropriate rabies prevention procedures and wildlife testing (see A(f) below).

A. Regulations and reporting

a. Permits: check with state and federal officials on laws and permit requirements for hospitalizing wildlife; if you do not have these permits, stabilize the animal and transport it to a permitted facility as soon as possible. Table 14-2 summarizes which agencies have authority over which wildlife species.
b. Species reporting: check with state or provincial wildlife officials for a list of reportable endangered, threatened, or listed species; these will vary by location.
c. Illegal activity: report injuries caused by illegal activities such as confirmed poisonings, illegal possession, or gunshot wounds to nongame species to local or federal wildlife authorities.
d. Reportable diseases: reportable or foreign animal diseases diagnosed in wildlife should be reported to the USDA-APHIS area veterinarian in charge (https://www.aphis.usda.gov/aphis/ourfocus/animalhealth/contact-us).
e. Banded birds: band numbers on federally banded birds should be reported to the U.S. Geological Survey Bird Banding Laboratory (https://www.pwrc.usgs.gov/BBL/bblretrv/).
f. Advise the public not to approach rabies vector species and to contact local wildlife authorities instead. In addition, bats should never be handled bare-handed. If a rescuer has handled a rabies vector species, report any potential rabies exposure (bite or contact with saliva through broken skin or mucous membranes) to the local health department. If a bat is removed from a room with a child, a sleeping person, or a mentally handicapped person, contact the local health department for guidance on rabies testing.

B. Patient background

a. Is the "orphan" truly an orphan? If not, return the animal to the nest or site where it was found. Human scent will not cause rejection of the young by the parents.
   - Many fledgling birds normally spend time on the ground before gaining full flight ability. The parents will continue to feed and guard the fledgling during this time.
   - Adult rabbits and deer normally leave their young unattended for much of the day. The mother will return to the site where the offspring were left to reunite, often hours later. Check for a "milk line" in the abdomen of young rabbits to determine if they were recently fed.
b. Get precise information. When was the animal found? Exact location? Circumstances? Has any medical or supportive care been provided?
c. The rescue location of many herptile species is particularly important, as they have high site fidelity.
d. Obtain the rescuer's name, address, and phone number in case further details are required.

C. Initial patient triage

a. What is medically wrong with the animal? Can it be treated, survive the rehabilitation period (sometimes months), and be released to the wild? Check with experienced wildlife veterinarians if you are unsure. In many cases, euthanasia is the most humane treatment option. The practitioner should be familiar with the release criteria in *Standards for Wildlife Rehabilitation* before embarking on treatment.
b. Address life-threatening problems first. ABC: Check that the *airway* is clear, the animal is *breathing,* and *cardiac beat and pulse* are present. The pulse of a bird can be most easily found over the ventral elbow.
c. Control hemorrhage. Apply direct pressure to hemorrhage sites, including those of broken blood feathers. Plucking broken flight feathers is painful and can cause follicle damage. Use topical epinephrine, cautery, and ligation if needed.

TABLE 14-1 Checklist for the Care of Sick, Injured, or Orphaned Wildlife. (cont'd)

d. Assess for shock. Evaluate neonates for hypoglycemia and hypothermia. Clinical signs include cold extremities, pale and tacky mucous membranes, and rapid heart rate. Treat with fluids and supplemental heat if needed; treat hypoglycemia with intravenous or oral dextrose. Treat hyperthermia with fluids and place the patient in a cool place; spray limbs with cool water or use isopropyl alcohol on the legs and foot pads. Cooling should be executed judiciously to prevent hypothermia.

e. Perform a full examination once the patient is stable. To minimize patient stress, the examination may need to be delayed, limited to a cursory exam, or done in stages.

- If possible, determine the species, sex, life stage, body condition, and weight. Species identification is crucial for proper husbandry, including diet type and presentation, and housing requirements.
- Is a zoonotic disease or infectious disease a concern? Isolate the patient if necessary. See Table 14-9 for more information on zoonoses of native wildlife.

D. Develop a treatment and supportive care plan

a. Assume patients are at least 5% dehydrated at the time of admission even if no signs of dehydration are present; this ensures mild dehydration is not neglected. Clinical signs of dehydration suggest a more severe state (often ≥6%) and should be corrected accordingly.

- Provide hydrating solutions and electrolyte support for the first 24 to 48 hours parenterally (Normasol, LRS, 0.9% saline) or orally with a multispecies electrolyte solution (e.g., Pedialyte [Abbott], or Bounce Back [Manna Pro]).
- Continue to treat if ongoing fluid losses occur.
- Most birds, herptiles, and mammals can be triaged with fluids based on an assumed maintenance rate of 60-80 mL/kg/day, 10-25 mL/kg/day, and 60-80 mL/kg/day, respectively.

b. Provide supplemental heat to neonates at 80-90°F (27-32°C). Incubators are often ideal, as they provide a warm, humid environment. Heating pads may be beneficial if an incubator is not available but should be kept on low to prevent thermal burns, with enough space for the animal to move away from the heat source to prevent overheating. Wrapped hot water bottles and heated rice pouches are also good options, but water bottles and rice bags must be monitored and reheated as necessary.

c. Treat and prevent infection. Open wounds should be thoroughly cleaned and may require antimicrobial therapy, particularly if the injury was inflicted by a domestic cat.

d. Provide analgesia and antiinflammatory medications as needed. Wild animals are often stoic in nature and may not demonstrate classic signs of pain. However, pain management is critical for successful management of trauma and other painful conditions in these species. In general, a condition that would be considered painful in a human or pet should be considered painful in a wild animal and managed accordingly. Nonsteroidal antiinflammatory drugs are useful for soft tissue injuries, head trauma, and spinal trauma. Steroid use, especially in birds, is controversial and generally not recommended. Opioids are useful for severe soft tissue injuries and fractures.

e. Develop a nutritional plan. The nutritional needs of wild animals vary considerably by species. It is neither practical nor cost effective for veterinary hospitals to stock the myriad food items and formulas required to provide a balanced diet to all orphaned and injured wild animals that may present for care. Therefore, the veterinarian is encouraged to transfer the wild animal to a permitted rehabilitator as soon as possible. If an animal cannot be transferred for an extended period of time, a rehabilitator should be contacted for milk replacer information for nursing mammals and food options for nestling birds. Tables 14-10 and 14-12 list common natural food items for independent wild animals. Natural history guides and other wildlife specific literature can be referenced for additional information.[b] Calculate the calories needed for each day's feeding based on the metabolic energy coefficient (MEC or kcals/24hr), where W = weight in kg.

- Placental mammals: MEC = 70 x $W^{.75}$
- Opossums: MEC = 49 x $W^{.75}$
- Birds <100g: MEC = 129 x $W^{.75}$
- Birds >100g: MEC = 78.3 x $W^{.75}$
- Reptiles: MEC = 10 x $W^{.75}$
- Adjust caloric need based on animal's condition:
  1. Debilitated adult: MEC × 3
  2. Healthy young: MEC × 4
  3. Debilitated young: MEC × 5

Continued

TABLE 14-1 Checklist for the Care of Sick, Injured, or Orphaned Wildlife. (cont'd)

Ideally, animals should be rehydrated before offering food. In some cases (e.g., stable young animals and hummingbirds), food should be offered in conjunction with rehydration to prevent hypoglycemia. Young mammals and birds should not be offered water until their eyes are open or they are out of the nest, respectively. Emaciated animals may need special diets (Emeraid Nutritional Care System [Lafeber]; Carnivore and Critical Care [Oxbow]) to allow enterocytes to recover. When in doubt, err on the side of gradual introduction of food to prevent overfeeding.

f. Neonatal mammals must be stimulated to urinate and defecate by gently brushing anal and genital areas with moist cotton or tissue after each feeding.

g. Determine appropriate housing. The main goals are safety and stress reduction for the animal by preventing noise and visual stimulation. In general, minimize contact with people and avoid contact with domestic animals. Wildlife should not be housed near (i.e., within sight, sound, or smell of) domestic animals or other wildlife that might be natural predators or competitors. Short-term housing options include aquariums, popup mesh enclosures, portable kennels, and cage banks. Perches, natural foliage, and hide boxes can be added to encourage natural behavior and allow the animal a safe place to retreat. Young animals may require supplemental heat.

E. Rehabilitation.

a. Contact the National Wildlife Rehabilitators Association (NWRA; 320-230-9920; www.nwrawildlife.org), the International Wildlife Rehabilitation Council (IWRC; 866-871-1869; https://theiwrc.org/), or state wildlife rehabilitation associations to find a rehabilitator near you.

b. Transfer the animal to a qualified permitted rehabilitator for continued care.

c. Rehabilitators are often familiar with animal nutrition and natural history and can provide initial supportive care recommendations.

F. Release criteria.

a. An animal must meet the following criteria to be released to the wild:
- Initial illness or injury is resolved with no risk of recurrence.
- Exhibits no sign of active disease or injury obtained while in captivity.
- Can recognize and interact appropriately with its own species and is capable of reproducing.
- Can recognize and effectively avoid predators.
- Is able to find food by foraging or hunting in the wild. This requires adequate vision and locomotive skills appropriate to that species.
- Is acclimated to current outdoor temperatures.
- Displays species-appropriate behavior (not improperly imprinted) and the fight or flight behavioral response.
- Must be the correct age to evade predators and survive independently (unless being reunited/renested).
- Possess pelage or plumage that is adequate for that species to survive, including waterproof pelage/plumage sufficient for that species.
- Has received a prerelease exam and any testing necessary to ensure it is healthy at the time of release.

b. Animals should be released at the original site of capture unless conservation efforts or safety considerations dictate otherwise. Animals should be released in a natural environment and habitat suitable for survival but away from traffic, people, and pets. The habitat must be within carrying capacity for the species. Diurnal species should be released in the morning and nocturnal species at dusk. Local and state laws regarding release of rabies vector species, deer, and nonindigenous wildlife should be checked prior to releasing these species.

c. Animals that cannot be returned to the wild for any reason should be euthanized unless they can be legally placed in permitted educational, breeding, or research programs.

[a]Although this outline is intended to provide general guidelines for the care of injured wildlife, the veterinarian is strongly encouraged to transfer these animals to an experienced permitted wildlife rehabilitator as soon as possible and/or to contact rehabilitators if questions arise. In addition, any individual working with wildlife should check with state and federal officials on permit requirements.

[b]For information on nutritional management of captive wildlife, see Poisson K, Weiss R, eds. *Wildlife Rehabilitation: A Comprehensive Approach*. Eugene, OR: The IWRC; 2016.

TABLE 14-2 Agencies Regulating Specific Taxa of Wildlife.[18,35]

Species	U.S. Regulatory Agency Responsible	Canadian Regulatory Agency Responsible
Endangered species: all taxa	USFWS (U.S. Fish & Wildlife Service)	CWS
Birds: migratory	USFWS, state wildlife agency	CWS, provincial wildlife agency
Birds: non-migratory	State wildlife agency	Provincial wildlife agency
Mammals: terrestrial	State wildlife agency	Provincial wildlife agency
Marine mammals: sea otters, manatees, walruses, polar bears	USFWS	DFO (Department of Fisheries and Oceans)
Marine mammals: seals, sea lions, cetaceans (whales, dolphins, porpoise)	NMFS (National Marine Fisheries Service)	DFO
Reptiles: sea turtles	NMFS	DFO
Reptiles: others	State wildlife agency	Provincial wildlife agency

TABLE 14-3 General Exceptions to the Migratory Bird Treaty Act.[18,35]

Licensed veterinarians who are not rehabilitation permit holders – may temporarily possess, stabilize, or euthanize sick and injured migratory birds, but must transfer birds to a federally permitted rehabilitator within 24 hours after stabilization (if a permitted rehabilitator is not found, the veterinarian must contact the Regional Migratory Bird Permit Office to obtain authorization to continue to possess the bird).

- Must contact local USFWS Ecological Services Office (http://offices.fws.gov) immediately upon receiving a threatened or endangered migratory bird species.
- May euthanize and dispose of migratory birds in accordance with the code for rehabilitation permits (Title 50 CFR Part 21.31).
- Must keep records of all migratory birds that die or are euthanized while under care; records to include species, injury, date of acquisition, date of death, cause of death.

Public Citizens – under these conditions, may humanely remove trapped migratory birds, including endangered species, from the interior of a structure if the bird is posing a health threat, is attacking humans or posing a threat to human safety because of its activities, poses a threat to commercial interests, or may become injured itself.

- Humane methods of capture must be used; adhesive traps are prohibited. Use of falconry birds to remove a trapped bird is prohibited. Causing the death of a trapped bird or using techniques likely to cause death is prohibited.
- If death occurs, the carcass must be disposed of immediately.
- The bird must be immediately released into a suitable habitat unless it is exhausted, ill, injured, or orphaned.
- If the bird is not releasable for the reasons stated above, the property owner must contact a federally permitted rehabilitator.
- Bald or golden eagles may not be removed without a permit.
- A federally permitted migratory bird rehabilitator must assist in the removal of an active nest with eggs or nestlings.
- All actions must comply with state and local regulations and ordinances.

TABLE 14-4 Considerations for Developing a Wildlife Policy in Private Practice.[1,3,5,16,35,51,53,54,56,57,59]

1. General considerations[35]
   All veterinary clinics should have a wildlife policy to ensure injured and orphaned wildlife receive timely care, regulatory and public health guidelines are followed, and a consistent message is presented to the public regarding the practice's willingness to see wildlife. Wildlife policies do not need to be complicated but should consider the time and resources the practice has available.
2. Treating injured and orphaned wildlife[3,53,54]
   Depending on the comfort level and expertise of the veterinarians and staff, the clinic may decide to see only certain types of wildlife, may treat to stabilize and transfer, or admit only severely injured animals for humane euthanasia. Whether or not the practitioner chooses to treat wildlife, a referral list should be available with wildlife-related contacts. This list should include veterinarians who treat wildlife, permitted wildlife rehabilitators, game wardens, wildlife biologists, animal control officers, public health offices, and state or provincial and federal wildlife agencies. It may be advantageous to build a network of volunteer transporters able to quickly move the wild animal to an appropriate location for initial or additional treatment.
3. Legalities (see Table 14-2)
4. Preparedness and safety[35]
   The practice should have the necessary restraint devices, enclosures, and experienced veterinarians and staff to provide treatment and supportive care to wildlife. The practice should also have space to house wildlife away from domestic animals, even if wildlife will only be on site for a few hours. Biosecurity and biosafety measures should be in place to prevent the spread of potential infectious diseases or parasites. Personal protective equipment should be on site and appropriate for the species. Additional considerations include disease reservoir or vector status of the animal, rabies immunization and titers of staff, and general safety for staff, clients, domestic patients, and the public.
5. VCPR (Veterinary Client Patient Relationship)[35,59]
   A VCPR between the practitioner and the wildlife rehabilitator should be agreed upon before wildlife are treated. This agreement should provide a clear mutual understanding of the division of responsibilities consistent with state or provincial laws regarding the practice of veterinary medicine. This agreement should contain these six components:
   a. The veterinarian has sufficient knowledge of wildlife medicine to provide a general or preliminary diagnosis.
   b. The veterinarian has recently seen the wildlife patient(s) through visits to the rehabilitation premises or at the veterinarian's facility.
   c. The veterinarian has assumed the responsibility for any medical judgments regarding the health of wildlife patients and the need for medical treatments.
   d. If the veterinarian intends to keep and treat any animal for more than 24 hours, the veterinarian must justify the need for prolonged veterinary care, have the appropriate wildlife rehabilitation permit(s), or be listed as a subpermittee to a wildlife rehabilitator; in accordance with state, provincial, and federal regulations.
   e. The veterinarian is available for followup in case of adverse reactions or failure of the regimen of therapy.
   f. Any agreement must abide by the laws and regulations governing the practice of veterinary medicine where and if they apply to wildlife rehabilitation.
6. Euthanasia[1,5,16,51,56,57]
   Injured wildlife may require humane euthanasia to alleviate pain and suffering due to injuries that are either severe or not conducive to release or placement in an education program. Euthanasia of wild animals should be conducted according to the AVMA Guidelines on Euthanasia or the AAZV Guidelines for the Euthanasia of Nondomestic Animals. Wildlife authorities should be contacted if a wild animal is fitted with a band, transmitter, tag, or other identification device. Carcasses should be disposed of in accordance with local regulations. Animals euthanized with pentobarbital should never be disposed of in a manner that makes the carcass accessible to scavenging and subsequent secondary barbiturate toxicosis. All carcasses, parts, and feathers from bald eagles and golden eagles must be sent to the National Eagle Repository. According to the Migratory Bird Treaty Act, it is illegal to keep carcasses, parts, and feathers from any migratory bird without an appropriate federal permit. Wildlife remains may be legally transferred to natural history museums.

TABLE 14-4 Considerations for Developing a Wildlife Policy in Private Practice. (cont'd)

7. Indications for euthanasia[35]
   Euthanasia should be considered for any animal:
   - whose injuries carry a poor prognosis for release (injuries will not resolve to the extent that the animal would be able to have a good life in the wild);
   - whose disease(s) may put personnel or other animals at serious risk;
   - whose injuries or illness require extended treatment and extensive care that would likely prolong that animal's stress and discomfort or might compromise the care of other animals through the use of time and resources;
   - that is nonreleasable and becomes self-mutilating in captivity or whose demeanor is otherwise not suitable for life in captivity.

TABLE 14-5 Recommendations for Safe Restraint of Native Wildlife.[4,7,9,17,23,27,29,33,37,38,44,47,50]

To ensure the safety of the handler and of the animal itself, it is imperative to understand and prepare for an animal's defense mechanisms. Additionally, wild animals may carry a variety of infectious and parasitic diseases that may present a health risk to veterinary staff, clients, the public, and domestic patients. A primary barrier (medical gloves) should be worn when handling wild animals.

Neonatal and juvenile mammals

Most young mammals can be safely handled awake with medical gloves +/- leather gloves and a towel. In general, scruffing wild animals is not recommended, as it does not provide adequate immobilization to prevent bites. Instead, older, more fractious juveniles should be restrained by grasping the head around the back of the neck with one hand and grasping the dorsal pelvis with the other hand. Additional species-specific recommendations are listed below.

Badgers, bobcats, lynx, raccoons, river otters

Subadult and adult animals can be dangerous and difficult to manually restrain. Thus, they often need to be sedated or anesthetized for safe handling using a squeeze cage, netting, or a syringe pole.

Coyotes, foxes

Subadult and adult animals are often easily subdued awake with a large blanket and leather gloves. A muzzle may be used during the procedure for added safety. Sedation and/or gas anesthesia may also be implemented for these species using a syringe pole while restraining the animal with a "Y" pole or manual restraint.

Skunks

Limit handling in this species to avoid being sprayed from the musk glands. Wear eye protection when handling. For young animals, attempt to drape a towel or plastic sheet over the animal and tuck the tail between the hind legs to decrease the possibility of being sprayed. Light pressure on the back (to prevent arching) also reduces spraying. Restrain older juveniles and adults with sedation and/or gas anesthesia.

Opossums

Subadult and adult animals can often be manually restrained with leather gloves and a towel by placing one hand under the ventrum to support the body and grasping the base of the tail with the other hand. Do not lift an opossum by the tail. Sedation and/or gas anesthesia may also be used.

Rabbits and hares

Subadult and adult animals can be manually restrained with a towel and light gloves. The animal's head should be covered with the towel before handling to reduce stress and the hindlimbs restrained so that the patient cannot kick and injure its back. Avoid overhandling; anesthetize for prolonged restraint.

Continued

TABLE 14-5 Recommendations for Safe Restraint of Native Wildlife. (cont'd)

Rodents
Subadult and adult animals should be handled with heavy leather gloves to protect against very sharp teeth. Nets may be useful for initial restraint of larger rodents. Porcupines can be manually restrained with leather gloves and a towel by placing one hand under the ventrum to support the body and grasping the base of the tail with the other hand in a cranial to caudal motion.
Insectivorous bats
All bats should be handled with medical gloves under light leather gloves, regardless of the animal's age. Place the bat gently in a soft cloth and cover. Expose portions of the bat to perform a physical exam. Cotton-tipped applicators are useful to assist with examinations.
Birds of prey (raptors)
Birds of prey should be handled with appropriately sized leather gloves. Raptors will use their talons for primary defense but may also use their beaks. A large sheet or towel should be placed over the animal's entire body and the feet securely restrained before removing it from the enclosure. The cloth should cover the head and drape over both wings to prevent flapping. A hood may be useful for some patients to reduce stress and struggling. Vulture defense includes regurgitation; keeping the patient's neck extended will reduce regurgitation efforts.
Passerines, woodpeckers, doves, etc.
Most of these species can be safely restrained using medical gloves and a small pillowcase with the fore- and middle fingers on either side of the bird's head and the bird's back pressed to the palm of the hand, taking care not to compress the neck or body and compromise respirations. Patients may become stressed or overheat with handling. Watch the patient closely and perform procedures in stages if needed.
Waterfowl, pelagic, and wading birds
Most of these species can be safely restrained using medical gloves and a towel. Bare hands are inappropriate for waterfowl, pelagic birds, and other species that require perfect waterproofing of the feathers. Waterfowl and large wading birds should be restrained by securing the legs with one hand, tucking the bird's body between the handler's side and the arm restraining the legs, and securing the head and neck with the opposite hand. Both the handler and the examiner should wear goggles and/or face shields for eye protection when working with long-billed birds such as herons and loons.
Snakes
Nonvenomous snakes may be restrained by grasping the head just behind the mandibles and securing the body with the other hand. An additional handler is needed for every 3-4 feet of snake to support the spine. Venomous snakes should be restrained only by experts using snake hooks and tongs to handle, and clear plastic tubes for restraint.
Chelonians
Chelonians may scratch or bite. Nonaggressive species may be restrained with medical gloves by grasping the sides of the shell between the front and back legs. Larger turtles, especially snapping turtles, require a hand under the caudal third of the plastron and the other hand grasping the tail or the caudal carapace. Do not lift a turtle by the tail. Snapping turtles can extend the head and neck two-thirds their body length caudally. A toilet plunger can be placed over a snapping turtle's head to reduce the risk of biting.
Lizards
Most lizards can be safely restrained wearing medical gloves by placing the index finger and thumb around the base of the mandibles to secure the head and prevent biting. The other hand should restrain the hind legs and tail. Never grab a lizard by the tail, especially in species with tail autonomy. To calm lizards, a vagal response can be created by placing cotton balls over the eyes and securing with bandage material.
Amphibians
Amphibians should only be briefly handled with nonpowdered, nonlatex gloves. Tadpoles are sensitive to nitrile and latex; vinyl gloves rinsed with nonchlorinated water should be used when handling tadpoles or cleaning their enclosures.

TABLE 14-6 Chemical Restraint/Anesthetic Agents Used in Select Wild Mammals.[a,6,11–14,20,21,24,25,26,39,42,45,46,48,60,61]

Agent	Dosage	Species/Comments
Acepromazine	0.1 mg/kg IM[25]	Beavers, porcupines
	0.5-2.5 mg/kg IM[25]	Prairie dogs
Alfaxalone (Alfaxan, Jurox)	1.5 mg/kg IV[48]	Most species
	5-10 mg/kg IM[48]	Most species
Atipamezole (Antisedan, Zoetis)	Give same volume IM as medetomidine and dexmedetomidine	Dexmedetomidine and medetomidine reversal
Atropine sulfate	0.03-0.05 mg/kg SC[42]	Most species/preanesthetic dose; may not be effective in lagomorphs and some rodents
Butorphanol (B)/ azaperone (A)/ medetomidine (Me) (Zoopharm)	(B) 0.51-0.65 mg/kg + (A) 0.17-0.22 mg/kg) + (Me) 0.2-0.26 mg/kg IM or 0.024 mL/kg if using combined formulation[46]	Beavers/sedation for minor procedures; surgical plane of anesthesia not achieved
	(B) 0.6 mg/kg + (A) 0.2 mg/kg) + (Me) 0.2 mg/kg IM[61]	Black bears
Dexmedetomidine (Dexdomitor, Zoetis)	Most species/generally insufficient alone to produce sedation in most wild mammals; combine with opioids and/or benzodiazepines; see ketamine for combinations	
Dexmedetomidine (De)/ butorphanol (B)	(De) 10-20 µg/kg + (B) 0.2 mg/kg IM[45]	Canids, felids, procyonids
Diazepam (available as a 1 mg/mL oral solution)	0.1-1 mg/kg PO, IM[25]	Beavers, porcupines
	0.5-2 mg/kg PO, SC, IM[6]	Bats
	1-2.5 mg/kg PO, IM, IP[25]	Prairie dogs
Flumazenil	0.01-0.05 mg/kg IM, IV, IO; repeat q1h prn[42]	Midazolam reversal; if using 5 mg/mL midazolam and 0.1 mg/mL flumazenil, use 2 × the volume of midazolam given
Glycopyrrolate	0.01 mg/kg SC, IM[25]	Beavers, porcupines/preanesthetic dose
	0.01-0.02 mg/kg SC, IM[25]	Prairie dogs/preanesthetic dose
Ketamine	—	Combinations frequently used by the authors; most can be followed by intubation and inhalant anesthetic drugs if general anesthesia is required; concentrated formulations of ketamine (200 mg/mL), butorphanol (30-50 mg/mL), and medetomidine (10 or 20 mg/mL) are available from compounding pharmacies and are advised for larger mammals; sustained release (SR) products are also available from compounding pharmacies
	30-100 mg/kg SC[6]	Bats
Ketamine (K)/ medetomidine (Me)	(K) 2-5 mg/kg + (Me) 0.04-0.1 mg/kg IM[21]	Carnivores

Continued

TABLE 14-6 Chemical Restraint/Anesthetic Agents Used in Select Wild Mammals. (cont'd)

Agent	Dosage	Species/Comments
Ketamine (K)/ medetomidine (Me)/ butorphanol (B)	(K) 2-4 mg/kg + (Me) 0.02 mg/kg + (B) 0.04-0.2 mg/kg IM[21]	Carnivores/deepen anesthesia with isoflurane for invasive procedures (wait at least 40 min after ketamine is administered before reversing medetomidine or dexmedetomidine)
Ketamine (K)/ dexmedetomidine (De)	(K) 2.6-5 mg/kg + (De) 0.048-0.056 mg/kg IM[14]	Fox
Ketamine (K)/midazolam (Mi)	(K) 18-25 mg/kg + (Mi) 0.20 mg/kg IM[39]	Mustelids
Ketamine (K)/ dexmedetomidine (De)/ midazolam (Mi)	(De) 0.1 mg/kg + (K) 30 mg/kg + (Mi) 0.75 mg/kg IM[20]	Squirrels
Ketamine (K)/xylazine (X)	(K) 3-4 mg/kg + (X) 2 mg/kg IM[11]	Cervids
	(K) 6.6 mg/kg + (X) 3.3 mg/kg IM[61]	Ursids
Midazolam	0.1-0.5 mg/kg IM[25]	Beavers, porcupines
	0.2-0.5 mg/kg IM, IV[21]	Carnivores/preanesthetic or sedative
	1-2 mg/kg IM, IP[25]	Prairie dogs
Propofol	—	Reduce dose with hypoproteinemia; supplemental oxygen recommended; induces profound respiratory depression; be prepared to ventilate
	3-7 mg/kg IV slowly to effect[42]	Carnivores
	0.1-0.6 mg/kg/min constant rate infusion[24]	Carnivores/sedation at lower doses; light anesthesia at higher doses
Xylazine	2-3 mg/kg IM[12]	Cervids
Zolazepam-tiletamine (Telazol)	3-7 mg/kg IM[13]	Ursids
Zolazepam-tiletamine (Telazol) (T)/medetomidine (Me)	(T) 1.54-2.3 mg/kg + (Me) 0.03-0.045 mg/kg IM[26]	Ursids
Zolazepam-tiletamine (Telazol) (T)/ dexmedetomidine (De)	(T) 0.94-1.0 mg/kg + (De) 33.05-35.25 μ/kg IM[16a]	Cervids

[a]Additional drug doses for other classes of wild animals may be found in other chapters of this formulary.

TABLE 14-7 Acceptable Methods for Euthanizing Wildlife.[a,1,5,19,32,35]

Chemical Methods of Euthanasia

Pentobarbital sodium

Species	Amphibians, reptiles, birds, mammals
Status	Recommended, considered the gold standard for animal euthanasia, license required

Potassium chloride

Species	Amphibians, reptiles, birds, mammals
Status	Conditionally acceptable; should only be used when animal is in a deep plane of anesthesia

TABLE 14-7 Acceptable Methods for Euthanizing Wildlife. (cont'd)

T–61 (mixture of embutramide, mebozonium [mebenzonium] iodide, and tetracaine hydrochloride) [Available in Canada, not in US]

Species	Amphibians, reptiles, birds, mammals
Status	Acceptable if administered by intravenous injection by trained personnel

Inhalant Methods of Euthanasia

Anesthetic gases: isoflurane, methoxyflurane, sevoflurane

Species	Amphibians, reptiles, birds, mammals
Status	Conditionally acceptable; acceptable in small animals <7 kg (15 lb); should be followed by other recommended methods to ensure death

Carbon dioxide (CO_2)

Species	Terrestrial reptiles, birds, mammals
Status	Conditionally acceptable—gradual fill recommended; bats, diving animals, and young animals may be more resistant

Physical Methods of Euthanasia

Gunshot

Species	Amphibians, reptiles, birds, mammals
Status	Conditionally acceptable; human safety and licensing concerns

Blunt force trauma to the head/stunning

Species	Amphibians, reptiles, birds, mammals
Status	Conditionally acceptable in small, thin-skulled animals when more direct and conventional methods are unavailable

Pithing

Species	Amphibians, reptiles
Status	Conditionally acceptable; is commonly used as a secondary method of euthanasia in reptiles following an accepted primary euthanasia protocol

Decapitation

Species	Amphibians, reptiles, birds, small mammals
Status	Conditionally acceptable; should be followed by pithing in amphibians and reptiles; appropriate for emergency euthanasia in remote locations

Cervical dislocation

Species	Reptiles, small birds, small mammals, all <200 g
Status	Conditionally acceptable; training required; prior sedation/general anesthesia is preferred

Thoracic compression

Species	Small birds and mammals
Status	Conditionally acceptable following primary anesthesia; three-point cardiac compression alone might be acceptable in small birds

Exsanguination

Species	Amphibians, reptiles, birds, mammals
Status	Conditionally acceptable; never acceptable on a conscious animal

[a]Additional methods of euthanasia for certain classes of wildlife may be found in other chapters of this formulary.

TABLE 14-8 Recommendations for Venipuncture Sites in Native Wildlife.[23,25,27,41,50]

Species	Notes
Carnivores	Jugular, cephalic, medial or lateral saphenous vein
Opossums	Lateral or ventral tail, cephalic or saphenous vein; pouch vein in females
Lagomorphs	Jugular, cephalic, medial or lateral saphenous vein
Rodents	Jugular, cephalic, medial or lateral saphenous, ventral or lateral tail vein; very small rodents often require cranial vena cava venipuncture under anesthesia
Birds of prey	Right jugular, medial metatarsal (use caution around talons), or basilic vein
Passerines, woodpeckers, doves, etc.	Right jugular, basilic, or medial metatarsal vein
Waterfowl, pelagic, and wading birds	Medial metatarsal vein preferred; basilic or right jugular vein also options
Insectivorous bats	Jugular, cephalic, or uropatagial vein; may require anesthesia for safe collection; consider volume needed vs. volume safe to collect
Snakes	Jugular vein (insert needle parallel to the ribs and at 9 ventral scales cranial to the heart), ventral tail vein, or heart in snakes >200 g (previous experience recommended; place snake in dorsal recumbency and insert needle under abdominal scale at 45° angle caudal to heart); venomous snakes should only be handled by professionals
Chelonians	Jugular vein, subcarapacial sinus, tail, brachial, or femoral vein; jugular vein accessed with neck in full extension and may require sedation; collection from the jugular vein least likely to result in lymph contamination
Lizards	Ventral tail, jugular, or ventral abdominal vein
Amphibians	Ventral abdominal, facial (maxillary)/musculocutaneous, or sublingual vein in larger animals

TABLE 14-9 Common Zoonoses of Native Wildlife.[28,30,43,52,58]

Disease	Etiology	Common Hosts	Transmission	Symptoms in Humans
Mycoses				
Aspergillosis	*Aspergillus fumigatus*	Birds	Airborne; inhalation of spores during necropsy	Respiratory disorders in immune-compromised individuals
Dermatophytosis (ringworm)	*Microsporum* spp., *Trichophyton* spp., *Epidermophyton floccosum*	Mammals, reptiles	Direct contact	Dermatitis

TABLE 14-9 Common Zoonoses of Native Wildlife. (cont'd)

Disease	Etiology	Common Hosts	Transmission	Symptoms in Humans
Systemic mycoses (blastomycosis, coccidioidomycosis, cryptococcosis, histoplasmosis)	*Blastomyces dermatidis, Coccidiodes immitis, Histoplasma capsulatum, Cryptococcus neoformans*	Birds, bats	Inhalation of spores; dried feces	Pulmonary disease; dyspnea; lethargy; cough; other organs eventually affected
Viruses				
Avian influenza	Avian influenza virus (H1, H5, H7)	Birds	Direct contact; inhalation of bodily secretions	Influenza-like
Hantaviral pulmonary syndrome (+/- renal failure)	*Hantavirus (*Bunyaviridae*); Sin Nombre* virus	Rodents	Inhalation from dried feces and urine	Fever; diarrhea; myalgia; vomiting; abdominal pain; tachypnea; tachycardia
Newcastle disease	Avian paramyxovirus-1	Birds (esp. juvenile cormorants and gulls)	Direct contact; inhalation of bodily secretions	Conjunctivitis; mild influenza-like symptoms
Rabies	Rhabdovirus	Warm-blooded vertebrates (RVS spp. vary by location)	Contact with saliva (bites) or neural tissue	Neurological signs
SARS-CoV-2	Coronavirus	Mustelids; possibly felids, canids, bats	Airborne; inhalation of bodily secretions	Fever; respiratory; GI
Parasitic				
Acariasis (mange)	*Sarcoptes* spp., *Cheyletiella* spp., *Notoedres* spp.	Mammals	Direct contact	Pruritic dermatitis
Baylisascaris larva migrans	*Baylisascaris procyonis*	Raccoons	Fecal-oral	Neurological signs; ocular disease
Cryptosporidiosis	*Cryptosporidium parva*	Deer & rodents	Fecal-oral	GI; diarrhea
Hydatid disease (echinococcosis)	*Echinococcus* spp.	Canids	Fecal-oral	Cough; abdominal pain; vomiting; fever
Toxoplasmosis	*Toxoplasma gondii*	Felids	Fecal-oral	Fever; ague; encephalitis; congenital chorioretinitis; mental retardation

Continued

TABLE 14-9 Common Zoonoses of Native Wildlife. (cont'd)

Disease	Etiology	Common Hosts	Transmission	Symptoms in Humans
Bacterial				
Brucellosis	*Brucella* spp.	Seals, cervids	Direct contact	Septicemia; fever
Campylobacteriosis	*Campylobacter fetus* subspp.	Cervids, birds	Fecal-oral	Gastroenteritis
Chlamydiosis (psittacosis)	*Chlamydia psittaci*	Psittacines, pigeons, raptors, sea turtles	Inhalation of dried feces or respiratory secretions	Respiratory disorders; flulike symptoms
Leprosy	*Mycobacterium leprae*	Armadillos	Inhalation of dried feces or respiratory secretions	Skin lesions; peripheral neuropathy
Leptospirosis	*Leptospira interogans*	Seals, cervids, rodents, carnivores, sea turtles	Contact with infected urine	Flulike; septicemia; renal failure
Salmonellosis	*Salmonella* spp.	Mammals, birds, herptiles	Fecal-oral	Gastroenteritis
Tuberculosis	*Mycobacterium bovis* and *avium*	Cervids, birds	Direct contact, inhalation	Respiratory disease
Methicillin-resistant *Staphylococcus aureus* (MRSA)	*Staphylococcus aureus*	Most wildlife species	Direct contact	Local abscesses; septicemia
Tularemia	*Francisella tularensis*	Rodents, lagomorphs	Tick bites, wound infection, fecal-oral, inhalation	Flulike; skin ulcers; pneumonia; gastroenteritis
Bubonic plague; pneumonic plague	*Yersina pestis*	Squirrels, rats, prairie dogs, carnivores	Fleas, airborne, wound infection	Lymphadenopathy; pneumonia; fever
Indirect, vector-borne (possible infection via necropsy)				
Encephalitides (EEE, SLE, WEE, WNV)	Arboviruses	Mammals, birds	Mosquito bites	Influenzalike; neurologic
Lyme disease	*Borrelia burgdorferi*	Small mammals, deer, passerines	Tick bites	Fever; fatigue; rash (erythema migrans); joint aches
Rocky Mountain spotted fever	*Rickettsia rickettsia*	Rodents	Tick bites	Cyclic fever; +/- rash

TABLE 14-10 **Development and Natural Diets of Common Young Wild Bird Species.**[8,34]

Species	# of Broods	Incubation (days)	Age When Able to Fly	Postfledging Dependence on Parent(s)	Natural Foods
American crow	1	16-19	28-35 days	2-3 wk; stay in family group	Small vertebrates, insects, fruit, seeds
American kestrel	1	26-32	28-31 days	14 days	Insects, small vertebrates
American robin	2-3	12-14	14-16 days	7-14 days	Insects, fruit
Bald eagle	1	35	8-14 wk	4-11 wk	Fish, mammals, birds, carrion
Black vulture	1	38-39	4 wk	4-10 mo	Carrion, some live prey
Blue jay	1-2	16-18	17-21 days	up to 2 mo	Small vertebrates, insects, fruit, seeds
Canada goose	1	25-30	40-73 days	Remain in family groups	Grasses, grain, aquatic invertebrates
Catbird	1-2	12-13	10-11 days	7-14 days	Insects, fruit
Chickadee	1-2	11-13	13-17 days	10 days	Insects, seeds, fruit
Chimney swift	1	19-21	28-30 days	Remain in flock year-round	Insects
Chipping sparrow	2	11-14	8-12 days	3-4 wk; stay in family group all summer	Insects, seeds
Common grackle	1	13-14	16-20 days	1-3 days; then flock with other juveniles	Small vertebrates, insects, fruit, seeds
Downy woodpecker	1	12	20-25 days	Up to 3 wk	Insects
Eastern bluebird	2-3	12-14	16-20 days	3-4 wk	Insects, fruit
Great horned owl	1	26-35	63-70 days	Several mo	Mammals, birds, insects
House finch	3	12-14	11-19 days	2-3 wk; then flock w/other juveniles	Seeds, fruit, buds
House wren	1-2	12-15	12-18 days	7-14 days	Insects
Killdeer	1-2	24-28	25 days	Stay w/male parent up to 5 wk	Insects
Mallard	1	23-29	42-60 days	Remain in family groups	Seeds, grasses, aquatic invertebrates

Continued

TABLE 14-10 Development and Natural Diets of Common Young Wild Bird Species (cont'd)

Species	# of Broods	Incubation (days)	Age When Able to Fly	Postfledging Dependence on Parent(s)	Natural Foods
Mourning dove	1-2	14-15	12-13 days	7-10 days; then join juvenile flock	Seeds, grain
Northern mockingbird	1-3	14-15	12-13 days	2-4 wk	Insects, fruit
Northern cardinal	1-2	12-13	9-11 days	2-3 wk	Insects, seeds, fruit
Northern flicker	1-2	11-14	25-28 days	2-3 wk	Insects
Northern oriole	1	12-14	12-14 days	7-10 days	Insects, fruit, nectar
Osprey	1	34-42	49-60 days	2-10 wk	Fish
Red-shouldered hawk	1	33	32-45 days	6-8 wk	Mammals, herptiles, birds
Red-tailed hawk	1	28-35	42-46 days	7-8 wk	Mammals, herptiles, birds, insects
Ruby-throated hummingbird	1-2	11-14	14-28 days	Up to 34 days	Nectar, insects
Screech owl	1	21-30	27 days	6-8 wk	Small vertebrates, insects
Song sparrow	2-3	12-13	9-16 days	21-30 days	Insects, seeds
Tufted titmouse	1-2	13-14	15-18 days	3-4 wk; stay in family groups in winter	Insects, seeds, fruit
Turkey vulture	1	38-40	9-12 wk	2-3 wk	Carrion
Wood duck	1	28-37	56-70 days	Left alone after 5 wk	Aquatic invertebrates, seeds

TABLE 14-11 Age Determination of Common Young Wild Mammals.[34,49]

Species	Age	Description
Badger	Birth	90-100 gm
	4 wk	Teeth erupt
	5 wk	Eyes open
	2-3 mo	Weaning begins
	5-6 mo	Weaned

TABLE 14-11 Age Determination of Common Young Wild Mammals. (cont'd)

Species	Age	Description
Bat	Birth	5-15 gm, 10 cm long
	2 days	Eyes open
	3-4 wk	Can fly
	6 wk	Weaned
	10 wk	Adult size
Beaver	Birth	Furred, eyes open, incisors present, 450 gm, 40 cm long
	16 days	Weaned
	21 days	Fully independent
	1 mo	Come out of den
	6 wk	2 kg
	2 yrs	Leave adults at this time
Bobcat	Birth	283-368 gm
	11-14 days	Eyes open, deciduous incisors and canines erupt
	17-21 wk	Permanent incisors and canines erupt
Chipmunk	Birth	Blind, hairless, 2-3 gm, 6 cm long
	4-6 days	Body hair begins to appear
	7-21 days	Incisors erupt
	8 days	Stripes appear
	1 mo	Eyes open, 28 gm, 14 cm long
	5-6 wk	Above ground
	6 wk	Fully independent
Cottontail rabbit	Birth	Naked or fine hair, 20-25 gm, 4-5 cm long
	4-5 days	Eyes and ears open, able to hop and squeak
	7 days	Fully furred
	13-16 days	Leave nest but return occasionally for a few days
	16 days	Weaned, 10-12 cm long
	21 days	Fully independent
	1 mo	Full set of teeth
Coyote	Birth	Blind, brown-gray, wooly fur, 250-300 gm
	8-14 days	Eyes open
	2-3 wk	Deciduous incisors and canines erupt
	8 wk	Weaned
Fox, gray	Birth	Blackish skin, naked, 100 gm
	9 days	Eyes open, fuzzy fur begins
	2-3 wk	Deciduous incisors and canines erupt
	4 wk	Hair growth
	7-8 wk	Weaned
	16 wk	Milk teeth lost, releasable

Continued

TABLE 14-11 Age Determination of Common Young Wild Mammals. (cont'd)

Species	Age	Description
Fox, red	Birth	Naked, 100 gm
	8-9 days	Eyes open, fuzzy fur begins
	2-3 wk	Deciduous incisors and canines erupt
	4-5 wk	Weaned
	7 wk	Pale yellowish-brown
	8-9 wk	Pale reddish-brown
	16-20 wk	Reddish, milk teeth lost, releasable
Ground squirrel (13-lined)	Birth	Naked, eyes & ears closed, 14-18 gm
	1 wk	28-30 gm
	10-14 days	Hair begins to appear
	3 wk	Lower incisors erupt, covered with hair, ears open
	4 wk	Eyes open
	5 wk	Upper incisors erupt
	6 wk	Can curl tail
	8-9 wk	Weaned, 140 gm, bushy tail
	11 wk	Releasable
Groundhog (woodchuck)	Birth	Blind, naked, wrinkled, pink skin, 22-30 gm, 10 cm long
	1 wk	Skin pigmented
	2 wk	Covering of short black hair
	3 wk	Begin to crawl
	4 wk	Eyes open, weaning begins; come to opening of den
	5 wk	Can whistle, look like adults
	6 wk	Weaned; venture outside den
Lynx	Birth	197-211 gm
	11-14 days	Eyes open, deciduous incisors and canines erupt
	17-21 wk	Permanent incisors and canines erupt
Muskrat	Birth	Blind, naked, 20 gm, 10 cm long
	7 days	Covered with coarse fur
	14-16 days	Eyes open
	3-4 wk	Weaned
Opossum	Birth	Naked, 13 gm, 10-20 mm long
	17 days	Whiskers & nose hairs present; genitalia visible
	29 days	Blond abdominal hairs
	33 days	Pigmentation at base of tail
	40 days	Blue-grey on upper neck & shoulders, 4-5 cm long
	43 days	Body hair begins on back
	48 days	Pigmentation on entire body
	55 days	Mouth open

TABLE 14-11 Age Determination of Common Young Wild Mammals. (cont'd)

Species	Age	Description
Opossum (cont'd)	58-72 days	Eyes open, 6-10 cm long
	60 days	Short, dark guard hairs on body, first premolar emerges
	70 days	Leave pouch for short time, >10 cm long
	75 days	Upper incisors & canines appear, begin weaning, 12 cm long
	81-87 days	12-16 cm long
	87-92 days	Produce clicking noises
	96-100 days	Fully weaned, 100-120 gm
Raccoon	Birth	60-75 gm
	2 wk	Mask fully furred
	18-24 days	Eyes & ears open, 250-300 gm
	3 wk	Tail rings prominent
	4 wk	Deciduous incisors erupt, begin walking
	6 wk	Guard hairs appear, 600 gm
	7 wk	Weaning begins, 700 gm
	16 wk	Weaning complete
River otter	Birth	128 gm
	1 wk	266 gm
	2 wk	515 gm
	3 wk	660-900 gm
	4 wk	Eyes open
	7 wk	Walking unsteadily
	8 wk	Eating solid food
Skunk	3-5 wk	Eyes open
	4 wk	Musk glands developed
	8 wk	Weaned
Squirrel, tree	Birth	Naked, eyes & ears closed, 14-18 gm
	1 wk	28-30 gm
	10-14 days	Hair begins to appear
	3 wk	Lower incisors erupt, covered with hair, ears open
	4 wk	Eyes open
	5 wk	Upper incisors erupt
	6 wk	Ears open, can curl tail
	8-9 wk	Weaned, bushy tail
	11 wk	Releasable

TABLE 14-12 Reproduction and Dietary Information for Common Wild Mammals.[34,49]

Species	Breed	Gestation	Birth	Litter/yr	#/Litter	Leave Den	Nurse	Natural Foods
Beaver	Jan-Feb	128 days	Apr-Jun, peak May	1	1-8, avg 3-4	At birth, but occupy den w/ parents for 2 yr	Mostly at night	Bark & twigs of various trees
Chipmunk	Apr, Jul, Aug	31 days	1st in May; 2nd in Aug or Sep	2	3-5	8 wk	Daylight	Nuts, seeds, berries, insects
Cottontail rabbit	Jan-Sep, peak Mar-Aug	26-28 days	Feb-Oct, peak Apr-Aug	6-8	3-9, avg 5	10 days	Night	Grasses, fruits, nuts, vegetables
Coyote	Jan-Apr	63 days	Mar-Jun	1	1-12, avg 5-7	1 mo	Dawn & dusk	Mammals, birds, snakes, fruit
Fox, red	Late Dec-Mar	49-56 days	Mar-Apr	1	4-9	1 mo	Night, dawn, & dusk	Fruit, small mammals
Groundhog (woodchuck)	Mar-May, peak Apr	31-32 days	Apr-Jun, peak May	1	2-7, avg 4-5	9-11 wk	Early morning, late afternoon	Grasses, peas, clover, lettuce, apples
Muskrat	Feb-Aug, peak Apr	22-30 days	Mar-Sep	2-3, avg 2	1-11, avg 4-7	15 days	Mostly evening, also daytime	Mussels, fish, frogs, insects, vegetation
Opossum	Jan-Oct, peak Feb-Mar	12-13 days	Feb-Nov	1-3, avg 1	5-25, avg 9	3 mo	Night	Carrion, insects, fish, nuts, eggs, fruits
Porcupine	Sept-Oct	7 mo	Apr-May	1	1	3-4 mo	Night	Vegetation, bark
Raccoon	Jan-Mar, peak Feb	63 days	Mar-Jun, peak Apr-May	1	1-7, avg 3-4	2 mo	Night	Fruits, nuts, frogs, mice
Skunk	Feb-Mar	63-75 days	May	1	2-10, avg 4-6	6-8 wk	Night	Mice, frogs, eggs, fish, grubs, fruit
Squirrel, grey	May-Jun, Dec-Jan, peak Jan & Jun	44 days	Feb-Mar, peak Mar-Jul	1-2	3-5	7-8 wk	Midmorning & midafternoon	Nuts, seeds, fruit, insects, various woods
Squirrel, red	Feb-Mar, Jun-Jul	38 days	Apr-May, Aug-Sep	2	2-7	7-8 wk	Daylight	Seeds, nuts, eggs, fungi
White-tailed deer	Sept-Feb, peak Nov	190-210 days	Late May-early Jun	1	1-3	At birth	Variable	Wild crabapple, leaves, grasses, wood

TABLE 14-13 Recommendations for Meat Withdrawal Times in Game Species.[2,10,22,36,40,55,59]

Drug use in wild animals is considered extralabel and as such is regulated by the Food and Drug Administration (FDA) through the Animal Medicinal Drug Use Clarification Act (AMDUCA). This act is divided into food-producing animals and non-food-producing animals. Drug residues in game animals are a potential public health risk to those who consume the meat. Wild game mammals include deer, antelope, rabbit, squirrel, opossum, raccoon, nutria, or muskrat, and nonaquatic reptiles such as land snakes. Wild game birds include waterfowl (ducks and geese), pheasants, partridge, quail, grouse, doves, snipes, and pigeons.

Practitioners need to be aware of potential meat withdrawal times (defined as the time between drug administration and when the meat can safely be consumed by a human) when administering drugs to game species during or just before established hunting and trapping seasons. Practitioners should check the Food Animal Residue Avoidance Database (FARAD) for guidance on drug administration in game species that could be consumed. Very few pharmacokinetic studies have been done in wildlife; therefore, wildlife should not be released until at least the recommended meat withdrawal time for cattle has elapsed. If a game animal cannot be held until the meat withdrawal time has passed, it should be identified with a unique number and warning that the meat should not be consumed. Permission to tag wildlife may also require permission from state, provincial, or federal authorities.

Some drugs may never be used in food-producing animals at any time. These include: chloramphenicol, clenbuterol, diethylstilbestrol, dimetridazole, ipronidazole, metronidazole, other nitromidazoles, furazolidone, nitrofurazone, glycopeptides, and fluoroquinolones. Adamantanes and neuraminidase inhibitors are prohibited in wild game birds.

Aminoglycosides should not be used in wildlife species due to prolonged tissue persistence (often >6 mo) and lack of data on residue depletion. Most cephalosporins, nitroimidazoles, and synthetic penicillins are not licensed for use in food animals and therefore should be used judiciously if the animal may be hunted for food.

The following is a list of recommended withdrawal times for select drugs used in wildlife.

Agent	Meat Withdrawal Time (days)	Agent	Meat Withdrawal Time (days)
Acepromazine	14	Naloxone	30
Atipamezole	14	Naltrexone	30
Diazepam	14	Penicillin (long-acting)	21
Diprenorphine	30	Tolazoline	30
Etorphine	30	Xylazine	30
Ivermectin	49	Yohimbine	30
Ketamine	3	Zolazepam and tiletamine (1:1)	14
Medetomidine	14		

TABLE 14-14 Resources for Training in Wildlife Medicine.

Cornell Wildlife Health Lab—https://cwhl.vet.cornell.edu/resources/training-materials
A variety of free videos on wildlife diseases, necropsy and sampling techniques, wildlife forensics, biosecurity, and more.

IWRC Wildlife Rehabilitation Courses—https://theiwrc.org/courses
On-line courses in wildlife rehabilitation topics (nutrition, fluid therapy, bandaging, etc.) beginning at $55. In-person training courses are also available for multiple attendees.

Lafeber Vet Wildlife Care—https://lafeber.com/vet/video/?fwp_topics=wildlife-rehabilitation
Webinars and short on-demand videos on basic techniques available free to Lafeber Vet members. Topics include: wildlife triage, critical care, anesthesia, necropsy, and more.

National Wildlife Rehabilitators Association—https://nwrawildlife.org
Courses and publications available on topics related to wildlife rehabilitation, wildlife medicine, and more. NWRA also offers a symposium in late February or early March each year.

The Raptor Academy—https://raptor.umn.edu/programs-and-events/raptor-academy
A comprehensive selection of webinars and self-study opportunities at $35 each for those working with raptors, including anatomy & physiology, physical exam, medical care, bandaging, nutrition, and more.

Wildlife Care Academy—https://wildlifeacademy.org/
Webinars and on-demand courses beginning at $15, including wildlife rehabilitation, wildlife medicine, outreach and communications, education, administration, and more.

TABLE 14-15 Websites of Wildlife Health Organizations and Related Information.

National Wildlife Rehabilitators Association—http://www.nwrawildlife.org

International Wildlife Rehabilitation Council—http://theiwrc.org/

USGS National Wildlife Health Center—http://www.nwhc.usgs.gov/

U.S. Fish and Wildlife Service—http://www.fws.gov/

Southeastern Cooperative Wildlife Disease Study—http://vet.uga.edu/scwds

Birds of North America Online—https://birdsna.org/Species-Account/bna/home

World Organization for Animal Health—http://www.oie.int/

National Association of State Public Health Veterinarians—http://www.nasphv.org/

REFERENCES

1. American Veterinary Medical Association (AVMA). 2020. *AVMA Guidelines on Euthanasia.* Available at: https://www.avma.org/sites/default/files/2020-01/2020_Euthanasia_Final_1-15-20.pdf. Accessed Nov 22, 2020.
2. American Veterinary Medical Association (AVMA). *Guidelines for Veterinary Prescription Drugs.* Available at: https://www.avma.org/resources-tools/avma-policies/guidelines-veterinary-prescription-drugs. Accessed Nov 22, 2020.
3. American Veterinary Medical Association (AVMA). *Wildlife Decision Tree.* Available at: https://www.avma.org/sites/default/files/2019-11/WildlifeDecisionTree_1.pdf. Accessed Nov 22, 2020.

4. Arent LR. *Raptors in Captivity*. Blaine, WA: Hancock House Publishers; 2007.
5. Baer CK, ed. *Guidelines for Euthanasia of Nondomestic Animals*. Yulee, FL: American Association of Zoo Veterinarians; 2006. Available at: https://www.aazv.org/page/441. Accessed 4 Oct 2020.
6. Barnard SM, ed. *Bats in Captivity Volume 1—Biological and Medical Aspects*. Washington, DC: Logos Press; 2009:493–558.
7. Beckwith S. Rehabilitation of orphan river otters. *Proc Nat Wildl Rehab Symp*. 2003;21:51–60.
8. Billerman SM, Keeney BK, Rodewald PG, et al., eds. *Birds of the World*. Ithaca, NY: Cornell Laboratory of Ornithology; 2020. Available at https://birdsoftheworld.org/bow/home. Accessed Nov 23, 2020.
9. Cashins SD, Alford RA, Skerratt LF. Lethal effect of latex, nitrile, and vinyl gloves on tadpoles. *Herp Rev*. 2008;39:298–301.
10. Cattet M. A *CCWHC Technical Bulletin: Drug Residues in Wild Meat—Addressing a Public Health Concern*: Canadian Cooperative Wildlife Health Centre: Newsletter & Publications; 2003: Paper 46.
11. Caulkett N. Anesthesia for North American cervids. *Can Vet J*. 1997;38:389–390.
12. Caulkett N, Arnemo J. Cervids (Deer). In: West G, Heard D, Caulkett N, eds. *Zoo Animal & Wildlife Immobilization and Anesthesia*. 2nd ed. Ames, IA: Wiley Blackwell; 2014:823–829.
13. Caulkett N, Fahlman A. Ursids (Bears). In: West G, Heard D, Caulkett N, eds. *Zoo Animal & Wildlife Immobilization and Anesthesia*. 2nd ed. Ames, IA: Wiley Blackwell; 2014:599–606.
14. Chirife AD, Cevidanes A, Millán J. Effective field immobilization of Andean fox (*Lycalopex culpaeus*) with ketamine-dexmedetomidine and antagonism with atipamezole. *J Wildl Dis*. 2020;56:447–451.
15. Clayton LA, et al. Natural history and medical management of amphibians. In: Hernandez SM, Barron HW, Miller EA, et al., eds. *Medical Management of Wildlife Species*. Hoboken, NJ: Wiley Blackwell; 2020:383–395.
16. Cornell Waste Management Institute. *US Mortality and Butcher Waste Disposal Laws*. Available at: http://compost.css.cornell.edu/mapsdisposal.html. 2014. Accessed Nov 27, 2020.
16a. Costa G, Musicò M, Spadola F, et al. Comparison of tiletamine-zolazepam combined with dexmedetomidine or xylazine for chemical immobilization of wild fallow deer (*Dama dama*). *J Zoo Wildl Med*. 2021;52(3):1009–1012.
17. Derrell CJ, Olfert ED. Rodents. In: Fowler ME, ed. *Zoo and Wild Animal Medicine*. 2nd ed. Philadelphia, PA: WB Saunders Co; 1986:727–747.
18. Duerr R, Whittington J. Legal responsibilities and restrictions on veterinarians working with wildlife. *Wildl Rehab Bull*. 2017;35(1):25–37.
19. Engilis A, Engilis IE, Paul-Murphy J. Rapid cardiac compression: an effective method of avian euthanasia. *Condor*. 2018;120:617–621.
20. Eshar D, Beaufrére H. Anesthetic effects of dexmedetomidine-ketamine-midazolam administered intramuscularly in five-striped palm squirrels (*Funambulus pennantii*). *Am J Vet Res*. 2019;80:1082–1088.
21. Fontenot DK. Exotic carnivore restraint, anesthesia and analgesia. *Proc Am Assoc Zoo Vet Annu Pre-Conf*. 2009:1–7.
22. Food Animal Residue Avoidance Databank (Farad). Available at: http://www.farad.org/. Accessed Nov 27, 2020.
23. Fowler ME, Miller RE, eds. *Zoo and Wild Animal Medicine*. 5th ed. St. Louis, MO: WB Saunders; 2003.
24. Hawkins MG, Pascoe PJ. Anesthesia, analgesia, and sedation of small mammals. In: Quesenberry KE, Orcutt CJ, Mans C, et al., eds. *Ferrets, Rabbits, and Rodents: Clinical Medicine and Surgery*. 4th ed. St. Louis, MO: Elsevier; 2021:536–558.
25. Heard DJ. Rodents. In: West G, Heard D, Caulkett N, eds. *Zoo Animal & Wildlife Immobilization and Anesthesia*. 2nd ed. Ames, IA: Wiley Blackwell; 2014:893–903.
26. Jeong DH, Yang JJ, Seok SH, et al. Immobilization of Asiatic black bears (*Ursus thibetanus*) with medetomidine-zolazepam-tiletamine in South Korea. *J Wildl Dis*. 2017;53:636–641.

27. Johnson-Delaney CA. What every veterinarian needs to know about Virginia opossums. *Exot DVM*. 2005;6:38–43.
28. Koopmans M. SARS-CoV-2 and the human-animal interface: outbreaks on mink farms. *Lancet Infect Dis*. 2020.
29. Lafeber Company (Cornell, IL). Available at: http://lafebervet.com. Accessed Oct 4, 2020.
30. Leveque NW, ed. *Zoonosis Updates from the Journal of Veterinary Medicine*. Schaumburg, IL: American Veterinary Medical Association; 1995.
31. Luther E. *Answering the Call of the Wild*. Toronto, ON: Toronto Wildlife Center; 2010.
32. McRuer D. Euthanasia in wildlife rehabilitation. *Wildl Rehab Bull*. 2018;36(1):6–17.
33. McRuer DL, Barron HW. Personal observations. 2016.
34. Miller EA, ed. *Quick Reference*. 3rd ed. St. Cloud, MN: National Wildlife Rehabilitators Association (NWRA); 2006.
35. Miller EA, Schlieps J, eds. *Standards for Wildlife Rehabilitation*. Bloomington, MN: National Wildlife Rehabilitators Association (NWRA); 2021.
36. Miller EA, Goodman M, Cox S. *NWRA Wildlife Formulary*. 4th ed. St. Cloud, MN: National Wildlife Rehabilitators Association (NWRA); 2017.
37. Mitchell MA, Tully TN Jr., eds. *Manual of Exotic Pet Practice*. St. Louis, MO: Elsevier; 2009.
38. Moore AT, Joosten S, eds. *Principles of Wildlife Rehabilitation*. 2nd ed. St. Cloud, MN: National Wildlife Rehabilitators Association (NWRA); 2002.
39. Mortenson JA, Moriarty KM. Ketamine and midazolam anesthesia in Pacific martens (*Martes caurina*). *J Wildl Dis*. 2015;51:250–254.
40. Needham ML, Webb AI, Baynes RE, et al. Current update on drugs for game bird species. *J Am Vet Med Assoc*. 2007;231(10):1506–1508.
41. Norton TM, Allender MA, et al. Natural history and medical management of terrestrial and aquatic chelonians. In: Hernandez SM, Barron HW, Miller EA, et al., eds. *Medical Management of Wildlife Species*. Hoboken, NJ: Wiley Blackwell; 2020:363–381.
42. Plumb DC. *Plumb's Veterinary Drug Handbook*. 9th ed. Ames, IA: Wiley-Blackwell; 2018.
43. Pruitt A. Zoonoses. In: Poisson K, Weiss R, eds. *Wildlife Rehabilitation: A Comprehensive Approach*. Eugene, OR: The IWRC; 2016:63–80.
44. Reed-Smith J, Ball J. *North American River Otter Husbandry Notebook*. 2nd ed. Grand Rapids, MI: John Ball Zoological Garden; 2001.
45. Rosenhagen N. *Personal observation*. 2020.
46. Roug A, Talley H, Davis T, et al. A mixture of butorphanol, azaperone and medetomidine for the immobilization of American beavers *(Castor canadensis)*. *J Wildl Dis*. 2018;54:617–621.
47. Samour JH, ed. *Avian Medicine*. 3rd ed. St. Louis, MO: Elsevier; 2016.
48. Schott R. Triaging the wildlife patient. *Proc Student Chap Am Vet Med Assoc Symp*. 2015.
49. Schwartz CW, Schwartz ER. *The Wild Animals of Missouri*. Columbia, MO: University of Missouri Press and Missouri Department of Conservation; 1981.
50. Scott DE. *Raptor Medicine, Surgery and Rehabilitation*. Boston, MA: CABI; 2016.
51. *Secondary Pentobarbital Poisoning in Wildlife*. Available at: https://www.fws.gov/mountain-prairie/poison.pdf. Accessed Oct 4, 2020.
52. Souza MJ. Human safety and zoonoses. In: Hernandez SM, Barron HW, Miller EA, et al., eds. *Medical Management of Wildlife Species*. Hoboken, NJ: Wiley Blackwell; 2020:11–21.
53. State and Territorial Fish and Wildlife Offices. Available at: https://www.fws.gov/offices/statelinks.html. Accessed Oct 4, 2020.
54. State and Territorial Public Health Offices. Available at: https://www.cdc.gov/publichealthgateway/healthdirectories/healthdepartments.html. Accessed 4 Oct 2020.
55. United States Department of Health and Human Services. *Food Code*. College Park, MD; 2013. Available at: https://www.fda.gov/media/87140/download. Accessed Nov 29, 2020.
56. United States Fish and Wildlife Service. *Migratory Bird Treaty Act*. Available at: https://www.fws.gov/birds/policies-and-regulations/laws-legislations/migratory-bird-treaty-act.php. Accessed Oct 4, 2020.

57. United States Fish and Wildlife Service. *National Eagle Repository*. Available at: https://www.fws.gov/eaglerepository/. Accessed Oct 4, 2020.
58. Wardyn SE, Kauffman LK, Smith TC. Methicillin-resistant *Staphylococcus aureus* in central Iowa wildlife. *J Wildl Dis*. 2012;48(4):1069–1073.
59. Western Association of Fish and Wildlife Agencies. *A Model Protocol for Purchase, Distribution and Use of Pharmaceuticals in Wildlife*. Available at: https://www.dfw.state.or.us/wildlife/docs/WWHC_DRUG_PROTOCOL2009.pdf. Accessed Nov 27, 2020.
60. Whittington JK, Rosenhagen N, et al. General principles of emergency care. In: Hernandez SM, Barron HW, Miller EA, et al., eds. *Medical Management of Wildlife Species*. Hoboken, NJ: Wiley Blackwell; 2020:29–44.
61. Williamson RH, Muller LI, Blair CD. The use of ketamine-xylazine or butorphanol-azaperone-medetomidine to immobilize American black bears (*Ursus americanus*). *J Wildl Dis*. 2018;54:503–510.

Chapter 15 **Select Topics for the Exotic Animal Veterinarian**

Julie Swenson | Jeffrey R. Applegate, Jr.

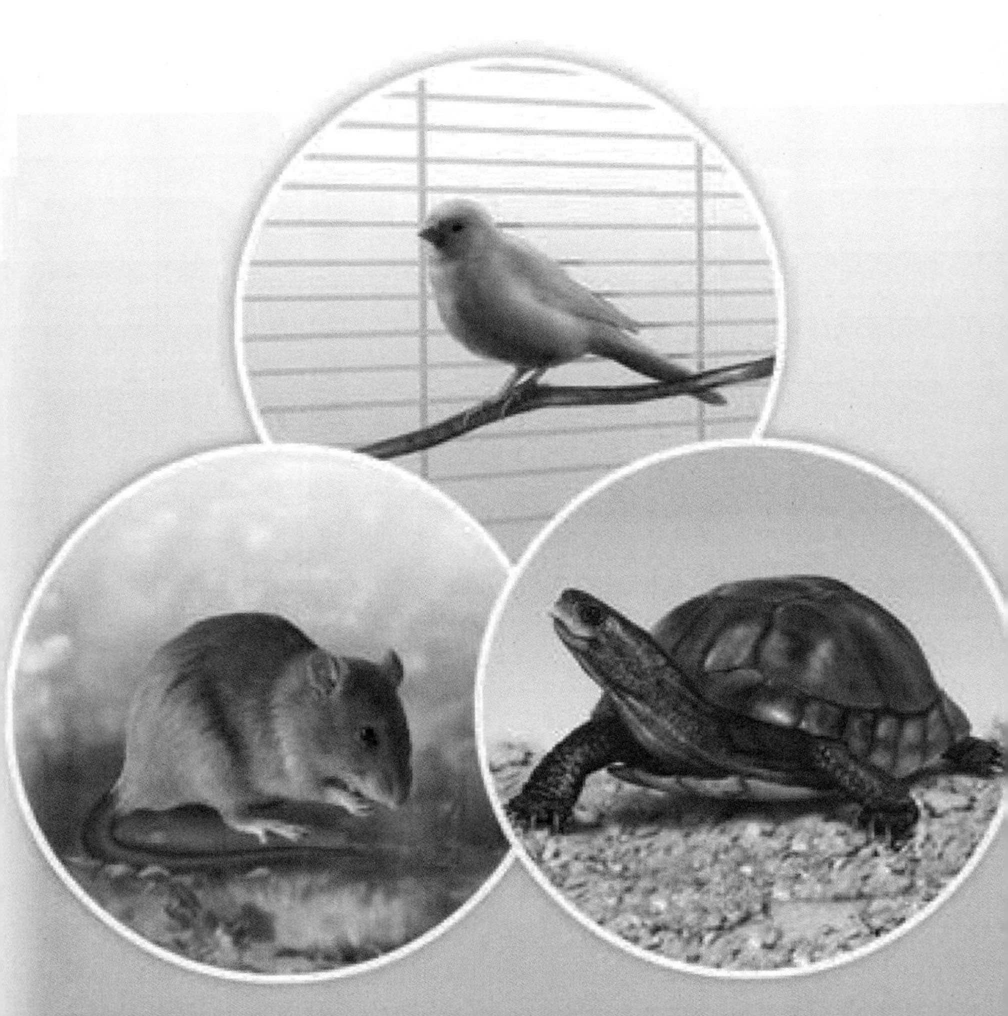

TABLE 15-1 Classification of Select Antimicrobials Used in Exotic Animal Medicine.

Class	Antimicrobial Agent
Aminocyclitols	Spectinomycin
Aminoglycosides	Amikacin
	Gentamicin
	Kanamycin
	Neomycin
	Streptomycin
	Tobramycin
β-lactamase inhibitors	Ampicillin/sulbactam
	Piperacillin/tazobactam
	Amoxicillin/clavulanate
	Ticarcillin/clavulanate
Carbapenems	Imipenem
	Meropenem
Cephalosporins, first-generation	Cefadroxil
	Cefazolin
	Cephalexin
Cephalosporins, third-generation	Cefixime
	Cefovecin
	Cefpodoxime
	Cefotaxime
	Ceftazidime
	Ceftiofur
Cephalosporins, fourth-generation	Cefepime
	Cefpirome
	Cefquinome
Chloramphenicol (or its derivative)	Chloramphenicol
	Florfenicol
Diaminopyrimidine	Ormetoprim
	Trimethoprim
Diaminopyrimidine/sulfas	Ormetoprim/sulfadimethoxine
	Trimethoprim/sulfadiazine
	Trimethoprim/sulfamethoxazole
Fluoroquinolones	Ciprofloxacin
	Danofloxacin
	Difloxacin

Continued

TABLE 15-1 Classification of Select Antimicrobials Used in Exotic Animal Medicine. (cont'd)

Class	Antimicrobial Agent
	Enrofloxacin
	Marbofloxacin
	Orbifloxacin
	Pradofloxacin
Lincosamides	Clindamycin
	Lincomycin
	Pirlimycin
Macrolides	Clarithromycin
	Erythromycin
	Tildipirosin
	Tilmicosin
	Tylosin
	Tylvalosin
Azalides	Azithromycin
	Gamithromycin
Ketolides	Telithromycin
Triamilides	Tulathromycin
Nitroimidazole	Metronidazole
	Ronidazole
Penicillins, benzyl	Benzathine penicillin G
	Procaine penicillin G
Penicillins, extended-spectrum	
Aminopenicillins	Amoxicillin
	Ampicillin
Antipseudomonal penicillins	
Carboxypenicillins	Carbenicillin
	Ticarcillin
Piperazine penicillins	Piperacillin
Quinolones	Nalidixic acid
Sulfonamides	Sulfachlorpyridazine
	Sulfadiazine
	Sulfadimethoxine
	Sulfamethazine
	Sulfamethoxazole
	Sulfaquinoxaline

TABLE 15-1 Classification of Select Antimicrobials Used in Exotic Animal Medicine. (cont'd)

Class	Antimicrobial Agent
Sulfonamides (cont'd)	Sulfathiazole
	Sulfisoxazole
Tetracyclines	Chlortetracycline
	Doxycycline
	Minocycline
	Oxytetracycline
	Tetracycline

TABLE 15-2 General Efficacy of Select Antimicrobial Agents Used in Exotic Animals.[a]

Infectious Agent	Antimicrobial Agent
Gram-positive bacteria	
Gram-positive bacteria (in general)	Aminoglycosides (select) (amikacin, gentamicin) Azalides (i.e., azithromycin) Cephalosporins Chloramphenicol Erythromycin Florfenicol Fluoroquinolones (note: poor activity against most *Streptococcus* spp.) Lincosamides Macrolides Penicillins Tetracyclines
Staphylococcus spp. (excluding methicillin resistant *Staphylococcus*)	Aminoglycosides (select) (amikacin, gentamicin) Azithromycin Cephalosporins (cefovecin, cefpodoxime) Chloramphenicol/florfenicol Clindamycin Fluoroquinolones Lincosamides Macrolides Penicillin/β-lactamase inhibitor (amoxicillin/clavulanate, ampicillin/sulbactam, piperacillin/tazobactam, ticarcillin/clavulanate) Trimethoprim/sulfas
Streptococcus spp.	Azithromycin Cephalosporins Chloramphenicol/florfenicol Clindamycin Lincosamides Macrolides Penicillins Tetracyclines Trimethoprim/sulfas

Continued

TABLE 15-2 General Efficacy of Select Antimicrobial Agents Used in Exotic Animals. (cont'd)

Infectious Agent	Antimicrobial Agent
Clostridium spp. and other anaerobes	Azithromycin Cephalosporins (cefotetan, cefoxitin) Chloramphenicol Clindamycin Erythromycin Florfenicol Lincomycin Metronidazole[b] Penicillins Tetracyclines
Gram-negative bacteria	
Enterobacterales (in general)	Aminoglycosides (amikacin, gentamicin) Azalides Carbapenems Cephalosporins (third-/fourth-generation) Fluoroquinolones Penicillins (extended-spectrum) Trimethoprim/sulfas
Campylobacter spp.	Amoxicillin Azithromycin Ceftriaxone Chloramphenicol Clindamycin Doxycycline Erythromycin Fluoroquinolones Furazolidone Gentamicin Neomycin
Pasteurella spp.	Aminoglycosides (amikacin, gentamicin) Ceftiofur Chloramphenicol/florfenicol Erythromycin Fluoroquinolones Macrolides Penicillins Sulfonamides Tetracyclines Trimethoprim/sulfas
Pseudomonas spp. (often resistant)	Aminoglycosides (frequently in combination with a β-lactam) Carbapenems Ceftazidime and fourth-generation cephalosporins (frequently in combination with an aminoglycoside) Fluoroquinolones Penicillins (carbenicillin, ticarcillin; frequently in combination with an aminoglycoside)
Salmonella spp. (note: highly variable resistance patterns depending on the serotype)	Aminoglycosides Chloramphenicol Fluoroquinolones Penicillins Trimethoprim/sulfas

TABLE 15-2 General Efficacy of Select Antimicrobial Agents Used in Exotic Animals. (cont'd)

Infectious Agent	Antimicrobial Agent
Gram-negative bacteria (cont'd)	
Chlamydia	Azithromycin Enrofloxacin (vs. some species) Erythromycin Tetracyclines (doxycyline)
Mycoplasma spp.	Azithromycin Chloramphenicol Clindamycin Enrofloxacin Lincosamides Macrolides Tetracyclines

[a]This table is intended to serve as a general guideline for selecting antimicrobial agents; it has some broad guidelines and, of course, doesn't account for resistance within specific isolates.
[b]Effective vs. most obligate anaerobes; inactive vs. most aerobic bacteria or facultative anaerobes.

TABLE 15-3 Antimicrobial Therapy Used in Exotic Animals According to Site of Infection.[a,b]

Site of Infection	Antimicrobial Agent
Bacteremia, septicemia	
Aerobic bacteria	Aminoglycoside with a penicillin or cephalosporin
	Cephalosporins (third-generation)
	Fluoroquinolone with amoxicillin
	Penicillins (penicillin, amoxicillin, amoxicillin/clavulanate, ampicillin/sulbactam)
Anaerobic bacteria	Azithromycin
	Cefoxitin, cefotetan
	Chloramphenicol
	Clindamycin
	Florfenicol
	Metronidazole
	Penicillin
Soft tissue infection	Azithromycin
	Cephalosporins
	Clindamycin or metronidazole (vs. anaerobes)
	Fluoroquinolones
	Fluoroquinolone with metronidazole (vs. polymicrobial aerobic and anaerobic infections)
	Penicillin/β-lactamase inhibitor (amoxicillin/clavulanate)
	Tetracyclines
	Trimethoprim/sulfas

Continued

TABLE 15-3 Antimicrobial Therapy Used in Exotic Animals According to Site of Infection. (cont'd)

Site of Infection	Antimicrobial Agent
Respiratory tract	Azithromycin
	Cephalosporins
	Chloramphenicol
	Clindamycin
	Enrofloxacin (vs. *Mycoplasma*, etc.)
	Florfenicol
	Macrolides (vs. *Mycoplasma*)
	Metronidazole (vs. anaerobes)
	Penicillins
	Tetracyclines (vs. *Mycoplasma* and *Chlamydia*)
	Trimethoprim/sulfas
Alimentary tract	Amoxicillin
	Cephalosporins
	Fluoroquinolones
	Metronidazole (vs. anaerobes)
	Neomycin
	Tetracyclines
	Trimethoprim/sulfas
Skin	Amoxicillin/clavulanate
	Azithromycin
	Cephalosporins
	Clindamycin
	Erythromycin
	Fluoroquinolones
	Lincomycin
	Trimethoprim/sulfas
Bone and/or joint	Aminoglycosides (for joints)
	Azithromycin
	Cephalosporins
	Cephalosporins (third-generation) with clindamycin (vs. anaerobes)
	Clindamycin
	Fluoroquinolones
	Lincosamides
	Penicillins (extended-spectrum)
	Penicillins with clindamycin (vs. anaerobes)

TABLE 15-3 Antimicrobial Therapy Used in Exotic Animals According to Site of Infection. (cont'd)

Site of Infection	Antimicrobial Agent
Urinary tract	Cephalosporins (cefadroxil, cefazolin, cephalexin)
	Fluoroquinolones
	Penicillins (amoxicillin, amoxicillin/clavulanate, ampicillin)
	Sulfisoxazole
	Tetracyclines (other than doxycycline)
	Trimethoprim/sulfas
Central nervous system	Azithromycin
	Cephalosporins (third-generation) (excluding cefovecin, cefpodoxime)
	Chloramphenicol (encephalitis)
	Florfenicol
	Fluoroquinolones (meningitis)
	Metronidazole (vs. anaerobes)
	Penicillins (in cases of inflammation)
	Trimethoprim/sulfas
Reproductive tract	Amoxicillin/clavulanate
	Chloramphenicol
	Clindamycin (vs. anaerobes)
	Fluoroquinolones
	Florfenicol
	Trimethoprim/sulfas

[a]Definitive therapy should be based on bacterial culture and antimicrobial susceptibility, and host species involved.
[b]Modified from: Carpenter JW, ed. *Exotic Animal Formulary.* 5th ed. St. Louis, MO: Elsevier, 2018; Papich MG. *Papich Handbook of Veterinary Drugs.* 5th ed. St. Louis, MO: Elsevier, 2020; Plumb DC, ed. *Plumb's Veterinary Drug Handbook.* 9th ed. Ames, IA: Wiley Blackwell, 2018.

TABLE 15-4 Antimicrobial Combination Therapies Commonly Used in Exotic Animals.[a]

Antimicrobial Agent	Combination Agents
Aminoglycosides[b] (amikacin, gentamicin)	Cephalosporins, clindamycin, fluoroquinolones, lincomycin, metronidazole, penicillins (amoxicillin, ampicillin, carbenicillin, piperacillin, ticarcillin), trimethoprim/sulfas
Amoxicillin	Clavulanate
Ampicillin	Sulbactam
Cephalosporin	Aminoglycosides,[b] clindamycin, fluoroquinolones, metronidazole
Clindamycin	Aminoglycosides, cephalosporins (third-generation), enrofloxacin, penicillins

Continued

TABLE 15-4 Antimicrobial Combination Therapies Commonly Used in Exotic Animals. (cont'd)

Antimicrobial Agent	Combination Agents
Fluoroquinolones (enrofloxacin, ciprofloxacin, marbofloxacin)	Aminoglycosides,[b] cephalosporins (third-generation), clindamycin, metronidazole, penicillins (extended-spectrum)
Lincomycin	Aminoglycosides,[b] spectinomycin
Metronidazole	Amikacin, azithromycin, carbenicillin, cefazolin, cefotaxime, chloramphenicol, enrofloxacin, gentamicin, marbofloxacin, others as indicated
Ormetoprim	Sulfadimethoxine
Penicillins (ampicillin, carbenicillin, piperacillin)	Aminoglycosides,[b] fluoroquinolones
Penicillins, early generation	Aminoglycosides,[b] third-generation cephalosporins, fluoroquinolones
Ticarcillin	Clavulanate
Trimethoprim	Sulfadiazine, sulfamethoxazole
Tylosin	Oxytetracycline

[a]Indicated when combination is advantageous in definitive therapy to treat polymicrobial infections or to broaden empiric coverage.
[b]Generally amikacin; occasionally gentamicin.

TABLE 15-5 Select Laboratories Conducting Exotic Animal Diagnostic Procedures.[a]

Laboratory	Select Tests/Procedures
Animal Health Diagnostic Center College of Veterinary Medicine Cornell University PO Box 5786 Ithaca, NY 14852 USA (607) 253-3900 ahdc.vet.cornell.edu	General: Chemistry, hematology, clotting panels, histopathology, microbiology, necropsy, parasitology, virology Avian: *Chlamydia, Cryptosporidium, Giardia, Mycobacterium, Mycoplasma,* infectious bronchitis virus, infectious bursal disease, influenza virus, paramyxovirus, West Nile virus, viral isolation, blood lead/zinc Mammal: Ferret enteric coronavirus, ferret influenza virus, mink enteric coronavirus, ferret adrenal testing Reptile: *Cryptosporidium, Salmonella*
Antech Diagnostics 10 Executive Boulevard Farmingdale, NY 11735 USA (800) 745-4725 (West) (800) 872-1001 (East) (800) 341-3440 (Canada) antechdiagnostics.com	General: Chemistry, electrophoresis, hematology, microbiology, virology Avian: *Mycoplasma, Chlamydia, Aspergillus,* polyomavirus, psittacine beak and feather disease virus, West Nile virus, sex determination, blood lead/zinc Mammal: *Pasteurella, Encephalitozoon, Treponema, Toxoplasma,* ferret adrenal panel, distemper virus, Aleutian disease virus Reptile: *Mycoplasma*
Animal Genetics 3382 Capital Circle NE Tallahassee, FL 32308 USA (800) 514-9672 animalgenetics.com	Avian: *Bordetella, Chlamydia, Mycobacterium, Salmonella, Aspergillus, Candida, Cryptosporidium, Giardia,* paramyxovirus, pigeon circovirus, polyomavirus, psittacine beak and feather disease virus, herpes virus, influenza virus, West Nile virus, Pacheco's disease, sex determination

TABLE 15-5 Select Laboratories Conducting Exotic Animal Diagnostic Procedures. (cont'd)

Laboratory	Select Tests/Procedures
Avian & Exotic Animal Clin Path Labs 2712 North Highway 68 Wilmington, OH 45177 USA (937) 383-3347 (800) 350-1122 avianexoticlab.com	General: Chemistry, electrophoresis, hematology, histopathology, microbiology, parasitology, toxicology, virology Avian: *Chlamydia, Salmonella, Aspergillus, Histoplasma, Cryptosporidium, Giardia, Sarcocystis,* adenovirus, influenza virus, Pacheco's disease, paramyxovirus, polyomavirus, West Nile virus, blood iron/lead/zinc Mammal: Heartworm testing, *Toxoplasma,* distemper virus Reptiles/amphibians: *Cryptosporidium, Giardia,* chytrid, inclusion body disease, ophidian paramyxovirus
Avian and Wildlife Laboratory Division of Comparative Pathology University of Miami School of Medicine 1611 NW 12th Avenue Miami, FL 33136 USA (305) 585-6303 cpl.med.miami.edu	General: Chemistry, electrophoresis, hematology Avian: *Aspergillus, Chlamydia, Cryptosporidium,* Pacheco's virus, polyomavirus, psittacine beak and feather disease virus, sex determination Mammal: CAR bacillus, *Clostridium piliforme, Mycoplasma, Pasteurella, E. cuniculi,* guinea pig adenovirus, coronavirus, Kilham's rat virus, lymphocytic choriomeningitis virus, mouse hepatitis virus, minute virus of mice, pneumonia virus of mice, parainfluenza virus 3, parvovirus, rotavirus, Sendai virus, Theiler's murine encephalomyelitis virus
Diagnostic Center for Population and Animal Health Michigan State University 4125 Beaumont Road Lansing, MI 48910 USA (517) 353-1683 animalhealth.msu.edu	General: Chemistry, hematology, histopathology, microbiology, necropsy, protein electrophoresis, toxicology, virology Avian: *Chlamydia, Mycobacterium, Mycoplasma, Aspergillus, Cryptosporidium, Salmonella,* Newcastle disease virus, infectious bronchitis virus, infectious laryngotracheitis virus, influenza virus, West Nile virus, blood lead Mammal: *Cryptosporidium, Giardia, Salmonella,* Aleutian disease virus, ferret enteric coronavirus, ferret rotavirus Reptiles/amphibians: *Mycoplasma, Salmonella, Cryptosporidium*
Diagnostic Laboratory Service College of Veterinary Medicine University of Tennessee 2407 River Drive Knoxville, TN 37996 USA (865) 974-8387 vetmed.tennessee.edu/vmc/dls	General: Chemistry, endocrinology, hematology, histopathology, microbiology, necropsy, parasitology, toxicology, virology Avian: *Chlamydia, Mycobacterium, Mycoplasma, Aspergillus, Cryptosporidium*, sex determination Mammal: *Giardia*, influenza A virus, ferret adrenal panel, rabbit adrenal panel Reptiles/amphibians: *Mycoplasma, Cryptosporidium*, herpesvirus, ophidian paramyxovirus, ranavirus
Georgia Veterinary Diagnostic Laboratories College of Veterinary Medicine University of Georgia 501 DW Brooks Drive Athens, GA 30602 USA (706) 542-5568 vet.uga.edu/dlab/	General: Chemistry, hematology, histopathology, microbiology, necropsy, parasitology, toxicology, virology Avian: *Chlamydia, Mycobacterium, Mycoplasma, Salmonella, Aspergillus, Cryptosporidium, Plasmodium,* herpesvirus, influenza virus, Newcastle disease virus, West Nile virus, Pacheco's disease Mammal: *Bordetella, Clostridium* (toxin panel), *Francisella tularensis, Helicobacter, Lawsonia, Mycobacteria, Mycoplasma, Pasteurella, Salmonella, Treponema, Encephalitozoon,* herpesvirus, influenza A virus, lymphocytic choriomeningitis virus, morbiliviruses, mouse hepatitis virus, mouse reoviruses, murine norovirus, paramyxovirus, pneumonia virus of mice, rabies virus, rodent parvoviruses, Sendai virus, simian virus 5, Tyzzer's disease Reptiles/amphibians: *Cryptosporidium, Mycoplasma, Salmonella,* adenovirus, herpesvirus, ranavirus Aquatic: Aquatic bacterial and fungal cultures (including *Mycobacterium* and *Mycoplasma*)

Continued

TABLE 15-5 Select Laboratories Conducting Exotic Animal Diagnostic Procedures. (cont'd)

Laboratory	Select Tests/Procedures
Kansas State Veterinary Diagnostic Laboratory College of Veterinary Medicine Kansas State University 1800 Denison Avenue Manhattan, KS 66506 USA (866) 512-5650 ksvdl.org	General: Chemistry, hematology, histopathology, microbiology, necropsy, parasitology, protein electrophoresis, toxicology, virology Avian: *Bordetella, Chlamydia, Salmonella, Aspergillus, Cryptosporidium,* influenza virus, Newcastle disease virus, West Nile virus, blood lead Mammal: *Francisella tularensis, Lawsonia, Giardia, Cryptosporidium,* influenza virus, rabies virus Reptiles/amphibians: *Salmonella*
National Veterinary Services Laboratory USDA-APHIS-VS-NVSL PO Box 844 Ames, IA 50010 USA (515) 337-7266 aphis.usda.gov/aphis/ourfocus/animalhealth/lab-info-services/	General: Microbiology, virology Avian: *Avibacterium paragallinarum, Bordetella, Chlamydia, Mycobacterium, Mycoplasma, Ornithobacterium rhinotracheale, Pasteurella, Salmonella,* adenoviruses, avian pox virus, chicken anemia virus, duck viral enteritis virus, encephalomyelitis virus, goose parvovirus, herpesviruses, infectious bronchitis virus, infectious bursal disease, infectious laryngotracheitis, influenza virus, Marek's disease, metapneumovirus, nephritis virus, paramyxoviruses, reovirus, rotavirus, West Nile virus Mammal: *Francisella tularensis* Aquatic: Various bacterial and viral testing options for aquaculture (contact lab for arrangements)
Northwest ZooPath 654 West Main Street Monroe, WA 98272 USA (360) 794-0630 zoopath.com	General: Pathology
Research Associates Laboratory 14556 Midway Road Dallas, TX 75224 USA (972) 960-2221 vetdna.com	General: Microbiology, virology Avian: *Bartonella, Bordetella, Chlamydia, Cryptosporidium, Helicobacter, Mycobacterium, Mycoplasma, Salmonella, Aspergillus, Candida,* avian gastric yeast, *Giardia,* plasmodium, adenoviruses, circoviruses, duck enteritis virus, herpesviruses, Marek's disease, polyomavirus, poxvirus, psittacine beak and feather disease virus, sex determination Mammal: *Anaplasma, Babesia, Bartonella, Bordetella, Brucella, Campylobacter, Chlamydia, Clostridium, Coxiella, E. coli, Ehrlichia, Francisella tularensis, Helicobacter, Lawsonia intracellularis, Pasteurella, Mycobacterium, Mycoplasma, Candida, Cryptosporidium, Encephalitozoon, Entamoeba, Enterocytozoon, Giardia, Hepatozoon, Plasmodium, Sarcocystis, Spironucleus, Toxoplasma,* Aleutian disease, astrovirus, distemper virus, ferret epizootic catarrhal enteritis, hantavirus, hepatitis E virus, lymphocytic choriomeningitis virus, myxomavirus, orthopoxvirus, rabies virus, West Nile virus Reptiles/amphibians: *Campylobacter, Clostridium, Mycobacterium, Mycoplasma, Pasteurella; Salmonella, Aspergillus, Candida, Chrysosporium*-related fungi, chytrid fungus (chytridiomycosis [i.e., *Batrachochytrium dendrobatidis*]), *Cryptosporidium, Entamoeba, Giardia, Plasmodium, Spironucleus,* arenavirus, atadenovirus, herpesviruses, iridovirus, fibropapillomatosis, ophidian paramyxovirus, ranavirus, sunshine virus, West Nile virus Aquatic: Bacterial, viral, and parasitic testing (see website for extensive list)

TABLE 15-5 Select Laboratories Conducting Exotic Animal Diagnostic Procedures. (cont'd)

Laboratory	Select Tests/Procedures
Texas Veterinary Medical Diagnostic Laboratory Texas A&M University 1 Sippel Road College Station, TX 77843 USA (979) 845-3414 (888) 646-5623 tvmdl.tamu.edu	General: Chemistry, hematology, histopathology, microbiology, necropsy, protein electrophoresis, toxicology, virology Avian: *Chlamydia, Mycobacterium, Mycoplasma, Salmonella, Aspergillus, Cryptosporidium,* avian encephalomyelitis virus, duck enteritis virus, infectious bronchitis virus, infectious bursal disease virus, infectious laryngotracheitis virus, influenza virus, paramyxoviruses, reovirus, reticuloendotheliosis virus, West Nile virus, blood lead/zinc/iron Mammal: *Bordetella, E. coli, Mycoplasma, Salmonella, Cryptosporidium, Giardia*, distemper virus, rabies virus Reptiles/amphibians: *Mycoplasma, Salmonella, Cryptosporidium*
Veterinary Medical Diagnostic Lab College of Veterinary Medicine University of Missouri PO Box 6023 Columbia, MO 65205 USA (573) 882-6811 vmdl.missouri.edu	General: Histopathology, microbiology, necropsy, toxicology, virology Avian: *Bordetella, Chlamydia, Mycoplasma, Ornithobacterium rhinotracheale, Salmonella, Cryptosporidium,* avian encephalitis virus, hemorrhagic enteritis virus, infectious bronchitis virus, influenza virus, Newcastle disease virus, rotavirus, blood lead/zinc
Veterinary Molecular Diagnostics, Inc. 5989 Meijer Drive, Suite 5 Milford, OH 45150 USA (513) 576-1808 vmdlabs.com	General: Molecular diagnostics Avian: *Bordetella, Chlamydia, Mycobacterium, Mycoplasma, Aspergillus,* avian gastric yeast, adenovirus, bornavirus, circoviruses, coronavirus, polyomavirus, psittacine beak and feather disease virus, psittacine herpes virus, West Nile virus, sex determination Mammal: *Campylobacter, Helicobacter, Lawsonia, Encephalitozoon,* Aleutian disease virus, epizootic catarrhal enteritis virus Reptiles/amphibians: *Cryptosporidium, Mycoplasma,* bearded dragon atadenovirus
Wisconsin Veterinary Diagnostic Laboratory University of Wisconsin 455 Easterday Lane Madison, WI 53706 USA (608) 262-5432 (800) 608-8387 wvdl.wisc.edu	General: Histopathology, microbiology, necropsy, virology Avian: *Bordetella, Chlamydia, Mycoplasma, Salmonella, Cryptosporidium,* avian encephalitis virus, duck viral enteritis virus, infectious bronchitis virus, infectious bursal disease virus, infectious laryngotracheitis virus, influenza virus, paramyxovirus, pneumovirus, polyomavirus, poxvirus, psittacine herpes virus, turkey hemorrhagic enteritis virus, West Nile virus Reptiles/amphibians: *Mycoplasma, Salmonella*
Zoo/Exotic Pathology Service Part of: ZNLabs 525 E 4500 S F200 Salt Lake City, UT 84107 USA (800) 426-2099 zooexoticpathologyservice.evetsites.net	General: Pathology

Continued

TABLE 15-5 Select Laboratories Conducting Exotic Animal Diagnostic Procedures. (cont'd)

Laboratory	Select Tests/Procedures
Zoologix, Inc 9811 Owensmouth Avenue Suite 4 Chatsworth, CA 91311 USA (818) 717-8880 zoologix.com	General: Molecular diagnostics Avian: *Avibacterium paragallinarum, Bordetella, Chlamydia, Mycobacterium, Mycoplasma, Ornithobacterium rhinotracheale, Salmonella, Aspergillus, Candida, Atoxoplasma, Cryptosporidium, Plasmodium,* adenovirus, bornavirus, circovirus, herpesvirus, infectious bronchitis virus, infectious bursal disease virus, infectious laryngotracheitis virus, influenza virus, Newcastle disease virus, Pacheco's disease, polyomavirus, poxvirus, psittacine beak and feather disease virus, reovirus, West Nile virus Mammal: *Bordetella, Campylobacter, E. coli, Francisella tularensis, Helicobacter, Lawsonia intracellularis, Mycobacterium, Mycoplasma, Pasteurella, Salmonella, Giardia, Treponema,* Aleutian disease virus, hantavirus, lymphocytic choriomeningitis virus, mink enteritis virus, monkeypox, mouse adenovirus, mouse cytomegaloviruses, mouse hepatitis virus, mouse minute virus, mouse norovirus, mouse parvovirus, mouse polyoma virus, mouse pox virus, mouse rotavirus, pneumonia virus of mice, rabbit fibroma virus, rabies virus, rat coronavirus, reovirus, rotavirus, Sendai virus, sialodacryoadenitis virus, Tyzzer's disease Reptiles/amphibians: *Mycobacterium, Mycoplasma, Salmonella,* chytrid fungus (chytridiomycosis [i.e., *Batrachochytrium dendrobatidis*]), *Cryptosporidium,* ranavirus
Zoo Medicine Service College of Veterinary Medicine University of Florida PO Box 100126 Gainesville, FL 32610 USA (352) 392-4700 (ext. 5700) labs.vetmed.ufl.edu	General: Consensus polymerase chain reaction (PCR) and sequencing Reptiles/amphibians: *Chlamydiales, Mycobacterium, Mycoplasma,* coccidia, *Cryptosporidium,* microsporidians, pentastomids, adenoviruses, arenaviruses, astroviruses, erythrocytic iridoviruses, ferlaviruses, herpesviruses, orthoreoviruses, papillomaviruses, paramyxoviruses, poxviruses, ranaviruses, rhabdoviruses

[a]Websites accessed on October 1, 2020.

TABLE 15-6 Professional Associations for Veterinarians Interested in Exotics.[a]

Organization	Website
American Association of Wildlife Veterinarians	aawv.net
American Association of Zoo Veterinarians	aazv.org
American Board of Veterinary Practitioners	abvp.com
American College of Zoological Medicine	aczm.org
American Society of Laboratory Animal Practitioners	aslap.org
Association of Amphibian and Reptilian Veterinarians	arav.org
Association of Avian Veterinarians	aav.org
Association of Exotic Mammal Veterinarians	aemv.org

TABLE 15-6 Professional Associations for Veterinarians Interested in Exotics. (cont'd)

Organization	Website
Association of Primate Veterinarians	primatevets.org
Association of Sugar Glider Veterinarians	asgv.org
Association of Zoo Veterinary Technicians	azvt.org
British Veterinary Zoological Society	bvzs.org
Canadian Association of Zoo and Wildlife Veterinarians	cazwv.org
European Association of Zoo and Wildlife Veterinarians	eazwv.org
Honey Bee Veterinary Consortium	hbvc.org
International Association for Aquatic Animal Medicine	iaaam.org
National Wildlife Rehabilitators Association	nwrawildlife.org
World Aquatic Veterinary Medical Association	wavma.org

[a]Websites accessed on October 1, 2020.

TABLE 15-7 Exotic Animal Online Resources for Practitioners.[a]

Site Name	Website	Description
American Society for the Prevention of Cruelty to Animals	aspca.org	Contains an Animal Poison Control Center and general pet care guidelines
Amphibian Diseases Knowledgebase	arwh.org/amphibian-dz-knowledgebase	Australian page focusing on current information on amphibian diseases
Animal Diversity Web	animaldiversity.org	Taxonomic site from the University of Michigan Museum of Zoology
Avibase	avibase.bsc-eoc.org	Searchable database with taxonomic information and photographs of the world's bird species
BioOne	bioone.org	Resource database collection of bioscience research journals; contains multiple peer-reviewed exotic journals
The Colyer Institute	colyerinstitute.org	Center for the study of oral disease and nutrition in exotic animals
Convention on International Trade in Endangered Species	cites.org	International agreement between governments concerning the international trade of wild animals and plants
Dental Anatomy	www.vivo.colostate.edu/hbooks/pathphys/digestion/pregastric/dentalanat.html	Includes information and images of dental anatomy of rabbits and rodents (from Colorado State University)
Diseases of Research Animals (DORA)	dora.missouri.edu	Teaching resources from the University of Missouri regarding diseases seen in species commonly kept for research purposes

Continued

TABLE 15-7 Exotic Animal Online Resources for Practitioners. (cont'd)

Site Name	Website	Description
Exotic DVM	exoticdvm.com	Veterinary forum for the care of companion exotic animals
Exotic Pet Vet Net	exoticpetvet.net	Website of veterinary articles from exotic veterinarians
The Humane Society	humanesociety.org	Includes care sheets for many exotic species
International Union for the Conservation of Nature	iucn.org	Organization dedicated to finding pragmatic solutions to environment and development challenges; produces the IUCN Red List of Threatened Species
International Veterinary Information System	ivis.org	Online veterinary book publisher with free access to multiple online books
An Introduction to Ratite Ranching and Medicine	instruction.cvhs.okstate.edu/kocan/ostrich/ostbk2a1.htm	Online book of ratite medicine from Oklahoma State University
Lafeber Vet	lafeber.com/vet/	Online resources for various clinical topics and species specific care sheets
Medirabbit	medirabbit.com	Rabbit medicine articles and video demonstrations
The Merck Veterinary Manual[b]	merckvetmanual.com	*Merck Veterinary Manual* online including exotic animals with normal physiological parameters
Oxbow Vet Connect	oxbowanimalhealth.com/vet-connect	Online resource for various clinical topics and disease and case reviews
PubMed	pubmed.gov	Digital archive of the US National Library of Medicine; contains multiple peer-reviewed exotic journals
Species 360 (formerly International Species Information System)	species360.org	Global network of animal management professionals
USDA APHIS	aphis.usda.gov/aphis/ourfocus/animalhealth/	United States Department of Agriculture, Animal Plant Health Inspection Service
Veterinary Information Network	vin.com	Member-based network of veterinary consultants; large bank of information on zoo and exotic animals
Veterinary Partner	veterinarypartner.com	Partner to the Veterinary Information Network, contains information and handouts for clients concerning medical diseases
VETgirl	vetgirlontherun.com	Subscription-based multimedia service offering RACE-approved, online continuing education
World Organization for Animal Health (OIE)	oie.int	Intergovernmental organization responsible for improving animal health worldwide

[a]Websites accessed on October 1, 2020.
[b]Merck is referred to as MSD internationally.

TABLE 15-8 Captive Husbandry Websites for Owners of Exotic Animals.[a]

Category	Site Name	Website	Description
Invertebrates	Bee Informed Partnership	beeinformed.org	Website providing information to help beekeepers make management decisions
Aquatics	Fish Lore	fishlore.com	Tropical fish, freshwater aquarium, and saltwater aquarium information website
	Fish Tank Guide	fish-tank-guide.com	Website including information on basic tank care, fish care, and medical information; also contains some species-specific information on common aquarium fish
	Goldfish Information Page	goldfish.nova.org	Includes husbandry and care information for goldfish hobbyists
	International Fancy Guppy Association	ifga.org	Association dedicated to the Fancy Show Guppy; contains general starter information and medical information on guppies
Reptiles and amphibians	Bearded Dragon Care	beardeddragoncare.net	Website dedicated to provide bearded dragon care information to pet lizard owners
	Boa Tips	boatips.com	Website for pet snakes; includes husbandry and care articles as well as species-specific information and photographs
	Box Turtle Care and Conservation	boxturtlesite.info	Website for natural history and captive care of box turtles
	Canadart	canadart.org	Canadian forums for the discussion of care of dart frogs
	Chameleon Care and Information Center	chameleoninfo.com	Website devoted to chameleons; includes husbandry and care articles
	Dendrobates.org	dendrobates.org	Website concerning natural history of poison dart frogs
	Frog Pets	frogpets.com	Website devoted to care and husbandry associated with keeping frogs as pets
	Green Iguana Society	green-iguana.info	Society dedicated to providing quality information on iguana care; contains husbandry and care articles as well as some medical information
	Lizard Landscapes	lizard-landscapes.com	Website with husbandry and care information for multiple species of reptiles; also contains information on building cage landscapes

Continued

TABLE 15-8 Captive Husbandry Websites for Owners of Exotic Animals. (cont'd)

Category	Site Name	Website	Description
	The Lizard Lounge	the-lizard-lounge.com	Website containing husbandry and care information as well as taxonomy, photographs, natural history, and medical information on multiple species of lizards
	Melissa Kaplan's Herp Care Collection	anapsid.org	Website containing husbandry and care articles on amphibians, reptiles, and invertebrates
	Poison Dart Frogs	poisondartfrog.co.uk	Website containing husbandry and care information on *Dendrobates* species
	Reptile Web	reptilesweb.com	A world reptile and amphibian information center; contains husbandry and care information for reptiles, amphibians, and invertebrates
	Tortoise Trust	tortoisetrust.org	Website with information on turtles and tortoises, including species care sheets and husbandry articles
	World Chelonian Trust	chelonia.org	Website with information on turtles and tortoises, including species care sheets and chelonian taxonomy
Avian	African Love Bird Society	africanlovebirdsociety.org	Association dedicated to keeping, breeding, and showing of love birds; contains husbandry and care information along with information on the nine species
	American Budgerigar Society	abs1.org	Society for information about keeping, breeding, and exhibiting budgerigars
	American Dove Association	americandoveassociation.com	Association for dove enthusiasts; contains husbandry and care information along with information on the different species
	American Federation of Aviculture	afabirds.org	Nonprofit organization whose purpose is to represent all aspects of aviculture and to educate the public about keeping and breeding birds in captivity
	American Ostrich Association	ostriches.org	Association to establish the standards for the highest quality American ostrich products to ensure the long-term viability of the industry

TABLE 15-8 Captive Husbandry Websites for Owners of Exotic Animals. (cont'd)

Category	Site Name	Website	Description
Avian (cont'd)	Foraging For Parrots	foragingforparrots.com	Website on how to make foraging toys for psittacine birds
	International Cockatiel Association	cockatiels.org/ica/	Society dedicated to providing information on the proper care, handling, maintenance, and breeding of cockatiels
	National Finch and Softbill Society	nfss.org	Society dedicated to promoting the enjoyment of keeping and breeding finches and softbills
	Organization of Professional Aviculturists	opabirds.org	Organization that represents the interests of professional aviculturalists
	Parrot A.L.E.R.T.	parrotalert.org	Website for reporting lost and found parrots; also includes husbandry articles
	Parrot Outreach Society	parrotoutreachsociety.org	Society dedicated to helping birds find homes; includes basic bird care articles
	World Parrot Trust	parrots.org	Organization to promote survival of all parrot species in the wild and to advocate for the welfare of individual birds in our homes
Mammal	American Fancy Rat and Mouse Association	afrma.org	Association to promote and encourage the breeding and exhibition of fancy rats and mice for show and pets
	American Ferret Association	ferret.org	Association to promote the domestic ferret as a companion animal through public education via shows, newsletters, legislative education, and other venues
	American Gerbil Society	agsgerbils.org	Society providing support and education to breeders, caregivers, and gerbil enthusiasts
	American Rabbit Breeders Association	arba.net	Association dedicated to the promotion, development, and improvement of the domestic rabbit and guinea pig
	Cheeky Chinchilla	cheekychinchillas.com	Husbandry and care information for chinchillas
	Gerbil Care	gerbilcare.org	Husbandry and care information for gerbils
	Guinea Lynx	guinealynx.info	Husbandry and care information for guinea pigs
	Hamster Hideout	hamsterhideout.com	Husbandry and care information for hamsters

Continued

TABLE 15-8 Captive Husbandry Websites for Owners of Exotic Animals. (cont'd)

Category	Site Name	Website	Description
Mammals (cont'd)	Hamsterific	hamsterific.com	Husbandry and care information for hamsters
	House Rabbit Society	rabbit.org	Society that rescues rabbits from animal shelters and educates the public on rabbit care and behavior
	International Hedgehog Association	hedgehogclub.com	Association to educate the public in the care and betterment of hedgehogs
	My House Rabbit	myhouserabbit.com	Website celebrating house rabbits and educating the public about rabbit care and behavior
	Pet Hamster Care	pethamstercare.com	Husbandry and care information for hamsters
	Rat Guide	ratguide.com	A layman's guide to health, medication use, breeding, and responsible care of pet rats
	Sugar Glider	sugarglider.com	Husbandry and care information for sugar gliders
	Weasel Words	weaselwords.com	Husbandry and care information for ferrets

[a]Websites accessed on October 1, 2020.

TABLE 15-9 Emergency Drug Doses (in mL) Commonly Used in Exotic Animals.[a]

Emergency Drug			Gerbils, Hamsters, Mice, Rats								Guinea Pigs, Chinchillas		
Drug	**Concentration**	**Route**	**25 g**	**50 g**	**75 g**	**100 g**	**125 g**	**150 g**	**250 g**	**500 g**	**0.5 kg**	**1 kg**	**1.5 kg**
Epinephrine	0.01 mg/mL	IV, IM, IO	0.01	0.02	0.02	0.03	0.04	0.05	0.08	0.15	0.15	0.3	0.45
Atropine	0.54 mg/mL	IM, SC	0.03	0.04	0.06	0.07	0.09	0.11	0.19	0.37	0.37	0.74	1.11
Glycopyrrolate	0.2 mg/mL	IM, SC	0.01	0.01	0.01	0.01	0.02	0.02	0.03	0.05	0.05	0.1	0.15
Dexamethasone-SP	4 mg/mL	IV, IM	0.03	0.06	0.09	0.13	0.16	0.19	0.32	0.63	0.63	1.25	1.87
Doxapram	20 mg/mL	IV, SC	0.02	0.03	0.04	0.05	0.07	0.08	0.13	0.25	0.25	0.5	0.75
Diazepam	5 mg/mL	IV, IM, IO	0.01	0.03	0.05	0.06	0.08	0.09	0.15	0.3	0.3	0.6	0.9
Furosemide	5 mg/mL	IV, IM, SC	0.02	0.04	0.06	0.08	0.1	0.12	0.2	0.4	0.4	0.8	0.12

Emergency Drug			Rabbits							Ferrets			
Drug	**Concentration**	**Route**	**0.5 kg**	**1 kg**	**1.5 kg**	**2 kg**	**3 kg**	**4 kg**	**5 kg**	**0.5 kg**	**1 kg**	**1.5 kg**	**2 kg**
Epinephrine	1 mg/mL	IV, IM, IO	0.5	1.0	1.5	2.0	3.0	4.0	5.0	0.1	0.2	0.3	0.4
Atropine	0.54 mg/mL	IM, SC	0.5	0.9	1.4	1.9	2.8	3.7	4.6	0.05	0.1	0.15	0.2
Glycopyrrolate	0.2 mg/mL	IM, SC	0.05	0.1	0.15	0.2	0.3	0.4	0.5	0.03	0.05	0.08	0.1
Dexamethasone-SP	4 mg/mL	IV, IM	0.25	0.5	0.75	1.0	1.5	2.0	2.5	1.0	2.0	3.0	4.0
Doxapram	20 mg/mL	IV, SC	0.13	0.25	0.38	0.5	0.75	1.0	1.3	0.05	0.1	0.15	0.2
Diazepam	55 mg/mL	IV, IM, IO	0.3	0.6	0.9	1.2	1.8	2.4	3.0	0.2	0.4	0.6	0.8
Furosemide	50 mg/mL	IV, IM, SC	0.04	0.08	0.12	0.16	0.24	0.32	0.4	0.04	0.08	0.12	0.16
Diphen-hydramine	50 mg/mL	IV, IM	—	—	—	—	—	—	—	0.02	0.04	0.06	0.08

Continued

TABLE 15-9 Emergency Drug Doses (in mL) Commonly Used in Exotic Animals. (cont'd)

Emergency Drug			Avian (Psittacine Birds)										
Drug	Concentration	Route	0.05 kg	0.1 kg	0.2 kg	0.3 kg	0.4 kg	0.5 kg	0.6 kg	0.7 kg	0.8 kg	0.9 kg	1.0 kg
Epinephrine	1 mg/mL	IV, IM, IO	0.05	0.1	0.2	0.3	0.4	0.5	0.6	0.7	0.8	0.9	1.0
Atropine	0.54 mg/mL	IM, SC	0.05	0.09	0.19	0.28	0.37	0.46	0.56	0.65	0.74	0.83	0.93
Doxapram	20 mg/mL	IV, IM, IO	0.05	0.1	0.2	0.3	0.4	0.5	0.6	0.7	0.8	0.9	1.0
Dexamethasone-SP	4 mg/mL	IV, IM	0.05	0.1	0.2	0.3	0.4	0.5	0.6	0.7	0.8	0.9	1.0
Ca gluconate	100 mg/mL	IV, IM	0.05	0.1	0.2	0.3	0.4	0.5	0.6	0.7	0.8	0.9	1.0
Diazepam	5 mg/mL	IV, IM, IO	0.01	0.02	0.04	0.06	0.08	0.1	0.12	0.14	0.16	0.18	0.2
Emergency Drug			**Reptiles**										
Drug	**Concentration**	**Route**	**0.1 kg**	**0.25 kg**	**0.5 kg**	**0.75 kg**	**1 kg**	**2 kg**	**3 kg**	**4 kg**	**5 kg**	**6 kg**	**7 kg**
Atropine	0.54 mg/mL	IV, IM, SC	0.01	0.02	0.04	0.06	0.07	0.15	0.22	0.3	0.37	0.44	0.52
Glycopyrrolate	0.2 mg/mL	IV, IM	0.01	0.02	0.03	0.04	0.05	0.1	0.15	0.2	0.25	0.3	0.35
Dexamethasone-SP	4 mg/mL	IV, IM	0.01	0.02	0.03	0.05	0.06	0.13	0.19	0.25	0.31	0.38	0.44
Diazepam	5 mg/mL	IV, IM, ICe	0.05	0.12	0.25	0.38	0.5	1.0	1.5	2.0	2.5	3.0	3.5
Ca gluconate	100 mg/mL	IV, IO, SC	0.1	0.3	0.5	0.75	1.0	2.0	3.0	4.0	5.0	6.0	7.0

[a]Modified from Kottwitz J, Kelleher S. Emergency drugs: quick reference chart for exotic animals. *Exotic DVM.* 2003;5.5:23-25.

TABLE 15-10 Fluid Solutions Used in Exotic Animal Medicine.

Solution Type	Solution	Na^+ (mmol/L)	K^+ (mmol/L)	Cl^- (mmol/L)	Ca^{++} (mEq/L)	Mg^{++} (mEq/L)	Buffer (mEq/L)	Osmolality (mOsm/L)	pH
Crystalloids	Ringer's solution	147	4	156	4	0	0	310	5-7.5
	Lactated Ringer's solution	130	4	109	3	0	28 (lactate)	275	6-7.5
	0.9% NaCl	154	0	154	0	0	0	308	4.5
	5% dextrose	0	0	0	0	0	0	252	4-6.5
	2.5% dextrose/0.45% NaCl	77	0	77	0	0	0	280	4.5
	Plasma-Lyte	140	5	98	0	3	27 (acetate) 23 (gluconate)	294	4-6.5
	Normosol-R	140	5	98	0	3	27 (acetate) 23 (gluconate)	294	6.6
Colloids	Dextran 6% and 0.9% NaCl	154	0	154	0	0	0	310	3-7.0
	Hetastarch	154	0	154	0	0	0	309	5.5
	Pentastarch	154	0	154	0	0	0	326	5.0

TABLE 15-11 Common Abbreviations Used in Prescription Writing.

a.c.	before meals	o.d (OD)	right eye
a.d.	right ear	o.s. (OS)	left eye
ad lib	at pleasure	o.u. (OU)	both eyes
adm	administer	oz	ounce
aq	water	p.c.	after meals
a.s.	left ear	PO (p.o.)	per os
a.u.	both ears	prn (p.r.n.)	as needed
bid (b.i.d.) (BID)	twice a day	q. (q)	every
c.	with	q.d. (QD)	every day
cap(s)	capsule(s)	q4h	every 4 hours, etc.
cc	cubic centimeter	q24h	once a day
disp	dispense	qid (q.i.d.) (QID)	four times a day
fl oz	fluid ounce	q.o.d. (QOD)	every other day
g (gm)	gram	q.s.	a sufficient quantity
gr	grain	®	trademarked name
gtt(s)	drop(s)	SC (SQ)	subcutaneously
h (hr)	hour	Sig:	instructions to patient
h.s.	at bedtime	sol'n	solution
IM	intramuscularly	stat	immediately
inj	inject	susp	suspension
IP	intraperitoneally	tab(s)	tablet(s)
IV	intravenously	Tbs	tablespoon
kg	kilogram	tid (t.i.d.) (TID)	three times a day
lb	pound	tsp	teaspoon
mg	milligram	ut dict.	as directed
mL	milliliter		

TABLE 15-12 Common Weight, Liquid Measure, Length, Percentage, and Milliequivalent Conversions.

Weights

1 milligram (mg) = 1000 micrograms (mcg orig) = 0.015 grain
1 grain (gr) = 64.8 mg (≈ 65 mg)
1 gram (g) = 15.43 grains (≈ 15 grains) = 1000 mg
1 kilogram (kg) = 1000 g = 2.2 lb
1 ounce (oz) = 28.35 g
1 pound (lb) = 454 g = 16 oz = 0.45 kg
2.2 pound = 1 kg

Liquid Measures

1 drop = 0.05 (1/20) milliliter (mL)
1 cubic centimeter (cc) = 1 mL
1 liter (L) = 1000 mL
1 teaspoon (tsp) = 5 mL
1 tablespoon (Tbs) = 15 mL
1 fluid ounce (fl oz) = 29.57 mL (≈ 30 mL)
1 pint = 473.2 mL (≈ 473 mL)
1 quart = 2 pints = 32 fl oz = 0.946 L
1 gallon = 4 quarts = 3.785 L
1 cup = 8 fl oz = 237 mL = 16 Tbs

Linear Measures

1 millimeter (mm) = 0.039 inches (in)
1 centimeter (cm) = 0.39 in
1 meter (m) = 39.37 in
1 inch (in) = 2.54 cm
1 foot (ft) = 30.48 cm
1 yard (yd) = 91.44 cm

Percentage Equivalents

0.1% solution = 1 mg per mL
1% solution = 10 mg per mL
10% solution = 100 mg per mL

Milliequivalents

1 mEq Na = 23 mg Na = 58.5 mg NaCl
1 g Na = 2.54 g NaCl = 43 mEq Na
1 g NaCl = 0.39 g Na = 17 mEq Na
1 mEq K = 39 mg K = 74.5 mg KCl
1 g K = 1.91 g KCl = 26 mEq K
1 g KCl = 0.52 g K = 13 mEq K
1 mEq Ca = 20 mg Ca
1 g Ca = 50 mEq Ca
1 mEq Mg = 0.12 g $MgSO_4 \times 7H_2O$
1 g Mg = 10.2 g $MgSO_4 \times 7H_2O$ = 82 mEq Mg

TABLE 15-13 Equivalents of Celsius (Centigrade) and Fahrenheit Temperature Scales.[a]

°C	°F	°C	°F	°C	°F
0	32.0	17	62.6	34	93.2
1	33.8	18	64.4	35	95.0
2	35.6	19	66.2	36	96.8
3	37.4	20	68.0	37	98.6
4	39.2	21	69.8	38	100.4
5	41.0	22	71.6	39	102.2
6	42.8	23	73.4	40	104.0
7	44.6	24	75.2	41	105.8
8	46.4	25	77.0	42	107.6
9	48.2	26	78.8	43	109.4
10	50.0	27	80.6	44	111.2
11	51.8	28	82.4	45	113.0
12	53.6	29	84.2	46	114.8
13	55.4	30	86.0	47	116.6
14	57.2	31	87.8	48	118.4
15	59.0	32	89.6	49	120.2
16	60.8	33	91.4	50	122.0

[a]Conversions: $°C = 5/9 \times (°F - 32)$; $°F = 9/5 \times (°C) + 32$.

TABLE 15-14 System of International (SI) Units of Hematology Commonly Used in Exotic Animal Medicine.[a]

Component	Conventional (USA) Units	SI Unit
Hemoglobin (Hgb)	g/dL	× 10 g/L
Red blood cells (RBC)	$\times 10^6$/µL	$\times 10^{12}$/L
Reticulocytes	%	%
Mean corpuscular volume (MCV)	fL	fL
Mean corpuscular Hgb (MCH)	Pg	Pg
Mean corpuscular Hgb concentration (MCHC)	g/dL	× 10 g/L
Platelets	$\times 10^3$/µL	$\times 10^9$/L
White blood cells (WBC)	$\times 10^3$/µL	$\times 10^9$/L
Neutrophils (segmented)	$\times 10^3$/µL	$\times 10^9$/L
Neutrophils (bands)	$\times 10^3$/µL	$\times 10^9$/L
Lymphocytes	$\times 10^3$/µL	$\times 10^9$/L
Monocytes	$\times 10^3$/µL	$\times 10^9$/L
Eosinophils	$\times 10^3$/µL	$\times 10^9$/L
Basophils	$\times 10^3$/µL	$\times 10^9$/L

[a]Adapted from *Veterinary Laboratory Medicine: Interpretation and Diagnosis,* Meyer DH, Harvey JW, 3rd ed., 2004, with permission from Elsevier.

TABLE 15-15 System of International (SI) Units Conversion Factors of Clinical Chemistries Commonly Used in Exotic Animal Medicine.[a]

Component	Conventional (USA) Units	Conversion Factor (x)	SI Unit
Albumin	g/dL	10	g/L
Alkaline phosphatase	U/L	1.0	IU/L
ALT (SGPT)	U/L	1.0	IU/L
Ammonia (NH_3)	µg/dL	0.5871	µmol/L
Amylase	U/L	1.0	IU/L
AST (SGOT)	U/L	1.0	IU/L
Bilirubin	mg/dL	17.10	µmol/L
Calcium	mg/dL	0.2495	mmol/L
Carbon dioxide	mEq/L	1.0	mmol/L
Chloride	mEq/L	1.0	mmol/L
Cholesterol	mg/dL	0.02586	mmol/L
Copper	µg/dL	0.16	µmol/L
Cortisol	µg/dL	27.59	nmol/L
Creatine kinase	U/L	1.0	IU/L
Creatinine	mg/dL	88.40	µmol/L
Fibrinogen	mg/dL	0.01	g/L
Glucose	mg/dL	0.05551	mmol/L
Iron	µg/dL	0.1791	µmol/L
Lipase			
Sigma Tietz	U/dL	280	IU/L
Cherry-Crandall	U/L	1.0	IU/L
Lipid, total	mg/dL	0.01	g/L
Magnesium	mEq/L	0.5	mmol/L
Osmolality	mOsm/kg	1.0	mmol/kg
Phosphate (as inorganic P)	mg/dL	0.3229	mmol/L
Potassium	mEq/L	1.0	mmol/L
Protein (total)	g/dL	10	g/L
Sodium	mEq/L	1.0	mmol/L
Thyroxine (T_4)	µg/dL	12.87	nmol/L
Triglycerides	mg/dL	0.011	mmol/L
Tri-iodothyronine (T_3)	µg/dL	15.6	nmol/L
Urea nitrogen	mg/dL	0.3570	mmol/L[b]
Uric acid	mg/dL	59.48	µmol/L

[a]Adapted from Meyer DH, Harvey JW. *Veterinary Laboratory Medicine: Interpretation and Diagnosis,* 3rd ed., 2004; with permission from Elsevier.

[b]Urea.

TABLE 15-16 Select Compounding Pharmacies.[a]

State	City	Name	Website	Phone
AR	Conway	US Compounding Pharmacy	uscompounding.com	800-718-3588
AZ	Scottsdale	Diamondback Drugs (now merged with Wedgewood pharmacy)	wedgewoodpharmacy.com	877-357-6613
	Phoenix	Roadrunner Pharmacy	roadrunnerpharmacy.com	877-518-4589
CA	Bakersfield	Precision Pharmacy	precisionpharmacy.com	877-734-3338
	Bellflower	B&B Pharmacy and Health Care Center	bbpharmacy.com	562-866-8363
	Costa Mesa	Creative Compounding Pharmacy	creative compounding.com	714-627-5600
	Encino	Valley Drug and Compounding	valleydrugcompounding.com	818-788-0635
	La Habra	Central Drugs Compounding Pharmacy	centraldrugsrx.com	877-447-7077
	Los Angeles	American Health Solutions Pharmacy	ahsrx.com	310-838-7422
	Merced	Valley Prescription and Compounding Pharmacy	valleyrxandcompounding.com	209-722-5765
	San Rafael	Golden Gate Veterinary Pharmacy	ggvcp.pharmacy	415-455-5590
CO	Monument	Monument Pharmacy	monumentpharmacy.com	800-595-7565
CT	Southington	Beacon Compounding Pharmacy	beaconcompounding.com	860-628-3972
DE	Newark	Save Way Pharmacy	savewaypharmacy.com	302-369-5520
FL	Gainesville	Westlab Pharmacy	westlabpharmacy.com	352-373-8111
IL	Chicago	Braun PharmaCare	braunrx.com	773-549-0634
	Naperville	Martin Avenue Pharmacy	martinavenue.com	630-355-6400
IN	Fort Wayne	Fort Wayne Custom Rx	fwcustomrx.com	260-490-3447
KS	Arkansas City	Taylor Drug	taylordrug.net	800-567-3733
	Lenexa	Midwest Compounders Pharmacy	mwcpharmacy.com	888-245-3012
	Overland Park	Stark Pharmacy	starkpharmacy.com	913-345-3800
MA	Scituate	Animal Pharm, LLC	animalpharmllc.com	866-544-3010
MI	Saginaw	Healthway Compounding Pharmacy	healthwayrx.com	866-883-8868
MN	Saint Peter	Soderlund Village Drug	drugstoremuseum.com	800-603-8196

TABLE 15-16 Select Compounding Pharmacies. (cont'd)

State	City	Name	Website	Phone
MO	Jackson	Horst Pharmacy	horstpharmacy.com	800-640-5940
NE	Ord	Good Life Pharmacy	goodliferx.com	800-752-5694
NH	Littleton	Eastern States Compounding Pharmacy	easternstatescompounding.com	603-444-0094
NJ	Swedesboro	Wedgewood Pharmacy	wedgewoodpharmacy.com	800-331-8272
NY	Canandaigua	Animal Pharmacy	animalpharmacy.net	800-663-5261
	Cross River	Cross River Pharmacy and Compounding Center	crossriverpharmacy.com	914-763-3152
	Jamestown	Pharmacy Innovations	pharmacyinnovations.net	716-720-5121
OH	Cincinnati	Tri-State Compounding Pharmacy	tristaterx.com	513-624-7333
	Avon, Perrysburg, and Sandusky	Buderer Drug	budererdrug.com	440-934-3100, 419-873-2800, 419-627-2800
OR	Tualatin	Northwest Compounders	northwestcompounders.com	800-968-0742
PA	Hatboro	Philadelphia Professional Compounding Agency	ppcpharmacy.com	215-672-8552
RI	South Kingstown	Bayview Pharmacy	bayviewrx.com	401-284-4505
TN	Cordova	Regel PharmaLab	regelpharmalab.com	866-907-3435
TX	Houston	BCP Veterinary Pharmacy	bcpvetpharm.com	800-481-1729
UT	Sandy	Meds for Vets	medsforvets.com	833-633-4838
VA	Alexandria	Alexandria Medical Arts Pharmacy & Compounding Lab	amapharmacy.com	703-549-4350
WA	Bellevue	Custom Prescriptions	custom-prescriptions.com	425-289-0347
WI	Milwaukee	Pet Apothecary	petapothecary.com	414-247-8633

[a]Websites accessed on October 1, 2020.

TABLE 15-17 Compounding Resources.[a]

Name	Contact	Description
AVMA Compounding FAQs	Website: Avma.org/KB/Resources/FAQs/Pages/Compounding-FAQs.aspx	FAQ regarding veterinary compounding
Compounding Today	Website: compoundingtoday.com	Several databases including flavoring recommendations by species, requires a login but does offer a 14-day free trial
Fagron	Website: us.fagron.com	Compounding bases and flavorings
FDA Compounding Resources	Website: fda.gov/animal-veterinary/unapproved-animal-drugs/animal-drug-compounding	Information regarding legal requirements for compounding
Flavorx	Website: flavorx.com	In-house compounding kits
Humco	Website: humco.com	Compounding supplies
Medisca	Website: medisca.com	Compounding flavors and recipes
Trissel's Stability of Compounded Formulations, 6th ed.[b]	Publisher: American Pharmacists Association	Monographs on various commonly compounded drugs
U.S. Pharmacopeial Convention	Website: usp.org/usp-healthcare-professionals/compounding	Compounding standards and resources

[a]Websites accessed on October 20, 2020.
[b]Trissel LA. *Trissel's Stability of Compounded Formulations*. 6th ed. Washington, DC: American Pharmacists Association, 2018.

TABLE 15-18 Select Toxins and Dangerous Substances in Exotic Animal Medicine.

Taxa	Substance	Species Affected	Condition
Avian	Aflatoxin	Northern bobwhites	Immunosuppression, hepatopathy[25]
	Avocado (persin)	Psittacine birds	Pericardial effusion, organ congestion[15,20,35]
	Chocolate (theobromine, caffeine)	Psittacine birds	Mucoid feces, heptotoxicity, renal toxicity, pulmonary congestion, death[13,20]
	Crown vetch (*Coronilla baria*)	Budgerigars	Tachypnea, neurologic signs, weakness, tremors, incoordination[5,20]
	Cyanobacterium	Snail kites	Avian vacuolar myelinopathy (AVM)[9]
	Diclofenac (NSAID)	Vultures	Renal failure[35]
	Iron	Toucans (*Rhamphastos*), lories and lorikeets (*Loriinae*)	Poor plumage, anorexia, lethargy, ascites, dyspnea, death; hepatopathy[20]

TABLE 15-18 Select Toxins and Dangerous Substances in Exotic Animal Medicine. (cont'd)

Taxa	Substance	Species Affected	Condition
Avian (cont'd)	*Kalanchoe* sp. (house plant)	Chickens	Ataxia, muscle tremors, seizure, death[20]
	Lead	Psittacine birds, passerine birds, Anseriformes, raptors, others	Neurological, hemaglobinuria, ocular pathologies[6,11,20,35]
	Polysulfated glycosaminoglycans (PSGAGs)	Various species	Acute hemorrhage[1]
	Polytetrafluoroethylene (PTFE)	Psittacine birds, others	Pulmonary pathology[20,35]
	Rodenticides	Various species	Anemia, death; increased plasma calcium, renal necrosis[17,32]
	Tea tree oil	Cockatiel	Hepatopathy[33]
	Vitamin A	Lorikeets, cockatiels	Various infectious and non-infectious associated pathologies[27]
	Vitamin B_6	Gyrfalcons	Hepatic necrosis[29]
	Zinc	Psittacine birds, various species	Nonspecific signs, PU/PD, diarrhea, regurgitation[20,35]
Reptiles and Amphibians	Acetaminophen	Monitors, pythons, tree snakes	Death[2,7,12,23]
	Chlorhexidine soak	Red-bellied short-necked turtles	Intoxication[21]
	Firefly (*Photinus*)	Bearded dragons	Gaping, dyspnea, cardiotoxicity[12,16,19]
	Ivermectin	Chelonians	Lethargy, paralysis, coma, death[12]
	Lead	Snapping turtle, various species	Lethargy, anorexia, neuromuscular dysfunction[3,12]
	Tetrodotoxin	Caiman	Lethargy, coma[34]
	Vitamin A	Various species	Skin sloughing[12]
	Vitamin D	Various species	Hypercalcemia[12]
	Zinc	Various species	Lethargy, anorexia[12]
Small Mammals	Aflatoxin	Rabbits, guinea pigs, chinchillas	Hepatotoxicity, renal degeneration[14,18,22,24,28]
	Antibiotics, per os • Amoxicillins • Cephalosporins • Clindamycin • Erythromycin • Lincomycin • Penicillins	Rabbits, hystricomorph rodents	Dysbiosis, eneritis[18]

Continued

TABLE 15-18 Select Toxins and Dangerous Substances in Exotic Animal Medicine. (cont'd)

Taxa	Substance	Species Affected	Condition
Mammals (cont'd)	Fipronil (Frontline)	Rabbits	Neurological, death[8,18]
	Lead	Rabbits, guinea pigs, chinchillas	Neurological[18,26,30,31]
	Rodenticides	Rabbits, guinea pigs, chinchillas, ferrets	Anticoagulant; effects may last up to 20 days[18]
	Tiletamine/zolazepam	Rabbits	Nephrotoxicity, urinary casts[4,10,18]

REFERENCES

1. Anderson K, Garner MM, Reed HH, et al. Hemorrhagic diathesis in avian species following intramuscular administration of polysulfated glycosaminoglycan. *J Zoo Wildl Med.* 2013;44(1):93–99.
2. Avery ML, Eisemann JD, Keacher KL, et al. Acetaminophen and zinc phosphide for lethal management of invasive lizards *Ctenosaura similis*. *Curr Zool.* 2011;57:625–629.
3. Borkowski R. Lead poisoning and intestinal perforations in a snapping turtle (*Chelydra serpentina*) due to fishing gear ingestion. *J Zoo Wildl Med.* 1997;28(1):109–113.
4. Brammer DW, Doerning BJ, Chrisp CE, et al. Anesthetic and nephrotoxic effects of Telazol in New Zealand white rabbits. *Lab Anim Sci.* 1991;41(5):432–435.
5. Campbell TW. Crown vetch (*Coronilla varia*) poisoning in a budgerigar (*Melopsittacus undulatus*). *J Avian Med Surg.* 2006;20(2):97–100.
6. Carneiro MA, Oliveira PA, Brandão R, et al. Lead poisoning due to lead-pellet ingestion in griffon vultures (*Gyps fulvus*) from the Iberian peninsula. *J Avian Med Surg.* 2016;30(3):274–279.
7. Clark L, Savarie PJ, Shivik JA, et al. Efficacy, effort, and cost comparisons of trapping and acetaminophen-baiting for control of brown treesnakes on Guam. *Hum-Wildl Interact.* 2012;6:222–236.
8. Cooper PE, Penaliggon J. Use of Frontline spray on rabbits. *Vet Rec.* 1997;140:535–536.
9. Dodd SR, Haynie RS, Williams SM, et al. Alternate food-chain transfer of the toxin linked to avian vacuolar myelinopathy and implications for the endangered Florida snail kite (*Rostrhamus sociabilis*). *J Wildl Dis.* 2016;52(2):335–344.
10. Doerning BJ, Brammer DW, Chrisp CE, et al. Anesthetic and nephrotoxic effects of tiletamine/zolazepam in rabbits. *Lab Anim Sci.* 1990;40(5):562.
11. Eid R, Guzman DSM, Keller KA, et al. Choroidal vasculopathy and retinal detachment in a bald eagle (*Haliaeetus leucocephalus*) with lead toxicosis. *J Avian Med Surg.* 2016;30(4):357–363.
12. Fitzgerald KT, Martínez-Silvestre A. Toxicology. In: Divers S, Stahl S, eds. *Mader's Reptile and Amphibian Medicine and Surgery*. 3rd ed. St. Louis, MO: Elsevier; 2019:977–991.
13. Gartrell BD, Reid C. Death by chocolate: a fatal problem for an inquisitive wild parrot. *NZ Vet J.* 2007;55(3):149–151.
14. González Pereyra ML, Carvalho ECQ, Tissera JL, et al. An outbreak of acute aflatoxicosis on a chinchilla (*Chinchilla lanigera*) farm in Argentina. *J Vet Diagn Invest.* 2008;20(6):853–856.
15. Grant R, Basson PA, Booker HH, et al. Cardiomyopathy caused by avocado (*Persea americana* Mill) leaves. *J S Afr Vet Assoc.* 1991;62(1):21–22.
16. Higbie C, Carpenter JW. Diagnostic Challenge: Lucibufagin toxicity in a pet bearded dragon (*Pogona vitticeps*). *J Exot Pet Med.* 2014;23(3):301–304.

17. Hydock KL, DeClementi C, Fish PH. Second-generation anticoagulant rodenticide poisoning in a captive Andean condor (*Vultur gryphus*). *J Avian Med Surg*. 2017;31(3):256–261.
18. Johnston MS. Clinical toxicosis of domestic rabbits. *Vet Clin North Am Exot Anim Pract*. 2008;11:315–326.
19. Knight M, Glor R, Smedley SR, et al. Firefly toxicosis in lizards. *J Chem Ecol*. 1999;25:1981–1986.
20. Lightfoot TL, Yeager JM. Pet bird toxicity and related environmental concerns. *Vet Clin North Am Exot Anim Pract*. 2008;11:229–259.
21. Lloyd ML. Chlorhexidine toxicosis in a pair of red-bellied short-necked turtles, *Emydura subglosa*. *Bull Assoc Rept Amph Vet*. 1996;6(4):6–7.
22. Makkar HPS, Singh B. Aflatoxicosis in rabbits. *J Appl Rabbit Res*. 1991;14:218–221.
23. Mauldin RRE, Savarie PJ. Acetaminophen as an oral toxicant for Nile monitor lizards (*Varanus niloticus*) and Burmese pythons (*Python molurus bivittatus*). *Wildl Res*. 2010;37:215–222.
24. Mehotra ML, Khanna RS. Aflatoxicosis in angora rabbits. *Indian Vet J*. 1973;50:620–622.
25. Moore DL, Henke SE, Fedynich AM, et al. Acute effects of aflatoxin on northern bobwhites (*Colinus virginianus*). *J Wildl Dis*. 2013;49(3):568–578.
26. O'Tuama LA, Kim CS, Gatzy JT, et al. The distribution of inorganic lead in guinea pig brain and neural barrier tissues in control and lead-poisoned animals. *Toxicol Appl Pharmacol*. 1976;36(1):1–9.
27. Park F. Vitamin A toxicosis in a lorikeet flock. *Vet Clin of North Am Exot Anim Pract*. 2006;9(3):495–502.
28. Penev G, Kotev-Penev LJ, Kocic' B, et al. Aflatoxicosis of the liver in the guinea pigs. *Infettive e Parassitarie*. 1990;42(8):629–630.
29. Samour J, Perlman J, Kinne J, et al. Vitamin B_6 (pyridoxine hydrochloride) toxicosis in falcons. *J Zoo Wildl Med*. 2016;47(2):601–608.
30. Sawmy S. Lead toxicosis in a rabbit. *Vet Times*. 2016;46(22):12–14.
31. Swartout MS, Gerken DF. Lead-induced toxicosis in two domestic rabbits. *J Am Vet Med Assoc*. 1987;191(6):717–719.
32. Swenson J, Bradley GA. Suspected cholecalciferol rodenticide toxicosis in avian species at a zoological institution. *J Avian Med Surg*. 2013;27(2):136–147.
33. Vetere A, Bertocchi M, Pelizzone I, et al. Acute tea tree oil intoxication in a pet cockatiel (*Nymphicus hollandicus*): a case report. *BMC Vet Res*. 2020;16(29).
34. Williams BL, Powers LV, Garner MM. A pufferfish (*Tetradon nigroviridis*) available in the common pet trade harbors lethal concentrations of tetrodotoxin: a case study of poisoning in a cuvier's dwarf caiman (*Paleosuchus palpebrosus*). *J Zoo Wildl Med*. 2016;47(2):676–680.
35. Wismer T. Advancements in diagnosis and management of toxocologic problems. In: Speer BL, ed. *Current Therapy in Avian Medicine and Surgery*. St. Louis, MO: Elsevier; 2016:589–599.

Index

Note: Page numbers followed by *t* indicate tables.

C

D

G

K

L

M

O

Q

U

V